PENNSYLVANIA COLLEGE OF TECHNOLOGY LIBRARY

5 0608 01183488 3

DISCARDED

D0846551

Newman and Carranza's

CLINICAL PERIODONTOLOGY

for the **Dental Hygienist**

Michael G. Newman, DDS, FACD
Professor Emeritus, Section of Periodontics
School of Dentistry
University of California
Los Angeles, California

Lory Laughter, RDH, MS
Assistant Professor, Department of Periodontics/Dental Hygiene Director
Arthur A. Dugoni School of Dentistry
University of the Pacific
San Francisco, California

Gwendolyn Essex, RDH, RDHAP, MS, EdD
Clinical Professor, Preventive and Restorative Dental Sciences
School of Dentistry
University of California, San Francisco
San Francisco, California

Satheesh Elangovan, BDS, DSc, DMSc
Professor, Department of Periodontics
The University of Iowa College of Dentistry and Dental Clinics
Iowa City, Iowa

ELSEVIER

MAR 12 2021

Madigan Library
Pennsylvania College
of Technology

One College Avenue
Williamsport, PA 17701-5799

Elsevier
3251 Riverport Lane
St. Louis, Missouri 63043

NEWMAN AND CARRANZA'S CLINICAL PERIODONTOLOGY FOR
THE DENTAL HYGIENIST

ISBN: 978-0-323-70841-8

Copyright © 2021 by Elsevier, Inc. All rights reserved.

No part of this publication may be reproduced or transmitted in any form or by any means, electronic or mechanical, including photocopying, recording, or any information storage and retrieval system, without permission in writing from the publisher. Details on how to seek permission, further information about the Publisher's permissions policies and our arrangements with organizations such as the Copyright Clearance Center and the Copyright Licensing Agency, can be found at our website: www.elsevier.com/permissions.

This book and the individual contributions contained in it are protected under copyright by the Publisher (other than as may be noted herein).

Notice

Practitioners and researchers must always rely on their own experience and knowledge in evaluating and using any information, methods, compounds or experiments described herein. Because of rapid advances in the medical sciences, in particular, independent verification of diagnoses and drug dosages should be made. To the fullest extent of the law, no responsibility is assumed by Elsevier, authors, editors or contributors for any injury and/or damage to persons or property as a matter of products liability, negligence or otherwise, or from any use or operation of any methods, products, instructions, or ideas contained in the material herein.

Library of Congress Control Number: 2020931484

Content Strategists: Joslyn Dumas and Kelly Skelton
Senior Content Development Specialist: Ann Ruzycka Anderson
Publishing Services Manager: Julie Eddy
Senior Project Manager: Rachel E. McMullen
Design Direction: Bridget Hoette

Printed in China

Last digit is the print number: 9 8 7 6 5 4 3 2 1

Working together
to grow libraries in
developing countries

www.elsevier.com • www.bookaid.org

Michael G. Newman, DDS, FACD

Dr. Michael G. Newman is the author of *Newman and Carranza's Clinical Periodontology,* 13th edition. Dr. Newman graduated from the University of California, Los Angeles (UCLA), College of Letters and Sciences with a degree in psychology. He completed his dental training at the UCLA School of Dentistry in 1972. Dr. Newman received a Certificate in Periodontics and Oral Medicine at the Harvard School of Dental Medicine and a Certificate in Oral Microbiology from the Forsyth Dental Institute under the mentorship of Dr. Sigmund Socransky. He is a Diplomate of the American Board of Periodontology and Professor Emeritus at the UCLA School of Dentistry. Dr. Newman is a fellow and past president of the American Academy of Periodontology. In 1975, he won the Balint Orban Memorial Prize from the American Academy of Periodontology. He has been in private practice of periodontics for more than 25 years. In 2007, Dr. Newman received the Gold Medal, the highest honor bestowed by the American Academy of Periodontology. Dr. Newman has published more than 260 abstracts, journal articles, and book chapters and has coedited nine textbooks. He has served as an ad hoc reviewer for the National Institute of Dental and Craniofacial Research, was a consultant to the Council on Scientific Affairs of the American Dental Association, and is a reviewer for numerous scientific and professional journals and governmental research organizations.

Professor Newman has lectured throughout the world to both dentist and dental hygienist audiences. Topics include: microbiology, antimicrobials, evidence-based methodology, risk factors, and diagnostic strategies for periodontal disease; clinical outcomes assessments; real-world evidence; and big data analytics. He has a strong interest in applied science and the transfer of new technology for practical use. He is a coauthor of the first online digital app simulation on a periodontal procedure. Dr. Newman is a consultant to major dental and pharmaceutical companies throughout the world. He is the founding editor-in-chief emeritus of the *Journal of Evidence-Based Dental Practice (JEBDP).* He was the associate editor of the *International Journal of Oral and Maxillofacial Implants.*

Lory Laughter, RDH, MS

Lory completed her BS at Idaho State University and her MS in Dental Hygiene at the University of California, San Francisco (UCSF). She has been a published author for dental hygiene journals as well as peer-reviewed research. Lory is currently an Assistant Professor and Dental Hygiene Program Director at University of the Pacific, Arthur A. Dugoni School of Dentistry. She presents continuing education nationally on topics of inflammation, insulin resistance, and the oral/systemic link.

Gwendolyn Essex, RDH, RDHAP, MS, EdD

Dr. Gwen Essex is a clinical professor at the University of California, San Francisco (UCSF) School of Dentistry, and has been contributing to dental hygiene and dental education for over 20 years. A graduate of the UCSF dental hygiene program, Dr. Essex continued her education to earn both Master of Science and Doctorate of Education degrees with emphasis on health sciences and learning and instruction, respectively. Empowering dental hygiene clinicians to work to the full extent of their education and licensing is a long-time passion, and contributing to this text intended to provide the science and clinical implications to dental hygienists furthers this goal.

Satheesh Elangovan, BDS, DSc, DMSc

Dr. Satheesh Elangovan completed his dental training from Tamil Nadu Dr. MGR Medical University, India. He subsequently received Doctor of Science degree from Boston University and combined Doctor of Medical Science degree in Oral Biology and a certificate in Periodontology from Harvard University. He is a Diplomate of the American Board of Periodontology and a Professor of Periodontics at the University of Iowa College of Dentistry and Dental Clinics. At the University of Iowa, he holds secondary appointments in the departments of Biomedical Engineering and Pharmaceuticals & Translational Therapeutics. His research focuses on biomaterials and bone tissue engineering, and evidence-based dentistry. He has published or presented more than 150 articles, abstracts, multimedia contributions, and book chapters. He has received several national honors and awards in the past for both his teaching and research efforts. He is currently on the editorial board of the *Journal of Dental Education* and recently served as an associate editor of *Newman and Carranza's Clinical Periodontology,* 13th edition, for which he also serves as an online editor.

EDITORIAL BOARD

Emily Boge, MPA, RDH, CDA
Dental Administrative Chair
Hawkeye Community College
Waterloo, Iowa

Irina F. Dragan, DMD, MS
Assistant Professor
Tufts University School of Dental Medicine
Boston, Massachusetts

Georgios A. Kotsakis, DDS, MS
Associate Professor
University of Texas Health Science Center at San Antonio
San Antonio, Texas

Chun-Teh Lee, DDS, MS, DMSc
Assistant Professor
University of Texas Health Science Center at Houston
Houston, Texas

CONTRIBUTORS

Sara Hughes, MBE, EdD, MA, BSc, PFHEA, NTFHEA, IHPE
Associate Dean for Education and
   Student Affairs
Professor of Preventive & Restorative
   Dental Sciences
University of California, San Francisco
San Francisco, California

Candice Kiefer, RDH, MS
Assistant Professor
University of Pittsburgh School of
   Dental Medicine
Pittsburgh Pennsylvania

Michael Le, DDS, PhD
Assistant Professor, Preventive &
   Restorative Dental Sciences
University of California, San Francisco
San Francisco, California

Peter Loomer, BSc, DDS, PhD, MRCD(C), FACD
Professor and Dean
School of Dentistry
University of Texas Health Science
   Center at San Antonio
San Antonio, Texas

PREFACE

With the help of Elsevier's advanced technology and high standards of quality, a recognized team of editors and editorial board members have developed the most comprehensive periodontal resource available for dental hygienists, *Newman and Carranza's Clinical Periodontology for the Dental Hygienists.* The book's Evolve Resources site includes a Test Bank, PowerPoint slides, and an image collection for instructors, and practice quizzes and informational videos for students. No other resource offers such a comprehensive approach to providing high-quality content for the expanding roles of the dental hygienists.

Since publication of the first edition of the parent of *Newman and Carranza's Clinical Periodontology* book in 1953, periodontology has made tremendous advancements. Scientific analysis of periodontal tissues and the elucidation of mechanisms and causes of disease have extended far beyond histology and physiology into the realm of cellular and molecular biologic understanding.

Implant dentistry has become a major component of periodontology, and this book offers a wide coverage of important treatment modalities that are relevant to the practice of dental hygiene.

New therapeutic goals and clinical techniques, based on an improved understanding of disease and healing, have facilitated better outcomes and brought us closer to achieving the ultimate goal of optimal periodontal health and function. Today, reconstruction and regeneration of lost periodontal structures, replacement of compromised teeth with implants, and creation of aesthetic results are integral parts of clinical practice.

The multifaceted, complex task of producing a first edition required the collaboration of numerous experts from various fields, and their contributions are invaluable. We know that this new first edition will be a useful and fundamental resource for dental hygienists and will contribute to the continuous progress of our profession.

ACKNOWLEDGMENTS

Newman and Carranza's Clinical Periodontology for the Dental Hygienists will become a trusted and valuable periodontics resource for students, academicians, scientists, and clinicians.

Dr. Satheesh Elangovan, a long-time collaborator with Dr. Newman, contributed greatly with his hands-on involvement in every aspect of producing this book.

Lory Laughter and Gwen Essex contributed not only as the "eyes and ears" of the dental hygiene community but also as true partners from the beginning of this big editorial project. They provided significant input, editing, original writing, commentary, and insights ensuring that all content of this first edition was relevant, important, and useful.

It is also important to recognize the many contributors of the parent book. We express our deep gratitude to all those contributors whose expertise, ideas, and efforts built the original book/resource over the years. Many scientists and clinicians have shared their wisdom and expertise in previous editions as associate editors, section editors, and contributors, though some of their names no longer appear.

Our appreciation goes to Elsevier and particularly to Joslyn Dumas, Ann Anderson, and Rachel McMullen. Their expertise and detailed attention to every word and every concept contributed greatly to producing a quality book and a truly useful website.

CONTENTS

VIDEO CONTENTS

All videos can be found on the Evolve Resources site.

The Historical Background of Periodontology[a]

CHAPTER OUTLINE

Gingival and periodontal diseases have afflicted humans since the dawn of history. Studies in paleopathology have indicated that destructive periodontal disease, as evidenced by bone loss, affected early humans in such diverse cultures as ancient Egypt and early pre-Columbian America. The earliest historical records that involve medical topics reveal an awareness of periodontal disease and the need for treatment. Almost all early writings that have been preserved have sections or chapters dealing with oral diseases, and periodontal problems comprise a significant amount of space in these writings. Calculus and systemic disease were frequently postulated as causes of periodontal disorders.

However, methodic and carefully reasoned therapeutic discussions did not exist until the Arabic surgical treatises of the Middle Ages. Modern treatment, with illustrated text and sophisticated instrumentation, did not develop until the time of Pierre Fauchard during the 18th century.

EARLY CIVILIZATIONS

Oral hygiene was practiced by the Sumerians, the Babylonians, and the Assyrians; this included gingival massage in combination with various herbal medications.[25,33]

Periodontal disease was the most common of all diseases found in the embalmed bodies of the ancient Egyptians.[7,44] The Ebers papyrus contains many references to gingival disease and offers a number of prescriptions for strengthening the teeth and gums.[14]

The medical works of ancient India and China devote significant space to oral and periodontal problems and oral hygiene,[47] and they describe gingival inflammations, periodontal abscesses, and gingival ulcerations.[12,21] The early Hebrews also recognized the importance of oral hygiene. Many pathologic conditions of the teeth and their surrounding structures are described in the Talmudic writings.

THE CLASSICAL WORLD

Among the ancient Greeks, Hippocrates of Cos (460-377 BC), the father of modern medicine, discussed the function and eruption of the teeth and the etiology of periodontal disease. He believed that inflammation of the gums could be caused by accumulations of "pituita" or calculus, with gingival hemorrhage occurring in cases of persistent splenic maladies.[10,27]

Among the Romans, Aulus Cornelius Celsus (25 BC-50 AD) referred to diseases that affect the soft parts of the mouth and their treatment, including oral hygiene. Paul of Aegina (625-690 AD) wrote that tartar deposits must be removed with either scrapers or a small file and that the teeth should be carefully cleaned after the last meal of the day.[41]

THE MIDDLE AGES

The decline and fall of the Roman Empire that plunged Europe into an age of darkness was accompanied by the rise of Islam and the golden age of Arabic science and medicine. The Arabic treatises derived their information from Greek medical treatises, but many refinements and novel approaches were added, particularly in surgical specialties.[45]

Albucasis (936-1013) was born and lived in Moorish Spain. His 30-volume medical encyclopedia, called al-Tasrif, was translated into Latin during the 12th century, and it was the medical text used in European universities until the 17th century. The contributions of Albucasis to dentistry and periodontology were outstanding achievements.[1] He had a clear understanding of the major etiologic role of calculus deposits, and he described the techniques of scaling the teeth with the use of a set of instruments that he developed (Fig. 1.1), splinting loose teeth with gold wire, and filing gross occlusal abnormalities.

Avicenna (980-1037) was possibly the greatest of the Persian physicians. His Canon, a comprehensive treatise on medicine, was in continuous use for almost 600 years. Avicenna used an extensive "materia medica" for oral and periodontal diseases and rarely resorted to surgery.[3]

[a]Adapted from the following chapter of Newman and Carranza's Clinical Periodontology, 13th edition: Introduction: The Historical Background of Periodontology, by Gerald Shklar and Fermin A. Carranza.

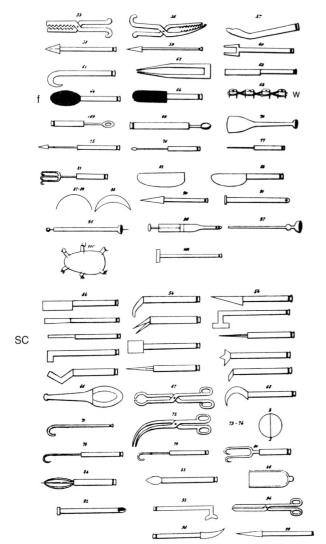

Fig. 1.1 Illustration of Albucasis' periodontal instruments, showing scalers *(sc)*, files *(f)*, and the wiring of loose teeth *(w)*.

THE RENAISSANCE

During the Renaissance—with the rebirth of classical scholarship, the development of scientific thought and medical knowledge, and the flowering of art, music, and literature—significant contributions were made to anatomy and surgery.

Albucasis' work was expanded during the 15th century by the Turkish author Serefeddin Sabuncuoglu (1385-1468), who included illustrations of the surgical removal of hypertrophic and swollen gingiva and lingual frenum (Fig. 1.2). "Drug treatment should be initiated if there are swollen gums, mobile teeth, and pus formation. If there is no response, surgical treatment should be performed. A tube is placed on the gums. A hot cautery is inserted into the cannula, and the gingival tissue is cauterized. If this is correctly applied, the adjacent teeth will be warm."

Paracelsus (1493-1541) developed an interesting and unusual theory of disease: the doctrine of calculus. Paracelsus recognized the extensive formation of tartar on the teeth and related this to toothache. He considered toothache to be comparable to the pain produced by calculus in other organs, such as the kidneys.[39]

Fig. 1.2 Illustration by Serefeddin Sabuncuoglu Showing Gingival Cauterization. (From Abulcasis and redrawn by Professor Ilter Uzel, Turkey.)

Andreas Vesalius (1514-1564), who was born in Brussels, taught at the University of Padua and wrote a magnificent book about anatomy that included many excellent illustrations.[48] Bartholomeus Eustachius (1520-1574) of Rome was another outstanding anatomist who wrote a small book about dentistry, *Libellus de Dentibus* ("A Little Treatise on the Teeth"), which contained 30 chapters.[16] This was the first original book about the teeth, and it included a description of the periodontal tissues as well as information about the diseases of the mouth, their treatment modalities, and the rationale for treatment. For the treatment of periodontitis, Eustachius recommended both the scaling of calculus and the curettage of granulation tissue so that actual reattachment of the gingival and periodontal tissues could take place.

The Frenchman Ambroise Paré (1509-1590) was the outstanding surgeon of the Renaissance, and his contributions to dental surgery included gingivectomy for hyperplastic gingival tissues.[40] He also understood the etiologic significance of calculus and used a set of scalers to remove hard deposits on the teeth.

The first book in the common language of German that was specifically devoted to dental practice was entitled *Artzney Buchlein* or *Zene Artzney* ("Medicine of the Teeth"), and was published in Leipzig in 1530.[2] It contains three chapters devoted to periodontal problems, including a crude concept of systemic and local factors in the etiology of periodontal disease. The presence of local infective agents or "worms" is also mentioned.

In this text, a variety of ointments, which are often astringent in nature, is suggested, and the binding of loose teeth to sound ones with silk or gold thread is recommended. Cauterizing the gingiva with a hot iron is mentioned.

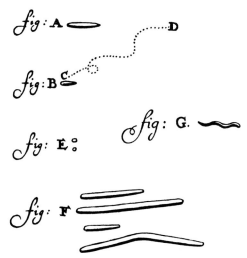

Fig. 1.3 Leeuwenhoek's Drawing of Oral Spirochetes, Bacilli, and Other Microorganisms.

Fig. 1.4 Frontispiece of Fauchard's Book Entitled *The Surgeon Dentist* (1746 edition).

The Italian physician, mathematician, and philosopher Girolamo Cardano (1501-1576) appears to have been the first to differentiate among the types of periodontal disease. In a publication dated 1562, he mentions one type of disease that occurs with advancing age and leads to progressive loosening and loss of teeth as well as a second very aggressive type that occurs in younger patients.[26] It was not until late in the 20th century that this classification was rediscovered and became widely accepted.

Anton van Leeuwenhoek (1632-1723) of Delft, Holland, was a layman, but he had an inquisitive mind and a hobby of grinding lenses that allowed him to develop the microscope. He used it to discover microorganisms, cellular structure, blood cells, sperm, and various other microscopic structures, including the tubular structure of dentin.[9,13] Using material from his own mouth, Leeuwenhoek first described oral bacterial flora, and his drawings offered a reasonably good presentation of oral spirochetes and bacilli (Fig. 1.3). He even performed antiplaque experiments involving the use of strong vinegar in his own mouth and in vitro on bacteria in a dish.[13]

THE 18TH CENTURY

Modern dentistry essentially developed in 18th-century Europe, particularly France and England. Pierre Fauchard, who was born in Brittany in 1678, is rightly regarded as the father of the dental profession as we know it. His book, *The Surgeon Dentist*, which was published in 1728, covered all aspects of dental practice, including restorative dentistry, prosthodontics, oral surgery, periodontics, and orthodontics (Fig. 1.4).[17] Fauchard described in detail his periodontal instruments and the scaling technique for using them (Fig. 1.5).

John Hunter (1728-1793), who was the most distinguished anatomist, surgeon, and pathologist of 18th-century England, wrote an excellent treatise on dentistry entitled *The Natural History of the Human Teeth*.[30] He offered remarkably clear illustrations of the anatomy of the teeth and their supporting structures, and he described the features of periodontal diseases.

1   4   2   5   3

Fig. 1.5 The five types of instruments used by Fauchard for detaching tartar from the teeth: *1*, chisel; *2*, parrot beak; *3*, graver; *4*, convex blade; and *5*, Z-shaped hook.

A contemporary of Hunter, Thomas Berdmore (1740-1785), was considered the outstanding dentist in England. In 1770, he published a book that had several chapters devoted to periodontal problems.[4]

THE 19TH CENTURY

Leonard Koecker (1785-1850) was a German-born dentist who practiced in Baltimore. In a paper in 1821, he mentioned the careful removal of tartar and the need for oral hygiene by the patient, recommending that it be performed in the morning and after every meal with the use of an astringent powder and a toothbrush, with care taken to place "the bristles … into the spaces of the teeth." Koecker was an early advocate of the "odontogenic focal infection" theory, and he recommended the extraction of all severely involved teeth and roots, including all unopposed molars, to prevent systemic infections.[35]

Levi Spear Parmly (1790-1859) was a New Orleans, Louisiana-based dentist who is considered the father of oral hygiene and the inventor of dental floss.[11,18]

During the mid-19th century, John W. Riggs (1811-1885) was the leading authority on periodontal disease and its treatment in the United States; in fact, at the time, periodontitis was known as "Riggs' disease." Riggs graduated from the Baltimore College of Dental Surgery in 1854 and practiced in Hartford, Connecticut, where he died on November 11, 1885. Riggs seems to have been the first individual to limit his practice to periodontics and can therefore be considered the first specialist in this field. Riggs' publications, however, are limited. In an 1876 paper, Riggs was a strong proponent of the so-called conservative approach to periodontal therapy; he developed the concept of oral prophylaxis and prevention, advocated for the cleanliness of the mouth, and opposed surgery, which at the time consisted of gingival resection.[43]

Riggs and his disciples had great influence on the dental profession. Among Riggs' followers were L. Taylor, D.D. Smith, R.B. Adair, and W.J. Younger. The instruments designed by Younger[57] and later modified by his student Robert Good were used widely until well beyond the middle of the 20th century.

Several major developments in medical science occurred during the second half of the 19th century and started the era that can be called *modern medicine*, which includes dentistry.[9,36] The first was the discovery of anesthesia by Horace Wells (1813-1848) of Hartford, Connecticut, in 1845 and by William Morton (1819-1868) of Boston, Massachusetts, in 1846, who discovered the general anesthetic effects of nitrous oxide and ether, respectively. *Local anesthesia* was developed by the Vienna ophthalmologist Carl Köller (1857-1944), who produced anesthesia of the eye with drops of cocaine. Procaine (Novocaine) was developed in 1905 by the Munich chemists Alfred Einhorn and Richard Willstädter. Later, with the addition of adrenaline, which was discovered separately in the United States by Jokichi Takamine and Thomas Bell Aldrich, local anesthesia was born.[29]

The second scientific breakthrough was made by the French chemist Louis Pasteur (1822-1895), who established the *germ theory of disease*. Subsequently, the German physician Robert Koch (1843-1910), in a series of brilliant investigations, discovered the microorganism that causes the cattle disease, anthrax, and the bacterial etiology of tuberculosis and cholera.

The concepts of Pasteur were transferred to clinical and surgical practice by Joseph Lister (1827-1912) of England, and thus the era of antisepsis—and later, asepsis—in surgery was born. Anesthesia and antisepsis made possible extraordinary advances in surgical techniques.

Pasteur, Koch, and their collaborators and followers—Elie Metchnikoff, Emile Roux, Paul Ehrlich, Emil von Behring, Shibasaburo Kitasato, and many others—discovered the bacterial etiologies of numerous diseases (e.g., pneumonia, puerperal fever, diphtheria, meningitis, plague, dysentery, syphilis) and gave birth

to two sciences that became basic to periodontics: bacteriology and immunology.

A third scientific finding that changed the practice of dentistry in general and of periodontics in particular was the *discovery of radiographs* by the German physicist Wilhelm Röntgen (1845-1923; also written as *Roentgen*). Röntgen's discovery was made in 1895 at the University of Würzburg and was purely a basic science finding, but it was immediately taken up by physicians and dentists, and it proved to be a crucial development in periodontics and many other areas of medicine and dentistry.

Also during the late 19th century, studies by Rudolph Virchow (1821-1902), Julius Cohnheim (1839-1884), Elie Metchnikoff (1845-1916), and others had started to reveal the microscopic changes that occur during inflammation.[8,9] This resulted in an understanding of the pathogenesis of periodontal disease on the basis of histopathologic studies. The Russian N.N. Znamensky described the complex interaction of local and systemic factors in the etiology of periodontal disease. His observations and concepts were summarized in 1902 in a classic paper in which he described the presence in inflamed gingivae of a cellular infiltrate that extends deeper as the disease progresses, thereby causing the bone resorption associated with multinucleated cells (osteoclasts) and Howship lacunae (Fig. 1.6).[58]

The first individual to identify bacteria as the cause of periodontal disease appears to have been the German dentist Adolph Witzel (1847-1906).[23,56] The first true oral microbiologist, however, was the American Willoughby D. Miller (1853-1907), whose professional activities took place in Berlin, where he embarked on a research career that introduced modern bacteriology principles to

Fig. 1.6 Microscopic Features of Periodontal Disease as Presented by Znamensky.

dentistry. Although his greatest accomplishments were in caries research, in his classic book, *The Microorganisms of the Human Mouth,* which was published in 1890, he described the features of periodontal disease and considered the role of predisposing factors, irritational factors, and bacteria in its etiology. He believed that the disease was not caused by a specific bacterium but by a complex array of various bacteria that are normally present in the oral cavity. This constitutes what was later known as the *nonspecific plaque hypothesis,* which went unchallenged for seven decades.[23,37]

Bacterial plaque was described by J. Leon Williams (1852-1932), an American dentist who practiced in London and who, in 1897, described a gelatinous accumulation of bacteria adherent to the enamel surface in relation to caries.[55] In 1899, G.V. Black (1836-1915) coined the term *gelatinous microbic plaque.*[5]

Salomon Robicsek (1845-1928) was born in Hungary and practiced dentistry in Vienna. He developed a surgical technique that consisted of a scalloped, continuous gingivectomy excision that exposed the marginal bone for subsequent curettage and remodeling.[46]

The first description in 1901 of a possible role of trauma from occlusion and bruxism in periodontal disease is generally attributed to the Austrian dentist Moritz Karolyi (1865-1945), who also recommended its correction by grinding occlusal surfaces and preparing bite plates.[34]

Necrotizing Ulcerative Gingivitis

Necrotizing ulcerative gingivitis had been recognized during the 4th century BC by Xenophon, who mentioned that Greek soldiers were affected with "sore mouth and foul-smelling breath." In 1778, Hunter described the clinical features of this disease and differentiated it from scurvy and chronic periodontitis.

Hyacinthe Jean Vincent (1862-1950),[23,49] a French physician working at the Pasteur Institute in Paris, and Hugo Carl Plaut (1858-1928)[42] in Germany described the spirillum and fusiform bacilli associated with what later became known as *Vincent's angina.* In 1904, Vincent described the presence of these organisms in ulceronecrotic gingivitis.[50]

THE 20TH CENTURY

During the first third of the 20th century, periodontics flourished in central Europe, with two major centers of excellence: Vienna and Berlin.[22]

Vienna

The Vienna school developed the basic histopathologic concepts on which modern periodontics was built. The major representative from this group was Bernhard Gottlieb (1885-1950), who published extensive microscopic studies of periodontal disease in human autopsy specimens (Fig. 1.7).[19] His major contributions appeared in the German literature during the 1920s, and they described the attachment of the gingival epithelium to the tooth, the histopathology of inflammatory and degenerative periodontal disease, the biology of the cementum, active and passive tooth eruption, and traumatic occlusion. A book published in 1938 by Gottlieb and Orban presented a complete review

Fig. 1.7 Bernhard Gottlieb (1885-1950). (From Gold SI: *J Clin Periodontol* 12:171, 1985.)

Fig. 1.8 Balint J. Orban (1899-1960). (From *J Periodontol* 31:266, 1960.)

in English of the concepts developed by Gottlieb and his coworkers in Vienna.[24]

A younger contemporary of Gottlieb's in Vienna was Balint J. Orban (1899-1960) (Fig. 1.8), who carried out extensive histologic studies on periodontal tissues. These studies serve as the basis for much of current therapy. Other members of the Viennese school were Rudolph Kronfeld (1901-1940), Joseph P. Weinmann (1889-1960), and Harry Sicher (1889-1974). All of these scientists emigrated to the United States during the 1930s and contributed greatly to the progress of American dentistry.

Berlin

The Berlin group consisted mostly of clinical scientists who developed and refined the surgical approach to periodontal

Fig. 1.9 Robert Neumann (1882-1958). (Courtesy Dr. Steven I. Gold, New York.)

Fig. 1.10 Surgical Procedure Advocated by Robert Neumann During the Early Part of the 20th Century. *Top,* After raising a mucoperiosteal flap, its edge is trimmed with scissors to leave a scalloped outline. *Bottom,* Osseous recontouring with burs. (From Gold SI: *J Periodontol* 53:456, 1982.)

therapy. Prominent in this group were Oskar Weski and Robert Neumann (Fig. 1.9).

Weski (1879-1952) carried out pioneering studies that correlated radiographic and histopathologic changes in patients with periodontal disease.[53] He also conceptualized the periodontium as being formed by the cementum, gingiva, periodontal ligament, and bone, and he gave it the name *paradentium;* this was later changed for etymologic reasons to *parodontium,* which is a term that is still used in Europe.

Neumann (1882-1958), in a book published in 1912[38] (with new editions in 1915, 1920, and 1924), described the principles of periodontal flap surgery, including osseous recontouring as it is currently known (Fig. 1.10).[20] Other clinicians who described flap surgery at the beginning of the 20th century were Leonard Widman of Sweden (1871-1956)[54] and A. Cieszynski of Poland. A bitter controversy developed among Widman, Cieszynski, and Neumann during the 1920s with regard to the priority of describing the periodontal flap.

The United States and Other Countries

In the United States before World War II, important contributions to periodontal surgery were made by A. Zentler, J. Zemsky, G.V. Black, O. Kirkland, A.W. Ward, A.B. Crane, H. Kaplan, and others. In 1923, Ward introduced the surgical pack under the trade name Wondr-Pak.[51]

The nonsurgical approach was championed by Isadore Hirschfeld (1882-1965) of New York, who wrote classic papers about oral hygiene,[28] local factors, and other topics. In 1913, Alfred Fones (1869-1938) opened the first school for dental hygienists in Bridgeport, Connecticut.[9]

In other countries, H.K. Box (Canada); M. Roy and R. Vincent (France); R. Jaccard and A.-J. Held (Switzerland); F.A. Carranza, Sr, and R. Erausquin (Argentina); W.W. James, A. Counsell, and E.W. Fish (Great Britain); and A. Leng (Chile) are well known

for their important contributions. Probably the most comprehensive book about periodontics published during the first half of the 20th century was *El Paradencio, Su Patologia y Tratamiento,* which was written by the Uruguayan F.M. Pucci in 1939.

Focal Infection

The concept of systemic diseases originating in dental and oral infections had been mentioned in the Assyrian clay tablets (7th century BC), by Hippocrates (460-370 BC), in the Babylonian Talmud (3rd century AD), and by Girolamo Cardano and the German Walter Hermann Ryff during the 16th century.[29,52] During the 19th century, Benjamin Rush (a famous physician and one of the signers of the American Declaration of Independence) in 1818 and Leonard Koecker in 1828 recognized the role of oral sepsis in rheumatic and other diseases. Later during the 19th century, W.D. Miller also mentioned oral infections as the cause of many diseases.[37]

In a paper published in 1900[31] and a decade later in a lecture at McGill University in Montreal, Quebec, Canada,[32] William Hunter (1861-1937), a British physician, indicted dentistry as being the cause of oral sepsis, which in turn caused rheumatic and other chronic diseases. This idea was taken up by Billings, Rosenow, and many others, who advocated the extraction of all teeth with periodontal or periapical infections to prevent systemic diseases. This led to the wholesale extraction of teeth and the removal of the tonsils.

The focal infection theory fell into disrepute when it was found that extractions failed to eliminate or reduce the systemic diseases to which the infected teeth were supposed to be linked.[15] However, the concept was revisited during the 1990s, this time with a more solid research foundation.

Dental Implants

The replacement of human teeth with implants has been attempted for centuries. Skulls with metal or stone implants have been found in a Gallo-Roman necropolis in France and dated from the 2nd century AD; they were also found in a mandible of Mayan origin dated about 600 AD.[9]

In 1806, the Italian M. Maggiolo attempted to place solid-gold roots in human jaws. Later during the 19th century, several other investigators used porcelain and metallic implants. During the first half of the 20th century, several attempts were made to use elaborate surgical techniques and complicated constructs of gold and other precious metals. Microscopic investigations were begun to address the tissue response to various metals.

In 1939, A.E. Strock of Harvard University started implanting cobalt–chromium (Vitallium) screws into tooth sockets. After World War II, numerous attempts were made with different materials and shapes of implants, including tantalum twisted spiral (Formiggini), Vitallium tree shaped (Lee), acrylic tooth root replica (Hodosh), Vitallium double helical spiral (Chércheve), tantalum tripodal pins (Scialom), tantalum vent-plant and titanium blade (Linkow), and vitreous carbon.[9]

During the 1950s, the Swedish orthopedic surgeon Per-Ingvar Bränemark developed a technique that involved the use of titanium screw-shaped intraosseous implants. This proved to be quite successful, and it was gradually adopted by the dental profession after the 1982 international conference in Toronto, Ontario, Canada. The success and predictability of Bränemark's technique are attributed to the achievement of direct contact between vital bone and the implant surface without intervening soft tissue; this phenomenon was later termed *osseointegration.*[6] Numerous variations of the Bränemark concept were presented by A. Kirsch, G.A. Niznick, A. Schroeder, and others, and they are widely used at present.

After World War II

The United States and Scandinavia took leading roles in basic and clinical periodontal research during and after the 1950s, with major advances made in the fields of experimental pathology, microbiology, immunology, and therapy.

In the United States, five individuals led the efforts to advance our understanding of disease processes and the technical approaches needed to address them: Irving Glickman (1914-1972) (Fig. 1.11), Henry M. Goldman (1911-1991), Balint J. Orban (1899-1960) (see Fig. 1.7), Sigurd P. Ramfjord (1911-1997), and Helmut A. Zander (1912-1991). In the clinical area, the influence of John Prichard (1907-1990) and Saul Schluger (1908-1990)

Fig. 1.11 Irving Glickman (1914-1972).

Fig. 1.12 Jens Waerhaug (1907-1980). (From *J Clin Periodontol* 7:534, 1980.)

led to new concepts and new directions in the pursuit of clinical success and excellence.

The leading figure of the Scandinavian group was Jens Waerhaug (1907-1980) (Fig. 1.12) of Oslo, Norway, whose dissertation entitled *The Gingival Pocket* (1952) and whose lifetime of research opened a new era in the understanding of the biology of the periodontium and the management of periodontal problems.

The next generations centered their attention more on the role of microorganisms and the host response, including its defensive and destructive aspects. Their contributions, as well as those of their predecessors, are documented in this book.

Several workshops and international conferences have summarized existing knowledge regarding the biologic and clinical aspects of periodontology. Worthy of mention are those that were conducted in 1951, 1966, 1977, 1989, 1996, 1999, and 2008, which were cosponsored and published by the American Academy of Periodontology.

The American Academy of Periodontology, which was founded in 1914 by two female periodontists, Grace Rogers Spalding (1881-1953) and Gillette Hayden (1880-1929), has become the leader in organized periodontics. Its monthly scientific publication, *Journal of Periodontology,* presents all current advances in this discipline. In Europe, the periodontal societies have joined to form the European Federation of Periodontology, which meets regularly at the Europerio meeting. Their official publication is *Journal of Clinical Periodontology.* Other scientific periodontal journals in English include *Journal of Periodontal Research, Periodontology 2000,* and *International Journal of Periodontics and Restorative Dentistry.* With regard to journals in other languages, *Journal de Parodontologie* (France), *Periodoncia* (Spain), and *Journal of the Japanese Association of Periodontology* deserve mention.

Periodontal education in the United States has also grown during the second half of the 20th century, and most dental schools have separate and independent units for teaching and research in this discipline. Periodontics was recognized as a specialty of dentistry by the American Dental Association in 1947. The first university-based programs for the training of specialists in periodontics were begun in several universities (e.g., Columbia, Michigan, Tufts) during the late 1940s; these 1-year programs expanded to 2-year programs about 10 years later. In 1995, the American Academy of Periodontology mandated that all postgraduate periodontal programs increase to a 3-year curriculum because of the increased knowledge in periodontics and the expansion of the scope of periodontics to include the placement of dental implants and the administration of conscious sedation. Currently in the United States, more than 50 periodontal graduate programs are based in universities and hospitals.

REFERENCES

 References for this chapter are found on the companion website.

PART 1

Evidence-Based Practice

Evidence-Based Decision Making[a]

Every day, dental care professionals make decisions about clinical care. It is important that these decisions incorporate the best available scientific evidence to maximize the potential for successful patient care outcomes. It is also important for readers of this book to have the background and skills necessary to evaluate information they read and hear about. These evaluative skills are as important as learning facts and clinical procedures. *The ability to find, discriminate, evaluate, and use information is the most important skill that can be learned as a professional and lifelong learner.* Becoming excellent at this skill will provide a rewarding and fulfilling professional career.

BACKGROUND AND DEFINITION

Using evidence from the medical literature to answer questions, direct clinical action, and guide practice was pioneered at McMaster University, Ontario, Canada, in the 1980s. As clinical research and the publication of findings increased, so did the need to use the medical literature to guide practice. The traditional clinical problem-solving model based on individual experience or the use of information gained by consulting authorities (colleagues or textbooks) gave way to a new methodology for practice and restructured the way in which more effective clinical problem solving should be conducted. This new methodology was termed *evidence-based medicine* (EBM).[12]

> ### KEY DEFINITIONS
>
> **Evidence:** Evidence is considered the synthesis of all valid research that answers a specific question and that, in most cases, distinguishes it from a single research study.[2]
>
> **Evidence-based medicine:** The integration of the best research evidence with our clinical expertise and our patient's unique values and circumstances.[31]
>
> **Evidence-based dentistry:** An approach to oral health care that requires the judicious integration of systematic assessments of clinically relevant scientific evidence, relating to the patient's oral and medical condition and history, with the clinician's expertise and the patient's treatment needs and preferences.[4]

[a]Adapted from the following chapter of Newman and Carranza's Clinical Periodontology, 13th edition: Chapter 1: Evidence-Based Decision Making, by Jane L. Forrest, Syrene A. Miller, Greg W. Miller, Satheesh Elangovan, and Michael G. Newman.

The use of evidence to help guide clinical decisions is not new. However, the following aspects of EBM are new:

- The methods of generating high-quality evidence, such as randomized controlled trials (RCTs) and other well-designed methods
- The statistical tools for synthesizing and analyzing the evidence (systematic reviews [SRs] and meta-analysis [MA])
- The ways of accessing evidence (electronic databases) and applying it (evidence-based decision making [EBDM] and practice guidelines)[9,10]

These changes have evolved along with the understanding of what constitutes the evidence and how to minimize sources of bias, quantify the magnitude of benefits and risks, and incorporate patient values.[13] "In other words, evidence-based practice is not just a new term for an old concept and as a result of advances, practitioners need (1) more efficient and effective online searching skills to find relevant evidence and (2) critical appraisal skills to rapidly evaluate and sort out what is valid and useful and what is not."[28]

EBDM is the formalized process and structure for learning and using the skills for identifying, searching for, and interpreting the results of the best scientific evidence, which is considered in conjunction with the clinician's experience and judgment, the patient's preferences and values, and the clinical and patient circumstances when making patient care decisions. Translating the EBDM process into action is based on the abilities and skills identified in Box 2.1.[31]

PRINCIPLES OF EVIDENCE-BASED DECISION MAKING

The use of current best evidence does not replace clinical expertise or input from the patient, but rather provides another dimension to the decision-making process,[11,16,19] which is also placed in context with the patient's clinical circumstances (Fig. 2.1). It is this decision-making process that we refer to as "evidence-based decision making" and is not unique to medicine or any specific health discipline; it represents a concise way of referring to the application of evidence to clinical decision making.

EBDM focuses on solving clinical problems and involves two fundamental principles, as follows[13]:

BOX 2.1   Skills and Abilities Needed to Apply an Evidence-Based Decision-Making Process[31]

1. Convert information needs and problems into clinical questions so that they can be answered.
2. Conduct a computerized search with maximum efficiency for finding the best external evidence with which to answer the question.
3. Critically appraise the evidence for its validity and usefulness (clinical applicability).
4. Apply the results of the appraisal, or evidence, in clinical practice.
5. Evaluate the process and your performance.

From Straus SE, Glasziou P, Richardson WS, Haynes RB: *Evidence-based medicine: How to practice and teach EBM*, ed 5, Edinburgh, 2019, Elsevier.

Fig. 2.1 Evidence-Based Decision Making. (Copyright Jane L. Forrest, reprinted with permission.)

1. Evidence alone is never sufficient to make a clinical decision.
2. Hierarchies of quality and applicability of evidence exist to guide clinical decision making.

EBDM is a structured process that incorporates a formal set of rules for interpreting the results of clinical research and places a lower value on authority or custom. In contrast to EBDM, traditional decision making relies more on intuition, unsystematic clinical experience, and pathophysiologic rationale.[13]

Evidence-Based Dentistry

Since the 1990s, the evidence-based movement has continued to advance and is widely accepted among the health care professions, with some refining the definition to make it more specific to their area of health care. The American Dental Association (ADA) has defined evidence-based dentistry (EBD) as "an approach to oral health care that requires the judicious integration of systematic assessments of clinically relevant scientific evidence, relating to the patient's oral and medical condition and history, with the clinician's expertise and the patient's treatment needs and preferences."[4] They also have established the ADA Center for Evidence-Based Dentistry (ebd.ada.org) to facilitate the integration of EBD into clinical practice.

The ADA's definition is now incorporated into the Accreditation Standards for Dental Education Programs.[3] Dental hygiene schools are expected to develop specific core competencies that focus on the need for graduates to become critical thinkers, problem solvers, and consumers of current research findings to enable them to become lifelong learners. The accreditation standards require learning EBDM skills so that dental hygiene graduates are competent in being able to find, evaluate, and incorporate current evidence into their decision making.[3]

KEY FACT

Patient Problem or Population, Intervention, Comparison, and Outcome(s)
The first step in evidence-based decision making is asking the right question. The key is to frame a question that is simple and at the same time highly specific to the clinical scenario. Dissecting the question that you want to ask into its components—problem or population (P), intervention (I), comparison group (C) and outcomes (O)—and then combining them will facilitate a thorough and precise evidence search.[31]

EVIDENCE-BASED DECISION-MAKING PROCESS AND SKILLS

The growth of evidence-based practice has been made possible through the development of online scientific databases such as MEDLINE (PubMed) and Internet-based software, along with the use of computers and mobile devices, for example, smart phones, that enable users to quickly access relevant clinical evidence from almost anywhere. This combination of *technology* and *good evidence* allows health care professionals to apply the benefits from clinical research to patient care.[29] EBDM recognizes that clinicians can never be completely current with all conditions, medications, materials, or available products, and it provides a mechanism for assimilating current research findings into everyday practice to answer questions and stay informed with regard to innovations in dentistry. Translating the EBDM process into action is based on the abilities and skills identified in Box 2.1.[31] This is illustrated clearly in a real patient case scenario (management of a patient with trauma-related avulsion and luxation of teeth) that is introduced in Case Scenario 2.1 (Figs. 2.2 and 2.3) and used throughout the chapter. *Avulsion* and *luxation* are terms used to describe trauma-related displacement of tooth from its socket.

Asking Good Questions: The Patient Problem or Population, Intervention, Comparison, and Outcome(s) Process

Converting information needs and problems into clinical questions is a difficult skill to learn, but it is fundamental to evidence-based practice. The EBDM process almost always begins with a patient question or problem. A "well-built" question should include four parts that identify the patient problem or population *(P)*, intervention *(I)*, comparison *(C)*, and outcome(s) *(O)*, referred to as patient problem or population, intervention, comparison, and outcome(s) (PICO).[31] Once these four

CASE SCENARIO 2.1

Clinical Application of Evidence-Based Decision Making

The clinician received a call from the parents of a 13-year-old female patient who had been struck in the face with a softball. She was being examined by paramedics in a town 30 minutes north of the dental office. The paramedics cleared the patient of any head or neck injury and other medical issues and informed the dentist that dental trauma was her primary injury. The dentist and his assistant met the parents and the patient at the office 45 minutes following the dental trauma. The patient's teeth remained in her mouth following the incident. Fig. 2.2A shows the initial examination of the patient. The preference of the patient and her parents was to "do anything to keep the teeth." After the site was cleaned and irrigated, it was apparent that there was complete avulsion of the maxillary right central incisor from the socket and lateral luxation of the maxillary left central and lateral incisors. In addition, there was alveolar bone fracture partially encasing the roots of the maxillary left central and lateral incisors (see Fig. 2.2B.) The clinician replanted the teeth and reapproximated the gingival tissue with sutures (see Fig. 2.2C). A stable and accurate ribbond and flowable composite splint were placed (see Fig. 2.2D), and a radiograph was taken (see Fig. 2.2E).

Radiographic Examination

The radiograph shows reimplantation of maxillary central incisors and left lateral incisor in correct socket location and confirmed proper reapproximation of the alveolar bone that was fractured with maxillary left central and lateral incisors. The stent also is apparent in this radiograph showing the splinting of the displaced teeth.

Due to the difficulty of splint placement and not wanting to risk displacing the teeth or breaking the splint prematurely, the clinician was hesitant to proceed with endodontic treatment until he had access to dependable information. The dentist had two questions regarding the treatment of the patient. He needed to determine the optimal timing of the pulp extirpation and splinting that would result in the best outcome and prognosis for healing. Fig. 2.3 diagrams the decision-making pathway from telephone call to resolution.[24]

components are clearly and succinctly identified, the following format can be used to structure the question:

"For a patient with _____ (P), will _____ (I) as compared with _____ (C) increase/decrease/provide better/in doing _____ (O)?"

The formality of using PICO to frame the question serves two key purposes, as follows:

1. PICO forces the clinician to focus on what he or she and the patient believe to be the most important single issue and outcome.

2. PICO facilitates the next step in the process, the computerized search, by identifying key terms that will be used in the search.[31]

The conversion of information needs into a clinical question is demonstrated using Case Scenario 2.1 Two separate PICO questions were written as follows:

1. For a patient with replanted avulsed and luxated teeth (P), will early pulp extirpation (complete removal of dental pulp) (10 to 14 days) (I) as compared with late pulp extirpation (past 14 days) (C) increase the likelihood of successful tooth integration and functional periodontal healing and decrease

the likelihood of resorption and ankylosis (direct fusion of root of a tooth with the surrounding bone) (O)?

2. For a patient with replanted avulsed and luxated teeth (P), will short-term splinting (stabilizing a tooth by physically connecting it with adjacent teeth) (7 to 14 days) (I) as compared with long-term splinting (2 to 4 weeks) (C) increase the likelihood of successful tooth integration and functional periodontal healing and decrease the development of resorption and ankylosis (O)?

PICO directs the clinician to clearly identify the problem, results, and outcomes related to the specific care provided to that patient. This, in turn, helps identify the search terms that should be used to conduct an efficient search. It also allows identification of the type of evidence and information required to solve the problem, as well as considerations for measuring the effectiveness of the intervention and the application of the EBDM process. Thus EBDM supports continuous quality improvements through measuring outcomes of care and self-reflection.

Before conducting a computerized search, it is important to have an understanding of the types of research study methodologies and the appropriate methodology that relates to different types of clinical questions. The methodology, in turn, relates to the levels of evidence. Table 2.1 shows these relationships.

Becoming a Competent Consumer of the Evidence

Evidence typically comes from studies related to questions about treatment and prevention, diagnosis, etiology and harm, and disease prognosis, as well as from questions about the quality and economics of care. Evidence is considered the synthesis of all valid research that answers a specific question and that, in most cases, distinguishes it from a single research study.[15] Once synthesized, evidence can help inform decisions about whether a method of diagnosis or a treatment is effective relative to other methods of diagnoses or other treatments and under what circumstances. The challenge in using EBDM arises when only one research study is available on a particular topic. In these cases, individuals should be cautious in relying on the study because it can be contradicted by another study, or it may test only efficacy and not effectiveness. This underscores the importance of staying current with the scientific literature because the body of evidence evolves over time as more research is conducted. Another challenge in using EBDM occurs when the limited research available is weak in quality or poorly conducted. In these cases, one may rely more heavily on clinical experience and patients' preferences and values than on the scientific evidence (see Fig. 2.1).

Sources of Evidence

The two types of evidence-based sources are primary and secondary, as follows:

- *Primary sources* are original research studies and publications that have not been filtered or synthesized, such as an RCT or cohort study.
- *Secondary sources* are synthesized studies and publications of the already-conducted primary research. These include clinical practice guidelines (CPGs), SRs, MAs, and evidence-based article reviews and protocols. This terminology is often

Fig. 2.2 (A) Initial examination of the patient. (B) Trauma site following irrigation. (C) Replantation of avulsed and luxated teeth. (D) Replanted and splinted teeth. (E) Radiograph after placement of the splint (Copyright Greg W. Miller, DDS, reprinted with permission.)

Fig. 2.3 Decision-Making Pathway From Telephone Call to Resolution. *ADA*, American dental association; *DARE*, database of abstracts of review of effectiveness; *PICO*, patient problem or population, intervention, comparison, and outcome(s). (Copyright Greg W. Miller, DDS, reprinted with permission.)

TABLE 2.1	Type of Question Related to Type of Methodology and Levels of Evidence		
Type of Question	**Methodology of Choice[27]**		**Question Focus[22]**
Therapy, prevention	MA or SR of randomized controlled trials SR of cohort studies		Study effect of therapy or test on real patients; allows for comparison between intervention and control groups; largest volume of evidence-based literature
Diagnosis	MA or SR of controlled trials (prospective cohort study) *Controlled trial* (Prospective: compare tests with a reference or "gold standard" test)		Measures reliability of a particular diagnostic measure for a disease against the "gold standard" diagnostic measure for the same disease
Etiology, causation, harm	MA or SR of cohort studies *Cohort study* (Prospective data collection with formal control group)		Compares a group exposed to a particular agent with an unexposed group; important for understanding prevention and control of disease
Prognosis	MA or SR of inception cohort studies *Inception cohort study* (All have disease but free of the outcome of interest) *Retrospective cohort*		Follows progression of a group with a particular disease and compares with a group without the disease

MA, Meta-analysis; *SR*, systematic review.

confusing to individuals new to the EBDM approach because, although SRs are *secondary* sources of evidence, they are considered a higher level of evidence than a *primary* source, such as an individual RCT.

Both primary and secondary sources can be found by conducting a search using such biomedical databases as MEDLINE (accessed through PubMed), EMBASE, and Database of Abstracts of Review of Effectiveness (DARE). Other sources of secondary evidence, such as CPGs, clinical recommendations, parameters of care, position papers, academy statements, and critical summaries related to dental practice can be found on the websites of professional organizations and journals as listed in Table 2.2.

Levels of Evidence

As previously mentioned, one principle of EBDM is that hierarchies of evidence exist to guide decision making. At the top of the hierarchy for therapy are CPGs (Fig. 2.4). These are systematically developed statements to assist clinicians and patients about appropriate health care for specific clinical circumstances.[8] CPGs should be based on the best available scientific evidence, typically from MAs and SRs, which put together all that is known about a topic in an objective manner. The level and quality of the evidence are then analyzed by a panel of experts who formulate the CPGs. Thus, guidelines are intended to translate the research into practical application.

Guidelines also will change over time as the evidence evolves, thereby underscoring the importance of keeping current with the scientific literature. One example of this is the change in the American Heart Association guidelines for the prevention of

TABLE 2.2	**Sources of Secondary Evidence**
Sources	**Websites**
American Academy of Pediatric Dentistry (AAPD): 2017-2018 definitions, oral health policies, and clinical practice guidelines	http://www.aapd.org/policies
American Academy of Periodontology (AAP): Clinical and scientific papers[1]	https://www.perio.org/resources-products/clinical-scientific-papers.html
American Dental Association (ADA), Center for Evidence-Based Dentistry	http://ebd.ada.org
American Heart Association (AHA): Prevention of bacterial endocarditis, recommendations	http://circ.ahajournals.org/content/116/15/1736.full.pdf+html?sid=ada268bd-1f10-4496-bae4-b91806aaf341
Centers for Disease Control and Prevention (CDC): Guidelines and recommendations	http://www.cdc.gov/OralHealth/guidelines.htm
Cochrane Collaboration: A nonprofit organization dedicated to producing systematic reviews as a reliable and relevant source of evidence about the effects of health care for making informed decisions.[7]	http://www.cochrane.org Cochrane Oral Health Group: http://ohg.cochrane.org
Journal: *Evidence-Based Dentistry*	http://www.nature.com/ebd/index.html
Journal: *Journal of Evidence-Based Dental Practice*	http://www.jebdp.com

Fig. 2.4 Hierarchy of Research and Levels of Clinical Evidence. (Image Copyright 2012 JL Forrest, SA Miller: National Center for Dental Hygiene Research & Practice.)

infective endocarditis related to the need for premedication before dental and dental hygiene procedures.[5] Before the 2007 guidelines, the last update was in 1997, and before then, eight updates were added to the primary regimens for dental procedures since the original guideline was first published in 1955. In the 2007 update, the rationale for revising the 1997 document was provided, notably that the prior guidelines were largely based on expert opinion and a few case-controlled studies. With more research conducted, the ability now existed to synthesize those findings to provide a more objective body of evidence on which to base recommendations.[5]

If a CPG does not exist, other sources of preappraised evidence (critical summaries, critically appraised topics [CATs], SRs, MAs, or reviews of individual research studies) are available to help stay current. MAs and SRs have strict protocols to reduce bias and the synthesis of research from more than one study. These reviews provide a summary of multiple research studies that have investigated the same specific question. SRs use explicit criteria for retrieval, assessment, and synthesis of evidence from individual RCTs and other well-controlled methods. SRs facilitate decision making by providing a clear summary of the current state of the existing evidence on a specific topic. SRs provide a way of managing large quantities of information,[25] thus making it easier to stay up to date with new research.

MA is a statistical process used when the data from the individual studies in the SR can be combined into one analysis. When data from these studies are pooled, the sample size and power usually increase. As a result, the combined effect can increase the precision of estimates of treatment effects and exposure risks.[25]

SRs and MAs are followed, respectively, by individual RCT studies, cohort studies, case–control studies, and then studies not involving human subjects.[27] In the absence of scientific evidence, the consensus opinion of experts in appropriate fields of research and clinical practice is used (see Fig. 2.4). This hierarchy of evidence is based on the concept of causation and the need to control bias.[21,22] Although each level may contribute to the total body of knowledge, "not all levels are equally useful for making patient care decisions."[22] In progressing up the pyramid, the number of studies and, correspondingly, the amount of available literature decrease, while at the same time their relevance to answering clinical questions increases.

Evidence is judged on its rigor of methodology, and the level of evidence is directly related to the type of question asked, such as those derived from issues of therapy or prevention, diagnosis, etiology, and prognosis (see Table 2.1). For example, the highest level of evidence associated with questions about therapy or prevention is from CPGs based on MAs and/or SRs of RCT studies. However, the highest level of evidence associated with questions about prognosis is from CPGs based on MAs and/or SRs of inception cohort studies.[27] Because the two case scenario questions are related to prognosis, the highest level of evidence for them is a CPG based on MAs and/or SRs of inception cohort studies. If no CPG is found, then the next highest level would be a critical summary of an MA or SR of cohort studies. In the event that a critical summary is not found, MAs or SRs of cohort

studies followed by individual cohort studies provide the next highest levels of evidence.

Knowing what constitutes the highest levels of evidence and knowing how to apply evidence-based filters are skills that are necessary to search the literature with maximum efficiency.[22] By using filters, one can refine the search to limit the citations to publication types such as practice guidelines, MAs, SRs, RCTs, and clinical trials, the highest levels of evidence.

Searching for and Acquiring the Evidence

PubMed is designed to provide access to both primary and secondary research from the biomedical literature. PubMed provides free access to MEDLINE, the National Library of Medicine's premier bibliographic database covering the fields of medicine, nursing, dentistry, veterinary medicine, the health care system, and the preclinical sciences. MEDLINE contains bibliographic citations and author abstracts from more than 5200 biomedical journals published in the United States and 80 other countries. The database contains more than 22 million citations dating back to 1966, and it adds more than 520,000 new citations each year.[26]

It is often helpful to identify the appropriate terminology when searching PubMed. This is done by using the Medical Subject Heading (MeSH) database. It provides the definition of terms and illustrates how the terms are indexed in MEDLINE. The PICO terms from the question can be typed into the MeSH database to maximize searching efficiency. For example, by typing "avulsed tooth" into the MeSH database, a term from the case scenario, it is learned that the MeSH term is "tooth avulsion." It is defined as partial or complete displacement of a tooth from its alveolar support. It is commonly the result of trauma. It also is learned that "tooth luxation" links to the MeSH term "tooth avulsion." This informs the searcher that "tooth avulsion" is the best term to use for the search because it encompasses both avulsed and luxated teeth.[23]

Using PubMed's Clinical Queries feature, one can quickly pinpoint a set of citations that will potentially provide an answer to the question being posed. Although online databases provide quicker access to the literature, knowing how databases filter information and having an understanding of how to use search terms and database features allow a more efficient search to be conducted.

Because two focused clinical (PICO) questions were generated from the clinical case, two separate searches were conducted, one for each PICO question. In addition to PubMed, several other databases were used to find high levels of evidence. These included the Database of Abstracts of Reviews of Effects (https://www.crd.york.ac.uk/CRDWeb/), the National Guideline Clearinghouse (http://www.guideline.gov), the ADA Center for Evidence-Based Dentistry website (http://ebd.ada.org), the American Academy of Pediatric Dentistry website (www.aapd.org), and the American Association of Endodontists (www.aae.org), resulting in several relevant references.

When searching for evidence, the PICO question guides the search (Table 2.3).[4,6] By using key terms identified in the PICO question and combining them using the Boolean operators "OR" and "AND," relevant articles can be narrowed to a manageable number.

TABLE 2.3 Search Terms for Each Patient Problem or Population, Intervention, Comparison, and Outcome(s) Question

PICO Question 1 Search Terms		PICO Question 2 Search Terms
Tooth avulsion (MeSH)[23] OR Tooth replantation (MeSH)[23]	**P**	Tooth avulsion (MeSH)[23] OR Tooth replantation (MeSH)[23]
Pulp extirpation OR Root canal therapy (MeSH)[23]	**I**	Splints (MeSH)[23]
(Same intervention as above; however, timing is the real comparison, so that is the factor in the final article selection.)	**C**	(Same intervention as above; however, timing is the real comparison, so that is the factor in the final article selection)
Tooth integration OR Functional periodontal healing OR Root resorption (MeSH)[23] OR Tooth ankylosis (MeSH)[23]	**O** These terms were used as inclusion criteria and were not used when searching PubMed because only a few number of systematic reviews and guidelines were found just using the P, I, and C terms	Tooth integration OR Functional periodontal healing OR Root resorption (MeSH)[23] OR Tooth ankylosis (MeSH)[23]

MeSH, Medical Subject Heading (database); *PICO,* patient problem or population, intervention, comparison, and outcome(s).

The first search used the terms "(tooth avulsion OR tooth replantation) AND (pulp extirpation OR root canal therapy)." This resulted in 590 papers. Studies were limited to practice guidelines, MAs, and SRs by using each of these three filters separately so that each of these types of studies could be identified. The findings included four practice guidelines, including those of the American Association of Endodontists and the International Association of Dental Traumatology, one critical summary of an SR, and one SR. The second search used the terms "(tooth avulsion OR tooth replantation) AND splints." This resulted in 340 papers. Again, studies were limited to practice guidelines, MAs, and SRs by using the filter for each publication type separately. Relevant results included four practice guidelines from the International Association of Dental Traumatology and Pediatric Dentistry, one MA, and one SR. Fig. 2.3 provides a detailed review of the decision-making steps in this case and the outcomes.[24]

The articles that were selected as relevant research included each aspect of the PICO question. Inclusion criteria included the following: The patient population studied had to have replanted avulsed or luxated teeth; the research studied the intervention for each of the two PICO questions, pulp extirpation and splint duration, respectively; and the research measured at least one of the outcomes of tooth integration, functional periodontal healing, or the levels of resorption or ankylosis. To reduce the requirement of critical appraisal, the search also looked for critical summaries of the SRs that were found.

Appraising the Evidence

After identifying the evidence gathered to answer a question, it is important to have the skills to understand the evidence found. In all cases, it is necessary to review the evidence, whether it is a CPG, MA, SR, or an original study, to determine whether the methods were conducted rigorously and appropriately. International evidence-based groups have made this easier by developing appraisal forms and checklists that guide the user

TABLE 2.4 Examples of Critical Analysis Guides

Guide	Purpose
CONSORT (Consolidated Standards of Reporting Trials) statement[3] http://www.consort-statement.org	To improve the reporting and review of RCTs
PRISMA (Preferred Reporting Items for Systematic Reviews and Meta-analyses) http://www.prisma-statement.org	To improve the reporting and review of SRs
CASP (Critical Appraisal Skills Program)[9] http://www.casp-uk.net	To review RCTs, SRs, and several other types of studies

RCTs, Randomized controlled trials; *SRs,* systematic reviews.

through a structured series of "YES/NO" questions to determine the validity of the individual study or SR. Table 2.4 provides the names and websites of three different guides that can be used for critical analysis.

Common Ways Used to Report Results

Once the results are determined to be valid, the next step is to determine whether the results and potential benefits (or harms) are important. Straus and colleagues[31] identified the clinically useful measures for each type of study. For example, in determining the magnitude of therapy results, we would expect articles to report the control event rate (CER), the experimental event rate (EER), the absolute and relative risk reduction (ARR or RRR), and number needed to treat (NNT). The NNT provides the number of patients (e.g., surfaces, periodontal pockets) who would need to be treated with the experimental treatment or intervention to achieve one additional patient (surfaces, periodontal pockets) who has a favorable response. Another way of assessing evidence is presented in Chapter 3, which introduces 12 tools that may be useful in assessing causality in clinical sciences.

In appraising the evidence found for the case scenario, the first research study retrieved that answered the first PICO question was a well-conducted SR published in *Dental Traumatology* in 2009.[17] Results indicated an association between pulp extirpations performed after 14 days following replantation and the development of inflammatory resorption. A corresponding critical summary also was found.[30] This evidence was consistent with the 2007 clinical guidelines from the International Association of Dental Traumatology for pulp extirpation within 10 to 14 days of replantation.[14]

The Practice Guideline on the Management of Acute Dental Trauma from the American Academy of Pediatric Dentistry answered the second PICO question. It recommended a "flexible splint for 1 week" for avulsed teeth. However, for lateral luxation, an additional 2 to 4 weeks may be needed when there is breakdown of marginal bone.[2] In addition, a well-conducted SR about splinting duration reported inconclusive evidence of an association between short-term splinting and an increased likelihood of functional periodontal healing, acceptable healing, or decreased development of replacement resorption.[18] The study found no evidence to contraindicate the current guidelines and suggested that the likelihood of successful periodontal healing after replantation was unaffected by splinting duration. Although this SR excluded studies of luxated teeth, it is still applicable to the patient. It concluded that dentists should continue to use the currently recommended splinting periods when replanting avulsed permanent teeth, pending future research to the contrary.[18] Consistent with previous reviews, another SR on splinting luxated, avulsed, and root-fractured teeth reported that "the types of splint and the fixation period are generally not significant variables when related to healing outcomes."[20] These two SRs were appraised using the Critical Appraisal Skills Program (CASP) form for appraising reviews (see Table 2.4).

Applying the Evidence: Evidence-Based Dentistry in Action

Throughout this chapter, the EBDM process has illustrated the application of evidence in clinical decision making. The clinician used the EBDM process to answer two clinical questions. Several relevant resources were incorporated into the decision-making process and the treatment of the patient. The clinician performed pulp extirpations on the avulsed and luxated teeth within the recommended time period of 10 to 14 days (Fig. 2.5A). Healing at 2 weeks post trauma is seen in Fig. 2.5B. The clinician also removed the splint within the recommended time frame for luxated teeth of 2 to 4 weeks. The evidence, in combination with clinical experience, helped provide care for this patient that resulted in the best possible prognosis given the extent of the patient's dental trauma. It also allowed the patient to keep her own teeth, which incorporated the patient preferences aspect of the EBDM process. Fig. 2.5C shows the patient at 4 weeks post

trauma; Fig. 2.5D shows the patient at 12 weeks; and Fig. 2.5E shows the patient 2 years post trauma.

Evaluating the Outcomes

The final steps in the EBDM process are to evaluate the effectiveness of the intervention and clinical outcomes and to determine how effectively the EBDM process was applied. For example, one question to ask in evaluating the effectiveness of the intervention is, "Did the selected intervention or treatment achieve the desired result?" In this specific case, the answer is yes.

EBDM is a valuable tool that guides practice decisions to achieve optimal results. In the case of tooth avulsion, the key PICO questions were established to identify research that studied the outcomes of reducing the risk of root resorption and tooth ankylosis and increasing periodontal healing. In using the EBDM process, providers can be confident that they have the most current and relevant evidence available on which to base treatment decisions, provide the best treatment, and improve the possibility of a successful outcome.

Using an EBDM approach requires understanding new concepts and developing new skills. In addition to evaluating patient care outcomes, another aspect of evaluation is in using the EBDM process. Questions that parallel each step in the EBDM process can be asked in evaluating self-performance. For example, "How well was the search conducted to find appropriate and relevant evidence to answer the question?" As with most learning, time and practice are essential to mastering new techniques.

CHAPTER HIGHLIGHTS

- Evidence-based decision making (EBDM) provides clinicians the skills to find, efficiently filter, interpret, and apply research findings so that what is known is reflected in the care provided.
- EBDM takes time and practice to learn to use.
- When mastered, EBDM is an efficient way for clinicians to stay current, and it maximizes the potential for successful patient care outcomes.

CONCLUSION

An EBDM approach closes the gap between clinical research and the realities of practice by providing dental hygienists the skills to find, efficiently filter, interpret, and apply research findings so that what is known is reflected in the care provided. This approach assists clinicians in keeping current with conditions that a patient may have by providing a mechanism for addressing gaps in knowledge to provide the best care possible.

As EBDM becomes standard practice, individuals must be knowledgeable about what constitutes the evidence and how it is reported. Understanding evidence-based methodology and distinctions among different types of articles allows the clinician to better judge the validity and relevance of reported findings.

Fig. 2.5 (A) Periapical radiograph following pulp extirpations. (B) Healing at 2 weeks post trauma. (C) Healing at 4 weeks post trauma. (D) Healing at 12 weeks post trauma. (E) Patient 2 years post trauma (Copyright Greg W. Miller, DDS, reprinted with permission.)

To assist practitioners with this endeavor, SRs and MAs are being conducted to answer specific clinical questions and support the development of CPGs. Journals devoted to evidence-based practice are being published to alert readers about important advances in a concise and user-friendly manner. By integrating good science with clinical judgment and patient preferences, clinicians enhance their decision-making ability and maximize the potential for successful patient care outcomes.

REFERENCES

 References for this chapter are found on the companion website.

3

Critical Thinking: Assessing Scientific Evidence[a]

🌐 For online-only content on tools for assessing scientific evidence, please visit the companion website.

CHAPTER OUTLINE

Between 1950 and 2016, 2290 scientific articles were published with the terms "periodontal diseases" and "antibacterial agents" as Medical Subject Headings. Which of these articles provide information that is clinically relevant? Are those articles that are clinically relevant selected and accurately summarized in educational courses, textbooks, or systematic reviews? Relying completely on authority to ensure that this happens can be dangerous.

Einstein purportedly said that "his own major scientific talent was his ability to look at an enormous number of experiments and journal articles, select the very few that were both correct and important, ignore the rest, and build a theory on the right ones."[4] Most evidence-based clinicians aspire to the same goal when evaluating clinical evidence. In this search for good evidence, a "baloney detection kit"[43] can be helpful to separate salesmanship from science and suggestive hints from unequivocal evidence. This chapter introduces 12 tools that may be useful in assessing causality in clinical sciences.

TOOLS FOR ASSESSING SCIENTIFIC EVIDENCE

Be Skeptical

Of all machines ours is the most complicated and inexplicable.

—*Thomas Jefferson*

Evidence on how to cure, manage, or prevent chronic diseases is notoriously contradictory, inconsistent, and unreliable. Mark Twain reminded people to be careful when reading health books because one may die of a misprint.[42] Powerful forces conspire to deliver a preponderance of misleading results:

1. Identifying a successful treatment for chronic diseases can be challenging. It has been estimated that less than 0.1% of all investigated treatments are effective. Because the odds of identifying successful interventions for chronic diseases are so small, most so-called effective treatments identified in small clinical trials turn out to be non-effective or harmful when they are evaluated in rigorously conducted pivotal trials.

2. Chronic diseases can be complex and include both environmental and genetic causes. The "obvious" causes of disease, such as tobacco and sugars for periodontitis, are often ignored.[30] As a result of such biased epidemiologic research, incomplete and mistaken understandings of chronic disease etiology can lead to a cascade of wrong turns in the exploration of possible diagnosis, prognosis, and treatment.

   Poor scientific methodology is a common problem permeating most of the evidence that surrounds us.

3. Finally, the possibility needs to be considered that no magic bullets exist against certain noxious aspects of civilized lifestyles. The experiences so far with finding prescriptions as protection against harmful lifestyles have been largely disastrous.

   These factors may all be at play in periodontics, thus suggesting that skepticism is required in the evaluation of scientific evidence.

Do Not Trust Biologic Plausibility

Born but to die, and reasoning but to err.

—*Alexander Pope*

Because of an incomplete understanding of biology, the use of deductive reasoning for clinical decisions may be dangerous. For thousands of years, deductive reasoning largely failed to lead to medical breakthroughs. In evidence-based medicine, evidence that is based on deductive inference is classified as level 5, which is the lowest level of evidence available. Unfortunately, much of our knowledge on how to prevent, manage, and treat chronic periodontitis depends largely on deductive reasoning.

---

[a]Adapted from the following chapter of Newman and Carranza's Clinical Periodontology, 13th edition: Chapter 2: Critical Thinking, by Philippe P. Hujoel.

CLINICAL CORRELATION

The Dietary Guidelines for Americans dropped their recommendation to floss because of the lack of scientific evidence. Dental floss has been recommended by oral hygiene companies and the dental profession based on the following biologic plausibility argument: dental plaque causes dental caries; floss removes dental plaque. Therefore, flossing will lower the risk of dental caries. Such reasoning is no longer accepted as evidence for effectiveness in the 21st century.

KEY FACT

Biologic plausibility will increasingly become an unacceptable rationale to recommend dental treatments.

What Level of Controlled Evidence Is Available?

Development of Western science is based on two great achievements: the invention of a formal logical system (in Euclidean geometry) by the Greek philosophers, and the discovery of the possibility to find out causal relationships by systematic experiment (during the Renaissance).

—*Albert Einstein*

Rational thought requires reliance on either deductive reasoning (biologic plausibility) or systematic experiments (sometimes referred to as inductive reasoning). Galileo is typically credited with the start of systematic experimentation in physics. Puzzlingly, it took until the latter half of the 20th century before systematic experiments became part of clinical research. Three systematic experiments are now routine in clinical research: the case-control study, the cohort study, and the RCT. In the following brief descriptions of these three systematic experimental designs, the term *exposure* refers to a suspected etiologic factor or an intervention, such as a treatment or a diagnostic test, and the term *endpoint* refers to the outcome of disease, quality-of-life measures, or any type of condition that may be of interest in clinical studies.

1. *RCT.* Individuals or clusters of individuals are randomly assigned to different exposures and monitored longitudinally for the endpoint of interest. An association between the exposure and the endpoint is present when frequency of the endpoint occurrence differs among the exposure groups. The RCT is the "gold standard" design in clinical research. In evidence-based medicine, RCTs, when properly executed, are referred to as level 1 evidence and the highest (best) level of evidence available.

2. *Cohort study.* Exposed individuals are compared with non-exposed individuals and monitored longitudinally for the occurrence of the primary endpoint of interest. An association between the exposure and endpoint is present when the frequency of endpoint occurrences differs between exposed and nonexposed individuals. A cohort study is often considered the optimal study design in nonexperimental clinical research (i.e., for those study designs where randomization may not be feasible). In evidence-based medicine, cohort studies, when properly executed, are referred to as level 2 evidence.

3. *Case-control study.* Cases (individuals with the endpoint of interest) are compared with controls (individuals without the endpoint of interest) with respect to the prevalence of the exposure. If the prevalence of exposure differs between cases and controls, an association between the exposure and the endpoint is present. In a case-control study, it is challenging to select cases and controls in an unbiased manner and to obtain reliable information on possible causes of disease that occurred in the past. The case-control study is the most challenging study design to use for obtaining reliable evidence. As a result, in evidence-based medicine, case-control studies, when properly executed, are considered the lowest level of evidence.

All three study designs permit us to study the association between the exposure and the endpoint. This association can be represented schematically as follows:

Exposure → Endpoint

An important challenge in the assessment of controlled evidence is determining whether the association identified (→) is causal. Criteria used to assess causality include factors such as the assessment of temporality, the presence of a pre-trial hypothesis, and the size or strength of the reported association. Unlike deductive reasoning, in which associations are either true or false, such absolute truths cannot be achieved with systematic experiments. Conclusions based on controlled study designs are always surrounded by a degree of uncertainty, a frustrating limitation to real-world clinicians who have to make yes/no decisions.

Did the Cause Precede the Effect?

You can't change the laws of physics, Captain.

—*"Scotty" in Star Trek*

In 2001, a study published in the *British Medical Journal* suggested that retroactive prayer shortened hospital stays in patients with bloodstream infection.[29] The only problem was that patients were already dismissed from the hospital when the nonspecified prayer to the nonspecified deity was made. To most scientists, findings in which the effect (shorter hospital stay) precedes the cause (the prayer) are impossible, and this provides an unequivocal example of a violation of correct temporality; the effect preceded the hypothesized cause. In chronic disease research, it is often challenging to disentangle temporality, and fundamental questions regarding temporality often remain disputed.

Vigorous investigation of temporality is a key aspect in scientific investigation.

Temporality is the only criterion that needs to be satisfied for claiming causality; the cause needs to precede the effect. In periodontal research, almost all studies relating plaque or specific infections to periodontal diseases suffer from unclear temporality.[30] Are observed microbial profiles the result or the cause of periodontitis? No cohort studies in adults have established that an infectious cause precedes the onset of chronic periodontitis.[30] Unequivocal establishment of temporality is an essential element of causality and can be surprisingly difficult to establish for chronic diseases, including periodontal diseases.

No Betting on the Horse After the Race Is Over

Predictions are difficult, especially about the future.

—*Niels Bohr*

One of the most pervasive cancers in clinical research is the inability of researchers to stick to a hypothesis. Science is about formulating a specific hypothesis, testing it in a clinical experiment, and accepting the findings for what they are. Not only does this rarely happen, but also, powerful forces sometimes actively try to prevent regulations that would enforce such scientific behavior.

An essential characteristic of science is that hypotheses or ideas predict observations, not that hypotheses or ideas can be fitted to observations. This essential characteristic of scientific enterprise—prediction—is often lost in medical and dental research when poorly defined prestudy hypotheses result in convoluted data-generated ideas or hypotheses that fit the observed data. It has been reported that even for well-organized studies with carefully written protocols, investigators often do not remember which hypotheses were defined in advance, which hypotheses were data derived, which hypotheses were "a priori" considered plausible, and which were unlikely.[52]

What Is a Clinically Relevant Pretrial Hypothesis?

Clinically relevant questions are designed to have an impact on improving patients' outcomes. Usually, clinically relevant questions share four important characteristics of the pretrial hypothesis: (1) a clinically relevant endpoint (referred to as the outcome in the populations/people/patient/problem, intervention(s), comparison, and outcome (PICO) question), (2) relevant exposure comparisons (referred to as the Intervention and the Control in the PICO question, (3) a study sample representative of real-world clinical patients (should be representative of the Patient defined in the PICO question), and (4) small error rates.

Clinically Relevant Endpoint

An endpoint is a measurement related to a disease process or a condition and is used to assess the exposure effect. Two different types of endpoints are recognized. True endpoints are tangible outcomes that directly measure how a patient feels, functions, or survives[45]; examples include tooth loss, death, and pain. Surrogate endpoints are intangible outcomes used as a substitute for true endpoints[15]; examples include blood pressure and probing depths of periodontal pockets. Treatment effects on surrogates do not necessarily translate into real clinical benefit (Table 3.1).

TABLE 3.1   Examples of Potentially Misleading Surrogates[a]

Disease or Condition	Experimental Treatment	Control Treatment	Effect on Surrogate Endpoint	Effect on True Endpoint	Misleading Conclusion	Reference
AIDS	Immediate zidovudine	Delayed zidovudine	Significant increase of 30–35 CD4 cells/mm^3	No change in incidence of AIDS, AIDS-related complex, or survival	False-positive	46
Osteoporosis	Fluoride	Placebo	Significant increase of 16% in bone mineral density of lumbar spine	Nonvertebral fracture rates increased by 85%	False-positive	
Lung cancer	ZD1839 (Iressa)	Placebo	Dramatic tumor shrinkage in 10% of patients	No effect	False-positive	48
Aphthous ulcers	Thalidomide	Placebo	Although thalidomide expected to decrease TNF-α production, significant increase of 4.4 pg/mL in TNF-α production occurred, suggesting harm	Pain diminished and ability to eat improved	False-negative	21
Edentulism dentures	Implant-supported	Conventional dentures	No impact on chewing cycles	Improved oral health–related quality of life	False-negative	3
Prostate cancer	Radical prostatectomy	Watchful waiting	Substantial elimination of tumor mass	No effect on overall mortality risk	False-positive	45
Advanced colorectal cancer	5-FU + LV	5-FU	23% of patients had 50% or greater reduction in tumor volume	No effect on overall survival	False-positive	26
Periodontitis	Surgery	Scaling	Mean pocket depth reduced by 0.5 mm	Effect on tooth loss or quality of life unknown	?	20

[a]For some examples, the experimental treatment led to improvements in surrogate endpoints, whereas the true endpoint was either unaffected or worsened (a false-positive conclusion). For other examples, the experimental treatment had no impact or worsened the surrogate endpoint, whereas the true endpoint improved (a false-negative conclusion).
AIDS, Acquired immunodeficiency syndrome; *5-FU*, 5-fluorouracil; *LV*, leucovorin; *TNF-α*, tumor necrosis factor-alpha.

Reliance on surrogate endpoints in clinical trials has led to widespread use of deadly medications, and such disasters have prompted minor changes in the drug approval process.[39] Most major causes of human disease (e.g., cigarette smoking) were identified through studies using true endpoints. A first requirement for a clinically relevant study is the pretrial specification of a true endpoint.

Common and Relevant Comparisons

The more prevalent a studied exposure, the more relevant the clinical question. A clinically relevant comparison implies the absence of comparator bias, which is defined as the presence of contrived or unethical control groups.[31] Providing the control subjects with less than the standard dose of the standard treatment and providing a control therapy that avoids the real clinical questions are examples of clinically irrelevant research. Similarly, the presence of a placebo treatment instead of "no" treatment in clinical trials can be critical given the large therapeutic effects that can be obtained by proper attention and care in medical settings. For instance, the absence of placebo controls in fluoride varnish trials for primary teeth raises serious doubts whether fluoride varnish has an effect above and beyond what would be observed with just a placebo. In case-control or cohort studies, the measurement and characterization of exposures (e.g., mercury, fluoride, chewing tobacco) can be difficult and imprecise, thus making answers to the questions almost unavoidably imprecise.

Representative Study Sample

The larger the discrepancy between the typical subjects enrolled in clinical studies and the patient you seek to treat, the more questionable the applicability of the study's conclusions becomes. When cholesterol-lowering drugs provided a small benefit in middle-aged men with abnormally high cholesterol levels, it was concluded that those benefits "could and should be extended" to other age groups and women with "more modest elevations" of cholesterol levels.[46] Findings on blood lipids and heart disease that were derived mostly from Polish immigrants in the Framingham Study were generalized to a much more diverse population. An antidepressant that was approved for use in adults was widely prescribed for children, with unexpected, serious consequences.[1]

Ideally, clinical trials should use simple entry criteria in which the enrolled patients reflect the real-world clinical practice situation as closely as possible. Legislation has been enacted to reach this goal. In 1993, US policy ensured the recruitment of women and minority groups in clinical trials.[8] A US policy for the inclusion of children in clinical studies was then set into law in 1998. Experiments with long lists of inclusion and exclusion criteria can be expensive recipes for failure because they can lead to study subjects who are unrepresentative of most real-world clinical patients.

Small Type I and Type II Error Rates

The type I error rate is the likelihood of concluding that an effect exists when in truth no effect exists. The type I error rate is set by the investigator, and common values are 1% or 5%. The type II error rate is the likelihood of concluding that no effect exists when in truth an effect does exist. The type II error rate is typically set by the investigator at 10% or 20%. The

complement of the type II error rate (i.e., 1—type II error rate) is referred to as the power of the study. The likelihood of a false-positive or false-negative result depends, in addition to the type I and II error rates, on the likelihood that the treatment under investigation is truly effective. This last component is obviously not under the investigator's control, and yet it determines the likelihood of making correct conclusions. For chronic diseases, in which the likelihood of identifying effective treatments or true causes is low, the false-positive rate can be high even when the type I error rate is low. Clinically relevant studies require small type I and type II error rates to minimize false-positive and false-negative conclusions.[24]

🌐 Size Does Matter

Chronic hepatitis B infection increased the chances for liver cancer by more than 23,000%.[5] Proximity to electromagnetic radiation increased the chance for leukemia in children by 49%.[50] Periodontitis in populations with smokers increased the chance for coronary heart disease by 12%.[21] No one doubts the causality of the association between chronic hepatitis B infection and liver cancer, but the role of periodontitis in coronary heart disease or electromagnetic radiation in childhood leukemia remain controversial. Why? To a large extent, the size of the association drives the interpretation of causality.

The larger an association, the less likely it is to be caused by bias, and the more likely it is to be causal.

One simple way to calculate the size of the association is to calculate an odds ratio. The odds of an event represent the probability that an event happens divided by the probability that an event does not happen.

The size of the odds ratio ranges between 0 and infinity. An odds ratio of 1 indicates the absence of an association, and if the two-by-two table is set up with the reference cell (poor outcome exposure of interest) in the left-hand side of the top data row, an odds ratio larger than 1 means a harmful effect (e.g., periodontitis increases the odds of a fatal myocardial infarction by 20%), and an odds ratio smaller than 1 means a protective effect (e.g., penciclovir decreases the odds of failed lesion healing by day 6 by 38%).

The confidence interval is the range of numbers between the upper confidence limit and the lower confidence limit. The confidence interval contains the true odds ratio with a certain predetermined probability (e.g., 95%). In a properly executed randomized trial, a conclusion of causality is typically made if the 95% confidence interval does not include the possibility of "no association" (e.g., odds ratio = 1). For example, because the 95% confidence interval for the odds ratio associated with penciclovir use is 0.52 to 0.73 and does not include 1, the effect can be referred to as "statistically significant." For the chronic periodontitis–myocardial infarction example, the 95% confidence interval ranges from 0.25 to 5.72, includes 1, and is therefore referred to as "statistically insignificant."

CLINICAL CORRELATION

Periodontitis during pregnancy was reported to increase the risk for preterm low birth weight eightfold.[14]

🌐 Is a Better Alternative Explanation Available?

No amount of experimentation can ever prove me right; a single experiment can prove me wrong.

—*Albert Einstein*

When you have eliminated the impossible, whatever remains, however improbable, must be the truth.

—*Sir Arthur Conan Doyle*

Dozens of epidemiologic studies appeared to support the hypothesis that β-carotene intake lowered lung cancer risk. However, RCTs provided unequivocal evidence to the contrary. What went wrong? Different explanations that worked as well or better may have been inadequately explored. Possibly, smoking was not adequately considered as an alternative explanation and led to a misunderstanding of the health effects of β-carotene.[14,44] Similarly, a systematic review of epidemiologic studies appeared to support the hypothesis that chronic periodontitis caused low birth weight.[51] In contrast, however, a systematic review of RCTs suggested that the periodontitis–low birth weight theory may be dead.[49] Why was epidemiology misleading? Again, different explanations may have been inadequately explored. More efforts may have been expended toward proving associations by ignoring common causal factors rather than disproving associations. The highest goal of a scientist is the attempt to refute, disprove, and vigorously explore factors and alternative hypotheses that may "explain away" the observed association.[9] The efforts at refuting smoking and nutrition as potential confounders in periodontics have been minimal and may have led to a significant waste of clinical research resources.

For a factor (i.e., a potential confounder) to explain away an observed association, two criteria need to be fulfilled. First, the factor must be related to the exposure, but not necessarily in a causal way. Second, the factor must be causally related to the outcome and must not be in the causal pathway. If both criteria are satisfied, the factor is referred to as a confounder, and confounding is said to be present. For example, smoking satisfied the criteria for a confounder in the β-carotene–lung cancer association because (1) cigarette smokers consumed less β-carotene than nonsmokers and (2) smoking caused lung cancer. Confounding is often represented schematically (Fig. 3.1).

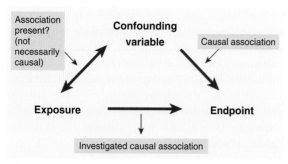

Fig. 3.1 Schematic representation of the two necessary criteria for a variable to induce spurious associations (i.e., to be a confounding variable). The confounding variable has to be associated with the exposure and causally linked to the outcome. When both criteria are satisfied, confounding is said to be present.

In randomized studies, confounding is typically not an issue because randomization balances known and unknown confounders across the compared groups with a high degree of certainty. In epidemiologic studies, in which no randomization is present, three questions related to confounding need to be considered in the assessment of the causality, as addressed next. The questions include: Were all important confounders identified? How accurately were confounders measured? And, was the statistical modeling of the confounders appropriate?

> **KEY FACT**
>
> Single epidemiologic studies reporting large odds ratios are unreliable.

> **CLINICAL CORRELATION**
>
> Epidemiologic evidence has suggested that periodontal patients who comply with periodontal maintenance procedures lose fewer teeth.[22]

🌐 Was the Study Properly Randomized?

It is often taken for granted that randomization is properly performed in RCTs. This is unfortunately not the case. Attempts by physicians to circumvent randomization are not isolated events; they used to be part of an endemic problem stemming from ignorance.[36]

Randomization can be a counterintuitive process because it (1) creates heterogeneity, (2) takes control over treatment assignment away from the physician, and (3) leads to apparently illogical situations in which patients who are randomly assigned to a treatment but are refusing compliance are still analyzed as if they received the treatment. Although randomization was a radical innovation introduced for agriculture, some have suggested that it is doubtful whether it would have ever been widely introduced into medicine (and subsequently dentistry) if not for a confluence of factors surrounding the end of World War II in Great Britain. Because of the revolutionary nature of randomization, fundamental misunderstandings of this process remained prevalent until recently. In 1994, about one-third of the clinical trials published in elite medical journals apparently did not ensure that patients are assigned to different treatments by chance.[36] The majority of reported periodontal trials failed to convince reviewers that (1) the studies were properly randomized, (2) randomization was concealed, or (3) randomized patients were accounted for.[33] Tampering with the delicate process of randomization can quickly, according to Ronald Fisher, a statistician and geneticist, turn an experiment into an experience.

When to Rely on Nonrandomized Evidence

Randomize the first patient.

—*Thomas Chalmers*

To tell the truth, all of the discussion today about the patient's informed consent still strikes me as absolute rubbish.

—*Sir Austin Bradford Hill*

Scores of epidemiologic studies reported evidence that hormone replacement therapy provided benefits to postmenopausal women. Despite this "strong" evidence from "leading" researchers, and despite the opposition on ethical grounds to begin a placebo-controlled trial, the Women's Health Initiative trial was initiated. The "miracle" of hormone replacement therapy was shown to lead to increased breast cancer risk, dementia, myocardial infarction, and stroke. This example illustrates the need for randomized studies and for questioning well-established and widely accepted beliefs based on numerous epidemiologic studies. Nonetheless, the initiation of randomized trials can become difficult because of ethical considerations and expensively large sample sizes.

Ethical principles dictate that proposed interventions do more good than harm, that the populations in whom the study will be conducted will benefit from the findings, that informed consent is obtained from enrolled subjects, and that a genuine uncertainty exists with respect to treatment efficacy. The interpretation of these ethical principles is largely determined by culture and era. Ethical principles also play an important role in determining which clinical questions are sufficiently important to warrant the conduct of an RCT.

Sample size requirements represent another consideration that may prevent the conduct of RCTs. The smaller the rate at which endpoints occur in an RCT, the larger the required sample size will be. For rare events, such as bacterial endocarditis subsequent to a dental procedure or HIV conversion after exposure to an HIV-contaminated dental needle, RCTs may never be possible because the required sample sizes are in the hundreds of thousands or millions of subjects.

In addition to both ethical and practical reasons, powerful political issues can surround the decision to initiate clinical trials. It has been pointed out that specialists are unlikely to support clinical trials that evaluate their main source of income.[38] This observation for medical specialties may also hold for periodontics. Although dental professional organizations commonly claim that periodontal disease is a major cause of tooth loss, evidence indicates that standard periodontal therapy is not effective at reducing tooth loss. Hopefully, well-designed and well-conducted studies in the future will allow us to compare different treatments effectively. Unequivocal evidence requires the conduct of rigorously designed and executed RCTs. The absence of RCT evidence for important and answerable clinical questions can be frustrating to those who seek reliable, evidence-based practice guidelines.

Did the Investigators Take Into Account the Placebo or Nocebo Effects?

I never knew any advantage from electricity in (the treatment of) palsies that was permanent. And how far the apparent temporary advantage might arise from the exercise in the patient's journey, and coming daily to my house, or from the spirits given by the hope of success, enabling them to exert more strength in moving their limbs, I will not pretend to say.

—*Benjamin Franklin*[48]

Sham or mock surgical procedures have been used to evaluate whether implanting human fetal tissue in the brain decreases symptoms of Parkinson disease, whether surgical lavage and debridement decrease pain in arthritic knee joints,[34] whether mammary artery ligation improves heart disease outcomes,[11] and whether alveolar trephination relieves the pain of acute apical periodontitis.[18,35]

What motivates clinical investigators to subject patients to surgical risks and yet knowingly provide no hypothesized benefits to those patients? A partial answer to this question lies in a phenomenon known as placebo or nocebo effects: the beneficial or harmful effects that patients may experience by participating in a study, by patient–physician interaction, by the patient's anticipation for improvement, or by the patient's desire to please the physician. One group of researchers suspects that the placebo or nocebo effect may be related to the balance of the parasympathetic and sympathetic nervous system, which could explain both placebo and nocebo effects.[27] Without mock surgical procedures, it would be impossible to tell whether the improvements observed in clinical trials are caused by the placebo effects associated with the surgical procedures or by the hypothesized active ingredient of the surgery itself.

Two studies have quantified the placebo effect. In the first study, the magnitude of the placebo effect was estimated by evaluating patients' responses to ineffective treatments.[41] Five treatments were identified as ineffective (all these treatments had been abandoned by the medical profession and at least one controlled study confirmed their ineffectiveness). With these ineffective treatments, good to excellent treatment responses were observed in 45% to 90% of the patients, a powerful placebo effect indeed. In the second study, placebo interventions (pharmacologic placebo, physical, or psychological interventions) were compared with true "no-treatment" interventions.[19] A significant placebo effect was observed for pain, the condition that was evaluated in the largest number of trials and that had the largest number of evaluated participants.

Placebo effects can reliably be estimated only when clinical trials randomly assign patients to a placebo treatment and no treatment. Such studies are rare. Some systematic reviews may provide a hint at the magnitude of placebo effects. One systematic review of 133 studies reported that the fluoride effect on caries was significantly larger when a no-treatment control group was used versus when a placebo control group was used.[32] One possible interpretation for these differences is a placebo effect: the placebo lowered caries rates, possibly through the re-equilibrating of parasympathetic and sympathetic nervous activity, which may influence factors such as improved saliva flow. Other explanations, such as the scientific quality of the studies, may, of course, also be responsible for such observed differences, especially for pain. Overall, sufficient evidence is available to suggest that placebo effects can be real and measurable, and that the magnitude of the placebo effect may depend on the treatment under study and the type of outcome evaluated.

🌐 Was Protection in Place Against Conflict of Interest?

In evidence-based medicine, the data from clinical research remain largely esoteric and of no real-world significance if the evidence fails to be translated into clinical practice. Spinal fusion, vertebroplasty, and arthroscopic surgery for knee pain have all shown noneffectiveness in clinical trials, yet these trials had no impact on clinical practice. In some instances, the use of surgical procedures actually increased after a demonstration of noneffectiveness.[25,28] Such discrepancies between clinical practice and science have been, in part, attributed to "perverse financial incentives."[25]

Can one trust clinical recommendations regarding a novel, noninvasive cardiac bypass operation by a physician who has a $100 million stake in the procedure that he or she is recommending? Is it possible that financial stakes are preventing physicians from disclosing a 10-fold increased mortality risk? Can one trust guidelines establishing sharply lowered lipid levels while knowing that eight of the nine panel experts have financial connections to the manufacturers of lipid-lowering drugs? Is it possible that panelists are picked for ideology?[6] Can one trust clinical guidelines published by professional dental organizations? The answers to these questions are not straightforward and, in general, are discussed under the heading of "conflicts of interest."

Conflict of interest has been defined as "a set of conditions in which professional judgment concerning a primary interest (such as patient's welfare or validity of research) tends to be unduly influenced by a secondary interest."[2] A common secondary interest is financial but can include others, such as religious or scientific beliefs, ideologic or political beliefs, or academic interests (e.g., promotion).

Some examples of how conflicts of interests can bias evidence can be found on the companion website.

Protection against potential conflict of interest is an important aspect of clinical research. Mandatory registration of clinical trials helps. The appointment of independent data and safety monitoring boards for trial monitoring provides protection against biases. Policy regulations established by journals, academic institutions, and governments can further decrease the impact of perceived conflicts of interests. For instance, all the work that has been done toward establishing registries of RCTs helps in decreasing biases.

Conflict of interest issues may be just as prevalent in dental research as in other medical areas dealing with chronic disease. In 2002, an article published in a leading dental journal ended up on the cover of the *New York Times*.[37] In part, the reason was a perceived conflict of interest; the article did not disclose that funding for the study came from an advertising company. Disclosure of conflict of interest is often poorly enforced, and some dental journals do not have regulations in place to reveal potential conflicts of interest of authors. Such situations (1) make it challenging for clinicians to recognize the potential for conflicts of interest, (2) may reduce trust in dental journals, and (3) may affect the scientific integrity of dental research.

CONCLUSION

Lessons learned from other chronic disease areas also apply to the evaluation of evidence in the periodontal disease research arena. Randomization and confounding are as important in periodontal research as they are in cancer research. Work remains to be done to integrate evidence-based thinking into clinical practice. One challenging task is to lessen the excessive reliance on biologic plausibility in determining both research priorities and patient management and to transition to clinical thinking that is based on controlled clinical observations. Maybe, however, the most challenging task for the dental profession to eliminate this bias will be to comply with the Institute of Medicine guideline, largely to exclude experts from writing clinical guidelines.[23] Although the 12 discussed tools for assessing evidence do not cover all necessary tools, or maybe even the most important tools, it is hoped that they provide a useful starting point for the further exploration of the issues and principles involved in the conduct of systematic experiments in periodontal disease research.

REFERENCES

 References for this chapter are found on the companion website.

Biologic Basis of Periodontology

4

Anatomy, Structure, and Function of the Periodontium[a]

 For online-only content on the gingival epithelium, the alveolar process, and the attachment apparatus, please visit the companion website.

The normal periodontium provides the support necessary to maintain teeth in function. It consists of four principal components: gingiva, periodontal ligament, cementum, and alveolar bone. Each of these periodontal components is distinct in its location, tissue architecture, biochemical composition, and chemical composition, but all of these components function together as a single unit. Research has revealed that the extracellular matrix components of one periodontal compartment can influence the cellular activities of adjacent structures. Therefore the pathologic changes that occur in one periodontal component may have significant ramifications for the maintenance, repair, or regeneration of other components of the periodontium.[18]

This chapter first discusses the structural components of the normal periodontium; it then describes their development, vascularization, innervation, and functions.

ORAL MUCOSA

The *oral mucosa* consists of the following three zones:
1. The gingiva and the covering of the hard palate, termed the *masticatory mucosa* (the *gingiva* is the part of the oral mucosa that covers the alveolar processes of the jaws and surrounds the necks of the teeth)

2. The dorsum of the tongue, covered by *specialized mucosa*
3. The oral mucous membrane lining the remainder of the oral cavity

GINGIVA

Clinical Features

In an adult, normal gingiva covers the alveolar bone and tooth root to a level just coronal to the cementoenamel junction. The gingiva is divided anatomically into *marginal, attached,* and *interdental areas*. Although each type of gingiva exhibits considerable variation in differentiation, histology, and thickness according to its functional demands, all types are specifically structured to function appropriately against mechanical and microbial damage.[7] In other words, the specific structure of different types of gingiva reflects each one's effectiveness as a barrier to the penetration by microbes and noxious agents into the deeper tissue.

Marginal Gingiva

The marginal or unattached gingiva is the terminal edge or border of the gingiva that surrounds the teeth in collar-like fashion (Figs. 4.1 and 4.2).[6] In approximately 50% of cases, it is demarcated from the adjacent attached gingiva by a shallow linear depression called the *free gingival groove*.[6] The marginal gingiva is usually approximately 1 mm wide, and it forms the soft-tissue wall of the gingival sulcus. The most apical point of the marginal gingival scallop is called the *gingival zenith*. Its apicocoronal and mesiodistal dimensions vary between 0.06 and 0.96 mm.[170]

[a]Adapted from the following chapter of Newman and Carranza's Clinical Periodontology, 13th edition: Chapter 3: Anatomy, Structure, and Function of the Periodontium, by Joseph P. Fiorellini, David Kim, and Yu-Cheng Chang.

Fig. 4.1 Normal Gingiva in a Young Adult. Note the demarcation (mucogingival line) *(arrows)* between the attached gingiva and the darker alveolar mucosa.

Fig. 4.3 Mean Width of the Attached Gingiva in the Human Permanent Dentition.

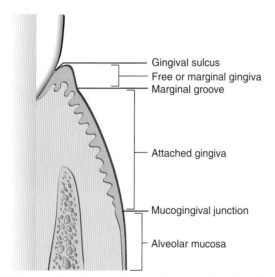

Gingival sulcus
Free or marginal gingiva
Marginal groove

Attached gingiva

Mucogingival junction

Alveolar mucosa

Fig. 4.2 Diagram Showing the Anatomic Landmarks of the Gingiva.

Gingival Sulcus

The gingival sulcus is the shallow crevice or space around the tooth bounded by the surface of the tooth on one side and the epithelium lining the free margin of the gingiva on the other side. It is V-shaped and barely permits the entrance of a periodontal probe. The clinical determination of the depth of the gingival sulcus is an important diagnostic parameter. Under absolutely normal or ideal conditions, the depth of the gingival sulcus is 0 mm or close to 0 mm.[104] These strict conditions of normalcy can be produced experimentally only in germ-free animals or after intense and prolonged plaque control.[13,49]

In clinically healthy human gingiva, a sulcus of some depth is found. The depth of this sulcus, as determined in histologic sections, has been reported as 1.8 mm, with variations from 0 to 6 mm[194]; other studies have reported 1.5 mm[288] and 0.69 mm.[91] The clinical evaluation used to determine the depth of the sulcus involves the introduction of a metallic instrument (i.e., the

periodontal probe) and the estimation of the distance it penetrates (i.e., the probing depth). The histologic depth of a sulcus does not need to be exactly equal to the depth of penetration of the probe. The penetration of the probe depends on several factors, such as probe diameter, probing force, and level of inflammation.[92] Consequently, the probing depth is not necessarily exactly equal to the histologic depth of the sulcus. The so-called probing depth of a clinically normal gingival sulcus in humans is 2 to 3 mm (see Chapter 30).

Attached Gingiva

The attached gingiva is continuous with the marginal gingiva. It is firm, resilient, and tightly bound to the underlying periosteum of alveolar bone. The facial aspect of the attached gingiva extends to the relatively loose and movable alveolar mucosa; it is demarcated by the *mucogingival junction* (see Fig. 4.2).

The *width of the attached gingiva* is another important clinical parameter.[7] It is the distance between the mucogingival junction and the projection on the external surface of the bottom of the gingival sulcus or the periodontal pocket. It should not be confused with the *width of the keratinized gingiva,* although this also includes the marginal gingiva (see Fig. 4.2).

The width of the attached gingiva on the facial aspect differs in different areas of the mouth.[40] It is generally greatest in the incisor region (i.e., 3.5 to 4.5 mm in the maxilla, 3.3 to 3.9 mm in the mandible) and narrower in the posterior segments (i.e., 1.9 mm in the maxillary first premolars and 1.8 mm in the mandibular first premolars) (Fig. 4.3).[6]

Because the mucogingival junction remains stationary throughout adult life,[4] changes in the width of the attached gingiva are caused by modifications in the position of its coronal portion. The width of the attached gingiva increases by the age of 4 years and in supraerupted teeth.[5] On the lingual aspect of the mandible, the attached gingiva terminates at the junction of the lingual alveolar mucosa, which is continuous with the mucous membrane that lines the floor of the mouth. The palatal surface of the attached gingiva in the maxilla blends imperceptibly with the equally firm and resilient palatal mucosa.

Interdental Gingiva

The interdental gingiva occupies the gingival embrasure, which is the interproximal space beneath the area of tooth contact. The interdental gingiva can be pyramidal, or it can have a "col" shape. In the former, the tip of one papilla is located immediately beneath the contact point; the latter presents a valley-like depression that connects a facial and lingual papilla and that conforms to the shape of the interproximal contact (Figs. 4.4 and 4.5).[62] The shape of the gingiva in a given interdental space depends on the presence or absence of a contact point between the adjacent teeth, the distance between the contact point and the osseous crest,[259] and the presence or absence of some degree of recession. Fig. 4.6 depicts the variations in normal interdental gingiva.

The facial and lingual surfaces are tapered toward the interproximal contact area, whereas the mesial and distal surfaces are slightly concave. The lateral borders and tips of the interdental papillae are formed by the marginal gingiva of the adjoining teeth. The intervening portion consists of attached gingiva (Fig. 4.7). If a diastema is present, the gingiva is firmly bound over the interdental bone to form a smooth, rounded surface without interdental papillae (Fig. 4.8).

Microscopic Features

Microscopic examination reveals that gingiva is composed of the overlying stratified squamous epithelium and the underlying central core of connective tissue. Although the epithelium is predominantly cellular in nature, the connective tissue is less cellular and composed primarily of collagen fibers and ground substance. These two tissues are considered separately. (A detailed description of gingival histology can be found in Schroeder HE: *The periodontium*, New York, 1986, Springer-Verlag; and in Biological structure of the normal and diseased periodontium, *Periodontol 2000* 13:1, 1997.)

Gingival Epithelium

General aspects of gingival epithelium biology. Historically, the epithelial compartment was thought to provide only a physical

Fig. 4.4 Site of Extraction Showing the Facial and Palatal Interdental Papillae and the Intervening Col *(Arrow).*

Fig. 4.5 Faciolingual Section of a Monkey Showing the Col Between the Facial and Lingual Interdental Papillae. The col is covered with nonkeratinized, stratified squamous epithelium.

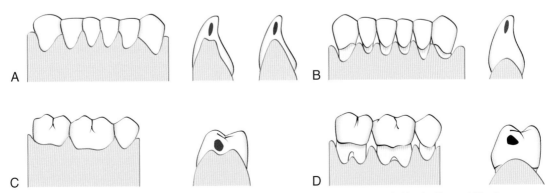

Fig. 4.6 A Diagram That Compares Anatomic Variations of the Interdental Col in the Normal Gingiva *(Left Side)* and After Gingival Recession *(Right Side).* (A and B) Mandibular anterior segment, facial and buccolingual views, respectively. (C and D) Mandibular posterior region, facial and buccolingual views, respectively. Tooth contact points are shown with black marks in the lower individual teeth.

Fig. 4.7 Interdental Papillae *(Arrow)* With a Central Portion Formed by the Attached Gingiva. The shape of the papillae varies according to the dimension of the gingival embrasure. (Courtesy Dr. Osvaldo Costa.)

Fig. 4.8 An Absence of Interdental Papillae and Col Where the Proximal Tooth Contact Is Missing. (Courtesy Dr. Osvaldo Costa.)

BOX 4.1 Functions and Features of Gingival Epithelium

Functions
Mechanical, chemical, water, and microbial barrier
Signaling functions

Architectural Integrity
Cell-cell attachments
Basal lamina
Keratin cytoskeleton

Major Cell Type
Keratinocyte

Other Cell Types
Langerhans cells
Melanocytes
Merkel cells

Constant Renewal
Replacement of damaged cells

Cell-Cell Attachments
Desmosomes
Adherens junctions
Tight junctions
Gap junctions

Cell–Basal Lamina
Synthesis of basal lamina components
Hemidesmosome

Modified from Dale BA: Periodontal epithelium: a newly recognized role in health and disease. *Periodontol* 30:71, 2002.

barrier to infection and the underlying gingival attachment. However, currently we believe that epithelial cells play an active role in innate host defense by responding to bacteria in an interactive manner,[67] which means that the epithelium participates actively in responding to infection, in signaling further host reactions, and in integrating innate and acquired immune responses. For example, epithelial cells may respond to bacteria by increased proliferation, the alteration of cell-signaling events, changes in differentiation and cell death, and, ultimately, the alteration of tissue homeostasis.[67] To understand this new perspective of the epithelial innate defense responses and the role of epithelium in gingival health and disease, it is important to understand its basic structure and function (Box 4.1).

The gingival epithelium consists of a continuous lining of stratified squamous epithelium. There are three different areas that can be defined from the morphologic and functional points of view: the oral or outer epithelium, the sulcular epithelium, and the junctional epithelium.

The principal cell type of the gingival epithelium—as well as of other stratified squamous epithelia—is the *keratinocyte*. Other cells found in the epithelium are the clear cells or nonkeratinocytes, which include the Langerhans cells, the Merkel cells, and the melanocytes.

The main function of the gingival epithelium is to protect the deep structures while allowing for a selective interchange with the oral environment. This is achieved via the proliferation and differentiation of the keratinocytes. The *proliferation* of keratinocytes takes place by mitosis in the basal layer and less frequently in the suprabasal layers, in which a small proportion of cells remain as a proliferative compartment while a larger number begin to migrate to the surface.

Differentiation involves the process of keratinization, which consists of progressions of biochemical and morphologic events that occur in the cell as they migrate from the basal layer (Fig. 4.9). The main morphologic changes include the following: (1) the progressive flattening of the cell with an increasing prevalence of tonofilaments; (2) the couple of intercellular junctions with the production of keratohyalin granules; and (3) the disappearance of the nucleus (see Schroeder[229] for further details).

A complete keratinization process leads to the production of an *orthokeratinized* superficial horny layer similar to that of the skin, with no nuclei in the stratum corneum and a well-defined stratum granulosum (Fig. 4.10). Only some areas of the outer gingival epithelium are orthokeratinized; the other gingival areas are covered by parakeratinized or nonkeratinized epithelium[45]

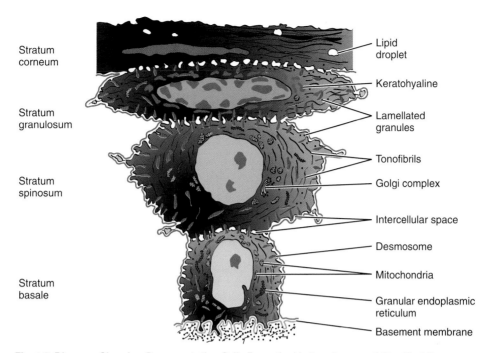

Stratum corneum — Lipid droplet

Keratohyaline

Stratum granulosum — Lamellated granules

Tonofibrils

Stratum spinosum — Golgi complex

Intercellular space

Desmosome

Mitochondria

Stratum basale — Granular endoplasmic reticulum

Basement membrane

Fig. 4.9 Diagram Showing Representative Cells From the Various Layers of Stratified Squamous Epithelium as Seen by Electron Microscopy. (Modified from Weinstock A: In Ham AW: *Histology,* ed 7, Philadelphia, 1974, Lippincott.)

Fig. 4.10 (A) Scanning electron micrograph of keratinized gingiva showing the flattened keratinocytes and their boundaries on the surface of the gingiva (×1000). (B) Scanning electron micrograph of the gingival margin at the edge of the gingival sulcus showing several keratinocytes about to be exfoliated (×3000). (From Kaplan GB, Pameijer CH, Ruben MP: *J Periodontol* 48:446, 1977.)

and are considered to be at intermediate stages of keratinization. These areas can progress to maturity or dedifferentiate under different physiologic or pathologic conditions.

In *parakeratinized epithelia,* the stratum corneum retains pyknotic nuclei, and the keratohyalin granules are dispersed rather than giving rise to a stratum granulosum. The *nonkeratinized*

epithelium (although cytokeratins are the major component, as in all epithelia) has neither granulosum nor corneum strata, whereas superficial cells have viable nuclei.

Nonkeratinocyte cells are present in gingival epithelium as in other malpighian epithelia. *Melanocytes* are dendritic cells located in the basal and spinous layers of the gingival epithelium.

Fig. 4.11 Pigmented Gingiva of Dog Showing Melanocytes *(M)* in the Basal Epithelial Layer and Melanophores *(C)* in the Connective Tissue (Glucksman Technique).

Fig. 4.13 Normal Human Gingiva Stained With the Periodic Acid–Schiff Histochemical Method. The basement membrane *(B)* is seen between the epithelium *(E)* and the underlying connective tissue *(C)*. In the epithelium, glycoprotein material occurs in cells and cell membranes of the superficial hornified *(H)* and underlying granular layers *(G)*. The connective tissue presents a diffuse, amorphous ground substance and collagen fibers. The blood vessel walls stand out clearly in the papillary projections of the connective tissue *(P)*.

Fig. 4.12 Human Gingival Epithelium, Oral Aspect. Immunoperoxidase technique showing Langerhans cells.

They synthesize melanin in organelles called *premelanosomes* or *melanosomes* (Fig. 4.11).[61,227,251]

Langerhans cells are dendritic cells located among keratinocytes at all suprabasal levels (Fig. 4.12). They belong to the mononuclear phagocyte system (reticuloendothelial system) as modified monocytes derived from the bone marrow. They contain elongated granules, and they are considered macrophages with possible antigenic properties.[72] Langerhans cells have an important role in the immune reaction as antigen-presenting cells for lymphocytes. They contain g-specific granules (Birbeck granules), and they have marked adenosine triphosphatase activity. They are found in the oral epithelium of normal gingiva and in smaller amounts in the sulcular epithelium; they are probably absent from the junctional epithelium of normal gingiva.

Merkel cells are located in the deeper layers of the epithelium; they harbor nerve endings, and they are connected to adjacent cells by desmosomes. They have been identified as tactile perceptors.[187]

The epithelium is joined to the underlying connective tissue by a *basal lamina* 300 to 400 Å thick and lying approximately 400 Å beneath the epithelial basal layer.[146,234,253] The basal lamina consists of lamina lucida and lamina densa. Hemidesmosomes of the basal epithelial cells abut the lamina lucida, which is mainly composed of the glycoprotein laminin. The lamina densa is composed of type IV collagen.

The basal lamina, which is clearly distinguishable at the ultrastructural level, is connected to a reticular condensation of the underlying connective tissue fibrils (mainly collagen type IV) by the anchoring fibrils.[182,212,256] Anchoring fibrils have been measured at 750 nm in length from their epithelial end to their connective tissue end, where they appear to form loops around collagen fibers. The complex of basal lamina and fibrils is the periodic acid–Schiff–positive and argyrophilic line observed at the optical level (Fig. 4.13).[236,257] The basal lamina is permeable to fluids, but it acts as a barrier to particulate matter.

Structural and metabolic characteristics of different areas of gingival epithelium. The epithelial component of the gingiva shows regional morphologic variations that reflect tissue adaptation to the tooth and alveolar bone.[230] These variations include the oral epithelium, the sulcular epithelium, and the junctional epithelium. The oral epithelium and the sulcular epithelium are largely protective in function, whereas the junctional epithelium serves many more roles and is of considerable importance in the regulation of tissue health.[18] It is currently recognized that epithelial cells are not passive bystanders in the gingival tissues; rather, they are metabolically active and capable of reacting to external stimuli by synthesizing a number of cytokines, adhesion molecules, growth factors, and enzymes.[18]

The degree of gingival keratinization diminishes with age and the onset of menopause,[198] but it is not necessarily related to the different phases of the menstrual cycle.[130] Keratinization of the oral mucosa varies in different areas in the following order: palate (most keratinized), gingiva, ventral aspect of the tongue, and cheek (least keratinized).[180]

Fig. 4.14 Variations in the Gingival Epithelium. (A) Keratinized. (B) Nonkeratinized. (C) Parakeratinized. Horny layer *(H)*, granular layer *(G)*, prickle cell layer *(P)*, basal cell layer *(Ba)*, flattened surface cells *(S)*, and parakeratotic layer *(Pk)*.

Fig. 4.15 Scanning Electron Microscopic View of the Epithelial Surface Facing the Tooth in a Normal Human Gingival Sulcus. The epithelium *(Ep)* shows desquamating cells, some scattered erythrocytes *(E)*, and a few emerging leukocytes *(L)*. (×1000.)

Fig. 4.16 Epon-Embedded Human Biopsy Specimen Showing a Relatively Normal Gingival Sulcus. The soft-tissue wall of the gingival sulcus is made up of the oral sulcular epithelium *(ose)* and its underlying connective tissue *(ct)*, whereas the base of the gingival sulcus is formed by the sloughing surface of the junctional epithelium *(je)*. The enamel space is delineated by a dense cuticular structure *(dc)*. A relatively sharp line of demarcation exists between the junctional epithelium and the oral sulcular epithelium *(arrow)*, and several polymorphonuclear leukocytes *(pmn)* can be seen traversing the junctional epithelium. The sulcus contains red blood cells that resulted from the hemorrhage that occurred at the time of biopsy. (×391; inset ×55.) (From Schluger S, Youdelis R, Page RC: *Periodontal disease,* ed 2, Philadelphia, 1990, Lea & Febiger.)

Oral (outer) epithelium. The oral or outer epithelium covers the crest and outer surface of the marginal gingiva and the surface of the attached gingiva. On average, the oral epithelium is 0.2 to 0.3 mm in thickness. It is keratinized or parakeratinized, or it may present various combinations of these conditions (Fig. 4.14). However, the prevalent surface is parakeratinized.[32,45,284] The oral epithelium is composed of four layers: stratum basale (basal layer), stratum spinosum (prickle cell layer), stratum granulosum (granular layer), and stratum corneum (cornified layer).

Sulcular epithelium. The sulcular epithelium lines the gingival sulcus (Fig. 4.15). It is a thin, nonkeratinized stratified squamous epithelium without rete pegs, and it extends from the coronal limit of the junctional epithelium to the crest of the gingival margin (Fig. 4.16). It usually shows many cells with hydropic degeneration.[32]

Despite these morphologic and chemical characteristics, the sulcular epithelium has the potential to keratinize if it is reflected and exposed to the oral cavity[44,48] or if the bacterial flora of the sulcus is totally eliminated.[50] Conversely, the outer epithelium loses its keratinization when it is placed in contact with the tooth.[50] These findings suggest that the local irritation of the sulcus prevents sulcular keratinization.

The sulcular epithelium is extremely important; it may act as a semipermeable membrane through which injurious bacterial products pass into the gingiva and through which tissue fluid from the gingiva seeps into the sulcus.[266] However, unlike the junctional epithelium, the sulcular epithelium is not heavily infiltrated by polymorphonuclear neutrophil leukocytes, and it appears to be less permeable.[18]

Junctional epithelium. The junctional epithelium consists of a collar-like band of stratified squamous nonkeratinizing epithelium. It is 3 to 4 layers thick in early life, but that number increases with age to 10 or even 20 layers. In addition, the junctional epithelium tapers from its coronal end, which may be 10 to 29 cells wide to 1 or 2 cells wide at its apical termination, which is located at the cementoenamel junction in healthy tissue. These cells can be grouped in two strata: the basal layer that faces the connective tissue and the suprabasal layer that extends to the tooth surface. The length of the junctional epithelium ranges from 0.25 to 1.35 mm (Fig. 4.17).

The junctional epithelium is formed by the confluence of the oral epithelium and the reduced enamel epithelium (REE) during tooth eruption. However, the REE is not essential for its formation; in fact, the junctional epithelium is completely restored after pocket instrumentation or surgery, and it forms around an implant.[150]

The junctional epithelium is attached to the tooth surface (epithelial attachment) by means of an internal basal lamina. It is attached to the gingival connective tissue by an external basal lamina that has the same structure as other epithelial–connective tissue attachments elsewhere in the body.[154,160]

The internal basal lamina consists of a lamina densa (adjacent to the enamel) and a lamina lucida to which hemidesmosomes are attached. Hemidesmosomes have a decisive role in the firm attachment of the cells to the internal basal lamina on the tooth surface.

Data suggest that the hemidesmosomes also act as specific sites of signal transduction and thus may participate in the regulation of gene expression, cell proliferation, and cell differentiation.[133] Organic strands from the enamel appear to extend into the lamina densa.[255] The junctional epithelium attaches to afibrillar cementum that is present on the crown (usually restricted to an area within 1 mm of the cementoenamel junction)[232] and root cementum in a similar manner.

Histochemical evidence for the presence of neutral polysaccharides in the zone of the epithelial attachment has been reported.[271] Data also have shown that the basal lamina of the junctional epithelium resembles that of endothelial and epithelial cells in its laminin content but differs in its internal basal lamina, which has no type IV collagen.[141,222] These findings indicate that the cells of the junctional epithelium are involved in the production of laminin and play a key role in the adhesion mechanism.

Fig. 4.17 Eruption Process in Cat's Tooth. (A) Unerupted tooth. Dentin *(D)*, remnants of enamel matrix *(E)*, reduced enamel epithelium *(REE)*, oral epithelium *(OE)*, and artifact *(a)*. (B) Erupting tooth forming junctional epithelium *(JE)*. (C) Completely erupted tooth. Sulcus with epithelial debris *(S)*, cementum *(C)*, and epithelial rests *(ER)*.

The attachment of the junctional epithelium to the tooth is reinforced by the gingival fibers, which brace the marginal gingiva against the tooth surface. For this reason, the junctional epithelium and the gingival fibers are considered together as a functional unit referred to as the *dentogingival unit.*[157]

In conclusion, it is usually accepted that the junctional epithelium exhibits several unique structural and functional features that contribute to preventing pathogenic bacterial flora from colonizing the subgingival tooth surface.[204] First, junctional epithelium is firmly attached to the tooth surface, thereby forming an epithelial barrier against plaque bacteria. Second, it allows access of gingival fluid, inflammatory cells, and components of the immunologic host defense to the gingival margin. Third, junctional epithelial cells exhibit rapid turnover, which contributes to the host-parasite equilibrium and the rapid repair of damaged tissue. Some investigators have also indicated that the cells of the junctional epithelium have an endocytic capacity equal to that of macrophages and neutrophils and that this activity may be protective in nature.[57]

Development of gingival sulcus. After enamel formation is complete, the enamel is covered with REE, which is attached to the tooth by a basal lamina and hemidesmosomes.[155,254] When the tooth penetrates the oral mucosa, the REE unites with the oral epithelium and transforms into the junctional epithelium. As the tooth erupts, this united epithelium condenses along the crown, and the ameloblasts, which form the inner layer of the REE (see Fig. 4.17), gradually become squamous epithelial cells. The transformation of the REE into a junctional epithelium proceeds in an apical direction without interrupting the attachment to the tooth. According to Schroeder and Listgarten,[232] this process takes between 1 and 2 years.

The junctional epithelium is a continually self-renewing structure, with mitotic activity occurring in all cell layers.[155,254] The regenerating epithelial cells move toward the tooth surface and along it in a coronal direction to the gingival sulcus, where they are shed (Fig. 4.18).[22] The migrating daughter cells provide a continuous attachment to the tooth surface. The strength of the epithelial attachment to the tooth has not been measured.

The gingival sulcus is formed when the tooth erupts into the oral cavity. At that time, the junctional epithelium and the REE form a broad band that is attached to the tooth surface from near the tip of the crown to the cementoenamel junction. The gingival sulcus is the shallow, V-shaped space or groove between the tooth and the gingiva that encircles the newly erupted tip of the crown. In the fully erupted tooth, only the junctional epithelium persists. *The sulcus consists of the shallow space that is coronal to the attachment of the junctional epithelium and bounded by the tooth on one side and the sulcular epithelium on the other. The coronal extent of the gingival sulcus is the gingival margin.*

Renewal of gingival epithelium. The oral epithelium undergoes continuous renewal. Its thickness is maintained by a balance between new cell formation in the basal and spinous layers and the shedding of old cells at the surface. The mitotic activity exhibits a 24-hour periodicity, with the highest and lowest rates occurring in the morning and evening, respectively.[255] The mitotic rate is higher in nonkeratinized areas and increased in gingivitis, without significant gender differences. Opinions differ with regard

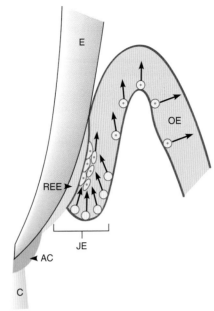

Fig. 4.18 Junctional Epithelium on an Erupting Tooth. The junctional epithelium *(JE)* is formed by the joining of the oral epithelium *(OE)* and the reduced enamel epithelium *(REE)*. Afibrillar cementum *(AC)* is sometimes formed on enamel after the degeneration of the REE. The arrows indicate the coronal movement of the regenerating epithelial cells, which multiply more rapidly in the JE than in the OE. *E,* Enamel; *C,* root cementum. A similar cell turnover pattern exists in the fully erupted tooth. (Modified from Listgarten MA: *J Can Dent Assoc* 36:70, 1970.)

to whether the mitotic rate is increased[159,160,178] or decreased[15] with age.

With regard to junctional epithelium, it was previously thought that only epithelial cells facing the external basal lamina were rapidly dividing. However, evidence indicates that a significant number of the cells (e.g., the basal cells along the connective tissue) are capable of synthesizing deoxyribonucleic acid (DNA), thereby demonstrating their mitotic activity.[220,221] The rapid shedding of cells effectively removes bacteria that adhere to the epithelial cells and therefore is an important part of the antimicrobial defense mechanisms at the dentogingival junction.[204]

Gingival fluid (sulcular fluid). The value of the gingival fluid is that it can be represented as either a transudate or an exudate. The gingival fluid contains a vast array of biochemical factors, thereby offering its potential use as a diagnostic or prognostic biomarker of the biologic state of the periodontium in health and disease (see Chapter 15). It also contains components of connective tissue, epithelium, inflammatory cells, serum, and microbial flora that inhabit the gingival margin or the sulcus (pocket).[79]

In the healthy sulcus, the amount of gingival fluid is very small. During inflammation, the gingival fluid flow increases, and its composition starts to resemble that of an inflammatory exudate.[59] The main route of the gingival fluid diffusion is through the basement membrane, through the relatively wide intercellular spaces of the junctional epithelium, and then into the sulcus.[204] The gingival fluid is believed to do the following: (1) cleanse material from the sulcus; (2) contain plasma proteins that may improve adhesion of the epithelium to the tooth; (3) possess antimicrobial properties; and (4) exert antibody activity to defend the gingiva.

Gingival Connective Tissue

The major components of the gingival connective tissue are collagen fibers (approximately 60% by volume), fibroblasts (5%), vessels, nerves, and matrix (approximately 35%). The connective tissue of the gingiva is known as the *lamina propria,* and it consists of two layers: (1) a *papillary layer* subjacent to the epithelium that consists of papillary projections between the epithelial rete pegs; and (2) a *reticular layer* that is contiguous with the periosteum of the alveolar bone.

Connective tissue has a cellular compartment and an extracellular compartment composed of fibers and ground substance. Thus the gingival connective tissue is largely a fibrous connective tissue that has elements that originate directly from the oral mucosal connective tissue as well as some fibers (dentogingival) that originate from the developing dental follicle.[18]

The *ground substance* fills the space between fibers and cells; it is amorphous, and it has a high water content. It is composed of proteoglycans (mainly hyaluronic acid and chondroitin sulfate) and glycoproteins (mainly fibronectin). Glycoproteins account for the faint periodic acid–Schiff–positive reaction of the ground substance.[81] Fibronectin binds fibroblasts to the fibers and many other components of the intercellular matrix, thereby helping to mediate cell adhesion and migration. Laminin, which is another glycoprotein found in the basal lamina, serves to attach it to epithelial cells.

The three types of connective tissue fibers are collagen, reticular, and elastic. Collagen type I forms the bulk of the lamina propria and provides the tensile strength to the gingival tissue. Type IV collagen (argyrophilic reticulum fiber) branches between the collagen type I bundles, and it is continuous with fibers of the basement membrane and the blood vessel walls.[160]

The elastic fiber system is composed of oxytalan, elaunin, and elastin fibers distributed among collagen fibers.[56] Densely packed collagen bundles that are anchored into the acellular extrinsic fiber cementum just below the terminal point of the junctional epithelium form the connective tissue attachment. The stability of this attachment is a key factor in the limitation of the migration of junctional epithelium.[57]

Gingival fibers. The connective tissue of the marginal gingiva is densely collagenous, and it contains a prominent system of collagen fiber bundles called the *gingival fibers.* These fibers consist of type I collagen.[212] The gingival fibers have the following functions:

1. To brace the marginal gingiva firmly against the tooth
2. To provide the rigidity necessary to withstand the forces of mastication without being deflected away from the tooth surface
3. To unite the free marginal gingiva with the cementum of the root and the adjacent attached gingiva

The gingival fibers are arranged in three groups: gingivodental, circular, and transseptal.[145]

The *gingivodental fibers* are those on the facial, lingual, and interproximal surfaces. They are embedded in the cementum

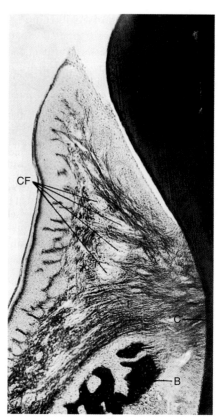

Fig. 4.19 Faciolingual section of marginal gingiva showing gingival fibers *(F)* that extend from the cementum *(C)* to the crest of the gingiva, to the outer gingival surface, and external to the periosteum of the bone *(B).* Circular fibers *(CF)* are shown in cross-section between the other groups. (Courtesy Sol Bernick.)

just beneath the epithelium at the base of the gingival sulcus. On the facial and lingual surfaces, they project from the cementum in a fanlike conformation toward the crest and outer surface of the marginal gingiva, where they terminate short of the epithelium (Figs. 4.19 and 4.20). They also extend externally to the periosteum of the facial and lingual alveolar bones, terminating in the attached gingiva or blending with the periosteum of the bone. Interproximally, the gingivodental fibers extend toward the crest of the interdental gingiva.

The *circular fibers* course through the connective tissue of the marginal and interdental gingivae and encircle the tooth in ringlike fashion.

The *transseptal fibers,* which are located interproximally, form horizontal bundles that extend between the cementum of the approximating teeth into which they are embedded. They lie in the area between the epithelium at the base of the gingival sulcus and the crest of the interdental bone, and they are sometimes classified with the principal fibers of the periodontal ligament.

Page and colleagues[197] described a group of *semicircular fibers* that attach at the proximal surface of a tooth immediately below the cementoenamel junction, go around the facial or lingual marginal gingiva of the tooth, and attach on the other proximal surface of the same tooth; they also discussed a group of *transgingival fibers* that attach in the proximal surface of one

Fig. 4.21 Section of Clinically Normal Gingiva Showing Some Degree of Inflammation, Which Is Almost Always Present Near the Base of the Sulcus.

Fig. 4.20 Diagram of the gingivodental fibers that extend from the cementum *(1)* to the crest of the gingiva, *(2)* to the outer surface, and *(3)* external to the periosteum of the labial plate. Circular fibers *(4)* are shown in cross-section.

tooth, traverse the interdental space diagonally, go around the facial or lingual surface of the adjacent tooth, again traverse the interdental space diagonally, and then attach in the proximal surface of the next tooth.

Tractional forces in the extracellular matrix produced by fibroblasts are believed to be responsible for generating tension in the collagen. This keeps the teeth tightly bound to each other and to the alveolar bone.

Cellular elements. The preponderant cellular element in the gingival connective tissue is the *fibroblast.* Numerous fibroblasts are found between the fiber bundles. Fibroblasts are of mesenchymal origin and play a major role in the development, maintenance, and repair of gingival connective tissue. As with connective tissue elsewhere in the body, fibroblasts synthesize collagen and elastic fibers as well as the glycoproteins and glycosaminoglycans of the amorphous intercellular substance. Fibroblasts also regulate collagen degradation through phagocytosis and the secretion of collagenases.

Fibroblast heterogeneity is now a well-established feature of fibroblasts in the periodontium.[225] Although the biologic and clinical significance of such heterogeneity is not yet clear, it seems that this is necessary for the normal functioning of tissues in health, disease, and repair.[18]

Mast cells, which are distributed throughout the body, are numerous in the connective tissue of the oral mucosa and the gingiva.[53,243,244,287] *Fixed macrophages* and *histiocytes* are present in the gingival connective tissue as components of the mononuclear phagocyte system (reticuloendothelial system) and are derived

from blood monocytes. *Adipose cells* and *eosinophils,* although scarce, are also present in the lamina propria.

In clinically normal gingiva, small foci of plasma cells and lymphocytes are found in the connective tissue near the base of the sulcus (Fig. 4.21). Neutrophils can be seen in relatively high numbers in both the gingival connective tissue and the sulcus. These inflammatory cells are usually present in small amounts in clinically normal gingiva.

Repair of gingival connective tissue. Because of the high turnover rate, the connective tissue of the gingiva has remarkably good healing and regenerative capacity. Indeed, it may be one of the best healing tissues in the body, and it generally shows little evidence of scarring after surgical procedures. This is likely caused by the rapid reconstruction of the fibrous architecture of the tissues.[177] However, the reparative capacity of gingival connective tissue is not as great as that of the periodontal ligament or the epithelial tissue.

Blood supply, lymphatics, and nerves. Microcirculatory tracts, blood vessels, and lymphatic vessels play an important role in the drainage of tissue fluid and in the spread of inflammation. In individuals with gingivitis and periodontitis, the microcirculation and vascular formation change greatly in the vascular network directly under the gingival sulcular epithelium and the junctional epithelium.[169]

Three sources of blood supply to the gingiva are (Figs. 4.22 and 4.23):

1. *Supraperiosteal arterioles* along the facial and lingual surfaces of the alveolar bone from which capillaries extend along the sulcular epithelium and between the rete pegs of the external gingival surface[8,76,112]: Occasional branches of the arterioles pass through the alveolar bone to the periodontal ligament or run over the crest of the alveolar bone.
2. *Vessels of the periodontal ligament,* which extend into the gingiva and anastomose with capillaries in the sulcus area.
3. *Arterioles,* which emerge from the crest of the interdental septa[83] and extend parallel to the crest of the bone to anastomose with vessels of the periodontal ligament, with capillaries in the gingival crevicular areas and vessels that run over the alveolar crest.

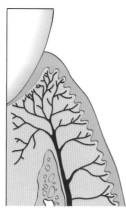

Fig. 4.22 Diagram of an arteriole penetrating the interdental alveolar bone to supply the interdental tissues *(left)* and a supraperiosteal arteriole overlying the facial alveolar bone, sending branches to the surrounding tissue *(right)*.

Fig. 4.24 Scanning Electron Microscopic View of the Gingival Tissues of Rat Molar Palatal Gingiva After the Vascular Perfusion of Plastic and the Corrosion of Soft Tissue. (A) Oral view of gingival capillaries: *t*, tooth; interdental papilla *(arrowhead)* (×180). (B) View from the tooth side. Note the vessels of the plexus next to the sulcular and junctional epithelium. The *arrowheads* point to vessels in the sulcus area with mild inflammatory changes. *g*, Crest of the marginal gingiva; *s*, bottom of the gingival sulcus; *pl*, periodontal ligament vessels. (×150.) (Courtesy NJ Selliseth and K Selvig, University of Bergen, Norway.)

Fig. 4.23 Blood Supply and Peripheral Circulation of the Gingiva. Tissues perfused with India ink. Note the capillary plexus parallel to the sulcus *(S)* and the capillary loops in the outer papillary layer. Note also the supraperiosteal vessels external to the bone *(B)*, which supply the gingiva, and a periodontal ligament vessel anastomosing with the sulcus plexus. (Courtesy Sol Bernick.)

Beneath the epithelium on the outer gingival surface, capillaries extend into the papillary connective tissue between the epithelial rete pegs in the form of terminal hairpin loops with efferent and afferent branches, spirals, and varices (Fig. 4.24; also see Fig. 4.23).[54,112] The loops are sometimes linked by cross-communications,[85] and flattened capillaries serve as reserve vessels when the circulation is increased in response to irritation.[98]

Along the sulcular epithelium, capillaries are arranged in a flat, anastomosing plexus that extends parallel to the enamel from the base of the sulcus to the gingival margin.[54] In the col area, a mixed pattern of anastomosing capillaries and loops occurs.

As mentioned previously, anatomic and histologic changes have been shown to occur in the gingival microcirculation of individuals with gingivitis. Prospective studies of the gingival vasculature in animals have demonstrated that, in the absence of inflammation, the vascular network is arranged in a regular, repetitive, and layered pattern.[54,215] By contrast, the inflamed gingival vasculature exhibits an irregular vascular plexus pattern, with the microvessels exhibiting a looped, dilated, and convoluted appearance.[215]

The role of the lymphatic system in removing excess fluids, cellular and protein debris, microorganisms, and other elements is important for controlling diffusion and the resolution of inflammatory processes.[167] The *lymphatic drainage of the gingiva* brings in the lymphatics of the connective tissue papillae.[237] It progresses into the collecting network external to the periosteum of the alveolar process and then moves to the regional lymph nodes, particularly the submaxillary group. In addition, lymphatics just beneath the junctional epithelium extend into the periodontal ligament and accompany the blood vessels.

Neural elements are extensively distributed throughout the gingival tissues. Within the gingival connective tissues, most nerve fibers are myelinated and closely associated with the blood vessels.[161] *Gingival innervation* is derived from fibers that arise from nerves in the periodontal ligament and from the labial, buccal, and palatal nerves.[30] The following nerve structures are present in the connective tissue: a meshwork of terminal argyrophilic fibers, some of which extend into the epithelium; Meissner-type tactile corpuscles; Krause-type end bulbs, which are temperature receptors; and encapsulated spindles.[14]

Correlation of Clinical and Microscopic Features

An understanding of the normal clinical features of the gingiva requires the ability to interpret them in terms of the microscopic structures that they represent.

Color

The color of the attached and marginal gingiva is generally described as "coral pink"; it is produced by the vascular supply, the thickness and degree of keratinization of the epithelium, and the presence of pigment-containing cells. The color varies and appears to be correlated with the cutaneous pigmentation. It is lighter in blond individuals with fair complexions than in dark-complexioned, dark-haired individuals (Fig. 4.25).

The attached gingiva is demarcated from the adjacent alveolar mucosa on the buccal aspect by a clearly defined mucogingival line. The alveolar mucosa is red, smooth, and shiny rather than pink and stippled. A comparison of the microscopic structure of the attached gingiva with that of the alveolar mucosa provides an explanation for the difference in appearance. The epithelium of the alveolar mucosa is thinner and nonkeratinized, and it contains no rete pegs (Fig. 4.26). The connective tissue of the alveolar mucosa is loosely arranged, and the blood vessels are more numerous.

Physiologic pigmentation (melanin). Melanin is a non–hemoglobin-derived brown pigment with the following characteristics:

- Melanin is responsible for the normal pigmentation of the skin, the gingiva, and the remainder of the oral mucous membrane.
- Melanin is present in all normal individuals (often not in sufficient quantities to be detected clinically), but it is absent or severely diminished in albinos.
- Melanin pigmentation in the oral cavity is prominent in black individuals (see Fig. 4.25).
- Ascorbic acid directly downregulates melanin pigmentation in gingival tissues.[245]

According to Dummett,[73] the distribution of oral pigmentation in black individuals is as follows: gingiva, 60%; hard palate, 61%; mucous membrane, 22%; and tongue, 15%. Gingival pigmentation occurs as a diffuse, deep-purplish discoloration or as irregularly shaped brown and light-brown patches. It may appear in the gingiva as early as 3 hours after birth, and it is often the only evidence of pigmentation.[73]

Oral repigmentation refers to the clinical reappearance of melanin pigment after a period of clinical depigmentation of the oral mucosa as a result of chemical, thermal, surgical, pharmacologic, or idiopathic factors.[74] Information about the repigmentation of oral tissues after surgical procedures

Fig. 4.25 (A) Clinically normal gingiva in a young adult. (B) Heavily pigmented (melanotic) gingiva in a middle-aged adult. *(From Glickman I, Smulow JB: Periodontal disease: clinical, radiographic, and histopathologic features, Philadelphia, 1974, Saunders.)*

Fig. 4.26 Oral Mucosa, Facial and Palatal Surfaces. The facial surface *(F)* shows the marginal gingiva *(MG),* the attached gingiva *(AG),* and the alveolar mucosa *(AM).* The *double line* marks the mucogingival junction. Note the differences in the epithelium and the connective tissue in the attached gingiva and the alveolar mucosa. The palatal surface *(P)* shows the marginal gingiva *(MG)* and the thick, keratinized palatal mucosa *(PM).*

is extremely limited, and no definitive treatment is offered at this time.

Size

The size of the gingiva corresponds with the sum total of the bulk of cellular and intercellular elements and their vascular supply. Alteration in size is a common feature of gingival disease.

Contour

The contour or shape of the gingiva varies considerably and depends on the shape of the teeth and their alignment in the arch, the location and size of the area of proximal contact, and the dimensions of the facial and lingual gingival embrasures.

The marginal gingiva envelops the teeth in collar-like fashion and follows a scalloped outline on the facial and lingual surfaces. It forms a straight line along teeth with relatively flat surfaces. On teeth with pronounced mesiodistal convexity (e.g., maxillary canines) or teeth in labial version, the normal arcuate contour is accentuated, and the gingiva is located farther apically. On teeth in lingual version, the gingiva is horizontal and thickened (Fig. 4.27). In addition, the gingival tissue biotype varies significantly. A thin and clear gingiva is found in one-third of the population and primarily in females with slender teeth with a narrow zone of keratinized tissue, whereas a clear, thick gingiva with a broad zone of keratinized tissue is present in two-thirds of the population and primarily in males.[70]

Shape

The shape of the interdental gingiva is governed by the contour of the proximal tooth surfaces and the location and shape of the gingival embrasures.

When the proximal surfaces of the crowns are relatively flat faciolingually, the roots are close together, the interdental bone is thin mesiodistally, and the gingival embrasures and interdental gingiva are narrow mesiodistally. Conversely, with proximal surfaces that flare away from the area of contact, the mesiodistal diameter of the interdental gingiva is broad (Fig. 4.28). The height of the interdental gingiva varies with the location of the proximal contact. Thus in the anterior region of the dentition, the interdental papilla is pyramidal in form, whereas the papilla is more flattened in a buccolingual direction in the molar region.

Consistency

The gingiva is firm and resilient and, with the exception of the movable free margin, tightly bound to the underlying bone. The collagenous nature of the lamina propria and its contiguity with the mucoperiosteum of the alveolar bone determine the firmness of the attached gingiva. The gingival fibers contribute to the firmness of the gingival margin.

Surface Texture

The gingiva presents a textured surface similar to that of an orange peel and is referred to as *stippled* (see Fig. 4.25). Stippling is best viewed by drying the gingiva. *The attached gingiva is stippled; the marginal gingiva is not.* The central portion of the interdental papillae is usually stippled, but the marginal borders are smooth. The pattern and extent of stippling vary among

Fig. 4.27 A Thickened, Shelflike Contour of Gingiva on a Tooth in Lingual Version Aggravated by Local Irritation Caused by Plaque Accumulation.

Fig. 4.28 Shape of the Interdental Gingival Papillae Correlated With the Shape of the Teeth and the Embrasures. (A) Broad interdental papillae. (B) Narrow interdental papillae.

individuals and among different areas of the same mouth.[107,215] Stippling is less prominent on lingual than facial surfaces and may be absent in some persons.

Stippling varies with age. It is absent during infancy, it appears in some children at approximately 5 years of age, it increases until adulthood, and it frequently begins to disappear during old age.

Microscopically, stippling is produced by alternate rounded protuberances and depressions in the gingival surface. The papillary layer of the connective tissue projects into the elevations, and the elevated and depressed areas are covered by stratified squamous epithelium (Fig. 4.29). The degree of keratinization and the prominence of stippling appear to be related.

Scanning electron microscopy has shown considerable variation in shape but a relatively constant depth of stippling. At low magnification, a rippled surface is seen, and this is interrupted by irregular depressions that are 50 μm in diameter. At higher magnification, cell micropits are seen.[61]

Stippling is a form of adaptive specialization or reinforcement for function. It is a feature of healthy gingiva, and the reduction or loss of stippling is a common sign of gingival disease. When the gingiva is restored to health after treatment, the stippled appearance returns.

The surface texture of the gingiva is also related to the presence and degree of epithelial keratinization. Keratinization is considered a protective adaptation to function. It increases when the gingiva is stimulated by toothbrushing. However, research on free gingival

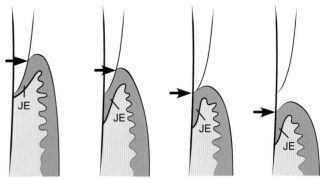

Fig. 4.30 Diagrammatic Representation of the Four Steps of Passive Eruption According to Gottlieb and Orban.[104] *1,* The base of the gingival sulcus *(arrow)* and the junctional epithelium *(JE)* are on the enamel. *2,* The base of the gingival sulcus *(arrow)* is on the enamel, and part of the junctional epithelium is on the root. *3,* The base of the gingival sulcus *(arrow)* is at the cementoenamel line, and the entire junctional epithelium is on the root. *4,* The base of the gingival sulcus *(arrow)* and the junctional epithelium are on the root.

Fig. 4.29 Gingival biopsy of the patient shown in Fig. 4.7 demonstrating alternate elevations and depressions *(arrows)* in the attached gingiva that are responsible for the stippled appearance.

grafts has shown that when connective tissue is transplanted from a keratinized area to a nonkeratinized area, it becomes covered by a keratinized epithelium.[139] This finding suggests a connective tissue–based genetic determination of the type of epithelial surface.

Position

The *position* of the gingiva is the level at which the gingival margin is attached to the tooth. When the tooth erupts into the oral cavity, the margin and sulcus are at the tip of the crown; as eruption progresses, they are seen closer to the root. During this eruption process, as described previously, the junctional epithelium, the oral epithelium, and the REE undergo extensive alterations and remodeling while maintaining the shallow physiologic depth of the sulcus. Without this remodeling of the epithelia, an abnormal anatomic relationship between the gingiva and the tooth would result.

Continuous tooth eruption. According to the concept of continuous eruption,[104] eruption does not cease when the teeth meet their functional antagonists; rather, it continues throughout life. Eruption consists of an active phase and a passive phase. *Active eruption* is the movement of the teeth in the direction of the occlusal plane, whereas *passive eruption* is the exposure of the teeth via apical migration of the gingiva.

This concept distinguishes between the anatomic crown (i.e., the portion of the tooth covered by enamel) and the anatomic root (i.e., the portion of the tooth covered by cementum) and between the clinical crown (i.e., the part of the tooth that has been denuded of its gingiva and projects into the oral cavity) and the clinical root (i.e., the portion of the tooth covered by periodontal tissues). When the teeth reach their functional antagonists, the gingival sulcus and the junctional epithelium

are still on the enamel, and the clinical crown is approximately two-thirds of the anatomic crown.

Gottlieb and Orban[104] believed that active and passive eruption proceed together. Active eruption is coordinated with attrition; the teeth erupt to compensate for tooth substance that has been worn away by attrition. Attrition reduces the clinical crown and prevents it from becoming disproportionately long in relation to the clinical root, thus avoiding excessive leverage on the periodontal tissues. Ideally, the rate of active eruption keeps pace with tooth wear, thereby preserving the vertical dimension of the dentition.

As teeth erupt, cementum is deposited at the apices and furcations of the roots, and bone is formed along the fundus of the alveolus and at the crest of the alveolar bone. In this way, part of the tooth substance lost by attrition is replaced by the lengthening of the root, and the socket depth is maintained to support the root.

Although originally thought to be a normal physiologic process, passive eruption is currently considered a pathologic process. Passive eruption is divided into the following four stages (Fig. 4.30):

Stage 1: The teeth reach the line of occlusion. The junctional epithelium and the base of the gingival sulcus are on the enamel.

Stage 2: The junctional epithelium proliferates so that part is on the cementum and part is on the enamel. The base of the sulcus is still on the enamel.

Stage 3: The entire junctional epithelium is on the cementum, and the base of the sulcus is at the cementoenamel junction. As the junctional epithelium proliferates from the crown onto the root, it does not remain at the cementoenamel junction any longer than at any other area of the tooth.

Stage 4: The junctional epithelium has proliferated farther on the cementum. The base of the sulcus is on the cementum, a portion of which is exposed. Proliferation of the junctional epithelium onto the root is accompanied by degeneration of the gingival and periodontal ligament fibers and their detachment from the tooth. The cause of this degeneration is not understood. At present, it is believed to be the result of chronic inflammation and therefore a pathologic process.

As noted, apposition of bone accompanies active eruption. The distance between the apical end of the junctional epithelium and the crest of the alveolus remains constant throughout continuous tooth eruption (i.e., 1.07 mm).[91]

Exposure of the tooth via the apical migration of the gingiva is called *gingival recession* or *atrophy.* According to the concept of continuous eruption, the gingival sulcus may be located on the crown, the cementoenamel junction, or the root, depending on the age of the patient and the stage of eruption. Therefore some root exposure with age would be considered normal and referred to as *physiologic recession.* Again, this concept is not accepted at present. Excessive exposure is termed *pathologic recession.*

PERIODONTAL LIGAMENT

The periodontal ligament is composed of a complex vascular and highly cellular connective tissue that surrounds the tooth root and connects it to the inner wall of the alveolar bone.[174] It is continuous with the connective tissue of the gingiva, and it communicates with the marrow spaces through vascular channels in the bone. Although the average width of the periodontal ligament space is documented to be approximately 0.2 mm, considerable variation exists. The periodontal space is diminished around teeth that are not in function and in unerupted teeth, but it is increased in teeth that have been subjected to hyperfunction.

Periodontal Fibers

The most important elements of the periodontal ligament are the *principal fibers,* which are collagenous and arranged in bundles and which follow a wavy course when viewed in longitudinal section (Fig. 4.31). The terminal portions of the principal fibers that are inserted into cementum and bone are termed *Sharpey fibers* (Fig. 4.32). The principal fiber bundles consist of individual fibers that form a continuous anastomosing network between tooth and bone.[25,58] Once embedded in the wall of the alveolus or in the tooth, Sharpey fibers calcify to a significant degree. They are associated with abundant noncollagenous proteins that are typically found in bone, and they have also been identified in tooth cementum.[33,131,174] Notable among these proteins are osteopontin and bone sialoprotein. These proteins are thought to contribute to the regulation of mineralization and to tissue cohesion at sites of increased biomechanical strain.[174]

Collagen is a protein that is composed of different amino acids, the most important of which are glycine, proline, hydroxylysine, and hydroxyproline.[51] The amount of collagen in a tissue can be determined by its hydroxyproline content. Collagen is responsible for the maintenance of the framework and the tone of tissue, and it exhibits a wide range of diversity.[80] There are at least 19 recognized collagen species encoded by at least 25 separate genes dispersed among 12 chromosomes.[80]

Collagen biosynthesis occurs inside the fibroblasts to form tropocollagen molecules. These aggregate into microfibrils that are packed together to form fibrils. Collagen fibrils have a

Fig. 4.31 Principal Fibers of the Periodontal Ligament Follow a Wavy Course When Sectioned Longitudinally. The formative function of the periodontal ligament is illustrated by the newly formed osteoid and osteoblasts along a previously resorbed bone surface *(left)* and the cementoid and cementoblasts *(right).* Note the fibers embedded in the forming calcified tissues *(arrows). V,* Vascular channels.

Fig. 4.32 Collagen Fibers Embedded in the Cementum *(Left)* and the Bone *(Right)* (Silver Stain). Note the Sharpey fibers within the bundle bone *(BB)* overlying the lamellar bone.

transverse striation with a characteristic periodicity of 64 μm; this striation is caused by the overlapping arrangement of the tropocollagen molecules. In collagen types I and III, these fibrils associate to form fibers; in collagen type I, the fibers associate to form bundles (Fig. 4.33).

Collagen is synthesized by fibroblasts, chondroblasts, osteoblasts, odontoblasts, and other cells. The several types of collagen are all distinguishable by their chemical composition, distribution, function, and morphology.[137] The principal fibers are composed mainly of collagen type I,[210] whereas reticular

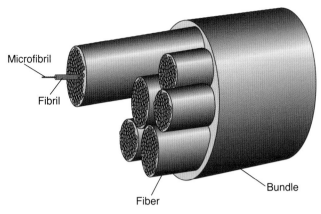

Fig. 4.33 Collagen Microfibrils, Fibrils, Fibers, and Bundles.

Fig. 4.35 Transseptal Fibers (f) at the Crest of the Interdental Bone.

Fig. 4.34 Diagram of the Principal Fiber Groups.

Fig. 4.36 Rat Molar Section Showing Alveolar Crest Fibers Radiating Coronally.

fibers are composed of collagen type III. Collagen type IV is found in the basal lamina.[211,213] The expression of type XII collagen during tooth development is timed with the alignment and organization of periodontal fibers and is limited in tooth development to cells within the periodontal ligament.[163] Type VI collagen has also been immunolocalized in the periodontal ligament and the gingiva.[82]

The molecular configuration of collagen fibers provides them with a tensile strength that is greater than that of steel. Consequently, collagen imparts a unique combination of flexibility and strength to the tissues.[137]

The principal fibers of the periodontal ligament are arranged in six groups that develop sequentially in the developing root: the transseptal, alveolar crest, horizontal, oblique, apical, and interradicular fibers (Fig. 4.34).

Transseptal fibers extend interproximally over the alveolar bone crest and are embedded in the cementum of adjacent teeth (Fig. 4.35). They are reconstructed even after destruction of the alveolar bone that results from periodontal disease. These fibers may be considered as belonging to the gingiva because they do not have osseous attachment.

Alveolar crest fibers extend obliquely from the cementum just beneath the junctional epithelium to the alveolar crest (Fig. 4.36). Fibers also run from the cementum over the alveolar crest and to the fibrous layer of the periosteum that covers the alveolar bone. The alveolar crest fibers prevent the extrusion of the tooth[52] and resist lateral tooth movements. The incision of these fibers during periodontal surgery does not increase tooth mobility unless significant attachment loss has occurred.[96]

Horizontal fibers extend at right angles to the long axis of the tooth from the cementum to the alveolar bone.

Oblique fibers, which constitute the largest group in the periodontal ligament, extend from the cementum in a coronal direction obliquely to the bone (see Fig. 4.34). They bear the brunt of vertical masticatory stresses and transform such stresses into tension on the alveolar bone.

The *apical fibers* radiate in a rather irregular manner from the cementum to the bone at the apical region of the socket. They do not occur on incompletely formed roots.

The *interradicular fibers* fan out from the cementum to the tooth in the furcation areas of multirooted teeth.

Other well-formed fiber bundles interdigitate at right angles or splay around and between regularly arranged fiber bundles. Less regularly arranged collagen fibers are found in the interstitial connective tissue between the principal fiber groups; this tissue contains the blood vessels, lymphatics, and nerves.

Although the periodontal ligament does not contain mature elastin, two immature forms are found: oxytalan and elaunin. The so-called oxytalan fibers[88,102] run parallel to the root surface in a vertical direction and bend to attach to the cementum[88] in the cervical third of the root. They are thought to regulate vascular flow.[87] An elastic meshwork has been described in the periodontal ligament[132] as being composed of many elastin lamellae with peripheral oxytalan fibers and elaunin fibers. Oxytalan fibers have been shown to develop de novo in the regenerated periodontal ligament.[218]

The principal fibers are remodeled by the periodontal ligament cells to adapt to physiologic needs[264,294] and in response to different stimuli.[276] In addition to these fiber types, small collagen fibers associated with the larger principal collagen fibers have been described. These fibers run in all directions and form a plexus called the *indifferent fiber plexus*.[242]

Cellular Elements

Four types of cells have been identified in the periodontal ligament: connective tissue cells, epithelial rest cells, immune system cells, and cells associated with neurovascular elements.[26,27]

Connective tissue cells include fibroblasts, cementoblasts, and osteoblasts. Fibroblasts are the most common cells in the periodontal ligament; they appear as ovoid or elongated cells oriented along the principal fibers, and they exhibit pseudopodia-like processes.[209] These cells synthesize collagen and possess the capacity to phagocytose "old" collagen fibers and degrade them[264] via enzyme hydrolysis. Thus collagen turnover appears to be regulated by fibroblasts in a process of intracellular degradation of collagen that does not involve the action of collagenase.[24]

Phenotypically distinct and functionally different subpopulations of fibroblasts exist in the adult periodontal ligament. They appear to be identical at both the light and electron microscopic levels,[114] but they may have different functions, such as the secretion of different collagen types and the production of collagenase.

Osteoblasts, cementoblasts, osteoclasts, and odontoclasts are also seen in the cemental and osseous surfaces of the periodontal ligament.

The *epithelial rests of Malassez* form a latticework in the periodontal ligament and appear as either isolated clusters of cells or interlacing strands (Fig. 4.37), depending on the plane in which the microscopic section is cut. Continuity with the

Fig. 4.37 Epithelial Rests of Malassez. (A) Erupting tooth in a cat. Note the fragmentation of the Hertwig epithelial root sheath giving rise to epithelial rests located along and close to the root surface. (B) Human periodontal ligament with rosette-shaped epithelial rests *(arrows)* lying close to the cementum *(C)*.

junctional epithelium has been suggested in experimental animals.[105] The epithelial rests are considered remnants of the Hertwig root sheath, which disintegrates during root development (see Fig. 4.37A).

Epithelial rests are distributed close to the cementum throughout the periodontal ligament of most teeth; they are most numerous in the apical area[206] and the cervical area.[278,279] They diminish in number with age[247] by degenerating and disappearing or by undergoing calcification to become cementicles. The cells are surrounded by a distinct basal lamina, they are interconnected by hemidesmosomes, and they contain tonofilaments.[24]

Although their functional properties are still considered to be unclear,[258] the epithelial rests are reported to contain keratinocyte growth factors, and they have been shown to be positive for tyrosine kinase A neurotrophin receptor.[90,280,290] In addition, epithelial rests proliferate when stimulated,[260,265,274] and they participate in the formation of periapical cysts and lateral root cysts.

The *defense cells* in the periodontal ligament include neutrophils, lymphocytes, macrophages, mast cells, and eosinophils. These cells, as well as those associated with neurovascular elements, are similar to the cells found in other connective tissues.

Ground Substance

The periodontal ligament also contains a large proportion of ground substance that fills the spaces between fibers and cells. This substance consists of two main components: *glycosaminoglycans,* such as hyaluronic acid and proteoglycans; and *glycoproteins,* such as fibronectin and laminin. It also has a high water content (i.e., 70%).

The cell surface proteoglycans participate in several biologic functions, including cell adhesion, cell-cell and cell-matrix interactions, binding to various growth factors as coreceptors, and cell repair.[291] For example, fibromodulin (a small proteoglycan rich in keratan sulfate and leucine) has been identified in bovine periodontal ligament.[282] The most comprehensive study of the proteoglycans in periodontal ligament was performed with the use of fibroblast cultures of human ligament.[148]

The periodontal ligament may also contain calcified masses called *cementicles,* which are adherent to or detached from the root surfaces (Fig. 4.38).

Cementicles may develop from calcified epithelial rests; around small spicules of cementum or alveolar bone traumatically displaced into the periodontal ligament; from calcified Sharpey fibers; and from calcified, thrombosed vessels within the periodontal ligament.[179]

Functions of Periodontal Ligament

The functions of the periodontal ligament are categorized as physical, formative and remodeling, nutritional, and sensory.

Physical Functions

The physical functions of the periodontal ligament entail the following:

1. Provision of a soft-tissue "casing" to protect the vessels and nerves from injury by mechanical forces
2. Transmission of occlusal forces to the bone

Fig. 4.38 Cementicles in the Periodontal Ligament. One is lying free and the other is adherent to the tooth surface.

3. Attachment of the teeth to the bone
4. Maintenance of the gingival tissues in their proper relationship to the teeth
5. Resistance to the impact of occlusal forces (i.e., shock absorption)

Resistance to impact of occlusal forces (shock absorption). Two theories pertaining to the mechanism of tooth support exist: the tensional theory and the viscoelastic system theory.

The tensional theory of tooth support states that the principal fibers of the periodontal ligament are the major factor in supporting the tooth and transmitting forces to the bone. When a force is applied to the crown, the principal fibers first unfold and straighten, and they then transmit forces to the alveolar bone, thereby causing an elastic deformation of the bony socket. Finally, when the alveolar bone has reached its limit, the load is transmitted to the basal bone. Many investigators find this theory insufficient to explain available experimental evidence.

The viscoelastic system theory states that the displacement of the tooth is largely controlled by fluid movements, with fibers having only a secondary role.[31,43] When forces are transmitted to the tooth, the extracellular fluid passes from the periodontal ligament into the marrow spaces of the bone through the foramina in the cribriform plate. These perforations of the cribriform plate link the periodontal ligament with the cancellous portion of the alveolar bone; they are more abundant in the cervical third than in the middle and apical thirds (Fig. 4.39).

After the depletion of tissue fluids, the fiber bundles absorb the slack and tighten. This leads to a blood vessel stenosis. Arterial back pressure causes ballooning of the vessels and passage of the blood ultrafiltrates into the tissues, thereby replenishing the tissue fluids.[31]

Transmission of occlusal forces to bone. The arrangement of the principal fibers is similar to that of a suspension bridge or a hammock. When an axial force is applied to a tooth, a tendency toward displacement of the root into the alveolus occurs. The oblique fibers alter their wavy, untensed pattern, assume their full length, and sustain the major part of the axial force.

TABLE 4.1	Thickness of the Periodontal Ligaments of 172 Teeth From 15 Human Subjects			
	Average of Alveolar Crest (mm)	Average of Midroot (mm)	Average of Apex (mm)	Average of Tooth (mm)
Ages 11–16 years	0.23	0.17	0.24	0.21
83 teeth from 4 jaws				
Ages 32–50 years	0.20	0.14	0.19	0.18
36 teeth from 5 jaws				
Ages 51–67 years	0.17	0.12	0.16	0.15
35 teeth from 5 jaws				
Age 24 years (1 case)	0.16	0.09	0.15	0.13
18 teeth from 1 jaw				

Modified from Coolidge ED: The thickness of the human periodontal membrane. *J Am Dent Assoc* 24:1260, 1937.

Fig. 4.39 Foramina Perforating the Lamina Dura of a Dog Jaw.

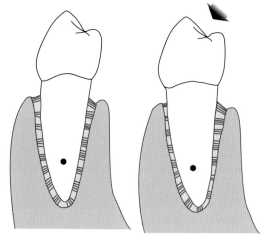

Fig. 4.40 *Left,* Diagram of a mandibular premolar in a resting state. *Right,* When a force is exerted on the tooth—in this case, in faciolingual direction *(arrow)*—the tooth rotates around the fulcrum or axis of rotation *(black circle on root)*. The periodontal ligament is compressed in areas of pressure and distended in areas of tension.

When a horizontal or tipping force is applied, two phases of tooth movement occur. The first is within the confines of the periodontal ligament, and the second produces a displacement of the facial and lingual bony plates.[69] The tooth rotates about an axis that may change as the force is increased.

The apical portion of the root moves in a direction that is opposite to the coronal portion. In areas of tension, the principal fiber bundles are taut rather than wavy. In areas of pressure, the fibers are compressed, the tooth is displaced, and a corresponding distortion of bone exists in the direction of root movement.[202]

In single-rooted teeth, the axis of rotation is located in the area between the apical third and the middle third of the root (Fig. 4.40). The root apex[183] and the coronal half of the clinical root have been suggested as other locations of the axis of rotation. The periodontal ligament, which has an hourglass shape, is narrowest in the region of the axis of rotation[65,144] (Table 4.1). In multirooted teeth, the axis of rotation is located in the bone between the roots (Fig. 4.41). In compliance with the physiologic mesial migration of the teeth, the periodontal ligament is thinner on the mesial root surface than on the distal surface.

Formative and Remodeling Function

Periodontal ligament and alveolar bone cells are exposed to physical forces in response to mastication, parafunction, speech, and orthodontic tooth movement.[172] Cells of the periodontal ligament participate in the formation and resorption of cementum and bone, which occur during physiologic tooth movement, during the accommodation of the periodontium to occlusal forces, and during the repair of injuries.

Variations in cellular enzyme activity are correlated with the remodeling process.[93-95] Although applied loads may induce vascular and inflammatory reactive changes in periodontal ligament cells, current evidence suggests that these cells have a mechanism to respond directly to mechanical forces via the activation of various mechanosensory signaling systems, including adenylate cyclase, stretch-activated ion channels, and via changes in cytoskeletal organization.[172]

Cartilage formation in the periodontal ligament, although unusual, may represent a metaplastic phenomenon in the repair of this ligament after injury.[20]

The periodontal ligament is constantly undergoing remodeling. Old cells and fibers are broken down and replaced by new ones, and mitotic activity can be observed in the fibroblasts and the endothelial cells.[184] Fibroblasts form the collagen fibers,

Fig. 4.41 Microscopic View of a Rat Molar Subjected to Occluso-horizontal Forces. Note the alternating widened and narrowed areas of the periodontal ligament as the tooth rotates around its axis of rotation. The axis of rotation is in the interradicular space.

and the residual mesenchymal cells develop into osteoblasts and cementoblasts. Therefore the rate of formation and the differentiation of osteoblasts, cementoblasts, and fibroblasts affect the rate of formation of collagen, cementum, and bone.

Radioautographic studies with radioactive thymidine, proline, and glycine indicate a high turnover rate of collagen in the periodontal ligament. The rate of collagen synthesis is twice as fast as that in the gingiva and four times as fast as that in the skin, as established in the rat molar.[249] A rapid turnover of sulfated glycosaminoglycans in the cells and amorphous ground substance of the periodontal ligament also occurs.[21] It should be noted that most of these studies have been performed in rodents and that information about primates and humans is scarce.[231]

Nutritional and Sensory Functions

The periodontal ligament supplies nutrients to the cementum, bone, and gingiva by way of the blood vessels, and it also provides lymphatic drainage as discussed later in this chapter. In relation to other ligaments and tendons, the periodontal ligament is highly vascularized tissue; almost 10% of its volume in the rodent molar is blood vessels.[35,173] This relatively high blood vessel content may provide hydrodynamic damping to applied forces as well as high perfusion rates to the periodontal ligament.[172]

The periodontal ligament is abundantly supplied with sensory nerve fibers that are capable of transmitting tactile, pressure, and pain sensations via the trigeminal pathways.[14,30] Nerve bundles pass into the periodontal ligament from the periapical area and through channels from the alveolar bone that follow the course of the blood vessels. The bundles divide into single myelinated fibers, which ultimately lose their myelin sheaths and end in one of four types of neural termination: (1) free endings, which have a treelike configuration and carry pain sensation; (2) Ruffini-like

mechanoreceptors, which are located primarily in the apical area; (3) coiled Meissner corpuscles and mechanoreceptors, which are found mainly in the midroot region; and (4) spindle-like pressure and vibration endings, which are surrounded by a fibrous capsule and located mainly in the apex.[87,165]

Regulation of Periodontal Ligament Width

Some of the most interesting features of the periodontal ligament in animals are its adaptability to rapidly changing applied force and its capacity to maintain its width at constant dimensions throughout its lifetime.[173] These are important measures of periodontal ligament homeostasis that provide insight into the function of the biologic mechanisms that tightly regulate the metabolism and spatial locations of the cell populations involved in the formation of bone, cementum, and periodontal ligament fibers. In addition, the ability of periodontal ligament cells to synthesize and secrete a wide range of regulatory molecules is an essential component of tissue remodeling and periodontal ligament homeostasis.[172]

CEMENTUM

Cementum is the calcified, avascular mesenchymal tissue that forms the outer covering of the anatomic root. The two main types of cementum are acellular (*primary*) and cellular (*secondary*) cementum.[103] Both consist of a calcified interfibrillar matrix and collagen fibrils.

The two main sources of collagen fibers in cementum are Sharpey fibers (*extrinsic*), which are the embedded portion of the principal fibers of the periodontal ligament[213] and which are formed by the fibroblasts, and fibers that belong to the cementum matrix (*intrinsic*), which are produced by the cementoblasts.[239] Cementoblasts also form the noncollagenous components of the interfibrillar ground substance, such as proteoglycans, glycoproteins, and phosphoproteins. Proteoglycans are most likely to play a role in regulating cell-cell and cell-matrix interactions, both during normal development and during the regeneration of the cementum.[17] In addition, immunohistochemical studies have shown that the distribution of proteoglycans is closely associated with the cementoblasts and the cementocytes.[1,2]

The major proportion of the organic matrix of cementum is composed of type I (90%) and type III (approximately 5%) collagens. Sharpey fibers, which constitute a considerable proportion of the bulk of cementum, are composed of mainly type I collagen.[205] Type III collagen appears to coat the type I collagen of the Sharpey fibers.[16]

Acellular cementum is the first cementum formed; it covers approximately the cervical third or half of the root, and it does not contain cells (Fig. 4.42). This cementum is formed before the tooth reaches the occlusal plane, and its thickness ranges from 30 to 230 μm.[247] Sharpey fibers make up most of the structure of acellular cementum, which has a principal role in supporting the tooth. Most fibers are inserted at approximately right angles into the root surface and penetrate deep into the cementum, but others enter from several different directions. Their size, number, and distribution increase with function.[122] Sharpey fibers are completely calcified, with the mineral crystals oriented parallel

Fig. 4.42 Acellular Cementum *(AC)* Showing Incremental Lines Running Parallel to the Long Axis of the Tooth. These lines represent the appositional growth of cementum. Note the thin, light lines running into the cementum perpendicular to the surface; these represent the Sharpey fibers of the periodontal ligament *(PL)*. D, Dentin. (×300.)

Fig. 4.43 Cellular Cementum *(CC)* Showing Cementocytes Lying Within the Lacunae. Cellular cementum is thicker than acellular cementum. The evidence of incremental lines also exists, but they are less distinct than in the acellular cementum. The cells adjacent to the surface of the cementum in the periodontal ligament *(PL)* space are cementoblasts. *D*, Dentin. (×300.)

to the fibrils as in dentin and bone, except in a 10- to 50-μm–wide zone near the cementodentinal junction, where they are only partially calcified. The peripheral portions of Sharpey fibers in actively mineralizing cementum tend to be more calcified than the interior regions, according to evidence obtained by scanning electron microscopy.[136] Acellular cementum also contains intrinsic collagen fibrils that are calcified and irregularly arranged or parallel to the surface.[231]

Cellular cementum, which is formed after the tooth reaches the occlusal plane, is more irregular and contains cells (cementocytes) in individual spaces (lacunae) that communicate with each other through a system of anastomosing canaliculi (Fig. 4.43). Cellular cementum is less calcified than the acellular type.[123] Sharpey fibers occupy a smaller portion of cellular cementum and are separated by other fibers that are arranged either parallel to the root surface or at random. Sharpey fibers may be completely or partially calcified, or they may have a central, uncalcified core surrounded by a calcified border.[134,239]

Both acellular cementum and cellular cementum are arranged in lamellae separated by incremental lines parallel to the long axis of the root (see Figs. 4.42 and 4.43). These lines represent "rest periods" in cementum formation, and they are more mineralized than the adjacent cementum.[214] In addition, the loss of the cervical part of the REE at the time of tooth eruption may place portions of mature enamel in contact with the connective tissue, which then will deposit an acellular and afibrillar type of cementum over the enamel.[156]

On the basis of these findings, Schroeder[132,133] has classified cementum as follows:

- Acellular afibrillar cementum contains neither cells nor extrinsic or intrinsic collagen fibers, except for a mineralized ground substance. Acellular afibrillar cementum is a product of cementoblasts and found as coronal cementum in humans, with a thickness of 1 to 15 μm.
- Acellular extrinsic fiber cementum is composed almost entirely of densely packed bundles of Sharpey fibers and lacks cells. Acellular extrinsic fiber cementum is a product of fibroblasts and cementoblasts. It is found in the cervical third of roots in humans, but it may extend farther apically. Its thickness is between 30 and 230 μm.
- Cellular mixed stratified cementum is composed of extrinsic (Sharpey) and intrinsic fibers, and it may contain cells. Cellular mixed stratified cementum is a coproduct of fibroblasts and cementoblasts. In humans, it appears primarily in the apical third of the roots and apices and in furcation areas. Its thickness ranges from 100 to 1000 μm.
- Cellular intrinsic fiber cementum contains cells but no extrinsic collagen fibers. Cellular intrinsic fiber cementum is formed by cementoblasts, and, in humans, it fills the resorption lacunae.

Intermediate cementum is a poorly defined zone near the cementodentinal junction of certain teeth that appears to contain cellular remnants of the Hertwig sheath embedded in a calcified ground substance.[77,152]

Inorganic content of cementum (hydroxyapatite; $Ca_{10}[PO_4]_6[OH]_2$) is 45% to 50%, which is less than that of bone (65%), enamel (97%), or dentin (70%).[298] Opinions differ with regard to whether the microhardness increases[188] or decreases

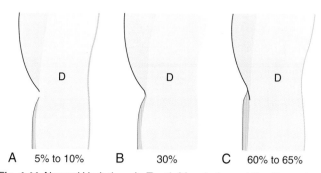

Fig. 4.44 Normal Variations in Tooth Morphology at the Cementoenamel Junction. (A) Space between the enamel and the cementum with the dentin *(D)* exposed. (B) End-to-end relationship of enamel and cementum. (C) Cementum overlapping the enamel.

with age,[281] and no relationship has been established between aging and the mineral content of cementum.

Permeability of Cementum

In very young animals, acellular cementum and cellular cementum are very permeable and permit the diffusion of dyes from the pulp and the external root surface. In cellular cementum, the canaliculi in some areas are contiguous with the dentinal tubuli. The permeability of cementum diminishes with age.[36]

Cementoenamel Junction

The cementum at and immediately subjacent to the *cementoenamel junction* is of particular clinical importance in root-scaling procedures. Three types of relationships involving the cementum may exist at the cementoenamel junction.[189] In approximately 60% to 65% of cases, cementum overlaps the enamel (Fig. 4.44); in approximately 30%, an edge-to-edge butt joint exists; and in 5% to 10%, the cementum and enamel fail to meet. In the last case, gingival recession may result in accentuated sensitivity as a result of exposed dentin.

Cementodentinal Junction

The terminal apical area of the cementum where it joins the internal root canal dentin is known as the *cementodentinal junction.* When root canal treatment is performed, the obturating material should be at the cementodentinal junction. There appears to be no increase or decrease in the width of the cementodentinal junction with age; its width appears to remain relatively stable.[252] Scanning electron microscopy of the human teeth reveals that the cementodentinal junction is 2 to 3 μm wide. The fibril-poor layer contains a significant amount of proteoglycans, and fibrils intermingle between the cementum and the dentin.[292,293]

Thickness of Cementum

Cementum deposition is a continuous process that proceeds at varying rates throughout life. Cementum formation is most rapid in the apical regions, where it compensates for tooth eruption, which itself compensates for attrition.

The thickness of cementum on the coronal half of the root varies from 16 to 60 μm, which is about the thickness of a hair. It attains its greatest thickness (≤150 to 200 μm) in the apical

third and in the furcation areas. It is thicker in distal surfaces than in mesial surfaces, probably because of functional stimulation from mesial drift over time.[68] Between the ages of 11 and 70 years, the average thickness of the cementum increases threefold, with the greatest increase seen in the apical region. Average thicknesses of 95 μm at the age of 20 years and of 215 μm at the age of 60 years have been reported.[297]

Abnormalities in the thickness of cementum may range from an absence or paucity of cellular cementum (i.e., cemental aplasia or hypoplasia) to an excessive deposition of cementum (i.e., cemental hyperplasia or hypercementosis).[151]

The term *hypercementosis* refers to a prominent thickening of the cementum. It is largely an age-related phenomenon, and it may be localized to one tooth or affect the entire dentition. As a result of considerable physiologic variation in the thickness of cementum among different teeth in the same person and also among different persons, distinguishing between hypercementosis and the physiologic thickening of cementum is sometimes difficult. Nevertheless, the excessive proliferation of cementum may occur with a broad spectrum of neoplastic and nonneoplastic conditions, including benign cementoblastoma, cementifying fibroma, periapical cemental dysplasia, florid cemento-osseous dysplasia, and other benign fibro-osseous lesions.[151]

Hypercementosis itself does not require treatment. It could pose a problem if an affected tooth requires extraction. In a multirooted tooth, sectioning of the tooth may be required before extraction.[19]

Cementum Resorption and Repair

Permanent teeth do not undergo physiologic resorption as primary teeth do. However, the cementum of erupted (as well as unerupted) teeth is subject to resorptive changes that may be of microscopic proportion or sufficiently extensive to present a radiographically detectable alteration in the root contour.

Microscopic cementum resorption is extremely common; in one study, it occurred in 236 of 261 teeth (90.5%).[117] The average number of resorption areas per tooth was 3.5. Of the 922 areas of resorption, 708 (76.8%) were located in the apical third of the root, 177 (19.2%) in the middle third, and 37 (4.0%) in the gingival third. Approximately 70% of all resorption areas were confined to the cementum without involving the dentin.

Cementum resorption may be caused by local or systemic factors, or it may occur without apparent etiology (i.e., idiopathic). Local conditions that cause cementum resorption include trauma from occlusion (Fig. 4.45)[193]; orthodontic movement[116,192,216]; pressure from malaligned erupting teeth, cysts, and tumors[143]; teeth without functional antagonists; embedded teeth; replanted and transplanted teeth[3,134]; periapical disease; and periodontal disease. Systemic conditions that are cited as predisposing an individual to or inducing cemental resorption include calcium deficiency,[135] hypothyroidism,[23] hereditary fibrous osteodystrophy,[268] and Paget disease.[217]

Cementum resorption appears microscopically as baylike concavities in the root surface (Fig. 4.46). Multinucleated giant cells and large mononuclear macrophages are generally found adjacent to cementum that is undergoing active resorption (Fig. 4.47). Several sites of resorption may coalesce to form a large

Fig. 4.45 Cemental Resorption Associated With Excessive Occlusal Forces. (A) Low-power histologic section of the mandibular anterior teeth. (B) High-power micrograph of the apex of the left central incisor shortened by the resorption of cementum and dentin. Note the partial repair of the eroded areas *(arrows)* and the cementicle at the upper right.

Fig. 4.46 Scanning electron micrograph of a root exposed by periodontal disease showing a large resorption bay *(R)*. Remnants of the periodontal ligament *(P)* and calculus *(C)* are visible. Cracking of the tooth surface occurs as a result of the preparation technique (×160). (Courtesy Dr. John Sottosanti, La Jolla, California.)

Fig. 4.47 Resorption of Cementum and Dentin. A multinuclear osteoclast in seen *(X)*. The direction of resorption is indicated by the arrow. Note the scalloped resorption front in the dentin *(D)*. The cementum is the darkly stained band at the upper and lower right. *P,* Periodontal ligament.

area of destruction. The resorptive process may extend into the underlying dentin and even into the pulp, but it is usually painless. Cementum resorption is not necessarily continuous and may alternate with periods of repair and the deposition of new cementum. The newly formed cementum is demarcated from the root by a deeply staining irregular line termed a *reversal line,* which delineates the border of the previous resorption. One study showed that the reversal lines of human teeth contain a few collagen fibrils and highly accumulated proteoglycans with mucopolysaccharides (glycosaminoglycans), and that fibril intermingling occurs only in some places between reparative cementum and resorbed dentin or cementum.[292,293] Embedded fibers of the periodontal ligament reestablish a functional relationship in the new cementum.

Cementum repair requires the presence of viable connective tissue. If epithelium proliferates into an area of resorption, repair will not take place. Cementum repair can occur in devitalized as well as vital teeth.

Histologic evidence demonstrates that cementum formation is critical for the appropriate maturation of the periodontium, both during development and during the regeneration of lost periodontal tissues.[224] In other words, a variety of macromolecules present in the extracellular matrix of the periodontium are likely to play a regulatory role in cementogenesis.[168]

The regeneration of cementum requires cementoblasts, but the origin of the cementoblasts and the molecular factors that regulate their recruitment and differentiation are not fully understood. However, research provides a better understanding; for example, the epithelial cell rests of Malassez are the only odontogenic epithelial cells that remain in the periodontium after the eruption of teeth, and they may have some function in cementum repair and regeneration under specific conditions.[113] The rests of Malassez may be related to cementum repair by activating their potential to secrete matrix proteins that have been expressed in tooth development, such as amelogenins, enamelins, and sheath proteins. Several growth factors have been shown to be effective in cementum regeneration, including members of the transforming growth factor superfamily (i.e., bone morphogenetic proteins), platelet-derived growth factor, insulin-like growth factor, and enamel matrix derivatives (Fig. 4.48).[138,224]

Ankylosis

Fusion of the cementum and the alveolar bone with obliteration of the periodontal ligament is termed *ankylosis*. Ankylosis occurs in teeth with cemental resorption, which suggests that it may represent a form of abnormal repair. Ankylosis may also develop after chronic periapical inflammation, tooth replantation, and occlusal trauma and around embedded teeth. This condition is relatively uncommon, and it occurs most frequently in the primary dentition.[175]

Exposure of Cementum to the Oral Environment

Cementum becomes exposed to the oral environment in cases of gingival recession and as a result of the loss of attachment in pocket formation. The cementum is sufficiently permeable to be penetrated in these cases by organic substances, inorganic ions, and bacteria. Bacterial invasion of the cementum occurs frequently in individuals with periodontal disease, and cementum caries can develop.

ALVEOLAR PROCESS

The alveolar process is the portion of the maxilla and mandible that forms and supports the tooth sockets (alveoli). It forms when the tooth erupts to provide the osseous attachment to the forming periodontal ligament; it disappears gradually after the tooth is lost.

Because the alveolar processes develop and undergo remodeling with tooth formation and eruption, they are tooth-dependent bony structures.[226] The size, shape, location, and function of the teeth determine their morphology. Interestingly, although the growth and development of the bones of the jaw determine the position of the teeth, a certain degree of repositioning of the teeth can be accomplished through occlusal forces and in response to orthodontic procedures that rely on the adaptability of the alveolar bone and the associated periodontal tissues.[250]

The alveolar process consists of the following:

1. An external plate of cortical bone is formed by haversian bone and compacted bone lamellae.
2. The inner socket wall of thin, compact bone called the *alveolar bone proper* is seen as the lamina dura in radiographs. Histologically, it contains a series of openings (i.e., the *cribriform plate*) through which neurovascular bundles link the periodontal ligament with the central component of the alveolar bone: the cancellous bone.
3. Cancellous trabeculae between these two compact layers act as supporting alveolar bone. The *interdental septum* consists of cancellous supporting bone enclosed within a compact border (Fig. 4.49).

In addition, the bones of the jaw include the basal bone, which is the portion of the jaw located apically but unrelated to the teeth (Fig. 4.50).

The alveolar process is divisible into separate areas on an anatomic basis, but it functions as a unit, with all parts interrelated in the support of the teeth. Figs. 4.51 and 4.52 show the

Fig. 4.48 A Clinical Human Histology Shows That New Cementum and New Periodontal Ligament Fiber Formed at a Previous Periodontal Defect Treated With Recombinant Human Platelet-Derived Growth Factor-BB With β-Tricalcium Phosphate. (Courtesy Dr. Daniel WK Kao, Philadelphia, Pennsylvania.)

Fig. 4.49 Mesiodistal Section Through the Mandibular Molars of a 17-Year-Old Girl Obtained at Autopsy. Note the interdental bony septa between the first and second molars. The dense cortical bony plates represent the alveolar bone proper (i.e., the cribriform plates) and are supported by cancellous bony trabeculae. The third molar is still in the early stages of root formation and eruption.

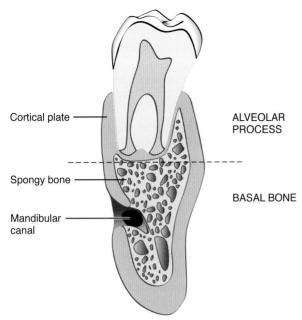

Fig. 4.50 Section Through a Human Jaw With a Tooth in Situ. The dotted line indicates the separation between the basal bone and the alveolar bone. (Redrawn from Ten Cate AR: *Oral histology: development, structure, and function*, ed 4, St Louis, 1994, Mosby.)

Labels on Fig. 4.50: Cortical plate, Spongy bone, Mandibular canal, ALVEOLAR PROCESS, BASAL BONE

Fig. 4.52 The Shape of the Roots and the Surrounding Bone Distribution in a Transverse Section of Maxilla and Mandible at the Midroot Level.

Labels on Fig. 4.52: Maxilla, Mandible

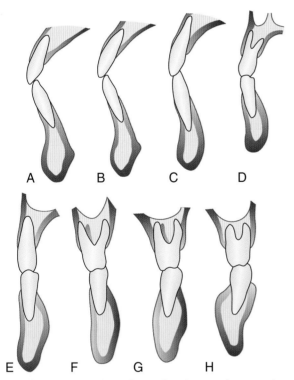

Fig. 4.51 Relative proportions of cancellous bone and compact bone in a longitudinal faciolingual section of (A) mandibular molars, (B) lateral incisors, (C) canines, (D) first premolars, (E) second premolars, (F) first molars, (G) second molars, and (H) third molars.

relative proportions of cancellous bone and compact bone that form the alveolar process. Most of the facial and lingual portions of the sockets are formed by compact bone alone; cancellous bone surrounds the lamina dura in apical, apicolingual, and interradicular areas.

Bone consists of two-thirds inorganic matter and one-third organic matrix. The inorganic matter is composed principally of the minerals calcium and phosphate, along with hydroxyl, carbonate, citrate, and trace amounts of other ions[100,101] such as sodium, magnesium, and fluorine. The mineral salts are in the form of hydroxyapatite crystals of ultramicroscopic size and constitute approximately two-thirds of the bone structure.

The organic matrix[75] consists mainly of collagen type I (90%),[184] with small amounts of noncollagenous proteins such as osteocalcin, osteonectin, bone morphogenetic protein, phosphoproteins, and proteoglycans.[208] Osteopontin and bone sialoprotein are cell-adhesion proteins that appear to be important for the adhesion of both osteoclasts and osteoblasts.[162] In addition, paracrine factors, including cytokines, chemokines, and growth factors, have been implicated in the local control of mesenchymal condensations that occur at the onset of organogenesis. These factors probably play a prominent role in the development of the alveolar processes.[250]

Although the alveolar bone tissue is constantly changing its internal organization, it retains approximately the same form from childhood through adult life. Bone deposition by osteoblasts is balanced by resorption by osteoclasts during tissue remodeling and renewal. It is well known that the number of osteoblasts decreases with aging; however, no remarkable change in the number of osteoclasts has ever been reported.[190]

Remodeling is the major pathway of bony changes in shape, resistance to forces, repair of wounds, and calcium and phosphate homeostasis in the body. Indeed, the coupling of bone resorption with bone formation constitutes one of the fundamental principles by which bone is necessarily remodeled throughout its life. Bone remodeling involves the coordination of activities of cells from two distinct lineages, the osteoblasts and the osteoclasts, which form and resorb the mineralized connective tissues of bone.[250]

The bone matrix that is laid down by osteoblasts is nonmineralized osteoid. While new osteoid is being deposited, the older osteoid located below the surface becomes mineralized as the mineralization front advances.

Fig. 4.53 **Rat Alveolar Bone.** This histologic view show two multinucleated osteoclasts in the Howship lacuna.

Bone resorption is a complex process that is morphologically related to the appearance of eroded bone surfaces (i.e., Howship lacunae) and large, multinucleated cells (osteoclasts) (Fig. 4.53). Osteoclasts originate from hematopoietic tissue[55,109,196] and are formed by the fusion of mononuclear cells of asynchronous populations.[140,200,263] When osteoclasts are active rather than resting, they possess an elaborately developed ruffled border from which hydrolytic enzymes are thought to be secreted.[277] These enzymes digest the organic portion of bone. The activity of osteoclasts and the morphology of the ruffled border can be modified and regulated by hormones such as parathyroid hormone (indirectly) and calcitonin, which has receptors on the osteoclast membrane.

Another mechanism of bone resorption involves the creation of an acidic environment on the bone surface, thereby leading to the dissolution of the mineral component of bone. This event can be produced by different conditions, including a proton pump through the cell membrane of the osteoclast,[34] bone tumors, and local pressure[196] translated through the secretory activity of the osteoclast.

Ten Cate[263] described the sequence of events in the resorptive process as follows:
1. Attachment of osteoclasts to the mineralized surface of bone
2. Creation of a sealed acidic environment through the action of the proton pump, which demineralizes bone and exposes the organic matrix
3. Degradation of the exposed organic matrix to its constituent amino acids via the action of released enzymes (e.g., acid phosphatase, cathepsin)
4. Sequestering of mineral ions and amino acids within the osteoclast

Notably, the cellular and molecular events involved in bone remodeling have a strong similarity to many aspects of

Fig. 4.54 **Deep Penetration of Sharpey Fibers Into Bundle Bone of a Rat Molar.**

inflammation and repair. The relationships among matrix molecules (e.g., osteopontin, bone sialoprotein, SPARC [secreted protein, acidic, rich in cysteine], osteocalcin), blood clotting, and wound healing are clearly evident.[250]

Cells and Intercellular Matrix

Osteoblasts, which are the cells that produce the organic matrix of bone, are differentiated from pluripotent follicle cells. Alveolar bone is formed during fetal growth by intramembranous ossification, and it consists of a calcified matrix with osteocytes enclosed within spaces called *lacunae.* The osteocytes extend processes into *canaliculi* that radiate from the lacunae. The canaliculi form an anastomosing system through the intercellular matrix of the bone, which brings oxygen and nutrients to the osteocytes through the blood and removes metabolic waste products. Blood vessels branch extensively and travel through the periosteum. The endosteum lies adjacent to the marrow vasculature. Bone growth occurs via the apposition of an organic matrix that is deposited by osteoblasts. Haversian systems (i.e., *osteons*) are the internal mechanisms that bring a vascular supply to bones that are too thick to be supplied only by surface vessels. These are found primarily in the outer cortical plates and the alveolar bone proper.

Socket Wall

The socket wall consists of dense, lamellated bone, some of which is arranged in haversian systems and bundle bone. *Bundle bone* is the term given to bone adjacent to the periodontal ligament that contains a great number of Sharpey fibers (Fig. 4.54).[285] It is characterized by thin lamellae arranged in layers parallel to the root, with intervening appositional lines (Fig. 4.55). Bundle bone is localized within the alveolar bone proper. Some Sharpey fibers are completely calcified, but most contain an uncalcified central core within a calcified outer layer.[239] Bundle bone is not unique to the jaws; it occurs throughout the skeletal system wherever ligaments and muscles are attached.

The cancellous portion of the alveolar bone consists of trabeculae that enclose irregularly shaped marrow spaces lined with a layer of thin, flattened endosteal cells. Wide variation occurs in the trabecular pattern of cancellous bone,[199] which is

Fig. 4.55 Bundle Bone Associated With the Physiologic Mesial Migration of the Teeth. (A) Horizontal section through the molar roots during the process of mesial migration (*left,* mesial; *right,* distal). (B) Mesial root surface showing osteoclasis of bone *(arrows).* (C) Distal root surface showing bundle bone that has been partially replaced with dense bone on the marrow side. *PL,* Periodontal ligament.

affected by occlusal forces. The matrix of the cancellous trabeculae consists of irregularly arranged lamellae separated by deeply staining incremental and resorption lines indicative of previous bone activity, with an occasional haversian system.

Cancellous bone is found predominantly in the interradicular and interdental spaces and in limited amounts facially or lingually, except in the palate. In the adult human, more cancellous bone exists in the maxilla than in the mandible.

Bone Marrow

In the embryo and the newborn, the cavities of all bones are occupied by red hematopoietic marrow. The red marrow gradually undergoes a physiologic change to the fatty or yellow inactive type of marrow. In the adult, the marrow of the jaw is normally of the latter type, and red marrow is found only in the ribs, sternum, vertebrae, skull, and humerus. However, foci of the red bone marrow are occasionally seen in the jaws, often accompanied by the resorption of bony trabeculae.[41] Common locations are the maxillary tuberosity, the maxillary and mandibular molar and premolar areas, and the mandibular symphysis and ramus angle, which may be visible radiographically as zones of radiolucency.

Periosteum and Endosteum

Layers of differentiated osteogenic connective tissue cover all of the bone surfaces. The tissue that covers the outer surface of bone is termed *periosteum,* whereas the tissue that lines the internal bone cavities is called *endosteum.*

The periosteum consists of an *inner layer* composed of osteoblasts surrounded by osteoprogenitor cells, which have the potential to differentiate into osteoblasts, and an *outer layer* rich in blood vessels and nerves and composed of collagen fibers and fibroblasts. Bundles of periosteal collagen fibers penetrate the bone, thereby binding the periosteum to the bone. The endosteum is composed of a single layer of osteoblasts and sometimes a small amount of connective tissue. The inner layer is the osteogenic layer, and the outer layer is the fibrous layer.

Cellular events at the periosteum modulate bone size throughout an individual's life span, and a change in bone size is probably the result of the balance between periosteal osteoblastic and osteoclastic activities. Little is currently known about the control of periosteal osteoblastic activity or the clinical importance of variations in periosteal bone formation.[195] Moreover, the nature and impact of periosteal bone resorption are virtually unexplored.

Interdental Septum

The interdental septum consists of cancellous bone that is bordered by the socket wall cribriform plates (i.e., lamina dura or alveolar bone proper) of approximating teeth and the facial and lingual cortical plates (Fig. 4.56). If the interdental space is narrow, the septum may consist of only the cribriform plate. In one study, for example, the space between the mandibular second premolars and first molars consisted of cribriform plate and cancellous bone in 85% of the cases and of only cribriform plate in the remaining 15%.[115] If the roots are too close together, an irregular "window" can appear in the bone between adjacent roots (Fig. 4.57). Between maxillary molars, the septum consisted of cribriform plate and cancellous bone in 66.6% of cases; it was composed of only cribriform plate in 20.8%, and it had a fenestration in 12.5%.[115]

Determining root proximity radiographically is important (see Chapters 31 and 33). The mesiodistal angulation of the crest of the interdental septum usually parallels a line drawn between the cementoenamel junctions of the approximating teeth.[208] The distance between the crest of the alveolar bone and the cementoenamel junction in young adults varies between 0.75 and 1.49 mm (average, 1.08 mm). This distance increases with age to an average of 2.81 mm.[91] However, this phenomenon may not be as much a function of age as of periodontal disease.

The mesiodistal and faciolingual dimensions and shape of the interdental septum are governed by the size and convexity of the crowns of the two approximating teeth, as well as by the position of the teeth in the jaw and their degree of eruption.[208]

Osseous Topography

The bone contour normally conforms to the prominence of the roots, with intervening vertical depressions that taper toward the margin (Fig. 4.58). Alveolar bone anatomy varies among patients and has important clinical implications. The height and

Fig. 4.56 Interdental Septa. (A) Radiograph of the mandibular incisor area. Note the prominent lamina dura. (B) Interdental septa between the mandibular anterior teeth shown in A. There is a slight reduction in bone height with widening of the periodontal ligament in the coronal areas. The central cancellous portion is bordered by the dense bony cribriform plates of the socket, which form the lamina dura around the teeth in the radiograph. Attachments for the mentalis muscle are seen between the canine and lateral incisors. (From Glickman I, Smulow J: *Periodontal disease: clinical, radiographic, and histopathologic features,* Philadelphia, 1974, Saunders.)

Fig. 4.57 Boneless "Window" Between Adjoining Close Roots of Molars.

Fig. 4.58 Normal That the Bone Contour Conforms to the Prominence of the Roots.

thickness of the facial and lingual bony plates are affected by the alignment of the teeth, the angulation of the root to the bone, and occlusal forces.

On teeth in labial version, the margin of the labial bone is located farther apically than it is on teeth that are in proper alignment. The bone margin is thinned to a knife edge, and it presents an accentuated arc in the direction of the apex. On teeth in lingual version, the facial bony plate is thicker than normal. The margin is blunt, rounded, and horizontal rather than arcuate. The effect of the root-to-bone angulation on the height of alveolar bone is most noticeable on the palatal roots of the maxillary molars. The bone margin is located farther apically on the roots, and it forms relatively acute angles with the palatal bone.[119] The cervical portion of the alveolar plate is sometimes considerably thickened on the facial surface, apparently as reinforcement against occlusal forces (Fig. 4.59).

Fenestration and Dehiscence

Isolated areas in which the root is denuded of bone and the root surface is covered only by periosteum and overlying gingiva are termed *fenestrations.* In these areas, the marginal bone is intact. When the denuded areas extend through the marginal bone, the defect is called a *dehiscence* (Fig. 4.60).

Such defects occur on approximately 20% of the teeth; they occur more often on the facial bone than on the lingual bone, they are more common on anterior teeth than on posterior teeth, and they are frequently bilateral. Microscopic evidence of lacunar resorption may be present at the margins. The cause of these defects is not clear. Prominent root contours, malposition, and

Fig. 4.59 Variations in the Cervical Portion of the Buccal Alveolar Plate. (A) Shelflike conformation. (B) Comparatively thin buccal plate.

Fig. 4.60 Dehiscence on the Canine and Fenestration of the First Premolar.

labial protrusion of the root in combination with a thin bony plate are predisposing factors.[78] Fenestration and dehiscence are important because they may complicate the outcome of periodontal surgery.

Remodeling of Alveolar Bone

In contrast with its apparent rigidity, alveolar bone is the least stable of the periodontal tissues, because its structure is in a constant state of flux. A considerable amount of internal remodeling takes place by means of resorption and formation, and this is regulated by local and systemic influences. Local influences include functional requirements on the tooth and age-related changes in bone cells. Systemic influences are probably hormonal (e.g., parathyroid hormone, calcitonin, vitamin D_3).

The remodeling of the alveolar bone affects its height, contour, and density and is manifested in the following three areas: adjacent to the periodontal ligament, in relation to the periosteum of the facial and lingual plates, and along the endosteal surface of the marrow spaces.

DEVELOPMENT OF THE ATTACHMENT APPARATUS

After the crown has formed, the stratum intermedium and the stellate reticulum of the enamel organ disappear. The outer and inner epithelia of the enamel organ remain and form REE. The apical portion of this constitutes the Hertwig epithelial root sheath, which will continue to grow apically and which determines the shape of the root. Before the beginning of root formation, the root sheath bends horizontally at the future cementoenamel junction, thereby narrowing the cervical opening and forming the epithelial diaphragm. The epithelial diaphragm separates the dental follicle from the dental papilla.

After root dentin formation begins, the Hertwig root sheath breaks up and partially disappears; the remaining cells form the epithelial clusters or strands known as the *epithelial rests of Malassez* (see Fig. 4.37A). In multirooted teeth, the epithelial diaphragm grows in such a way that tonguelike extensions develop horizontally, thereby leaving spaces for each of the future roots to form.

The role of the Hertwig epithelial root sheath in root development, especially as it relates to the initiation of cementogenesis, has become a focus of research.[270] On the basis of various studies, it is now generally accepted that there is a transient period of the secretion of proteins (e.g., bone sialoprotein, osteopontin, and amelin) by the cells of the Hertwig epithelial root sheath.[38,84] In addition, research shows that growth and differentiation factors may play roles in the development of the attachment apparatus of periodontal tissues. Pluripotent dental follicle cells have been shown to differentiate into osteoblasts, cementoblasts, and periodontal fibroblasts.[240]

Cementum

The rupture of the Hertwig root sheath allows the mesenchymal cells of the dental follicle to contact the dentin, where they start forming a continuous layer of cementoblasts. On the basis of immunochemical and ultrastructural studies, Thomas[269] and others[35,164] have speculated that cementoblasts can be of epithelial origin (i.e., the Hertwig root sheath), having undergone an epithelial mesenchymal transformation.

Cementum formation begins with the deposition of a meshwork of irregularly arranged collagen fibrils sparsely distributed in a ground substance or matrix called *precementum* or *cementoid.* This is followed by a phase of matrix maturation, which subsequently mineralizes to form cementum. Cementoblasts, which are initially separated from the cementum by uncalcified cementoid, sometimes become enclosed within the matrix and are trapped. After they are enclosed, they are referred to as *cementocytes,* and they will remain viable in a manner similar to that of osteocytes.

A layer of connective tissue known as the *dental sac* surrounds the enamel organ and includes the epithelial root sheath as it develops. The zone that is immediately in contact with the dental organ and continuous with the ectomesenchyme of the dental papilla is called the *dental follicle,*[261,262,265] and it consists of undifferentiated fibroblasts.

Periodontal Ligament

As the crown approaches the oral mucosa during tooth eruption, these fibroblasts become active and start producing collagen fibrils. They initially lack orientation, but they soon acquire an orientation that is oblique to the tooth. The first collagen bundles then appear in the region immediately apical to the cementoenamel junction and give rise to the gingivodental fiber groups. As tooth eruption progresses, additional oblique fibers appear and become attached to the newly formed cementum and bone. The transseptal and alveolar crest fibers develop when the tooth merges into the oral cavity. Alveolar bone deposition occurs simultaneously with periodontal ligament organization.[249]

The developing periodontal ligament and the mature periodontal ligament contain undifferentiated stem cells that retain the potential to differentiate into osteoblasts, cementoblasts, and fibroblasts.[171]

Alveolar Bone

Just before mineralization, osteoblasts start producing matrix vesicles. These vesicles contain enzymes (e.g., alkaline phosphatase) that help to jump-start the nucleation of hydroxyapatite crystals. As these crystals grow and develop, they form coalescing bone nodules, which, with fast-growing nonoriented collagen fibers, are the substructure of woven bone and the first bone formed in the alveolus. Later, through bone deposition, remodeling, and the secretion of oriented collagen fibers in sheets, mature lamellar bone is formed.[28,29]

The hydroxyapatite crystals are generally aligned with their long axes parallel to the collagen fibers, and they appear to be deposited on and within the collagen fibers in mature lamellar bone. In this way, bone matrix is able to withstand the heavy mechanical stresses applied to it during function.

The alveolar bone develops around each tooth follicle during odontogenesis. When a deciduous tooth is shed, its alveolar bone is resorbed. The succedaneous permanent tooth moves into place and develops its own alveolar bone from its own dental follicle. As the tooth root forms and the surrounding tissues develop and mature, alveolar bone merges with the separately developing basal bone, and the two become one continuous structure. Although alveolar bone and basal bone have different intermediate origins, both are ultimately derived from neural crest ectomesenchyme.

Mandibular basal bone begins mineralization at the exit of the mental nerve from the mental foramen, whereas the maxillary basal bone begins at the exit of the infraorbital nerve from the infraorbital foramen.

Physiologic Migration of the Teeth

Tooth movement does not end when active eruption is completed and the tooth is in functional occlusion. With time and wear, the proximal contact areas of the teeth are flattened, and the teeth tend to move mesially. This is referred to as *physiologic mesial migration.* By the age of 40 years, this process results in a reduction of approximately 0.5 cm in the length of the dental arch from the midline to the third molars. Alveolar bone is reconstructed in compliance with the physiologic mesial migration of the teeth. Bone resorption is increased in areas of pressure along the mesial surfaces of the teeth, and new layers of bundle bone are formed in areas of tension on the distal surfaces (see Fig. 4.55).

EXTERNAL FORCES AND THE PERIODONTIUM

The periodontium exists for the purpose of supporting teeth during function, and it depends on the stimulation that it receives from function for the preservation of its structure. Therefore a constant and sensitive balance is present between external forces and the periodontal structures.

Alveolar bone undergoes constant physiologic remodeling in response to external forces, particularly occlusal forces. Bone is removed from areas where it is no longer needed and added to areas where it is presently needed.

The socket wall reflects the responsiveness of alveolar bone to external forces. Osteoblasts and newly formed osteoid line the socket in areas of tension; osteoclasts and bone resorption occur in areas of pressure. Forces exerted on the tooth also influence the number, density, and alignment of cancellous trabeculae. The bony trabeculae are aligned in the path of the tensile and compressive stresses to provide maximal resistance to the occlusal force with a minimum of bone substance (Fig. 4.61).[99,246] When forces are increased, the cancellous bony trabeculae increase in number and thickness, and bone may be added to the external surface of the labial and lingual plates.

A study has shown that the presence of antagonists of occlusal force and the severity of periodontal disease increase the extension of periodontal tissue resorption.[66]

The periodontal ligament also depends on the stimulation provided by function to preserve its structure. Within physiologic limits, the periodontal ligament can accommodate increased function with an increase in width (Table 4.2), a thickening of its fiber bundles, and an increase in the diameter and number of Sharpey fibers. Forces that exceed the adaptive capacity of the periodontium produce injury called *trauma from occlusion.* Because trauma from occlusion can only be confirmed histologically, the clinician is challenged to use clinical and radiographic surrogate indicators in an attempt to facilitate and assist with its diagnosis[110] (see Chapter 24).

Fig. 4.61 Bony Trabeculae Realigned Perpendicular to the Mesial Root of a Tilted Molar.

TABLE 4.2 Comparison of Periodontal Width of Functioning and Functionless Teeth in a 38-Year-Old Man			
	AVERAGE WIDTH OF PERIODONTAL SPACE		
	Entrance of Alveolus (mm)	**Middle of Alveolus (mm)**	**Fundus of Alveolus (mm)**
Heavy Function	0.35	0.28	0.30
Left upper second bicuspid			
Light function	0.14	0.10	0.12
Left lower first bicuspid			
Functionless	0.10	0.06	0.06
Left upper third molar			

Modified from Kronfeld R: Histologic study of the influence of function on the human periodontal membrane. *J Am Dent Assoc* 18:1242, 1931.

When occlusal forces are reduced, the number and thickness of the trabeculae are reduced.[64] The periodontal ligament also atrophies and appears thinned; the fibers are reduced in number and density, disoriented,[11,207] and ultimately arranged parallel to the root surface (Fig. 4.62). This phenomenon is termed *disuse atrophy* or *afunctional atrophy*. With this condition, the cementum is either unaffected[64] or thickened, and the distance from the cementoenamel junction to the alveolar crest is increased.[203]

Decreased occlusal function causes changes in the periodontal microvasculature, such as the occlusion of blood vessels and a decrease in the number of blood vessels.[120] For example, Murrell and colleagues[186] reported that the application and removal of orthodontic force produced significant changes in blood vessel number and density; however, no evidence-based explanation exists for why the force stimulated such changes in the number of blood vessels.

Fig. 4.62 Atrophic periodontal ligament *(P)* of a tooth devoid of function. Note the scalloped edge of the alveolar bone *(B)*, which indicates that resorption has occurred. *C,* Cementum.

Orthodontic tooth movement is thought to result from site-specific bone remodeling in the absence of inflammation. It is well recognized that tensional forces will stimulate the formation and activity of osteoblastic cells, whereas compressive forces promote osteoclastic activity.[250]

VASCULARIZATION OF THE SUPPORTING STRUCTURES

The blood supply to the supporting structures of the tooth is derived from the inferior and superior alveolar arteries to the mandible and maxilla, and it reaches the periodontal ligament from three sources: apical vessels, penetrating vessels from the alveolar bone, and anastomosing vessels from the gingiva.[63]

The branches of the apical vessels supply the apical region of the periodontal ligament before the vessels enter the dental pulp. The transalveolar vessels are branches of the intraseptal vessels that perforate the lamina dura and enter the ligament. The intraseptal vessels continue to vascularize the gingiva; these gingival vessels in turn anastomose with the periodontal ligament vessels of the cervical region.[83]

The vessels within the periodontal ligament are contained in the interstitial spaces of loose connective tissue between the principal fibers, and they are connected in a netlike plexus that runs longitudinally and closer to the bone than the cementum (Figs. 4.63 and 4.64).[54] The blood supply increases from the incisors to the molars; it is greatest in the gingival third of single-rooted teeth, less in the apical third, and least in the middle; it is equal in the apical and middle thirds of multirooted teeth; it is slightly greater on the mesial and distal surfaces than on the facial and lingual surfaces; and it is greater on the mesial surfaces of the mandibular molars than on the distal surfaces.[33]

The vascular supply to the bone enters the interdental septa through nutrient canals together with veins, nerves, and

Fig. 4.64 Vascular Supply to the Periodontal Ligament in a Rat Molar as Viewed by Scanning Electron Microscopy After Perfusion With Plastic and Tissue Corrosion. Middle and apical areas of the periodontal ligament are shown with longitudinal blood vessels from the apex *(below)* to the gingiva *(above)*, perforating vessels entering the bone *(b)*, and many transverse connections *(arrowheads)*. Apical vessels *(a)* form a cap that connects with the pulpal vessels. (Courtesy NJ Selliseth and K Selvig, University of Bergen, Norway.)

Fig. 4.63 Vascular Supply of a Monkey Periodontium Perfused With India Ink. Note the longitudinal vessels in the periodontal ligament and the alveolar arteries passing through channels between the bone marrow *(M)* and the periodontal ligament. *D,* Dentin. (Courtesy Dr. Sol Bernick, Los Angeles, California.)

lymphatics. Dental arterioles, which also branch off the alveolar arteries, send tributaries through the periodontal ligament, and some small branches enter the marrow spaces of the bone through the perforations in the cribriform plate. Small vessels that emanate from the facial and lingual compact bone also enter the marrow and spongy bone.

The *venous drainage* of the periodontal ligament accompanies the arterial supply. Venules receive the blood through the abundant capillary network. In addition, arteriovenous anastomoses bypass the capillaries and are seen more frequently in apical and interradicular regions; their significance is unknown.

Lymphatics supplement the venous drainage system. Lymphatic channels that drain the region just beneath the junctional epithelium pass into the periodontal ligament and accompany the blood vessels into the periapical region.[42] From there, they pass through the alveolar bone to the inferior dental canal in the mandible or the infraorbital canal in the maxilla and then go on to the submaxillary lymph nodes.

REFERENCES

 References for this chapter are found on the companion website.

Aging and the Periodontium[a]

Increased health awareness and improvements in preventive dentistry have led to decreasing tooth loss for all age groups. The effects of this shift in tooth retention need to be considered carefully. In particular, increased life expectancy and greater health expectations may lead to changes in demand from older individuals for periodontal treatment and potentially a substantial increase in supportive periodontal therapy. Therefore an understanding of the impact of aging on the periodontium is critical. This chapter first reviews the literature concerning the fundamental aspects of aging on the periodontal tissues; broader aspects of aging are then examined and their possible effects on treatment outcomes discussed. The chapter has been updated following a detailed search of new research published since 2012.

The evidence base is not without problems, many of which make it difficult to draw conclusions about the effects of aging. Some of these problems include inconsistency with regard to the definition of a true "older" group, the inadequate exclusion of adults with systemic diseases that can modify study findings, and attempts to extrapolate results from animal research. For the purposes of this chapter, the effects of aging are limited to a narrow review of possible biologic and microbiologic changes. (For further information on the effects of aging on the dental and periodontal patient, the reader should consult Holm-Pedersen et al.[23]) The reader should be fully aware that this narrower scope excludes many important age-associated phenomena, including reductions in an individual's cognitive or motor function skills, which may have a direct impact on periodontal management. These issues are discussed more fully in Chapter 38. Several studies have reported associations between periodontitis and cognitive impairment and aging,[16,51] although whether these findings reflect causation or simply association remains unclear. These links are difficult to entangle because *"chronic inflammation is a prominent feature of aging and of age-related diseases."*[48]

> ### CLINICAL CORRELATION
>
> For a full understanding of aging and managing periodontal health, in addition to this chapter on biology, readers should understand aging more broadly, including, for instance, cognitive and motor function effects that could affect oral hygiene.

Since first writing this chapter in 1999, the volume of new research into aging and the periodontium has not increased substantially. Highly sensitive molecular and genomic techniques have been employed in related laboratory research, and these are starting to provide insight into age-associated effects. These approaches will likely prove fruitful in the future. Despite the limited data directly related to the periodontium, much effort and many resources have been used to research questions at least partially related to this topic. These include the effect of periodontal infection on general health and the impact of osteoporosis on periodontal status.

EFFECTS OF AGING ON THE PERIODONTIUM

Gingival Epithelium

Thinning and decreased keratinization of the gingival epithelium have been reported with age.[52] The significance of these findings could mean an increase in epithelial permeability to bacterial antigens, a decreased resistance to functional trauma, or both. If so, such changes may influence long-term periodontal outcomes. However, other studies have found no age-related differences in the gingival epithelium of humans or dogs.[8,25] Other reported changes with aging include the flattening of rete pegs and altered cell density. Conflicting data regarding the surgical regeneration times for gingival epithelium have been ascribed to problems with research methodology.[57]

The effect of aging on the location of the junctional epithelium has been the subject of much speculation. Some reports show migration of the junctional epithelium from its position in healthy individuals (i.e., on the enamel) to a more apical position on the root surface, with accompanying gingival recession.[8] However,

[a]Adapted from the following chapter of Newman and Carranza's Clinical Periodontology, 13th edition: Chapter 4: Aging and the Periodontium, by Ian Needleman.

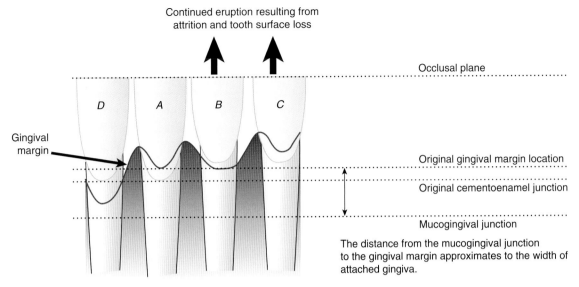

Continued eruption resulting from attrition and tooth surface loss

Occlusal plane

Gingival margin

Original gingival margin location

Original cementoenamel junction

Mucogingival junction

The distance from the mucogingival junction to the gingival margin approximates to the width of attached gingiva.

Fig. 5.1 Diagram Showing the Relationship of the Gingival Margin With the Crown and Root Surface. (A) Normal relationship with the gingival margin 1 to 2 mm above the cementoenamel junction. (B) Wear of the incisal edge and continued tooth eruption. The gingival margin remains in the same position as shown in A. Therefore the root surface is exposed, and clinical recession is evident. The width of the attached gingiva has not changed. (C) Wear of the incisal edge and continued tooth eruption. The gingival margin has moved with the tooth; therefore the entire dentogingival complex has moved coronally, with a resulting increase in the width of the attached gingiva. (D) No wear of incisal edge is evident. The gingiva has moved apically, and clinical recession is evident. The width of attached gingiva is reduced.

in other animal studies, no apical migration has been noted.[27] With continuing gingival recession, the width of the attached gingiva would be expected to decrease with age, but the opposite appears to be true.[2,3] Alternatively, the migration of the junctional epithelium to the root surface could be caused by the tooth erupting through the gingiva in an attempt to maintain occlusal contact with its opposing tooth (i.e., passive eruption) as a result of tooth surface loss from attrition (Fig. 5.1). The consensus is that gingival recession is not an inevitable physiologic process of aging, but rather that it can be explained by the cumulative effects of inflammation or trauma on the periodontium (Fig. 5.2)[6,8]; this is discussed in more detail later in this chapter. Changes in the apoptotic gene expression of gingival tissue with age have been reported in nonhuman primates.[19] This finding requires further research to understand its potential impact on gingival homeostasis and the pathogenesis of periodontal diseases.

> **KEY FACT**
>
> Gingival recession is not an inevitable consequence of aging but is the cumulative result of trauma or periodontitis.

Gingival Connective Tissue

Increasing age results in coarser and denser gingival connective tissues.[59] Qualitative and quantitative changes in collagen have been reported. These changes include an increased rate of conversion of soluble to insoluble collagen, increased mechanical

strength, and increased denaturing temperature. These results indicate increased collagen stabilization caused by changes in the macromolecular conformation.[49] Not surprisingly, an increased collagen content has been found in the gingivae of older animals, despite a lower rate of collagen synthesis decreasing with age.[8,57]

Periodontal Ligament

Changes in the periodontal ligament that have been reported with aging include decreased numbers of fibroblasts and a more irregular structure, thereby paralleling the changes seen in the gingival connective tissues.[8,49,57] Other findings include decreased organic matrix production, decreased epithelial cell rests, and increased amounts of elastic fiber.[57] Conflicting results have been reported for changes in the width of the periodontal ligament in human and animal models. Although true variation may exist, this finding probably reflects the functional status of the teeth in the studies: the width of the space will decrease if the tooth is unopposed (i.e., hypofunction) or increase with excessive occlusal loading.[57] Both scenarios can be anticipated as a result of tooth loss in this population. These effects may also explain the variability in studies that have reported qualitative changes within the periodontal ligament.

Recognition that the periodontal ligament has an important role in alveolar bone metabolism has led to an increased interest in investigating this role in relation to the maintenance of periodontal health and the pathogenesis of periodontitis. One approach to investigating this role is to examine mediators of bone homeostasis, such as receptor activator of nuclear factor-κB ligand (RANKL) and osteoprotegerin (OPG). RANKL is

Fig. 5.2 Three Scenarios Illustrating the Variation of the Position of the Gingival Margin With Age. (A) Overeruption with recession in an older individual (i.e., a 68-year-old woman) with generalized recession and a history of previously treated periodontitis. Note some overeruption of the lower anterior teeth and wear of teeth related to oral hygiene measures. (B) Radiographs of the patient shown in A. (C) Overeruption without recession in an older individual (i.e., a 72-year-old woman) with no periodontitis but marked lower incisor tooth wear and overeruption. Note how the gingival margin has migrated coronally with the erupting teeth. (D) Extensive recession in a younger individual (i.e., a 32-year-old man) with marked recession and no history of periodontitis. The recession has resulted from a combination of anatomically thin tissues and toothbrush-related trauma.

widely recognized for its role in activating osteoclasts, whereas OPG antagonizes RANKL binding, thereby helping to maintain balance. The interplay of cytokines—and, in particular, the interleukin family—has also been extensively researched in periodontal pathogenesis. Some of the interleukins are potent mediators of inflammation (e.g., IL-1), whereas others have been shown to down-regulate this process (e.g., IL-4, IL-10). Therefore evaluating the balance between these homeostatic processes would seem to be of great merit when assessing possible negative changes in the periodontium. Such a strategy appears to be predictive of hard tissue destruction among individuals with rheumatoid arthritis.[15] Findings comparing periodontal ligament cells in older individuals (i.e., >60 years old) with those of younger individuals (i.e., 15 to 20 years old) have suggested greater gene expression for proinflammatory cytokines.[7] This finding has been reported more widely as an age-associated change, although it is unclear whether it is a cause or an effect.[41] However, in addition to increased IL-1 and IL-6 expression, OPG was also increased, which suggests that increased OPG may be a homeostatic response to the up-regulation of inflammation.[7] If this homeostatic mechanism was effective, it may explain why an increase in inflammation did not result in greater tissue damage with age. Periodontal ligament cell proliferation was decreased with age, thereby suggesting an impairment of repair potential, although such an impact does not appear to be manifested clinically.[58] Further research investigating periodontal ligament cells from individuals

diagnosed with periodontitis will be important to understand the potentially important relationship between aging and periodontal ligament cells.

Cementum

Some consensus regarding the effect of aging on cementum exists. An increase in cemental width is a common finding; this increase may be 5 to 10 times wider than in those of younger age.[8] This finding is not surprising because deposition continues after tooth eruption. The increase in width is greater apically and lingually.[57] Although cementum has limited capacity for remodeling, an accumulation of resorption bays explains the finding of increasing surface irregularity.[20]

Alveolar Bone

Reports of morphologic changes in alveolar bone mirror age-related changes in other bony sites. Specific to the periodontium are findings of a more irregular periodontal surface of bone and the less-regular insertion of collagen fibers.[57] Although age is a risk factor for the bone mass reductions in individuals with osteoporosis, it is not causative and, therefore, should be distinguished from physiologic aging processes.[24] Overriding the diverse observations of bony changes with age is the important finding that the healing rate of bone in extraction sockets appears to be unaffected by increasing age.[4] Indeed, the success of osseointegrated dental implants, which relies on intact bone healing responses, does not appear to be age related.[9] However, balancing this view is the observation that bone graft preparations (i.e., decalcified freeze-dried bone) from donors who were more than 50 years old possessed significantly less osteogenic potential than graft material from younger donors.[50] The possible significance of this phenomenon for normal healing responses needs to be investigated.

Bacterial Plaque

Dental plaque biofilm accumulation has been suggested to increase with age.[22] This may be explained by the increase in hard tissue surface area as a result of gingival recession and the surface characteristics of the exposed root surface as a substrate for plaque formation as compared with enamel. Other studies have shown no difference in plaque quantity with age. This contradiction may reflect the different age ranges of experimental groups as variable degrees of gingival recession and root surface exposure. For supragingival plaque, no real qualitative differences have been shown for plaque composition.[22] With regard to subgingival plaque, one study showed subgingival flora to be similar to normal flora, whereas another study reported increased numbers of enteric rods and pseudomonads in older adults.[37,55] Mombelli[35] suggested caution when interpreting this finding because of the increased oral carriage of these species among older adults. It has been speculated that a shift occurs in the importance of certain periodontal pathogens with age, specifically including an increased role for *Porphyromonas gingivalis* and a decreased role for *Aggregatibacter actinomycetemcomitans*. However, differentiating true age-related effects from the changes in ecologic determinants for periodontal bacteria will be difficult.

Another approach to investigating microbiology consists of conducting intervention studies and examining the impact on the microflora. Among individuals who were 60 to 75 years old, the prevalence of *P. gingivalis*, *Treponema forsythia*, *Treponema denticola*, *A. actinomycetemcomitans*, and *Prevotella intermedia* was high and was not clearly related to probing depth.[45] The finding of high levels of the organisms could have been related to the sample of individuals: the participants were mostly those with low incomes and with no recent dental care. Long-term use (i.e., 5 years) of a 0.12% chlorhexidine mouthrinse did not promote reductions in the proportions of the organisms in individuals experiencing alveolar bone loss as compared with the placebo mouthrinse, possibly because the mouthrinse routine may have been less frequent than daily.[45]

Immune and Inflammatory Responses

Advances in the study of the effects of aging on the immune response (i.e., immunosenescence) have altered the understanding of this phenomenon. In particular, more recent studies have set tighter controls on excluding individuals with systemic conditions known to affect the immune response. As a result, age has been recognized as having much less effect on the alteration of the host response than previously thought.[31] Differences between younger and older individuals can be demonstrated for T and B cells, cytokines, and natural killer cells, with increased inflammatory-type (M1) macrophage subset gene expression (in a nonhuman primate model),[18] but not for polymorphonuclear

cells. McArthur[31] concluded the following: "Measurement of indicators of immune and inflammatory competency suggested that, within the parameters tested, there was no evidence for age-related changes in host defenses correlating with periodontitis in an elderly (65 to 75 years) group of individuals, with and without disease." Laboratory studies have shown age-related changes in the expression of proinflammatory mediators,[11] innate immunity,[21] and major histocompatibility complex II (MHC II) pathway gene expression,[17] with the potential to alter the pathology of periodontal diseases or antimicrobial function. However, the relevance of these findings to the clinical situation has not been demonstrated. Age-related differences in the inflammatory response among individuals with gingivitis have been clearly demonstrated and are discussed later in this textbook.

In relation to systematic inflammatory responses, C-reactive protein (CRP) is an acute phase protein that is widely regarded as a marker of inflammatory burden and response to bacterial infection.[53] In an investigation of serum CRP levels among individuals who were 60 to 75 years old and comparing individuals with progressive periodontitis with those with stable disease, CRP levels were increased in people with progressive periodontitis and no other systemic conditions.[56] This finding may indicate that inflammatory burden can be investigated with the use of CRP, although growing evidence indicates that CRP alone may not be as reliable a marker in older people.[46]

A further modulator of the immune and inflammatory responses is nutrition. Interest in this field is increasing rapidly as part of both medicine and periodontology.[10] Nutrition has been studied extensively in geriatric medicine due to the nutritional intake changes that occur with age. The impact of nutrition as a potential risk factor for periodontal diseases and their progression is, therefore, of interest. Emerging data suggest a negative association of serum folate with periodontitis. After controlling for major known confounders, lower serum folate levels in dentate adults who are more than 60 years old are associated with greater levels of periodontitis.[61] These cross-sectional data cannot demonstrate causality alone, but the recognized relationship between folate protection and chronic inflammatory diseases (e.g., cardiovascular disease[33]) offers biologic plausibility to a potential relationship that merits further investigation with prospective studies.

Although many contradictions exist, a survey of the literature demonstrates that some age-related changes are evident in the periodontium and the host response. Whether these changes are significant in the alteration of the progression of periodontal diseases or the response of an older adult to periodontal treatment is examined next.

EFFECTS OF AGING ON THE PROGRESSION OF PERIODONTAL DISEASES

In a classic experimental gingivitis study, subjects were rendered free of plaque and inflammation through frequent professional cleaning. After this was achieved, the subjects abstained from oral hygiene measures for periods of 3 weeks to allow gingivitis to develop.[30] In this experimental model, a comparison of developing gingivitis between younger and older individuals demonstrated a greater inflammatory response in older subjects, both in humans and in dogs.[8,12,13,22] In the older age group (i.e., 65 to 80 years), the findings included a greater amount of infiltrated connective tissue, increased gingival crevicular fluid flow, and an increased gingival index.[12,13] Other studies have not demonstrated differences between subjects; this finding may be related to smaller differences between the ages of the younger and older experimental groups.[60] Intriguingly, even at the baseline level of excellent gingival health before the commencement of plaque accumulation, differences may exist between groups, with older individuals demonstrating more inflammation.[12,13]

The phrase "getting long in the tooth" expresses a widespread belief that age is inevitably associated with an increased loss of connective tissue attachment. However, this observation may equally reflect cumulative exposure to a number of potentially destructive processes. These exposures may include plaque-associated periodontitis, long-term mechanical trauma from toothbrushing, and iatrogenic damage from unfavorable restorative dentistry or repeated scaling and root planing. The effects of these exposures act in one direction only (i.e., an increased loss of attachment).

In an attempt to differentiate the effects of age from these other processes, several studies have been designed to eliminate confounding issues and to address more clearly the question of age as a risk factor for periodontitis. A *risk factor* is defined as "any characteristic, behavior, or exposure with an association to a particular disease. The relationship is not necessarily causal in nature. … Some risk factors, if causal, can be modified to reduce one's risk of initiation or progression of disease, such as smoking or improved oral hygiene … while other factors cannot be modified, such as genetic factors."[14] The conclusions from these studies are strikingly consistent and show that the effect of age is either nonexistent or provides a small and clinically insignificant increased risk of loss of periodontal support.[29,34,38,42,43] Indeed, in comparison with the odds ratio of 20.52 for poor oral hygiene status and periodontitis, the odds ratio for age was only 1.24,[1] and smoking was much more influential than age.[38] Therefore age has been suggested to be not a true risk factor but rather a background or associated factor for periodontitis.[42] In addition, the clarification of a genetic basis for susceptibility to severe forms of periodontitis underlines the overriding importance of plaque, smoking, and susceptibility in explaining most of the variations in periodontal disease severity among individuals.[26] Nevertheless, a longitudinal study of essentially untreated periodontitis in an older adult (≥70 years old) Japanese population indicated that 296 of 394 individuals (75%) had a least one site with 3 mm or more loss of attachment over a 2-year period.[39] Smoking and a baseline attachment level of 6 mm or more were significantly associated with disease progression. A more recent study modeling the transition of periodontal health states over a 2-year period estimated that the risk of transitioning from health to gingivitis was overall reduced by 3% with age.[32] Each year of age increase was associated with a 2% decreased risk of such a transition. Furthermore, increased age was not statistically associated with an increased risk of transitioning from health or gingivitis to periodontitis.

AGING AND THE RESPONSE TO TREATMENT OF THE PERIODONTIUM

The successful treatment of periodontitis requires both meticulous home plaque control by the patient and meticulous supragingival and subgingival debridement by the therapist.[36] Unfortunately, only a few studies have directly compared such an approach among patients of different age groups. The few studies that have done so clearly demonstrate that, despite the histologic changes in the periodontium with aging, no differences in response to nonsurgical or surgical treatment have been shown for periodontitis.[5,28,58] However, if plaque control is not ideal, the continued loss of attachment is inevitable. Furthermore, without effective periodontal therapy, the progression of disease may be faster with increasing age.[44] Attempts to increase plaque control by chemical means have also been reported.[54]

A purely biologic or physiologic review indicates that aging has some impact on the structure and function of the periodontium, as well as on the immune response and the nature of either supragingival or subgingival plaque. However, these changes have a negligible impact on an individual's responsiveness to treatment. Aging may affect other aspects of the management of periodontal health (e.g., the risk of root caries[47]; see Chapter 38), and the resulting difficulties should not be underestimated. One study identified greater compliance with supportive maintenance among older individuals as compared with younger patients.[40]

> ### KEY FACT
>
> The biologic effects of aging have either no impact or a minimal impact on an individual's response to periodontal treatment. However, other factors may have a profound impact, including cognitive and motor skills as well as medical history.

A Case Scenario is found on the companion website www.expert consult.com.

REFERENCES

 References for this chapter are found on the companion website.

6

Classification of Diseases and Conditions Affecting the Periodontium[a]

CHAPTER OUTLINE

Our understanding of the causes and pathogenesis of oral diseases and conditions changes continually with increased scientific knowledge. In light of this fact, a classification can be most consistently defined by the differences in the clinical manifestations of diseases and conditions: they are clinically consistent and require little (if any) clarification by laboratory testing. Since the 1999 World Workshop in Periodontics, classification of periodontal diseases is based on their extent (generalized versus localized), severity (slight, moderate, or severe), rate of progression (aggressive versus chronic), and localization (i.e., contained within the gingiva, as in gingivitis, or further involving periodontal bone loss, as in periodontitis). The existing definitions encompass the best available way to universally define a spectrum of diseases affecting the periodontal tissues and to guide therapeutic approaches. Nonetheless, the disease state is dynamic, and the appropriate diagnosis for an individual can change over time. For instance, a patient diagnosed with existing periodontitis who undergoes successful periodontal therapy may be classified as having a healthy but reduced periodontium (with slight, moderate, or severe attachment loss) at the reevaluation. Subsequently, if the same individual presents with gingival inflammation without signs of further attachment loss at a future appointment, the appropriate diagnosis would be "gingivitis on a reduced periodontium." Depending on their future compliance with home care and maintenance visits, patients may progress to periodontitis or maintain a healthy but reduced periodontium. The case example highlights the importance of conceptualizing the dynamic nature of inflammatory diseases that affect the periodontium while appreciating the importance of commonly accepted definitions for periodontal diseases. If a case of gingivitis on a reduced periodontium relapses into

periodontitis, the prognosis of the affected teeth will depend on the preexisting attachment loss.

The classification presented in this chapter presents the overall classification system that was proposed at the 1999 International Workshop for a Classification of Periodontal Diseases and Conditions (Box 6.1) and details the changes that occurred in the more recent 2018 Classification of Periodontal Diseases and Conditions. Each disease or condition is explored where clarification is needed. In each case, the reader is referred to pertinent reviews on the subject and specific chapters within this book that discuss the topics in more detail.

2018 PERIODONTAL DISEASE CLASSIFICATION SYSTEM

Health care is constantly evolving. As new diagnostic strategies and therapeutic approaches are being developed, so do the options for characterizing and classifying diseases. In 1999, a classification system for diseases and conditions that affect the periodontium was introduced by the International Workshop for a Classification of Periodontal Diseases and Conditions, which has served our profession well for 19 years. Since then, periodontology has made major advances over the past two decades. Therefore in 2017 the American Academy of Periodontology and the European Federation of Periodontology convened 170 periodontal experts from around the world to develop updated definitions for periodontal health, gingival disease, periodontitis, periodontal manifestations of systemic diseases, and peri-implant diseases.[10]

These redefined classifications (especially for periodontitis), are intended to provide a more precise diagnosis characterized by a multidimensional staging and grading system while still being user-friendly to clinicians. In this new classification, staging will be predominately determined by the severity of the disease at time of presentation:

- Stages 1 through 4 will be assigned according to the degree of clinical attachment loss (CAL), amount of bone loss, probing depth, presence of infrabony bony defects, furcation

---

[a]Adapted from the following chapter of Newman and Carranza's Clinical Periodontology, 13th edition: Chapter 5: Classification of Diseases and Conditions Affecting the Periodontium by James E. Hinrichs and Georgios A. Kotsakis.

BOX 6.1 **1999 Classification of Periodontal Diseases and Conditions**

Gingival Diseases
    Plaque-induced gingival diseases[a]
    Non-plaque–induced gingival lesions
Chronic Periodontitis[b]
    Localized
    Generalized
Aggressive Periodontitis
    Localized
    Generalized
Periodontitis as a Manifestation of Systemic Diseases
Necrotizing Periodontal Diseases
    Necrotizing ulcerative gingivitis
    Necrotizing ulcerative periodontitis
Abscesses of the Periodontium
    Gingival abscess
    Periodontal abscess
    Pericoronal abscess
Periodontitis Associated With Endodontic Lesions
    Endodontic-periodontal lesion
    Periodontal-endodontic lesion
    Combined lesion
Developmental or Acquired Deformities and Conditions
    Localized tooth-related factors that predispose to plaque-induced gingival diseases or periodontitis
    Mucogingival deformities and conditions around teeth
    Mucogingival deformities and conditions on edentulous ridges
    Occlusal trauma

[a]These diseases may occur on a periodontium with no attachment loss or on a periodontium with attachment loss that is stable and not progressing.
[b]Chronic periodontitis can be further classified based on extent and severity. As a general guide, extent can be characterized as localized (<30% of teeth involved) or generalized (>30% of teeth involved). Severity can be characterized based on the amount of clinical attachment loss (CAL) as follows: *slight* = 1 or 2 mm CAL, *moderate* = 3 or 4 mm CAL, and *severe* ≥5 mm CAL.
Data from Armitage GC: Development of a classification system for periodontal diseases and conditions. *Ann Periodontol* 4:1, 1999.

involvement, tooth mobility, and existing tooth loss due to periodontitis.

- Grades A through C will be designated according to the risk of progressive periodontitis associated with systemic disease status, exposure to smoking, level of metabolic control of diabetes, historic rate of progression, and other individualized risk predictors.

One major addition to the periodontal classification system is the introduction of a new category for peri-implant conditions that are stratified as peri-implant health, peri-implant mucositis, or peri-implantitis (Fig. 6.1). Peri-implant health is clinically characterized by the absence of visual signs of inflammation and lack of bleeding on probing. In contrast, peri-implant mucositis exhibits visual signs of inflammation and/or bleeding on probing but without loss of supportive or marginal bone. Peri-implantitis is a pathologic condition with inflammation and/or bleeding on probing accompanied by progressive loss of supportive bone. Furthermore, based on ample evidence that hard- and soft-tissue ridge profiles are diminished following tooth loss, these peri-implant hard- and soft-tissue deficiencies are currently included in the classification under the broader category of Peri-implant Diseases and Conditions. The magnitude of such ridge deficiencies may be related to a history of severe periodontitis, traumatic extraction, root fractures, endodontic complications, pneumatization of the maxillary sinus, and others.

Periodontal Health, Gingival Diseases, and Conditions

The new periodontal classification establishes a definition for a widely accepted but not previously defined state—that of periodontal health. This is a major improvement from earlier classifications because it becomes emphatically evident that periodontal health is much more than the mere absence of disease, which is consistent with the World Health Organization's definition of health.[11] On a molecular level, periodontal health is consistent with well-regulated immune surveillance and maintenance of homeostasis. Clinically, periodontal health is

Fig. 6.1 Illustration of the Overall Similarities and Differences Between the 1999 and 2018 Disease Classifications. (Data from the American Academy of Periodontology and the European Federation of Periodontology.)

determined by the absence of signs of inflammation but also necessitates the absence of patient-perceived symptoms of disease. For instance, a periodontium with no evidence of attachment loss and negative bleeding on probing cannot be defined as healthy if the person in the dental chair complains of halitosis and papillary swelling. It cannot be overstated that as clinicians we best serve a person by treating him or her and not the findings of a metal probe.

The current definition of periodontal health further clarifies what was previously empirically referred to as a "reduced periodontium," (i.e., a periodontium with previous loss of structural alveolar support and clinical findings of attachment loss). Thus the definition of periodontal health is broadened to encompass health on an intact or reduced periodontium. In the former case, periodontal health is consistent with the absence of detectable attachment and/or bone loss and physiologic bone levels range from 1.0 to 3.0 mm apical to the cementoenamel junction (CEJ). In the latter case, periodontal health may be established as a result of therapy for periodontitis or as a result of surgical interventions to manage other conditions affecting the periodontium, such as crown lengthening procedures (Table 6.1). The aforementioned procedures will lead to attachment loss, but the probing depths will be within the normal range and therefore termed as reduced but healthy periodontium. If gingivitis occurs in a reduced periodontium, which is characterized by the return of bacterially induced inflammation with no evidence of progressive attachment loss, it is currently accepted that this puts the person at increased risk of recurrent periodontitis. Gingivitis is clinically diagnosed based on signs and symptoms such as bleeding while brushing, blood in saliva, gingival swelling, redness, tenderness, edema, and halitosis. This overarching theme of incorporating risk factors and their management in clinical practice towards a more "personalized dentistry" approach is being emphasized heavily in this new classification.

Periodontitis

The 1999 classification established four descriptors for periodontitis that have been widely accepted: *Extent*, *Severity*, *Rate of Progression*, and *Periodontitis*, (e.g., Generalized, Moderate, and Chronic Periodontitis). Extensive discussion of this classification scheme follows in this chapter. A fundamental change took place in the 2018 classification grouping the "chronic" and "aggressive," the two descriptors of rate of progression of periodontitis, under a single category of "periodontitis." Consequently, the remaining descriptors where "extent" and "severity." Although "extent" remained as a descriptor of periodontitis (generalized, localized, or molar-incisor pattern), the "severity of disease" was replaced by two new dimensions: staging and grading.

Staging and grading are not diagnoses. A diagnosis of periodontitis is determined first, with staging and grading providing supplemental information that helps to determine treatment complexity and prognosis. Staging describes the complexity of each case and incorporates the following elements[10]:
- Severity of the disease
- Tooth loss due to periodontitis
- Management complexity of the patient's periodontal condition
- Overall oral rehabilitation needs

Staging is based on a full-mouth diagnosis and is *not* subdivided into different severity levels for different parts of the mouth (Table 6.2). Staging is designed to give information about the whole mouth, relative to the severity and complexity of the patient's periodontal status. The stage will also inform the clinician of the initial difficulty and complexity of required treatment. Although staging is not equivalent to severity, based on the determinants of each periodontitis stage it is expected that the majority of cases of mild to moderate periodontitis will typically be either Stage I or Stage II, whereas severe periodontitis will typically be either Stage III or Stage IV. The staging system is designed to highlight the patient's most severe areas of destruction, and it considers the single interdental site with the maximum attachment loss as one of its determinants. Determining the tooth loss number should include those teeth planned for extraction due to periodontitis as part of active therapy.

Stage I periodontitis (mild disease)
- Probing depths ≤4 mm.
- Interdental CAL ≤1 to 2 mm.
- Horizontal bone loss.
- Will require nonsurgical treatment.

TABLE 6.1 Different Scenarios of Periodontal Health

Parameters	Intact Periodontium	Reduced Periodontium Nonperiodontitis Patient (Example: Tooth Brush Trauma Induced Generalized Gingival Recession)	Successfully Treated Stable Periodontitis Patient (e.g., Patient With a Past History of 4 Quadrants of Osseous Surgery)
Probing attachment loss	No	Yes	Yes
Probing pocket depths (assuming no pseudo pockets)	≤3 mm	≤3 mm	≤4 mm (no site greater than 4 mm with BOP)
Bleeding on probing (BOP) %	<10	<10	<10
Radiographic bone loss	No	Possible	Yes

Adapted from Chapple ILC, Mealey BL, Van Dyke TE, et al: Periodontal health and gingival diseases and conditions on an intact and a reduced periodontium: Consensus report of workgroup 1 of the 2017 World Workshop on the Classification of Periodontal and Peri-Implant Diseases and Conditions. *J Periodontol* 89(Suppl 1):S74–S84, 2018, with permission.

TABLE 6.2 Key Periodontitis Staging Elements

Periodontitis		Stage I	Stage II	Stage III	Stage IV
Severity	Clinical Attachment Loss	1–2 mm	3–4 mm	≥5 mm	≥5 mm
	Radiographic Bone Loss	Coronal third of the root	Coronal third of the root	Middle or apical third of the root	Middle or apical third of the root
	Tooth loss due to periodontitis	No tooth loss		≤4 teeth	≥5 teeth
Complexity		• PD ≤4 mm • Mostly horizontal bone loss	• PD ≤5 mm • Mostly horizontal bone loss	In addition to Stage II: • PD ≥6 mm • Vertical bone loss ≥3 mm • Class II or III furcation involvement • Moderate ridge defects	In addition to Stage II: • Need for complex rehabilitation due to: masticatory dysfunction, tooth mobility, bite collapse, pathologic migration, <20 remaining teeth
Extent and Distribution		- Localized (<30% of the teeth involved) - Generalized (≥30% of the teeth involved) - Molar-incisor pattern			

Adapted from Tonetti MS, Greenwell H, Kornman KS: Staging and grading of periodontitis: Framework and proposal of a new classification and case definition. *J Periodontol* 89(Suppl 1):S159–S172, 2018, with permission.

• No posttreatment tooth loss expected.
• The patient has a good prognosis.
Stage II periodontitis (moderate disease)
• Probing depths ≤5 mm.
• Interdental CAL ≤3 to 4 mm.
• Horizontal bone loss.
• Will require nonsurgical *and* may be surgical treatment.
• No posttreatment tooth loss is expected.
• The patient has a good prognosis.
Stage III periodontitis (severe disease)
• Probing depths ≥6 mm.
• Interdental CAL ≥5 mm.
• May have vertical bone loss and/or furcation involvement of Class II or III.
• Will require initial nonsurgical treatment followed most probably by surgical treatments.
• Potential for tooth loss from 0 to 4 teeth.
• Complexity of implant and/or restorative treatment is increased and may require multispecialty treatment.
• The patient has a fair prognosis.
Stage IV periodontitis (very severe disease)
• Probing depths ≥6 mm.
• Interdental CAL ≥5 mm.
• May have vertical bone loss and/or furcation involvement of Class II or III.
• Less than 20 teeth may be present.
• Potential for tooth loss of five or more teeth.
• Patients will require initial nonsurgical treatment followed by advanced surgical treatment and/or regenerative therapy, including augmentation treatment to facilitate implant therapy.
• Very complex implant and/or restorative treatment may be needed usually requiring multispecialty treatment.
• The patient has a questionable prognosis going into maintenance.

Grading

Grading provides the likelihood of posttreatment disease progression, and it can change along the way because it depends on the state of the patient at the time of examination. In essence, grading is this dimension of the new classification that enables clinicians to incorporate individual characteristics into the diagnosis and related treatment plans. These include history-based and/or anticipated rate of periodontitis progression, presence and control of risk factors, and general health modifiers (Table 6.3).

The designations of grading are[10]:
• **A**, slow or no progression.
• **B**, moderate progression.
• **C**, rapid progression.

Incorporating grading in clinical practice will likely require some modifications as compared with the previously established 1999 classification scheme. For example, the rate of radiographic bone loss/CAL can be directly assessed via longitudinal radiographic evaluation or review of clinical measurements from successive examinations. This is indeed the "gold standard" approach for grading periodontitis but not always feasible due to that lack of documentation or multiple providers. As a result, the 2018 classification recommends that the percentage of bone loss as per the individual's age group is considered. For example, when reclassifying a case of Generalized Severe Chronic Periodontitis (Fig. 6.2A and B) staging becomes a more straightforward task, because it is dependent upon current clinically presentation, which is a cross-sectional observation. In other words, staging of periodontitis determines the case's current complexity that is related to its initial management, whereas grading is used to incorporate a temporal characterization of the disease progress in order to assess risk.

In the case presented in Fig. 6.2, staging could be classified as Stage III based on the interdental CAL exceeding 5 mm at the deepest site, the extent of bone loss, and the loss of fewer

TABLE 6.3	**Key Periodontitis Grading Elements**				
	Progression		**Grade A:** **Slow Rate**	**Grade B:** **Moderate Rate**	**Grade C:** **Rapid Rate**
Primary criteria (direct evidence should be used when available)	Direct evidence of progression	Radiographic bone loss or CAL	No loss over 5 years	<2 mm over 5 years	≥2 mm over 5 years
	Indirect evidence of progression	% bone loss/age	<0.25	0.25–1	>1
		Case phenotype	Heavy biofilms with low levels of destructions	Destruction commensurate with biofilm deposits	Destruction inconsistent with biofilm deposits; clinical patterns suggestive of periods of rapid progression and/or early onset
Grade modifiers	Risk factors	Smoking	Nonsmoker	<10 cigarettes/day	≥10 cigarettes/day
		Diabetes	Nondiabetic	Diabetic with HbA$_{1c}$ <7%	Diabetic with HbA$_{1c}$ ≥7%

CAL, Clinical attachment loss.
Adapted from Tonetti MS, Greenwell H, Kornman KS: Staging and grading of periodontitis: framework and proposal of a new classification and case definition. *J Periodontol* 89(Suppl 1):S159–S172, 2018, with permission.

Tooth Number	2			3			4			5			6		
(B) CAL	6	4	5	5	3	3	3	2	3	3	3	3	5	5	3
CEJ-GM	0	0	0	0	1	0	0	0	0	0	1	0	0	1	0
PD & BOP	6	4	5	5	2	3	3	2	3	3	2	3	5	4	3
(L) PD & BOP	7	8	6	5	3	7	5	6	6	4	5	3	4	3	3
CEJ-GM	0	0	0	0	0	0	0	0	0	0	0	0	0	0	0
CAL	7	8	6	5	3	7	5	6	6	4	5	3	4	3	3

Fig. 6.2 (A) Clinical case of generalized severe chronic periodontitis. The *green box* demarcates a region showing local factor (calculus) accumulation in the mandibular incisor area; (B) Radiographic images of the anterior sextants reveal moderate to severe horizontal bone loss consistent and a maximum interdental attachment loss exceeding 5 mm. Reclassification of this case requires consideration of the relative rate of disease progression in addition to clinical and radiographic measurements.

than four teeth. However, determining grading requires consideration of the rate of progression of disease as well as consideration of underlying risk factors. For educational purposes let us consider that the patient presented in Fig. 6.2 is self-referred and there is no access to previous examination or radiographic records. The person's age is 51 years, and the bone loss is approximately 30%. A simple calculation of percentage bone loss/age equals to 0.69, which puts the patient at grade B rate of progression. Of course, modifiable risk factors, such as smoking and glycemic control, have to be considered and could further modify the rate of progression, which highlights the need for careful medical history review and frequent updates.

Peri-Implant Diseases and Conditions

Peri-implant diseases and conditions is a newly established category in the Periodontal classification. This category was introduced in response to the overwhelming evidence that peri-implantitis is a prevalent entity worldwide. This first ever classification includes a breakdown of these diseases and conditions into four subcategories[6]:

- Peri-implant Health
- Peri-implant Mucositis
- Peri-implantitis
- Peri-implant Soft- and Hard-Tissue Deficiencies

Clinically, peri-implant health is characterized by an absence of visual signs of inflammation and bleeding on probing, and consistent with the periodontal health definition it can exist around implants that have experienced some loss of bone support. Admittedly, however, implants behave fundamentally different than teeth do due to their different surface properties and attachment apparatus. Once the implant surface (e.g., titanium, zirconium, or various alloys) is exposed to the oral environment, the maintenance of health becomes more challenging as compared with natural teeth. Another important distinction between teeth and implants is that in the latter case, establishing a range of probing depths compatible with peri-implant health is challenging. For instance, Fig. 6.3 illustrates how implant positioning is often dictated by local anatomic factors and existing conditions, such as ridge resorption and thus varies largely between implants and teeth, as well as among implants. Therefore relative change becomes the most accurate measure of pathologic changes. It cannot be emphasized enough that dentists who place implants need to consistently record peri-implant clinical measurements at the time of implant loading that will serve as baseline for monitoring future changes. When the peri-implant examination reveals changes in comparison to baseline, then the classification requires discriminating between peri-implant mucositis and peri-implantitis through a thorough peri-implant evaluation (Fig. 6.4).

The distinctive difference between a diagnosis of peri-implant mucositis and peri-implantitis is the presence of bone loss in peri-implantitis. Both diseases are associated with visual inflammatory changes in the peri-implant soft tissues combined with bleeding on probing and/or suppuration. Furthermore, increasing probing pocket depths as compared with measurements obtained at placement of the restoration are much more common in peri-implantitis rather than peri-implant mucositis. However, due to the changes in probe resistance during peri-implant inflammation, increasing probing depths may also be encountered in peri-implant mucositis. Progressive bone loss in relation to the radiographic bone level assessment at 1 year following the delivery of the definitive restoration is the diagnostic sign that bares most weight for diagnosing peri-implantitis. Importantly, in the absence of initial radiographs and probing depths, radiographic evidence of bone loss, (3 mm or greater) and/or probing depths (6 mm or greater) in conjunction with profuse bleeding represents peri-implantitis (Fig. 6.5).

Mucogingival Deformities and Conditions

A major change that occurred in the classification of mucogingival deformities and conditions is the incorporation of classification of Mucogingival Recessions by Cairo et al.[8] This classification that supersedes previous recession classification that were descriptive is an evidence-based approach for classifying recessions according to the predictability of recession coverage based on contemporary periodontal plastic surgery procedures. The cornerstone of this classification scheme is the assessment of the interedental tissues adjacent to the recession defects. Its

Fig. 6.3 Note the Discrepancy in the Position of the Implant Platform as Compared to the Cementoenamel Junction/Crown Margin of the Adjacent Teeth.

Peri-implant evaluation

Probing	**Radiograph**	**Visual inspection**
Presence of profuse (line or drop) bleeding and/or suppuration on probing and an increase in probing depths compare to baseline.	Presence of bone loss beyond crestal bone level changes resulting from the intial remodeling.	Visual inspection demonstrating the presence of peri-implant signs of inflammation: red as opposed to pink, swollen tissues as opposed to no swelling, soft as opposed to firm tissue consistency

Fig. 6.4 Key Components of Peri-Implant Evaluation.

validity and reliability have been clinically tested and support its use. The classification of recession defects according to Cairo et al. encompasses three recession types:

Recession Type 1 (RT1):

- Gingival recession with no loss of interproximal attachment. Interproximal CEJ is clinically not detectable at both mesial and distal aspects of the tooth.

Recession Type 2 (RT2):

- Gingival recession associated with loss of interproximal attachment. The amount of interproximal attachment loss is less than or equal to the buccal attachment loss.

Recession Type 3 (RT3):

- Gingival recession associated with loss of interproximal attachment. The amount of interproximal attachment loss is higher than the buccal attachment loss.

Notably, the predictability of recession coverage shrinks with ascending recession type classification (Fig. 6.6). Also important to remember is the lack of consideration given to mucogingival junction and interdental radiographic bone level in this classification.

Fig. 6.5 A Case of Peri-Implantitis During Surgical Intervention. Note the multiple exposed threads of the implant body that are denuded of bone. Also note the peri-implant bony socket following the explantation of a mobile implant.

1999 PERIODONTAL DISEASE CLASSIFICATION SYSTEM

Gingival Diseases

Dental Plaque–Induced Gingival Diseases

Gingivitis that is associated with retained dental plaque is the most common form of gingival disease (Fig. 6.7). Box 6.2 outlines the classifications of gingival diseases. These diseases may occur on a periodontium with no attachment loss or on a periodontium with attachment loss that is stable and not progressing (i.e., reduced periodontium). What separates gingivitis from periodontitis is the containment of the inflammatory lesion within the gingiva in the former. As such, gingivitis is not associated with progressive attachment loss. This is not to say that gingivitis is solely associated with teeth showing no attachment loss (Fig. 6.8). Gingivitis can also be diagnosed in the gingiva of periodontitis-affected teeth that have previously lost attachment but that have been successfully treated with periodontal therapy to prevent any further attachment loss. In these treated cases, where gingival inflammation recurs around teeth with existing attachment loss due to a history of treated periodontitis, the appropriate diagnosis would be gingivitis on a reduced periodontium. This implies that gingivitis may be the diagnosis for inflamed gingival tissues associated with a tooth with no previous attachment loss or with a tooth that has previously undergone attachment and bone loss (i.e., with reduced periodontal support) and is not currently losing attachment or bone, even though gingival inflammation is present. Clinical attachment levels and radiographic records are needed to establish this diagnosis.

> **KEY FACT**
>
> Gingivitis may be the diagnosis for inflamed gingival tissues associated with a tooth without previous attachment loss or with a tooth that has previously undergone attachment and bone loss (i.e., with reduced periodontal support) but is not currently losing attachment, even though gingival inflammation is present. In the latter case the appropriate definition would be "gingivitis on a reduced periodontium."

Fig. 6.6 A Clinical Case With Extensive Facial Gingival Recession of the Maxillary Canines but Excellent Tissue Integrity in the Papillary Areas Is Being Illustrated. Root coverage can be predictably achieved in recession type 1 defects as illustrated here in a case treated via single, contoured, subepithelial connective tissue autografts.

Fig. 6.7 (A) Plaque-related gingivitis depicts marginal and papillary inflammation, with 1- to 4-mm probing depths and generalized zero clinical attachment loss, except recession in tooth #28. (B) Radiographic images of the patient.

Fig. 6.8 Maxillary Second Molar Exhibits Mild Inflammation at Mesial-Palatal Surface. However, the clinical attachment loss has been stable for 15 years after apical positioned flap and periodontal maintenance, which is consistent with remission. The appropriate diagnosis is gingivitis on a reduced periodontium.

Gingivitis associated with dental plaque only. Plaque-induced gingival disease is the result of an interaction between the microorganisms found in the dental plaque biofilm and the inflammatory host response. A cause-and-effect relationship between microbial plaque and gingivitis has been elegantly demonstrated by a classic experiment demonstrating that the cessation of oral hygiene consistently leads to the manifestation of gingivitis within 2 to 3 weeks in healthy adults.[23] Clinical gingivitis is histologically characterized by a dense infiltrate of lymphocytes and other mononuclear cells, fibroblast alterations, increased vascular permeability, and continuing loss of collagen in response to the microbial challenge. However, the alveolar bone is not affected. Microbial plaque is thus considered to be the primary etiologic factor for gingivitis. The severity and duration of the inflammatory response interaction can be altered by the modifying local (see Chapter 12) or systemic modifying factors (see Chapters 13 and 14). Gingivitis is fully reversible in otherwise healthy persons within weeks following the removal of local factors and reduction of the microbial load around the teeth. As noted earlier, gingivitis is rapidly established in cases of generalized or localized inefficient plaque removal. Therefore it is crucial that patients are instructed in oral hygiene to maintain long-term gingival health.

Gingival diseases modified by systemic factors. Systemic factors that contribute to gingivitis—such as the endocrine changes associated with puberty (Fig. 6.9), the menstrual cycle, pregnancy (Fig. 6.10A), and diabetes—may exacerbate the gingival inflammatory response to plaque.[22,33] This altered response appears to result from the effects of systemic conditions on the host's cellular and immunologic functions, but the primary etiologic factor is still considered to be microbial plaque. One example of altered host response due to systemic factors is apparent during pregnancy, when the incidence and severity of gingival inflammation may increase even in the presence of low levels of plaque.

CLINICAL CORRELATION

Increased estrogen and progesterone levels in pregnant women during their third trimester have been associated with increased severity of gingivitis via substituting nutrient needs for certain oral bacteria and stimulating their proliferation. One species that has been specifically associated with gingivitis during pregnancy is *Prevotella intermedia*.

BOX 6.2 Gingival Diseases (According to 1999 Classification)

Dental Plaque–Induced Gingival Diseases

These diseases may occur on a periodontium with no attachment loss or with attachment loss that is stable and not progressing.

I. Gingivitis associated with dental plaque only
   A. Without local contributing factors
   B. With local contributing factors (see Box 6.4)
II. Gingival diseases modified by systemic factors
   A. Associated with endocrine system
      1. Puberty-associated gingivitis
      2. Menstrual cycle–associated gingivitis
      3. Pregnancy associated
         a. Gingivitis
         b. Pyogenic granuloma
      4. Diabetes mellitus–associated gingivitis
   B. Associated with blood dyscrasias
      1. Leukemia-associated gingivitis
      2. Other
III. Gingival diseases modified by medications
   A. Drug-influenced gingival diseases
      1. Drug-influenced gingival enlargements
      2. Drug-influenced gingivitis
         a. Oral contraceptive–associated gingivitis
         b. Other
IV. Gingival diseases modified by malnutrition
   A. Ascorbic acid deficiency gingivitis
   B. Other

Non-Plaque–Induced Gingival Lesions

I. Gingival diseases of specific bacterial origin
   A. *Neisseria gonorrhoeae*
   B. *Treponema pallidum*
   C. *Streptococcus* species
   D. Other
II. Gingival diseases of viral origin
   A. Herpesvirus infections
      1. Primary herpetic gingivostomatitis
      2. Recurrent oral herpes
      3. Varicella zoster
   B. Other

III. Gingival diseases of fungal origin
   A. *Candida* species infections: generalized gingival candidiasis
   B. Linear gingival erythema
   C. Histoplasmosis
   D. Other
IV. Gingival lesions of genetic origin
   A. Hereditary gingival fibromatosis
   B. Other
V. Gingival manifestations of systemic conditions
   A. Mucocutaneous lesions
      1. Lichen planus
      2. Pemphigoid
      3. Pemphigus vulgaris
      4. Erythema multiforme
      5. Lupus erythematosus
      6. Drug induced
      7. Other
   B. Allergic reactions
      1. Dental restorative materials
         a. Mercury
         b. Nickel
         c. Acrylic
         d. Other
      2. Reactions attributable to the following:
         a. Toothpastes or dentifrices
         b. Mouth rinses or mouthwashes
         c. Chewing gum additives
         d. Foods and additives
      3. Other
VI. Traumatic lesions (factitious, iatrogenic, or accidental)
   A. Chemical injury
   B. Physical injury
   C. Thermal injury
VII. Foreign body reactions
VIII. Not otherwise specified

Data from Holmstrup P: Nonplaque-induced gingival lesions. *Ann Periodontol* 4:20, 1999; and Mariotti A: Dental plaque-induced gingival diseases. *Ann Periodontol* 4:7, 1999.

In blood dyscrasias (e.g., leukemia), the reduced number of immunocompetent lymphocytes in the periodontal tissues is associated with increased edema, erythema, and bleeding of the gingiva, as well as gingival enlargement that may be associated with the swollen, spongy gingival tissues caused by the excessive infiltration of malignant blood cells (Fig. 6.11).

Gingival diseases modified by medications. Gingival diseases that are modified by medications include gingival overgrowth due to anticonvulsant drugs such as phenytoin, immunosuppressive drugs such as cyclosporine (Fig. 6.12), and calcium channel blockers such as nifedipine (Fig. 6.13), verapamil, diltiazem, and sodium valproate.[14,24,33] The development and severity of gingival enlargement in response to medications is patient specific and may be influenced by uncontrolled plaque accumulation as well as by elevated hormonal levels. The increased use

of oral contraceptives by premenopausal women has also been previously associated with a higher incidence of gingival inflammation and gingival enlargement. Although this fact stood true for earlier contraceptive formulations, existing contraceptives that include more modest doses of active ingredients are not commonly associated with gingival inflammation.

Gingival diseases modified by malnutrition. Gingival diseases modified by malnutrition have received attention because of clinical descriptions of bright red, swollen, and bleeding gingiva associated with severe ascorbic acid (vitamin C) deficiency or scurvy.[24] Various nutrients, such as long chain omega-3 fatty acids, have been found to have immunomodulatory properties, whereas others act to ameliorate the destructive effects of reactive oxygen species (ROS) functioning as ROS scavengers. Nonetheless, the available evidence to support a clinically impactful role for mild nutritional deficiencies in the development or severity of gingival inflammation in humans is limited. Data have shed light on the implication of increased dietary carbohydrate intake on gingivitis, in addition to its known causal role on the occurrence of dental caries.[19]

Non-Plaque–Induced Gingival Lesions

Oral manifestations of systemic conditions that produce lesions in the tissues of the periodontium are less common than plaque-induced gingivitis. This category mainly encompasses lesions of autoimmune or idiopathic etiology that can manifest in the gingiva. Benign mucous membrane pemphigoid is an example of a non-plaque–induced lesion associated with sloughing gingival tissues, which leave painful ulcerations of the gingiva

(Fig. 6.14). In pemphigoid, autoimmune antibodies are targeted at the basement membrane, and histologically the destruction resembles a subepithelial blister (see Fig. 6.14C and D). Case Scenario 6.2 depicts gingival recession accompanied by a mucosal lesion located on the gingiva manifesting with a white lacy pattern with characteristic striations.

Gingival diseases of specific bacterial origin. Gingival diseases of this category are attributed to specific bacteria that cause characteristic lesions in the gingiva. *Neisseria gonorrhoeae* and *Treponema pallidum* that can be transferred as a result of sexually transmitted diseases such as gonorrhea and syphilis, respectively, cause characteristic lesions in the gingiva.[34,38] Refer to the online references for further description.

Gingival diseases of viral origin. Gingival diseases of viral origin may be caused by a variety of deoxyribonucleic acid and ribonucleic acid viruses, with the most common being the herpesviruses. A case example of herpetic stomatitis is demonstrated in Fig. 6.15A and B. Herpetic lesions are not uncommon and develop as intraoral blisters, usually grouped together, that quickly burst, leaving minuscule ulcerations. Lesions are frequently related to the reactivation of latent viruses, especially as a result of reduced immune function. The oral manifestations of viral

Fig. 6.9 A 13-Year-Old Female With Hormone-Exaggerated Marginal and Papillary Inflammation, With 1- to 4-mm Probing Depths Yet Minimal Clinical Attachment Loss. (A) Facial view. (B) Lingual view.

Fig. 6.11 A 12-Year-Old Female With a Primary Medical Diagnosis of Leukemia That Exhibits Swollen/Spongy Gingiva.

Fig. 6.10 (A) Clinical image of pyogenic granuloma in a 27-year-old pregnant female. (B) Histologic image depicts dense inflammatory infiltrate and prominent vessels.

Fig. 6.12 Clinical Images of a 9-Year-Old Male With Severe Gingival Overgrowth Secondary to Heart Transplant and Cyclosporine Therapy.

Fig. 6.13 Clinical Images of Gingival Overgrowth Following Use a of Calcium Channel Blocker to Control Hypertension.

Fig. 6.14 A 62-Year-Old Female With Benign Mucous Membrane Pemphigoid. (A and B) Clinical image with sloughing epithelial surface. (C) Hematoxylin and eosin stain depicting separation of epithelium from connective tissue. (D) Immunofluorescent-labeled antibodies to basement membrane.

Fig. 6.15 (A and B) A 29-year-old male with primary herpetic infection and severe gingival inflammation. (C and D) Six weeks post systemic acyclovir.

infection have been comprehensively reviewed.[18,37] Viral gingival diseases are treated with topical or systemic antiviral drugs (see Fig. 6.15C and D).

CLINICAL CORRELATION

Unlike other herpetic recurrences, varicella zoster virus (VZV) usually manifests with a prodrome of tingling, itching, burning, or a unilateral numbness at the affected dermatome. These symptoms are followed by moderate to severe pain shortly after initiation and are very important for differential diagnosis.

Gingival diseases of fungal origin. Gingival diseases of fungal origin are relatively uncommon in immunocompetent individuals, but they occur more frequently in immunocompromised individuals and in those with disturbed microbiota by the long-term use of broad-spectrum antibiotics.[18,38,39] The most common oral fungal infection is candidiasis (*Candida albicans* is often implicated). Candidiasis can also be seen under prosthetic devices, in individuals using topical steroids, and in individuals with decreased salivary flow, increased salivary glucose, or decreased salivary pH. A generalized candidal infection may manifest as white patches on the gingiva, tongue, or oral mucous membrane that can potentially be removed with gauze and leave a red, bleeding surface. In human immunodeficiency virus (HIV)-seropositive persons, candidal infection may present as continuous erythematous stripe of the attached gingiva; this has been referred to as *linear gingival erythema* or *HIV-associated gingivitis* (see Chapter 28).

Gingival diseases of genetic origin. Gingival diseases of genetic origin may involve the tissues of the periodontium and have been described in detail.[1] One of the most clinically evident conditions is *hereditary gingival fibromatosis*, which exhibits

autosomal dominant or (rarely) autosomal recessive modes of inheritance. The gingival enlargement may completely cover the teeth, delay eruption, and present as an isolated finding; alternatively, it may be associated with several more generalized syndromes.

Gingival manifestations of systemic conditions. Gingival manifestations of systemic conditions may appear as desquamative lesions, ulcerations of the gingiva, or both.[18,32,38] Allergic reactions that manifest with gingival changes are uncommon but have been observed in association with several restorative materials (Fig. 6.16A), toothpastes, mouthwashes, chewing gums (Fig. 6.17), and foods (see Box 6.2). Histologic traits of biopsies from gingival allergic reactions include a dense infiltrate of eosinophilic cells (see Fig. 6.16B and C).

Traumatic lesions. Traumatic lesions may be self-inflicted and *factitious* in origin, which means that they are intentionally or unintentionally produced by artificial means (Fig. 6.18). Other examples of traumatic lesions include toothbrush trauma that results in gingival ulceration, recession, or both.

CLINICAL CORRELATION

Individuals who perform aggressive horizontal brushing are often found to have gingival recession or cervical abrasion on the teeth quadrants contralateral to their dominant hand.

Iatrogenic trauma (i.e., induced by the clinician or health professional) to the gingiva may also lead to a gingival lesion. Such trauma may be caused directly (i.e., via use of dental instruments) or by the induction of cement or preventive or restorative materials (Fig. 6.19A). Peripheral ossifying fibroma may develop in response to the embedment of a foreign body (see Fig. 6.19B

Fig. 6.16 (A) Localized pronounced gingival inflammation secondary to nickel allergy. (B and C) Biopsy depicts dense infiltrate of plasma cells.

Fig. 6.17 Generalized Severe Allergic Response of Gingiva as a Result of Additive in Chewing Gum.

Fig. 6.18 Self-Inflicted Gingival Dehiscence Induced via Patient's Fingernail.

and C). Self-inflicted *accidental damage* to the gingiva may also occur as a result of minor burns from hot foods and drinks.[18]

Foreign body reactions. Foreign body reactions lead to localized inflammatory conditions of the gingiva and are caused by the introduction of foreign material into the gingival connective tissues through breaks in the epithelium.[18] Common examples are the introduction of amalgam into the gingiva during the placement of a restoration, the extraction of a tooth, or an endodontic apicoectomy with retrofill leaving an amalgam tattoo (Fig. 6.20A), with resultant metal fragments observed during biopsies (see Fig. 6.20B); abrasives may also be introduced during polishing procedures.

Periodontitis

Periodontitis is defined as "an inflammatory disease of the supporting tissues of the teeth caused by specific microorganisms or groups of specific microorganisms, resulting in progressive destruction of the periodontal ligament and alveolar bone with increased probing depth formation, recession, or both."[42] The clinical feature that distinguishes periodontitis from gingivitis is the presence of clinically detectable attachment loss as a result of inflammatory destruction of the periodontal ligament and alveolar bone. This loss is often accompanied by periodontal pocket formation and changes in the density and height of the subjacent alveolar bone. In some cases, recession of the marginal

Fig. 6.19 (A) Proliferative gingival overgrowth secondary to impaction of foreign body. (B) Histology of peripheral ossifying fibroma. (C) Higher magnification of image in part B. (D) Four weeks post excisional biopsy.

Fig. 6.20 (A) Gingival pigmentation associated with previous apicoectomy and amalgam retro-fill. (B) Biopsy depicts metal fragments.

gingiva may accompany attachment loss, thereby masking ongoing disease progression if only probing depth measurements are taken without measurements of clinical attachment levels.

KEY FACT

Probing depth measurement alone is inadequate for an assessment of periodontitis. Clinical attachment loss (CAL) is usually assessed by adding the extent of gingival recession to the probing depth measurement to estimate the total extent of tissue loss from the cementoenamel junction (CEJ) of the tooth. However, when recession is not visible, it is essential that height of the marginal gingiva coronal to the CEJ be determined and that measurement subtracted from the probing depth to establish the extent of CAL. The measurement of clinical attachment around a tooth provides insights on the history and extent of periodontal destruction around the tooth. One common pitfall of clinical periodontal examination is the direct translation of probing depths as clinical attachment levels when the gingival margin lies above the CEJ, leading to an overestimation of attachment levels.

KEY FACT

In the American Academy of Periodontology and European Federation of Periodontology (AAP/EFP) 2018 classification of periodontal diseases, a multidimensional staging and grading system will be introduced to subclassify periodontitis disease entities. The severity of periodontal disease at the time of presentation and the complexity of disease management will dictate the staging, while grading offers additional information, including the rate of past progression of the disease and the risk for future progression.

Although many classifications of the different clinical manifestations of periodontitis have been presented since the late 1990s, consensus workshops in North America in 1989[9] and in Europe in 1993[4] identified that periodontitis may present in early-onset, adult-onset, and necrotizing forms (Table 6.4). In addition, the AAP consensus concluded that periodontitis may be associated with systemic conditions (e.g., diabetes, HIV) and that some forms of periodontitis may be refractory to conventional therapy.

TABLE 6.4	Classification of the Various Forms of Periodontitis	
Classification	**Forms of Periodontitis**	**Disease Characteristics**
AAP World Workshop in Clinical Periodontics, 1989[5]	Adult periodontitis	Age of onset >35 years Slow rate of disease progression No defects in host defenses
	Early-onset periodontitis (may be prepubertal, juvenile, or rapidly progressive)	Age of onset <35 years Rapid rate of disease progression Defects in host defenses Associated with specific microflora
	Periodontitis associated with systemic disease	Systemic diseases that predispose to rapid rates of periodontitis Diseases: diabetes, Down syndrome, HIV infection, Papillon-Lefèvre syndrome
	Necrotizing ulcerative periodontitis	Similar to acute necrotizing ulcerative gingivitis but with associated clinical attachment loss
	Refractory periodontitis	Recurrent periodontitis that does not respond to treatment
European Workshop in Periodontology, 1993[3]	Adult periodontitis	Age of onset: fourth decade of life Slow rate of disease progression No defects in host response
	Early-onset periodontitis	Age of onset: before fourth decade of life Rapid rate of disease progression Defects in host defense
	Necrotizing periodontitis	Tissue necrosis with attachment and bone loss
AAP International Workshop for Classification of Periodontal Diseases, 1999[2]	Chronic periodontitis Aggressive periodontitis Periodontitis as a manifestation of systemic diseases	See Box 6.3

AAP, American Academy of Periodontology; *HIV*, human immunodeficiency virus.

Early-onset disease was distinguished from adult-onset disease by the age of onset (<35 years of age was set as an arbitrary separation of diseases), the rate of disease progression, and the presence of alterations in host defenses. The early-onset diseases were more aggressive, occurred in individuals younger than 35 years old, and were associated with defects in host defenses. Adult forms of disease were slowly progressive, became clinically more evident during the fourth decade of life, and were not associated with defects in host defenses. In addition, early-onset periodontitis was subclassified into prepubertal, juvenile, and rapidly progressive forms with localized or generalized disease distributions.

Extensive clinical and basic scientific research involving these disease entities has been performed in many countries, and emerging information has provided support for the unification of many of the preexisting disease categories.[12,22,41] In particular, supporting evidence was lacking for the distinct classifications of adult periodontitis, refractory periodontitis, and the various different forms of early-onset periodontitis as outlined by the AAP Workshop for the International Classification of Periodontal Diseases in 1999[4] (see Table 6.4). It has been observed that chronic periodontal destruction caused by the accumulation of local factors (e.g., plaque, calculus) can occur before the age of 35 years and that the aggressive disease seen in young patients may be independent of age and instead have a familial (genetic) association. With respect to refractory periodontitis, little evidence supports the theory that this condition is indeed a distinct clinical entity. The causes of continued loss of clinical attachment and

alveolar bone after periodontal therapy are currently poorly defined and apply to many disease entities. In addition, clinical data from the medical community emerged to support the belief that forms of periodontitis that were collectively referred to as prepubertal periodontitis were in fact representing periodontitis as a manifestation of distinct systemic diseases, such as in leukocyte adhesion deficiency syndromes. As a result, the AAP held an International Workshop for the Classification of Periodontal Diseases in 1999 to further refine the classification system with the use of current clinical and scientific data.[4] The resulting classification of the different forms of periodontitis was simplified to describe three general disease forms: chronic periodontitis, aggressive periodontitis, and periodontitis as a manifestation of systemic disease (see Table 6.4 and Box 6.3).

Since the establishment of the currently accepted 1999 classification, a taskforce commissioned by the AAP proposed an update to the existing classification scheme in 2015, which was further changed in the more recent 2018 Classification as mentioned previously.[2] The update focused on suggestions to address the challenges in clinical documentation of attachment level changes and the distinction between chronic and aggressive periodontitis. In particular, the AAP task force recommended the consideration of probing depth levels, in addition to attachment levels, in determining the severity of periodontitis to avoid overestimation. The classification of diseases and conditions of the periodontium discussed in this chapter will focus on the currently accepted 1999 classification with references to the AAP update when appropriate.

BOX 6.3   Periodontitis (According to 1999 Classification)

The disease periodontitis can be subclassified into the following three major types based on clinical, radiographic, historical, and laboratory characteristics.

Chronic Periodontitis

The following characteristics are common to patients with chronic periodontitis:

- Prevalent in adults but can occur in children.
- Amount of destruction consistent with local factors.
- Associated with a variable microbial pattern.
- Subgingival calculus frequently found.
- Slow-to-moderate rate of progression with possible periods of rapid progression.
- Possibly modified by or associated with the following:
  - Systemic diseases such as diabetes mellitus and human immunodeficiency virus infection.
  - Local factors predisposing to periodontitis.
  - Environmental factors such as cigarette smoking and emotional stress.

Chronic periodontitis may be further subclassified into localized and generalized forms and characterized as mild, moderate, or severe based on the common features described previously and the following specific features:

- Localized form: <30% of teeth involved.
- Generalized form: >30% of teeth involved.
- Mild: 1–2 mm clinical attachment loss (CAL).
- Moderate: 3–4 mm CAL.
- Severe: ≥5 mm CAL.

Aggressive Periodontitis

The following characteristics are common to patients with aggressive periodontitis:

- Otherwise clinically healthy patient (note the distinction with periodontitis as a manifestation of systemic disease).
- Rapid attachment loss and bone destruction.
- Familial aggregation of diseased individuals.
  The following characteristics are common but not universal:
- Amount of microbial deposits inconsistent with disease severity.
- Increased levels of *Actinobacillus actinomycetemcomitans*.
- Abnormalities in phagocyte function.
- Hyper-responsive macrophages, producing increased prostaglandin E_2 (PGE_2) and interleukin-1β (IL-1β).
- In some cases, self-arresting disease progression.

Aggressive periodontitis may be further classified into localized and generalized forms based on the common features described here and the following specific features.

Localized Form

- Circumpubertal onset of disease.
- Localized first molar or incisor disease with proximal attachment loss on at least two permanent teeth, one of which is a first molar.
- Robust serum antibody response to infecting agents.

Generalized Form

- Usually affecting persons under 30 years of age (however, may be older).
- Generalized proximal attachment loss affecting at least three teeth other than first molars and incisors.
- Pronounced episodic nature of periodontal destruction.
- Poor serum antibody response to infecting agents.

Periodontitis as a Manifestation of Systemic Diseases

Periodontitis may be observed as a manifestation of the following systemic diseases:

1. Hematologic disorders
   a. Acquired neutropenia
   b. Leukemias
   c. Other
2. Genetic disorders
   a. Familial and cyclic neutropenia
   b. Down syndrome
   c. Leukocyte adhesion deficiency syndromes
   d. Papillon-Lefèvre syndrome
   e. Chédiak-Higashi syndrome
   f. Histiocytosis syndromes
   g. Glycogen storage disease
   h. Infantile genetic agranulocytosis
   i. Cohen syndrome
   j. Ehlers-Danlos syndrome (types IV and VIII autosomal dominant)
   k. Hypophosphatasia
   l. Other
3. Not otherwise specified

Data from Flemmig TF: Periodontitis. *Ann Periodontol* 4:32, 1999; Kinane DF: Periodontitis modified by systemic factors. *Ann Periodontol* 4:54, 1999; and Tonetti MS, Mombelli A: Early-onset periodontitis. *Ann Periodontol* 4:39, 1999.

Chronic Periodontitis

Chronic periodontitis is the most common form of periodontitis[12]; Box 6.3 includes the characteristics of this form of periodontitis. Chronic periodontitis is most prevalent in adults, but it can also be observed in children. Different classification schemes have confirmed or discarded the age range of more than 35 years to separate chronic versus aggressive periodontitis. According to the existing definition, persons younger than 35 years may exhibit a rate of progression of disease consistent with the definition of chronic periodontitis. Nonetheless, epidemiologic evidence supports the suggestion that persons younger than 25 years at disease onset are likely to exhibit aggressive periodontitis. Intraoral radiographs along with periodontal charting records are of paramount importance to the documentation of disease onset and rate of progression.

Chronic periodontitis is associated with the accumulation of plaque and calculus. It generally has a slow to moderate rate of disease progression, but periods of more rapid destruction may also be observed. Increases in the rate of disease progression may be caused by the impact of local, systemic, or environmental factors that may influence the normal host–bacteria interaction. Local factors may influence plaque accumulation (Box 6.4), whereas systemic diseases (e.g., diabetes mellitus and HIV) may influence the host's defenses, and environmental factors (e.g., cigarette smoking and stress) may influence the response of the host to plaque accumulation. Chronic periodontitis may occur as a localized disease in which less than 30% of evaluated teeth demonstrate attachment and bone loss, or it may occur as generalized when more than 30% of teeth are affected.

BOX 6.4 Developmental or Acquired Deformities and Conditions (According to 1999 Classification)

Localized Tooth-Related Factors That Modify or Predispose to Plaque-Induced Gingival Diseases or Periodontitis
1. Tooth anatomic factors
2. Dental restorations or appliances
3. Root fractures
4. Cervical root resorption and cemental tears

Mucogingival Deformities and Conditions Around Teeth
1. Gingival or soft tissue recession
   a. Facial or lingual surfaces
   b. Interproximal (papillary)
2. Lack of keratinized gingiva
3. Decreased vestibular depth
4. Aberrant frenum or muscle position
5. Gingival excess
   a. Pseudopocket
   b. Inconsistent gingival margin
   c. Excessive gingival display
   d. Gingival enlargement (see Box 6.2)
   e. Abnormal color

Mucogingival Deformities and Conditions on Edentulous Edges
1. Vertical and/or horizontal ridge deficiency
2. Lack of gingiva or keratinized tissue
3. Gingival or soft tissue enlargements
4. Aberrant frenum or muscle position
5. Decreased vestibular depth
6. Abnormal color

Occlusal Trauma
1. Primary occlusal trauma
2. Secondary occlusal trauma

Data from Blieden TM: Tooth-related issues. *Ann Periodontol* 4:91, 1999; Halmon WW: Occlusal trauma: effect and impact on the periodontium. *Ann Periodontol* 4:102, 1999; and Pini Prato GP: Mucogingival deformities. *Ann Periodontol* 4:98, 1999.

KEY FACT

Chronic periodontitis is classified by extent and severity of disease, such as generalized (extent), moderate (severity) chronic periodontitis.

Chronic periodontitis can be further classified on the basis of its extent and severity. The severity of disease has been traditionally determined as either slight/mild (1 to 2 mm of loss; Fig. 6.21), moderate (3 to 4 mm of loss; Fig. 6.22), or severe (≥5 mm of loss; Fig. 6.23) on the basis of the amount of CAL (see Box 6.3). Clinical attachment levels provide important benefits over probing depth alone to monitor disease progression using the CEJ as a fixed reference point. In fact, probing depth levels only have poor to moderate sensitivity for predicting attachment level changes overtime. Nonetheless, clinical experience has revealed that oftentimes measurement of clinical attachment levels in practice may prove to be erroneous. The most common

error occurs in the case of sites without gingival recession, whereby the location of the gingival margin is coronal to the CEJ. If the clinician in such a case records only the probing depth without charting the location of the CEJ (often charted as "positive recession" in electronic periodontal charts), the resulting attachment levels will be erroneously recorded as being equal to the probing depth. To prevent such an overestimate of disease, it has been suggested that clinicians consider that mild periodontitis be associated with probing depths of less than 4 mm, moderate periodontitis with probing depths of 5 to 6 mm, and severe periodontitis with probing depths of 7 mm or greater. However, probing depths alone should not be used to classify periodontitis without simultaneous consideration of clinical attachment levels and radiographic bone loss.

KEY FACT

In the AAP/EFP 2018 classification of periodontal diseases, one of the major changes that will be implemented is avoidance of a separate category of "aggressive periodontitis." Both chronic and aggressive periodontitis disease entities will be grouped together and will be simply called *periodontitis*.

Aggressive Periodontitis

Aggressive periodontitis differs from the chronic form primarily by the rapid rate of disease progression seen in an otherwise healthy individual (Figs. 6.24 and 6.25). The absence of large accumulations of plaque and calculus, with a positive family history of aggressive disease, is suggestive of a genetic trait[30,41] (see Box 6.3). This form of periodontitis was previously classified as early-onset periodontitis (see Table 6.4) and therefore still includes many of the characteristics previously identified with the localized and generalized forms of early-onset periodontitis. Although the clinical presentation of aggressive disease appears to be universal, the causative factors involved are not always consistent. Box 6.3 outlines additional clinical, microbiologic, and immunologic characteristics of aggressive disease that may be present. As was previously described for early-onset disease, aggressive forms of periodontitis usually affect young individuals during or shortly after puberty and may be observed during the second and third decades of life (i.e., 10 to 30 years of age). The disease may be localized, as previously described for localized juvenile periodontitis, or generalized, as previously described for generalized juvenile periodontitis and rapidly progressive periodontitis (see Table 6.4). Box 6.3 describes the common features of the localized and generalized forms of aggressive periodontitis.

FLASH BACK

Recall that chronic periodontitis is also categorized by the extent of *localized* or *generalized* disease according to the percentage of teeth involved with 30% of teeth being the cutoff between the two categories. Importantly, there is a distinct difference in the use of these definitions in the context of aggressive periodontitis. For aggressive periodontitis, the localized form is recognized to have a specific clinical phenotype, which is typically limited to incisor and first molar teeth.

Fig. 6.21 (A) Clinical image of plaque-related slight/early chronic periodontitis with 1- to 2-mm clinical attachment loss in 40-year-old female. (B) Radiographic images of the patient.

Fig. 6.22 (A) Clinical image of plaque-related moderate chronic periodontitis with 3- to 4-mm clinical attachment loss in a 53-year-old male smoker. (B) Radiographic images of the patient.

Fig. 6.23 (A) Clinical image of plaque-related severe/advanced chronic periodontitis with >5 mm clinical attachment loss in a 47-year-old female. (B) Radiographic images of the patient.

Fig. 6.24 (A) Clinical image of plaque-related aggressive moderate periodontitis with 1- to 7-mm pocket depth (PD) and 3- to 4-mm clinical attachment loss in a 31-year-old male. (B) Radiographic images of the patient.

Fig. 6.25 (A) Clinical image of plaque-related aggressive severe periodontitis with 3- to 13-mm PD and 7- to 15-mm clinical attachment loss in a 32-year-old male. (B) Radiographic images of the patient.

Periodontitis as a Manifestation of Systemic Disease

Several hematologic and genetic disorders have been associated with the development of periodontitis in affected individuals[21,22] (see Box 6.3). The clinical manifestation of many of these disorders appears at an early age and may be confused with aggressive forms of periodontitis depicting rapid attachment loss and the potential for early tooth loss.

More information on periodontitis as a manifestation of systemic diseases can be found on the companion website.

CLINICAL CORRELATION

When monogenic diseases are encountered, consanguinity can be a common finding particularly in certain ethnic cultures where it is socially acceptable. Appropriate genetic counseling is advisable. In addition, when the diagnosis for the proband (the first offspring for whom disease is noted) is established, it is crucial that the siblings are carefully examined for prompt diagnosis of additional cases.

Medication-Related Osteonecrosis of the Jaw

Medication-related osteonecrosis of the jaw (MRONJ) is an updated term that has replaced the phrase bisphosphonate-related osteonecrosis of the jaw (BRONJ). Bisphosphonates (BPs) are pyrophosphate analogues with a high affinity for hydroxyapatite crystals. They inhibit osteoclast-mediated bone resorption and play a key role in the management of osteolytic bone disorders,

Fig. 6.26 Exposed Bone on Buccal Lower Premolar and Molar in Medication-Related Osteonecrosis of the Jaw Patient Following Extraction of the First Molar. (Courtesy Dr. Vivek Thumbigere Math, Minneapolis.)

including osteoporosis, Paget disease, bone metastasis, and multiple myeloma.[36] However, their prolonged use is associated with MRONJ.[17]

The American Association of Oral and Maxillofacial Surgeons (AAOMS) defined MRONJ as "exposed bone in the maxillofacial area occurring in the absence of head and neck irradiation and showing no evidence of healing for at least 8 weeks after identification in patients treated with BP therapy"[3] (Figs. 6.26 and 6.27). To date, the true incidence of, causes of, and risk factors for the development of MRONJ are largely unknown. An overwhelming proportion (i.e., 97%) of the reported cases are related

Fig. 6.27 Medication-Related Osteonecrosis of the Jaw Patient With Exposed Bone on Lingual Aspect of Lower Premolar and Molar Following Root Canal Treatment. (Courtesy Dr. Vivek Thumbigere Math, Minneapolis.)

Fig. 6.28 (A) Ulcerative gingivitis illustrating sloughing of marginal gingiva. (B) Phase-contrast microscopy reveals spirochetes in subgingival plaque sample.

Fig. 6.29 (A) Necrotizing ulcerative periodontitis with severe clinical attachment loss in a 28-year-old male infected with human immunodeficiency virus. (B) Spirochetes noted on surface of sloughed epithelial cells.

to the high-dose intravenous BP given to patients with cancer. However, a small fraction (i.e., 3%) has been reported in patients with osteoporosis and patients with Paget disease who are receiving oral BP.[17] The estimated incidence of MRONJ in patients with osteoporosis who are receiving oral BP is approximately 0.7 per 100,000 persons/years of exposure.[3] The incidence of MRONJ among patients with cancer who are receiving intravenous BP ranges from 0.72% to 7.4%.[17]

MRONJ lesions may be asymptomatic, or they may present with pain, purulent discharge, swelling, tooth mobility, and paresthesia, culminating in a reduced ability to eat and speak. MRONJ occurs most frequently in the mandible (65%), followed by the maxilla (26%) and both jaws (95%).[43] The frequency of MRONJ is higher in the posterior region of the jaw. Among patients who develop MRONJ, approximately 60% of cases occur after an invasive dental procedure (e.g., tooth extraction), whereas 40% develop spontaneously.[40] Radiographic evaluation is usually inconclusive for early lesions. In advanced cases, a poorly defined moth-eaten radiolucency is noted with radiopaque sequestra.

Currently, there is no effective treatment for MRONJ.

The use of the term *MRONJ* was introduced to capture the rising number of osteonecrosis cases of the jaw that are associated with new types of medication, such as other antiresorptive (denosumab) and antiangiogenic therapies, by the AAOMS in their 2014 update. Readers are referred to the position paper by the AAOMS for additional information on MRONJ.[3]

Necrotizing Periodontal Diseases

The clinical characteristics of necrotizing periodontal diseases may include (but are not limited to) ulcerated and necrotic papillary and marginal gingiva that is covered by a yellowish white or grayish slough or pseudomembrane, blunting and cratering of the papillae, bleeding on provocation or spontaneous bleeding, pain, and fetid breath. These diseases may be accompanied by fever, malaise, and lymphadenopathy, although these characteristics are not consistent. Two forms of necrotizing periodontal disease have been described: *necrotizing ulcerative gingivitis (NUG)*

(Fig. 6.28) and *necrotizing ulcerative periodontitis (NUP)* (Fig. 6.29). NUG was previously classified as "gingival disease" or "gingivitis" because CAL is not a consistent feature. NUP has been classified as a form of "periodontitis" because attachment loss is present. Nonetheless, NUP cases are almost exclusively reported in immunocompromised persons. Both NUG and

NUP have been determined to constitute a separate group of diseases that have *tissue necrosis* as a primary clinical feature (see Box 6.1).

Necrotizing Ulcerative Gingivitis

The clinical and causative characteristics of NUG[35] are described in detail in Chapter 19. The defining characteristics of NUG are its bacterial cause, necrotic lesion, and predisposing factors, such as psychologic stress, smoking, and immunosuppression. In addition, malnutrition may be a contributing factor in developing countries. NUG is usually seen as an acute lesion that responds well to antimicrobial therapy in combination with professional plaque and calculus removal as well as improved oral hygiene.

Necrotizing Ulcerative Periodontitis

NUP differs from NUG in that the loss of clinical attachment and alveolar bone is a consistent feature originating from the proximal region.[29] The characteristics of NUP are described in detail in Chapter 27. NUP may be observed among HIV seropositive individuals with low CD4 counts. Clinical manifestations include local ulceration and the necrosis of gingival tissue with the exposure and rapid destruction of underlying bone, as well as spontaneous bleeding and severe pain. HIV+ persons with NUP are 20.8 times more likely to have CD4+ cell counts of less than 200 cells/mm[3] of peripheral blood as compared with those without NUP, which suggests that immunosuppression is a major contributing factor. NUP has also been associated with severe malnutrition in developing countries. More aggressive cases of necrotizing stomatitis exhibit tissue necrosis beyond the confines of the periodontium to include other oral tissues, such as the hard palate.

KEY FACT

Necrotizing stomatitis is a serious inflammatory condition that develops in systemically compromised individuals and is characterized by soft-tissue necrosis that extends beyond the gingiva, with potential bony sequestrum formation. This disease entity is now included in the AAP/EFP 2018 classification of periodontal disease.

Abscesses of the Periodontium

A periodontal abscess is a localized purulent infection of periodontal tissues, and it is classified by its tissue of origin as gingival, periodontal, or pericoronal abscesses.[26] The clinical characteristics of abscesses are discussed in Chapter 41.

Periodontitis Associated With Endodontic Lesions

The classification of lesions that affect the periodontium and the pulp is based on the sequence of the disease process.

Endodontic-Periodontal Lesions

Pulpal necrosis precedes periodontal changes in endodontic-periodontal lesions. A periapical lesion that originates with pulpal infection and necrosis may drain to the oral cavity through the periodontal ligament, resulting in the destruction of the periodontal ligament and the adjacent alveolar bone. This may present clinically as a localized, deep, periodontal probing depth that extends to the apex of the tooth (Fig. 6.30A). If the endodontic infection is left untreated in such cases, an extensive alveolar ridge defect may occur (see Fig. 6.30B and C), thereby necessitating reconstructive surgery (see Fig. 6.30D) before the placement of implants and prostheses (Fig. 6.31) to reestablish a functional and aesthetic outcome. Pulpal infection may also drain through accessory canals, especially in the area of the furcation, which may lead to furcal involvement through the loss of clinical attachment and alveolar bone.

CLINICAL CORRELATION

In early stages of primary endodontic lesions, root canal therapy may be the only treatment necessary to restore the periodontal apparatus.

Periodontal-Endodontic Lesions

It is more uncommon for periodontal disease to lead to endodontic disease than vice versa. In a periodontal-endodontic lesion, the bacterial infection from a periodontal pocket leads to loss of attachment, and root exposure then spreads to the pulp, resulting in pulpal necrosis. In the case of advanced periodontal disease, the infection may reach the pulp through the apical foramen. Nonetheless, existing studies have shown that although scaling and root planing remove cementum and underlying dentin, they may lead to dentine hypersensitivity but not to irreversible pulpitis.

Combined Lesions

Combined lesions occur when pulpal necrosis and a periapical lesion occur on a tooth that is also periodontally involved. An intrabony defect that communicates with a periapical lesion of pulpal origin results in a combined periodontal-endodontic lesion.

In all cases of periodontitis associated with endodontic lesions, the endodontic infection should be controlled before the definitive management of the periodontal lesion begins, especially when regenerative or bone-grafting techniques are planned.[27] Tooth prognosis in combined lesions highly depends on the outcome of the periodontal treatment.

Developmental or Acquired Deformities and Conditions

Localized Tooth-Related Factors That Modify or Predispose Individuals to Plaque-Induced Gingival Diseases or Periodontitis

In general, localized tooth-related factors contribute to the initiation and progression of periodontal disease through the enhancement of plaque accumulation or the prevention of effective plaque removal via normal oral hygiene measures.[7] These factors fall into the four subgroups outlined in Box 6.4.

Tooth anatomic factors. Tooth anatomic factors are associated with malformations of tooth development or tooth location.

Fig. 6.30 (A and C) Clinical images of extensive loss of alveolar ridge secondary to periapical endodontic lesion. (B) Computed tomography (CT) scan depicts alveolar bone loss. (D) CT image of regenerated ridge via allogenic bone graft, tenting screw, and membrane.

Fig. 6.31 Same Patient Depicted in Fig. 6.27. (A and B) Computed tomography scans of regenerated ridge with implants placed in areas 7, 9, and 10. (C and D) Clinical images of implant-supported bridge.

Fig. 6.32 (A and B) Clinical images of fistula tract. (C) Root fracture. (D) Resultant alveolar ridge defect.

Anatomic factors (e.g., cervical enamel projections, palatal grooves, enamel pearls) have been associated with CAL, especially in furcation areas. Cervical enamel projections are found on 15% to 24% of mandibular molars and on 9% to 25% of maxillary molars, and strong associations have been observed with furcation involvement.[25] Palatogingival grooves, which are found primarily on maxillary incisors, are observed in 8.5% of the population and are associated with increased plaque accumulation and clinical attachment as well as bone loss. Proximal root grooves on incisors and maxillary premolars also predispose individuals to plaque accumulation, inflammation, and the loss of clinical attachment and bone.

Tooth location is considered important for the initiation and development of disease. Misaligned teeth predispose individuals to plaque accumulation with resultant inflammation in children, and they may predispose adults to CAL, especially when they are associated with poor oral hygiene habits. Open interproximal contacts that contribute to food impaction have been associated with an increased loss of attachment.[20]

Dental restorations and appliances. Dental restorations or appliances are frequently associated with the development of gingival inflammation. Restorations placed deep in the sulcus or within the junctional epithelium may impinge on the biologic width resulting in inflammation and the loss of clinical attachment and bone. Contour of a complete crown restoration can affect plaque retention with flat surfaces being more hygienic as compared with convex restorations exhibiting increased bulk of material at the cervical region.

Root fractures. Root fractures may be associated with endodontic or restorative procedures as well as traumatic forces (Fig. 6.32A to C) and may lead to periodontal involvement through the apical migration of plaque along the fracture line (see Fig. 6.32D).

FLASH BACK

Vertical root fractures involving both the pulp and periodontal ligament (PDL) are true combined endodontic-periodontal lesions.

Cervical root resorption and cemental tears. Invasive cervical resorption (ICR) (as noted on the cone beam computed tomography scans shown in Fig. 6.33A and B) and cemental tears may lead to periodontal destruction when the lesion communicates with the oral cavity and allows bacteria to migrate subgingivally. The atraumatic removal of teeth with progressed cervical resorption lesions and the reconstruction of resultant ridge defects with bone grafts, dental implants, and prostheses are viable solutions for such defects (Fig. 6.34). Avulsed teeth that are reimplanted frequently develop ankylosis and cervical root resorption many years after reimplantation. If the patient is still in the phase of skeletal growth, decoronation may be the treatment of choice for ridge preservation. In adults with completed skeletal growth, atraumatic removal of such ankylosed teeth, followed by ridge reconstruction and placement of implants and prosthesis, is a viable treatment option in adults (see Fig. 6.34).

Mucogingival Deformities and Conditions Around the Teeth

Mucogingival deformity is a generic term used to describe the mucogingival junction and its relationship to the gingiva (Fig. 6.35), the alveolar mucosa, and frenula muscle attachments. A mucogingival deformity is a significant departure from the normal shape of the gingiva and the alveolar mucosa, and it may involve the underlying alveolar bone. Mucogingival surgery and periodontal plastic and aesthetic surgery correct defects in the morphology, position, or amount of gingiva.

Fig. 6.33 (A and B) Computed tomography scans reveal severe cervical root resorption of maxillary central incisors and periapical abscess. (C) Crowns fractured because of resorption. (D) Biopsy of soft tissue from resorption.

Fig. 6.34 (A) Posttreatment clinical image of same patient depicted in Fig. 6.30 with implant-supported crowns and veneers on laterals. (B and C) Computed tomography scans of bone grafts and implants replacing central incisors lost as the result of severe cervical root resorption.

Fig. 6.35 (A) Mucogingival defect depicted by recession. (B) Defects extend into alveolar mucosa and lack keratinized gingiva.

Fig. 6.36 (A) Mucogingival ridge defect from floor of mouth to vestibular fornix. (B) Partial thickness flap with vestibular deepening. (C) Placement of free gingival graft. (D) Reestablishment of vestibular depth and keratinized attached gingiva.

Fig. 6.37 (A) Clinical image of edentulous ridge defect. (B) Pretreatment computed tomography (CT) image of defect. (C) Reconstructed ridge using ramus block graft. (D) CT scan of grafted site.

Fig. 6.38 (A) Clinical image of ridge 6 months after grafting. (B) Placement of implants in area of teeth #23 and #26. (C) Porcelain fused to metal (PFM) crowns for maxillary incisors and implant-supported bridge from teeth #23 to #25.

Mucogingival Deformities and Conditions of the Edentulous Ridges

Mucogingival deformities, such as a lack of stable keratinized gingiva between the vestibular fornices and the floor of the mouth (Fig. 6.36A), may require soft-tissue grafting and vestibular deepening before prosthodontic reconstruction (see Fig. 6.36B to D). Alveolar bone defects in edentulous ridges (Fig. 6.37A and B) usually require corrective surgery (see Fig. 6.37C and D) to restore form and function before the placement of implants and prostheses to replace missing teeth (Fig. 6.38).[31]

Occlusal Trauma

The causes of trauma from occlusion and the effect of this trauma on the periodontium[13] are discussed in detail in Chapter 48.

To view the **updated AAP/EFP 2018 classification system,** visit the companion website.

Case Scenarios 6.1 to 6.7 are found on the companion website.

REFERENCES

 References for this chapter are found on the companion website.

Fundamentals in the Methods of Periodontal Disease Epidemiology[a]

CHAPTER OUTLINE

THE NEED FOR EPIDEMIOLOGY

The World Health Organization (WHO) defines epidemiology as "the study of the distribution and determinants of health-related states or events (including disease), and the application of this study to the control of diseases and other health problems." Distinct study designs are employed to examine the distribution of periodontal diseases in populations and to determine its etiology and its association with other diseases; the ultimate goal is to determine evidence-driven preventive and therapeutic strategies. "Periodontal [gum] diseases, including gingivitis and destructive periodontal disease, are serious infections."[55] This 2009 statement from a professional dental organization reflected the dominating belief accepted since the 1960s that bacteria cause periodontal conditions.[15] This bacterial dogma had several consequences. Clinical management and research became largely focused on vaccines, microbial diagnosis, antimicrobials, antibiotics, dental plaque, and immunology. Clinical diagnoses that did not fit the infection paradigm (e.g., periodontal atrophy) were eliminated from some periodontal disease classifications, and it was hypothesized that periodontal infections caused systemic diseases.

But are periodontal diseases really infectious diseases? A reliable answer to this question requires epidemiologic evidence. This chapter focuses on the role of epidemiology in the study of human diseases. *Case-control studies* and *cohort studies* are two epidemiologic study designs that identify common causes of chronic disease, such as smoking, ionizing radiation, hepatitis B, and high blood pressure. *Randomized controlled trials* are study designs that assess the diagnosis, management, and prognosis of chronic diseases and that either confirm or refute the suspected causes of disease identified in case-control or cohort studies. Prostate surface antigen screening, polio vaccination, and hormone replacement therapy are examples of diagnoses and treatments for chronic diseases that were evaluated by means of randomized controlled trials.

---

[a]Adapted from the following chapter of Newman and Carranza's Clinical Periodontology, 13th edition: Chapter 6: Fundamentals in the Methods of Periodontal Disease Epidemiology, by Philippe P. Hujoel and Georgios A. Kotsakis.

STUDY DESIGNS

Epidemiologic study designs fall within two broad categories: observational and interventional studies. As the terms imply, assigning a study to one of these categories depends on whether the investigators assess the efficacy of an intervention (interventional) or whether the intervention is not under control of the investigators (observational). Examples of interventional studies in oral health research are randomized clinical trials and nonrandomized clinical trials. Examples of observational studies are cross-sectional studies, cohort studies, and case-control studies.

Some of the essential characteristics of epidemiologic studies are that they are conducted in humans, there is a control or a comparison group, and clinically relevant endpoints are evaluated. Such studies are available to support the direct effects that oral bacteria have on reversible gingival inflammation (i.e., gingivitis).[56] In contemporary practice, the strength of scientific evidence is formally ranked based on the study design. One widely used level of evidence classification by the Oxford Center for Evidence-Based Medicine (http://www.cebm.net/wp-content/uploads/2014/06/CEBM-Levels-of-Evidence-2.1.pdf) generally considers animal studies (i.e., mechanism-based reasoning) as having the lowest level of evidence to impact clinical thinking, whereas systematic reviews of randomized controlled trials are generally considered as having the highest available level of evidence.

SYSTEMATIC REVIEW VERSUS EXPERT OPINION

A systematic review is considered a form of secondary research that aims to screen the entire breadth of information on a selected topic, identify relevant research studies, and summarize their findings. The key difference between an expert opinion review and a systematic review is that the latter is more objective in the sense that it intends to summarize the available body of literature inclusively and not based on the author's opinion about which studies are noteworthy or impactful. It goes without saying that systematic reviews are considered to be high level and are often used to guide clinical decision-making, but the clinicians should be aware that their conclusions suffer from the shortcomings of the included studies.

FLASH BACK

Recall that well-designed interventional studies generally are higher level than observational studies.

The emerging epidemiologic evidence regarding the cause of periodontal diseases suggests that factors such as cigarette smoking, sugar, cereals, and chronic diseases such as diabetes could be primary causes of periodontal disease.[4,17,47] Notably, the 2004 US Surgeon General report concluded that the evidence was sufficient to infer a causal relationship between smoking and periodontitis.[57] Organizations such as the WHO suggest that periodontal disease prevention be made an integral part of programs that focus on tobacco control, diet, and physical activity, which are also shared risk factors with other prevalent chronic diseases such as cardiovascular diseases.[40] Regardless of your current beliefs about the causes of periodontal disease, becoming familiar with the epidemiologic methodology may be important in order to judge this emerging evidence independently and critically.

Measuring the Occurrence of Conditions or Diseases

The fundamental tools of epidemiology are simple sums and divisions that reflect how many individuals or sites either have or develop a particular condition or disease.

The *prevalence* is the sum of all examined individuals or sites that exhibit the condition or disease of interest divided by the sum of the number of individuals or sites examined. The prevalence can range from 0% (no one has the condition or disease of interest) to 100% (everyone has the condition or disease of interest).

As an example of prevalence, the Centers for Disease Control and Prevention reported on the prevalence of individuals with at least one periodontal pocket depth of 4 mm or deeper. It was reported that, from 1988 to 1994, a little more than 1 in 5 Americans had such a condition, for a prevalence of a little more than 20%; from 1999 to 2004, only 1 in 10 Americans fell into this category,[11] for a prevalence of around 10%. These findings suggest a more than 50% decline in the prevalence of pocket depths greater than or equal to 4 mm for adults between the ages of 20 and 64 years, which occurred over approximately a decade. These epidemiologic data confirm another report of declining destructive periodontal disease prevalence in the United States.[5] Such information about prevalence measures of periodontal conditions may have implications for human resource needs in the United States and may provide clues with respect to the causative factors that drive such changes. Many countries do not have prevalence surveillance systems,[40] which makes it difficult to determine whether these trends observed in the United States are isolated events or part of a more general trend.

The *risk* is the probability that an individual or site will develop a particular condition or disease during follow-up. The risk for a condition or a disease is a number that ranges between 0% and 100%. The simplest way to estimate risk is to have a fixed number of persons or sites at risk at some defining moment (i.e., time zero [t_0]). Individuals or sites within individuals are followed up over time after this defining moment. After a follow-up period (i.e., from t_0 to t_n), the risk can be calculated as the proportion of persons or sites in which the clinical outcome of interest develops during the follow-up period. Because the risk is estimated as a proportion, it is without dimension, and it ranges between 0 and 1. When a risk is reported, it should be accompanied by a specific time period to which it is applied. A 5% risk for death may be considered small when it refers to a 20-year period but may be large when it refers to a 3-month period.

As an example, consider concerns about occupational human immunodeficiency virus (HIV) infection among dentists. It has been reported that the risk for developing an HIV infection within the year subsequent to an accidental needle stick with HIV-contaminated blood is 0.3%. Such a statistic has an intuitive appeal and can be related to patients or colleagues. A risk of 0.003 (0.3%) indicates that for every 1000 individuals who have an accidental HIV-contaminated needle stick, 3 are expected to develop an HIV infection within a year of the event.

The *odds* for an event is the probability that an event occurred divided by the probability that an event did not occur. Whereas probability is a value that has to range between 0 and 1, odds values range from 0 to infinity. If the probability for observing an event is small, then the odds and the probability are almost identical. For example, if the probability for a vertical root fracture after an endodontic procedure is 0.001, then the odds are 0.001/0.999 or 0.001001. Odds are commonly reported in studies because they are often easier to estimate with statistical models than probabilities. For example, the odds for developing an HIV infection after an accidental needle stick with HIV-contaminated blood are 0.003 (0.003/0.997).

Incidence rates are an alternative measure to describe disease occurrence. One example of an incidence rate is the speedometer in a car that displays at any given time the number of kilometers being traveled per hour. In clinical trials or epidemiology, the rate reflects the number of disease occurrences per person-time or site-time. The disease rate is a ratio in which the numerator is the number of subjects or sites diagnosed with the disease of interest and the denominator is the sum of the time at risk over all subjects or sites in the population.

INCIDENCE VERSUS PREVALENCE

Recall that prevalence is the proportion of a population found to have a condition at a given point in time (e.g., 9% of the US population had severe periodontitis in the 2009–2010 NHANES survey), while incidence is the probability that a disease will occur in a previously healthy population over a period of time (e.g., the incidence of peri-implantitis for patients with mandibular overdentures is 17% after 5 years).

Incidence rates—as opposed to the previously introduced measures of disease occurrence—imply an element of time. The denominator in the incidence rate has time as the dimension. Thus the dimension of incidence rate is 1/time. This dimension is often referred to as "person-time" or "site-time" to distinguish the time summation from ordinary clock-time. The magnitude

Fig. 7.1 Rate of tooth loss per 1000 tooth-years as a function of maximum probing depth per tooth in a cohort of 1021 patients between the ages of 40 and 65 years under periodontal specialist care for destructive periodontal disease. (Data from Hujoel PP, Cunha-Cruz J, Selipsky H, et al. Abnormal pocket depth and gingival recession as distinct phenotypes. *Periodontol 2000.* 2005;39:22–29.)

of the incidence rate can vary between 0 and infinity. When there are no new disease onsets during the study period, the incidence rate is 0. When every person observed dies instantaneously at the start of the study (and thus the sum of the time periods is 0), then the incidence rate is infinity.

An example of the application of rates is provided in Fig. 7.1, in which the number of teeth lost per 1000 tooth-years is plotted as a function of the maximum probing depth at the start of follow-up. The plot suggests a nonlinear relationship between maximum pocket depth and tooth loss, with a substantial increase in tooth loss rate for teeth that have periodontal pockets of 7 mm or deeper.

For the study of risk, the population studied is usually limited to those individuals at risk for the outcome of interest. Thus, if the outcome of interest is a disease, the following subjects are excluded from the cohort: persons who already have the disease, persons who have immunity to the disease, and persons who are biologically incapable of developing the disease.

Periodontal Measures Typically Recorded Clinically

A periodontal examination can measure various characteristics of the periodontium. Dental records of periodontal patients typically contain information about the teeth that are present, missing, or impacted as well as measurable information about the periodontal status of those teeth. Information such as clinical probing depth, bleeding on probing, gingival recession, mobility of teeth, and the presence of furcation involvements can be charted. In addition, some clinicians may collect information about the presence of gingivitis by evaluating the color and form of the gingival tissues. These measures can be complemented with radiographic examinations that may provide information about marginal bone levels.

Two common measures of gingival inflammation are the gingival index (GI) and bleeding on probing.[19] The GI was proposed in 1963 as a method for assessing the severity and quantity of gingival inflammation.[32,33] With this particular index, only gingival tissues are assessed. Each of the four gingival areas of the tooth (i.e., facial, mesial, distal, and lingual) are assessed for inflammation and rated as normal gingiva (a score of 0) to severely inflamed gingiva with a tendency to spontaneously bleed (a score of 3). Gingiva that is mildly inflamed but without bleeding on probing is given a score of 1, whereas moderately inflamed gingiva with bleeding is given a score of 2. The scores can be averaged for each patient to provide patient means. Alternatively, site-specific analyses can relate local and patient-specific factors to the GI that is measured at individual sites.[10]

BLEEDING ON PROBING VERSUS GINGIVAL INDEX

In clinical settings the term *gingival index* is often misused in lieu of bleeding on probing (BOP). According to the existing nomenclature, gingival index is a categorical index that assesses the severity of gingival inflammation on a scale from 0 to 3. On the other hand, BOP is a binary index (Yes/No) that determines whether a site is bleeding on probing or not. The two should not be confused.

Commonly used measures of periodontal tissue destruction include mean probing depth, mean attachment loss, and mean recession level.[24] The clinical protocols regarding how such mean values are collected and calculated can vary considerably. One example of how such values can be ascertained clinically is described in the National Institute of Dental and Craniofacial Research "periodontal destruction" examination.[38] This examination includes an assessment of periodontal attachment loss[43] as the distance in millimeters from the cemento-enamel junction to the bottom of the gingival sulcus. This distance was measured at the facial and mesiofacial sites of teeth in a randomly selected maxillary and mandibular quadrant with the use of the indirect measurement method developed by Ramfjord.[43]

SENSITIVITY VERSUS SPECIFICITY

Sensitivity is defined as the number of diseased patients who are correctly identified as having disease—that is, the diagnostic marker leads to a minimum number of false negative diagnoses. *Specificity* is defined as the number of healthy persons who are correctly determined to not have the disease—that is, the diagnostic marker leads to a minimum number of false positive diagnoses.

True and Surrogate Measures of the Periodontal Condition

The epidemiology of true and surrogate endpoints of periodontal disease do not necessarily coincide. *True endpoints* are tangible outcomes that directly measure how a patient feels, functions, or survives.[13] True endpoints include oral health–related quality-of-life measurements[29,35,51] and self-reported problems, such as a positive answer to the following question: "When you brush or floss your teeth, do you notice bleeding that is both regular and that involves spitting blood-stained saliva?" *Surrogate endpoints* are intangible to the patient.[54] Surrogate endpoints in periodontal research include anatomic measures (e.g., probing depth), measures of inflammation (e.g., bleeding), microbiologic measures, and immunologic measures.[10] Surrogate endpoints are often objective, because they can be measured by the clinician (rather than relying on self-report by patients) or by laboratory methods.

Surrogate endpoints can be misleading when the goal is to provide reliable information about clinical decisions related to diagnosis, etiology, treatment, or prognosis. One periodontal example is the use of systemic antibiotics that may have a beneficial impact on attachment gain[15] but a potential increased risk for tooth loss.[8]

More information on the Challenges of Obtaining Epidemiologic Measures of Periodontal Conditions and Diseases will be found in the companion website.

TABLE 7.1 Examples of Periodontal Randomized Controlled Trials		
Periodontal Treatment	**Outcome**	**Sample Size**
Scaling and root planing for pregnant women[36]	Infants with low birth weights	823
Biphasic calcium phosphate ceramic[39]	Clinical attachment level	137

TABLE 7.2 Examples of Periodontal Cohort Studies		
Periodontal Exposure	**Outcome**	**Sample Size**
Periodontal disease and tooth loss[25]	Coronary heart disease	51,529
Gingivitis[7]	Tooth loss	>500

PERIODONTAL ENDPOINT EXAMPLES:

True endpoints: Tooth loss, patient's quality of life, and oral function

Surrogate endpoints: Probing depths, bleeding on probing, microbial measures

---

EPIDEMIOLOGIC STUDY DESIGNS

The essence of epidemiology and clinical epidemiology is to relate measures of disease occurrence to suspected causes or interventions. Can the dramatic drop in destructive periodontal disease prevalence in the United States be attributed to a change in smoking prevalence? Can the presence of particular microbiologic species around a tooth be related to the risk of future tooth loss? Can the rate of tooth loss in a sample of elderly patients be related to the use of an antimicrobial rinse? With an evidence-based approach, these questions can be most reliably answered by three epidemiologic study designs. As mentioned earlier in this chapter, these study designs (in order of decreasing reliability) are the randomized controlled trial, the cohort study, and the case-control study.

Randomized Controlled Trials

Randomized controlled trials in periodontics typically assign patients or some teeth within a patient randomly to a treatment. Patients are then monitored, and subsequent outcomes are assessed. Table 7.1 provides two examples of randomized controlled trials.

The randomized controlled trial is the only study design that can provide a probabilistic basis for the making of a causal inference between an intervention and an outcome. Reliable inference regarding the causality of associations can be obtained if the delicate machinery of clinical trial design and analysis is strictly respected. For example, there needs to be a pretrial hypothesis that specifies the endpoint, the treatments to be compared, the patient population, and the degree of required precision. Other factors that are important for obtaining reliable answers include a secure randomization process, the masking of patients and

clinicians, the presence of an independent data and safety monitoring board, and strict adherence to the pretrial hypothesis, which must include an intent-to-treat analysis. Trials with exquisite attention to detail are referred to as *definitive trials,* and they are rare in any field, including periodontal research. Definitive trials are required to provide reliable answers about treatment efficacy. Most of the trials published in the literature are in the category of exploratory trials. These trials typically do not report a pretrial hypothesis, and they conclude that the intervention was successful when compared to the control.[20] These are almost always false-positive conclusions.[21]

Cohort Studies

Cohort studies can also be referred to as *exposure-based study designs.* Subjects who are free of the disease of interest are classified with respect to an exposure (e.g., cigarette smoking, diabetes) and followed longitudinally for the assessment of periodontal outcomes. Table 7.2 provides two examples of cohort studies.

Cohorts can be defined by a geographic area, records, exposure status, or a combination of different criteria. In one study of the causal factors of edentulism, the population of interest was defined as the inhabitants of the town of Tecumseh, Michigan. Persons within this community were examined in 1959 as part of a community-wide health study. Twenty-eight years later, a subset of these patients was reexamined to study the risk factors for edentulism.[38] Some natural disease history studies of destructive periodontal disease have been conducted on the basis of geographic location. Examples include the Norwegian Longitudinal Study,[1] the Veterans Administration Longitudinal Study,[28] and the Sri Lanka study.[2] A cohort can be defined by records (e.g., schools, health insurance plans, unions, industries, professional organizations). Many cohort studies of periodontal disease outcomes are performed in patients who belong to a particular dental insurance company[9] or to a professional group.[26] Finally, cohorts can be defined on the basis of a specific exposure. For example, different levels of fluoride concentrations in the water supply have been used for the definition of cohorts.

Case-Control Studies

Case-control studies are typically referred to as *outcome-based study designs*. Persons with a condition or outcome of interest (i.e., cases) are compared with persons without a condition of interest (i.e., controls) with respect to the history of the suspected causal factors. Many people intuitively think along the lines of a case-control study when evaluating disease causes. For example, if an individual suffers from food poisoning after a party, he or she is likely to compare past food intake with those individuals who did *not* experience food poisoning. Similarly, if one is diagnosed with a serious illness, a common reaction is to ask, "Why me?" This is usually followed by a comparison of one's history of exposures with those of other individuals who did *not* develop the serious illness. The primary goal of a case-control study is to find out what *past* exposures or factors are different between patients with a disease versus those without the disease. Table 7.3 provides two examples of case-control studies.

For example, the case definition for a myocardial infarction in a case-control study of the relationship between dental health and acute myocardial infarction was as follows[2]:
1. Symptoms start within 36 hours before the admission
2. No prior myocardial infarction
3. Residing in Helsinki or an immediate neighborhood
4. Age <60 years for men and <65 years for women
5. Blood samples available at admission and at 4 weeks

In a case-control study, the *controls* should be at risk for developing the investigated disease and come from the same population that generated the cases. For example, if the investigated disease is root caries, the controls should be at risk for developing root caries (i.e., have exposed root surfaces) and originate from the same population that generated the cases that have root caries.

 More information on determining causality from epidemiological studies will be found on the companion website.

Suspected Modifiable Causative Factors for Periodontal Disease
Tobacco Smoking

Tobacco smoking is recognized by several organizations as one of the primary drivers of periodontal disease epidemiology.[4] Many criteria for causality have been satisfied,[14] and smoking cessation has been shown to slow the progression of periodontal disease.[27,28,41] The strong impact of tobacco smoking on periodontal disease has the potential to induce spurious causal associations in other suspected risk factors for periodontal disease.

For example, smoking is a risk factor for both type 2 diabetes[58] and periodontal disease, thereby making associations between type 2 diabetes and periodontal disease susceptible to biases. To obtain reliable inferences about causal factors other than smoking, studies of periodontal disease epidemiology may need to be restricted to those who have never smoked.

Nutrition

Several studies have demonstrated relationships between periodontal disease and a variety of medical conditions that center on carbohydrate metabolism, including intake of dietary carbohydrates, exercise, obesity, prediabetes, and diabetes. A systematic review of randomized controlled trials involving carbohydrates suggested that the increased intake of fermentable carbohydrates may cause an increase in gingivitis.[20] Two systematic reviews suggested that diabetes was a risk factor for destructive periodontal disease.[47,50]

Dental Plaque

Several systematic reviews have provided evidence that chemotherapeutic and mechanical plaque control will reduce gingival inflammation. Essential oils[3] and cetylpyridinium-chloride–containing mouth rinses[16] may reduce gingival inflammation. Interdental brushes may reduce dental plaque, bleeding, and probing pocket depth.[52] Power-driven toothbrushes may be more effective than manual toothbrushes for removing plaque and reducing inflammation.[49] Self-performed dental flossing may not be effective for reducing plaque and gingival inflammation.[3] Although these systematic reviews provide evidence about the role of dental plaque in gingival inflammation, they do not necessarily suggest that dental plaque is the primary cause of gingival inflammation.[18] Stomach acids may cause heartburn, and antacids may be effective at eliminating heartburn symptoms. However, this evidence does not make stomach acids a primary cause of heartburn. The primary cause of heartburn may, for instance, be a gluten allergy, and thus, the cure of the heartburn requires the elimination of gluten from the diet. Antacids can be considered a palliative that is needed as long as the primary cause has not been identified.

Neither is there reliable evidence that gingival inflammation precedes destructive periodontal disease. There is no reliable randomized controlled trial evidence that oral hygiene has a beneficial impact on the prevention of periodontal destruction.[21,23]

The Cause of Periodontal Disease for the Patient Sitting in Your Chair

In clinical epidemiology, in a court of a law, and in modern-day clinical practice, uncertainty regarding the "cause" is an important consideration when discussing causality. The term *attributable risk percentage* is used to express the probability that a disease is caused by a suspected causative agent. For example, in a smoker with lung cancer, there may be a 20% probability that the lung cancer was caused by a factor other than smoking (e.g., radon). In an obese person with diabetes, there may be a 10% chance that obesity played no role in the onset of diabetes. For a worker with leukemia in the nuclear industry, there may be an 80% chance that the leukemia was not caused by the low-level

TABLE 7.3	Examples of Periodontal Case–Control Studies	
Case–Control Criteria	**Investigated Risk Factors**	**Sample Size**
Destructive periodontal disease[34]	Smoking	177
Acute myocardial infarction[42]	Dental health	202

protracted radiation exposures. One can almost never determine with certainty what caused a particular condition or disease to appear in a patient; all one can do is assign probabilities to the likelihood that a particular causal factor was responsible for the disease diagnosed in the patient. Destructive periodontal disease and periodontal inflammation are no exception to this general rule of uncertainty for determining a disease's cause. As a result, diagnostic names (e.g., plaque-induced gingival disease, non-plaque-induced inflammatory gingival lesions[30]) can be considered misnomers, because such names imply diagnostic certainty that lead to circular reasoning.[2] The principle of diagnostic uncertainty is also important when it comes to the diagnosis of periodontal conditions.

DIAGNOSIS

Periodontal Conditions Versus Periodontal Diseases

Disease is defined as an attribute or a characteristic of a person, and *diagnosis* is the clinician's belief that the person has the attribute.[53] The WHO defined disease as those adverse health consequences that include physical or psychological impairment, activity restrictions, and role limitations.[53] Certain periodontal conditions have been associated with such adverse consequences, and thus, certain periodontal conditions qualify as diseases according to the WHO's definition. In one study, about 1 in 5 patients who presented to a periodontal specialist reported that their teeth, gums, or dentures had an impact fairly often or very often on either eating; relaxing; avoiding going out; or feeling self-conscious, pain, or discomfort. In this same study, 4 out of 10 patients rated their oral health as fair or poor.[8] Other studies have shown that gingival conditions (e.g., necrotizing ulcerative gingivitis, attachment loss in high school students) are similarly related to oral health–related quality of life.[31]

An important thing to consider during periodontal diagnosis is to determine which periodontal conditions can be diagnosed as "diseased." Can a patient with a couple of sites with 1 or 2 mm of attachment loss be classified in this way? What about a patient with such subtle gingival inflammation that the majority of clinicians would not notice the inflammation and that even highly trained clinical examiners agree poorly about the presence of gingivitis? Disagreement regarding such questions is one of the reasons that the prevalence of gingivitis and destructive periodontal disease can range widely, depending on which reference levels are considered to be the cutoff for normal as compared with diseased.

Diagnostic Tests Available to Assess Periodontal Conditions

Diagnostic tests for periodontal disease can include anatomic measures of tissue destruction, such as probing pocket depth and clinical attachment loss; measures of gingival inflammation, such as redness, suppuration, bleeding, bleeding on probing, elevated gingival temperature, and gingival crevicular fluid markers; radiographic measures of bone destruction and tooth mobility; and microbiologic measures. These test results—in combination with factors such as age, dental history, and systemic conditions—can be translated into a distinct set of periodontal diagnoses.

REFERENCES

 References for this chapter are found on the companion website.

Periodontal Disease Pathogenesis and Genetics

CHAPTER OUTLINE

Understanding periodontal pathogenesis is key to improving management strategies for this common, complex disease. The first challenge is to understand exactly what is meant by the term *pathogenesis*. According to *Merriam Webster's Collegiate Dictionary,* the word "pathogenesis" is defined as "the origination and development of a disease." Essentially, this refers to the step-by-step processes that lead to the development of a disease, which result in a series of changes in the structure and function of, in this case, the periodontium. In broad terms, the pathogenesis of a disease is the mechanism by which a causative factor (or factors) causes the disease. The word itself is derived from the Greek roots *pathos* (meaning "suffering") and *genesis* (meaning "generation or creation").

During the 1970s, the role of plaque as the sole causative factor for periodontitis was unquestioned. In those days, nonsurgical treatment was in its infancy, and most treatment options involved surgery (e.g., gingivectomy for the treatment of shallower pockets, access flap surgery for the treatment of deeper sites). Looking back, it becomes clear that the treatment strategies used during a given time period entirely depend on the prevailing understanding of pathogenesis at that particular point in time. It is therefore very likely that the management options that we take for granted now will change again in the future. This is to be welcomed because a progressive clinical discipline such as periodontology that is well founded in science and with benefit to the patient as its primary value should strive to improve therapeutic strategies in parallel with continued discovery.

CLINICIAN'S CORNER

Why Is Studying Periodontal Pathogenesis Important?
Pathogenesis refers to the processes that cause disease. In periodontitis, bacteria in the biofilm stimulate an immune–inflammatory response that causes the tissue damage that we recognize clinically as periodontitis. Understanding the disease processes is important because it may lead to the development of improved treatment strategies.

Periodontal disease results from a complex interplay between the subgingival biofilm and the host immune–inflammatory events that develop in the gingival and periodontal tissues in response to the challenge presented by the bacteria. The tissue damage that results from the immune–inflammatory response is recognized clinically as periodontitis. Gingivitis precedes periodontitis, but it is clear that not all cases of gingivitis progress to periodontitis. In gingivitis, the inflammatory lesion is confined to the gingiva; however, with periodontitis, the inflammatory processes extend to additionally affect the periodontal ligament and the alveolar bone. The net result of these inflammatory changes is the breakdown of the fibers of the periodontal ligament, resulting in clinical loss of attachment together with resorption of the alveolar bone.

During the 1970s and 1980s, bacterial plaque was generally considered to be preeminent as the cause of periodontitis. It was clear (as it is now) that poor oral hygiene results in increased plaque accumulation, and it was accepted that this, in turn, resulted in periodontal disease. However, this model failed to

---

ªNote: In the 2018 Classification of Periodontal and Peri-Implant Diseases and Conditions, "chronic periodontitis" and "aggressive periodontitis" disease categories are grouped under a single category called "periodontitis," and are further characterized based on a multidimensional staging and grading system. In this chapter, the term "aggressive periodontitis" is still used because the related studies were conducted before the 2018 classification. Readers are referred to Chapter 6 for detailed discussion on periodontal disease classification.

take into account observations such as the finding that there are many individuals with poor oral hygiene who do not develop advanced periodontal disease, and conversely, some individuals, despite good oral hygiene and compliance with periodontal treatment protocols, present with advanced and progressing periodontitis. These findings were confirmed by the work of Löe and colleagues,[117] who studied Sri Lankan tea laborers who had no access to dental care and who could be divided into three main categories: (1) individuals (≈8% of the population studied) who had rapid progression of periodontal disease, (2) those (≈81%) who had moderate progression of such disease, and (3) those (≈11%) who demonstrated no progression of periodontal disease beyond gingivitis. All patients in this population displayed abundant plaque and calculus deposits, so clearly susceptibility to disease is influenced by more than just presence of dental plaque. The causative role of bacteria in the biofilm is clear in that the bacteria initiate and perpetuate the inflammatory responses that develop in the gingival tissues. However, the main determinant of susceptibility to disease is the nature of the immune–inflammatory responses themselves. It is paradoxical that these defensive processes, which are protective by intent (i.e., to prevent the ingress of the bacteria and their products into the tissues), result in the majority of tissue damage that leads to the clinical manifestations of disease.

Periodontal disease is therefore a unique clinical entity. It is not an infection in the classic sense of the word. With many infections, a single infective organism causes the disease (e.g., human immunodeficiency virus, syphilis, tuberculosis), and the identification of that organism can provide the basis for the diagnosis. With periodontal disease, many species are identifiable in the periodontal pocket, and it is impossible to conclude that a single species or even a group of species causes periodontal disease. Many of the species that are considered important in periodontal pathogenesis may predominate in deep pockets because the pocket is a favorable environment in which they can survive (i.e., it is warm, moist, and anaerobic, with a ready supply of nutrients). Many of the unique features of periodontitis are derived from the anatomy of the periodontium, in which a hard, nonshedding surface (the tooth) is partly embedded within the body (within connective tissue), crosses an epithelial surface, and is partly exposed to the outside world (within the confines of the mouth). The bacteria that colonize this surface are effectively outside of the body (although they are in the gingival crevice or pocket), yet the inflammatory response that develops is located within the body (i.e., within the tissues). These factors add complexity to our understanding of the role of the biofilm and the immune–inflammatory responses that are part of periodontal tissue breakdown.

HISTOPATHOLOGY OF PERIODONTAL DISEASE

To understand periodontal pathogenesis better, it is important to have an appreciation of the histology of clinically healthy tissues, as well as of inflamed gingival and periodontal tissues. Even gingival tissues that clinically would be considered to be noninflamed and healthy always have evidence of inflammatory responses occurring at the microscopic level. This is normal

given the chronic low-grade challenge presented by the subgingival biofilm. The low-grade inflammatory response that results is not detectable macroscopically at the clinical level, but it is an essential protective mechanism for combating the microbial challenge and for preventing bacteria and their products from infiltrating tissues and causing tissue damage. Our current understanding of susceptibility to periodontitis suggests that individuals who are susceptible to the disease mount an excessive or dysregulated immune–inflammatory response for a given bacterial challenge that leads to increased tissue breakdown as compared with those individuals who have a more normal inflammatory response.

Clinically Healthy Gingival Tissues

Clinically healthy gingival tissues appear pink, are not swollen or inflamed, and are firmly attached to the underlying tooth and bone, with minimal bleeding on probing (BOP). The dentogingival junction is a unique anatomic feature that functions to attach the gingiva to the tooth. It has an epithelial portion and a connective tissue portion, both of which are of fundamental importance for periodontal pathogenesis. The epithelial portion can be divided into three distinct epithelial structures: the gingival epithelium, the sulcular epithelium, and the junctional epithelium (Fig. 8.1). These epithelial structures are in continuity with each

Fig. 8.1 Histologic Appearance of Healthy Gingiva. A photomicrograph of a demineralized tooth with the gingival tissues in situ (hematoxylin and eosin staining, low magnification). Cementoenamel junction *(A)*. Enamel space *(ES)*. Gingival health is characterized by the organization of the epithelium into distinct zones; junctional epithelium *(A and B)*, sulcular epithelium *(B and C)*, free gingiva *(C and D)*, and attached gingiva *(D and E)*. The gingival connective tissue is composed of densely packed, organized, and interlacing collagen bundles. A few scattered inflammatory cells are present but no significant inflammatory cell infiltrate.

BOX 8.1   Characteristics of the Epithelial Component of the Dentogingival Unit

Gingival Epithelium
- Stratified squamous keratinized and parakeratinized epithelium
- Continuous with the sulcular epithelium at the gingival crest/gingival margin
- Covers the gingiva and forms the clinically visible gingival tissues
- Covers both the free and attached gingival tissues

Sulcular Epithelium
- Stratified squamous epithelium
- Nonkeratinized
- Faces the tooth surface but is not attached to it
- Forms the soft tissue lining of the gingival sulcus or the periodontal pocket

Junctional Epithelium
- Forms the epithelial attachment between the gingiva and the tooth
- Nonkeratinized
- Forms the floor of the sulcus/pocket
- Wraps around the tooth like a collar in health following the morphology of the cementoenamel junction
- Wider at the floor of the sulcus (i.e., 15–30 cells thick) and tapers apically to 3–4 cells thick
- Composed of layers of flattened squamous cells oriented parallel to the tooth surface
- Surface cells attach to the tooth surface through hemidesmosomes
- Basal lamina differs from other basal laminae that oppose connective tissue in that type IV collagen is absent

other, but they have distinct structures and functions, as indicated in Box 8.1.

Readers are referred to the online material for a detailed discussion of epithelial and connective tissue structures. Online materials for this chapter are found on the companion website www.expertconsult.com.

Even in clinically healthy gingiva, the gingival connective tissue contains at least some inflammatory cells, particularly neutrophils. Neutrophils continually migrate through the connective tissues and pass through the junctional epithelium to enter the sulcus or pocket. These findings were reported in the classic investigations of the histology of periodontal disease reported by Page and Schroeder in 1976.[148] This low-grade inflammation occurs in response to the continued presence of bacteria and their products in the gingival crevice. There is a continuous exudate of fluid from the gingival tissues that enters the crevice and flows out as gingival crevicular fluid (GCF). In addition to the continuous migration of neutrophils through the gingival tissues, lymphocytes and macrophages also accumulate. The presence of leukocytes in the connective tissues results from the chemotactic stimulus created by the subgingival biofilm and bacterial products, as well as from the chemoattractant factors produced by the host.

In clinically healthy tissues, this steady-state equilibrium between low-grade inflammation in the tissues and the continual presence of the bacterial biofilm may persist for many years or indeed for the lifetime of the individual. Overt clinical signs of gingivitis (i.e., redness, swelling, and BOP) do not develop because

of several innate and structural defense mechanisms, including the following:

- The maintenance of an intact epithelial barrier (the junctional and sulcular epithelium)
- The outflow of GCF from the sulcus (dilution effect and flushing action)
- The sloughing of surface epithelial cells of the junctional and sulcular epithelium
- The presence of neutrophils and macrophages in the sulcus that phagocytose bacteria
- The presence of antibodies in the GCF

However, if plaque accumulation increases, then inflammation and the classic clinical signs of gingivitis may develop. Although the development of gingivitis in response to the accumulation of plaque is fairly predictable, research has identified that a spectrum of responses may be observed, with some individuals developing more pronounced gingival inflammation for a given plaque challenge and others developing minimal gingival inflammation.[190] These observations underscore the importance of variations in host responses among individuals in terms of gingival inflammatory responses. The host's immune–inflammatory response is fundamental for determining which individuals may progress to developing periodontitis. The challenge that this presents clinically is that we do not yet know enough about susceptibility to periodontitis to identify these individuals before they actually develop signs of disease.

Histopathology of Gingivitis and Periodontitis

The development of gingivitis can be clearly observed from a clinical perspective. In addition, the changes that occur within the tissues are very obvious when examined under a microscope. In broad terms, infiltration of the connective tissues by numerous defense cells, particularly neutrophils, macrophages, plasma cells, and lymphocytes, is noted. As a result of the accumulation of these defense cells and the extracellular release of their destructive enzymes, disruption of the normal anatomy of the connective tissues occurs and causes collagen depletion and subsequent proliferation of the junctional epithelium. Vasodilation and increased vascular permeability lead to increased leakage of fluid out of the vessels and facilitate the passage of defense cells from the vasculature into the tissues, thus resulting in enlargement of the tissues, which appear erythematous and edematous (i.e., the clinical appearance of gingivitis). These changes are all reversible if the bacterial challenge is substantially reduced by improved oral hygiene.

The landmark studies of Page and Schroeder[148] described the histologic changes that occur in the gingival tissues as the *initial, early, established,* and *advanced* gingival lesions (Box 8.2). These are *histologic descriptions only,* and they should not form part of a clinical diagnosis. Moreover, these classic descriptions are primarily based on findings in experimental animals. The histologic appearances of gingivitis and periodontitis are shown in Figs. 8.2 and 8.3, respectively.

Readers are referred to the online material for a detailed discussion of the four histological stages proposed by Page and Schroeder. Online materials for this chapter are found on the companion website.

BOX 8.2 Key Features of the Histologic Stages of Gingivitis and Periodontitis

Initial Lesion (Corresponds With Clinically Healthy Gingival Tissues)

- Slightly elevated vascular permeability and vasodilation
- Gingival crevicular fluid flows out of the sulcus
- Migration of leukocytes, primarily neutrophils, in relatively small numbers through the gingival connective tissue, across the junctional epithelium, and into the sulcus

Early Lesion (Corresponds With Early Gingivitis That Is Evident Clinically)

- Increased vascular permeability, vasodilation, and gingival crevicular fluid flow
- Large numbers of infiltrating leukocytes (mainly neutrophils and lymphocytes)
- Degeneration of fibroblasts
- Collagen destruction that results in collagen-depleted areas of the connective tissue
- Proliferation of the junctional and sulcular epithelium into collagen-depleted areas

Established Lesion (Corresponds With Established Chronic Gingivitis)

- Dense inflammatory cell infiltrate (i.e., plasma cells, lymphocytes, and neutrophils)
- Accumulation of inflammatory cells in the connective tissues
- Elevated release of matrix metalloproteinases and lysosomal contents from neutrophils
- Significant collagen depletion and proliferation of epithelium
- Formation of pocket epithelium that contains large numbers of neutrophils

Advanced Lesion (Marks the Transition From Gingivitis to Periodontitis)

- Predominance of neutrophils in the pocket epithelium and in the pocket
- Dense inflammatory cell infiltrate in the connective tissues (primarily plasma cells)
- Apical migration of junctional epithelium to preserve an intact epithelial barrier
- Continued collagen breakdown that results in large areas of collagen-depleted connective tissue
- Osteoclastic resorption of alveolar bone

Note: These classic descriptions are primarily based on findings in experimental animals, and the correlation with the clinical situation in humans is approximate.
Adapted from Page RC, Schroeder HE: Pathogenesis of inflammatory periodontal disease: a summary of current work. *Lab Invest* 33:235–249, 1976.

Fig. 8.2 A Series of Photomicrographs Illustrating the Histologic Appearance of Gingivitis (Hematoxylin and Eosin Staining). In all cases, the tooth is to the left side of the image. (A) Low magnification of the gingiva demonstrates hyperplastic junctional and sulcular epithelium with a dense inflammatory cell infiltrate in the adjacent connective tissue. (B) Medium magnification of the epithelial–connective tissue interface shows numerous intraepithelial inflammatory cells along with intercellular edema. The connective tissue contains dilated capillaries (hyperemia), and a dense inflammatory cell infiltrate is noted. (C) High magnification shows neutrophils and small lymphocytes transiting the sulcular epithelium.

INFLAMMATORY RESPONSES IN THE PERIODONTIUM

The molecules that play a role in the pathogenesis of periodontitis can be broadly divided into two main groups: those derived from the subgingival microbiota (i.e., microbial virulence factors) and those derived from the host immune–inflammatory response. In terms of the relative importance of each, it is now clear that most of the tissue breakdown results from the host's inflammatory processes.

Fig. 8.3 Histologic Appearance of Periodontitis. A photomicrograph of adjacent demineralized teeth with the interproximal gingiva and periodontium in situ (hematoxylin and eosin staining, low magnification). The root of the tooth on the *right* is coated with a layer of dental biofilm or calculus, and attachment loss is noted with the formation of a periodontal pocket *(P)*. The periodontium is densely inflamed, and alveolar bone *(AB)* loss produces a triangular defect in addition to vertical bone loss. The base of the pocket *(BP)* is apical to the alveolar bone crest *(BC)*; this is called an *infrabony periodontal pocket.* (From Soames JV, Southam JC: *Oral pathology,* ed 4, Oxford, 2005, Oxford University Press.)

Microbial Virulence Factors

The subgingival biofilm initiates and perpetuates inflammatory responses in the gingival and periodontal tissues. The subgingival bacteria also contribute directly to tissue damage by the release of noxious substances, but their primary importance in periodontal pathogenesis is that of activating immune–inflammatory responses that, in turn, result in tissue damage, which may well be beneficial to the bacteria located within the periodontal pocket by providing nutrient sources.

Lipopolysaccharide

Lipopolysaccharides (LPSs) are large molecules composed of a lipid component (lipid A) and a polysaccharide component. They are found in the outer membrane of gram-negative bacteria, they act as endotoxins (LPS is frequently referred to as *endotoxin*), and they elicit strong immune responses in animals. LPSs are highly conserved in gram-negative bacterial species, a finding that reflects their importance in maintaining the structural integrity of the bacterial cells. Immune systems in animals have evolved to recognize LPS through Toll-like receptors (TLRs), a family of cell surface molecules that are highly conserved in animal species ranging from *Drosophila* (a genus of fruit flies) to humans, thereby reflecting their importance in innate immune responses.[30] TLRs

are cell surface receptors that recognize *microbe-associated molecular patterns* (MAMPs), which are conserved molecular structures located on pathogens. TLR-4 recognizes LPS from gram-negative bacteria and functions as part of a complex of cell surface molecules, including CD14 and MD-2 (also known as *lymphocyte antigen 96*). The interaction of this CD14/TLR-4/MD-2 complex with LPS triggers a series of intracellular events, the net results of which are the increased production of inflammatory mediators (most notably cytokines) and the differentiation of immune cells (e.g., dendritic cells) for the development of effective immune responses against the pathogens. LPS is of key importance for initiating and sustaining inflammatory responses in the gingival and periodontal tissues. *Porphyromonas gingivalis* has an atypical form of LPS that is recognized by both TLR-2 and TLR-4.[40,48]

BIOLOGIC PROPERTIES OF LIPOPOLYSACCHARIDE
- Located in the outer membrane of gram-negative bacteria
- Fundamental for maintaining structural integrity of the bacteria
- Elicits a strong response from animal immune systems
- Interacts with the CD14/TLR-4/MD-2 receptor complex on immune cells such as macrophages, monocytes, dendritic cells, and B cells, with resulting release of proinflammatory mediators such as cytokines from these cells

---

A component of gram-positive cell walls, lipoteichoic acid also stimulates immune responses, although less potently than LPS. Lipoteichoic acid signals through TLR-2. Both LPS and lipoteichoic acid are released from the bacteria present in the biofilm and stimulate inflammatory responses in the tissues, thereby resulting in increased vasodilation and vascular permeability, the recruitment of inflammatory cells by chemotaxis, and the release of proinflammatory mediators by the leukocytes that are recruited to the area.

Bacterial Enzymes and Noxious Products

Plaque bacteria produce several metabolic waste products that contribute directly to tissue damage. These include noxious agents such as ammonia (NH_3) and hydrogen sulfide (H_2S), as well as short-chain carboxylic acids such as butyric acid and propionic acid. These acids are detectable in GCF and are found in increasing concentrations as the severity of periodontal disease increases. These substances have profound effects on host cells (e.g., butyric acid induces apoptosis in T cells, B cells, fibroblasts, and gingival epithelial cells).[104,105,177] The short-chain fatty acids may aid *P. gingivalis* infection through tissue destruction, and they may also create a nutrient supply for the organism by increasing bleeding into the periodontal pocket. The short-chain fatty acids also influence cytokine secretion by immune cells, and they may potentiate inflammatory responses after exposure to proinflammatory stimuli such as LPS, interleukin-1β (IL-1β), and tumor necrosis factor alpha (TNF-α).[135]

Plaque bacteria produce proteases, which are capable of breaking down structural proteins of the periodontium such as collagen, elastin, and fibronectin. Bacteria produce these proteases to digest proteins and thereby provide peptides for bacterial nutrition. Bacterial proteases disrupt host responses, compromise tissue integrity, and facilitate the microbial invasion of the tissues. *P.*

gingivalis produces two classes of cysteine proteases that have been implicated in periodontal pathogenesis. These are known as *gingipains*, and they include the lysine-specific gingipain Kgp and the arginine-specific gingipains RgpA and RgpB. The gingipains can modulate the immune system and disrupt immune–inflammatory responses, thus potentially leading to increased tissue breakdown.[151] Gingipains can reduce the concentrations of cytokines in cell culture systems,[7] and they digest and inactivate TNF-α.[27] The gingipains can also stimulate pro-inflammatory cytokine secretion through the activation of protease-activated receptors (PARs).

Microbial Invasion

Microbial invasion of the periodontal tissues has long been a contentious topic.[12] In histologic specimens, bacteria (including cocci, filaments, and rods) have been identified in the intercellular spaces of the epithelium.[53] Periodontal pathogens such as *P. gingivalis* and *Aggregatibacter actinomycetemcomitans* have been reported to invade the gingival tissues,[32,77,163] including the connective tissues.[164] *Fusobacterium nucleatum* can invade oral epithelial cells, and bacteria that routinely invade host cells may facilitate the entry of noninvasive bacteria by coaggregating with them (Fig. 8.4).[50] It has also been shown that *A. actinomycetemcomitans* can invade epithelial cells and persist intracellularly.[52] The clinical relevance of these various findings is unclear, however, and more recent studies have reported that although species such as *P. gingivalis* can be found located within the tissues, they are mainly within the epithelium, and it is unusual for the bacteria to reach the connective tissue until extensive tissue destruction has occurred, and even then it is as a result of inflammation rather than "invading" bacteria.[12]

CLINICAL CORRELATION

Is Bacterial Invasion of the Tissues a Valid Concept, and Does It Have Implications for Therapy?
Good evidence indicates that certain species of subgingival bacteria are able to invade epithelial cells, thereby providing a shelter from the host defenses (and also highlighting the important role of epithelium in host defenses by release of cytokines to activate inflammatory responses). However, invasion of the deeper connective tissues by live bacteria such as *Porphyromonas gingivalis* seems to occur (if it occurs!) at a much later stage in advanced disease, probably as a result of inflammation and resultant tissue destruction. Reports of bacteria present in the tissues (described as a "reservoir of infection") have sometimes been used to justify the use of antibiotics for treatment of periodontitis as a means to try to eliminate those organisms that are located in the tissues and that are therefore "protected" from mechanical disruption by root surface debridement. However, until the clinical relevance of the presence of bacteria in the tissues is better defined, it is inappropriate to make clinical treatment decisions (e.g., whether to use adjunctive systemic antibiotics) on this premise alone.

Fimbriae

The fimbriae of certain bacterial species, particularly *P. gingivalis*, may also play a role in periodontal pathogenesis. *P. gingivalis* fimbriae stimulate immune responses, such as IL-6 secretion,[106,141] and the major fimbrial structural component of *P. gingivalis*, FimA, has been shown to stimulate nuclear factor (NF)-κB and IL-8 in a gingival epithelial cell line through TLR-2.[6] Monocytes are also stimulated by *P. gingivalis* FimA, secreting IL-6, IL-8, and TNF-α.[51] *P. gingivalis* fimbriae also interact with complement receptor-3 (CR-3) to activate intracellular signaling pathways that inhibit IL-12 production mediated by TLR-2 signaling.[69]

Fig. 8.4 Invasion of Epithelial Cells by *Fusobacterium nucleatum*. In both images, a single epithelial cell is shown being penetrated by invading *F. nucleatum* bacteria; three or four bacteria are evident in (A), and one bacterium is evident in (B). (A) The ruffled surface of the epithelial cells (multiple small fingerlike projections that are much smaller than the *F. nucleatum* bacteria) is likely to be an artifact. (B) *F. nucleatum* may facilitate the colonization of epithelial cells by bacteria that are unable to adhere or invade directly as evidenced by the single coccoid bacterium *(Streptococcus cristatus)* that has coaggregated with the *F. nucleatum* bacterium as it penetrates the epithelial cell. (A and B, Courtesy Dr. A.E. Edwards, Imperial College, London, UK; Dr. J.D. Rudney, Bath University, Bath, UK; and Dr. T.J. Grossman, the University of Minnesota, Minneapolis, MN.)

This may be of clinical relevance because IL-12 is important in the activation of natural killer (NK) cells and CD8+ cytotoxic T cells, which themselves may be important in killing *P. gingivalis*–infected host cells, such as epithelial cells. Indeed, the blockade of the CR-3 receptor promotes IL-12–mediated clearance of *P. gingivalis* and negates its virulence.[69] Bacterial fimbriae are therefore important for modifying and stimulating immune responses in the periodontium.

Bacterial Deoxyribonucleic Acid and Extracellular Deoxyribonucleic Acid

Bacterial deoxyribonucleic acid (DNA) stimulates immune cells through TLR-9, which recognizes hypomethylated CpG regions of the DNA.[102] (CpG sites are regions of DNA at which a cytosine nucleotide is found next to a guanine nucleotide, separated by a phosphate molecule, which links the C and G nucleotides together, hence "CpG".) Extracellular DNA (eDNA) is a ubiquitous constituent of all biofilms and of particular interest in biofilms associated with chronic diseases such as periodontitis.[86] eDNA is derived from the chromosomal DNA of bacteria in biofilms, and the majority of eDNA is released after bacterial cell lysis.[2,185] However, evidence also indicates that eDNA secretion may occur from bacterial cells by mechanisms that are independent of cell lysis.[70,158] The significance of this finding is not yet clear, but such "donated" DNA may be used by bacterial species as a means of increasing genetic diversity (if taken up by other bacteria), thereby contributing to antigenic variation and the spread of antibiotic resistance, and they may also modulate the host immune response. Thus eDNA may function as a source of genetic information for naturally transformable bacteria in the biofilm[196] or as a stimulus for host immunity. Perhaps more important, it is becoming increasingly clear that eDNA plays a number of important roles in biofilm integrity and formation on hard and soft tissues in the oral cavity. These include roles in adhesion and biofilm formation, protection against antimicrobial agents, and nutrient storage, as well as genetic exchange, and it is possible that eDNA may ultimately prove to be an important target for biofilm control.[86]

Host-Derived Inflammatory Mediators

The inflammatory and immune processes that develop in the periodontal tissues in response to the long-term presence of the subgingival biofilm are protective by intent but can result in considerable tissue damage, thereby leading to the clinical signs and symptoms of periodontal disease. It is paradoxical that the host response causes most of the tissue damage, although this is not unique to periodontal disease. For example, the tissue damage that occurs in the joints in patients with rheumatoid arthritis results from prolonged and excessive inflammatory responses, and it is characterized by the increased production of many of the cytokines that are also known to be important in periodontal pathogenesis. In the case of rheumatoid arthritis, the initiating factor is an autoimmune response to structural components of the joint; in periodontitis, the initiating factor is the subgingival biofilm. In both cases, the destructive inflammatory events are remarkably similar, although the pathogenesis varies as a result of the different anatomy. Key types of mediators

that orchestrate the host responses in periodontitis are summarized in the following subsections.

Cytokines

Cytokines play a fundamental role in inflammation, and they are key inflammatory mediators in periodontal disease.[155] They are soluble proteins, and they act as messengers to transmit signals from one cell to another. Cytokines bind to specific receptors on target cells and initiate intracellular signaling cascades that result in phenotypic changes in the cell by altered gene regulation.[18,183] Cytokines are effective in very low concentrations, they are produced transiently in the tissues, and they primarily act locally in the tissues in which they are produced. Cytokines are able to induce their own expression in either an autocrine or paracrine fashion, and they have pleiotropic effects (i.e., multiple biologic activities) on a large number of cell types. (Autocrine signaling means that the autocrine agent [in this case cytokines] binds to receptors on the cell that secreted the agent, whereas paracrine signaling affects other nearby cells.) Simply put, cytokines bind to cell surface receptors and trigger a sequence of intracellular events that lead ultimately to the production of protein by the target cell that alters that cell's behavior and could result in, for example, the increased secretion of more cytokines in a positive feedback loop.

Cytokines are produced by a large number of cell types, including infiltrating inflammatory cells (e.g., neutrophils, macrophages, lymphocytes), as well as resident cells in the periodontium (e.g., fibroblasts, epithelial cells). Cytokines signal, broadcast, and amplify immune responses, and they are fundamentally important for regulating immune–inflammatory responses and for combating infections. They have profound biologic effects that also lead to tissue damage with chronic inflammation; the prolonged and excessive production of cytokines and other inflammatory mediators in the periodontium leads to the tissue damage that characterizes the clinical signs of the disease. For example, cytokines mediate connective tissue and alveolar bone destruction through the induction of fibroblasts and osteoclasts to produce proteolytic enzymes (i.e., MMPs) that break down structural components of these connective tissues.[11]

Significant overlap and redundancy exist in the functions of individual cytokines. Cytokines do not act in isolation; rather, they function in flexible and complex networks that involve both proinflammatory and antiinflammatory effects and that bring together aspects of both innate and acquired immunity.[8] Cytokines play a key role at all stages of the immune response in periodontal diseases.[155]

Prostaglandins

The prostaglandins (PGs) are a group of lipid compounds derived from arachidonic acid, a polyunsaturated fatty acid found in the plasma membrane of most cells. Arachidonic acid is metabolized by cyclooxygenase-1 and 2 (COX-1 and COX-2) to generate a series of related compounds called the *prostanoids*, which include the PGs, the thromboxanes, and the prostacyclins. PGs are important mediators of inflammation, particularly prostaglandin E_2 (PGE_2), which results in vasodilation and induces cytokine production by a variety of cell types. COX-2 is up-regulated by

IL-1β, TNF-α, and bacterial LPS, thus resulting in increased production of PGE_2 in inflamed tissues. PGE_2 is produced by various types of cells and most significantly in the periodontium by macrophages and fibroblasts. PGE_2 results in the induction of MMPs and osteoclastic bone resorption, and it has a major role in contributing to the tissue damage that characterizes periodontitis.

Matrix Metalloproteinases

MMPs are a family of proteolytic enzymes that degrade extracellular matrix molecules such as collagen, gelatin, and elastin. They are produced by a variety of cell types, including neutrophils, macrophages, fibroblasts, epithelial cells, osteoblasts, and osteoclasts. The names and functions of key MMPs are shown in Table 8.1. The nomenclature of MMPs has been based on the perception that each enzyme has its own specific substrate; However, it is now appreciated that MMPs usually degrade multiple substrates, with significant substrate overlap among individual MMPs.[72]

MMPs are secreted in a latent form (inactive) and are activated by the proteolytic cleavage of a portion of the latent enzyme. This is achieved by proteases, such as cathepsin G, produced by neutrophils. MMPs are inhibited by proteinase inhibitors, which have antiinflammatory properties. Key inhibitors of MMPs found in the serum include the glycoprotein α_1-antitrypsin and α_2-macroglobulin, a large plasma protein produced by the liver that is capable of inactivating a wide variety of proteinases. Inhibitors of MMPs that are found in the tissues include the tissue inhibitors of metalloproteinases (TIMPs), which are produced by many cell types; the most important in periodontal disease is TIMP-1.[19]

MMPs are also inhibited by the tetracycline class of antibiotics, which has led to the development of a subantimicrobial formulation of doxycycline as an adjunctive systemic drug treatment for periodontitis. Doxycycline, like all the tetracyclines, possesses the ability to down-regulate MMPs, and this was recognized as representing a potential novel treatment strategy for periodontitis. The subantimicrobial formulation has been shown to inhibit collagenase activity in the gingival tissues and GCF of patients with chronic periodontitis,[63] and some clinical trials have investigated the clinical effect of using this formulation of doxycycline as an adjunct to periodontal therapy.[153]

TABLE 8.1 Classification of Matrix Metalloproteinases

Group	Enzyme	Name
Collagenases	MMP-1	Collagenase 1, fibroblast collagenase
	MMP-8	Collagenase 2, neutrophil collagenase
	MMP-13	Collagenase 3
Gelatinases	MMP-2	Gelatinase A
	MMP-9	Gelatinase B
Stromelysins	MMP-3	Stromelysin 1
	MMP-10	Stromelysin 2
	MMP-11	Stromelysin 3
Matrilysins	MMP-7	Matrilysin 1, pump-1
	MMP-26	Matrilysin 2
Membrane-type MMPs	MMP-14	MT1-MMP
	MMP-15	MT2-MMP
	MMP-16	MT3-MMP
	MMP-17	MT4-MMP
	MMP-24	MT5-MMP
	MMP-25	MT6-MMP
Others	MMP-12	Macrophage elastase
	MMP-19	—
	MMP-20	Enamelysin

MMPs, Matrix metalloproteinases; *MT,* membrane type.
Adapted from Hannas AR, Pereira JC, Granjeiro JM, et al: The role of matrix metalloproteinases in the oral environment. *Acta Odontol Scand* 65:1–13, 2007.

PROPERTIES OF KEY TYPES OF INFLAMMATORY MEDIATORS IN PERIODONTITIS

Cytokines	Proteins that transmit signals from one cell to another
	Bind to cell surface receptors to trigger production of protein by the cell
	There are proinflammatory and antiinflammatory cytokines.
	A key proinflammatory cytokine is interleukin-1β, which up-regulates inflammatory responses and is produced by multiple cell types in the periodontium.
Prostaglandins	Lipid compounds derived from arachidonic acid
	Prostaglandin E_2 (PGE_2) is a key inflammatory mediator, stimulating production of other inflammatory mediators and cytokine production.
	PGE_2 also stimulates bone resorption and plays a key role in periodontitis progression.
Matrix metalloproteinases (MMPs)	A group of enzymes that break down structural proteins of the body
	MMPs include collagenases, which break down collagen.
	Key MMPs in periodontitis include MMP-8 and MMP-9, which are produced by neutrophils as they migrate through the periodontal tissues, thus contributing to periodontal tissue breakdown.

Role of Specific Inflammatory Mediators in Periodontal Disease

Interleukin-1 Family Cytokines

The IL-1 family of cytokines comprises at least 11 members, including IL-1α, IL-1β, IL-1 receptor antagonist (IL-1Ra), IL-18, and IL-33.[155]

IL-1β plays a key role in inflammation and immunity; it is closely linked to the innate immune response, and it induces the synthesis and secretion of other mediators that contribute to inflammatory changes and tissue damage. For example, IL-1β stimulates the synthesis of PGE_2, platelet-activating factor, and nitrous oxide, thereby resulting in vascular changes associated with inflammation and increasing blood flow to the site of infection or tissue injury. IL-1β is mainly produced by monocytes, macrophages, and neutrophils and also by other cell types such as fibroblasts, keratinocytes, epithelial cells, B cells, and osteocytes.[42] IL-1β increases the expression of ICAM-1 on endothelial cells and stimulates the secretion of the chemokine CXCL8 (IL-8), thereby stimulating and facilitating the infiltration of neutrophils into the affected tissues. IL-1β also synergizes with other proinflammatory cytokines and PGE_2 to induce bone resorption. IL-1β has a role in adaptive immunity; it regulates the development of antigen-presenting cells (APCs) (e.g., dendritic cells), stimulates IL-6 secretion by macrophages (which, in turn, activates B cells), and has been shown to enhance the antigen-mediated stimulation of T cells.[14] GCF concentrations of IL-1β are increased at sites affected by gingivitis[74] and periodontitis,[108] and tissue levels of IL-1β correlate with clinical periodontal disease severity.[178] Studies in experimental animals have shown that IL-1β exacerbates inflammation and alveolar bone resorption.[105] It is clear from the multiplicity of studies that have investigated this cytokine that IL-1β plays a fundamental role in the pathogenesis of periodontal disease.[110]

IL-1α is primarily an intracellular protein that is not normally secreted and that therefore is not usually found in the extracellular environment or in the circulation.[46] Unlike IL-1β, biologically active IL-1α is constitutively expressed and likely mediates inflammation only when it is released from necrotic cells, thus acting as an "alarmin" to signal the immune system during cell and tissue damage.[17] The precise role of IL-1α in periodontal pathogenesis is not well defined, although studies have reported elevated IL-1α levels in GCF and gingival tissues in patients with periodontitis.[156] IL-1α is a potent bone-resorbing factor involved in the bone loss that is associated with inflammation.[181] It is possible that the measured level of IL-1α in gingival tissues represents intracellular IL-1α that has been released from damaged or necrotic cells, and it is probable that IL-1α plays a role in periodontal pathogenesis, possibly as a signaling cytokine (signaling tissue damage) and contributing to bone resorptive activity.

IL-1Ra has structural homology to IL-1β, and it binds to the IL-1 receptor (IL-1R1). However, the binding of IL-1Ra does not result in signal transduction; therefore, IL-1Ra antagonizes the action of IL-1β.[45] IL-1Ra is important for the regulation of inflammatory responses, and it can be considered an antiinflammatory cytokine. IL-1Ra levels have been reported to be elevated in the GCF and tissues of patients with periodontal disease, thereby suggesting that it has a role in immunoregulation in cases of periodontitis.[160]

Readers are referred to the online material for a detailed discussion of other interleukin family of cytokines. Online materials for this chapter are found on the companion website.

IL-33, which is also known as IL-1F11, is of interest because, uniquely among the IL-1 cytokines, it stimulates the production of Th2 cytokines (e.g., IL-5, IL-13), it activates Th2 cells, and it plays a role in mast cell development and function.[1,78,98,128,167] IL-33 is mainly found in nonimmune cells such as bronchial and arterial smooth muscle cells and epithelial cells from the

bronchus.[167] It is constitutively expressed in the endothelial cells of small and large blood vessels, in the fibroblastic reticular cells of lymphoid tissues, and in epithelial cells.[28,129] Our knowledge of the expression of IL-33 in myeloid immune cells and of any role in periodontitis pathogenesis is very limited. However, it has been reported that IL-33 activates Th2 cells[167] and is chemoattractant for these cells.[98] Given that Th2 cells are likely to play a role in the destructive phases of periodontal disease and that the balance of T-cell subsets is an important factor in determining disease progression,[59] IL-33 may yet prove to play a role in periodontal pathogenesis.

Tumor necrosis factor α. TNF-α is a key inflammatory mediator in periodontal disease, and it shares many of the cellular actions of IL-1β.[66] It plays a fundamental role in immune responses, it increases neutrophil activity, and it mediates cell and tissue turnover by inducing MMP secretion. TNF-α stimulates the development of osteoclasts and limits tissue repair by the induction of apoptosis in fibroblasts. TNF-α is secreted by activated macrophages, as well as by other cell types, particularly in response to bacterial LPS. The proinflammatory effects of TNF-α include the stimulation of endothelial cells to express selectins that facilitate leukocyte recruitment, the activation of macrophage IL-1β production, and the induction of PGE_2 by macrophages and gingival fibroblasts.[146] TNF-α—although possessing similar activity to IL-1β—has a less potent effect on osteoclasts, and it is present at lower levels in inflamed gingival tissues than IL-1β.[179] GCF levels of TNF-α increase as gingival inflammation develops, and higher levels are found in individuals with periodontitis.[66,74]

Interleukin-6 and Related Cytokines

The cytokines in this group—which include IL-6, IL-11, leukemia-inhibitory factor (LIF), and oncostatin M—share common signaling pathways through signal transducers gp 130.[75] IL-6 is the most extensively studied of this group, and it has pleiotropic proinflammatory properties.[94] IL-6 secretion is stimulated by cytokines such as IL-1β and TNF-α, and it is produced by a range of immune cells (e.g., T cells, B cells, macrophages, dendritic cells), as well as resident cells (e.g., keratinocytes, endothelial cells, fibroblasts).[193] IL-6 is also secreted by osteoblasts, and it stimulates bone resorption and the development of osteoclasts.[85,103] IL-6 is elevated in the cells, tissues, and GCF of patients with periodontal disease.[58,113] IL-6 may have an influence on monocyte differentiation into osteoclasts and a role in bone resorption in patients with periodontal disease.[142] IL-6 also has a key role in regulating the proliferation and differentiation of B cells and T cells, particularly the Th17 subset.[94] IL-6 therefore has an important role in periodontal pathogenesis, although less than that of IL-1β or TNF-α.

IL-6 also has many activities outside of the immune system, such as in the cardiovascular and nervous systems. It has an important role in hematopoiesis and in signaling the production of C-reactive protein (CRP) in the liver. Furthermore, IL-6 stimulates T-cell differentiation and function, and it is important in the regulation of the balance of T-cell subsets, particularly the activation of Th17 cells (a subset of T cells that produce IL-17) and their balance with regulatory T cells (T_{reg} cells).[15]

Prostaglandin E₂

The cells primarily responsible for PGE$_2$ production in the periodontium are macrophages and fibroblasts. PGE$_2$ levels are increased in the tissues and in GCF at sites undergoing periodontal attachment loss. PGE$_2$ induces the secretion of MMPs, as well as osteoclastic bone resorption, and it contributes significantly to the alveolar bone loss seen with periodontitis. PGE$_2$ release from monocytes from patients with severe or aggressive periodontitis is greater than that from monocytes from patients who are periodontally healthy.[57,140] A large body of evidence has demonstrated the importance of PGE$_2$ in periodontal pathogenesis, and given that PGs are inhibited by nonsteroidal antiinflammatory drugs (NSAIDs), researchers have investigated the use of NSAIDs as potential host–response modulators in the management of periodontal disease.[199,200] However, daily administration for extended periods is necessary for the periodontal benefits to become apparent, and NSAIDs are associated with significant unwanted side effects, including gastrointestinal (GI) problems, hemorrhage (from impaired platelet aggregation resulting from inhibition of thromboxane formation), and renal and hepatic impairment. NSAIDs are therefore not indicated as adjunctive treatments for the management of periodontitis.

The PGs, including PGE$_2$, are derived from the COX pathway of arachidonic acid metabolism. The two main isoforms of the COX enzyme are COX-1 and COX-2. COX-1 is constitutively expressed and has antithrombogenic and cytoprotective functions. COX-2 is induced after stimulation with various cytokines, growth factors, and LPS. The inhibition of COX-1 by nonselective NSAIDs results in the majority of the unwanted side effects associated with NSAID usage, such as GI ulceration and impaired hemostasis. The induction of COX-2 results in the production of elevated quantities of PGs (e.g., PGE$_2$); therefore, the inhibition of COX-2 by NSAIDs that selectively inhibit COX-2 results in a reduction of inflammation without the unwanted effects commonly seen after long-term NSAID use. Preliminary studies in animal models have shown that selective COX-2 inhibitors slowed alveolar bone loss,[16,79] and human studies confirmed that PG production in the periodontal tissues was modified.[194] However, in a dramatic and unfortunate development, the selective COX-2 inhibitors were later identified to be associated with significant and life-threatening adverse events, thereby resulting in several of these drugs being withdrawn from the market.[49] The selective COX-2 inhibitors therefore cannot be considered as adjunctive treatments for periodontal disease.

Matrix Metalloproteinases

MMPs are a family of zinc-dependent enzymes that are capable of degrading extracellular matrix molecules, including collagens.[19,162] MMPs play a key role in periodontal tissue destruction and are secreted by the majority of cell types in the periodontium, including fibroblasts, keratinocytes, endothelial cells, osteoclasts, neutrophils, and macrophages. In healthy tissues, MMPs are mainly produced by fibroblasts, which produce MMP-1 (also known as *collagenase-1*), and these have a role in the maintenance of the periodontal connective tissues. The transcription of genes coding for MMPs is up-regulated by cytokines such as IL-1β

and TNF-α.[119] MMP activity is regulated by specific endogenous TIMPs and serum gps such as α-macroglobulins, which form complexes with active MMPs and their latent precursors.[159] TIMPs are produced by fibroblasts, macrophages, keratinocytes, and endothelial cells; they are specific inhibitors that bind to MMPs in a 1:1 stoichiometry.[72] MMPs are also produced by some periodontal pathogens, such as *A. actinomycetemcomitans* and *P. gingivalis,* but the relative contribution of these bacterially derived MMPs to periodontal pathogenesis is small. Most MMP activity in the periodontal tissues is derived from infiltrating inflammatory cells.

Readers are referred to the online material for a further discussion of MMPs. Online materials for this chapter are found on the companion website.

Chemokines

Chemokines are cytokine-like molecules that are characterized by their chemotactic activity.[30] This activity gave rise to the term *chemokine* (i.e., they are chemotactic cytokines). Chemokines orchestrate leukocyte recruitment in physiologic and pathologic conditions,[21] so they are important for periodontal pathogenesis, which results in the chemotactic migration of neutrophils through the periodontal tissues toward the site of the bacterial challenge in the periodontal pocket.[176] Chemokines play a key role in neutrophil recruitment and the recruitment of other adaptive and innate immune cells to the site of immune and inflammatory responses. The chemokines are divided into two subfamilies according to structural similarity: the CC subfamily and the CXC subfamily.[174] The chemokine CXCL8, which is more familiarly known as IL-8, has been demonstrated to be localized in the gingival tissues in areas of plaque accumulation and in the presence of neutrophilic infiltration,[187] and it has also been found in GCF.[121] Interaction between bacteria and keratinocytes results in the up-regulation of IL-8 and ICAM-1 expression in the gingival epithelium and the development of a chemotactic gradient of these molecules in the gingiva, thereby stimulating neutrophil migration into the tissues and the gingival sulcus.[186,189] Similar chemotactic gradients are also present in the gingiva of periodontally healthy individuals; this suggests a role for this process in the maintenance of periodontal health and supports the findings of infiltrating neutrophils being present even in clinically healthy tissues.[188]

It is becoming clear that chemokines play an important role in leukocyte migration in periodontal disease. CCL2 and CCL5 (also known as *regulated on activation, normal T-cell expressed and secreted* [RANTES]) play a role in macrophage migration, and CCL3 (also known as *macrophage inflammatory protein-1α* [MIP-1α]) and CXCL10 play a role in T-cell migration in inflamed periodontal tissues.[176] Chemokines play important roles in immune responses, repair, and inflammation, and they regulate osteoclast activity by influencing myeloid cell differentiation into osteoclasts, which may be of particular importance in the context of periodontitis.

Antiinflammatory Cytokines

The balance between proinflammatory and antiinflammatory events is crucial for determining disease progression, and it is now clear that individual cytokines do not act in isolation but rather as part of complex networks of mediators that have different functional activities. Antiinflammatory cytokines include IL-10, TGF-β, IL-1Ra, IL-1F5, and possibly IL-1F10.

The IL-10 family of cytokines has multiple pleiotropic effects and possesses immunosuppressive properties.[34,36] IL-10 is produced by T_{reg} cells, monocytes, and B cells, and it suppresses cytokine secretion by Th1 cells, Th2 cells, monocytes, and macrophages. The role of IL-10 in periodontal disease has been minimally studied, but animal models support that IL-10 down-regulates inflammatory responses. For example, IL-10 knockout mice are more susceptible to alveolar bone loss than wild-type mice.[165] IL-10 is also present in GCF and periodontal tissues.[80]

TGF-β is a growth factor that functions as a cytokine and has immunoregulatory roles, such as the regulation of T-cell subsets and the action of T_{reg} cells, and it also plays a role in repair and regeneration.[201] It has multifunctional roles in various cellular functions, including angiogenesis, the synthesis of the extracellular matrix, apoptosis, and the inhibition of cell growth. TGF-β levels are higher in the GCF and periodontal tissues of patients with periodontitis and gingivitis than in patients who are periodontally healthy.[71]

LINKING PATHOGENESIS TO CLINICAL SIGNS OF DISEASE

Advanced forms of periodontal disease are characterized by the symptoms of tooth mobility, tooth loss, and tooth migration. These result from the loss of attachment between the tooth and its supporting tissues after the breakdown of the inserting fibers of the periodontal ligament and the resorption of alveolar bone. Having reviewed the histopathology and the inflammatory processes that develop in the periodontal tissues as a result of prolonged accumulation of dental biofilm, it is now necessary to link these changes to the structural damage that occurs in the periodontium, thereby leading to the well-defined signs of disease.

Even clinically healthy tissues demonstrate signs of inflammation when histologic sections are examined. For example, transmigrating neutrophils are evident in clinically healthy gingival tissues moving toward the sulcus for the purpose of eliminating bacteria. If the inflammation becomes more extensive, then vasodilation and increased vascular permeability lead to edema of the tissues, as well as erythema, thereby causing gingival swelling and a slight deepening of the sulcus and further compromising plaque removal. The increased infiltration of inflammatory cells (particularly neutrophils) and the breakdown of collagen result in the development of collagen-depleted areas below the epithelium; as a result, the epithelium proliferates to maintain tissue integrity.

The epithelium provides a physical barrier to impede the ingress of bacteria and their products; therefore, the disruption of the epithelial barrier can lead to further bacterial invasion and inflammation. Antimicrobial peptides (AMPs), which are also called *defensins,* are expressed by epithelial cells, and gingival epithelial cells express two human β-defensins (hBD-1 and hBD-2). Furthermore, a cathelicidin class AMP, LL-37, which is found in the lysosomes of neutrophils, is also expressed in gingiva. These AMPss are important for determining the outcomes of the host–pathogen interactions at the epithelial barrier.[197] The epithelium is therefore more than simply a passive barrier: it also has an active role in innate immunity.[39] Epithelial cells in the junctional and sulcular epithelium are in constant contact with bacterial products and respond to these products by secreting chemokines (e.g., IL-8, CXCL8) to attract neutrophils, which migrate up the chemotactic gradient toward the pocket. Epithelial cells are therefore active in responding to infection and signaling further host responses.

If the bacterial challenge persists, the cellular and fluid infiltrate continues to develop, and neutrophils and other inflammatory cells soon occupy a significant volume of the inflamed gingival tissues. Neutrophils are key components of the innate immune system, and they play a fundamental role in maintaining periodontal health, despite the constant challenge presented by the plaque biofilm.[134] Neutrophils are protective leukocytes that phagocytose and kill bacteria, and deficiencies in neutrophil functioning result in increased susceptibility to infections in general, as well as periodontal disease.[109] Neutrophils also release large quantities of destructive enzymes (e.g., MMPs) as they migrate through the tissues (particularly MMP-8 and MMP-9), a process that results in the breakdown of structural components of the periodontium and the development of collagen-depleted areas. Neutrophils also release their potent lysosomal enzymes, cytokines, and reactive oxygen species (ROS) extracellularly, thereby causing further tissue damage.[89] Neutrophil hyperactivity in periodontitis has also been suggested, which leads to the overproduction of damaging ROS and other mediators.[55] Patients with periodontitis have been reported to have neutrophils that demonstrate enhanced enzymatic activity and that produce increased levels of ROS.[122,123] However, it is not yet clear whether the enhanced responsiveness of neutrophils is the result of the innate properties of the neutrophils in certain individuals, of priming by cytokines or bacteria, or of a combination of these factors. It is certainly clear, however, that the extracellular release of lysosomal enzymes contributes to continued tissue damage and collagen depletion in the periodontal tissues. The degeneration of fibroblasts limits opportunities for repair, and the epithelium continues to proliferate apically, thus deepening the pocket further; the pocket is then rapidly colonized by the subgingival bacteria.

The very first steps in the development of the pocket result from a combination of factors, including the detachment of cells at the coronal aspect of the junctional epithelium, whereas cells at the apical aspect migrate apically into the collagen-depleted areas; intraepithelial cleavage occurs within the junctional epithelium.[115,170,180] Epithelial tissues do not have their own blood supply and must rely on the diffusion of nutrients from the underlying connective tissues. Thus, as the epithelium proliferates and thickens, necrosis of epithelial cells that are more distant from the connective tissues can lead to intraepithelial clefts and splits, which also contribute to the early stages of pocket formation.

CLINICIAN'S CORNER

How Does a Pocket Develop?

The bacterial biofilm causes inflammation in the gingival tissues that causes swelling, and therefore the sulcus deepens slightly. The inflammatory response may subsequently spread to the deeper tissues and is characterized by infiltration by defense cells and breakdown of collagen in the connective tissues. The junctional epithelium migrates apically to maintain an intact epithelial barrier, and thus the sulcus becomes deeper again and is now referred to as a pocket. Bacteria in the biofilm proliferate apically, exploiting and perpetuating this environmental niche. The bacteria are never completely eradicated by the host response, and thus they continue to provoke an immune–inflammatory response, leading to progressing tissue breakdown, continued apical migration of the junctional epithelium, resorption of alveolar bone, and gradual deepening of the pocket.

A cycle of chronic inflammation is therefore established in which the presence of subgingival bacteria drives inflammatory responses in the periodontal tissues; this is characterized by infiltration by leukocytes, the release of inflammatory mediators and destructive enzymes, connective tissue breakdown, and the breakdown and proliferation of the epithelium in an apical direction. The junctional and pocket epithelia become thin and ulcerated and bleed more readily, a condition that results in BOP. The bacteria in the pocket are never fully eliminated because they are effectively outside the body, but their continued presence drives the destructive inflammatory response in the periodontal tissues. Attempts at effective oral hygiene are rendered more difficult by the deepening of the pocket, and the cycle continues.

Alveolar Bone Resorption

As the advancing inflammatory front approaches the alveolar bone, osteoclastic bone resorption commences.[33] This is a protective mechanism to prevent bacterial invasion of the bone, but it ultimately leads to tooth mobility and even tooth loss. The resorption of alveolar bone occurs simultaneously with the breakdown of the periodontal ligament in the inflamed periodontal tissues. Two critical factors determine whether bone loss occurs: (1) the concentration of inflammatory mediators in the gingival tissues must be sufficient to activate the pathways that lead to bone resorption; and (2) the inflammatory mediators must penetrate to within a critical distance of the alveolar bone.[66]

Histologic studies have confirmed that the bone resorbs so that a width of noninfiltrated connective tissue of about 0.5 to 1.0 mm overlying the bone is always present.[195] It has also been demonstrated that bone resorption ceases when at least a 2.5-mm distance is present between the site of bacteria in the pocket and the bone.[149] Osteoclasts are stimulated by proinflammatory cytokines and other mediators of inflammation to resorb the bone, and the alveolar bone "retreats" from the advancing inflammatory front. Osteoclasts are multinucleated cells that are formed from osteoclast progenitor cells and macrophages, and osteoclastic bone resorption is activated by a variety of mediators (e.g., IL-1β, TNF-α, IL-6, PGE$_2$).[131] Other mediators that also stimulate bone resorption include LIF, oncostatin M, bradykinin, thrombin, and various chemokines.[110]

Receptor Activator of Nuclear Factor-κB Ligand and Osteoprotegerin

A key system for controlling bone turnover is the receptor activator of the NF-κB (RANK)/RANK ligand (RANKL)/osteoprotegerin (OPG) system. RANK is a cell surface receptor expressed by osteoclast progenitor cells, as well as by mature osteoclasts. RANKL is a ligand that binds to RANK and is produced as either a membrane-bound or secreted protein by a range of cells, including fibroblasts, osteoblasts, mesenchymal cells, and T- and B-lymphocytes. OPG is the inhibitor of RANKL and functions as a decoy receptor—that is, it binds to RANKL and prevents it from interacting with RANK. OPG is secreted primarily by osteoblasts, fibroblasts, and bone marrow stromal cells. The binding of RANKL to RANK results in osteoclast differentiation and activation, and thus bone resorption. The balance between RANKL and OPG activity (often referred to as the *RANKL:OPG ratio*) can therefore determine bone resorption or bone formation.

IL-1β and TNF-α regulate the expression of RANKL and OPG, and T cells express RANKL, which binds directly to RANK on the surfaces of osteoclast progenitors and osteoclasts, thereby resulting in cell activation and differentiation to form mature osteoclasts. In individuals with periodontitis, elevated levels of proinflammatory cytokines (e.g., IL-1β, TNF-α) and increasing numbers of infiltrating T cells result in the activation of osteoclasts by RANK, which results in alveolar bone loss. It has been reported that levels of RANKL are higher and that levels of OPG are lower in sites with active periodontal breakdown as compared with sites with healthy gingiva.[37] In addition, GCF RANKL/OPG ratios are higher in periodontitis than in healthy tissue.[23] It is clear that alterations in the relative levels of these key regulators of osteoclasts play a key role in the bone loss that characterizes periodontal disease.

RANK/RANKL/OPG SYSTEM

RANK (receptor activator of nuclear factor-κB)	Cell surface receptor on osteoclast progenitor cells
RANKL (RANK ligand)	Cytokine-like molecule that is the ligand for RANK (i.e., binds to RANK) and causes maturation into fully98888z differentiated osteoclasts
OPG (osteoprotegerin)	Cytokine-like molecule that binds to RANKL and inhibits the interaction between RANKL and RANK

The RANK/RANKL/OPG signaling pathway plays a key role in regulating bone resorption. RANKL binds to RANK and stimulates osteoclast differentiation and activation. OPG antagonizes this action by binding to RANKL and preventing it from binding to RANK. The ratio of RANKL to OPG is important, with studies reporting higher levels of RANKL and lower levels of OPG in patients with advanced periodontitis compared with healthy controls.

RESOLUTION OF INFLAMMATION

Inflammation is an important defense mechanism to combat the threat of bacterial infection, but inflammation also results in tissue damage associated with the development and progression of most chronic diseases associated with aging, including periodontal disease.[191,192] It is becoming evident that the resolution of inflammation (i.e., "turning off" inflammation) is an active process that is regulated by specific mechanisms that restore homeostasis (see Chapter 10). It is possible that controlling or augmenting these mechanisms may lead to the development of new treatment strategies for managing chronic diseases such as periodontitis.[90] The resolution of inflammation is an active process that results in a return to homeostasis, and it is mediated by specific molecules, including a class of endogenous, proresolving lipid mediators that includes the lipoxins, resolvins, and protectins.[171]

IMMUNE RESPONSES IN PERIODONTAL PATHOGENESIS

The immune system is essential for the maintenance of periodontal health, and it is central to the host response to periodontal pathogens. However, if the immune response is dysregulated, inappropriate, persistent, or excessive in some way, then damaging chronic inflammatory responses such as those observed in periodontal disease can ensue. The immune response to plaque bacteria involves the integration at the molecular, cellular, and organ level of elements that are often categorized as being part of the innate immune system or the adaptive immune system. It is now widely appreciated that immune responses are complex biologic networks in which pathogen recognition, innate immunity, and adaptive immunity are integrated and mutually dependent.[54] This complex network is flexible and dynamic, with aspects of positive and negative regulation, as well as feedback control; signals are amplified and broadcast, which leads to diverse effector functions. Furthermore, the immune system is integrated with other systems and processes, including the nervous system, hematopoiesis, and hemostasis, as well as elements of tissue repair and regeneration.[132]

Observational studies of periodontal tissues and investigations of animal models and cell and tissue systems have allowed us to identify aspects of the immune response that are relevant to periodontitis.[101,148] Immune responses, which underpin periodontal disease, have unique facets that must be considered before we can truly rationalize the detailed information that we have about individual immune cell functions and their responses to specific periodontal pathogens. Thus we need to understand how the polymicrobial biofilm (as opposed to individual species of periodontal pathogens) interacts with host immune defenses. We also need to appreciate specific immunologic properties that relate to the unique anatomy of the periodontium, to understand how immune responses contribute to the dynamic aspects of periodontal disease and its various clinical courses, and to gain a comprehension of how elements of host immunity contribute to tissue destruction, resolution, repair, and regeneration.

Innate Immunity

Defenses against infection include a wide range of mechanical, chemical, and microbiologic barriers that prevent pathogens from invading the cells and tissues of the body. Saliva, GCF, and the epithelial keratinocytes of the oral mucosa all protect the underlying tissues of the oral cavity and the periodontium. The commensal microbiota (e.g., in dental biofilm) may also be important for providing protection against infection by pathogenic microorganisms through effective competition for resources and ecologic niches and also by stimulating protective immune responses. The complex microanatomy of the periodontium, including the diversity of specialized epithelial tissues, presents many interesting challenges for the study of the immunopathogenesis of periodontal disease.

If bacterial products enter the tissues, then the cellular and molecular elements of the innate immune response are activated. The term *innate immunity* refers to the elements of the immune response that are determined by inherited factors (and therefore "innate"), that have limited specificity, and that are "fixed" in that they do not change or improve during an immune response or as a result of previous exposure to a pathogen. The recognition of pathogenic microorganisms and the recruitment of effector cells (e.g., neutrophils) and molecules (e.g., the complement system) are central to effective innate immunity. Innate immune responses are orchestrated by a broad range of cytokines, chemokines, and cell surface receptors, and the stimulation of innate immunity leads to a state of inflammation. If innate immune responses fail to eliminate infection, then the effector cells of adaptive immune responses (lymphocytes) are activated. It is increasingly appreciated that the immune response functions as a network of interacting molecular and cellular elements in which innate immunity and adaptive (antigen-specific) immunity work together toward a common purpose. Aspects of innate immunity that are relevant to periodontal disease are now considered.

Innate Immunity	Adaptive Immunity
Refers to nonspecific defense mechanisms that act as barriers to infection. Components include: • Barriers to infection such as skin, mucosa, acid pH in the stomach • Antimicrobial molecules such as lysozyme, antimicrobial peptides • Immune system cells such as neutrophils and macrophages that kill infecting organisms • Receptors (e.g., Toll-like receptors) that recognize pathogen-derived molecules and activate immune–inflammatory responses • Antigen presentation to activate adaptive immune responses	Refers to antigen-specific immune responses. Components include: • Recognition of specific molecules on infecting organisms at the species and strain level • Cellular immune responses focused on defense from intracellular pathogens (e.g., viruses), involving cytokines from T helper cells, macrophages, and natural killer cells • Humoral immune responses focused on defense from extracellular pathogens (e.g., bacteria), involving B cells that differentiate into antibody-producing plasma cells

Innate and adaptive immunity do not function in isolation; close integration exists between the innate and adaptive arms of the immune response.

Saliva

Saliva that is secreted from the three major salivary glands (i.e., parotid, submandibular, and sublingual), as well as from the numerous minor salivary glands, has an important role in the maintenance of oral and dental health. The action of shear forces

TABLE 8.2   Constituents of Saliva That Contribute to Innate Immunity

Saliva Constituent	Host Defense Function
Antibodies (e.g., immunoglobulin A)	Inhibit bacterial adherence, promote agglutination
Histatins	Neutralize lipopolysaccharides, inhibit destructive enzymes
Cystatins	Inhibit bacterial growth
Lactoferrin	Inhibits bacterial growth
Lysozyme	Lyses bacterial cell walls
Mucins	Inhibits bacterial adherence, promotes agglutination
Peroxidase	Neutralizes bacterial hydrogen peroxide

associated with saliva flow is important for preventing the attachment of bacteria to the dentition and oral mucosal surfaces. Human saliva also contains numerous molecular components that contribute to host defenses against bacterial colonization and periodontal disease (Table 8.2). These components include molecules that nonspecifically inhibit the formation of the plaque biofilm by inhibiting adherence to oral surfaces and promoting agglutination (e.g., mucins), those that inhibit specific virulence factors (e.g., histatins that neutralize LPS), and those that inhibit bacterial cell growth (e.g., lactoferrin) and that may induce cell death.[61,107] Saliva also contains specific immunoglobulin A (IgA) antibodies to periodontal pathogens that target specific antigens and which inhibit bacterial adherence.

Epithelial Tissues

The epithelial tissues play a key role in host defense because they are the main site of the initial interactions between plaque bacteria and the host, and they are also the site of the invasion of microbial pathogens. The keratinized epithelium of the sulcular and gingival epithelial tissues provides protection for the underlying periodontal tissue in addition to acting as a barrier against bacteria and their products.[13,169] By contrast, the junctional epithelium has significant intercellular spaces, it is not keratinized, and it exhibits a higher cellular turnover rate. These properties render the junctional epithelium permeable, thereby allowing for the inward movement of microbes and their products and the outward movement of GCF and the cells and molecules of innate immunity. Furthermore, the spaces between the cells of the junctional epithelium widen with inflammation, which results in increased GCF flow.[169]

At the cellular and molecular levels, most in vitro studies of epithelial cell responses to periodontal bacteria have been carried out in primary gingival epithelial cells or various immortalized cell lines derived from oral epithelial tissue; these studies have provided insight into host cell responses to periodontal bacteria.[4,68,71,202] Epithelial cells also constitutively express AMPs (e.g., hBDs, LL-37), and the synthesis and secretion of these molecules is up-regulated in response to periodontal bacteria. Neutrophils are also a source of AMPs (i.e., α-defensins). AMPss are small, polycationic peptides that disrupt bacterial cell membranes and thereby directly kill bacteria with broad specificity.

The different categories of AMPs are defined on the basis of structural homology. The α-defensins (e.g., human neutrophil peptides 1 through 4) are expressed by neutrophils and as such are commonly found in GCF. The hBDs (e.g., hBDs 1 through 3) are expressed in the gingival epithelial cells, the salivary glands, and the tongue, as well as in immune cells (e.g., macrophages, dendritic cells); some hBDs are constitutively expressed, and others are expressed only in response to cytokines and bacterial products (e.g., gingipains of *P. gingivalis*).[4,39] A third class of AMPs are the cathelicidins, of which LL-37 is expressed in high levels in the junctional epithelium. Like the hBDs, LL-37 has a widespread expression pattern in the mouth; it is found in the salivary glands, the tongue, and the leukocytes as well as in the connective tissue. AMPs have more recently assumed greater importance because it has been recognized that they have a wider role in regulating innate and adaptive immune responses to infection.[43] Thus these molecules have chemokine-like activity in that they stimulate the chemotaxis of a range of leukocytes involved in innate and acquired immunity. AMPs also stimulate mast cell degranulation and cytokine production, and they likely have a role in wound healing through their effect on keratinocyte differentiation. Furthermore, some interest has been expressed in their possible role in therapy for oral inflammatory diseases.[43]

Epithelial cells that are directly stimulated with bacterial components and cytokines can produce MMPs, which contribute to a loss of connective tissue. Epithelial cells also secrete a range of cytokines in response to periodontal bacteria (e.g., *P. gingivalis*, *A. actinomycetemcomitans*, *F. nucleatum*, *Prevotella intermedia*), which signal immune responses. These include the proinflammatory cytokines IL-1β, TNF-α, and IL-6, as well as the chemokine IL-8 (CXCL8) and the monocyte chemoattractant protein-1 (MCP-1), which serve to signal neutrophil and monocyte migration from the vasculature into the periodontal tissue. In some (but not all) experimental systems, *P. gingivalis* has been shown to inhibit IL-8; it has been suggested that this may result in a temporary local immune suppression in the periodontium and facilitate the accumulation and invasion of pathogenic periodontal bacteria and the initiation of periodontitis.[41,68] *P. gingivalis* is an example of one periodontal pathogen with a range of virulence factors that affect host immune defenses,[68,106] as indicated in Table 8.3.

Gingival Crevicular Fluid

GCF originates from the postcapillary venules of the gingival plexus. It has a flushing action in the gingival crevice, but it also likely functions to bring the blood components (e.g., neutrophils, antibodies, complement components) of the host defenses into the sulcus.[67] The flow of GCF increases in inflammation, and neutrophils are an especially important component of GCF in periodontal health and disease.[101]

Pathogen Recognition and Activation of Cellular Innate Responses

If plaque bacteria and their products penetrate the periodontal tissues, specialized "sentinel cells" of the immune system recognize their presence and signal protective immune responses. These cells include macrophages and dendritic cells, which express a range of

TABLE 8.3 Virulence Factors of _Porphyromonas gingivalis_ That Interact With the Immune System

Virulence Factor	Effect on Immune System
Proteases (gingipains)	Degradation of signaling molecules (CD14) and cytokines (e.g., interleukin-1β, interleukin-6)
Cell invasion capabilities	Inhibition of interleukin-8 secretion
Lipopolysaccharides	Antagonism of the stimulatory effects of lipopolysaccharides from other species; no up-regulation of E-selectin
Fimbriae	Inhibition of interleukin-12 secretion in macrophages
Cell surface polysaccharides	Resistance to complement
Short-chain fatty acids	Induction of apoptosis in host cells

pattern recognition receptors (PRRs) that interact with MAMPs. The activation of PRRs activates innate immune responses to provide immediate protection, and adaptive immunity is also activated with the aim of establishing a sustained antigen-specific defense. Excessive and inappropriate or dysregulated immune responses lead to chronic inflammation and the concomitant tissue destruction associated with periodontal disease.

A glossary of terms relevant to periodontal immunobiology is presented in eTable 8.3, which can be accessed on the companion website.

Neutrophil Function

Neutrophils are the "professional" phagocytes that are critical to the clearance of bacteria that invade host tissues.[134] Neutrophils are present in clinically healthy gingival tissues, and they migrate through the intercellular spaces of the junctional epithelium into the sulcus.[98,169] This is part of a "low-grade defense" against plaque bacteria, and it is necessary to prevent infection and periodontal tissue damage.[169] The importance of neutrophils to the maintenance of periodontal health is demonstrated clinically by the observations of severe periodontitis in patients with neutrophil defects.[134]

A small proportion (1% to 2%) of the intercellular spaces in healthy junctional epithelium is occupied by neutrophils (and other leukocytes at various stages of differentiation), but this can increase to 30% with even modest inflammation. In the inflammatory state, changes to the local vasculature occur in the gingiva: high endothelial venules develop from the postcapillary venules of the gingival plexus, which facilitates leukocyte emigration and increases the flow of GCF into the pocket.[169]

Neutrophils migrate from the gingival plexus to the extravascular connective tissue and then into the junctional epithelium through the basement membrane. The presence of a layer of neutrophils in the junctional epithelium forms a host defense barrier between subgingival biofilm and the gingival tissue. At the molecular level, the interaction of adhesion molecules (e.g., ICAM-1) on endothelial and epithelial cells with β2 integrins on neutrophils facilitates neutrophil migration. Indeed, evidence from immunohistochemistry studies indicate the existence of

gradients of IL-8 (a "chemotactic gradient"), as well as gradients of ICAM-1, which direct the neutrophils from the vasculature into the tissues and toward the junctional epithelium.[188] The migration of neutrophils contributes to the disruption of the junctional epithelium by the degradation of the basement membrane through protease release and the action of ROS. An aspect of neutrophil-mediated immunity is the formation of neutrophil extracellular traps (NETs).[198] NETs constitute a highly conserved antimicrobial strategy in which decondensed nuclear DNA and associated histones are extruded from the neutrophil, thus forming weblike strands of DNA in the extracellular environment. These strands, in conjunction with AMPs, facilitate the extracellular killing of microorganisms that become trapped within the NETs. The potential role of NETs in periodontal pathogenesis is an area of ongoing research.

Adaptive Immunity

Adaptive immunity has evolved to provide a focused and intense defense against infections that overwhelm innate immune responses. Adaptive immunity is particularly important as ecologic, social, and demographic changes—which alter susceptibility to existing and emerging infective microorganisms—outpace the natural evolution of biologic systems. Furthermore, the development of effective vaccination is, along with the identification of antibiotics, perhaps one of the greatest triumphs of medical science; this success is based on knowledge of the elements and principles of adaptive immunity.

Adaptive immunity contrasts with innate immunity with regard to the dynamic of the underlying cellular and molecular responses: adaptive immunity is slower and reliant on complex interactions between APCs and T and B lymphocytes. A key element is the antigen specificity of the responses that facilitates the specific targeting of a diverse range of effector elements, including cytotoxic T cells and antibodies. Another facet is the ability of adaptive immune responses to improve during exposure to antigen and on subsequent reinfection events.[26] Our current understanding suggests that the cellular and molecular elements of adaptive immunity are more diverse than those of innate immunity, and although a role for many of these factors in periodontal disease has been identified, our knowledge is far from complete. The importance of adaptive immune responses in periodontal pathogenesis is endorsed by histologic studies of established lesions in periodontal disease.[101,148] The population of leukocytes in the periodontium in gingivitis (i.e., the early stages of responses to the plaque biofilm) and in stable periodontal lesions (i.e., those in which tissue destruction is apparently not progressing) has been reported to be dominated by T cells, and these cells are clustered mainly around blood vessels. Cell surface marker studies suggest that these cells are activated but not proliferating.[60] In addition, a predominance of the helper T-cell subset (i.e., CD4-expressing T cells) over the cytotoxic T-cell subset (i.e., CD8-expressing T cells) is observed. These T cells are considered to be proactively maintaining tissue homeostasis in the presence of the microbial challenge of the plaque biofilm.[60] By contrast, in active (progressing) periodontitis, B cells and plasma cells predominate and are associated with pocket formation and the progression of disease.

Antigen-Presenting Cells

Central elements of the activation and function of T cells and B cells are the presentation of antigen by specialized APCs to T cells and the development of a specific cytokine milieu that influences the development of T cells with particular effector functions. APCs detect and take up microorganisms and their antigens, after which they may migrate to lymph nodes and interact with T cells to present antigen. The periodontium contains a number of APCs, including B cells, macrophages, and at least two types of dendritic cells (i.e., dermal dendritic cells and Langerhans cells).[38] It is increasingly recognized that the engagement of PRRs (and in particular TLRs) by MAMPs from pathogenic microorganisms is not only central to signaling innate immunity in the form of cytokine up-regulation but also a critical element of the activation of APCs and the elaboration of T-cell effector function. Thus TLR activation increases the expression of costimulatory molecules on APCs, which are critical to the interaction of these cells with T cells. In addition, TLR activation enhances antigen uptake and processing. Different APCs process and present antigens by different pathways and mechanisms, and this variation is one of the factors—along with the presence of specific combinations of cytokines—that influences the phenotype of T-cell effector function produced during specific immune responses.[60]

T Cells

Several different subsets of thymic lymphocytes (i.e., T cells) develop in the bone marrow and thymus and migrate to the peripheral tissues to participate in adaptive immune responses. The expression of the cell surface molecules (CD4 or CD8) or particular T-cell antigen receptors ($\alpha\beta$ or $\gamma\delta$) broadly defines functional T-cell subsets that emerge from the thymus. The role of T cells in periodontal disease has been established through immunohistologic studies of diseased tissues.[173] CD4+ helper T cells are the predominant phenotype in the stable periodontal lesion, and it is thought that alterations in the balance of effector T-cell subsets within the CD4+ population may lead to progression toward a destructive, B-cell–dominated lesion.[60] CD4+ T-cell subsets are defined on the basis of their phenotypic characteristics and effector functions. The nature of the APCs, which present antigen to cognate T-cell receptors on T cells, and the presence of specific combinations of cytokines and chemokines locally influence the nature of the CD4+ T-cell effector subset that develops from naive T cells (Fig. 8.5). CD4+ T-cell subsets are defined by the expression of specific transcription factors, and their functional characteristics are associated with their cytokine secretion profile.

The best-defined functional subsets of CD4+ T cells are the Th1 and Th2 cells, and a dynamic interaction between Th1 and Th2 cells may provide, in part, an explanation for fluctuations in disease activity and the progression of periodontal disease (Box 8.3). Th1 cells secrete IFN-γ, which activates cell-mediated immunity (i.e., macrophages, NK cells, and CD8+ cytotoxic T cells) against pathogenic microorganisms. The activation of macrophages promotes phagocytosis and killing of microbial pathogens, whereas NK cells and CD8+ T cells are cytotoxic T cells that kill infected host cells. Conversely, Th2 cells regulate humoral (antibody-mediated) immunity and mast cell activity

BOX 8.3 The T-Helper 1/T-Helper 2 Concept of Periodontal Disease Progression

A dynamic interaction between T-helper 1 (Th1) and T-helper 2 (Th2) cells represents a possible explanation for aspects of the fluctuations in disease activity and clinical progression seen with periodontal disease. It has been hypothesized that a strong innate response results in interleukin-12 synthesis (e.g., by tissue macrophages) that leads to a Th1 response that provides protective cell-mediated immunity that would be manifested as a "stable" periodontal lesion. Conversely, a poor innate response would lead to reduced interleukin-12, which would permit the development of Th2 responses and lead to the activation of B cells; this, in turn, would mediate a destructive lesion, possibly through enhanced B-cell–derived interleukin-1β.[60,172] However, definitive evidence to support associations of Th1 and Th2 cells with different clinical presentations of periodontal disease has been difficult to obtain. Investigators have suggested that this is a result of variations among experimental studies, which have differed with respect to the material that has been used, the definitions of disease stages, the experimental designs, and analytic methods used.[56,60,172] In addition, in general terms, the Th1/Th2 dichotomy does not explain all aspects of the regulation of adaptive immune responses. More recently, other T-cell subsets have been identified and defined. For example, regulatory T cells secrete interleukin-10 and transforming growth factor beta and thereby suppress immune responses. Th17 cells have a proinflammatory action through the secretion of interleukin-17, a cytokine that synergizes with interleukin-1β and tumor necrosis factor α. Therefore, although it is widely accepted that Th1 and Th2 cells are likely to be important in the immunopathogenesis of periodontal disease, it is increasingly recognized that the Th1/Th2 model alone is probably inadequate to explain the role of T cells in this process.

through the secretion of the cytokines IL-4, IL-5, and IL-13. Thus the predominance of Th2 cells leads to a B-cell response. The B-cell response may be protective, for example, as a result of the production of specific antibodies that would serve to clear tissue infections through interaction with the complement system and by enhancing neutrophil phagocytosis. However, B cells are also a source of proinflammatory cytokines that contribute to tissue destruction.

T_{reg} cells have an immunosuppressive action that is mediated by the secretion of TGF-β and that is important to the prevention of autoimmune disease. These cells are increased in periodontitis lesions and may therefore have a role in disease pathogenesis.[130] Certain lines of evidence suggest that the pathogenesis of periodontal disease may involve some elements of autoimmunity.[60] For example, immunologic cross-reactivity occurs between HSP60 expressed on human cells and the GroEL molecule of *P. gingivalis*, and specific serum antibodies and antigen-specific T cells to these molecules have been detected in periodontal disease. Similarly, autoantibodies and specific T cells against other host (i.e., self) molecules, such as type I collagen, have been identified in periodontal disease.

Th17 cells comprise another subset of T cells, and they have a proinflammatory action that is important in immune responses against extracellular infections mediated by the cytokine IL-17. Infections with a diverse range of pathogens have been shown to activate strong Th17 cell responses, and Th17 cells are thought to provide a substantial inflammatory response to clear microorganisms that Th1/Th2 cells have failed to eradicate. IL-17 has a number of activities in common with IL-1β and TNF-α, and it

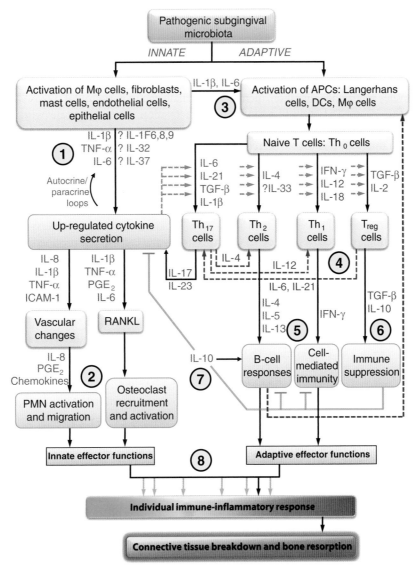

Fig. 8.5 Cytokine Networks in Periodontal Diseases. Schematic to illustrate the multiple interactions between cytokines and cellular functions in periodontal diseases. *(1)* Resident and infiltrating cells in the periodontium respond to microbe-associated molecular patterns signaling through pattern-recognition receptors by the production of cytokines as an early step in innate immune responses. Cytokine up-regulation is sustained by autocrine and paracrine feedback loops. (Note: *Question marks* indicate more speculative suggestions about the role of specific cytokines in periodontal pathogenesis than are known at present.) *(2)* Up-regulated cytokine activity leads to vascular changes, polymorphonuclear leukocyte *(PMN)* activation and migration, and, ultimately, osteoclastogenesis and osteoclast activation. *(3)* Cytokines produced in innate responses contribute to the activation of antigen-presenting cells *(APCs)*. These present specific antigens to naive CD4+ T cells *(Th0 cells)*, which differentiate into CD4+ effector T cells (e.g., T-helper cells *[Th1, Th2, Th17]*, and T-regulatory *[Treg] cells*) according to the local cytokine milieu (as indicated by the groups of *four parallel horizontal gray dashed arrows*). For example, Th0 cells differentiate into Th17 cells under the influence of interleukin-6 *(IL-6)*, IL-21, transforming growth factor beta *(TGF-β)*, and IL-1β. (APCs are also activated by B cells, which are themselves activated at a later stage in the cytokine network [indicated by the *brown dashed arrow at the right edge of the figure*]; this is an example of the complexities of sequential feedback loops that develop). *(4)* Th1 and Th2 cells have a relatively stable phenotype, but other T-cell subsets can exhibit functional plasticity under the influence of different cytokine environments (indicated by *purple dashed arrows*). For example, Th17 cells can develop into Th1 cells under the influence of IL-12 and into Th2 cells under the influence of IL-4. *(5)* Different T-cell subsets are associated with various cytokine secretion profiles that regulate different aspects of immune responses and that contribute to up-regulated cytokine activity. For example, Th1 cells secrete interferon gamma *(IFN-γ)* (which activates cell-mediated immunity), and Th2 cells regulate antibody-mediated (humoral) immunity through the secretion of cytokines IL-4, IL-5, and IL-13. Cytokines produced by different T-cell subsets increase their further secretion in positive feedback loops and also inhibit the development of other T-cell subsets (e.g., IL-4 from Th2 cells inhibits Th1 development, and IFN-γ from Th1 cells inhibits Th2 T-cell subsets). *(6)* Treg cells secrete TGF-β and IL-10, which have immunosuppressive functions. For example, IL-10 suppresses Th1 and Th2 responses, as well as cells of monocyte/macrophage lineage *(Mφ)* and dendritic cell *(DC)* function, and it also down-regulates cytokine production in various cells (i.e., Th1 cells, Th2 cells, PMNs, and natural killer cells). (Suppressive effects are indicated by *flat-ended green lines.*) *(7)* IL-10 functions as a regulatory mediator, but it can also exhibit other activities (e.g., the activation of B cells). The different aspects of IL-10 biology (i.e., immunosuppressive vs. immunostimulatory) likely depend on the local cytokine environment. These dual roles of IL-10 are indicated by the *green (inhibitory) line* and the *black (stimulatory) arrow.* *(8)* The sum total of innate and adaptive effector functions results in an immune–inflammatory response, the precise nature of which will vary from person to person (as indicated by the *multiple gray arrows,* with some patients being more susceptible to disease than others), as well as over time within an individual. In this case, the *black arrow* indicates an individual who has a proinflammatory response that leads to connective tissue breakdown and bone resorption. *ICAM-1,* intercellular adhesion molecule-1; *PGE₂,* prostaglandin E₂; *RANKL,* receptor activator of nuclear factor-κB ligand; *TNF-α,* tumor necrosis factor alpha. (Reproduced with permission from Kinane DF, Preshaw PM, Loos BG: Host-response: understanding the cellular and molecular mechanisms of host-microbial interactions—consensus of the Seventh European Workshop on Periodontology. *J Clin Periodontol* 38[Suppl 11]:44–48, 2011.)

has a synergistic activity with these cytokines, particularly TNF-α. IL-17 induces proinflammatory cytokine expression (including IL-1β and TNF-α) in macrophages, stimulates chemokine expression, and thereby activates neutrophil infiltration. Increasing evidence indicates a role of IL-17 and Th17 cells in periodontal disease.[56] IL-17 has been detected in periodontal tissues at sites of advanced disease. IL-17 induces IL-6 and IL-8 secretion by gingival fibroblasts and also up-regulates MMP-1 and MMP-3 in these cells. IL-17 also induces IL-1β and TNF-α secretion from macrophages and gingival epithelial cells. In a mouse model of periodontitis induced by *P. gingivalis*, IL-17 receptor deficiency (IL-17RA knockouts) resulted in increased susceptibility to alveolar bone loss, thereby suggesting a protective role of IL-17 in bone homeostasis, possibly by an effect on neutrophil function.

Cytokines produced by differentiated T-cell subsets feed back to stimulate differentiation and to sustain the activity of the cells from which they are derived (i.e., in a positive feedback loop). Simultaneously, they inhibit the development of other competing subsets. For example, IL-4 from Th2 cells inhibits the development of Th1 cells, and IFN-γ from Th1 cells inhibits Th2 cells.

It is increasingly appreciated that individual CD4+ T-cell clones—after they have encountered antigen and differentiated in response under the influence of a specific cytokine environment (i.e., a milieu)—may not be terminally differentiated cells. Rather, functional flexibility appears to exist between T-cell subsets and in particular within the memory T-cell population (see Fig. 8.5). For example, Th17 and T$_{reg}$ cells can interconvert, depending on the local concentrations of cytokines such as IL-6, IL-23, and TGF-β.[182] It is thought that the plethora of functional subsets of T cells, their anatomic location, and their ability to switch phenotype are reflections of the requirement for effective responses against diverse pathogens.

The complexities of the interactions between cellular and molecular aspects of innate and adaptive immune functioning are presented in Fig. 8.5. It is clear that multiple proinflammatory and antiinflammatory pathways, positive and negative feedback loops, and agonists and antagonists all play a role in determining the nature of the immune–inflammatory response to the bacterial challenge and the degree of tissue damage that is experienced. Furthermore, the nature of the inflammatory response varies among individuals; this could explain why certain people appear to be more susceptible to periodontitis than others.

CLINICIAN'S CORNER

What Makes a Person Susceptible to Periodontitis?
We have all seen patients with good oral hygiene yet advanced periodontitis and, conversely, patients with poor oral hygiene who may have gingivitis or mild periodontitis but who do not develop advanced periodontitis. It is clear that immune functioning and inflammatory responses are highly complex processes that vary from person to person. Our understanding is that the sum total of all the immune–inflammatory events in the periodontal tissues (which are also influenced by environmental factors such as smoking or diabetes) is the main determinant of how much tissue damage occurs in response to the challenge presented by the bacterial biofilm. This tissue damage is what we recognize clinically as disease. Our challenge for the future is to learn how to identify susceptible patients at a much earlier stage in the disease process, before tissue damage occurs.

Antibodies

Specific antibodies are produced in response to the bacterial challenge in periodontal disease and are the endpoint of B-cell activation. Commensurate with the appearance of antibodies against bacterial antigens is the appearance of differentiated plasma cells. High levels of antibodies appear in GCF (in addition to those in the circulation), and these are produced locally by plasma cells in periodontal tissues.[9] Antibodies to periodontal pathogens are primarily IgG, with few IgM or IgA types produced.

Many species of oral bacteria elicit a polyclonal B-cell response (with the consequent production of specific antibodies against those bacteria). However, these responses augment responses against nonoral bacteria and may lead to the production of autoantibodies (e.g., antibodies against collagen and connective tissue proteins), which may contribute to tissue destruction in periodontal disease.[9,60] The incidence and levels of specific serum and GCF IgG antibodies are raised in chronic periodontitis, a finding suggesting that local and peripheral generation of antibodies may be important in the immune response to periodontal pathogens. Antibodies (i.e., IgA) to periodontal pathogens are also found in saliva. Variations in the levels of specific antibodies to different species in different clinical presentations suggest differences in pathogenesis. For example, antibodies to *A. actinomycetemcomitans* of the IgG$_2$ subclass predominate in aggressive periodontitis.[166]

Other *P. gingivalis* molecules (i.e., fimbriae and hemagglutinin) also act as antigens. Specific antibodies are also generated by serotype-specific carbohydrate antigens (e.g., capsular polysaccharide of *P. gingivalis*, carbohydrate of *A. actinomycetemcomitans* LPS). The subclass distribution of antibodies is influenced by cytokines that are derived from monocytes.[166] For example, IgG$_2$ production is regulated by IL-1α, IL-1β, and PGE$_2$ from monocytes as well as by platelet-activating factor from neutrophils. PGE$_2$ and platelet-activating factor indirectly induce Th1 responses and therefore IFN-γ, which stimulates IgG$_2$ production. Individuals with aggressive periodontitis have monocytes that are hyperresponsive to LPS and that produce elevated quantities of PGE$_2$.[9] *A. actinomycetemcomitans* is commonly associated with aggressive periodontitis, which induces IL-12 production that regulates NK cells and Th1 cells. These cells are a source of IFN-γ, which, in turn, regulates IgG$_2$.

Some studies have reported an effect of treatment on levels of specific antibodies to periodontal pathogens. For example, plaque removal reduces the titers of antibodies to *P. gingivalis* and *A. actinomycetemcomitans* in serum, GCF, and saliva.[9] Some studies have observed a transient increase in antibody titers after treatment, which may be due to the release of antigens into the tissue and circulation.

The significance of antibodies in periodontitis is not clear. It is not known whether these antibodies have a protective function or whether they participate in disease pathogenesis. Although some evidence indicates a correlation between clinical parameters of disease and titers of specific antibodies to periodontal pathogens, other studies report an inverse correlation of antibody levels and avidity with periodontal destruction. In addition, specific antibodies to periodontal pathogens are found in healthy individuals, as well as in persons with periodontal disease.

CONCEPT OF HOST SUSCEPTIBILITY

The immune and inflammatory processes that result from the challenge presented by the subgingival biofilm are complex and are mediated by a large number of proinflammatory and anti-inflammatory cytokines and enzymes that function as a network of mediators with overlapping roles and activity (see Fig. 8.5). Immune responses to the bacterial challenge do not occur in isolation, but rather take place in the context of other host and environmental factors that influence these responses and thereby determine the progression of disease. Certain risk factors increase susceptibility to periodontal disease, particularly smoking[138] and diabetes[154]; these are considered elsewhere in this book.

A feature of human development and evolution has been that quantitative and qualitative differences exist in immune responses among individuals.[76] Indeed, infectious agents (e.g., bacteria) exert evolutionary selection pressures on the species that they infect. This may be relevant in periodontal disease, and some studies have confirmed that immune cells from patients with periodontal disease secrete higher quantities of proinflammatory cytokines than do cells from persons who are periodontally healthy.[183] Cytokine profiles are also different in those individuals with immune-mediated diseases as compared with healthy control subjects.

These observations have led to the concept of the "hyperinflammatory" or "hyperresponsive" trait in which certain individuals possess a hyperinflammatory phenotype that accounts for their increased susceptibility to chronic inflammatory conditions such as periodontitis.[31] Such a trait may also underpin shared susceptibility between conditions such as periodontitis and cardiovascular disease or diabetes. However, at present, it is not possible to identify with certainty those patients who are hyperresponders. The hyperresponder concept was originally proposed in the context of the responsiveness of monocytes to LPS challenge; this suggests that patients with disease possess an individual hyperresponsive monocytic trait that is characterized by elevated levels of inflammatory mediators released from monocytes in response to bacterial challenge.[140] It is likely that many reasons contribute to disease variations among individuals, such as variations in immune responses, pathogenesis, and the plaque biofilm; this situation results in an uneven disease experience in the population.

Fig. 8.6 is a schematic illustration of how increasing bacterial challenge can result in differing levels of inflammatory response according to the response profile of an individual patient.[140] Most individuals would be considered normal, and for a given bacterial challenge, they would produce a certain level of inflammatory mediators in the periodontal tissues. For those who are hyperresponders, the same bacterial challenge results in a greater inflammatory response, which over time would result in increased tissue breakdown, earlier presentation of the clinical signs of disease, and a clinical interpretation of having increased susceptibility to periodontitis. Those individuals who are hyporesponsive produce lower levels of inflammatory mediators and are therefore

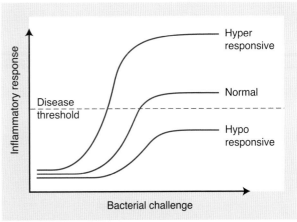

Fig. 8.6 Inflammatory Response Characteristics in Relation to Bacterial Challenge. A given bacterial challenge results in differing levels of inflammatory response according to the response profile of an individual. Most people are close to normal and produce a certain level of inflammatory mediators for a given challenge. Those who are hyperresponders generate an excessive inflammatory response for the same bacterial challenge and cross the threshold into active disease at an earlier stage. Those who are hyporesponsive produce lower levels of inflammatory mediators and, despite a significant bacterial challenge, may never develop advanced periodontitis. (Modified from Champagne CM, Buchanan W, Reddy MS, et al: Potential for gingival crevice fluid measures as predictors of risk for periodontal diseases. *Periodontol 2000* 31:167–180, 2003.)

somewhat resistant to the development of periodontitis, even though plaque may be present and they may have widespread gingivitis and/or mild periodontitis. The nature of the immune–inflammatory response is governed by genetic factors and environmental factors, and it may vary over time within the same individual (e.g., if environmental factors such as smoking status, stress, or systemic disease should change).[95]

A similar dose–response curve can also be expressed in the context of stable or progressing disease, and, as shown in Fig. 8.7, a certain level of bacterial challenge results in a moderate release of inflammatory cytokines, mediators, and enzymes. These mediators, together with the infiltrating defense cells, have a protective role to eliminate bacteria in the sulcus and do not trigger periodontal disease breakdown. Such a steady-state scenario may persist indefinitely. However, if something changes (e.g., the quantity or quality of the biofilm alters, or the host defenses alter as a result of a change in an environmental exposure), then the secretion of cytokines, prostanoids, MMPs, and other mediators may increase in the tissues, thereby leading to the histopathologic changes described previously and a transition to periodontitis. Thus a threshold exists between stable and active disease, and this varies from person to person. The dose–response curve for any individual can shift to the left or the right according to environmental changes. A shift to the left would result in an increase in the quantities of inflammatory mediators produced for a given bacterial challenge and potentially an exacerbation of disease; a shift to the right would have the opposite effect. In all cases, an increase in the bacterial challenge would have the tendency to increase the production of inflammatory mediators, which may tip the balance from a stable to a progressing periodontal lesion.

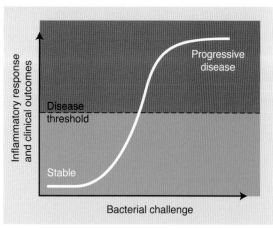

Fig. 8.7 Inflammatory Response Characteristics in Relation to an Individual's Threshold for Periodontitis. A certain level of bacterial challenge results in a moderate inflammatory response, which is protective by intent and may not be sufficient to transition to periodontal disease. This stable condition may persist for many years or even throughout the individual's lifetime. Changes in the bacterial burden (i.e., qualitative, quantitative, or both) or changes in the host response (e.g., as a result of a change in an environmental exposure) could result in an up-regulated inflammatory response characterized by marked cellular infiltrate and the increased secretion of inflammatory mediators leading to tissue damage and a transition from the stable situation to periodontitis. The location of the threshold between stable and active disease varies from person to person. In addition, the dose–response curve for any individual can shift to the left or the right in accordance with environmental changes. A shift to the left would result in an increased inflammatory response to a given bacterial challenge and potentially an exacerbation of disease. A shift to the right would have the opposite effect. (Modified from Champagne CM, Buchanan W, Reddy MS, et al: Potential for gingival crevice fluid measures as predictors of risk for periodontal diseases. *Periodontol 2000* 31:167–180, 2003.)

These are, of course, simplistic models to explain a highly complex phenomenon, and it is clear that cytokines and inflammatory mediators function in complicated networks (see Fig. 8.5).[93,155] Therefore, although increases and decreases in the absolute levels of cytokines have been reported in disease states, it is clear that the dysregulation of cytokine networks and other mediators is the key determinant of disease progression. Thus the relative proportions of mediators within inflammatory networks are fundamental to determining disease progression, and changes in these proportions are driven by inflammatory challenges and the genetic and environmental factors that govern how the host responds to such challenges.[99,147] Schematic illustrations to explain the pathogenesis of periodontal disease, such as presented in Fig. 8.5, can be useful; however, given the complexity of the disease processes, they are inevitably simplistic. Earlier models were very simplistic indeed, being essentially linear and suggesting that periodontitis resulted directly from the microbial challenge.[99] This concept influenced periodontal treatment over the decades and resulted in treatment strategies that focused primarily on the biofilm. Modern concepts of periodontal pathogenesis describe a host response that transitions from being proportionate and proresolving (in terms of resolving inflammation) to one that is disproportionate and nonresolving and ultimately self-destructive as chronic inflammation develops.

These changes occur in parallel with changes in the biofilm, the nature of which is influenced by the development of inflammation in the tissues, as it transitions from being health-promoting to dysbiosis, thus perpetuating the chronic inflammation.[124]

Increasing awareness of the importance of host factors in determining interindividual differences in disease progression has resulted in the realization that, although plaque bacteria initiate and perpetuate the inflammatory response, most of the tissue damage results from the host response, which is influenced by genetic factors, as well as environmental and acquired risk factors. Risk factors such as smoking alter the progression of the immune–inflammatory response and shift the balance toward increased periodontal breakdown.[87] This implies that the presence of plaque bacteria does not inevitably lead to tissue destruction, and this concept is supported by a large number of epidemiologic studies, which confirm that more advanced disease is usually confined to a minority of the population.[117]

Our improved understanding of the disease processes in periodontitis has led to the development of a biologic systems model for representing periodontal pathogenesis. This involves bacterial components, environmental factors, specific inflammatory mechanisms, and host–genetic variations that are associated with disease.[99] A biologic systems approach provides a framework for viewing the contributions and relative importance of all the components that contribute to the clinical presentation of disease. Thus, in the context of periodontal disease, such a system would include a person level, a genetic/epigenetic level, the biologic phenotype, and, ultimately, the clinical phenotype (Fig. 8.8).[139] Such systems provide a more comprehensive view of the disease as a complex regulatory network in which aspects of the specific genetic factors, environmental exposures, and other modifying factors that an individual is exposed to determine the development of the disease state.

To summarize, it is clear that the subgingival bacteria initiate and perpetuate the immune–inflammatory responses in the periodontal tissues. These responses are characterized by classic signs of inflammation that are modified as a result of the unique anatomy of the periodontium and the dentogingival apparatus. The inflammatory events that develop in response to the bacterial challenge are protective by intent, but they result in the majority of tissue damage and breakdown that lead to the clinical signs of periodontitis. Individuals vary with regard to their susceptibility to periodontal disease and also in the threshold level at which a stable periodontal site progresses to an active site. Such variations are genetically determined, and they are also influenced by environmental risk factors (e.g., smoking), some of which are modifiable and some of which are not. The challenge for the future is to identify at-risk individuals who possess the hyperinflammatory trait so that disease can be prevented by careful management strategies before tissue loss has occurred.

GENETICS OF PERIODONTAL DISEASE RISK AND TREATMENT

It is now widely accepted that differences among individuals who are at risk for the development of most diseases (host susceptibility) have a substantial inherited component. Factors in

Fig. 8.8 A Biologic Systems Model of Periodontitis. The outermost level of this model is the *Person Level*, which represents an individual's unique characteristics as they are related to periodontitis. These include the compositional characteristics of the subgingival biofilm, as well as known risk factors and environmental exposures such as smoking and diabetes. The *Person Level* characteristics interact with the *Genetic/Epigenetic Level* characteristics, which include nonmodifiable factors such as age, sex, and genetic composition. Gene polymorphisms are known to be associated with periodontal disease, and epigenetics refers to changes in phenotype (i.e., clinical disease expression) caused by mechanisms other than changes in the underlying DNA sequence. Epigenetics can be defined as all the meiotically and mitotically inherited changes in gene expression that are not encoded in the DNA sequence itself. Epigenetic modifications are important permissive and suppressive factors for controlling the expressed genome through gene transcription. Two major epigenetic mechanisms are the posttranslational modification of histone proteins in chromatin and the methylation of DNA. The *Genetic/Epigenetic Level* characteristics influence the *Biologic Phenotype*, which is characterized by the specific immune–inflammatory responses (i.e., cellular and molecular events and the production of inflammatory mediators) that are associated with the *Clinical Phenotype* (i.e., the clinical presentation of the disease). This model reflects how different individuals with the same presentation (e.g., periodontitis) may have very different predisposing and risk factors. The model depicts the different biologic factors that underpin the development of periodontal disease in different individuals and that ultimately may be used to classify disease by the contribution provided to the clinical phenotype at each level. (Modified from Offenbacher S, Barros SP, Beck JD: Rethinking periodontal inflammation. *J Periodontol* 79:1577–1584, 2008.)

the environment (e.g., diet, smoking, preventive care, exposure to pathogens) interact with each person's genetic predisposition to determine his or her health outcomes. This complex combination of variables determines if and when a disease affects the person, how fast and how severely symptoms of the disease progress, and how the person responds to different treatments in terms of both side effects and the success of alternative therapies.

Most cases of periodontitis appear to fit this complex gene and environment model. With the exception of a handful of rare syndromes caused by mutations of single genes, evidence indicates that inherited variation in DNA has a role roughly equal to that of the environment in determining who remains periodontally healthy versus who is affected by this disease. This knowledge about genetics is necessary for the development of

"personalized" or "individualized" periodontal treatment strategies, an approach that is playing an increasingly important role in improving virtually all other areas of health care today. Opportunities for advanced study designs and next-generation DNA sequencing and other genomic technologies to improve the understanding of the inherited basis of periodontitis make it likely (although by no means certain) that genetic variation will become an important variable to be routinely considered by practicing dentists within the careers of dental students today. This is already starting to occur.

Searching for Answers in the Deoxyribonucleic Acid

It is known that the comparison of periodontitis in different populations across the globe is extremely challenging because of the lack of calibrated examiners and standardized disease definitions.[22] One of the most dramatic population differences in which data quality is not an issue is the observation that both localized and generalized forms of early-onset aggressive periodontitis occur about 10 times more frequently among African Americans as compared with Caucasians.[116] Human racial and ethnic groups often differ dramatically with regard to the frequency of mutations at genes that have major effects on disease risk. For example, cystic fibrosis is caused exclusively by recessive mutations in the CFTR gene, and it varies in frequency from 1 in 3000 Caucasians to 1 in 15,000 African Americans in the United States, whereas only 1 in 350,000 Japanese individuals are affected.[145] It is possible that the 10-fold higher prevalence of early-onset aggressive periodontitis in African Americans is caused by the elevated frequency of high-risk gene variants in this population. However, additional evidence is needed before such a conclusion can be drawn. Although comparative studies of different populations may provide clues as to possible genetic mechanisms underlying a disease, the environments of the populations may also be dissimilar in important ways. It is possible that variations in diet, exposure to pathogenic oral bacteria, or some unknown and unmeasured environmental factors could entirely explain the observed differences in the frequency of aggressive periodontitis among population groups. Until solid data confirm a genetic basis for population differences, we need to wait before drawing firm conclusions.

The comparison of disease occurrence or severity in identical (monozygotic) versus nonidentical (dizygotic) twins is a powerful method for distinguishing between effects caused by variation in genes versus factors in the environment. This requires us to make what is usually a reasonable assumption that the environments of pairs of identical twins are no more or less similar than the environments shared by pairs of nonidentical twins. If variation among individuals in disease susceptibility or severity is caused entirely by factors in the environment, then we expect pairs of identical twins to be no more similar to each other in terms of disease risk than pairs of nonidentical twins. All twins (whether identical or nonidentical) are expected to be more similar to their co-twins, on average, than to unrelated members of their local population because they were raised in the same family environment, with similar diets, microbial exposures, and so on. However, if genetic variation plays an important role in determining a certain trait, then genetically identical twin pairs will be more similar to each other than nonidentical twin pairs. This is because identical twins share 100% of the same genes, whereas nonidentical twin pairs share only 50% of their parents' genes on average. Genetic epidemiologists calculate a measure called *heritability* that is based on these correlations and that estimates the portion of all variation in the trait attributable to inherited genetic variation. Traits with variation that is determined entirely by differences in environmental exposures have heritabilities of 0.0, whereas traits with variation attributable solely to inherited genetic differences without any environmental influence have heritabilities of 1.0. Heritabilities are sometimes reported as a percentage that ranges from 0% to 100%.

Most human diseases and nondisease traits fall in the middle of this range, with heritability ranging between 0.25 and 0.75. For example, in one study, type 2 diabetes was estimated to have a heritability of 0.26, and abnormal glucose tolerance had a heritability of 0.61.[152] For it to be feasible to use the twin method with adequate statistical power, the disease has to be fairly common so that the researcher can recruit enough twin pairs in which at least one of the twins is affected by the disease. Not surprisingly, with regard to periodontal disease, only chronic periodontitis occurs frequently enough to have been studied using the twin design. Two twin studies of modest size (i.e., 110 and 117 pairs) have been reported, and these estimate the heritability of measures of chronic periodontitis to range between 40% and 80%, thereby clearly implicating genetic variation in disease risk.[125,126] Interestingly, a study of bacteria associated with periodontitis found no difference between identical versus nonidentical twins.[127] This suggests (at least for these twins, most of whom did not have severe periodontitis) that inherited variation in risk is not mediated by genes that influence the presence of specific bacteria in subgingival plaque. Another review also failed to find an association between single nucleotide polymorphisms (SNPs; pronounced "snips") at IL-1 or other host genes and the presence or counts of subgingival bacteria.[133] These studies were performed before today's high-throughput DNA sequencing technologies were fully available to study the microbiome in depth, however, and it remains to be seen whether sharing specific strains of the hundreds of oral microbial species may be related to host genetics.

Genetic Basis for Individual Differences in Disease Risk

A number of extremely rare conditions consistently include periodontitis among the array of clinical manifestations that define a syndrome. Many genetic syndromes involve mutations of single genes or larger chromosomal regions. However, a number of syndromes, such as fetal alcohol syndrome, are purely environmental in origin. Some of the syndromes that include periodontitis are caused by mutations in specific genes. For example, mutations in the cathepsin C gene have been shown to cause both Papillon–Lefèvre syndrome and Haim–Munk syndrome as well as some forms of nonsyndromic prepubertal periodontitis, and they may also be associated with a risk of aggressive periodontitis.[137] Periodontitis frequently occurs with some subtypes of Ehlers–Danlos syndrome, Kindler syndrome, Down syndrome

(trisomy 21), leukocyte adhesion deficiencies (Fig. 8.9), hypophosphatasia, two types of neutropenia, and aplasia of the lacrimal and salivary glands. A large triracial extended family demonstrated evidence of a single gene that caused both early-onset aggressive periodontitis and dentinogenesis imperfecta.

The gene has been mapped with the use of linkage to a chromosomal region that contains a dentin matrix protein gene.[118] Many of these conditions are so rare that few periodontists see even a single case during a lifetime of practice. However, dentists and hygienists should be aware that these single-gene conditions exist; they need to be prepared to extend clinical evaluations to close relatives and to seek the assistance of or to refer to appropriately trained genetic counselors or specialists if a patient's medical history or the presentation of multiple symptoms raises the possibility that he or she may be affected.

Using Genetics for Personalized Treatment

If individuals differ in susceptibility to a disease, especially if underlying the superficial signs and symptoms of a disease there really are etiologically distinct subtypes of disease pathogenesis, then the traditional medical model of "one size fits all" treatment may not be optimal. It is why the personalized treatment using genetic data is important and developing.

In dentistry, a test based on inherited genetic variation at the interleukin-1 alpha (IL-1α) and IL-1β cytokine genes was proposed as being able to predict the risk, progression, and severity of periodontitis. The test has been commercialized and has gone through multiple versions (PST, PerioPredict; today's version is called ILUSTRA). Although specific numbers are not available, the test does not appear to be widely used yet. A number of reviews of the large number of studies of the IL-1 gene polymorphisms (eTable 8.4 and Table 8.4) indicate that genetic variation at these loci may be associated with, at most, a modest effect on disease risk.[81,136] In 2007, Huynh-Ba and colleagues concluded that "there is insufficient evidence to establish if a positive IL-1 genotype status contributes to progression of periodontitis or treatment outcomes."[81] A similar lack of supporting evidence for the use of IL-1 genetic testing to predict implant success has also been reported.[3,82] A more recent meta-analysis of the available data suggested that these much-studied IL-1 polymorphisms have a small (odds ratio, ≈1.5) but significant effect on periodontitis risk, although only for chronic periodontitis in white populations.[91] However, it is essential to emphasize that because heritability for chronic periodontitis is estimated to be 50%,[126] the small effect of the IL-1 polymorphisms makes up at most a tiny fraction of the genetic component of risk for this disease.

CANDIDATE GENES POSSIBLY RELATED TO RISK OF PERIODONTITIS

- Interleukin (IL)-1 gene cluster (IL-1A, IL-1B, IL-1 receptor antagonist), IL-4, IL-6, and IL-10.
- TNF-α
- Leukocyte receptors for the constant (Fc) part of immunoglobulin (FcγR)
- Vitamin D receptor
- Pattern recognition receptor genes (TLRs, cluster of differentiation [CD]-14)
- Matrix metalloproteinase (MMP)-1

TABLE 8.4 Number of Independent Gene Association Reports for Aggressive Periodontitis and Chronic Periodontitis[a]

Gene Symbol[b]	AGGRESSIVE PERIODONTITIS				CHRONIC PERIODONTITIS		
	None[c]	Weak	Moderate	Strong	None	Weak	Moderate
CD14	3				7	5	
CDKN2BAS		1	1				
ESR1	1	1				2	
FCGR2A	8	1			12	3	
FCGR2B	2	1			2	1	
FCGR3A	7	1			7	3	
FCGR3B	3	8			11	2	2
FGB	1				1	2	
FPR1	4	4	1		2		
GLT6D1				1			
GSTM1		1				2	
HLA-A	3	11			2	5	
HLA-B	8	2			1	4	
HLA-C	8				1	2	
HLA-DQ	1	1			1	1	
HLA-DQB1	3	3			2		
HLA-DR	3	2			2	1	
HLA-DRB1	3	2			2	2	
HLA-DRB3/4/5	1	1			1	1	
IL-10	10	2			10	4	2
IL-1A	17	5			23	5	3
IL-1A.IL-1B	3	1			9	8	4
IL-1B	16	9	1		29	11	2
IL-1RN	10	2	1		10	3	1
IL-2	2				2	2	
IL-4	2	2			7	1	
IL-6	4	3	1		8	11	
IL-6R		1				1	
LTA					1	2	
LTF	1	3				1	
MMP1	2	1			5	3	
MMP9	1	1			1	3	
MPO						2	
NAT2						2	1
NOS3		1				1	
PTGS2			1			2	1
S100A8	1	2				1	
SERPINE1	1					2	1
TGFB1	1				4	3	
TLR4	6	1			12	1	1
TNF	13	1			17	6	
VDR	3	6			7	12	

[a]Only genes with two or more reports of association are included.
[b]Full gene names and a summary of knowledge about the gene's function can be found by typing the gene symbol into the search box at http://www.ncbi.nlm.nih.gov/gene.
[c]Strength of association is defined as follows: weak (P value of <.05 but ≥.001; if <50 cases are in the study, then the finding is considered weak, regardless of the P value); moderate (P value of <.001 but ≥.0001 or if <101 cases are in the study regardless of P value); strong (P value <.0001 and >250 cases in the study).

Fig. 8.9 Oral (A) and radiographic (B) appearance of a patient with leukocyte adhesion deficiency. The child was deficient in CD18 (i.e., leukocyte adhesion deficiency type I), which results in absent or severely reduced levels of the β2 integrin molecule. The patient suffered from recurrent infections of the middle ear, the tongue, and the perirectal areas as well as of the periodontium. (B, From Majorana A, Notarangelo LD, Savoldi E, et al: Leukocyte adhesion deficiency in a child with severe oral involvement. *Oral Surg Oral Med Oral Pathol Oral Radiol Endod* 87:691–694, 1999.)

As the benefits of individualized or personalized treatments that are optimally matched to the genome of each patient have been demonstrated for cancer and increasing numbers of other human diseases, interest has grown in applying this approach to dentistry.[100,157] The first major study that attempted to develop guidelines for individualized treatment has been reported.[62] This study involved 5117 adults between the ages of 34 and 55 years with no prior diagnosis of early periodontitis who were followed retrospectively for 16 years. The aim was to evaluate whether only a subset of high-risk patients really benefits from two versus only one preventive visit per year to avert tooth loss. The risk factors that were tested were smoking, diabetes, and the IL-1 composite genotype. The authors of the study concluded that all three risk factors predict which patients benefit from two preventive visits. They proposed the use of the IL-1 genetic test[83] to detect the IL-1 composite genotype, which, along with smoking and diabetic status, was looked at as a risk factor for progressive periodontitis. The study claimed that by reducing the preventive dental visits to one per year in so-called low-risk patients, $4.8 billion would be saved annually. However, an independent reanalysis of the findings[44] showed that of the three assessed risk factors, only diabetes and smoking had statistically significant effects on tooth extraction risk. This conclusion was supported by an independent critical commentary by a leading expert in the field of epidemiology.[84] Therefore it is clear that we lack consistent evidence to demonstrate the scientific validity or clinical utility, of the IL-1 genetic test that is commercially available as a periodontitis risk prediction tool.[83] This first major attempt to use a genetic test in mainstream dentistry continues to be an area of great controversy, and dentists will need to remain aware of the scientific consensus regarding such tests as these emerge in the future so that they can accurately advise patients on their use and limitations.

As genetic testing becomes widespread, especially if it is marketed through direct-to-consumer models, increasing responsibility will fall on clinicians to fully understand and counsel their patients about the implications of test results for their treatment options and their risk of developing various dental diseases in the future. Tests for diseases of the oral cavity may likely combine inherited polymorphisms with oral microbial profiles, and they might also include assays of gene expression or proteomic data measured in saliva or other oral tissues. Few dentists or hygienists practicing today have been educated to prepare themselves for these future challenges. This major shortfall of knowledge urgently needs to be addressed. This can be done by continually educating today's dental professionals about advances in knowledge of human genetics and the uses and potential misuses of genetic testing; by establishing multidisciplinary teams of health practitioners in which dentists and hygienists work closely with genetics counselors and medical geneticists; or by combining these approaches.

Case Scenarios are found on the companion website.

REFERENCES

 References for this chapter are found on the companion website.

Biofilm and Periodontal Microbiology and Molecular Biology[a,b]

For additional content on the criteria for the identification of periodontopathogens, Videos 9.1 to 9.5, and expanded discussions of the structure of a mature dental plaque biofilm; the initial adhesion or attachment of bacteria; colonization and plaque maturation; and interactions among dental plaque bacteria, bacterial transmission and translocation, viruses, host susceptibility, adhesive surface proteins and fibrils, and tissue-destruction–promoting factors, please visit the companion website.

CHAPTER OUTLINE

The human fetus inside the uterus is sterile, but as soon as it passes through the birth canal, it acquires vaginal and fecal microorganisms.[116,154] Within 2 weeks, a nearly mature *microbiota* is established in the gut of the newborn baby. After weaning (>2 years), the entire human microbiota is formed and comprises a very complex collection of hundreds of different types of bacteria with approximately 10^{14} microbial cells.[362] From this moment on, our body contains *1.3 to 10 times more bacteria* than human cells.[493] It has been estimated that, for a normal, healthy human being, the bacterial population comprises 2 kg of the total body weight. This is fascinating if one realizes that the average human brain weighs only about 1.4 kg.

[a]Adapted from the following chapters of Newman and Carranza's Clinical Periodontology, 13th edition: Chapter 8: Biofilm and Periodontal Microbiology, by Wim Teughels, Isabelle Laleman, Marc Quirynen, and Nicholas Jakubovics, and Chapter 9: Practical Molecular Biology of Host–Microbe Interactions by Chad M. Novince, Carlos Rossa Jr., and Keith L. Kirkwood.
[b]Note: In the 2018 Classification of Periodontal and Peri-Implant Diseases and Conditions, "chronic periodontitis" and "aggressive periodontitis" disease categories are grouped under a single category called "periodontitis" and are further characterized based on a multidimensional staging and grading system. In this chapter, the term "aggressive periodontitis" is still used because the related studies were conducted before the 2018 classification. Readers are referred to Chapter 6 for the detailed discussion on periodontal disease classification.

The colonization of the oral cavity also starts close to the time of birth (Fig. 9.1). Within hours after birth, the sterile oral cavity is colonized by low numbers of mainly facultative and aerobic bacteria.[521] At that time, the oral microbiota of newborns closely resembles the mother's vaginal microbiota or, for newborns delivered by cesarean section, the mother's skin microbiota.[116] From the second day, anaerobic bacteria can be detected in the infant's edentulous mouth.[133,462] The number of oral bacteria increases gradually as a result of exposure to external environmental microbial sources.[276,401,462] *Streptococcus salivarius* and *Streptococcus mitis* (Fig. 9.2A) have been identified as the first and most dominant oral microbes to colonize the oral cavity of newborn infants.[274,275,300] *Veillonella* spp. (see Fig. 9.2B), *Neisseria* spp., *Actinomyces* spp. (see Fig. 9.2C and D), and *Staphylococcus* spp. are also among the first colonizers of the oral cavity. After tooth eruption, a more complex oral microbiota is established. The species that colonize the teeth after eruption include *Streptococcus sanguinis* (see Fig. 9.2D), *Lactobacillus* spp. (see Fig. 9.2E), and *Streptococcus oralis*. Oral streptococci, including *S. oralis, Streptococcus anginosus*, mutans streptococci (*Streptococcus mutans* and *Streptococcus sobrinus*), and *Streptococcus gordonii* (see Fig. 9.2F) are commonly reported to be present after the first year of life.[70,75,321,401] In addition, anaerobes, including *Fusobacterium* spp. (see Fig. 9.2G) and *Prevotella* spp. (see Fig. 9.2H and I), can also be detected in young children.[70,276] In later childhood, the bacterial diversity and numbers in the oral cavity increase as more teeth erupt and provide more areas for the adherence and retention of bacteria.[51]

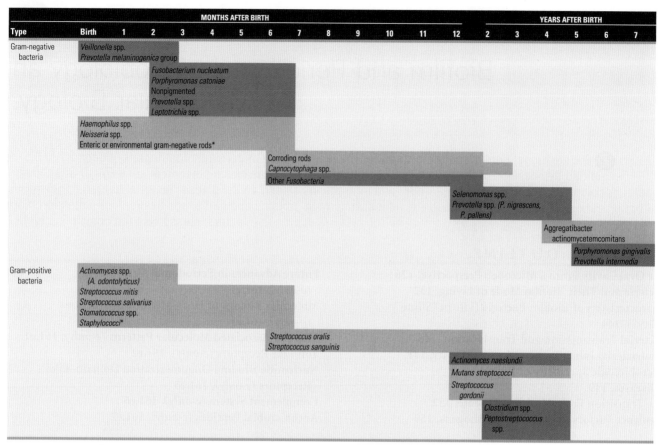

Fig. 9.1 Colonization of the Oral Cavity. Amenable periods for the establishment of the most frequent bacterial species or groups (prevalence, >25%) in infants' mouths. Anaerobic bacteria are indicated in green, and aerobic or facultative bacteria are indicated in orange. *Asterisk,* The prevalence of these bacteria decrease with age. (From Kononen E: Oral colonization by anaerobic bacteria during childhood: role in health and disease, *Oral Dis* 5:278, 1999; and Kononen E: Development of oral bacterial flora in young children, *Ann Med* 32:107, 2000.)

Because of the paucity of longitudinal studies, relatively little is known about the initial colonization of key microbes found in the oral cavity of children and adults.[300] It is estimated that the oral bacterial microbiome of adults encompasses approximately 700 commonly occurring species, approximately half of which can be present at any time in any individual.[38,395] When one thinks about bacteria, one almost immediately associates them with different pathologic conditions. However, most oral bacteria are harmless commensals under normal circumstances. This means that this microbiota lives in harmony with its host but that, under specific conditions (i.e., increased mass and/or pathogenicity, suppression of commensal or beneficial bacteria, and/or reduced host response), disease can occur. The importance of the commensal microbiota is clearly illustrated by the development of *Candida* infections when the normal oral microbiota is reduced, such as after a longer period of systemic antibiotic usage.[582] In addition, it has been shown that aggressive periodontitis is associated with a loss of colonization of *S. sanguinis*.[531] Conversely, investigators have shown in mice that the commensal microbiota is required for *Porphyromonas gingivalis*–induced bone loss.[3,107]

It is obvious that the periodontal microbiota is extremely complex. Because it both affects and is affected by the host, the oral environment, and periodontal treatment, a profound knowledge of periodontal microbiology is necessary.

THE ORAL CAVITY FROM A MICROBE'S PERSPECTIVE

With the exception of those microorganisms that are present in feces and in secretory fluids, all bacteria maintain themselves within their host by adhering to a surface. This principle also applies to the oral cavity. From an ecologic viewpoint, the oral cavity, which communicates with the pharynx, should be considered as an "open growth system" with an uninterrupted ingestion and removal of microorganisms and their nutrients.

KEY FACT

Most organisms can survive in the oropharynx only when they adhere to either the soft tissues or the hard surfaces. Otherwise, they may be removed by:
- Swallowing, mastication, or blowing the nose
- Tongue and oral hygiene implements
- The wash-out effect of the salivary, nasal, and crevicular fluid outflow
- The active motion of the cilia of the nasal and sinus walls

Fig. 9.2 Various Periodontal and Cariogenic Species Grown on Agar Plates. (A) *Streptococcus mitis* are gram-positive, fast-growing, facultatively anaerobic bacteria that are easy to culture on a blood-agar plate. A clear halo surrounding the colonies appears through hemolytic activity. (B) *Veillonella parvula* are anaerobic, gram-negative, small cocci. They form small transparent colonies (<1.0 mm) after 48 hours of incubation. (C) *Actinomyces viscosus* are microaerophilic to anaerobic gram-positive rods with possible branches (pseudomycelium). They form slimy, white, spherical colonies in 48 hours. (D) The typical colony morphology of *Streptococcus sanguinis (right)* and *Actinomyces odontolyticus (left)*. (E) *Lactobacillus* spp. typically grow on Rogosa agar as a sesame seed. (F) *Streptococcus gordonii* are facultative, anaerobic, gram-positive cocci. On a blood plate, colonies of 1 to 3 mm are formed within 48 hours. These bacteria are α-hemolytic, which results in the formation of a clear halo surrounding the colony. (G) This selective agar plate, which contains crystal violet and erythromycin (i.e., a CVE-agar plate), will allow *Fusobacterium nucleatum* to grow as a round, flat rhizoid, opaque purple colony. (H) A detailed picture of *Porphyromonas gingivalis* (green-brown colony) and *Prevotella intermedia* (black colony) on a classic nonspecific blood-agar plate. (I) *Prevotella nigrescens* forms like *P. intermedia*, a black pigmented colony on a blood agar plate. It is a strictly anaerobic bacterium with growth that is limited to an oxygen-free environment. (J) A detailed picture of *Parvimonas micra* (small white colony) next to *Porphyromonas gingivalis* (green-brown colony) on a classic nonspecific blood-agar plate. (K) A detailed picture of *Aggregatibacter actinomycetemcomitans* grown on a selective agar plate that contains tryptic soy, horse serum, bacitracin, and vancomycin (i.e., a TSBV-agar plate).

Continued

Fig. 9.2, cont'd (L) It is extremely difficult to culture *Treponema denticola* (spirochete) on an agar plate and therefore not possible to identify this bacteria with classic culture. A phase-contrast microscope, a dark-field microscope, or an electron microscope is often used to visualize this bacterium. Identification and quantification are possible only through DNA analysis. (M) On a selective agar plate that contains trypticase yeast extract, cystine, sucrose, and bacitracin (i.e., a TYCSB agar plate), *Streptococcus mutans* will grow as a sugar cube. (N) *Eubacterium nodatum* colony morphology strongly depends on its substrate. Its growth is very slow, and it is an obligate anaerobic gram-positive rod. (O) *Tannerella forsythia* organisms are fastidious bacteria that are therefore difficult to culture. This organism grows on a blood-agar plate as a smooth white colony with a faded edge. The bacteria are strictly anaerobic. (P) The typical colony morphology of *Streptococcus sobrinus* on TYCSB agar (colony with a white halo). (Q) *Capnocytophaga* are slowly growing bacteria that require an elevated carbon dioxide concentration for their growth. They are facultative anaerobic rods. (R) *Campylobacter rectus* grows on a Hammond plate as small, smooth, opaque, round colonies that are black. (S) *Eikenella corrodens* has a variable colony morphology and shows different biochemical and serologic reactions. Because of the difficult determination with classic culture, identification and quantification through DNA techniques are very suitable for this organism. *E. corrodens* cells are facultative, anaerobic, gram-negative rods. ([A] to [C], [F], [I], [L], [N], [O], [Q], and [S] Courtesy ADD Clinident, Malden, the Netherlands.)

Fig. 9.3 Epithelial Intercellular Spaces Containing Plaque. Scanning electron micrograph of epithelial intercellular spaces that contain bacterial plaque (B) enmeshed in a fibrin-like material. C, Epithelial cells; E, erythrocyte. The cells to the left show signs of necrosis. ×4000.

The ability of a bacterium to adhere to its host is crucial for the induction of infectious diseases, such as gingivitis or periodontitis.[444] Oral bacteria, and especially pathogenic bacteria, such as *Porphyromonas gingivalis* (see Fig. 9.2H and J) and *Aggregatibacter actinomycetemcomitans* (see Fig. 9.2K), have a large battery of virulence factors, one of which is the ability to adhere to hard intraoral surfaces and/or to the oral mucosae (Fig. 9.3).[82,84,152,510]

On the basis of physical and morphologic criteria, the oral cavity can be divided into *six major ecosystems* (also called *niches*), each of which has the following distinct ecologic determinants:

1. The intraoral and supragingival hard surfaces (teeth, implants, restorations, and prostheses)
2. Subgingival regions adjacent to a hard surface, including the periodontal/peri-implant pocket (characterized by the presence of crevicular fluid, the root cementum or implant surface, and the pocket epithelium)
3. The buccal palatal epithelium and the epithelium of the floor of the mouth
4. The dorsum of the tongue
5. The tonsils
6. The saliva

In health, a core set of microorganisms is almost universally present in these ecosystems. This core microbiome includes members of the phyla Firmicutes (*Streptococcus* spp., *Veillonella* spp., and *Granulicatella* spp.), Proteobacteria (*Neisseria* spp., *Campylobacter* spp., and *Haemophilus* spp.), Actinobacteria (*Corynebacterium* spp., *Rothia* spp., and *Actinomyces* spp.), Bacteroidetes (*Prevotella* spp., *Capnocytophaga* spp., and *Porphyromonas* spp.), and Fusobacteria (*Fusobacterium* spp.).[217,301,621]

Table 9.1 summarizes several publications that discuss the detection frequency of periodontopathogens in these different niches. Most species (with the exception of spirochetes) (see Fig. 9.2L) are able to colonize all of them. Some periodontopathogens

(e.g., *Fusobacterium nucleatum* [see Fig. 9.2G] and *Prevotella intermedia* [see Fig. 9.2H]) are involved in the etiology of tonsillitis, and most periodontopathogens are able to colonize the maxillary sinus.[56,577]

The soft tissue surfaces are actively involved in the process of bacterial adhesion and colonization.[214] They use a variety of mechanisms to prevent the adhesion of pathogenic organisms, with shedding being one of the most important.

CLINICIAN'S CORNER

Is It Necessary to Brush the Gums?

In essence, it is not. The epithelial cells are shed twice a day in a process known as *desquamation*, which is considered to be a natural cleansing mechanism. However, due to the morphology of the tongue and under removable prostheses, desquamated epithelial cells will not be flushed away by removal forces within the oral cavity. Brushing these areas may therefore be recommended.

In periodontal pockets, studies have shown high numbers of bacteria attached to pocket epithelial cells in vivo. Areas of gingival inflammation are characterized by an increased number of adhering bacteria.[121,569] These adhering bacteria can also infiltrate the pocket wall in relatively large numbers and reach the underlying stroma (Fig. 9.4).[142,337,471] In general, a positive correlation exists between the adhesion rate of pathogenic bacteria to different epithelia and the susceptibility of the affected patient to certain infections.[383]

Isogai and coworkers[225] reported a significantly lower adherence rate of *P. gingivalis* and *P. intermedia* strains to gingival epithelial cells in rats that were resistant to gingivitis as compared to susceptible rats. An in vitro study of cultured human pocket epithelial cells (Fig. 9.5) showed a similar tendency when patients who were resistant to periodontitis were compared with patients with severe periodontal breakdown.[429]

Bacteria also adhere to hard tissues. In the human body, teeth and nails are the only naturally occurring nonshedding surfaces. Artificial nonshedding surfaces of medical importance include prosthetic devices such as catheters, artificial joints, dental implants, and heart valves. From a microbiologic viewpoint, teeth and implants are unique for two reasons: (1) they provide a hard, nonshedding surface that allows for the development of extensive structured bacterial deposits; and (2) they form a unique ectodermal interruption. A special seal of epithelium (junctional epithelium) and connective tissue is present between the external environment and the internal parts of the body. The accumulation and metabolism of bacteria on these hard surfaces are considered the primary causes of caries, gingivitis, periodontitis, peri-implantitis, and, sometimes, bad breath.

In the periodontal pocket, different strategies contribute to bacterial survival, such as adhesion to the pocket epithelium and, when dentin is encountered, the colonization of the dentinal tubules.[421] The crevicular fluid, with its constant outflow, does not favor the maintenance of unattached bacteria in the periodontal pocket.

Investigators have suggested that teeth are the primary habitat for periodontopathogens, because soon after a full-mouth tooth

TABLE 9.1   Intraoral Habitats (Periodontal Pockets, Buccal Mucosa, Tongue, Saliva, Tonsils, and Supragingival Plaque) for Periodontopathogenic and Cariogenic Species

Authors	Infection	Age Group (n)	Species	No. of Positive Patients	DIFFERENT INTRAORAL NICHES					
					Periodontal Pockets	Buccal Mucosa	Tongue	Saliva	Tonsils	Supragingival Plaque
Asikainen et al., 1991	Periodontitis	Adult	A. a.	—	100%[a]	—	56%	72%	—	—
Petit et al., 1994	—	Child (45)	A. a.	5	4[b]	3	1	3	2	—
			P. g.	1	0	1	0	1	1	—
			P. i.	34	23	18	25	31	22	—
			Spi	13	6	0	7	3	1	—
Petit et al., 1994	Periodontitis	Adult (24)	A. a.	13	13[c]	11	11	11	5	—
			P. g.	18	18	14	7	10	11	—
			P. i.	24	24	22	23	23	23	—
			Spi	22	22	0	2	5	1	—
von Troil-Lindén et al., 1995	Periodontitis	Adult (10)	A. a.	—	6[c]	—	—	6	—	—
			P. g.	—	7	—	—	4	—	—
			P. i.	—	10	—	—	9	—	—
Danser et al., 1994	Periodontitis/E	Adult (8)	A. a.	2	2/—[d]	2/0	2/0	2/0	2/0	1/0
			P. g.	6	6/—	2/0	4/0	4/0	3/0	2/0
			P. i.	8	8/—	4/1	6/3	6/4	5/3	6/1
			Prev.	8	3/—	4/5	7/6	7/5	4/6	5/4
Danser et al., 1996	Periodontitis/R	Adult (15)	A. a.	11	9/4[e]	10/9	—	5/2	2/0	2/0
			P. g.	10	6/5	9/7	—	4/1	6/0	6/0
			P. i.	15	11/1	15/15	—	14/13	11/1	11/1
Gibbons and van Houte, 1975	—[f]	—	S. m.	—	?	<1[e]	<1	<1	—	0–50
			L.	—	?	<0.1	<0.1	<1	—	0–1

[a]Percentage of "specific" positive sites in positive patients.

[b]Number of "specific" positive sites in positive patients.

[c]Number of "specific" positive sites in patients with advanced periodontitis.

[d]Number of "specific" positive sites in positive patients before/after full-mouth extraction (e.g., two patients tested positive for A. a. before extraction, and no patients tested positive for A. a. after full-mouth extraction).

[e]Number of "specific" positive sites in positive patients before/after periodontal therapy including surgery (e.g., nine patients tested positive for A. a. before periodontal therapy as compared with only four patients after periodontal therapy).

[f]Percentage of total flora cultivable in anaerobically incubated agar in nonspecific patients as estimated from several studies.

A. a., Aggregatibacter actinomycetemcomitans; E, full-mouth extraction; L, Lactobacillus spp.; P. g., Porphyromonas gingivalis; P. i., Prevotella intermedia; Prev., Prevotella spp. (e.g., P. melaninogenica, P. denticola, P. loescheii, P. veroralis); R, periodontal therapy including surgery; S. m., Streptococcus mutans; Spi, spirochetes.

Fig. 9.4 Bacterial Penetration Into the Pocket Wall With Advanced Periodontitis. (A) Penetration through the pocket epithelium *(E)* and the basement lamina *(BL)* into the connective tissue *(CT)* *(arrows)*. *CF,* Collagen fibers. (B) Connective-tissue–associated bacteria *(arrows)* in a patient with advanced periodontitis. ([A] Courtesy Dr. R. Saglie. [A] and [B] From Nissengard RJ, Newman MG: *Oral microbiology and immunology,* ed 2, Philadelphia, 1994, Saunders.)

extraction in patients with severe periodontitis, key pathogens such as *A. actinomycetemcomitans* and *P. gingivalis* disappeared from the oral cavity, as determined by bacterial culturing techniques.[103] *P. intermedia* and other black-pigmented *Prevotella* spp. remained, but at lower detection frequencies and numbers (see Table 9.1).

The same applies to edentulous infants and wearers of full dentures in whom significant proportions of periodontopathogens have been recorded, with the exception of *A. actinomycetemcomitans* and *P. gingivalis.*[102,276] Therefore, teeth were considered as a "porte d'entrée" for periodontopathogens.

However, studies involving the use of molecular tools to detect and quantify oral bacteria seem to indicate that *A. actinomycetemcomitans* and *P. gingivalis* are not entirely eradicated after full-mouth extraction. They may remain colonizers of the oral cavity, but when teeth are lost, the relative numbers of these bacteria decrease.[433,435]

KEY FACT

Hard surfaces such as teeth and dental implants are very important habitats for oral pathogens. However, they are by far not the only habitats.

Fig. 9.5 *Porphyromonas gingivalis* **Adhesion Capacity Differences.** Microscopic confirmation of significant differences in the adhesion capacity of *P. gingivalis (small green dots)* to epithelial cells from (A) a resistant patient as compared with (B) a patient with severe periodontitis.

Fig. 9.6 Vertical Section Through a 4-Day Human Plaque Sample. An intraoral device designed for the in vivo generation of plaque biofilms on enamel was used. Confocal microscopy enabled the visualization of the section of plaque without the dehydration steps used in conventional histologic preparations. Notice the open fluid-filled channels *(arrows)* that traverse from the plaque surface through the bacterial mass (*M*; gray-white areas) to the enamel surface. An area in which the bacterial mass appears to attach to the enamel surface *(A)* is indicated. Scale bar = 25 μm. (From Wood SR, Kirkham J, Marsh PD, et al: Architecture of intact natural human plaque biofilms studied by confocal laser scanning microscopy, *J Dent Res* 79:21, 2000.)

Alternatively, cariogenic species were thought to be relatively restricted to solid surfaces (see Table 9.1). Therefore *S. mutans* (Fig. 9.2M) was often considered an *obligate periphyte*.[546] In some studies, this species was detected only from the time that the deciduous teeth erupted in the oral cavity.[71] In a longitudinal observation of adults with severe dental caries, the cariogenic species fell below detection level after full-mouth extraction but reappeared a few days after denture insertion.[72] On the basis of these reports and on their own observations, Caufield and Gibbons[76] concluded that most of the *S. mutans* cells in the saliva or on the tongue are derived from the biofilm present on the teeth and that the mucosae could not act as a reservoir for the infection of teeth by those organisms. These investigators suggested a "window of infectivity" for the acquisition of *S. mutans* at a mean age of 26 months (range, 9 to 44 months).[75] This observation has been supported by a few clinical studies, which showed that the initial colonization of *S. mutans* varied between 7 to 36 months, which is the time period that coincides with the eruption of the primary teeth.[10,70,144] Conversely, longitudinal studies by Wan and coworkers[583,584] and Law and Seow[299] showed that *S. mutans* colonization increased with the age of children, without any discrete window of infectivity. Clinical evidence now shows that *S. mutans* can be detected in the mouths of predentate children before the eruption of the first tooth.[356,583,585]

BACTERIA AND THEIR BIOFILM MODE OF LIVING

The importance of surfaces for microbial growth was recognized as early as the 1920s, when a number of workers independently noted that bacteria growing on glass slides submerged in soil were different from bacteria that could be cultured in broth.[298] However, it was not until around 50 years later that sessile microbial populations were considered to be sufficiently different from free-living microorganisms to merit their own name, and the term *biofilms* was coined (Figs. 9.6 and 9.7B and C). Biofilms

Fig. 9.7 Subgingival Plaque. (A) Diagram depicting the plaque–bacteria association between the tooth surface and the periodontal tissues. (B) Scanning electron photomicrograph of a cross-section of cementum *(C)* with attached subgingival plaque *(AP)*. The area shown is within a periodontal pocket. (C) Scanning electron micrograph of cocci and filaments associated with the surface of pocket epithelium in a case of marginal gingivitis. ×3000. (D) *Left,* Diagrammatic representation of the histologic structure of subgingival plaque. *Right,* Histologic section of subgingival plaque. *Arrow with box,* Sulcular epithelium. *White arrow,* Predominantly gram-negative unattached zone. *Black arrow,* Tooth surface. *Asterisk,* Predominantly gram-positive attached zone. (B, Courtesy Dr. J. Sottosanti, La Jolla, Calif.)

are composed of microbial cells encased within a matrix of extracellular polymeric substances, such as polysaccharides, proteins, and nucleic acids.

Biofilm bacteria are often up to 1000 times more resistant to antimicrobial agents than their planktonic counterparts.[13,133] Bacteria that grow in multispecies biofilms interact closely with neighboring cells. Sometimes, these interactions are mutually

beneficial, as is the case when one organism removes another's waste products and uses them as an energy source.

In other instances, bacteria compete with their neighbors by secreting antibacterial molecules such as inhibitory peptides (bacteriocins) or hydrogen peroxide (H_2O_2) (Video 9.1). In addition, the biofilm mode of growth facilitates cell–cell signaling and deoxyribonucleic acid (DNA) exchange between bacteria.

Subject 1   **Subject 2**   **Subject 3**

Fig. 9.8 Architecture of Oral Biofilms Formed on Enamel Discs in situ in Three Subjects. Biofilms were allowed to develop on the enamel surfaces mounted on healing abutments in the oral cavity for 7 days. The abutments were then removed, stained with BacLight Live/Dead (ThermoFisher Scientific, Waltham, Mass.) staining, and visualized using confocal laser scanning microscopy. (From Rabe P, Twetman S, Kinnby B, et al: Effect of fluoride and chlorhexidine digluconate mouthrinses on plaque biofilms, *Open Dent J* 31:106–111, 2015.)

Fig. 9.9 Clinical Picture of 10-Day-Old Supragingival Plaque. The first signs of gingival inflammation *(arrows)* are becoming visible.

It is clear that microbial ecology within biofilm communities is highly complex and that, in many cases, knowledge is only beginning to emerge.

Biofilms are heterogeneous: variations in biofilm structure exist within individual biofilms, between different types of biofilms, and between individuals (Fig. 9.8).[436] However, some structural features that are common to many biofilms have been noted. For example, biofilms frequently contain microcolonies of bacterial cells. Water channels are commonly found in biofilms, and these can form a primitive circulatory system that removes waste products and brings fresh nutrients to the deeper layers of the film. Surface structures, such as fronds, can dissipate the energy of fluid flowing over the biofilm and lead to the rapid blockage of vessels.[119] Mixed-species biofilms often have heterogeneity in the distribution of different species. Steep chemical gradients exist, such as those of oxygen or pH, and these produce distinct microenvironments within the biofilm.

Microbial populations on the surfaces of teeth (dental plaque) are excellent examples of biofilm communities (Fig. 9.9). The architecture of a dental plaque biofilm has many features in common with other biofilms. It is heterogeneous in structure, with clear evidence of open fluid-filled channels running through the plaque mass (see Fig. 9.6).[91,92,607] Nutrients make contact with the sessile (attached) microcolonies by diffusion from the water channels to the microcolony, rather than from the matrix. The bacteria exist and proliferate within the intercellular matrix through which the channels run. The matrix confers a specialized environment that distinguishes the bacteria that exist within the biofilm from those that are free floating; this is the so-called planktonic state in solutions, such as saliva or crevicular fluid. The biofilm matrix functions as a barrier. Substances produced by bacteria within the biofilm are retained and concentrated, which fosters metabolic interactions among the different bacteria.

The intercellular matrix consists of organic and inorganic materials derived from saliva, gingival crevicular fluid, and bacterial products.

Organic constituents of the matrix include polysaccharides, proteins, glycoproteins, lipid material, and DNA.[317] Albumin, which probably originates from crevicular fluid, has been identified as a component of the plaque matrix. The lipid material consists of debris from the membranes of disrupted bacterial and host cells, bacterial vesicles, and possibly food debris. *Glycoproteins* from the saliva are important components of the pellicle that initially coat a clean tooth surface, but they also become incorporated into the developing plaque biofilm. Polysaccharides produced by bacteria also contribute to the organic portion of the matrix. They play a major role in maintaining the integrity of the biofilm.

The *inorganic components* of plaque are predominantly calcium and phosphorus, with trace amounts of other minerals such as sodium, potassium, and fluoride. The source of inorganic constituents of supragingival plaque is primarily saliva. As the mineral content increases, the plaque mass becomes calcified to form calculus (Fig. 9.10). Calculus is frequently found in areas of the dentition adjacent to salivary ducts (e.g., the lingual surface of the mandibular incisors and canines, the buccal surface of the maxillary first molars), and this reflects the high concentration of minerals available from saliva in those regions. The inorganic

Fig. 9.10 Supragingival Calculus is Depicted on the Buccal Surface of the Maxillary Molars Adjacent to the Orifice of the Parotid Duct.

Fig. 9.11 Dark-Pigmented Deposits of Subgingival Calculus on the Distal Root of an Extracted Lower Molar.

components of subgingival plaque are derived from crevicular fluid (a serum transudate). The calcification of subgingival plaque also results in calculus formation (Fig. 9.11). Subgingival calculus is typically dark green or dark brown, which probably reflects the presence of blood products that are associated with subgingival hemorrhage.

The importance of these biofilms for oral diseases, such as dental caries and periodontitis—together with the relative ease with which tooth surface biofilms can be accessed—has caused dental plaque to be one of the most highly studied biofilm systems. It is anticipated that, by understanding the mechanisms involved in the accumulation of dental plaque and the transition from health to disease, it will be possible to improve our control over these processes and to restrict plaque-associated oral diseases further.

Structure of a Mature Dental Plaque Biofilm

Dental plaque (see Fig. 9.9) is clinically defined as a structured, resilient, yellow-grayish substance that adheres tenaciously to the intraoral hard surfaces, including removable and fixed restorations.[48] The tough extracellular matrix makes it impossible to remove plaque by rinsing or with the use of sprays. Plaque can thus be differentiated from other deposits that may be found on the tooth surface, such as materia alba and calculus. *Materia alba* refers to soft accumulations of bacteria, food matter, and tissue cells that lack the organized structure of dental plaque and that are easily displaced with a water spray. *Calculus* is a

TABLE 9.2 Differences Between Tooth Deposits

Materia Alba	Dental Plaque	Calculus
• White, cheese-like accumulation	• Resilient clear to yellow-grayish substance	• Hard deposit that forms via the mineralization of dental plaque
• Soft accumulation of salivary proteins, some bacteria, many desquamated epithelial cells, and occasional disintegrating food debris	• Primarily composed of bacteria in a matrix of salivary glycoproteins and extracellular polysaccharides	• Generally covered by a layer of unmineralized dental plaque
• Lacks an organized structure and is therefore not as complex as dental plaque	• Considered to be a biofilm	
• Easily displaced with a water spray	• Impossible to remove by rinsing or with the use of sprays	

hard deposit that forms via the mineralization of dental plaque and that is generally covered by a layer of unmineralized plaque (Table 9.2).

Dental plaque is composed primarily of microorganisms. One gram of plaque (wet weight) contains approximately 10^{11} bacteria.[489,513] The number of bacteria in supragingival plaque on a single tooth surface can exceed 10^9 cells. In a periodontal pocket, counts can range from 10^3 bacteria in a healthy crevice to more than 10^8 bacteria in a deep pocket. With the use of highly sensitive molecular techniques for microbial identification, it has been estimated that more than 750 distinct microbial phylotypes can be present as natural inhabitants of dental plaque.[1]

Any individual may harbor hundreds of different species. Next to bacteria, nonbacterial organisms can also be found in the dental plaque biofilm, including archaea, yeasts, protozoa, and viruses.[89,307]

CLINICIAN'S CORNER

Is It Possible to Remove Dental Plaque by Rinsing?
The biofilm nature of dental plaque means that it tenaciously adheres to surfaces. Therefore it cannot be removed by rinsing or sprays.

Dental plaque is broadly classified as supragingival or subgingival on the basis of its position on the tooth surface toward the gingival margin.
• *Supragingival plaque* is found at or above the gingival margin; when in direct contact with the gingival margin, it is referred to as *marginal plaque.*

Fig. 9.12 Plaque Formation. (A) One-day-old plaque. Microcolonies of plaque bacteria extend perpendicularly away from the tooth surfaces. (B) Developed supragingival plaque showing the overall filamentous nature and the microcolonies *(arrows)* that extend perpendicularly away from the tooth surface. The saliva–plaque interface is shown *(S)*. (C) A histologic section of plaque showing nonbacterial components such as white blood cells *(arrow)* and epithelial cells *(asterisk)* interspersed among bacteria *(B)*. (Courtesy Dr. Max Listgarten, Philadelphia, Pa.)

- *Subgingival plaque* is found below the gingival margin, between the tooth and the gingival pocket epithelium.

Supragingival plaque typically demonstrates the stratified organization of a multilayered accumulation of bacterial morphotypes (Fig. 9.12).[626] Gram-positive cocci and short rods predominate at the tooth surface, whereas gram-negative rods, filaments, and spirochetes predominate in the outer surface of the mature plaque mass.

In general, the subgingival microbiota differs in composition from the supragingival plaque, primarily because of the local availability of blood products and a low reduction–oxidation (redox) potential, which characterizes the anaerobic environment.

The environmental parameters of the subgingival region differ from those of the supragingival region. The gingival crevice or pocket is bathed by the flow of crevicular fluid, which contains many substances that bacteria may use as nutrients. Host inflammatory cells and mediators are likely to have considerable influence on the establishment and growth of bacteria in the subgingival region. Both morphologic and microbiologic studies of subgingival plaque reveal distinctions between the tooth-associated regions and the soft tissue–associated regions of subgingival plaque (see Fig. 9.7A to C).[312,369]

KEY FACT

The specific microbial composition and structure of dental biofilms are highly dependent on the region of the tooth and the local environmental parameters.

The tooth-associated cervical plaque that adheres to the root cementum does not markedly differ from that observed in gingivitis. At this location, filamentous microorganisms dominate, but cocci and rods also occur. This plaque is dominated by gram-positive rods and cocci, including *S. mitis, S. sanguinis, Actinomyces oris, Actinomyces naeslundii,* and *Eubacterium* spp. (see Fig. 9.2N). However, in the deeper parts of the pocket, the filamentous organisms become fewer in number; in the apical portion, they seem to be virtually absent. Instead, the microbiota is dominated by smaller organisms without a particular orientation.[312] The apical border of the plaque mass is separated from the junctional epithelium by a layer of host leukocytes, and the bacterial population of this apical-tooth–associated region shows an increased concentration of gram-negative rods (see Fig. 9.7D).

The layers of microorganisms that face the soft tissue lack a definite intermicrobial matrix and contain primarily gram-negative rods and cocci, as well as large numbers of filaments, flagellated rods, and spirochetes. Studies of plaque associated with crevicular epithelial cells indicate a predominance of species such as *S. oralis, S. intermedius, Parvimonas micra* (formerly *Micromonas micra* and *Peptostreptococcus micros*), *P. gingivalis, P. intermedia, Tannerella forsythia* (see Fig. 9.12), and *F. nucleatum*.[113,121] Host-tissue cells (e.g., white blood cells, epithelial cells) may also be found in this region (see Fig. 9.12C). Bacteria are also found within the host tissues, such as in the soft tissues (see Fig. 9.4), and within epithelial cells (Fig. 9.13), as well as in the dentinal tubules (Fig. 9.14).[470,471]

The composition of the subgingival plaque depends on the pocket depth. The apical part is more dominated by spirochetes, cocci, and rods, whereas in the coronal part, more filaments are observed.

The site specificity of plaque is significantly associated with diseases of the periodontium. Marginal plaque, for example, is of prime importance during the initiation and development of gingivitis. Supragingival plaque and tooth-associated subgingival plaque are critical in calculus formation and root caries, whereas tissue-associated subgingival plaque is important in the tissue destruction that characterizes different forms of periodontitis.

Fig. 9.13 Bacteria in Epithelial Cells. (A) to (C) Images of z-section no. 39 from a stack of 74 0.2-μm z-sections (×600; the scale bar in [A] also applies to [B] and [C]). Buccal epithelial cells in this field were double-labeled with (A) the EUB338 universal probe and (B) the *Aggregatibacter actinomycetemcomitans*–specific probe. The cell in the center of (A) contained a large mass of brightly fluorescent intracellular bacteria *(red arrow)*. Other cells in the field contained smaller bacterial masses (not marked). (B) A portion of the large mass labeled with the universal probe also hybridized with the *A. actinomycetemcomitans*–specific probe *(green arrow)*. Images from (A) and (B) were superimposed in (C) to confirm that bacteria labeled with both probes *(yellow arrow)* were adjacent to other bacteria labeled only with the universal probe *(red arrow)*. (D) Three-dimensional reconstruction of the same field. Bacteria recognized only by the universal probe are shown in solid red, whereas the colocalization of the *A. actinomycetemcomitans* and universal probes is depicted by a green wireframe over a red interior. Reconstructed buccal epithelial cell surfaces are presented in blue. The red and green colors are muted when bacterial masses are intracellular and brighter when bacteria appear to project out of the surface. The angle of view was rotated along the z-axis, and the image was zoomed. The large mass that appeared to have a lobular structure in z-section no. 39 was seen to be a cohesive unit that contained *A. actinomycetemcomitans* in direct proximity to other species *(red and green arrows)*. (From Rudney JD, Chen R, Sedgewick GJ: *Actinobacillus actinomycetemcomitans, Porphyromonas gingivalis,* and *Tannerella forsythensis* are components of a polymicrobial intracellular flora within human buccal cells, *J Dent Res* 84:59–63, 2005.)

Fig. 9.14 Scanning Electron Micrograph of Bacteria Within Dentinal Tubules.

Biofilms also establish on artificial surfaces exposed to the oral environment, such as prostheses and implants.

Accumulation of a Dental Plaque Biofilm

The process of plaque formation can be divided into several phases: (1) the formation of the pellicle on the tooth surface, (2) the initial adhesion/attachment of bacteria, and (3) colonization/plaque maturation.

Formation of the Pellicle

All surfaces in the oral cavity, including the hard and soft tissues, are coated with a layer of organic material known as the acquired pellicle. The pellicle on tooth surfaces consists of more than 180 peptides, proteins, and glycoproteins, including keratins, mucins, proline-rich proteins, phosphoproteins (e.g., statherin), histidine-rich proteins, and other molecules that can function as adhesion sites (receptors) for bacteria.[500,501,612] The salivary pellicle can be detected on clean enamel surfaces within 1 minute after their introduction into the mouths of volunteers.[199] By 2 hours, the pellicle is essentially in equilibrium between adsorption and detachment, although further pellicle maturation can be observed for several hours.

Transmission electron microscopy shows the pellicle to be composed of two layers: a thin basal layer that is very difficult to remove, even with harsh chemical and mechanical treatments; and a thicker globular layer, up to 1 μm or more, that is easier to detach.[199,200] From these observations, it can be concluded that dental enamel is permanently covered with an acquired pellicle from the moment that the teeth erupt.

Consequently, bacteria that adhere to tooth surfaces do not contact the enamel directly but interact with the acquired enamel pellicle. However, the pellicle is not merely a passive adhesion matrix. Many proteins retain enzymatic activity when they are incorporated into the pellicle, and some of these, such as peroxidases, lysozyme, and α-amylase, may affect the physiology and metabolism of adhering bacterial cells.[194,196-198]

In addition, a close ecologic relationship between the pellicle and its associated microbiology seems to exist. Walker and coworkers[581] reported that dental plaque samples produced in vitro biofilms only if the surface on which they were grown contained a salivary pellicle belonging to the patient who donated the plaque sample. No biofilm could be grown on a pellicle that came from a different subject.[581]

Initial Adhesion/Attachment of Bacteria

Colonization of a surface begins immediately after its introduction in the oral cavity. Colonizing bacteria can be detected within 3 minutes after the introduction of sterile enamel into the mouth.[195]

The initial steps of transport and interaction with the surface are essentially nonspecific (i.e., they are the same for all bacteria). The proteins and carbohydrates that are exposed on the bacterial cell surface become important when the bacteria are in loose contact with the acquired enamel pellicle. The specific interactions between microbial cell surface "adhesin" molecules and receptors in the salivary pellicle determine whether a bacterial cell will remain associated with the surface. Only a relatively small proportion of oral bacteria possess adhesins that interact with receptors in the host pellicle, and these organisms are generally the most abundant bacteria in biofilms on tooth enamel shortly after cleaning. Over the first 4 to 8 hours, the genus *Streptococcus* tends to dominate, usually accounting for >20% of bacteria present.[114,378,579] Other bacteria that commonly present at this time include species that cannot survive without oxygen (obligate aerobes), such as *Haemophilus* spp. and *Neisseria* spp., as well as organisms that can grow in the presence or absence of oxygen (facultative anaerobes), including *Actinomyces* spp. and *Veillonella* spp.[1,111] These species are considered the "primary colonizers" of tooth surfaces. The primary colonizers provide new binding sites for adhesion by other oral bacteria. The metabolic activity of the primary colonizers modifies the local microenvironment in ways that can influence the ability of other bacteria to survive in the dental plaque biofilm. For example, by removing oxygen, the primary colonizers provide conditions of low oxygen tension that permit the survival and growth of obligate anaerobes.

The initial steps in colonization of teeth by bacteria occur in three phases. Phase 1 is transport to the surface, phase 2 is initial reversible adhesion, and phase 3 is strong attachment. The reader is referred to the online material for a detailed discussion of these three phases.

Online materials for this chapter are found on the companion website.

Colonization and Plaque Maturation

The primary colonizing bacteria (Table 9.3) adhered to the tooth surface provide new receptors for attachment by other bacteria as part of a process known as *coadhesion*.[271] Together with the growth of adherent microorganisms, coadhesion leads to the development of microcolonies (Fig. 9.15) and eventually to a mature biofilm.

Cell–cell adhesion between genetically distinct oral bacteria also occurs in the fluid phase (i.e., in saliva). In the laboratory, interactions between genetically distinct cells in suspension result in clumps or coaggregates that are macroscopically visible (Fig. 9.16).

TABLE 9.3	Overview of Primary and Secondary Colonizers in Dental Plaque
Primary colonizers	*Streptococcus gordonii*
	Streptococcus intermedius
	Streptococcus mitis
	Streptococcus oralis
	Streptococcus sanguinis
	Actinomyces gerencseriae
	Actinomyces israelii
	Actinomyces naeslundii
	Actinomyces oris
	Aggregatibacter actinomycetemcomitans serotype a
	Capnocytophaga gingivalis
	Capnocytophaga ochracea
	Capnocytophaga sputigena
	Eikenella corrodens
	Actinomyces odontolyticus
	Veillonella parvula
Secondary colonizers	*Campylobacter gracilis*
	Campylobacter rectus
	Campylobacter showae
	Eubacterium nodatum
	Aggregatibacter actinomycetemcomitans serotype b
	Fusobacterium nucleatum spp. *nucleatum*
	Fusobacterium nucleatum spp. *vincentii*
	Fusobacterium nucleatum spp. *polymorphum*
	Fusobacterium periodonticum
	Parvimonas micra
	Prevotella intermedia
	Prevotella loescheii
	Prevotella nigrescens
	Streptococcus constellatus
	Tannerella forsythia
	Porphyromonas gingivalis
	Treponema denticola

Coaggregation is a direct interaction; it is distinct from agglutination, which occurs when cells are stuck together by molecules in solution. The reader is referred to the online material for a detailed discussion of coaggregation. Online materials for this chapter are found on the companion website www.expertconsult.com.

The significance of coaggregation in oral colonization has been documented in studies of biofilm formation in vitro as well as in animal model studies.[50,346]

Well-characterized interactions of secondary colonizers (see Table 9.3) with early colonizers include the coaggregation of *F. nucleatum* with *S. sanguinis*, *Prevotella loescheii* with *A. oris*, and *Capnocytophaga ochracea* with *A. oris*.[247,249,593-595] Streptococci show intrageneric coaggregation, which allows them to bind to the nascent monolayer of already bound streptococci.[216,267,379,502]

Secondary colonizers (see Table 9.3) such as *P. intermedia*, *P. loescheii*, *Capnocytophaga* spp., *F. nucleatum*, and *P. gingivalis* do not initially colonize clean tooth surfaces but rather adhere to bacteria that are already in the plaque mass.[270] The transition from early supragingival dental plaque to mature plaque growing below the gingival margin involves a shift in the microbial population from primarily gram-positive organisms to high numbers of gram-negative bacteria. Therefore, during the later stages of plaque formation, coaggregation among different gram-negative species is likely to predominate. Examples of these types of interactions are the coaggregation of *F. nucleatum* with *P. gingivalis* or *Treponema denticola* (see Fig. 9.2L).[258,266,272]

KEY FACT

Biofilm maturation is a highly specific event that involves a nonrandom aggregation of different bacteria.

Fig. 9.15 Dental Plaque. (A) and (B) When a single microorganism adheres to the tooth surface, it can start to multiply, and it slowly forms a microcolony of daughter cells. These views were taken after plaque formation on a plastic strip (e.g., as shown in Fig. 8.20) glued to a tooth surface.

Fig. 9.16 Coaggregation. Coaggregation between *Streptococcus gordonii* DL1 and *Actinomyces oris* MG1 in vitro. A monoculture of *S. gordonii* appears uniformly turbid. Microscopically, cells labeled with specific anti-DL1 antibodies (green) are in small chains or clumps. After the addition of *A. oris*, cells clump together to form macroscopic coaggregates *(yellow arrowhead)*. Under the microscope, *S. gordonii* (green) are evenly distributed throughout the coaggregates with *A. oris* (orange). Bar = 20 μm. (Image reproduced in part from Jakubovics NS, Gill SR, Iobst SE, et al: Regulation of gene expression in a mixed-genus community: stabilized arginine biosynthesis in *Streptococcus gordonii* by coaggregation with *Actinomyces naeslundii*, *J Bacteriol* 190:3646, 2008.)

An analysis of more than 13,000 plaque samples that looked for 40 subgingival microorganisms using a DNA-hybridization methodology defined color-coded "complexes" of periodontal microorganisms that tend to be found together in health or disease. The composition of the different complexes was based on the frequency with which different clusters of microorganisms were recovered, and the complexes were color coded for easy conceptualization (eFig. 9.2).[516] Interestingly, the early colonizers are either independent of defined complexes *(A. naeslundii, A. oris)* or members of the yellow (*Streptococcus* spp.) or purple complexes *(A. odontolyticus)* (see Fig. 9.2D). The microorganisms primarily considered secondary colonizers fell into the green, orange, and red complexes. The red complex consists of *P. gingivalis, T. forsythia,* and *T. denticola.* This complex is of particular interest because it is associated with bleeding on probing.[516] The existence of complexes of species in plaque is another reflection of bacterial interdependency in the biofilm environment.

Factors That Affect Supragingival Dental Plaque Formation

Clinically, early undisturbed plaque formation on teeth follows an exponential growth curve when measured planimetrically.[428]

During the first 24 hours, when starting with a clean tooth surface, plaque growth is negligible from a clinical viewpoint (i.e., <3% coverage of the vestibular tooth surface, which is an amount nearly undetectable clinically). This "lag time" is a result of the fact that the microbial population must reach a certain size before it can easily be detected by a clinician. During the following 3 days, coverage progresses rapidly to the point at which, after 4 days, an average of 30% of the total coronal tooth area will be covered with plaque (Video 9.2).

Several reports have shown that the microbial composition of the dental plaque will change, with a shift toward a more anaerobic and a more gram-negative flora, including an influx of fusobacteria, filaments, spiral forms, and spirochetes, when periodontal tissues are inflamed (Fig. 9.17). This was clearly illustrated in experimental gingivitis studies.[537,552] For example, using next-generation sequencing, the microbiota was shown to shift from baseline to a significantly different community within 1 week of withdrawing oral hygiene.[261] With this ecologic shift within the biofilm, a transition occurs from the early aerobic environment, which is characterized by gram-positive facultative species, to a highly oxygen-deprived environment, in which gram-negative anaerobic microorganisms predominate. Bacterial growth in older plaque is much slower than in newly formed

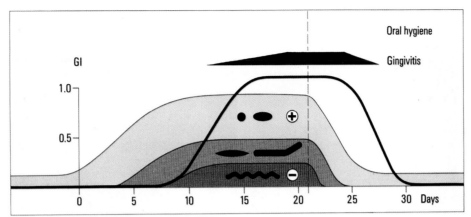

Fig. 9.17 Artistic Impression of the 1965 Published Classic Experimental Proof of the Bacterial Etiology of Gingivitis Using the Experimental Gingivitis Model. In plaque-free subjects with clinically noninflamed gingiva, plaque will slowly develop on the teeth when all mechanical plaque control is stopped. With time, the plaque composition changes. During the first few days, the plaque is mainly composed of gram-positive (+) cocci and rods. Later on, the composition is shifted toward more gram-negative species and more rods and filaments; finally, gram-negative (–) spirochetes appear (see morphotypes in *black*). Within a few days, mild gingivitis ensues (*black line;* gingival index [GI] of 1 according to Löe and Silness). From the moment that proper plaque control is reestablished (*vertical line*), the plaque composition returns to the initial situation, and the symptoms of gingivitis disappear. (From Löe H, Theilade E, Jensen SB: Experimental gingivitis in man, *J Periodontol* 36:177, 1965.)

Fig. 9.18 Typical Topography of Plaque Growth. Initial growth starts along the gingival margins and from the interdental spaces (i.e., areas protected from shear forces) to extend farther in a coronal direction. This pattern may fundamentally change, for example, if the tooth surface contains irregularities, such as those evident in Fig. 8.19.

Fig. 9.19 Surface Irregularities and Plaque Growth. Important surface irregularities (i.e., a crack on the central upper incisor, several small pits on the canine) are also responsible for the so-called individualized plaque growth pattern.

dental plaque, presumably because nutrients become limiting for much of the plaque biomass.[590]

Topography of Supragingival Plaque

Early plaque formation on teeth follows a typical topographic pattern (Fig. 9.18), with initial growth along the gingival margin and from the interdental spaces (i.e., the areas protected from shear forces). Later, a further extension in the coronal direction can be observed.[354,431] This pattern may change severely when the tooth surface contains irregularities that offer a favorable growth path (Fig. 9.19). Plaque formation may also originate from grooves, cracks, perikymata, or pits. Scanning electron microscopy studies clearly revealed that the early colonization of the enamel surface starts from surface irregularities in which bacteria shelter from shear forces, thereby permitting them the time needed to change from reversible to irreversible binding.

KEY FACT

Dental plaque growth starts at areas that are protected from shear forces such as the gingival margin, the interdental space, and along grooves, cracks, pits, and fissures.

By multiplication, the bacteria subsequently spread out from these starting-up areas as a relatively even monolayer. Surface irregularities are also responsible for the so-called individualized plaque growth pattern (see Fig. 9.19), which is reproduced in the absence of optimal oral hygiene.[354,355] This phenomenon illustrates the importance of surface roughness in plaque growth, which should lead to proper clinical treatment options.

A   Cellulose acetate

B   Teflon

Fig. 9.20 Photographs Showing the Clinical Impact of Surface Roughness and Surface Free Energy on De Novo Plaque Formation. (A) and (B) Two small strips were glued to the central upper incisors of a patient who refrained from oral hygiene for 3 days. Each strip was divided in two halves: a rough region (R_a 2.0 μm) located mesially and a smooth region (R_a 0.1 μm) located distally. (A) Cellulose acetate strip (medium surface free energy [sfe]: 58 ergcm^{-2}). (B) Teflon strip (low sfe: 20 ergcm^{-2}). Plaque was disclosed with 0.5% neutral red solution. The smooth regions show the decrease in biofilm formation because of the low sfe; the rough regions demonstrate the predominance of surface roughness (i.e., more plaque with no difference between the two surfaces), even with different sfe. (From Quirynen M, Listgarten MA: Distribution of bacterial morphotypes around natural teeth and titanium implants ad modum Brånemark, *Clin Oral Implants Res* 1:8, 1990.)

Surface Microroughness

Rough intraoral surfaces (e.g., crown margins, implant abutments, denture bases) accumulate and retain more plaque and calculus in terms of thickness, area, and colony-forming units.[421] Ample plaque also reveals an increased maturity or pathogenicity of its bacterial components, which is characterized by an increased proportion of motile organisms and spirochetes and/or a denser packing of them (Figs. 9.20 and 9.21). Smoothing an intraoral surface decreases the rate of plaque formation. Below a certain surface roughness ($R_a < 0.2$ μm), however, further smoothing does not result in an additional reduction in plaque formation.[43,422] There seems to be a threshold level for surface roughness ($R_a \approx 0.2$ μm) above which bacterial adhesion will be facilitated.[42] Although surface free energy and surface roughness are two factors that influence plaque growth, the latter predominates (see Figs. 9.20 and 9.21).

Individual Variables That Influence Plaque Formation

The rate of plaque formation differs significantly among subjects, and these differences may overrule surface characteristics. A distinction is often made between "heavy" (fast) and "light" (slow) plaque formers (Video 9.3).

A multiple regression analysis showed that the clinical wettability of the tooth surfaces, the saliva-induced aggregation of oral bacteria, and the relative salivary flow conditions around the sampled teeth explained 90% of the variation. Moreover, the saliva from light plaque formers reduced the colloidal stability of bacterial suspensions of, for example, *S. sanguinis*.[498]

> ### CLINICIAN'S CORNER
>
> **Do Some Patients Form Plaque Faster Than Others?**
> Yes, so-called heavy and light plaque formers exist. However, in both cases it takes days before the plaque is clinically visible. Patients cannot justify poor oral hygiene by being heavy plaque formers.

In a study by Zee and colleagues,[623] de novo plaque formation was followed on small enamel blocks that were bonded onto the teeth of slow and heavy plaque formers. After 1 day, the heavy plaque formers showed more plaque with a more complex supragingival structure. However, from days 3 to 14, no discernible differences were noted between both groups, except for a more prominent intermicrobial matrix in the group of fast growers. In another study by the same group of investigators, qualitative differences in the composition of the plaque between slow and rapid plaque formers were detected.[622] Rapid plaque formers demonstrated higher proportions of gram-negative rods (35% vs. 17%) in 14-day-old plaque. The inter-subject variation in plaque formation can also be explained by factors such as diet, chewing fibrous food, smoking, the presence of copper amalgam, tongue and palate brushing, the colloid stability of bacteria in the saliva, antimicrobial factors present in the saliva, the chemical composition of the pellicle, and the retention depth of the dentogingival area.[a]

---

[a]References 5, 8, 21, 223, 227, 494, 498, 499.

Fig. 9.21 Plaque Formation and Surface Roughness. (A) A small plastic strip, divided in half (a rough region [R_a 2.0 μm] located mesially and a smooth region [R_a 0.1 μm] located distally), had been glued to the central upper incisors of a patient who refrained from oral hygiene for 3 days. (B) and (C) After removal, the strip had been cut into small slices for microscopic evaluation. It is obvious that the rough part (C) contains a thicker plaque layer than the smooth part (B). The *arrow* shows the border between the rough and smooth surfaces. (From Quirynen M, Listgarten MA: Distribution of bacterial morphotypes around natural teeth and titanium implants ad modum Brånemark, *Clin Oral Implants Res* 1:8, 1990.)

Variation Within the Dentition

Within a dental arch, large differences in plaque growth rate can be detected. In general, early plaque formation occurs faster: in the lower jaw (as compared with the upper jaw); in molar areas; on the buccal tooth surfaces (as compared with palatal sites, especially in the upper jaw); and in the interdental regions (as compared with the buccal or lingual surfaces).[147,297,420]

Impact of Gingival Inflammation and Saliva

Several studies clearly indicate that early in vivo plaque formation is more rapid on tooth surfaces facing inflamed gingival margins than on those adjacent to healthy gingivae.[425,438,439] These studies suggest that the increase in crevicular fluid production enhances plaque formation. Probably some substances from this exudate (e.g., minerals, proteins, carbohydrates) favor both the initial adhesion and/or the growth of the early colonizing bacteria. In addition, it is known that, during the night, the plaque growth rate is reduced by around 50%.[431] This seems surprising because one would expect that reduced plaque removal and the decreased salivary flow at night would enhance plaque growth. The fact that the supragingival plaque obtains its nutrients mainly from the saliva appears to be of greater significance than the antibacterial activity of saliva.[68]

Impact of Patient's Age

Although older studies were contradictory, more recent reports clearly indicate that a subject's age does not influence de novo plaque formation. In a study by Fransson and colleagues,[143] no differences could be detected in de novo plaque formation between a group of young (20 to 25 years old) patients and a group of older (65 to 80 years old) subjects who abolished mechanical tooth cleaning measures for 21 days, neither in amount nor in composition.[143] This observation largely confirms data by Holm-Pedersen and colleagues[215] and data by Winkel and coworkers.[604] However, the developed plaque in the older patient group resulted in more severe gingival inflammation, which seems to indicate an increased susceptibility to gingivitis with aging.

Fig. 9.22 Lower Premolars and Molars From a Dental Student Who Refrained From Oral Hygiene for 100 Hours to Evaluate Undisturbed Plaque Formation. (A) Before dinner. (B) After dinner, which included fibrous foods. Nearly no reduction in plaque extension could be observed, thereby illustrating the absence of spontaneous plaque removal.

CLINICIAN'S CORNER

Do Older People Form More Plaque?
No, the rate of de novo plaque formation is similar in young and old patients. However, older patients may have less dexterity, which could explain larger amounts of plaque.

Spontaneous Tooth Cleaning

Many clinicians still think that plaque is removed spontaneously from the teeth, such as during eating. However, on the basis of the firm attachment between the bacteria and the surface, this seems unlikely. Even in the occlusal surfaces of the molars, plaque remains, even after chewing fibrous food (e.g., carrots, apples, chips). The inefficiency of the spontaneous plaque removal is neatly illustrated by the clinical pictures in Fig. 9.22, which were taken before and after dinner starting from 4 days of undisturbed plaque formation. Only negligible differences in plaque extent could be observed.

De Novo Subgingival Plaque Formation

It is technically impossible to record the dynamics of subgingival plaque formation in an established dentition for the simple reason that one cannot sterilize a periodontal pocket. Some early studies involving the use of culturing techniques examined the changes within the subgingival microbiota during the first week after mechanical debridement and reported an only partial reduction of around 3 logs (from 10^8 bacterial cells to 10^5 cells), followed by rapid regrowth toward nearly pretreatment levels (−0.5 log) within 7 days.[161,201,335] The fast recolonization was explained by several factors. A critical review of the effectiveness of subgingival debridement, for instance, revealed that a high proportion of treated tooth surfaces (5% to 80%) still harbored plaque and/or calculus after scaling. These remaining bacteria were considered the primary source for the subgingival recolonization.[408] Some pathogens penetrate the soft tissues or the dentinal tubules and eventually escape instrumentation (see Fig. 9.14).[7,157,463] In a beagle dog study, Leknes and colleagues[304] studied the extent of subgingival colonization in 6-mm pockets with smooth or rough root surfaces. These investigators also observed that smooth surfaces harbored significantly less plaque and concluded that subgingival irregularities shelter submerged microorganisms. Moreover, biopsies of the soft tissues showed an elevated proportion of inflammatory cells in the junctional epithelium (and the underlying connective tissue) facing the rough surfaces.[305] Finally, the same group reported higher rates of attachment loss around teeth with grooves in the root surface.[303]

The introduction of oral implants, especially of the two-stage type, provided a new experimental setup. When the transmucosal part of the implant (the abutment) is inserted on top of the osseointegrated endosseous part, a new "pristine" surface is created on which the intraoral translocation of bacteria can be investigated.[422] It has been demonstrated that a complex subgingival microbiota, including most periodontopathogens, is established within 1 week after abutment insertion. This is followed by a slow increase in the number of periodontopathogens.[146,434,435] Oral implants have also been used as a model to study the impact of surface roughness on subgingival plaque formation.[43,62,173,422,432,452] Smooth abutments ($R_a < 0.2$ μm) were found to harbor 25 times fewer bacteria than rough ones, with a slightly higher density of coccoid (i.e., nonpathogenic) cells. The subgingival microbiota was also largely dependent on the remaining presence of teeth and the degree of periodontitis in the remaining natural dentition (for a review, see reference 407). These observations highlight the importance of intraoral bacterial translocation for subgingival biofilms.

CHARACTERISTICS OF BIOFILM BACTERIA (LIFE IN "SLIME CITY")

Metabolism of Dental Plaque Bacteria

Most nutrients for dental plaque bacteria originate from saliva or gingival crevicular fluid, although the host diet provides an occasional but nevertheless important food supply. The transition from gram-positive to gram-negative microorganisms observed in the structural development of dental plaque is paralleled by a physiologic transition in the developing plaque.

The early colonizers (e.g., *Streptococcus* and *Actinomyces* spp.) use oxygen and lower the redox potential of the environment, which then favors the growth of anaerobic species.[112,580] Many of the gram-positive early colonizers use sugars as an energy source. The bacteria that predominate in mature plaque are

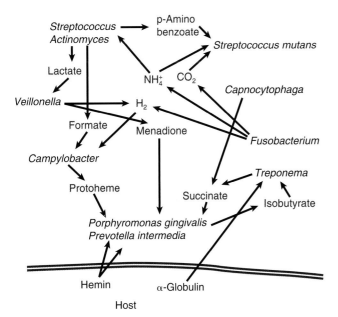

Fig. 9.23 Schematic Illustration of Metabolic Interactions Among Different Bacterial Species Found in Plaque and Between the Host and the Plaque Bacteria. These interactions are likely to be important to the survival of bacteria in the periodontal environment. CO_2, Carbon dioxide; H_2, hydrogen; NH^+_4, ammonium. (Data from Carlsson J: Microbiology of plaque associated periodontal disease. In Lindhe J, editor: *Textbook of clinical periodontology*, Munksgaard, 1983, Munksgaard International Publishers; Grenier D: Nutritional interactions between two suspected periodontopathogens, *Treponema denticola* and *Porphyromonas gingivalis*. *Infect Immun* 60:5298, 1992; Loesche WJ: Importance of nutrition in gingival crevice microbial ecology. *Periodontics* 6:245, 1968; and Walden WC, Hentges DJ: Differential effects of oxygen and oxidation-reduction potential on the multiplication of three species of anaerobic intestinal bacteria, *Appl Microbiol* 30:781, 1975.)

anaerobic and asaccharolytic (i.e., they do not break down sugars), and they use amino acids and small peptides as energy sources.[322]

Laboratory studies have demonstrated many metabolic interactions among the different bacteria found in dental plaque (Fig. 9.23). For example, lactate and formate are byproducts of the metabolism of streptococci and *Actinomyces* spp.; they may be used in the metabolism of other plaque microorganisms, including *Veillonella* spp. and *A. actinomycetemcomitans*.[61,127] Interestingly, the commensal bacterium *S. gordonii* have also been shown to provide electron acceptors that promote respiratory growth of *A. actinomycetemcomitans* in vivo during abscess formation.[528] The importance of this cross-respiration in dental plaque biofilms is not yet clear.

The growth of *P. gingivalis* is enhanced by metabolic byproducts produced by other microorganisms, such as succinate from *C. ochracea* or *T. denticola* and protoheme from *Campylobacter rectus* (see Fig. 9.2R).[167,168,345] In turn, *P. gingivalis* provides isobutyric acid that stimulates growth of *T. denticola*.[167] Overall, the total plaque population is more efficient than any one constituent organism at releasing energy from the available substrates.[600]

Metabolic interactions also occur between the host and the plaque microorganisms. The bacterial enzymes that degrade host proteins mediate the release of ammonia, which may be used by bacteria as a nitrogen source.[69] Hemin iron from the breakdown of host hemoglobin may be important in the metabolism of *P. gingivalis*.[52] Increases in steroid hormones are associated with significant increases in the proportions of *P. intermedia* found in subgingival plaque.[278] These nutritional interdependencies are probably critical to the growth and survival of microorganisms in dental plaque, and they may partly explain the evolution of the highly specific structural interactions observed among bacteria in plaque.

Communication Between Biofilm Bacteria

Bacterial cells do not exist in isolation. In a biofilm, bacteria have the capacity to communicate with each other. One example of this is quorum sensing, in which bacteria secrete a signaling molecule that accumulates in the local environment and triggers a response such as a change in the expression of specific genes once they reach a critical threshold concentration. The reader is referred to the online material for a detailed discussion of quorum sensing. Online materials for this chapter are found on the companion website www.expertconsult.com.

Interactions Among Dental Plaque Bacteria

Some evidence indicates from laboratory studies that nonpathogenic organisms in subgingival dental plaque can modify the behavior of periodontal pathogens. For example, long and short fimbriae of *P. gingivalis* are required for adhesion and biofilm formation. The expression of long fimbriae is down-regulated in the presence of *Streptococcus cristatus*, and short fimbriae are down-regulated by *S. gordonii*, *S. mitis*, or *S. sanguinis*.[311,397] Changes in bacterial physiology after transitions from monoculture to mixed-species communities may be quite wide ranging.

With the use of a proteomics approach to probe the phenotype of *P. gingivalis*, it has been shown that the expression of almost 500 *P. gingivalis* proteins is changed in model oral microbial communities that contain *S. gordonii* and *F. nucleatum*.[285] At present, it is not clear how these changes affect the interaction between *P. gingivalis* and the host.

In multispecies biofilms in which many bacteria are juxtaposed to cells of different species, interactions among genetically distinct microorganisms can be mutually beneficial (see Fig. 9.5A). However, many examples of competitive interactions between different bacteria exist (Fig. 9.24). For example, *S. mutans* produces antimicrobial peptides that have broad activity against bacteria in vitro.[283] Other oral streptococci compete with *S. mutans* by excreting the strongly oxidizing molecule H_2O_2.[283] In fact, *Streptococcus oligofermentans* can convert lactic acid produced by *S. mutans* into H_2O_2, which then kills the *S. mutans* cells.[555]

In subgingival biofilms, oxygen is scarce, and therefore H_2O_2 production by bacteria is lower. Oxidizing agents may be more important in the interaction between the host and the pathogen because reactive oxygen species are a major component of the neutrophil response to bacteria.

Another example of competitive interaction exists between streptococci and periodontopathogens. *S. sanguinis*, *S. salivarius*, and *S. mitis* have been shown to inhibit hard and soft tissue colonization of *A. actinomycetemcomitans* (Video 9.4), *P. gingivalis*, and *P. intermedia* in vitro.[504,550,571]

Fig. 9.24 Growth Inhibition Induced by Streptococci. The growth of *Prevotella intermedia* (black colonies) is inhibited by the presence of *Streptococcus mitis, Streptococcus salivarius,* and *Streptococcus sanguinis* (in the white holes). This is represented by a zone of no growth (halo) around the white holes. This is a typical example of growth inhibition induced by streptococci.

Biofilms and Antimicrobial Resistance

Bacteria growing in microbial communities adherent to a surface do not "behave" the same way as bacteria growing suspended in a liquid environment (i.e., in a planktonic or unattached state). For example, the resistance of bacteria to antimicrobial agents is dramatically increased in the biofilm.[13,92,207,416] Almost without exception, organisms in a biofilm are 1000 to 1500 times more resistant as compared with antibiotics in their planktonic state. The mechanisms of this increased resistance differ from species to species, from antibiotic to antibiotic, and for biofilms growing in different habitats.

It is generally accepted that the resistance of bacteria to antibiotics is affected by their nutritional status, growth rate, temperature, pH, and prior exposure to sub-effective concentrations of antimicrobial agents.[59,60,602] Variations in any of these parameters will lead to a varied response to antibiotics within a biofilm. An important mechanism of resistance appears to be the slower rate of growth of bacterial species in a biofilm, which makes them less susceptible to many but not all antibiotics.[23,57,92,610] The biofilm matrix, although not a significant physical barrier to the diffusion of antibiotics, does have certain properties that can retard antibiotic penetration. For example, strongly charged or chemically highly reactive agents can fail to reach the deeper zones of the biofilm because the biofilm acts as an ion-exchange resin that removes such molecules from solution.[155,539]

> ### KEY FACT
> The bacteria within biofilms are often up to 1000 times more resistant to antimicrobial agents than their planktonic counterparts.

In addition, extracellular enzymes such as β-lactamases, formaldehyde lyase, and formaldehyde dehydrogenase may become trapped and concentrated in the extracellular matrix, and as such inactivate some antibiotics (especially positively charged hydrophilic antibiotics).

Some antibiotics, such as the macrolides, which are positively charged but hydrophobic, are unaffected by this process.

"Super-resistant" bacteria were identified within a biofilm. These cells have multidrug resistance pumps that can extrude antimicrobial agents from the cell.[57] Because these pumps place the antibiotics outside of the outer membrane, the process offers protection against antibiotics that target, for example, cell wall synthesis. The penetration and efficacy of antimicrobials against biofilm bacteria are critical issues for the treatment of periodontal infections.

Antibiotic resistance may be spread through a biofilm via the intercellular exchange of DNA. The high density of bacterial cells in a biofilm facilitates the exchange of genetic information among cells of the same species and across species and even across genera. Conjugation (i.e., the exchange of genes through a direct interbacteria connection formed by a sex pilus), transformation (i.e., the movement of small pieces of DNA from the environment into the bacterial chromosome), plasmid transfer, and transposon transfer have all been shown to occur in biofilms.

BACTERIAL TRANSMISSION AND TRANSLOCATION

The transmission of pathogens from one *locus* to another is an important aspect of infectious diseases. In theory, such transmission may jeopardize the outcome of periodontal therapy; in addition, the transmission of pathogens from one person to another may be important in terms of disease transmission. The significance of such an intraoral transmission or of a vertical or horizontal transmission is, however, difficult to prove or to quantify.

One of the first questions in this regard is, "Are oral bacteria transmissible between humans?" Molecular fingerprinting techniques have clearly illustrated that periodontal pathogens are transmissible within members of a family (Fig. 9.25).[618]

This bacterial transmission between subjects (and even between animals and human beings) should not be confused with contagion (with the term *contagious* referring to the likelihood that a microorganism will be transmitted from an infected to an uninfected host to create disease). Asikainen and coworkers[24] used a genetic fingerprinting method called *arbitrarily primed-polymerase chain reaction* to genotype *A. actinomycetemcomitans* isolates from family members. In 11 of 12 families, these investigators found identical *A. actinomycetemcomitans* genotypes among family members. This finding suggests that the transmission of this microorganism occurs among family members. However, it was more often encountered that children carried a genotype identical to one of their parents than that spouses carried an identical genotype. This indicates that, in terms of *A. actinomycetemcomitans* transmission, vertical transmission is more important than horizontal transmission. Similar observations were made for the transmission of cariogenic species from mother to child.[263] The vertical or horizontal transmission of *P. gingivalis* has rarely been observed.[566]

The existence of an "intraoral" translocation of bacteria (i.e., from one niche to another) has been investigated more thoroughly. Intraoral transmission of bacteria was first examined in cariology.

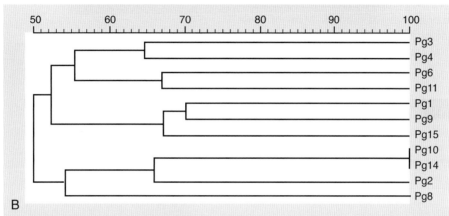

Fig. 9.25 *Porphyromonas gingivalis* **Strains.** (A) Band pattern of DNA isolated from multiple *Porphyromonas gingivalis* strains after pulsed-field gel electrophoresis. Lanes 1, 8, and 15 contain a reference strain of DNA (*Staphylococcus aureus*) cut with SmaI (a restriction endonuclease) in lanes 2 through 7 and 9 through 14; 12 different *P. gingivalis* strains are compared for their genetic similarity. (B) The genetic similarity is expressed in a dendrogram. Bacteria are considered genetically similar when their band patterns are 80% similar.

Loesche and coworkers[324] showed that streptomycin-resistant strains of *S. mutans* grown on a dental inlay were spontaneously transmitted to the neighboring teeth (probably via saliva) and could even reach the contralateral quadrant after transmission with a dental explorer. Previously, Edman and coworkers[125] had successfully implanted the previously mentioned species in two volunteers by means of inoculated dental flosses. Comparable observations have been made for periodontopathogens.

Christersson and coworkers[83] demonstrated a translocation of *A. actinomycetemcomitans* via periodontal probes in localized juvenile periodontitis patients. Although the colonization was only temporary, the question remained whether the colonization could not have become permanent if the site had offered more suitable growth conditions (e.g., a deep bleeding pocket, as frequently encountered immediately after initial periodontal therapy). It is well-established that colonization of an already established microbial niche by a new species is difficult because it is hampered by a variety of microbial interactions. Therefore, intraoral translocation to and the colonization of sterile surfaces may be different from the translocation and colonization of already colonized surfaces. Within the oral cavity, such sterile surfaces are not naturally occurring. However, at the moment of abutment placement on a dental implant, a sterile subgingival pocket is created. A large series of articles compared the microbiota in pockets around teeth with that found in peri-implant pockets in partially edentulous patients and reported a striking similarity.[a] Several studies have investigated the subgingival colonization of such "sterile" peri-implant pockets in partially edentulous patients.[146] The initial colonization of these pockets with periodontopathogens is completed within 1 week. After 2 weeks, only minor additional changes occur in this newly developed microbiota.[146,434,435] These additional changes mainly reflect changes in the numbers of species. On the basis of the previously mentioned similarities between the microbial populations associated with teeth and implants, it has been suggested that, at least in partially edentulous patients, teeth may act as a reservoir for the (re)colonization of the subgingival area around implants.

---

[a]References 17, 221, 222, 262, 264, 302, 306, 350, 360, 396, 427, 483.

This hypothesis was supported by Sumida and coworkers,[536] who detected similar intrasubject pulsed field gel electrophoresis patterns for *P. gingivalis* from teeth and implants (indicating that these locations contained precisely the same *P. gingivalis* strains) as compared with large inter-subject variations. The reader is referred to the online material for a detailed discussion of intraoral translocation. Online materials for this chapter are found on the companion website www.expertconsult.com.

NONBACTERIAL INHABITANTS OF THE ORAL CAVITY

Oral microbiology is often reduced to "oral bacteriology." However, the oral cavity comprises a much more diverse microbiota than merely a bacterial one. Viruses, fungi, archaea, and protozoa can be encountered in the oral cavity of humans. Many of these species can reside in the oral cavity in harmony with the host as commensals, similar to oral bacteria, but they can also cause several oral diseases.

> ### KEY FACT
>
> In addition to bacteria, viruses can be present in the mouth. Herpesviruses, human papillomaviruses, picornaviruses, and retroviruses can all contribute to the development of oral ulcers, tumors, mononucleosis, Sjögren syndrome, osteomyelitis, osteonecrosis, oral leukoplakia, and oral lichen planus.

Viruses

Viral diseases of the oral mucosa and the perioral region are often encountered in dental practice. Viruses are important ulcerogenic and tumorigenic agents of the human mouth. The finding of an abundance of mammalian viruses in periodontitis lesions may suggest a role for viruses in more oral diseases than previously recognized.[491] A more in-depth review can be found in two articles by Slots.[508,509]

In contrast to most bacteria, viruses replicate only when they are present within eukaryotic (animals, plants, protists, and fungi) or prokaryotic (bacteria and archaea) cells and not on their own. The extracellular virion particle ranges in size from 20 to 300 nm and consists of either DNA or ribonucleic acid (RNA) contained within a protective protein coat or capsid (Fig. 9.26).

The reader is referred to the online material for a detailed discussion of the role of viruses in periodontal diseases. Online materials for this chapter are found on the companion website www.expertconsult.com.

Fungi

Many fungal species have been isolated from the oral cavity. Most isolates are *Candida*, and the most prevalent species is *Candida albicans* (Fig. 9.27). Together with *C. albicans*, some of the most common opportunistic fungal candidal pathogens in humans are *C. tropicalis, C. glabrata, C. krusei, C parapsilosis, C. guilliermondii,* and *C. dubliniensis. Candida* spp. thrive in low-pH environments, and high *Candida* loads are associated with the presence of relatively low-diversity dental plaque that contains aciduric and acidogenic species such as *Streptococcus* spp. and

Fig. 9.26 Herpes Simplex Virus Type 1. Electron micrographic picture of herpes simplex virus type 1, enveloped *(left)* and naked capsids *(right)*. ×198,000. (From Fields BN, Knipe DM: In Fields BN, editors: *Virology,* New York, 1985, Raven Press.)

Fig. 9.27 Sample From the Palate of a Patient With Denture Stomatitis With Clear Candidal Mycelia Visualized Under a Phase-Contrast Microscope.

Lactobacillus spp.[281] In addition to *C. albicans, C. glabrata* is now emerging as an important agent in both mucosal and bloodstream infections.[309,410] The reader is referred to the online material for a detailed discussion of the role of fungi in periodontal diseases. Online materials for this chapter are found on the companion website www.expertconsult.com.

Protozoa

The mouth is the entry port for many parasites that have adapted to the human host. Only a few parasites affect the oral cavity, but an increasing body of literature indicates that oral protozoa are more common than previously appreciated.[37] Depending on the type of infection, the parasitic infectious agents can be divided into two categories: (1) those that induce local infections and (2) those that induce systemic infections with indirect effects on the oral cavity. The former group comprises saprophytes (e.g., *Entamoeba gingivalis, Trichomonas tenax*) (Fig. 9.28; Video 9.5), which have the potential to turn into opportunistic pathogens or free-living amoebas, which occasionally become invasive but are seldom clinically present. Protozoa tend to be seen in cases of poor oral hygiene and poor periodontal health. The reader is referred to the online material for a detailed discussion

Fig. 9.28 *Trichomonas* in Dental Plaque Visualized Under a Phase-Contrast Microscope.

of the role of parasites in periodontal diseases. Online materials for this chapter are found on the companion website www.expertconsult.com.

Archaea

Archaea are single-celled organisms that are as distinct from bacteria as they are from eukaryotes. The role of archaea in oral diseases is only beginning to be explored. The reader is referred to the online material for a detailed discussion of the role of archaea in periodontal diseases. Online materials for this chapter are found on the companion website www.expertconsult.com.

MICROBIOLOGIC SPECIFICITY OF PERIODONTAL DISEASES

Nonspecific Plaque Hypothesis

During the mid-1900s, periodontal diseases were thought to result from an accumulation of plaque over time, eventually in conjunction with a diminished host response and increased host susceptibility with age. This theory, which is called the *nonspecific plaque hypothesis*, was supported by epidemiologic studies that correlated both age and the amount of plaque with evidence of periodontitis.[328,465,485]

According to the nonspecific plaque hypothesis, periodontal disease results from the "elaboration of noxious products by the entire plaque flora."[323] When only small amounts of plaque are present, the noxious products are neutralized by the host. Similarly, large amounts of plaque would cause a higher production of noxious products, which would essentially overwhelm the host's defenses.

> **KEY FACT**
>
> Although the nonspecific plaque hypothesis has been discarded in favor of other etiologic hypotheses, most of the therapeutic interventions are still based on the principles of the nonspecific plaque hypothesis.

Several observations contradicted these conclusions: First, some individuals with considerable amounts of plaque and calculus, as well as gingivitis, never developed destructive periodontitis.

Furthermore, individuals who did present with periodontitis demonstrated considerable site specificity with regard to the pattern of disease. Some sites were unaffected, whereas advanced disease was found in adjacent sites. In the presence of a uniform host response, these findings were inconsistent with the concept that all plaque was equally pathogenic. Recognition of the differences in plaque at sites of different clinical statuses (i.e., disease versus health) led to a renewed search for specific pathogens in periodontal diseases and a conceptual transition from the nonspecific to the specific plaque hypothesis.[321,506,513]

Inherent to the nonspecific plaque hypothesis is the concept that the control of periodontal disease depends on the reduction of the total amount of plaque. The current standard treatment of periodontitis by debridement (nonsurgical or surgical) and oral hygiene measures still focuses on the removal of plaque and its products. Although the nonspecific plaque hypothesis has been discarded in favor of other etiologic hypotheses, most of the therapeutic interventions are still based on the basic principles of the nonspecific plaque hypothesis.

Specific Plaque Hypothesis

The specific plaque hypothesis underlines the importance of the qualitative composition of the resident microbiota. The pathogenicity of dental plaque depends on the presence of or an increase in specific microorganisms.[323] This concept encapsulates that plaque that harbors specific bacterial pathogens may provoke periodontal disease because key organisms produce substances that mediate the destruction of host tissues. The association of specific bacterial species with disease came about during the early 1960s, when the microscopic examination of plaque revealed that different bacterial morphotypes were found in healthy versus periodontally diseased sites (see Video 9.5). At about the same time, major advances were made in the techniques used to isolate and identify periodontal microorganisms. These included improvements in procedures to sample subgingival plaque, in the handling of samples to prevent killing the bacteria, and in the media used to grow the bacteria in the laboratory.[515] The results were a tremendous increase in the ability to isolate periodontal microorganisms and to achieve a considerable refinement in bacterial taxonomy.[284] Acceptance of the specific plaque hypothesis was spurred by the recognition of *A. actinomycetemcomitans* as a pathogen in localized aggressive periodontitis.[370,506] These advances led to a series of association studies focused on identifying specific periodontal pathogens by examining the microbiota associated with states of health and disease in cross-sectional and longitudinal studies.

The introduction of molecular methods for bacterial identification has greatly increased the power of association studies because we are no longer constrained by analyzing those bacteria that can be cultured (i.e., up to 50% of the total oral microbiota). For example, specific members of the phylum Synergistetes that have never been cultured in isolation show a clear association with periodontal disease.[574] Molecular identification techniques such as DNA checkerboard hybridization can identify and enumerate many different organisms simultaneously and are thus well suited to high-throughput studies (see eFig. 9.2). The association of Socranksy's "red complex" bacteria (*P. gingivalis, T. forsythia,* and

T. denticola) with periodontal disease was based on the analysis of 40 different bacteria in more than 13,000 plaque samples.[516] Nevertheless, disease association studies do not reveal whether the presence of specific bacteria *causes* or *correlates with* the presence of disease. In addition, these studies have shown that periodontal disease can occur even in the absence of defined "pathogens," such as red complex bacteria, and conversely, that "pathogens" may be present in the absence of disease.

Ecologic Plaque Hypothesis

During the 1990s, Marsh and coworkers[339] developed the "ecologic plaque hypothesis" as an attempt to unify the existing theories regarding the role of dental plaque in oral disease (Fig. 9.29). According to the ecologic plaque hypothesis, both the total amount of dental plaque and the specific microbial composition of plaque may contribute to the transition from health to disease. The health-associated dental plaque microbiota is considered to be relatively stable over time and in a state of dynamic equilibrium or "microbial homeostasis." The host controls subgingival plaque to some extent by a tempered immune response and low levels of gingival crevicular fluid flow. Perturbations to the host response may be brought about by an excessive accumulation of nonspecific dental plaque, by plaque-independent host factors (e.g., the onset of an immune disorder, changes in hormonal balance [e.g., during pregnancy], or by environmental factors [e.g., smoking, diet]).

Changes in the host status, such as inflammation, tissue degradation, and/or high gingival crevicular fluid flow, may lead to a shift in the microbial population in plaque. As a result of microenvironmental changes, the number of beneficial species may decrease, whereas the number of potentially pathogenic species increases. This gradual shift in the entire microbial community, known as *dysbiosis*, may result in a chronic disease state such as periodontitis.[35] The ecologic plaque hypothesis is entirely consistent with observations that disease-associated organisms are minor components of the oral microbiota in health; these organisms are kept in check by interspecies competition during microbial homeostasis. Disease is associated with the overgrowth of specific members of the dental plaque biofilm when the local microenvironment changes, but it is not necessarily the same species in each case. An important consideration of the ecologic plaque hypothesis is that therapeutic intervention can be useful on a number of different levels. Eliminating the etiologic stimulus—whether it is microbial, host, or environmental—will help to restore microbial homeostasis. Targeting specific microorganisms may be less effective because the conditions for disease will remain.

Keystone Pathogen Hypothesis and Polymicrobial Synergy and Dysbiosis Model

The keystone pathogen hypothesis indicates that certain low-abundance microbial pathogens can orchestrate inflammatory disease by remodeling a normally benign microbiota into a dysbiotic one. It may provide a novel conceptual basis for the development of targeted diagnostic and treatment modalities for complex dysbiotic diseases.[180,185]

Some evidence indicates that certain pathogens may trigger the disruption of microbial homeostasis, thereby leading to the development of periodontal disease, even when they are present only in low numbers. For example, specific pathogen-free mice exposed to *P. gingivalis* developed periodontal bone loss even when the pathogen was present in less than 0.1% of the total microbiota. Disease did not occur in the absence of other bacteria (i.e., in germ-free mice) or in mice lacking the C3a or C5a complement receptors. These data indicated that *P. gingivalis* subverts the host immune system and changes the microbial composition of dental plaque, ultimately leading to periodontal bone loss. On this basis, *P. gingivalis* was labeled a "keystone" pathogen; this means that it is an organism that is central to the disease process, even when it is at a relatively low abundance. The reader is referred to the online material for a detailed discussion of keystone pathogens. Online materials for this chapter are found on the companion website.

Complicating Factors

The identification of bacterial pathogens in periodontal diseases has been difficult because of a number of factors.[515] The periodontal microbiota is a complex community of microorganisms,

Fig. 9.29 Ecologic Plaque Hypothesis in Relation to Periodontal Diseases: Gingivitis and Periodontitis. The accumulation of plaque causes the inflammation of adjacent tissues (gingivitis) and other environmental changes that favor the growth of gram-negative anaerobes and proteolytic species, including periodontopathogens. The increased proportions of such species result in the destruction of periodontal tissues (i.e., periodontitis). E_h, Redox potential; *GCF*, gingival crevicular fluid. (From Marsh PD: Microbial ecology of dental plaque and its significance in health and disease, *Adv Dent Res* 8:263, 1994.)

many of which are still difficult or impossible to cultivate or identify. The chronic nature of periodontal disease has complicated the search for bacterial pathogens. It was previously thought that periodontal diseases progressed at a slow but steady rate.[319] However, epidemiologic studies established that the disease progresses at different rates, with alternating episodes of rapid tissue destruction and periods of remission (Fig. 9.30).[517] At this moment, by means of multilevel modeling, the linear and burst theories of periodontitis progression are considered to be manifestations of the same phenomenon: some sites improve, whereas others progress, and this occurs in a cyclic manner.[156] Identification of the microorganisms found during the different phases of the disease progression is technically challenging. The interpretation of microbiologic data is further complicated by the clinical classification of the disease status, an area that has undergone revisions.[20,570] Previous and perhaps current classifications involve the grouping of potentially different disease states as a result of difficulties with accurately distinguishing them clinically. It is important to recognize that groupings such as this may obscure microbiologic associations.

Periodontitis is currently considered a mixed infection. This has significant implications for both the diagnosis and the treatment of periodontitis. For the diagnosis, some clinicians evaluate the presence of up to 40 species, but it still is unclear whether some combinations of species are more pathogenic than others. The treatment is directed toward the eradication or reduction of the number of key periodontopathogens. Because several species may be involved, the appropriate use of antimicrobials (especially antibiotics) is extremely difficult to define, given that not all expected periodontopathogens are equally susceptible to the same antibiotic.

Microbiologic diagnostic tests indicated that the presence of periodontopathogens alone is not sufficient for the development of periodontitis. Because of the high sensitivity of these tests, several pathogens have been detected in periodontitis-free patients. Thus, merely the presence of pathogens is not sufficient for disease, and the amount of the pathogens plays a key role in relation to disease.[464] These observations have major clinical implications. First, the specificity of microbial detection is dramatically reduced (specificity in the sense that the presence of a specific pathogen means periodontitis). In other words, even though the result of a microbiologic analysis is positive, the patient can be without disease.[327] In addition, understanding the etiology becomes more complicated because the threshold level for periodontopathogens between health and disease is unknown and is obviously subject-dependent. Moreover, for several species, large intrastrain variations in genetic information have been detected (i.e., different genotypes), so that, in fact, genotypical information is necessary for pathogenicity assessment.[81,108,170,402] The quality of the host response also plays an essential role, but this cannot yet be correctly estimated. Finally, it may be questioned whether periodontopathogens are endogenous resident species or exogenous invaders. Indeed, the newer techniques have reported high detection frequencies of all pathogens in healthy subjects.[327,478] This has significant impact on the treatment strategies. For endogenous species, the endpoint of a therapy is the quantitative reduction of the species, whereas for

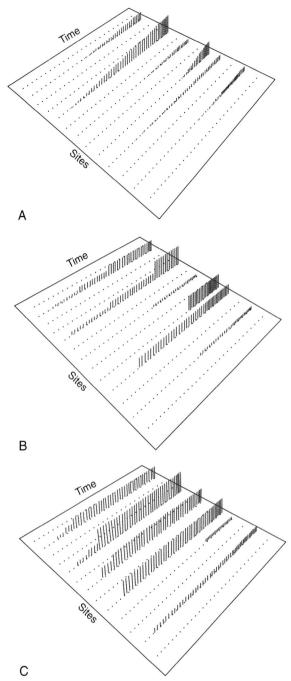

Fig. 9.30 Diagrammatic Representation of Possible Modes of Progression of Chronic Destructive Periodontal Diseases. Sites on the x-axis are plotted against time on the y-axis, and activity is shown on the z-axis. (A) Some sites show a progressive loss of attachment over time, whereas others show no destruction. The time of onset and the extent of destruction vary among sites. (B) Random burst model. Activity occurs at random in any site. Some sites show no activity, whereas others show one or several bursts of activity. The cumulative extent of destruction varies among sites. (C) Asynchronous multiple burst model. Several sites show bursts of activity over a finite period followed by prolonged periods of inactivity. Occasional bursts may occur infrequently at certain sites at later periods. Other sites show no periodontal disease activity at any time. The difference from the model shown in (B) is that in (C) the majority of destructive disease activity takes place within a few years of the individual's life. (Courtesy Drs. S. Socransky, A. Haffajee, and M. Goodson, [Boston] and J. Lindhe [Göteborg, Sweden].)

exogenous species, the endpoints are eradication and the prevention of reinfection.

It is currently impossible to alter the susceptibility of the host, so periodontal therapy must be focused on the reduction or elimination of periodontopathogens in combination with the reestablishment, often by surgical pocket elimination, of a more suitable (i.e., less anaerobic) environment for a more beneficial microbiota. Several studies have indicated that the presence of the previously mentioned periodontopathogens (that persist or are reestablished after treatment) is associated with a negative clinical outcome of periodontal treatment.[175,445,446] Because several species may be involved, the use of antimicrobials (especially antibiotics) is extremely difficult because antibiotic susceptibility is very diverse among periodontopathogens and often depends on the geographic region.[430,567]

It is obvious that several key questions still remain unanswered. Some researchers question whether the presence of specific microorganisms in the periodontal pocket is a cause or a consequence of disease.[518] Because most periodontopathogens are fastidious strict anaerobes, they may contribute little to the initiation of disease in shallow gingival pockets and instead be found only in deep periodontal pockets, which is their preferred habitat.

THE TRANSITION FROM HEALTH TO DISEASE

The oral microbial ecology is dynamic. The presence and numbers of particular microorganisms, even as a part of a community colonizing a niche in a human being, are controlled by the type and quantity of nutrients present (nutritional determinant), their ability to tolerate the specific physicochemical factors (physicochemical determinants), and their ability to cope with antimicrobial compounds (biologic determinants) or mechanical removal forces (mechanical determinants).[603] Although these determinants are well defined from a theoretical point of view, in practice, they overlap each other, especially in more complex environments (i.e., multispecies environments). Inherent to their biologic nature, bacteria interact with each other, with their environment, and vice versa. Therefore, the microbial ecology will change its composition, or the composition of the microbial

ecology will be changed when transitioning from a healthy status to a diseased status or vice versa. A change in the composition of a bacterial community as the result of external, nonmicrobial factors is termed *allogenic succession*. Smoking is a good example of such interaction. In *autogenic succession* (i.e., a change in the composition of a microbial community that arises from microbial activities), interbacterial and viral-bacterial interactions are involved.

KEY FACT

Transition from health to disease results from a complex interplay among the host, pathogenic bacteria, and commensal bacteria.

Early microscopic studies clearly demonstrated that the number and proportions of different subgingival bacterial morphotypes differ between healthy and diseased sites (Figs. 9.31 and 9.32; see Video 9.5).[313,506,513] The total number of bacteria, which was determined by microscopic counts per gram of plaque, was twice as high in periodontally diseased sites as compared with healthy sites.[513] Because considerably more plaque is found at diseased sites, this suggests that, in general, the total bacterial load in diseased sites is greater than that of healthy sites. Fewer coccal cells and more motile rods and spirochetes are found in diseased sites as compared with healthy sites.[313] Although this morphologic criterion can be of diagnostic value, one should remember that nearly all key periodontal pathogens (except *C. rectus* and spirochetes) are immobile rods, which adds to the confusion regarding the bacterial etiology of periodontal diseases. Culturing has shown that the microbiota in periodontally healthy sites consists predominantly of gram-positive facultative rods and cocci (approximately 75%).[506] The recovery of this group of microorganisms is decreased proportionally in gingivitis (44%) and periodontitis (10% to 13%). These decreases are accompanied by increases in the proportions of gram-negative rods, from 13% in health to 40% in gingivitis and 74% in advanced periodontitis.

The current concept regarding the etiology of periodontal diseases considers three groups of factors that determine whether

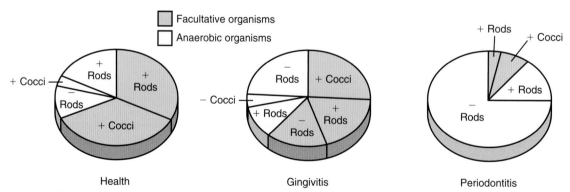

Fig. 9.31 Pie Charts Based on Culturing Studies That Represent the Relative Proportion of Different Morphotypes in Subgingival Samples in Cases of Periodontal Health, Gingivitis, and Periodontitis. A clear distinction is made between facultative species and obligate anaerobic species. Spirochetes are not included. +, Gram-positive; −, gram-negative.

Fig. 9.32 Phase-Contrast Micrographs of Plaque Samples. Phase-contrast micrographs of plaque samples from (A) a healthy patient and (B) a patient with periodontitis. Note the large rods and spirochetes in the periodontitis plaque sample.

active periodontal destruction will occur in a subject: a susceptible host, the presence of pathogenic species, and the absence or small proportion of so-called beneficial bacteria.[16,512,515,522,606] The clinical manifestations of periodontal destruction will result from a complex interplay among these etiologic agents. In general, small amounts of bacterial plaque can be controlled by the body's defense mechanisms without destruction; however, when dysbiosis happens (e.g., as a result of increased susceptibility, high bacterial load, or pathogenic infections), periodontal destruction could occur.[35]

Host Susceptibility

The susceptibility of the host is determined by genetic factors, as well as by environmental and behavioral factors, such as smoking, stress, and viral infections.

Genetic factors seem important for patients with so-called early-onset periodontitis, which is now referred to as aggressive periodontitis.[352] Reports regarding the familial nature of chronic forms of periodontitis are less conclusive. The aggregation of aggressive periodontitis within families is consistent with a genetic predisposition, although common environmental factors cannot be excluded (see Chapter 8).

Smoking is considered a behavioral factor and eventually an environmental factor. It dramatically increases host susceptibility to periodontal breakdown. Nevertheless, the exact nature of the relationship between periodontitis and smoking is unclear (see Chapter 11). Reports are conflicting regarding the effects of smoking on the oral microbiota. Some are in favor of an increased prevalence of *P. gingivalis, A. actinomycetemcomitans, T. forsythia, E. coli,* and *C. albicans* in smokers, whereas others report no difference.[47,177,417,537,563,565,619]

More recently, pyrosequencing revealed a lower subgingival taxonomic diversity in smokers as compared with nonsmokers.[40] Moreover, investigators showed that in smokers the ability to rebound from a dysbiotic state and reestablish a health-compatible community is impaired.[243] Smoking cessation, in contrast, can alter the subgingival biofilm and suggests a mechanism for improved periodontal health associated with smoking cessation.[145] Some evidence indicates that the epithelial cells of smokers are

more prone to colonization by respiratory pathogens. Depending on the bacterial strain, the relative increase in the number of adhering pathogens in smokers versus nonsmokers ranged from 40% up to 150%.[134,468] Cigarette smoke has been shown to modify the expression of *P. gingivalis* genes directly, including several virulence-associated genes.[27] After exposure to cigarette smoke extract, *P. gingivalis* cells induce a lower proinflammatory response than unexposed *P. gingivalis* cells.

Viral infections have been added to the list of factors that modify host susceptibility. HIV and herpesviruses are often associated with periodontal infections.

Increasing evidence suggests that emotional stress and negative life events can play an important role in the development and progression of periodontitis and that they may also modify the response to periodontal treatment. Stress associated with financial strain is a significant risk indicator for more severe periodontitis in adults (odds ratio: 2.24; confidence interval: 1.15 to 4.38).[153] Emotional and psychological loads can influence the immune system, and they will also alter oral health behaviors.[97] Both factors increase the susceptibility to periodontitis.

Racial factors have also been implicated in the differences in prevalence of early-onset periodontitis and in the frequency of detection of putative periodontopathogens.[32,320]

Pathogenic Bacteria

The second essential factor for disease initiation and progression is the presence of one or more pathogens of the appropriate clonal type and in sufficient numbers. Despite the difficulties inherent in characterizing the microbiology of periodontal diseases, a small group of pathogens is recognized because of their close association with disease. Obvious data support the designation of *A. actinomycetemcomitans, T. forsythia, T. denticola,* and *P. gingivalis* as key pathogens because they are strongly associated with periodontal disease status, disease progression, and unsuccessful therapy. For the following list of bacteria, moderate evidence for etiology has been reported, at least if their concentration passes a certain threshold level: *P. intermedia, Prevotella nigrescens* (see Fig. 9.2I), *C. rectus, P. micra* (see Fig. 9.2J), *F. nucleatum, Eubacterium nodatum* (see Fig. 9.2N), and various spirochetes.[16,512,515,522,606] The significance of the role of these key pathogens is largely based on epidemiologic data, the ability of these microorganisms to produce disease when inoculated in animals, and their capacity to produce virulence factors. However, the mere presence of putative periodontopathogens in the gingival crevice is not in itself sufficient to initiate or cause periodontal inflammation. An elevation in the relative proportion or number of these pathogens to reach a critical mass seems more crucial to mount an effective tissue-damaging process. Indeed, even in health, periodontopathogens are or can be present in the gingival crevice, albeit in low numbers, as members of the normal resident flora.[327] Table 9.4 gives a general overview of the detection frequency for most key pathogens in different forms of periodontal infections. It is immediately obvious that no black-or-white situation exists; there are no specific types of periodontitis for which any known pathogen is always present. This table also illustrates the difficulties with using the microbial composition to differentiate between different forms of periodontal infections.

Table 9.5 further highlights the complexity of the microbiology of periodontitis. Most periodontopathogens can also be detected in healthy subjects, with frequencies that range from 10% to 85%. It is obvious that this automatically reduces the specificity of microbiologic testing in periodontology.

However, technologic advancements such as next-generation sequencing have lengthened the list of bacterial species associated with periodontitis. Moderate evidence in the literature is suggested to support the association of 17 species of phylotypes from the phyla Bacteroidetes, Candidatus Saccharibacteria, Firmicutes, Proteobacteria, Spirochaetes, and Synergistetes.[405] The phylum Candidatus Saccharibacteria and the Archaea domain also seem to be associated with disease.[405] For more information, see Table 9.6.

Beneficial Species

The role of "beneficial" species is less obvious in the development of periodontal diseases.[453,515] These bacteria can affect the

TABLE 9.4   Prevalence of Microbial Species Associated With Various Clinical Forms of Periodontitis

Species	FORMS OF PERIODONTITIS		
	Chronic Periodontitis (%)	Localized Aggressive Periodontitis (%)	Aggressive Periodontitis (%)
Aggregatibacter actinomycetemcomitans	28.2	81.8	40.9
Porphyromonas gingivalis	53.8	13.3	79.6
Prevotella intermedia/nigrescens	50.2	53.4	71.4
Tannerella forsythia	50.6	0	50.8
Campylobacter rectus	40.3	12.5	47.8

O, Occasionally isolated.
From Haffajee AD, Socransky SS: Microbial etiological agents of destructive periodontal diseases, *Periodontol 2000* 5:78, 1994; and Mombelli A, Casagni F, Madianos PN: Can presence or absence of periodontal pathogens distinguish between subjects with chronic and aggressive periodontitis? A systematic review, *J Clin Periodontol* 29(Suppl 3):10, 2002.

TABLE 9.5   Prevalence of Key Pathogens in Healthy Subjects and Patients With Periodontitis

Species	PREVALENCE		SIGNIFICANCE OF DIFFERENCE	
	Health (%)	Periodontitis (%)	*P* Value	Odds Ratio[a]
Aggregatibacter actinomycetemcomitans	12.8	31.0	0.002	3.1
Porphyromonas gingivalis	10.6	59.5	<0.001	12.3
Prevotella intermedia/nigrescens	69.1	87.9	0.001	3.3
Tannerella forsythia	47.9	90.5	<0.001	10.4
Fusobacterium nucleatum	85.1	95.7	0.014	3.9
Parvimonas micra	67	94	<0.001	7.7
Campylobacter rectus	13.8	20.7	NS	1.6

[a]The ratio of the probability of developing the disease to the probability of nonoccurrence. For example,"3" means a threefold increased chance that the disease will develop if that species is present.
NS, Not significant.
From Van Winkelhoff, Loos BG, van der Reijden WA, et al: *Porphyromonas gingivalis, Bacteroides forsythus* and other putative periodontal pathogens in subjects with and without periodontal destruction, *J Clin Periodontol* 29:1023, 2002.

TABLE 9.6 Newly Identified Pathogens in the Etiology of Periodontitis for Which Three or More Studies Are Available

Phylum	Species	Gram	Culture Characteristics	No. of Studies
Bacteroidetes	*Bacteroidales* sp. oral taxon 274 HOT 274	–	a	3
	Porphyromonas endodontalis HOT 273	–	a	4
Firmicutes	*Eubacterium saphenum* HOT 759	+	a	5
	Mogibacterium timidum HOT 042	+	a	3
	Peptostreptococcus stomatis HOT 112	+	a	3
	Filifactor alocis HOT 539	+	a	5
	Anaeroblobus geminatus HOT 112	–	a	3
	Selenomonas sputigena HOT 151	–	a	5
	Enterococcus faecalis HOT 604	+	f	4
Proteobacteria	*Desulfobulbus* sp. oral taxon 041 HOT 041	/	/	3
Spirochaetes	*Treponema lecithinolyticum* HOT 653	–	a	4
	Treponema medium HOT 667	–	a	5
	Treponema vincentii HOT 029	–	a	3
Synergistetes	*Fretibacterium* sp. oral taxon 360 HOT 360	/	/	4
	Fretibacterium fastidiuosum HOT 363	–	a	3
Candidatus saccharibacteria	TM7 sp. oral taxon 356 HOT 356	/	/	3

/, Not yet cultivable; +, gram positive; –, gram negative; *a*, anaerobic; *f*, facultative anaerobic.
Data from Pérez-Chaparro PJ, Gonçalves C, Figueiredo LC, et al: Newly identified pathogens associated with periodontitis: a systematic review, *J Dent Res* 93:846–858, 2014.

pathogenic species in different ways and can thus modify the disease process as follows: (1) by passively occupying a niche that may otherwise be colonized by pathogens, (2) by actively limiting a pathogen's ability to adhere to appropriate tissue surfaces, (3) by adversely affecting the vitality or growth of a pathogen, (4) by affecting the ability of a pathogen to produce virulence factors, or (5) by degrading the virulence factors produced by the pathogen. The often-used textbook example of such a beneficial action is the effect of *S. sanguinis* (formerly known as *S. sanguis*) on *A. actinomycetemcomitans*.[557] *S. sanguinis* produces H_2O_2, which either directly or by host enzyme amplification can kill *A. actinomycetemcomitans*.[212] However, interactions between oral streptococci and *A. actinomycetemcomitans* are not so simple, and streptococci may actually promote the growth of *A. actinomycetemcomitans* by providing nutrients in the form of lactic acid and electron acceptors that enhance respiratory growth.[441,528] To obtain the benefits of oral streptococcal products without succumbing to H_2O_2, *A. actinomycetemcomitans* regulates the exopolysaccharide-degrading enzyme dispersin B to position itself at an optimal distance from streptococcal cells.[527] Although the so-called beneficial bacteria may be of importance for maintaining a healthy subgingival ecosystem, evidence is limited.[453] Despite rapidly increasing knowledge of periodontopathogen–host interactions, the role of beneficial microbiota in this crosstalk remains obscure. In periodontal microbiology, a bacterial strain is considered beneficial when its prevalence is high in periodontal health and low in diseased situations. It has been shown for other fields in microbiology that direct and indirect microbial interactions can suppress the emergence of pathogens.[55] The importance of the latter is evidenced within the oral cavity by the development of *Candida* infections when the

normal oral flora is reduced, such as after a period of systemic antibiotic usage.[582]

Because it has so far been impossible to alter the susceptibility of the host, periodontal therapy is necessarily focused on the reduction or elimination of periodontopathogens in combination with the reestablishment, often by surgical pocket elimination, of a more suitable (e.g., less anaerobic) environment for a more beneficial microbiota. Several studies have indeed indicated that the presence of the previously mentioned periodontopathogens (that have persisted or been reestablished after treatment) is associated with a negative clinical outcome of periodontal treatment.[95,176,445,446,516]

Taking all of this together, it is clear that the periodontal microbiota will shift when going from a periodontally healthy situation toward a periodontally diseased situation (Fig. 9.33).

When comparing the microbiota among conditions of health, gingivitis, and periodontitis, the following microbial shifts can be identified as health progresses to periodontitis:

- From gram-positive to gram-negative
- From cocci to rods (and, at a later stage, to spirochetes)
- From nonmotile to motile organisms
- From facultative anaerobes to obligate anaerobes
- From fermenting to proteolytic species

Periodontal Health

The recovery of microorganisms from periodontally healthy sites is lower as compared with diseased sites (Table 9.7). The bacteria associated with periodontal health are primarily gram-positive facultative species and members of the genera *Streptococcus* and *Actinomyces* (e.g., *S. sanguinis, S. mitis, A. oris, Actinomyces israelii, Actinomyces gerencseriae, Actinomyces viscosus*

Fig. 9.33 Vitality Stain of Subgingival Plaque. (A) Plaque derived from a healthy patient that primarily consists of cocci. (B) Plaque derived from a patient with periodontitis. Note the important morphologic differences from (A). Green bacteria are alive; red bacteria are dead.

[see Fig. 9.2C], *A. naeslundii*). Small proportions of gram-negative species are also found, most frequently *P. intermedia, F. nucleatum, F. nucleatum* spp. polymorphum, *F. periodonticum, Capnocytophaga* spp. *(C. gingivalis, C. ochracea,* and *C. sputigena), Neisseria* spp., and *Veillonella* spp. Microscopic analyses indicate that a few spirochetes and motile rods may also be present. On the basis of checkerboard DNA–DNA hybridization data, *Eubacterium saburreum, Propionibacterium acnes, S. anginosus, S. gordonii,* and *S. oralis* can also be considered as health-associated bacteria.[135,549,608,609]

Certain bacterial species have been proposed to be protective or beneficial to the host, including *S. sanguinis, Veillonella parvula* (see Fig. 9.2B), and *C. ochracea.* They are typically found in high numbers at periodontal sites that do not demonstrate attachment loss (inactive sites) but in low numbers at sites where active periodontal destruction occurs.[123,515] These species probably function to prevent the colonization or proliferation of pathogenic microorganisms. Clinical studies have shown that sites with high levels of *C. ochracea* and *S. sanguinis* are associated with a greater gain in attachment after therapy, thereby further supporting this concept.[515] A better understanding of plaque ecology and the interactions between bacteria and their products in plaque will undoubtedly reveal many other examples.

Gingivitis

The development of gingivitis has been extensively studied in a model system referred to as *experimental gingivitis* and initially described by Löe and coworkers.[321,552] Periodontal health is first established in human subjects via cleaning and rigorous oral hygiene measures that are followed by abstinence from oral hygiene for 21 days. After 8 hours without oral hygiene, bacteria may be found at concentrations of 10^3 to 10^4 per square millimeter of tooth surface, and they will increase in number by a factor of 100 to 1000 during the next 24-hour period.[520] After 36 hours, the plaque becomes clinically visible (see Video 9.2). The initial microbiota of experimental gingivitis (see Fig. 9.17) consists of gram-positive rods, gram-positive cocci, and

gram-negative cocci. The transition to gingivitis is evidenced by inflammatory changes; it is accompanied first by the appearance of gram-negative rods and filaments and then by spirochetal and motile microorganisms.[552]

The subgingival microbiota of dental-plaque–induced gingivitis (chronic gingivitis) differs from that of both health and chronic periodontitis (see Table 9.6).[261] It consists of roughly equal proportions of gram-positive (56%) and gram-negative (44%) species as well as facultative (59%) and anaerobic (41%) microorganisms.[506] It should be noted that the majority of predominant species in chronic periodontitis are already present in the gingivitis state, but mostly in small numbers.

Predominant gram-positive species include Streptococcus spp. *(S. sanguinis, S. mitis, S. intermedius, S. oralis, S. anginosus),* Actinomyces spp. *(A. oris, A. naeslundii), E. nodatum,* and *P. micra.* The gram-negative microorganisms are predominantly Capnocytophaga spp., Fusobacterium spp., Prevotella spp., *Campylobacter gracilis, Campylobacter concisus, V. parvula,* Haemophilus spp., and *Eikenella corrodens.* Both groups are commonly associated with gingivitis. The following gram-negative species are commonly found in periodontitis, and they are also associated with gingivitis but in fewer numbers: *P. gingivalis, T. forsythia, P. intermedia, C. rectus,* Treponema spp., and *A. actinomycetemcomitans* serotype a.[358,364,506] Pyrosequencing has identified additional taxa that are associated with gingivitis, including Leptotrichia spp. and Selenomonas spp.[220] In this study, Streptococcus spp. were more strongly associated with health than with gingivitis.

Pregnancy-associated gingivitis is an acute inflammation of the gingival tissues that is associated with pregnancy. This condition is accompanied by increases in steroid hormones in the crevicular fluid and dramatic increases in the levels of *P. intermedia* and *C. rectus,* which use the steroids as growth factors.[278,613]

Studies of gingivitis support the conclusion that disease development is associated with selected alterations in the microbial composition of dental plaque and not just the result of an accumulation of plaque. Gingivitis was generally thought to precede the development of chronic periodontitis; however, many individuals

TABLE 9.7 Summary of Bacterial Species Significantly Associated With Different Clinical Conditions Based on Culture, Polymerase Chain Reaction, and Checkerboard Data

Bacterial Species	Health	Gingivitis	Chronic Periodontitis	Localized Aggressive Periodontitis	Aggressive Periodontitis	Necrotizing Periodontal Diseases	Abscesses of the Periodontium	Peri-Implantitis
Actinomyces gerencseriae	X							
Actinomyces israelii	X							
Actinomyces naeslundii 1	X	X						
Actinomyces oris	X							
Actinomyces viscosus	X	X						X
Aggregatibacter actinomycetemcomitans				X				
Aggregatibacter actinomycetemcomitans high (leukotoxin clone)				X				
Aggregatibacter actinomycetemcomitans serotype a		X						
Aggregatibacter actinomycetemcomitans serotype b			X		X			
Campylobacter concisus		X						
Campylobacter gracilis					X			
Campylobacter rectus		X	X	X				X
Campylobacter showae					X			
Capnocytophaga gingivalis	X	X						
Capnocytophaga ochracea	X		X					
Capnocytophaga spp.	X	X	X	X				X
Capnocytophaga sputigena	X							
Eikenella corrodens		X	X	X				
Enterobacter spp.			X					
Eubacterium nodatum		X	X	X	X			X
Eubacterium saburreum	X						X	
Fusobacterium nucleatum		X	X	X		X	X	X

Continued

TABLE 9.7   Summary of Bacterial Species Significantly Associated With Different Clinical Conditions Based on Culture, Polymerase Chain Reaction, and Checkerboard Data—cont'd

Bacterial Species	Health	Gingivitis	Chronic Periodontitis	Localized Aggressive Periodontitis	Aggressive Periodontitis	Necrotizing Periodontal Diseases	Abscesses of the Periodontium	Peri-Implantitis
Fusobacterium periodonticum	X							
Fusobacterium polymorphum	X							
Haemophilus spp.		X						
Leptotrichia buccalis		X	X	X				
Neisseria spp.	X							
Parvimonas micra		X	X				X	X
Prevotella intermedia			X	X	X	X	X	X
Prevotella intermedia spirochetes		X						
Porphyromonas gingivalis			X	X	X		X	X
Prevotella nigrescens			X		X			
Propionibacterium acnes	X							
Pseudomonas aeruginosa								X
Selenomonas noxia			X					
Spirochetes			X	X	X	X	X	X
Staphylococcus aureus								X
Staphylococcus epidermidis								X
Streptococcus anginosus	X	X						
Streptococcus gordonii	X							
Streptococcus intermedius		X						
Streptococcus mitis	X	X						
Streptococcus oralis	X	X						
Streptococcus sanguinis	X	X						
Tannerella forsythia			X	X	X			X
Treponema denticola			X	X	X			X
Treponema spp.		X	X	X	X	X		X
Veillonella parvula	X	X						

demonstrate long-standing gingivitis that never advances to the destruction of the periodontal attachment.[58,318]

Chronic Periodontitis

Numerous forms of periodontal disease are found in adult populations, and they are characterized by different rates of progression (see Fig. 9.30) and different responses to therapy.[20] Studies in which untreated populations were examined over long time intervals indicate disease progression at mean rates that range from 0.05 mm to 0.3 mm of attachment loss per year (i.e., the gradual model).[58] When populations are examined over short time intervals, individual sites demonstrated short phases of attachment destruction interposed by periods of no disease activity (i.e., the burst model).[162] At this moment, by means of multilevel modeling, the linear and burst theories of periodontitis progression are considered to be manifestations of the same phenomenon: some sites improve whereas others progress, and this occurs in a cyclic manner.[156]

Microbiologic examinations of chronic periodontitis have been carried out in both cross-sectional and longitudinal studies; the latter have been conducted with and without treatment. These studies support the concept that chronic periodontitis is associated with specific bacterial agents. The microscopic examination of plaque from sites with chronic periodontitis has consistently revealed elevated proportions of spirochetes (see Video 9.5).[313,325] The cultivation of plaque microorganisms from sites of chronic periodontitis reveals high percentages of anaerobic (90%) gram-negative (75%) bacterial species (see Fig. 9.23 and Table 9.7).[505,506]

In patients with chronic periodontitis, the bacteria that are most often detected at high levels include *P. gingivalis, T. forsythia, P. intermedia, P. nigrescens, C. rectus, E.a corrodens* (see Fig. 9.2S), *F. nucleatum, A. actinomycetemcomitans* (often serotype b), *P. micra, E. nodatum, Leptotrichia buccalis, Treponema (T. denticola), Selenomonas* spp. (*S. noxia*), and *Enterobacter* spp.[a] The introduction of pyrosequencing techniques for microbial community analysis has provided additional sensitivity for detecting periodontal pathogens, although the broad picture has not changed. Unculturable organisms such as Synergistetes appear to correlate with periodontal disease, whereas high proportions of *Actinomyces* spp., *Rothia* spp., and *Streptococcus* spp. are correlated with health.[3,169] When periodontally active sites (i.e., with recent attachment loss) were examined in comparison with inactive sites (i.e., with no recent attachment loss), concentrations of *C. rectus, P. gingivalis, P. intermedia, F. nucleatum,* and *T. forsythia* were found to be elevated in the active sites.[122] Furthermore, detectable levels of *P. gingivalis, P. intermedia, T. forsythia, C. rectus,* and *A. actinomycetemcomitans* are associated with disease progression, and their elimination via therapy is associated with an improved clinical response.[85,122,175,511,597] Both *P. gingivalis* and *A. actinomycetemcomitans* are known to invade host tissue cells, which may be significant in aggressive forms of periodontitis.[73,82,471]

Studies have documented an association between chronic periodontitis and viral microorganisms of the herpesviruses group, most notably EBV-1 and hCMV.[89] Furthermore, the presence of subgingival EBV-1 and hCMV is associated with high levels of putative bacterial pathogens, including *P. gingivalis, T. forsythia, P. intermedia,* and *T. denticola.* These data support the hypothesis that viral infection may contribute to periodontal pathogenesis, but the potential role of viral agents remains to be determined.

The reader is referred to the online material for a detailed discussion of microbiota in aggressive periodontitis, necrotizing periodontal diseases, and abscesses of the periodontium. Online materials for this chapter are found on the companion website www.expertconsult.com.

Peri-Implantitis

The term *peri-implantitis* refers to an inflammatory process that affects the tissues around an already osseointegrated implant and that results in the loss of supporting bone.[20] Originally, this inflammatory process was thought to be associated (e.g., in animal studies, in cross-sectional and longitudinal observations in man) with a microbiota comparable to that of periodontitis (i.e., a high proportion of anaerobic gram-negative rods, motile organisms, and spirochetes), but this association does not necessarily prove a causal relationship.[426] Evidence suggests a lower degree of bacterial complexity in the peri-implant crevice.[288] Healthy peri-implant pockets are characterized by high proportions of coccoid cells, a low ratio of anaerobic-to-aerobic species, a low number of gram-negative anaerobic species, and low detection frequencies for periodontopathogens.[6,49,302,390] Implants with peri-implantitis reveal a microbiota that encompasses conventional periodontal pathogens (see Table 9.7), as well as the cariogenic bacterium *S. mutans.*[288,407] Species such as *A. actinomycetemcomitans, P. gingivalis, T. forsythia, P. micra, C. rectus, F. nucleatum, P. intermedia, T. denticola,* and *Capnocytophaga* are often isolated from failing sites, but they can also be detected around healthy peri-implant sites.[495] Other species, such as *Pseudomonas aeruginosa, Enterobacter* spp., *C. albicans,* and staphylococci, are also frequently detected around implants.[12] These organisms are uncommon in the subgingival area, but they have been associated with refractory periodontitis.[512] High proportions of *Staphylococcus aureus* and *S. epidermidis* on oral implants have been reported.[440] The relative resistance of these organisms to commonly used antibiotics suggests that their presence may represent an opportunistic colonization that is caused by systemic antibiotic therapy.[511]

However, some studies using open-ended microbial techniques suggest that the microbiota associated with peri-implantitis is not as similar as thought to that associated with periodontitis.[96,98,136,288,524,625] Some large-scale clinical follow-up studies seem to indicate that implant failures cluster within patients, with increased odd ratios for a second implant failure in patients who have already lost one implant.[564,598] These observations indicate that, within patients, systemic factors are important for the characterization of implant losses.

VIRULENCE FACTORS OF PERIODONTOPATHOGENS

It is clear that some organisms, such as *P. gingivalis, A. actinomycetemcomitans,* spirochetes, and *P. intermedia,* are strongly

---

[a]References 282, 291, 322, 364, 506, 514, 515, 545, 549, 608, 626.

associated with a number of periodontal diseases. However, periodontal disease never occurs in the absence of a complex microbiota, and it is often difficult (if not impossible) to determine precisely how different organisms contribute to an individual case of disease. In fact, the contributions of specific bacteria to disease may be unimportant according to the ecologic plaque hypothesis.

KEY FACT

The best-known virulence factors of periodontopathogens are adhesive surface proteins and fibrils, tissue destruction–promoting factors, and host immunity–evading strategies.

Targeting one or more "pathogens" will not necessarily cure disease, because other organisms with similar activities may take their place. Therefore, it may make sense to focus on the specific molecules that contribute to disease (virulence factors), rather than on the microorganisms that produce them. In fact, it is often difficult to separate the virulence determinants from the organisms that produce them. For example, adhesins are produced by commensal organisms, as well as by pathogens, yet only those adhesins that promote the attachment of a pathogenic organism could be considered virulence determinants. With this in mind, some of the known or putative virulence factors for periodontal disease are described in the following sections. The following are important:

1. Only a proportion of periodontal bacteria has ever been isolated, and is is almost certain that many other virulence factors are currently unknown.
2. Most of our understanding of virulence factors has come from studies of a very limited number of bacterial species and strains. It is far from clear that the molecules that have been studied in the greatest detail are truly representative of their classes.

Virulence factors of periodontal microorganisms can be subdivided as follows: (1) factors that promote colonization (adhesins), (2) toxins and enzymes that degrade host tissues, and (3) mechanisms that protect pathogenic bacteria from the host.

Adhesive Surface Proteins and Fibrils

To colonize the periodontal pocket, bacteria must adhere to cells or tissues in the region, such as teeth, the existing microbial biofilm, or the pocket epithelium. Bacterial cell surface structures provide the points of contact. Often these structures extend some distance from the cell surface. Fimbriae or pili are polymeric fibrils that are composed of repeating subunits that can extend several micrometers from the cell membrane. Pili were once thought to be unique to gram-negative bacteria, but they have now been identified in several gram-positive organisms, including streptococci and actinomyces.[336] Strains of *P. gingivalis* produce two types of fimbriae, which are known as the major fimbriae and the minor fimbriae.[189]

The major fimbriae are single-stranded filaments approximately 5 nm in diameter and up to 3 μm in length. The backbone of major fimbriae is a chain of repeating subunits of the 43-kDa FimA protein. Minor fimbriae are composed of a 67-kDa protein, Mfa1, and they extend approximately 0.1 to 0.5 μm from the cell surface.[19] Major and minor fimbriae interact with oral streptococci, such as *S. gordonii*. *P. gingivalis*, and *FimA* binds to glyceraldehyde-3-phosphate dehydrogenase, whereas Mfa1 interacts with the *S. gordonii* cell surface adhesin B.[332,398] Major fimbriae have also been shown to bind host extracellular matrix proteins fibronectin and type I collagen, salivary proline-rich proteins and statherin, and epithelial cells.[15,190,373] Extensive variation in the *fimA* gene that encodes the FimA fimbrial subunit has been observed, and six different genotypes have been designated (i.e., genotypes I, Ib, II, III, IV, and V).[131] Of these, genotypes II and IV are associated with periodontitis.[14,130] However, at present, no evidence indicates that fimbriae of genotypes II and IV are functionally distinct from other major fimbriae.

Tissue Destruction–Promoting Factors

Many bacterial proteins that interact with host cells are recognized by the immune system, and they may trigger immune responses. Fimbriae of *P. gingivalis* and *A. actinomycetemcomitans* are highly antigenic. Inflammation is a major contributor to tissue destruction in periodontal disease; this is considered separately in Chapter 8. However, some bacterial products directly promote tissue destruction in addition to modulating host immunity, with extracellular proteolytic enzymes being the most notable. Most of the tissue destruction in periodontal pockets is actually caused by host matrix metalloproteinases (MMPs), but bacterial proteases play important roles in activating the host enzymes.[165]

Bacterial proteolytic activity in dental plaque—and, in particular, trypsin-like protease activity—is closely correlated with clinical markers of periodontal disease.[382]

However, the bulk of the host tissue–degrading activity is restricted to a small number of these enzymes. In the case of *P. gingivalis*, three enzymes known as gingipains are responsible for at least 85% of the total proteolytic activity of the bacterium.[412]

The gingipains belong to the cysteine protease family, and they use an active-site cysteine residue for catalysis. Gingipains are classed as "Arg-gingipains" (RgpA and RgpB) or "Lys-gingipains" (Kgp) on the basis of their ability to cleave Arg-Xaa or Lys-Xaa peptide bonds (Xaa represents any amino acid). Gingipains are multifunctional proteins that play important roles in adhesion, tissue degradation, and the evasion of host responses.

Proteases are produced by *A. actinomycetemcomitans*, but these appear to be less important for the virulence of this organism than the leukotoxin (LtxA). LtxA is a member of the repeats-in-toxin family of proteins. These toxins act by delivering an adenylate cyclase domain into cells, which catalyzes the uncontrolled conversion of adenosine triphosphate to cyclic adenosine monophosphate.

Most strains of *A. actinomycetemcomitans* produce low levels of LtxA. However, some strains are regarded as hyper-leukotoxic because they express high levels of the transcript from the *ltxA* gene, thereby encoding LtxA. Hyper-leukotoxic strains include the JP2 clone of *A. actinomycetemcomitans*, which is uniquely associated with localized aggressive periodontitis.[206,357]

Fig. 9.34 Glycocalyx or Polysaccharide Capsule of *Porphyromonas gingivalis* Visualized With East Indian Ink Staining (clear halo).

Strategies for Evading Host Immunity

Pathogenic bacteria have many and varied strategies for evading or subverting the host immune system, including the following: (1) the production of an extracellular capsule, (2) the proteolytic degradation of host innate or acquired immunity components, (3) the modulation of host responses by binding serum components on the bacterial cell surface, and (4) the invasion of gingival epithelial cells. Selected examples of factors that mediate these processes are given in the following paragraphs.

Strains of *P. gingivalis* produce polysaccharide capsules (Fig. 9.34) that surround the outer membrane. Six different antigenic capsule types have been described on the basis of the differences in the polysaccharide K antigen.[293] In a mouse model, capsular strains of *P. gingivalis* produced a spreading type of infection, whereas acapsular strains tended to form more localized abscesses.[295] Most *P. gingivalis* isolates from periodontitis patients are encapsulated.[294] It is hypothesized that the capsule protects cells from the host immune system. However, protection against the complement system appears to be mediated primarily by a branched phosphomannan polysaccharide that is independent of the K antigen.[503]

Several periodontopathogens are resistant to complement-mediated phagocytosis, and it is thought that the proteolysis of complement components contributes to resistance to some extent. *P. gingivalis* gingipains have been shown to degrade complement components C3, C4, C5, and factor B.[411] More recently, a cysteine protease of *P. intermedia* called interpain A has also been shown to degrade C3.[413] In vitro, interpain A acts synergistically with gingipains to decrease the deposition of complement C3b.[413] These data fit with the hypothesis that periodontal disease processes are mediated by polymicrobial consortia rather than by individual periodontopathogens.

A novel mechanism for complement evasion has been identified in *A. actinomycetemcomitans*. This organism produces a 100-kDa protein on the outer membrane, Omp100 or ApiA, which mediates adhesion to and the invasion of host cells.[22,308] Mutants lacking ApiA were sensitized to killing by human serum: wild-type cells were almost completely resistant to 30% or 50% normal human serum, whereas 90% of ApiA mutant cells were killed. ApiA was shown to bind factor H, which is an inhibitor of the complement cascade.

Periodontal pathogens are notoriously difficult to completely eradicate. Despite aggressive antibacterial attacks from the host defenses and from clinical treatments, it is often impossible to prevent reinfection. One potential reservoir for periodontopathogens is inside gingival epithelial cells. *P. gingivalis* and *A. actinomycetemcomitans*, for example, can invade epithelial cells in vitro.[296,351] In vivo, *P. gingivalis*, *T. forsythia*, *P. intermedia*, *T. denticola*, and *A. actinomycetemcomitans* can be detected within the gingival epithelial cells of patients with periodontitis before and after periodontal therapy.[241] Adhesion to host cells is critical for invasion. However, it has been suggested that some factors may specifically control the ability of bacteria to invade cells. In *A. actinomycetemcomitans*, a screen for invasion-associated genes identified two loci, encoding ApiA (see previous paragraph) and ApiBC, which are related to known bacterial invasion proteins (invasins).[308] The ability of bacteria to invade cells may be influenced by their interactions with other organisms in the gingival sulcus. Thus, the coinfection of an epithelial cell line with *P. gingivalis* and a coaggregating strain of *F. nucleatum* resulted in increased invasion by *P. gingivalis* as compared with a monoculture control.[474] Coaggregation with *F. nucleatum* is mediated by the *P. gingivalis* capsular polysaccharide and lipopolysaccharide; therefore, these molecules may indirectly contribute to invasion.[457]

The reader is referred to the online material for a brief discussion on future advances in periodontal microbiology and a detailed discussion on the molecular biology of the host–microbe interactions. Online materials for this chapter are found on the companion website.

Case Scenarios are found on the companion website www .expertconsult.com.

REFERENCES

 References for this chapter are found on the companion website.

Resolution of Inflammation[a,b]

🌐 For additional content on systemic links, including type 2 diabetes, cardiovascular diseases, cancer, and pregnancy outcomes, please visit the companion website.

CHAPTER OUTLINE

INFLAMMATION

Inflammation is an essential biologic response observed across species with particular importance to human health and disease. The first description of a localized response to injury and infection that resembled signs of inflammation was recorded by the ancient Egyptian and Greek cultures. Four cardinal signs describing inflammation were identified. First was *rubor et tumor cum calore et dolore* (redness and swelling with heat and pain).[60] Then, in 1958, Virchow's investigations led to an understanding of the cellular basis of inflammation as a pathologic condition, and his observations led to the addition of a new cardinal sign, functio laesa (loss of organ/tissue function).[60]

More recently, advanced cellular and molecular mechanisms governing the fate of inflammation have been identified. The initiation of acute response is accepted to be a physiologic response occurring in vascularized tissues to defend the host and maintain homeostasis. Inflammation response is an active cellular and molecular response that aims to control challenge.[35] When activated, inflammation is protective to host tissues against stimuli, such as pathobionts, foreign bodies, toxic chemicals, and trauma.

As an initial and protective response to challenges presented by host tissues, inflammation is characterized by increased blood flow, vascular dilation, increased vascular permeability, and cellular recruitment. This response requires four biologic components: inflammation inducers, detecting sensors, downstream mediators, and target tissues. The type and degree of an inflammatory response are dependent on the nature of the trigger (e.g., bacterial, viral, parasitic, or chemical) and its duration.[34] With specific cellular and molecular cues, inducers will be detected by antigen first line of response and activate a cascade of events that are tightly regulated.

The major sensors for the inflammatory response are epithelial cells and innate immune cells that migrate to the injured site as well as resident stromal cells. Polymorphonuclear leukocytes or neutrophils (PMLs/PMNs) (named for their staining characteristics with hematoxylin and eosin) constitute the cellular arm of the first line of defense of the innate immune system. PMNs are phagocytes with potent oxidative and nonoxidative killing mechanisms that combat bacteria.[5] PMN infiltration is followed by the entry of mononuclear cells, monocytes, and activated macrophages into the inflammatory site that clears cellular debris, bacteria, and apoptotic PMNs by phagocytosis without prolonging inflammation. Together, innate cells trigger production of mediators that modulate the fate of inflammation. Neutrophils, macrophages, dendritic cells, and mast cells produce low–molecular weight proteins called cytokines that control initiation, maintenance, and regulation of the amplitude and duration of the inflammatory response.

In consequence, the production of communicating molecules such as inflammatory cytokines(e.g., interleukins [ILs]), chemokines (CXCs), and inflammatory lipid mediators (LMs) is key to signal an effective response.[8,9] A didactical, and hopefully functional, classification of mediators categorized the inflammatory molecules according to their functions in the context of activation (pro-) of inhibition (anti-) of inflammation. It

---

[a]Adapted from the following chapter of Newman and Carranza's Clinical Periodontology, 13th edition: Chapter 10: Resolution of Inflammation, by Marcelo Freire.

[b]Note: In the 2018 Classification of Periodontal and Peri-Implant Diseases and Conditions, "chronic periodontitis" and "aggressive periodontitis" disease categories are grouped under a single category called "periodontitis" and are further characterized based on a multidimensional staging and grading system. In this chapter, the term "aggressive periodontitis" is still used because the related studies were conducted before the 2018 classification. Readers are referred to Chapter 6 for the detailed discussion on periodontal disease classification.

is important to note the binary terminologies of pro- and antiinflammatory are more dynamic than first described. This complex relationship is controlled by the molecule concentration, the interaction with its receptors and other interactants, and finally, the time of production and activity. The binary view of a molecule's activity is still the convention and the accepted terminology, but it is crucial to contextualize these concepts. Pro-inflammatory mediators, for example, are produced locally in the tissues or systemically in the bloodstream (e.g., IL-1β, IL-6, tumor necrosis factor alpha [TNF-α], and PGE2). In response to the direct challenge or to the production of pro-inflammatory molecules, antiinflammatory cytokines control the response and maintain the reaction in check (e.g., IL-10, IL13, TGF-β, IL1RA).[52]

Although the inflammatory response is protective, unresolved inflammation is detrimental to tissue function, thereby promoting dysbiosis. Failure to resolve inflammation leads to chronic diseases, including inflammatory bowel syndrome, type 2 diabetes, cardiovascular diseases, Alzheimer disease, cancer, and periodontal diseases. Resolution of inflammation is an active biochemical mechanism regulated by mediators that switch gene expression, protein functions, and cells to return to homeostasis. Among the mediators that regulate this process, specialized pro-resolving mediators (SPMs) activate cells to start resolution. Thus, beneficial acute inflammation is spatially and temporally regulated by SPMs.[4,12,40,45,55]

KEY FACTS

Pro-resolution Versus Antiinflammation

Pro-resolution lipid mediators are fatty acids that are expressed endogenously to activate cells and tissues to control inflammation. Initiation of inflammation requires external and internal cellular signals, which, in turn, activates pro-resolution enzymes to produce lipid ligand signals. Upon interaction with a cellular receptor with lipid ligands, cells are activated to produce pro-resolution or antiinflammation. The stereospecificity guides the cell function to either suppress and/or pro-resolve. In antiinflammation, blocking and suppressing pathways that activate inflammation are the usual mechanism. In pro-resolution, specific lipids are able to activate cell switching from pro-inflammation to pro-resolution. For example, the endogenous mediators are able to enhance deficient phagocytosis seen in type 2 diabetes, increase chemotaxis in localized aggressive periodontitis (LAP), and prevent gingivitis. Thus, stimulating resolution either endogenously or therapeutically activates protective signals that prevent collateral damage and limit acute or continuous inflammation.

ACUTE INFLAMMATION IS SELF-LIMITED

To maintain homeostasis, a class switch activity of enzymes from pro-inflammation to pro-resolution controls temporal regulation of acute inflammation.[15,19] For many years, our understanding of inflammation was mostly on initiation as an active process, whereas termination (a.k.a. resolution) was thought to be a passive process with decay of inflammation (Fig. 10.1) until

Fig. 10.1 Acute Inflammation Is Self-Limited. In clinical scenarios of health, resident cells, molecular mediators, and tissues respond to injure effectively and return to homeostasis. If acute inflammation is unresolved, chronic inflammation and disease will establish. Tissue healing is effective when a class switch from pro-inflammation to pro-resolution is activated. *CXC motif,* Chemokine; *IL,* interleukin; *NF-κB,* nuclear factor kappa-B; *TNF-α,* tumor necrosis factor-α.

basic and translational studies from Drs. Charles Serhan and Thomas Van Dyke came to light that proved otherwise. Contrary to older beliefs, they showed that resolution is an active process and can only be initiated when enzymes produce bioactive pro-resolution lipids.[19,47,56]

In the context of acute inflammation initiation, locally produced lipid mediators, such as prostaglandins, prostacyclin, leukotrienes, and thromboxanes, regulate major processes and act as autacoids (short-lived molecules that act at the site of synthesis). These lipid mediators are synthesized in a sequence of enzymatic activation when arachidonic acid (AA) is released from the cell membrane due to trauma or via cell-cell communication. Structurally, most of the lipids of inflammation are eicosanoids (20-carbon chains) and act as endogenous precursors for biosynthesis of a chain of several molecules. In fact, the enzyme phospholipase A2 releases AA from the phospholipid membrane. This release constitutes the rate-determining step in the generation of eicosanoids produced by most phagocytic and immune cells.[31] AA is rapidly converted into various potent lipid mediators with specific functions in a cell-specific manner by cyclooxygenases (COXs), lipoxygenases (LOs), or epoxygenases to yield prostaglandins, leukotrienes, and endoperoxides, respectively. Readers are referred to the online material for a detailed discussion of SPM biosynthetic cascades. Online materials for this chapter are found on the companion website.

In addition to pro-inflammatory mediators that turn on inflammation, there is a separate set of lipid mediators that act as endogenous agonists to activate termination of inflammation by stimulating resolution.[43] The following sections provide a more detailed look at SPMs in the resolution of acute inflammation.

Specialized Pro-Resolving Mediators

Pro-resolution signals are activated mostly by resolvins, lipoxins, maresins, and protectins. Lipid mediator class-switches biosynthesize pro-resolution lipid mediators, such as lipoxin A4, eicosapentaenoic acid (EPA)–derived resolvins (i.e., RvE1, RvE2), and docosahexaenoic acid (DHA)–derived lipid mediators including D-series resolvins, protectins, and maresins (Fig. 10.2).[59] More details on the key pro-resolution mediators are given next.

Lipoxins

Derived from AA, lipoxins are natural pro-resolving molecules produced from endogenous fatty acids. Lipoxins have strong dual antiinflammatory and pro-resolution actions. Lipoxins A4 and B4 were first isolated and identified as inhibitors of PMN infiltration and stimulators of nonphlogistic (nonfever) recruitment of macrophages.[16,22,42] Three main pathways of lipoxin synthesis have been identified. In humans, sequential oxygenation of AA-derived lipids by 15-lipoxygenase and 5-lipoxygenase, followed by enzymatic hydrolysis, leads to LXA4, and LXB4 occurs in the mucosal tissues including the oral cavity, gastrointestinal tract, and airways. While in blood vessels, 5-lipoxygenase biosynthesizes LXA4 and 12-lipoxygenase in platelets produce LXB4. Lipoxin receptors are ubiquitously expressed by many cells, including neutrophils and monocytes. Aspirin triggers a third synthetic pathway. Aspirin promotes acetylation of COX-2 leading

Fig. 10.2 Chemical Structure of Pro-Resolution Lipid Mediators. Lipid mediator class switches yield lipoxins, eicosapentaenoic acid–derived E-series resolvins, and docosahexaenoic-acid derived D series resolvins, protectins, and maresins. *LXA4,* Lipoxin A4; *MaR1,* maresin 1; *PD1,* protectin D1; *RvE1,* resolvin E1.

to a change in COX-2 activity and the chirality of the products, which are termed *aspirin triggered lipoxins* (ATLs).[21] Cells that express COX-2 include vascular endothelial cells, epithelial cells, macrophages, and neutrophils.[51] In addition to the synthesis of lipoxin, aspirin also blocks prostaglandin synthesis by acetylation of COX-2 inhibiting inflammation.[39]

Resolvins

Resolvins are endogenous lipid mediators induced during the resolution phase of inflammation. These lipid mediators are biosynthesized from the essential ω-3 polyunsaturated fatty acids (EPA and DHA) derived from the diet. The two primary groups of the resolvin family have distinct chemical structures: E-series, obtained from EPA; and D-series, derived from DHA. Vascular endothelium produces E-series resolvins via aspirin-modified COX-2 that converts EPA to 18R-hydroperoxyeicoapentaenoic acid (18R-HPEPE) and 18S-hydroperoxyeicoapentaenoic acid (18S-HPEPE). Neutrophils are rapidly taken up by human monocytes and metabolized to RvE1 and RvE2 by 5-lipoxygenase. Resolvin E1 production increases in plasma of individuals taking aspirin or EPA, resulting in amelioration of clinical signs of inflammation.[32] Similarly, DHA-derived D-series resolvins have been shown to reduce inflammation by decreasing platelet–leukocyte adhesion, and aspirin-triggered DHA conversion produces molecules with dual antiinflammatory and pro-resolution function.[49]

The interaction between resolvins and specific receptors modulates the fate of innate immune cells and counter-regulates active inflammation. Selective target sites for resolvins are G-protein coupled receptors (GPCRs).[50] ERV1 receptor (also known as ChemR23 or CMKLR1) is a GPCR expressed on monocytes and dendritic cells. BLT1, a leukotriene receptor, is the resolvin E1 receptor on neutrophils. Upon selective binding to the receptors, RvE1 attenuates NF-κB signaling and production of proinflammatory cytokines including TNF-α.[7,37] D-series resolvins target GPR32 and ALX receptors[62] expressed on platelets and PMN. Activation of CB2 receptor leads to inhibition of P-selectin expression, decreasing PMN chemotaxis. Resolvins induce hallmark functions of resolution of inflammation, including decreasing neutrophil migration, phagocytosis of apoptotic cells, and increasing clearance of infection to activate tissue healing.[50]

Readers are referred to the online material for a discussion of protectins and maresins. Online materials for this chapter are found on the companion website.

> **KEY FACTS**
>
> - Resolution of inflammation is an active biochemical process regulated by a class switch of enzymes and lipid mediators.
> - A novel class of lipid mediators is known to modulate the resolution of inflammation; it consists of lipoxins, resolvins, maresins, and protectins.

UNRESOLVED CHRONIC INFLAMMATION IN PERIODONTAL DISEASES

The oral microbiome modulates oral and systemic immune development, and a physiologic interaction maintains the homeostatic response. Periodontal diseases are chronic inflammatory diseases initiated by dysbiosis and microbial biofilms.[11] In the case of gingivitis, acute inflammation is self-limited and reversible. When the etiologic factor and modifiers are "removed," the host returns to health. When stimuli persist, unresolved inflammation causes chronic lesions, loss of attachment, disease progression, and tissue loss. The host immune response functions as a protective mechanism, but continuous or exacerbated response risks the tissue integrity.[36]

Altered balance either from the microbiota or the host response (or both) allows the disease initiation and progression.[11,23]

Although plaque is an evident etiologic factor in gingivitis, in periodontitis the specificity or number of the pathogens has not explained the variability in individual host response. For many patients, periodontal destruction does not commensurate with biofilm deposits.[28] It is therefore possible that bacteria are not the primary factor of gingivitis-periodontitis transition. Whereas "plaque" is a traditional concept in etiology, the host presents multiple variations that provide increased susceptibility changing taxonomic composition of the plaque and metabolomic functions.[58] Resolution failure is a plausible explanation of this pathologic transition.

Classic studies in the 1980s showed that intake of antiinflammatory medications prevented the progression of periodontal disease.[27] Although this was promising, it is now clear that inflammation is an important biologic process, and complete suppression of its cascade influences the host entirely. Instead of suppressing the system, resolution aims to enhance "good" inflammation to terminate the disease process.[29,41] In fact, deficient phagocytosis is seen in aggressive forms of periodontitis and is reversed by resolution mediators.[18,24] Thus, host-derived etiology is now well accepted and is a target for future therapies.

In a clinical trial of patients with moderate to severe periodontitis, the actions of dietary supplementation of ω-3 polyunsaturated fatty acid (PUFA) and aspirin were evaluated. In patients taking the preceding supplements, in addition to scaling and root planing, significant improvements were noted in pocket depth reduction and clinical attachment level gain, with lower levels of inflammatory mediators in saliva compared to patients who underwent scaling and root planing alone.[14] Lipid mediators are considered excellent candidates for the prevention and treatment of periodontal diseases.

> **FLASH BACK**
>
> Bacteria have been recognized for years as the main etiologic factor for periodontal diseases. With advances in molecular immunology and genetics, inflammation and resolution pathways have been shown to play an integral role in the multifactorial pathogenesis of periodontal diseases.

THERAPEUTIC ACTIONS OF RESOLUTION MEDIATORS

Periodontal diseases, including gingivitis and periodontitis, are leukocyte-driven inflammatory conditions characterized by soft-tissue and osteoclasts-mediated bone loss.[28,36,53] Resolution mediators are needed to control and treat periodontal diseases. In animal models, restoration of tissue health by resolution lipids is initiated after acute response generates classic eicosanoids, prostanoids, and prostacyclins and leukotrienes. The synthesis of immune-resolvents by key enzymes that induce a class switch is partially known.[44] Thus return to homoeostasis is highly regulated by resolution pathways.

In human cells obtained from LAP, RvE1 and LXA4 treatment decreased neutrophil superoxide production in response to TNFα and the bacterial surrogate peptide marker N-formyl-methionyl-leucyl-phenylalanine by 80%.[18,25]

Evidence from animal studies demonstrated that overexpression of 15-lipoxygenase type I in rabbits increased endogenous levels of LXA4 protecting the host from developing periodontal disease. The application of LXA4 or RvE1 reversed bone loss in experimental periodontitis models of rabbits,[26] mini pigs,[57] or rats.[30] These preclinical models also demonstrated that shifts of periodontal microbiota in animals were associated with the resolution of inflammation induced by RvE1.[26,30,38] Hile no-animal model is a perfect fit for humans, as proof-of-principle, these concepts could be translated 0%.[18,25]

The potential for treatment of periodontal diseases with one or a combination of SPMs is clear, but it requires further investigation clinically. In one trial previously mentioned, scaling and root planing (SRP) with dietary supplementation of ω-3 PUFA and lower dose of aspirin reduced pocket depths and increased clinical attachment levels significantly when compared to SRP alone.[14] The clinical benefits were accompanied by lower levels of inflammatory mediators in saliva compared to SRP alone.[14]

CLINICAL IMPLICATIONS

- Inflammation is a biologic protective mechanism against injury.
- Acute inflammation seen in gingivitis is reversible and self-limited.
- Chronic inflammation in periodontitis has a failure of signals that activate resolution and return to homeostasis.
- Inflammation and resolution are connecting links with systemic disease (e.g., type 2 diabetes, cancer, and cardiovascular diseases) and periodontal diseases.

Tissue regeneration has also been a target of SPMs. Treatment with maresin 1 has been demonstrated to stimulate tissue regeneration in system models, including planaria models.[48] Consistently in periodontal disease models, lipoxin A4/ATL and resolvin E1 prevented connective tissue and bone loss. Treatment of experimental periodontitis with lipid mediators completely resolved inflammation and rescued tissue loss with the regeneration of periodontal tissues.[26,30,57] It has been suggested that defective endogenous resolution of inflammation underlies the inflammatory phenotype presented in chronic diseases and that exogenous therapeutic molecules rescue this phenotype. Pro-resolution lipid mediators play a role as natural molecules in the maintenance of homeostasis with promising potential as therapeutic agents in human diseases.[17,19]

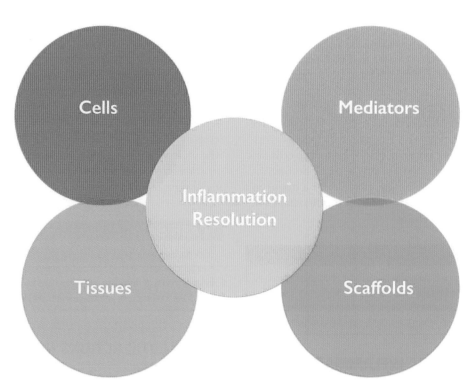

Fig. 10.3 Inflammation Resolution is a Key Component of Tissue Healing and Regeneration. Upon antigenic challenge, cells, tissue, vasculature, and mediators have to synchronize the host response to adequately remove triggers and protect the host prior to regeneration. Resolution of inflammation has main functions in the activation of cells to promote clearance, return to homeostasis, and together with the factors described promote tissue regeneration.

FINAL REMARKS

The role of acute inflammation is the protection of the host and the development of tissue integrity. The fate of this process is determined by the balance and magnitude of mediators and sensors that amplify the inflammatory process or control the restoration to normal health. It is now evident that the resolution of inflammation is modulated by SPMs. The selective interaction of the lipid mediators with GPCR receptors of innate immune cells induces the cessation of leukocyte infiltration; the return to normal levels of vascular permeability/edema; PMN death (mostly via apoptosis); and nonphlogistic infiltration of monocyte/macrophages and macrophage removal of apoptotic PMN, pathogens, and necrotic debris from the site. These cellular events lead to resolution with a return to pre-disease homeostasis. Unresolved inflammation is a hallmark of various human diseases, including diabetes, ulcerative colitis, rheumatoid arthritis, cancer, cardiovascular diseases, and periodontitis. The fate of acute inflammation determines the restoration to homeostasis versus disease establishment. Diseases associated with uncontrolled acute inflammation are characterized by a continuous release of histotoxic substances that results in local tissue damage, prolonged inflammatory response, and loss of function. In contrast, in health, the fate of inflammation is influenced by endogenous mediators, cells, tissue, and scaffolds to resolve the acute process and reestablish homeostasis, thereby promoting tissue healing and regeneration (Fig. 10.3).[3]

A Case Scenario is found on the companion website.

REFERENCES

 References for this chapter are found on the companion website.

Smoking and Periodontal Disease[a,b]

CHAPTER OUTLINE

THE SMOKING EPIDEMIC

Smoking is highly prevalent and can be considered an epidemic in both developed and developing nations. Smoking rates, however, have seen marked declines since the 1980s. Global estimated daily tobacco smoking prevalence rates (in individuals >15 years old) reduced from 41.2% in 1980 to 31.1% in 2012 for men and from 10.6% (1980) to 6.2% (2012) for women.[96] Despite this development, with population growth, the number of daily smokers worldwide has actually increased to just short of 1 billion people in 2012, upholding tobacco smoking's position as a major public health threat. Developed countries had their highest prevalence rates in those aged 30 to 34 years, whereas in developing countries the greatest prevalence was among those aged 45 to 49 years. The highest prevalence rates (male) are now often seen in developing countries (e.g., Bangladesh [44.4%], China [40.1%], Indonesia [57%]), although several developed countries also have similarly high rates (e.g., Russia [50.1%], Greece [40.8%], Japan [35.3%]).[96] The overall daily smoking prevalence rates for the United States were 15.5% in 2012 (17.2% for males, 14.3% for females).[96]

A Global Perspective

- As many as 6.25 trillion cigarettes are smoked annually across the globe.[96]
- Tobacco kills 6 million people each year.[147]
- Only 15% of people worldwide have access to smoking cessation services.[147]
- About 18% of people worldwide are protected by smoke-free laws.[147]

Smoking is harmful to almost every organ in the body and is associated with multiple diseases that reduce life expectancy and quality of life. Diseases associated with smoking include lung cancer, heart disease, stroke, emphysema, bronchitis, and cancers of the oral cavity, bladder, kidney, stomach, liver, and cervix. Approximately half of long-term smokers will die early as a result of smoking, and those who die before the age of 70 years will lose an average of 20 years of life.[37] Most deaths from smoking are due to lung cancer, chronic obstructive pulmonary disease, and coronary heart disease.

Tobacco smoke contains thousands of noxious chemicals, and it comprises a gaseous phase and a solid (particulate) phase. The gas phase contains carbon monoxide, ammonia, formaldehyde, hydrogen cyanide, and many other toxic and irritant compounds, including more than 60 known carcinogens such as benzo(a)pyrene and dimethylnitrosamine. The particulate phase includes nicotine, "tar" (itself made up of many toxic chemicals), benzene, and benzo(a)pyrene. Tar is inhaled with the smoke. In its condensate form, it is the sticky brown substance that stains fingers and teeth yellow and brown. Nicotine, which is an alkaloid, is found within the tobacco leaf and evaporates when the cigarette is lighted. It is quickly absorbed in the lungs, and it reaches the brain within 10 to 19 seconds. Nicotine is highly addictive. It causes a rise in blood pressure, increased heart and respiratory rates, and peripheral vasoconstriction.

---

[a]Adapted from the following chapter of Newman and Carranza's Clinical Periodontology, 13th edition: Chapter 12: Smoking and Periodontal Disease, by Philip M. Preshaw, Leandro Chambrone, and Richard Holliday.
[b]Note: In the 2018 Classification of Periodontal and Peri-Implant Diseases and Conditions, "chronic periodontitis" and "aggressive periodontitis" disease categories are grouped under a single category called "periodontitis," and are further characterized based on a multidimensional staging and grading system. In this chapter, the term "aggressive periodontitis" is still used, because the related studies were conducted before the 2018 classification. Readers are referred to Chapter 6 for the detailed discussion on periodontal disease classification.

CLINICIAN'S CORNER

Smokeless Tobacco

Smokeless tobacco products are becoming increasingly popular and exist in many different forms. Tobacco can be ground/grated and presented with salt and water as "moist snuff," which is usually delivered as a small tea-bag-like sachet placed under the lip. Alternatively, tobacco can be ground to a powder ("dry snuff") that is inhaled into the nasal cavity. Finally, tobacco can be coarsely cut (chewing tobacco) and placed into the cheek. Numerous smokeless tobacco varieties are popular in South Asian communities. The International Agency for Research on Cancer classifies smokeless tobacco as a cause of mouth, esophageal, and pancreatic cancer.[64]

Snus (or Swedish snuff) is a special type of smokeless tobacco that is popular in Sweden and increasingly the United States. It is banned across the rest of Europe. The manufacturers claim to use a special process to lower the levels of carcinogens in the product. Studies have shown a link to pancreatic cancer but not to mouth or lung cancer.[81]

All dental patients must be asked about their smoking status or tobacco usage. Current smoking status is the minimal information that must be recorded (e.g., "Patient is currently smoking *X* cigarettes per day"), but the importance of cumulative exposure to cigarette smoke means that it is more appropriate to record pack-years of smoking (Box 11.1). Readers are referred to the online material for a brief discussion on the biochemical tests used to assess smoking status. Online materials for this chapter are found on the companion website.

Smoking is a major risk factor for periodontitis, and it affects the prevalence, extent, and severity of disease. In addition, smoking has an adverse impact on the clinical outcome of nonsurgical and surgical therapy as well as the long-term success of implant placement. With 41.9% of periodontitis cases in the United States reported as being *attributable* to smoking (discussed next),[139] it is essential to understand the impact of smoking on the initiation, progression, and management of the disease. This chapter discusses the effects of smoking on the prevalence, severity, etiology, and pathogenesis of periodontal disease as well as its impact on treatment. The reader is referred to several excellent reviews of the topic for detailed results of specific studies.[1,27,54,70,71,97,98,112,140,145]

EFFECTS OF SMOKING ON THE PREVALENCE AND SEVERITY OF PERIODONTAL DISEASES

Gingivitis

Controlled clinical studies have demonstrated that, in human models of experimental gingivitis, the development of inflammation in response to plaque accumulation is reduced in smokers as compared with nonsmokers (Table 11.1).[19,33] In addition, cross-sectional studies have consistently demonstrated that smokers present with less gingival inflammation than nonsmokers.[12,13,17,105,106] These data suggest that smokers have a decreased expression of clinical inflammation in the presence of plaque accumulation as compared with nonsmokers. The microbiologic,

BOX 11.1 Challenge of Assessing Smoking Status

Current Smokers

Ask about current smoking and past smoking. Many smokers are trying to quit, and therefore simply asking how many cigarettes they are smoking today may not give an accurate assessment of their lifetime exposure (e.g., a patient who is currently smoking 5 cigarettes per day may have been smoking 40 cigarettes per day until yesterday, when he or she decided to cut down). Try to get an indication of the patient's approximate level of smoking (e.g., the average number of cigarettes per day for a certain number of years). It can also be useful to calculate the number of pack-years:

Pack-years = Number of packs smoked per day × Number of years of smoking

In other words, one pack-year is the cumulative exposure that corresponds with the smoking of one pack of 20 cigarettes per day for 1 year. For example, a smoker who has smoked 20 cigarettes per day for 15 years has 15 pack-years of smoking.

Former Smokers

Ask patients about their past smoking. Patients with periodontitis may have a significant smoking history that has had an impact on their periodontal status, even if they no longer smoke. Former smokers should always be congratulated for their achievement in quitting, but it is also very important to document the following:

- How much they used to smoke
- How many years they smoked
- When they quit

Is the Patient's Response Accurate?

The inaccurate or false reporting of smoking status is common; patients will tell you what they think you want to hear, or they may be embarrassed because they have not managed to cut down yet. Many patients report smoking 20 cigarettes per day, because this is the number of cigarettes in a pack in most countries, so 20 may be a convenient response rather than an accurate response. Cultural factors may also influence responses.[128]

When Is a Smoker Not a Smoker?

- Smokers have smoked ≥100 cigarettes in their lifetime and currently smoke.
- Former smokers have smoked ≥100 cigarettes in their lifetime and do not currently smoke.
- Nonsmokers have not smoked ≥100 cigarettes in their lifetime and do not currently smoke.

It must be noted that many periodontal research studies have not used these definitions, and this can sometimes make it difficult to interpret the studies, particularly in the context of what constitutes a former smoker. For example, from an exposure point of view, there is a big difference between someone who smoked 5 cigarettes per day for 10 years and who quit 30 years ago as compared with someone who smoked 40 cigarettes per day for 20 years and quit 6 months ago. It is always best in clinical practice to gather full information about each patient's smoking history.

immunologic, and physiologic factors that may account for this observation are discussed later.

Periodontitis

Although gingival inflammation in smokers appears to be reduced in response to plaque accumulation as compared with nonsmokers, an overwhelming body of evidence points to smoking as a major risk factor for increasing the prevalence and severity of

TABLE 11.1   Effects of Smoking on Gingivitis and Periodontitis

Periodontal Disease	Effects of Smoking
Gingivitis	↓Gingival inflammation and bleeding on probing
Periodontitis	↑Prevalence and severity of periodontal destruction ↑Pocket depth, attachment loss, and bone loss ↑Rate of periodontal destruction ↑Prevalence of severe periodontitis ↑Tooth loss ↑Prevalence with increased number of cigarettes smoked per day ↓Prevalence and severity with smoking cessation

↓, Decreased; ↑, increased.

BOX 11.2   Should We Change How We Manage Periodontal Disease?

Fact 1: Smoking is a major risk factor for periodontal disease.

Fact 2: According to the literature, smoking may be responsible for more than half of periodontitis cases among adults in the United States.[139]

Fact 3: Depending on the study, approximately 10%–15% of adults in most populations examined have advanced periodontitis.

Questions

- Would there be a benefit at the population level for periodontal health if all smokers in the population quit smoking today?
- Would dental professionals be able to more successfully manage periodontitis in smokers if we focused more on smoking cessation as a primary treatment strategy for managing periodontitis?

These questions are intended to be controversial. It is clear that smoking has a huge deleterious impact on periodontal status, and smoking cessation *must* be a core part of periodontal treatment in patients with periodontitis who smoke. The answer to the first question is almost certainly a resounding yes, but this probably will never be able to be tested. The answer to the second question is more difficult. Certainly, smokers with periodontitis must be educated about the harm that they are causing to their periodontal tissues, and they must be encouraged and helped to quit smoking. Treatment outcomes are improved among smokers who quit as compared with those who continue to smoke.[109]

Two Final Points (These Are Contentious and Designed to Stimulate Discussion)

- If more than half of the cases of periodontitis are attributable to smoking, then patients who smoke may be better served if dental professionals put more than half of their efforts into treating these patients via smoking cessation treatments (as opposed to other forms of periodontal therapy). Discuss!
- It is absurd for smokers in the Western world to worry about anything except stopping smoking.[103]

periodontal destruction. Multiple cross-sectional and longitudinal studies have demonstrated that pocket depth, attachment loss, and alveolar bone loss are more prevalent and severe in patients who smoke as compared with nonsmokers.[70,71,112,140] An assessment of the relationship between cigarette smoking and periodontitis was performed in more than 12,000 dentate individuals who were more than 18 years old as part of the Third National Health and Nutrition Examination Survey.[139] Periodontitis was defined as one or more sites with clinical attachment loss of 4 mm or greater and pocket depth of 4 mm or greater. Smoking status was defined with the use of criteria established by the Centers for Disease Control and Prevention (CDC) (see Box 11.1). Of the more than 12,000 individuals studied, 9.2% had periodontitis; this represented approximately 15 million cases of periodontitis in the United States. On average, smokers were four times as likely to have periodontitis as compared with persons who had never smoked after adjusting for age, gender, race/ethnicity, education, and income/poverty ratio. Former smokers were 1.7 times more likely to have periodontitis than persons who had never smoked. This study also demonstrated a dose–response relationship between cigarettes smoked per day and the odds of having periodontitis. In subjects smoking nine or fewer cigarettes per day, the odds for having periodontitis were 2.8, whereas subjects who smoked 31 or more cigarettes per day were almost 6 times more likely to have periodontitis. In former smokers, the odds of having periodontitis declined with the number of years since quitting. These data indicated that approximately 42% of periodontitis cases (6.4 million cases) in the U.S. adult population were attributable to current smoking and that approximately 11% (1.7 million cases) were attributable to former smoking. These data highlight the serious threat to dental public health posed by cigarette smoking and raise questions about the best methods for managing periodontitis in patients who smoke (Box 11.2).

These data are consistent with the findings of other cross-sectional studies performed in the United States and Europe. The odds ratio for periodontitis in current smokers has been estimated to range from as low as 1.5 to as high as 7.3 compared to nonsmokers, depending on the observed severity of periodontitis.[98] A meta-analysis of data from six such studies involving 2361 subjects indicated that current smokers were almost three times more likely to have severe periodontitis than nonsmokers.[97] The detrimental impact of long-term smoking on the periodontal and dental status of older adults has been clearly demonstrated. Older adult smokers are approximately three times more likely to have severe periodontal disease,[10,80] and the number of years of tobacco use is a significant factor in tooth loss, coronal root caries, and periodontal disease.[68,69]

Smoking has also been shown to affect periodontal disease severity in younger individuals. Cigarette smoking is associated with increased severity of generalized aggressive periodontitis in young adults,[127] and those who smoke are 3.8 times more likely to have periodontitis as compared with nonsmokers.[48] Longitudinal studies have demonstrated that young individuals who smoke more than 15 cigarettes per day showed the highest risk for tooth loss.[60] In addition, smokers are more than 6 times as likely as nonsmokers to demonstrate continued attachment loss.[65] Over a 10-year period, bone loss has been reported to be twice as rapid in smokers as in nonsmokers[20] and to proceed

TABLE 11.2 Barriers Against and Stimuli for the Provision of Smoking Cessation Advice by the Dental Team in Dental Practice

	Barriers	Stimuli
Professional characteristics	Perceived lack of efficacy or lack of confidence in giving the advice	Self-efficacy
	Concerns about disturbing the patient–clinician relationship	Positive attitude toward giving advice as part of health care provider role
	Lack of knowledge about how to give the correct advice	Training
	Belief that counseling is unnecessary or perception that advising patients is frustrating and has a low success rate	Self-belief
	Dental team member may be a smoker himself or herself	Dental team member needs to quit!
Practice organization	Lack of time	Task delegation
	No organizational support in the practice to deliver advice	Focus on helping smokers quit
Health care system	No reimbursement	Health care system changes to encourage healthier lifestyles
	No referral options for further help	Local availability of smoking cessation services

Adapted from Rosseel JP, Jacobs JE, Hilberink SR, et al: What determines the provision of smoking cessation advice and counselling by dental care teams? *Br Dent J* 206(7):E13, 2009.

more rapidly, even in the presence of excellent plaque control.[14] Less information is available about the effects of cigar and pipe smoking, but it appears that effects similar to those of cigarette smoking are observed with these forms of tobacco use.[5,40,41,78] The prevalence of moderate and severe periodontitis and the percentage of teeth with more than 5 mm of attachment loss were most severe in current cigarette smokers, but cigar and pipe smokers showed a severity of disease that was intermediate between that of current cigarette smokers and nonsmokers.[5] Tooth loss is also increased among cigar and pipe smokers as compared with nonsmokers.[78]

Former smokers have less risk for periodontitis than current smokers but more risk than nonsmokers, and the risk for periodontitis decreases with the increasing number of years since quitting smoking.[139] This suggests that the negative effects of smoking on the host are reversible with smoking cessation, and therefore that smoking cessation programs must be an integral component of periodontal education and therapy (Box 11.3 and Table 11.2). Several tobacco intervention approaches can be used

BOX 11.3 Helping Your Patients to Quit Smoking

Smoking cessation is a public health priority for governments around the world. Excellent online resources are available to provide information about the harmful effects of smoking and to help people to quit, including the following:

- http://www.cdc.gov/tobacco
- http://www.ash.org.uk
- http://smokefree.nhs.uk

Smoking cessation must be an integral part of the management of dental patients who smoke, and it is the responsibility of all dental health professionals to address this issue with their patients. The dental team is well placed to provide this treatment, because they see patients on a regular basis as part of ongoing routine dental management. Furthermore, interventions to help patients quit smoking in dental practices are effective, with quit rates of 15% to 20% as compared with approximately 5% in control groups.[119] The whole dental team should therefore be involved in smoking cessation, but this is not always the case. Why? Some of the barriers to providing smoking cessation counseling in the dental practice are shown in Table 12.2.

Various methods for helping patients to quit smoking in the dental environment have been described, and these are typically referred to as *brief intervention programs*. One such program[12] is known as the 5 As:

ASK Ask the patient about his or her smoking status (see Box 11.1).

This should be part of the medical history.

ADVISE Advise smokers of the associations between oral disease and smoking.

Be informative, honest, and helpful but not judgmental. The patient's response to this information will reveal his or her interest in quitting.

ASSESS Assess the patient's interest in and readiness to attempt smoking cessation.

Patients may not yet be in an action phase when it comes to quitting smoking, which is why it is always important to make these assessments every time you see the patient.

ASSIST Assist the patient with his or her quit attempt.

If you are trained, there are many techniques that can be used (see Box 11.4). Alternatively, assist the patient with seeking the help that he or she needs.

ARRANGE Arrange for a follow-up visit or a referral to professional smoking cessation services.

The most important aspect of this strategy is to keep in regular contact, particularly around the quit date and during the immediate period after the patient quits.

A simplified version of this is the 3 As. This is a *very brief intervention* and can be particularly useful for the dental team.[95,111] The intervention is designed to be used at every clinical contact, and its very brief nature may help overcome some of the barriers presented by dental practices (the duration is <30 s). The focus is taken away from advising smokers to stop and shifts to offering support. The "advise" step deliberately leaves out the health benefits of stopping smoking or the harms of smoking. This minimizes the duration of the intervention and helps to avoid a defensive reaction or developing anxiety in the patient. The 3 As technique is as follows:

ASK and record smoking status.

ADVISE how to stop.

ACT on the patient's response (prescribe, monitor, or refer).

Clearly, for the patient undergoing a comprehensive course of periodontal therapy, over several visits, there may be more opportunity to focus on the harms of smoking and the personal benefits of quitting.

when helping the patient deal with the physiologic factors (i.e., nicotine withdrawal symptoms) and the psychological factors associated with smoking cessation (Box 11.4).[99,116] Electronic cigarettes have also emerged and are being used by many smokers to help them quit (Box 11.5). However, the effects on oral health are yet to be established.

Beyond E-Cigarettes
The popularity of e-cigarettes took most people by surprise. But what's next?

"Heat-Not-Burn" Tobacco Products
These products heat tobacco to ~500°C, producing an inhalable aerosol.[24] Although not a new idea, they have received recent attention. One manufacturer introduced a product into the Japanese market in 2015, which has been popular, with the media reporting sales outstripping demand.

Water Pipes (Hookah, Shisha)
Popular in some communities, these are likely to carry significant negative health risks. A good summary is produced by the National Center for Smoking Cessation and Training (NCSCT).[94]

Nicotine Gels
These gels allow nicotine to be absorbed through the skin. Currently, they are not very popular.

EFFECTS OF SMOKING ON THE ETIOLOGY AND PATHOGENESIS OF PERIODONTAL DISEASE

The increased prevalence and severity of periodontal destruction associated with smoking suggests that the host–bacterial interactions normally seen with chronic periodontitis are altered, resulting in more extensive periodontal breakdown (Table 11.3). This imbalance between bacterial challenge and host response may be caused by changes in the composition of the subgingival biofilm (e.g., increases in the numbers and virulence of pathogenic organisms), changes in the host response to the bacterial challenge, or a combination of both.

Microbiology

Several studies have explored the possible changes in the subgingival microbiome caused by smoking. Earlier studies tended to show little difference between smokers and nonsmokers. For example, Preber and colleagues (1992) took plaque samples from deep pockets (i.e., ≥6 mm) in 142 patients and found no differences in the counts of *Aggregatibacter actinomycetemcomitans*, *Porphyromonas gingivalis*, and *Prevotella intermedia*.[108] In a similar study of 615 patients involving the use of immunoassay, the prevalence of *A. actinomycetemcomitans*, *P. gingivalis*, *P. intermedia*, and *Eikenella corrodens* was not found to be significantly different between smokers and nonsmokers.[134]

By contrast, other studies have demonstrated differences in the microbial composition of subgingival biofilm of smokers and nonsmokers. A study of 798 subjects with different smoking histories found that smokers had significantly higher levels of *Tannerella forsythia* and that smokers were 2.3 times more

---

BOX 11.4   Methods of Smoking Cessation

Willpower Alone
This is the least effective method of smoking cessation, with only 3% of smokers managing to quit after 12 months.[2]

Self-Help Materials
The provision of self-help materials can increase quit rates compared to no intervention, although only by a small amount.[53] When included with any other intervention, there was no additional benefit.

Brief Intervention Program in Primary Care
A brief advice intervention delivered by a physician or dental professional can increase the rate of quitting (12 months) by 40%–90%.[25,132] Assuming an unassisted quit rate of 3%, a brief intervention by a dental hygienist could increase the quit rates to 4.5%–6%. Although this cessation rate may seem low, if the dental team gave this brief advice to most of their smoking patients, a significant number of smokers in the whole population would be assisted to quit each year.

Nicotine Replacement Therapy
Nicotine replacement therapy (NRT) can increase the rate of quitting (12 months) by 50%–70%.[133] For example, in primary care settings in which brief advice is given, 12-month success rates can increase from around 5% to around 8% if NRT is also used. In an intensive setting such as a smoker's clinic, success rates increase from around 10% to up to 16%. NRT is not a magic cure, but it helps with cravings and withdrawal when a person quits smoking. Although NRT products do contain nicotine, they do not contain the toxic products such as tar and carbon monoxide that are found in cigarette smoke. NRT products include the following:
- Patches (available in different doses and worn for 16–24 h/day)
- Lozenges and gum (available in different flavors; should be chewed slowly to allow the nicotine to be absorbed through the mouth)
- Nasal spray (delivers nicotine solution via the nasal passages)
- Inhalator (a plastic mouthpiece with a supply of nicotine cartridges that fit on the end; nicotine is absorbed in the mouth by drawing on the inhalator like a cigarette).

Varenicline
A course of varenicline, at standard dose, can increase the rate of quitting (12 months) by 100%–150%.[22] Varenicline is a nicotine receptor partial agonist, and it aims to reduce both withdrawal symptoms and the pleasure people usually experience when they smoke.

Bupropion
Bupropion can increase the rate of quitting (12 months) by 50%–80%.[62] This medication is used as an antidepressant at higher doses, but it is effective for smoking cessation at lower doses. It is usually prescribed to be started 1–2 weeks before the quit date. There are serious potential drug interactions and unwanted effects.

Other Methods
Whatever works for the patient is good! In addition to combinations of the methods listed here, techniques for smoking cessation can include intensive counseling, motivational interviewing, cognitive behavioral therapy, hypnosis, and acupuncture. Many smokers are now also using e-cigarettes to help to quit smoking (see Box 11.5).

BOX 11.5 Electronic Cigarettes

Electronic cigarettes (e-cigarettes) are electronic devices that produce an aerosol that the user inhales. The e-cigarette contains a solution, often called an "e-liquid," which is drawn through a heating element to produce the aerosol. The process of using an e-cigarette (often referred to as *vaping*) closely resembles tobacco smoking, making e-cigarettes a particularly attractive alternative to smokers. In contrast, this similarity to cigarette smoking has produced much of the controversy and concerns around e-cigarettes.

What Is in the E-Liquid?
The e-liquid usually comprises three main components: diluents, nicotine, and flavorings. The diluents account for the majority of the solution and are usually propylene glycol or vegetable glycerin. Nicotine is included at a wide range of concentrations, the most popular strength in Great Britain being 13 to 18 mg/mL.[3] Nicotine-free e-liquids are available and used by approximately 10% of users (Great Britain).[3] Flavorings are often added, as both nicotine and the diluents are largely tasteless. The large range of flavors can generally be divided into three main groups: tobacco, fruit, and menthol/mint.

Are E-Cigarettes a Useful Smoking Cessation Aid?
E-cigarettes are a modern phenomenon introduced to the U.S. and European markets in 2006, with their popularly taking off in around 2011. The evidence base is continually growing with several ongoing clinical trials. A Cochrane Collaboration systematic review concluded that e-cigarettes helped smokers to stop smoking and showed particular promise in reducing cigarette consumption in smokers unwilling to quit (although further studies are needed to confirm this conclusion).[88]

Are E-Cigarettes Safe?
This has been the topic of many debates, and controversy still exists. Two substantial reports concluded that the hazard to health from long-term e-cigarette vapor inhalation was unlikely to exceed 5% of the harm from smoking tobacco.[87,120]

What Are the Oral Health Effects?
Very little has been published in this field. A handful of in vitro cell line studies have shown a variety of effects including cytotoxicity and DNA damage.[125,146,148] As with all in vitro studies, the clinical relevance is difficult to interpret, and unfortunately some of these studies are of questionable quality.[59] From a clinical perspective, e-cigarette vapor is likely to have different effects on the oral tissues when compared with the well-known effects of tobacco smoke. Interestingly, nicotine has been shown to be angiogenic[66] with wound-healing properties[85] and with potential intraoral applications.[114,115] Well-conducted clinical studies are required to enable us to appropriately inform patients about e-cigarette use.

How Are E-Cigarettes Regulated?
A range of regulatory approaches have been taken across the globe, from e-cigarettes being completely prohibited to being classified under general consumer product regulations.[24]

What Is the Bottom Line?
E-cigarettes are a consumer led bottom-up public health initiative that has taken the realms of research, public health, regulation, and industry by surprise. They are extremely popular with users (smokers/former smokers), with probably only a fraction of the health hazard of tobacco smoking. From a public health perspective, they have the potential to significantly reduce tobacco-related morbidity and mortality. The oral health risks are currently unknown but are likely to be less than those associated with tobacco smoking.

TABLE 11.3 Effects of Smoking on the Etiology and Pathogenesis of Periodontal Disease

Etiologic Factor	Effects of Smoking
Microbiology	Increased complexity of the microbiome and colonization of periodontal pockets by periodontal pathogens
Immune–inflammatory response	Altered neutrophil chemotaxis, phagocytosis, and oxidative burst ↑Tumor necrosis factor-α and prostaglandin E_2 in gingival crevicular fluid ↑Neutrophil collagenase and elastase in gingival crevicular fluid ↑Production of prostaglandin E_2 by monocytes in response to lipopolysaccharide
Physiology	↓Gingival blood vessels with ↑ inflammation ↓Gingival crevicular fluid flow and bleeding on probing with ↑ inflammation ↓Subgingival temperature ↑Time needed to recover from local anesthesia

↓, Decreased; ↑, increased.

likely to harbor *T. forsythia* as compared with nonsmokers and former smokers.[149] Of interest were observations that smokers did not respond to mechanical therapy as well as nonsmokers did; this was associated with increased levels of *T. forsythia*, *A. actinomycetemcomitans*, and *P. gingivalis* remaining in the pockets after therapy in the smoking group as compared with nonsmokers.[45,46,49,113]

Many discrepancies between the findings of microbiologic studies are a function of the methodology involved, including bacterial counts versus proportions or prevalence of bacteria, the number of sites sampled, and the pocket depths selected, the sampling technique, the disease status of the subject, and the methods of bacterial identification and data analysis. In an attempt to overcome some of these problems, one study sampled subgingival biofilm from all teeth with the exception of third molars in 272 adult subjects, including 50 current smokers, 98 former smokers, and 124 nonsmokers.[51] Using checkerboard DNA–DNA hybridization technology to screen for 29 different subgingival species, it was found that members of the orange and red complex species—including *Eikenella nodatum*, *Fusobacterium nucleatum* ss *vincentii*, *P. intermedia*, *Peptostreptococcus micros*, *Prevotella nigrescens*, *T. forsythia*, *P. gingivalis*, and *Treponema denticola*—were significantly more prevalent in current smokers than in nonsmokers and former smokers. The increased prevalence of these periodontal pathogens was caused by an increased colonization of shallow sites (pocket depth ≤4 mm), with no differences among smokers, former smokers, and nonsmokers in pockets 4 mm or greater. In addition, these pathogenic bacteria were more prevalent in the maxilla than the mandible. These data suggest that smokers have a greater extent of colonization by periodontal pathogens than nonsmokers or former smokers, which may increase the risk of periodontal disease progression.

Contemporary studies have drawn similar conclusions, with next-generation sequencing analysis of periodontally healthy smokers demonstrating a highly diverse, pathogen-rich, commensal-poor, anaerobic microbiome that is more similar to the microbiome observed in patients with advanced periodontitis than that which is observed in periodontally healthy nonsmokers, and which is primed for future development of periodontitis given appropriate ecologic and environmental changes.[86]

Immune–Inflammatory Responses

The immune response of the host to biofilm accumulation is essentially protective. In periodontal health, a balance exists between the bacterial challenge of the biofilm and the immune–inflammatory responses in the gingival tissues, with no resulting loss of periodontal support. By contrast, periodontitis is associated with an alteration in the host–bacterial balance that may be initiated by changes in the bacterial composition of the subgingival biofilm, changes in the host responses, other environmental changes, or a combination of these.

Smoking exerts a major effect on the immune–inflammatory response that results in an increase in the extent and severity of periodontal destruction. The deleterious effects of smoking appear to result from alterations in the immune–inflammatory response to bacterial challenge. The neutrophil is an important component of the host response to the bacterial challenge, and alterations in neutrophil number or function may result in localized and systemic infections. Critical functions of neutrophils include *chemotaxis* (directed locomotion from the bloodstream to the site of infection), *phagocytosis* (internalization of foreign particles such as bacteria), and *killing* via oxidative and nonoxidative mechanisms.

Neutrophils that are obtained from the peripheral blood, oral cavity, or saliva of smokers or that are exposed in vitro to whole tobacco smoke or nicotine have demonstrated functional alterations in chemotaxis, phagocytosis, and the oxidative burst.[38,74] In vitro studies of the effects of tobacco products on neutrophils have shown detrimental effects on cell movement as well as on the oxidative burst.[32,73,79,123,129] In addition, levels of antibody to the periodontal pathogens essential for phagocytosis and killing of bacteria, specifically immunoglobulin G_2, have been reported to be reduced in smokers as compared with nonsmokers with periodontitis,[23,47,49,136] thereby suggesting that smokers may have reduced protection against periodontal bacteria. By contrast, elevated levels of tumor necrosis factor–α have been demonstrated in the gingival crevicular fluid of smokers,[21] and elevated levels of prostaglandin E_2, neutrophil elastase, and matrix metalloproteinase-8 have also been found.[131] In vitro studies have also shown that exposure to nicotine increases the secretion of prostaglandin E_2 by monocytes in response to lipopolysaccharide.[101]

These data suggest that smoking alters the response of neutrophils to the bacterial challenge such that there are increases in the release of tissue-destructive enzymes, causing increased periodontal tissue destruction. However, the exact changes in the immunologic mechanisms involved in the rapid tissue destruction seen in smokers are not yet fully understood, and more research in this area is indicated.

Physiology

Previous studies have shown that certain clinical signs of inflammation (e.g., gingival redness, gingival bleeding) are less pronounced in smokers than in nonsmokers.[13,33] This may result from alterations in the vascular response of the gingival tissues. Although no significant differences in the vascular density of healthy gingiva have been observed between smokers and nonsmokers,[102] the response of the microcirculation to biofilm accumulation appears to be altered in smokers as compared with nonsmokers. With developing inflammation, increases in gingival crevicular fluid flow, bleeding on probing,[19] and gingival blood vessels[18] are lower in smokers than in nonsmokers. In addition, the oxygen concentration in healthy gingival tissues appears to be lower in smokers than in nonsmokers, although this condition is reversed in the presence of moderate inflammation.[52] Subgingival temperatures are lower in smokers than nonsmokers,[35] and recovery from the vasoconstriction caused by local anesthetic administration takes longer in smokers.[75,142] These data suggest that significant alterations are present in the gingival microvasculature of smokers as compared with nonsmokers and that these changes lead to decreased blood flow and decreased clinical signs of inflammation. This explains the long-observed phenomenon of a transient increase in gingival bleeding when a smoker quits; patients need to be warned about this phenomenon.

IS NICOTINE THE BAD GUY? The role of nicotine in the detrimental health effects seen in smokers has never been more relevant with the increasing popularity of novel nicotine delivery devices (e.g., e-cigarettes). Nicotine is not carcinogenic,[55,63] and it is now largely accepted that nicotine has likely been unfairly blamed. A classic quote, with reference to lung cancer, is "smokers smoke for nicotine but are killed by tar."[121] The potential role of nicotine in periodontitis development is less clear. Nicotine has been the subject of many in vitro investigations with oral cells. These studies often present conflicting results with regard to cellular viability and functions. For example, with regard to cellular viability, overall, the studies show that the harsher the conditions (e.g., higher concentrations of nicotine and longer durations of exposure), the more significant the detrimental effects of the nicotine on cell culture systems. Cellular viability has generally been shown to be unaffected[44,93,130] by nicotine concentrations in the range found in blood plasma (~36 ng/mL)[122] or the saliva of smokers (906 ng/mL).[42] Much higher nicotine concentrations can be found in the saliva of smokeless tobacco users (70 to 1560 µg/mL),[58] and studies with these nicotine concentrations demonstrate significant cellular toxicity in vitro.[6,31,138] Interestingly, cells derived from smokers and older donors demonstrated less sensitivity to nicotine.[31]

Clinical studies are required to determine the clinical relevance of these in vitro results.

EFFECTS OF SMOKING ON THE RESPONSE TO PERIODONTAL THERAPY

Nonsurgical Therapy

Numerous studies have indicated that current smokers do not respond as well to periodontal therapy as nonsmokers or former

TABLE 11.4 Effects of Smoking on the Response to Periodontal Therapy

Therapy	Effects of Smoking
Nonsurgical	↓ Clinical response to root surface debridement ↓ Reduction in probing depth ↓ Gain in clinical attachment levels ↓ Negative impact of smoking with ↑ level of plaque control
Surgery and implants	↓ Probing depth reduction and ↓ gain in clinical attachment levels after access flap surgery ↑ Deterioration of furcations after surgery ↓ Gain in clinical attachment levels, ↓ bone fill, ↑ recession, and ↑ membrane exposure after guided tissue regeneration ↓ Root coverage after grafting procedures for localized gingival recession ↓ Probing depth reduction after bone graft procedures ↑ Risk for implant failure and periimplantitis
Maintenance care	↑ Probing depth and attachment loss during maintenance therapy ↑ Disease recurrence in smokers ↑ Need for retreatment in smokers ↑ Tooth loss in smokers after surgical therapy

↓, Decreased; ↑, increased.

smokers do (Table 11.4). Most clinical research supports the observation that probing depth reductions are generally greater in nonsmokers than in smokers after nonsurgical periodontal therapy.[4,45,46,49,72,107,113] In addition, gains in clinical attachment as a result of nonsurgical treatment are less pronounced in smokers than in nonsmokers. In a study of patients with previously untreated advanced periodontal disease, nonsurgical therapy resulted in significantly greater mean reductions in probing depth and bleeding on probing in nonsmokers than in smokers when evaluated 6 months after the completion of therapy.[113] Mean probing depth reductions of 2.5 mm for nonsmokers and 1.9 mm for smokers were observed in pockets that averaged 7 mm or more before treatment. In another study, the nonsurgical management of pockets of 5 mm or greater showed that smokers had less probing depth reduction than nonsmokers after 3 months (1.29 mm vs. 1.76 mm) as well as less gain in clinical attachment levels.[45] When a higher level of oral hygiene was achieved as part of nonsurgical care, the differences in the resolution of 4- to 6-mm pockets between nonsmokers and smokers became clinically less significant.[107]

It can be concluded that smokers respond less well to nonsurgical therapy than do nonsmokers. With excellent plaque control, these differences may be minimized, but the emphasis is on truly excellent plaque control. When comparing current smokers with former smokers and nonsmokers, the former and nonsmoking subjects appear to respond equally well to nonsurgical care,[45] thereby reinforcing the need for patients to be informed of the benefits of smoking cessation.

Surgical Therapy and Implants

The less favorable response of the periodontal tissues to nonsurgical therapy that is observed in current smokers is also observed after surgical therapy. In a longitudinal comparative study of the effects of four different treatment modalities (coronal scaling, root planing, modified Widman flap surgery, and osseous resection surgery), smokers (with "heavy" defined as ≥20 cigarettes/day and "light" defined as ≤19 cigarettes/day) consistently showed less pocket reduction and less gain in clinical attachment as compared with nonsmokers or former smokers.[72] These differences were evident immediately after the completion of therapy and continued throughout 7 years of supportive periodontal therapy. Smoking has also been shown to have a negative impact on the outcomes of guided tissue regeneration,[141,143] the treatment of infra-bony defects by bone grafts,[118] and periodontal plastic surgery.[27,30]

Several meta-analyses have investigated the influence of smoking on the short- and long-term outcomes of implant therapy and have identified that smoking increases the risk of implant failure.[28,57,77,90,135] These studies used various definitions to define implant failure, including implant loss, implant bone loss, mobility, pain, and periimplantitis. Overall, the risk for implant failure in smokers appears to be approximately double the risk for failure in nonsmokers, and the risks appear to be higher in maxillary implants and when implants are placed in poor-quality bone. Smoking has also been shown to be a risk factor for periimplantitis, with a majority of studies showing a significant increase in peri-implant bone loss as compared with nonsmokers.[56] Collectively, these data indicate that implant failure is more common among smokers than nonsmokers. However, because numerous factors can influence implant success, further controlled clinical trials are needed to address the role of smoking as an independent variable in implant failure. Given the current evidence, all patients who are considering implant therapy should be informed about the benefits of smoking cessation and the risks of smoking for the development of periimplantitis and implant failure.

Maintenance Therapy

The detrimental effect of smoking on treatment outcomes appears to be long lasting and independent of the frequency of maintenance therapy. After four modalities of therapy (scaling, scaling and root planing, modified Widman flap surgery, and osseous surgery), maintenance therapy was performed by a hygienist every 3 months for 7 years.[72] Smokers consistently had deeper pockets than nonsmokers and less gain in attachment when evaluated each year for the 7-year period. Even with more intensive maintenance therapy given every month for 6 months after flap surgery,[126] smokers had deeper and more residual pockets than nonsmokers, although no significant differences in plaque or bleeding on probing scores were found. These data suggest that the effects of smoking on the host response and the healing characteristics of the periodontal tissues may have a long-term effect on pocket resolution in smokers, possibly requiring more intensive management during the maintenance phase. Smokers also tend to experience more periodontal breakdown than nonsmokers after therapy.[82,84] In studies of patients who failed to respond to periodontal therapy, approximately 90% of these poorly responding patients were smokers.[82,83]

A systematic review that assessed the potential predictors of tooth loss during long-term periodontal maintenance care demonstrated that, although oral health and the prevention of tooth loss were achieved in the majority of patients, the long-term outcomes were also influenced by smoking.[26] Tobacco smoking was positively associated with tooth loss even when regular recall maintenance care was performed (overall, smokers had a risk of losing their teeth that was up to 380% higher than that of nonsmokers).[26] Similarly, smoking has a detrimental effect on peri-implant tissue status, even when patients are under strict peri-implant preventive maintenance care. For instance, when comparing nonsmokers and light smokers (i.e., subjects who smoked <10 cigarettes per day), it was found that the majority of patients who experienced bone loss were smokers (88.9%), with an odds ratio of 39.64 (95% confidence interval, 8.62 to 182.27) for increased risk of bone loss.[34]

It is clear from these studies that (1) smokers may present with periodontal disease at an early age; (2) they may be difficult to treat effectively with conventional therapeutic strategies; (3) they may continue to have progressive or recurrent periodontitis; and (4) they may be at an increased risk of tooth loss or peri-implant bone loss, even when adequate maintenance control is established. For these reasons, smoking cessation counseling must be a cornerstone of periodontal therapy in smokers.

EFFECTS OF SMOKING CESSATION ON PERIODONTAL TREATMENT OUTCOMES

The effect of smoking cessation on periodontal status has been studied in a large number of cross-sectional and cohort observational studies, in which the periodontal status of smokers, former smokers, and nonsmokers is compared.[8,9,14-16,20,36,48,50,69,100,137,139] Similarly, periodontal treatment outcomes have been assessed in smokers, former smokers, and nonsmokers.[46,61,72,89,110,124] Collectively, these studies have demonstrated that smokers have significantly worse periodontal status (i.e., deeper probing depths, more attachment loss and bone loss) than either former smokers or nonsmokers and usually have poorer treatment outcomes. The periodontal status of former smokers is intermediate to that of current smokers and nonsmokers, and it appears to usually be closer to that of nonsmokers.

There are very few intervention studies of the effect of smoking cessation on periodontal treatment outcomes (i.e., studies in which smokers were helped to quit and in which the effect on periodontal status was assessed). Two short-term studies have indicated that smoking has a negative impact on the gingival vasculature and that these changes are reversible with smoking cessation.[91,92] Two interventional studies have assessed the impact of smoking cessation on outcomes after nonsurgical periodontal treatment.[109,117] The first study employed dental hygienists who were trained as smoking cessation advisers and who achieved a 20% quit rate at 12 months in a population of smokers who also had periodontitis. The hygienists used a variety of strategies to assist these smokers, including counseling, nicotine replacement

therapy, and bupropion. All of the patients received nonsurgical therapy as treatment for their periodontitis in addition to smoking cessation counseling. Those individuals who successfully quit smoking for the entire 12 months of the study had the best response to the periodontal treatment. The treatment responses in the nonquitters and the failed quitters (i.e., the "oscillators," who initially quit but then resumed smoking) were significantly poorer than those seen in the quitters, and they did not differ significantly from each other. The second study was a 12-month prospective single-blinded study in which smoking cessation advice, nicotine replacement therapy, and medication were provided at four consecutive appointments, once a week, by a multidisciplinary team that included doctors, psychologists, and a dentist, in addition to nonsurgical treatment of periodontitis.[117] The confirmed continuous quit rate at 12 months was 18.3%. At the end of the 12-month follow-up period, it was identified that the quitters had improved clinical attachment gain as compared with the nonquitters. In addition, a supplementary study that described a set of meta-analyses performed with individual patient data from these two trials reported a highly significant beneficial impact of quitting smoking, with quitters demonstrating 30% more sites with probing depth reductions of 2 mm or more as compared with nonquitters.[29] Equally, quitters had 22% fewer sites with residual probing depths of 4 mm or greater as compared with nonquitters at the end of the 12-month follow-up period.[29]

The benefit of smoking cessation on the periodontium is likely to be mediated through various pathways, such as a shift toward a less pathogenic microbiome, the recovery of the gingival microcirculation, and improvements in certain aspects of the immune–inflammatory responses. In support of this observation, in the interventional study described previously,[109] plaque samples were collected as the study progressed. It became clear that subgingival microbial profiles differed significantly between smokers and quitters at 6 and 12 months after smoking cessation.[43] At 6 and 12 months after treatment, the microbial community in smokers was similar to that observed at baseline (i.e., before periodontal treatment/smoking cessation counseling), whereas the quitters demonstrated significantly divergent profiles; changes in bacterial levels contributed to this shift. These data suggest a critical role for smoking cessation in the alteration of the subgingival biofilm. Further research is necessary to investigate the impact of smoking cessation on the immune–inflammatory mechanisms that drive tissue destruction in the periodontium.

In conclusion, smoking is a major risk factor for periodontitis, and smoking cessation should be an integral part of periodontal therapy among patients who smoke. Smoking cessation should be considered a priority for the management of periodontitis in smokers.

A Case Scenario is found on the companion website www .expertconsult.com.

REFERENCES

 Rneferences for this chapter are found on the companion website www.expertconsult.com.

12

The Role of Dental Calculus and Other Local Predisposing Factors[a]

CHAPTER OUTLINE

The primary cause of gingival inflammation is bacterial plaque bioflim. Other predisposing factors include calculus, faulty restorations, complications associated with orthodontic therapy, self-inflicted injuries, and the use of tobacco.

CALCULUS

Calculus consists of mineralized bacterial plaque that forms on the surfaces of natural teeth and dental prostheses.

Supragingival and Subgingival Calculus

Supragingival calculus is located coronal to the gingival margin and therefore is visible in the oral cavity. It is usually white or whitish yellow in color; hard, with a claylike consistency; and easily detached from the tooth surface. After removal, it may rapidly recur, especially in the lingual area of the mandibular incisors. The color is influenced by contact with substances such as tobacco and food pigments. It may be localized on a single tooth or group of teeth, or it may be generalized throughout the mouth.

> **KEY FACT**
>
> Mechanical removal of subgingival plaque biofilm and calculus is considered the fundamental cornerstone to the treatment of chronic periodontitis.

The two most common locations for the development of supragingival calculus are the buccal surfaces of the maxillary molars (Fig. 12.1) and the lingual surfaces of the mandibular anterior teeth (Fig. 12.2).[36]

Saliva from the parotid gland flows over the facial surfaces of the upper molars via the parotid duct, whereas the submandibular duct and the lingual duct empty onto the lingual surfaces of the lower incisors from the submaxillary and sublingual glands,

respectively. In extreme cases, calculus may form a bridge-like structure over the interdental papilla of adjacent teeth or cover the occlusal surface of teeth that are lacking functional antagonists.

Subgingival calculus is located below the crest of the marginal gingiva and is not visible on routine clinical examination. The location and the extent of subgingival calculus may be evaluated by careful tactile perception with a delicate dental instrument such as an explorer. Subgingival calculus is typically hard and dense; it frequently appears to be dark brown or greenish black in color (Fig. 12.3), and it is firmly attached to the tooth surface. Supragingival calculus and subgingival calculus generally occur together, but one may be present without the other. Microscopic studies demonstrate that deposits of subgingival calculus usually extend nearly to the base of periodontal pockets in individuals with chronic periodontitis but do not reach the junctional epithelium.

When the gingival tissues recede, subgingival calculus becomes exposed and is therefore reclassified as supragingival (Fig. 12.4A). Thus, supragingival calculus can be composed of both the initial supragingival calculus and previous subgingival calculus. A reduction in gingival inflammation and probing depths with a gain in clinical attachment can be observed after the removal of subgingival plaque and calculus (see Fig. 12.4B; see Chapter 45).

> **CLINICAL CORRELATION**
>
> A reduction in gingival inflammation and probing depths accompanied by a gain in clinical attachment can be expected following thorough removal of subgingival plaque and calculus.

Prevalence

Anerud and colleagues[4] observed the periodontal status of a group of Sri Lankan tea laborers and a group of Norwegian academicians for a 15-year period. The Norwegian population had ready access to preventive dental care throughout their lives, whereas the Sri Lankan tea laborers did not. The formation of supragingival calculus was observed early in life in the Sri Lankan individuals, probably shortly after the teeth erupted. The first areas to exhibit calculus deposits were the facial aspects of

[a]Adapted from the following chapter of Newman and Carranza's Clinical Periodontology, 13th edition: Chapter 13: The Role of Dental Calculus and Other Local Predisposing Factors, by James E. Hinrichs and Vivek Thumbigere-Math.

Fig. 12.1 Supragingival Calculus is Depicted on the Buccal Surfaces of Maxillary Molars Adjacent to the Orifice for the Parotid Duct.

Fig. 12.2 Extensive Supragingival Calculus is Present on the Lingual Surfaces of the Lower Anterior Teeth.

Fig. 12.3 Dark Pigmented Deposits of Subgingival Calculus are Shown on the Distal Root of an Extracted Lower Molar.

Fig. 12.4 (A) A 31-year-old white man with extensive supragingival and subgingival calculus deposits throughout his dentition is shown. (B) One year after receiving thorough scaling and root planing to remove supragingival and subgingival calculus deposits, followed by restorative care. Note the substantial reduction in gingival inflammation.

In contrast to the Sri Lankan group, the Norwegian academicians who received oral hygiene instructions and frequent preventive dental care throughout their lives exhibited a marked reduction in the accumulation of calculus. Approximately 80% of teenagers formed limited supragingival calculus on the facial surfaces of the upper first molars and the lingual surfaces of lower incisors. However, no additional calculus formation occurred on other teeth, and its presence did not increase with the individual's age.[4]

Both supragingival calculus and subgingival calculus may be seen on radiographs (see Chapter 31). Highly calcified interproximal calculus deposits are readily detectable as radiopaque projections that protrude into the interdental spaces (Fig. 12.5).

The sensitivity level of detecting calculus by radiographs is inconsistent.[27] The location of calculus does not indicate the bottom of the periodontal pocket, because the most apical plaque is not sufficiently calcified to be visible on radiographs.

FLASH BACK

Whereas the presence of subgingival calculus can be observed on dental radiographs, the sensitivity of such detection is inconsistent.

maxillary molars and the lingual surfaces of mandibular incisors. The deposition of supragingival calculus continued as individuals aged, and it reached a maximal calculus score when the affected individuals were 25 to 30 years old.

At this time, most of the teeth were covered by calculus, although the facial surfaces had less calculus than the lingual or palatal surfaces. Calculus accumulation appeared to be symmetric, and by the age of 45 years, these individuals had only a few teeth (typically the premolars) without calculus deposits. Subgingival calculus appeared first either independently or on the interproximal aspects of areas where supragingival calculus already existed.[4] By the age of 30 years, all surfaces of all teeth had subgingival calculus without any pattern of predilection.

Composition

Inorganic Content

Dental calculus is primarily composed of inorganic components (70% to 90%)[58] and the organic components constitute the rest. The major inorganic proportions of calculus are approximately

Fig. 12.5 A Bitewing Radiograph Illustrating Subgingival Calculus Deposits That are Depicted as Interproximal Spurs *(Arrows).*

TABLE 12.1 Calculus Versus Other Oral Hard Tissues	
Structure	**Inorganic Content (%)**[a]
Dental Calculus	70–90
Enamel	96
Dentin	45
Bone	60–70

[a]Organic components and water constitute the rest.

76% calcium phosphate (Ca$_3$[PO$_4$]$_2$), 3% calcium carbonate (CaCO$_3$), 4% magnesium phosphate (Mg$_3$[PO$_4$]$_2$), 2% carbon dioxide, and traces of other elements such as sodium, zinc, strontium, bromine, copper, manganese, tungsten, gold, aluminum, silicon, iron, and fluorine.[131,205] The percentage of inorganic constituents in calculus is similar to that of other calcified tissues of the body (Table 12.1).

At least two-thirds of the inorganic component is crystalline in structure.[102] The four main crystal forms and their approximate percentages are as follows: hydroxyapatite, 58%; magnesium whitlockite, 21%; octacalcium phosphate, 12%; and brushite, 9%.

Two or more crystal forms are typically found in a sample of calculus. Hydroxyapatite and octacalcium phosphate are detected most frequently (i.e., in 97% to 100% of all supragingival calculus) and constitute the bulk of the specimen. Brushite is more common in the mandibular anterior region, and magnesium whitlockite is found in the posterior areas. The incidence of the four crystal forms varies with the age of the deposit.[17]

FLASH BACK

The four main crystalline inorganic forms of calculus are hydroxyapatite, magnesium whitlockite, octacalcium phosphate, and brushite.

Organic Content

The organic component of calculus consists of a mixture of protein–polysaccharide complexes, desquamated epithelial cells, leukocytes, and various types of microorganisms.[115]

Between 1.9% and 9.1% of the organic component is carbohydrate, which consists of galactose, glucose, rhamnose, mannose, glucuronic acid, galactosamine, and sometimes arabinose, galacturonic acid, and glucosamine.[108,114,185] All of these organic components are present in salivary glycoprotein, with the exception of arabinose and rhamnose. Salivary proteins account for 5.9% to 8.2% of the organic component of calculus and include most amino acids. Lipids account for 0.2% of the organic content in the form of neutral fats, free fatty acids, cholesterol, cholesterol esters, and phospholipids.[109]

The composition of subgingival calculus is similar to that of supragingival calculus, with some differences. It has the same hydroxyapatite content but more magnesium whitlockite and less brushite and octacalcium phosphate.[166,190] The ratio of calcium to phosphate is higher in subgingival calculus, and the sodium content increases with the depth of periodontal pockets.[110] These altered compositions may be attributed to fact that the origin of subgingival calculus is plasma, whereas supragingival calculus is partially composed of salivary constituents. Salivary proteins present in supragingival calculus are not found in subgingival calculus.[12] Dental calculus, salivary duct calculus, and calcified dental tissues are similar in inorganic composition.

Attachment to the Tooth Surface

Differences in the manner in which calculus is attached to the tooth surface affect the relative ease or difficulty encountered during its removal. Four modes of attachment have been described:[93,174,179,213] (1) Attachment by means of an organic pellicle on cementum is depicted in Fig. 12.6, and attachment on enamel is shown in Fig. 12.7. (2) Mechanical locking into surface irregularities, such as caries lesions or resorption lacunae, is illustrated in Fig. 12.8. (3) Close adaptation of the undersurface of calculus to depressions or gently sloping mounds of the unaltered cementum surface[185] is shown in Fig. 12.9. (4) Penetration of bacterial calculus into cementum is shown in Figs. 12.10 and 12.11.

FLASH BACK

Four modes by which calculus may attach to cementum are (1) organic pellicle, (2) mechanical locking into surface irregularities, (3) close adaption to gentle depression or sloping mounts of unaltered cementum, and (4) bacterial penetration into cementum surface.

Formation

Calculus is *mineralized dental plaque.* The soft plaque is hardened by the precipitation of mineral salts, which usually starts between

Fig. 12.6 Calculus Attached to the Pellicle on the Enamel Surface and the Cementum. An enamel void *(E)* has been created during the preparation of the specimen. *C,* Cementum; *CA,* calculus; *P,* pellicle.

Fig. 12.8 Calculus *(CA)* Attached to a Cemental Resorption Area *(CR)* With Cementum *(C)* Adjacent to Dentin *(D).*

Fig. 12.7 Non-Decalcified Specimen With Calculus *(CA)* Attached to Enamel *(E)* Surface Just Coronal to the Cementoenamel Junction *(CEJ).* Note plaque *(P)* on the surface of the calculus; dentin *(D)* and cementum *(C)* are also identified. (Courtesy Dr. Michael Rohrer, Minneapolis, MN.)

Fig. 12.9 Undersurface of Subgingival Calculus *(C)* Previously Attached to the Cementum Surface *(S).* Note the impression of cementum mounds in the calculus *(arrows).* (Courtesy Dr. John Sottosanti, La Jolla, CA.)

Fig. 12.10 Subgingival Calculus *(C)* Embedded Beneath the Cementum Surface *(Arrows)* and Penetrating to the Dentin *(D),* Thereby Making Removal Difficult. (Courtesy Dr. John Sottosanti, La Jolla, CA.)

the 1st and 14th days of plaque formation. Calcification has been reported to occur within as little as 4 to 8 hours.[191] Calcifying plaques may become 50% mineralized in 2 days and 60% to 90% mineralized in 12 days.[130,168,178] All plaque does not necessarily undergo calcification. Early plaque contains a small amount of inorganic material, which increases as the plaque develops into calculus. Plaque that does not develop into calculus reaches a plateau of maximal mineral content within 2 days.[169] Microorganisms are not always essential in calculus formation, because calculus readily occurs in germ-free rodents.[65]

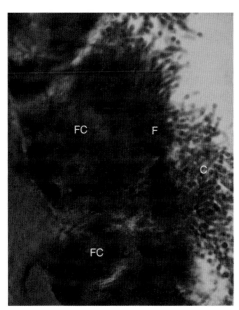

Fig. 12.11 Plaque and Calculus on the Tooth Surface. Note the spherical areas of focal calcification *(FC)* and the perpendicular alignment of the filamentous *(F)* organisms along the inner surface of plaque and cocci *(C)* on the outer surface.

KEY FACT

Calculus by itself does not contribute directly to gingival inflammation. Like other retentive factors such as open crown margin or an overhanging restoration, calculus retains dental plaque, which contributes to gingival inflammation.

Saliva is the primary source of mineralization for supragingival calculus, whereas the serum transudate called *gingival crevicular fluid* furnishes the minerals for subgingival calculus.[79,187] The calcium concentration or content in plaque is 2 to 20 times higher than in saliva.[17] Early plaque of heavy calculus formers contains more calcium, three times more phosphorus, and less potassium than that of noncalculus formers, suggesting that phosphorus may be more critical than calcium for plaque mineralization.[115] Calcification entails the binding of calcium ions to the carbohydrate–protein complexes of the organic matrix and the precipitation of crystalline calcium phosphate salts.[113] Crystals form initially in the intercellular matrix and on the bacterial surfaces and finally within the bacteria.[59,214]

The calcification of supragingival plaque and the attached component of subgingival plaque begins along the inner surface adjacent to the tooth structure. Separate foci of calcification increase in size and coalesce to form solid masses of calculus (see Fig. 12.11). For the initial mineralization process to occur, calcium phosphate supersaturation, certain membrane-associated components, and regulation of nuclear inhibitors are required.[81] Calcification may be accompanied by alterations in the bacterial content and staining qualities of the plaque. As calcification progresses, the number of filamentous bacteria increases, and the foci of calcification change from basophilic to eosinophilic. There is a reduction in the staining intensity of groups that exhibit a positive periodic acid–Schiff reaction.

Sulfhydryl and amino groups are also reduced and instead stain with toluidine blue, which is initially orthochromatic but becomes metachromatic and disappears.[201] Calculus is formed in layers, which are often separated by a thin cuticle that becomes embedded in the calculus as calcification progresses.[117]

The initiation of calcification and the rate of calculus accumulation vary among individuals, among tooth variety in the same dentition, and at different times in the same person.[131,194] On the basis of these differences, persons may be classified as *heavy, moderate,* or *slight* calculus formers or as noncalculus formers. The average daily increment in calculus formers is from 0.10% to 0.15% of dry weight calculus.[178,194] Calculus formation continues until it reaches a maximum, after which it may be reduced in amount. The time required to reach the maximal level has been reported to be between 10 weeks[34] and 6 months.[200]

The decline from maximal calculus accumulation, which is referred to as the *reversal phenomenon,* may be explained by the vulnerability of bulky calculus to mechanical wear from food and from the cheeks, lips, and tongue movement.

Theories Regarding the Mineralization of Calculus

The theoretical mechanisms by which plaque mineralizes is stratified into two categories.[132]

1. Mineral precipitation results from a local rise in the degree of saturation of calcium and phosphate ions, which may be brought about in several ways:
   - *A rise in the pH of the saliva causes the precipitation of calcium phosphate salts by lowering the precipitation constant.* The pH may be elevated by the loss of carbon dioxide and the formation of ammonia by dental plaque bacteria or by protein degradation during stagnation.[16,73]
   - Colloidal proteins in saliva bind calcium and phosphate ions and maintain a supersaturated solution with respect to calcium phosphate salts. With the stagnation of saliva, colloids settle out, and the supersaturated state is no longer maintained, thereby leading to the precipitation of calcium phosphate salts.[151,170]
   - Phosphatase liberated from dental plaque, desquamated epithelial cells, or bacteria precipitates calcium phosphate by hydrolyzing organic phosphates in saliva, thereby increasing the concentration of free phosphate ions.[204] Esterase is another enzyme that is present in the cocci and filamentous organisms, leukocytes, macrophages, and desquamated epithelial cells of dental plaque.[10] Esterase may initiate calcification by hydrolyzing fatty esters into free fatty acids. The fatty acids form soaps with calcium and magnesium that are later converted into the less-soluble calcium phosphate salts.
2. Seeding agents induce small foci of calcification that enlarge and coalesce to form a calcified mass.[134] This concept has been referred to as the *epitactic concept* or, more appropriately, as *heterogeneous nucleation.* The seeding agents in calculus formation are not known, but it is suspected that the intercellular matrix of plaque plays an active role.[116,130,214] The carbohydrate–protein complexes may initiate calcification by removing calcium from the saliva (chelation) and binding with it to form nuclei that induce the subsequent deposition of minerals.[113,196]

Role of Microorganisms in the Mineralization of Calculus

Mineralization of plaque generally starts extracellularly around both gram-positive and gram-negative organisms, but it may also start intracellularly.[98] Filamentous organisms, diphtheroids, and *Bacterionema* and *Veillonella* species have the ability to form intracellular apatite crystals (see Fig. 12.11). Mineralization spreads until the matrix and the bacteria are calcified.[59,215]

Bacterial plaque may actively participate in the mineralization of calculus by forming phosphatases, which change the pH of the plaque and induce mineralization,[42,113] but the prevalent opinion is that these bacteria are only passively involved[59,161,204] and are simply calcified with other plaque components. The occurrence of calculus-like deposits in germ-free animals supports this opinion.[65] However, other experiments suggest that transmissible factors are involved in calculus formation and that penicillin in the diets of some of these animals reduces calculus formation.[11]

Etiologic Significance

Distinguishing between the effects of calculus and plaque on the gingiva is difficult, because calculus is always covered with a nonmineralized layer of plaque.[169] A positive correlation between the presence of calculus and the prevalence of gingivitis exists,[155] but this correlation is not as great as that between plaque and gingivitis.[61] The initiation of periodontal disease in young people is closely related to plaque accumulation, whereas calculus accumulation is more prevalent in chronic periodontitis found in older adults.[61,105]

The incidence of calculus, gingivitis, and periodontal disease increases with age. It is extremely rare to find periodontal pockets in adults without at least some subgingival calculus being present, although the subgingival calculus may be of microscopic proportions.

Calculus does not contribute directly to gingival inflammation, but it provides a fixed nidus for the continued accumulation of bacterial plaque and its retention in close proximity to the gingiva (Fig. 12.12). Periodontal pathogens such as *Aggregatibacter actinomycetemcomitans*, *Porphyromonas gingivalis*, and *Treponema denticola* have been found within the structural channels and lacunae of supragingival and subgingival calculus.[135,136]

Subgingival calculus is likely to be the product rather than the cause of periodontal pockets. Plaque initiates gingival inflammation, which leads to pocket formation, and the pocket in turn provides a sheltered area for plaque and bacterial accumulation. The increased flow of gingival crevicular fluid associated with gingival inflammation provides the minerals that mineralize the continually accumulating plaque, resulting in the formation of subgingival calculus (Fig. 12.13). Over a 6-year period, Albandar and colleagues observed 156 teenagers with aggressive periodontitis.[2] They noted that areas with detectable subgingival calculus at the initiation of the study were much more likely to experience a loss of periodontal attachment than sites that did not initially exhibit subgingival calculus.

Although the bacterial plaque biofilm that coats the teeth is the main etiologic factor in the development of periodontal disease, the removal of subgingival plaque and calculus constitutes

Fig. 12.12 Calculus *(CA)* Penetrates the Tooth Surface and is Embedded Within the Cementum *(C)*. Note the plaque *(P)* attached to the calculus.

Fig. 12.13 Scanning Electron Microscope View of an Extracted Human Tooth Showing a Cross-Section of Subgingival Calculus *(C)* Separated *(Arrows)* from the Cemental Surface During Processing of the Specimen. Note the bacteria *(B)* attached to the calculus and the cemental surfaces. (Courtesy Dr. John Sottosanti, La Jolla, CA.)

the cornerstone of periodontal therapy. Calculus plays an important role in maintaining and accentuating periodontal disease by keeping plaque in close contact with the gingival tissue and by creating areas where plaque removal is impossible. Therefore, the dental hygienist must not only possess the clinical skill to remove the plaque and calculus, but they must also be very conscientious about performing this task.

Materia Alba, Food Debris, and Dental Stains

Materia alba is an accumulation of microorganisms, desquamated epithelial cells, leukocytes, and a mixture of salivary proteins and lipids, with few or no food particles; it lacks the regular internal pattern observed in plaque.[171] It is a yellow or grayish-white, soft, sticky deposit, and it is somewhat less adherent than dental plaque. The irritating effect of materia alba on the gingiva is caused by bacteria and their products.

Most food debris is rapidly liquefied by bacterial enzymes and cleared from the oral cavity by salivary flow and the mechanical action of the tongue, cheeks, and lips. The rate of clearance from the oral cavity varies with the type of food and the individual. Aqueous solutions are typically cleared within 15 minutes, whereas sticky foods may adhere for more than 1 hour.[100,199] Dental plaque is not a derivative of food debris, and food debris is not an important cause of gingivitis.[41,85]

Pigmented deposits on the tooth surface are called *dental stains*. Stains are primarily an aesthetic problem and do not cause inflammation of the gingiva. The use of tobacco products (Fig. 12.14), coffee, tea, certain mouthrinses, and pigments in foods can contribute to stain formation.[111,186]

OTHER PREDISPOSING FACTORS

Iatrogenic Factors

Deficiencies in the quality of dental restorations or prostheses are contributing factors to gingival inflammation and periodontal destruction. Inadequate dental procedures that contribute to the deterioration of the periodontal tissues are referred to as

Fig. 12.14 Tobacco Stains on the Apical Third of the Clinical Crown Caused by Cigarette Smoking.

iatrogenic factors. Iatrogenic endodontic complications that can adversely affect the periodontium include root perforations, vertical root fractures, and endodontic failures that may necessitate tooth extraction.[210,213] Immediate implant placement in conjunction with extraction can contribute to an excessive labial and apical position of the implant, whereby the blood supply of surrounding osseous and gingival tissues is compromised, yielding to gingival fenestration or dehiscence (Fig. 12.15).[192] In order to mitigate the risk of dental implant complications, evidence-based clinical guidelines encourage practitioners to consider cone-beam computed tomography (CBCT) for dental implant treatment planning while taking into account the cost, acceptable radiation dose, and risks versus benefits.[195]

Characteristics of dental restorations and removable partial dentures that are important to the maintenance of periodontal health include the location of the gingival margin for the restoration, the space between the margin of the restoration and the unprepared tooth, the contour of the restorations, the occlusion, the materials used in the restoration, the restorative procedure itself, and the design of the removable partial denture. These characteristics are described in this chapter as they relate to the etiology of periodontal disease.

Margins of Restorations

Overhanging margins of dental restorations contribute to the development of periodontal disease by (1) changing the ecologic balance of the gingival sulcus to an area that favors the growth of disease-associated organisms (predominantly gram-negative anaerobic species) at the expense of the health-associated organisms (predominantly gram-positive facultative species)[100] and (2) inhibiting the patient's access to remove accumulated plaque.

The frequency of overhanging margins on proximal restorations has varied in different studies from 16.5% to 75%.[19,57,78,141] A highly significant statistical relationship has been reported between marginal defects and reduced bone height.[19,66,78] Gilmore and Sheiham noted that persons with overhanging posterior restorations had an average of 0.22 mm reduced alveolar bone support adjacent to the surfaces with overhangs.[57] The removal of

Fig. 12.15 (A) A fenestration defect *(arrow)* is noted after placement of a dental implant too far labial and apical, yielding inadequate bone and blood supply to support the surrounding gingiva. (B) Radiograph of the malpositioned dental implant.

overhangs allows for the more effective control of plaque, thereby resulting in a reduction of gingival inflammation and a small increase in radiographic alveolar bone support (Fig. 12.16).[60,70,182]

The location of the gingival margin of a restoration is directly related to the health status of the adjacent periodontal tissues.[180] Numerous studies have shown a positive correlation between restoration margins located apical to the marginal gingiva and the presence of gingival inflammation.[57,75,84,158,182] Subgingival margins are associated with large amounts of plaque, more severe gingivitis, deeper pockets, and a change in the composition of the subgingival microflora that closely resembles the microflora noted in chronic periodontitis.[97] Even high-quality restorations with clinically perfect margins, if placed subgingivally, will increase plaque accumulation, gingival inflammation,[97,100,128,133,159,181] and the rate of gingival crevicular fluid flow.[13,62] Margins placed at the level of the gingival crest induce less severe inflammation, whereas supragingival margins are associated with a degree of periodontal health similar to that seen with nonrestored interproximal surfaces.[51,180]

Roughness in the subgingival area is considered to be a major contributing factor to plaque buildup and subsequent gingival inflammation.[180] The subgingival zone is composed of the margin of the restoration, the luting material, and the prepared and unprepared tooth surfaces. Sources of marginal roughness include grooves and scratches in the surface of acrylic resin, porcelain, or gold restorations (Fig. 12.17); separation of the restoration margin and the luting material from the cervical finish line, thereby exposing the rough surface of the prepared tooth (Fig. 12.18); dissolution and disintegration of the luting material between the preparation and the restoration, thereby leaving a space; and inadequate marginal fit of the restoration.[180] Subgingival margins typically have a gap of 20 to 40 µm between the margin of the restoration and the unprepared tooth.[177] Colonization of this gap by bacterial plaque undoubtedly contributes to the detrimental effect of margins placed in a subgingival environment (Fig. 12.19).

Retained Cement and Periimplantitis

Periimplantitis is an inflammatory disease of the tissues around dental implants resulting in progressive bone loss (Fig. 12.20A and B), whereas periimplant mucositis is a reversible inflammatory change of the soft tissues around implants without bone loss.[106]

Fig. 12.16 (A) Radiograph of an amalgam overhang on the distal surface of the maxillary second molar that is a source of plaque retention and gingival irritation. (B) Radiograph depicts the removal of excessive amalgam.

Fig. 12.18 After Cementation, Luting Material Prevents the Approximation of the Crown Margin and the Finishing Line, Thereby Leaving Part of the Prepared Tooth Uncovered (Area Between Arrowheads). (From Silness J: Fixed prosthodontics and periodontal health, Dent Clin North Am 24:317–329, 1980.)

Fig. 12.17 (A) Polished gold alloy crown demonstrating surface scratches. (B) Gold alloy crown that had been in the patient's mouth for several years has scratches filled with deposits. (From Silness J: Fixed prosthodontics and periodontal health, Dent Clin North Am 24:317–329, 1980.)

Fig. 12.19 A Void has Developed After Dissolution and Disintegration of the Luting Material. Spherical bodies are not identified. *C,* Crown; *R,* root. (From Silness J: Fixed prosthodontics and periodontal health, *Dent Clin North Am* 24:317–329, 1980.)

The prevalence of periimplantitis among implant-supported prostheses/restorations ranges from 28% to 56%.[217] The early diagnosis of this condition and its proper management are critical to the longevity of the implant and the supported prosthesis.

Complex microbiota colonize pristine periimplant crevices within a week after implant placement, and the microbiota associated with failing implants is significantly different from that of healthy implants.[22,74,101,153,167] Classic studies that explored the composition of the periimplant biofilm in disease have shown that periimplantitis is an infection that is dominated by gram-negative bacteria with many similarities to the microbiota that is responsible for the development of periodontal diseases, including *A. actinomycetemcomitans, P. gingivalis, Tannerella forsythia,* and *Fusobacterium* species.[153,160,167] The application of new microbiologic approaches has allowed for a broader characterization of the periimplant microbiome, which has led to the identification of periimplant-specific microbial lineages such as *Streptococcus mutans* and *Butyrivibrio fibrisolvens.*[96,126,167]

Fig. 12.20 (A) Radiograph of a moat-like bony defect at a periimplantitis site associated with retained cement and a crown that is not fully seated. (B) Moat-like bony defect and retained excessive cement. (C) The *arrow* points to visibly retained excessive cement between the crown margin and the abutment that prevents the full seating of the crown and leads to hyperocclusion. (Courtesy Dr. Emilie Vachon, Minneapolis, MN.) (D) Radiograph of a periimplantitis site shows bone loss associated with retained excessive cement *(arrow)*. (E) Retrieved implant restoration shows excessive cement remnants *(arrow)* on implant surface.

FLASH BACK

Periimplantitis is frequently associated with crowns exhibiting retained excessive luting cement.

A larger proportion of black-pigmented bacteria are found at periimplantitis sites in dentate patients as compared with edentulous patients. Presumably these periimplantitis infectious organisms arise from the sulcular microbiota of the natural dentition.[7] Consequently, it is critical that practitioners evaluate the patient's periodontal status and provide appropriate periodontal therapy in conjunction with implant rehabilitation.

Local factors such as retained residual cement or inadequate seating of the implant abutment or prosthesis can lead to bone loss around an implant (see Fig. 12.20C–E). In a retrospective study, Wilson found that 81% of the implants diagnosed with periimplantitis had residual cement associated with their cement-retained restorations.[207] The surgical removal of the residual cement resolved the infection and halted the periimplantitis in 74% of the implants. A deeper crown margin makes it more difficult to remove excess cement. The greatest amount of residual cement was noted when the crown margin was 2 or 3 mm below the gingival margin.[107]

CLINICAL CORRELATION

The deeper a subgingival crown margin is located, the higher the likelihood of poorer marginal integrity with accompanying gingival inflammation.

The possible adverse effect of traumatic occlusion on implants has been correlated with early implant failures.[124] However, the relationship between traumatic occlusion and periimplantitis is, to date, a controversial issue. In vivo experiments have shown that, in the absence of periimplant inflammation, the application of excessive occlusal stress leads to only minor alterations in the marginal bone level.[91] Alternatively, the application of excessive occlusal forces in the presence of plaque-induced inflammation can significantly increase the rate of bone loss around implant-supported restorations.[32]

Contours and Open Contacts

Overcontoured crowns and restorations tend to accumulate plaque and handicap oral hygiene measures in addition to possibly preventing the self-cleaning mechanisms of the adjacent cheek, lips, and tongue (Fig. 12.21).[6,94,129,208] Restorations that fail to reestablish adequate interproximal embrasure spaces are associated with papillary inflammation. Undercontoured crowns that lack a protective height of contour do not retain as much plaque as overcontoured crowns and therefore may not be as detrimental during mastication as once thought.[208]

CLINICAL CORRELATION

Overcontoured crowns are more detrimental to periodontal health than under-contoured crowns.

Fig. 12.21 (A) Inflamed marginal and papillary gingiva adjacent to an overcontoured porcelain-fused-to-metal crown on the maxillary left central incisor. (B) Radiograph of an ill-fitting porcelain-fused-to-metal crown.

The contour of the occlusal surface as established by the marginal ridges and related developmental grooves normally serves to deflect food away from the interproximal spaces. The optimal cervico-occlusal location for a posterior contact is at the longest mesiodistal diameter of the tooth, which is generally just apical to the crest of the marginal ridge. The integrity and location of the proximal contacts along with the contour of the marginal ridges and developmental grooves typically prevent interproximal food impaction. *Food impaction* is the forceful wedging of food into the periodontium by occlusal forces. As the teeth wear down, their originally convex proximal surfaces become flattened, and the wedging effect of the opposing cusp is exaggerated. Cusps that tend to forcibly wedge food into interproximal embrasures are known as *plunger cusps*. The interproximal plunger cusp effect may also be observed when missing teeth are not replaced and the relationship between the proximal contacts of adjacent teeth is altered. An intact proximal contact precludes the forceful wedging of food into the interproximal embrasure space, whereas a light or open contact is conducive to impaction.

FLASH BACK

Posterior teeth with open contact and food impaction exhibit greater probing depth and clinical attachment loss than contralateral control sites without food impaction.

The classic analysis of the factors that lead to food impaction was made by Hirschfeld,[72] who recognized the following factors: uneven occlusal wear, opening of the contact point as a result of loss of proximal support or from extrusion, congenital morphologic abnormalities, and improperly constructed restorations.

The presence of the previously mentioned abnormalities does not necessarily lead to food impaction and periodontal disease. A study of interproximal contacts and marginal ridge relationships[100] in three groups of periodontally healthy males revealed that 4.9% to 62.5% of the proximal contacts were defective and that 33.5% of adjacent marginal ridges were uneven.[140] However, greater probing depth and a loss of clinical attachment have been reported for sites that exhibited both an open contact and food impaction as compared with contralateral control sites without open contacts or food impaction.[80] Excessive anterior overbite is a common cause of food impaction on the lingual surfaces of the maxillary anterior teeth and the facial surfaces of the opposing mandibular teeth. These areas may be exemplified by attachment loss with gingival recession.

Materials

In general, restorative materials are not in themselves injurious to the periodontal tissues.[6,87] One exception to this may be self-curing acrylics (Fig. 12.22).[202]

Plaque that forms at the margins of restorations is similar to that found on adjacent nonrestored tooth surfaces. The composition of plaque formed on all types of restorative materials is similar, with the exception of that formed on silicate.[134] Although surface textures of restorative materials differ with regard to their capacity to retain plaque,[205] all can be adequately cleaned if they are polished and accessible to methods of oral hygiene.[137,183] The undersurface of pontics in fixed bridges should barely touch the mucosa. Access for oral hygiene is inhibited with excessive pontic-to-tissue contact, thereby contributing to plaque accumulation that will cause gingival inflammation and possibly the formation of pseudopockets.[49,180]

Design of Removable Partial Dentures

Several investigations have shown that, after the insertion of partial dentures, mobility of the abutment teeth, gingival inflammation, and periodontal pocket formation all increase.[18,29,173]

Fig. 12.22 Inflamed Palatal Gingiva Associated With a Maxillary Provisional Acrylic Partial Denture. Note the substantial difference in color of the inflamed gingiva adjacent to the premolars and the first molar as compared with the gingiva adjacent to the second molar.

This is because partial dentures favor the accumulation of plaque, particularly if they cover the gingival tissue. Partial dentures that are worn during both night and day induce more plaque formation than those worn only during the daytime.[18] These observations emphasize the need for careful and personalized oral hygiene instruction to avoid the harmful effects of partial dentures on the remaining teeth and the periodontium.[13] The presence of removable partial dentures induces not only quantitative changes in dental plaque[55] but also qualitative changes, thereby promoting the emergence of spirochetal microorganisms.[56]

Restorative Dentistry Procedures

The use of rubber dam clamps, matrix bands, and burs in such a manner as to lacerate the gingiva results in varying degrees of mechanical trauma and inflammation. Although such transient injuries generally undergo repair, they are needless sources of discomfort to the patient. The forceful packing of a gingival retraction cord into the sulcus to prepare the subgingival margins of a tooth or for the purpose of obtaining an impression may mechanically injure the periodontium and leave behind impacted debris that is capable of causing a foreign body reaction.

Malocclusion

The irregular alignment of teeth as found in cases of malocclusion may facilitate plaque accumulation and make plaque control more difficult. Several authors have found a positive correlation between crowding and periodontal disease,[28,144,189] whereas other investigators did not find such a correlation.[54] Uneven marginal ridges of contiguous posterior teeth have been found to have a low correlation with pocket depth, loss of attachment, plaque, calculus, and gingival inflammation.[89] Roots of teeth that are prominent in the arch (Fig. 12.23)—such as in a buccal or lingual version or that are associated with a high frenal attachment and small quantities of attached gingiva—frequently exhibit recession.[1,123]

The failure to replace missing posterior teeth may have adverse consequences on the periodontal support for the remaining teeth.[31] The following hypothetical scenario illustrates the possible ramifications of not replacing a missing posterior tooth. When the mandibular first molar is extracted, the initial change is a mesial drifting and tilting of the mandibular second and third molars with extrusion of the maxillary first molar. As the mandibular second molar tips mesially, its distal cusps extrude and act as plungers. The distal cusps of the mandibular second molar wedge between the maxillary first and second molars and open the contact by deflecting the maxillary second molar distally. Subsequently, food impaction may occur and may be accompanied by gingival inflammation with the eventual loss of the interproximal bone between the maxillary first and second molars. This example does not occur in all cases in which mandibular first molars are not replaced. However, the drifting and tilting of the remaining teeth with an accompanying alteration of the proximal contacts is generally a consequence of not replacing posterior teeth that have been extracted.

Tongue thrusting exerts excessive lateral pressure on the anterior teeth, which may result in the spreading and tilting of the anterior teeth (Fig. 12.24). Tongue thrusting is an important contributing factor to tooth migration and the development of an anterior

Fig. 12.23 (A) Lower incisor showing a prominent root with gingival recession and a lack of attached gingiva. (B) Appearance 3 months after the placement of a free gingival graft, which resulted in a gain in attached gingiva and a reduction in gingival recession.

Fig. 12.24 (A) Anterior open bite with flared incisors as observed in association with a habit of tongue thrusting. (B) Radiographs show severe periodontal destruction *(arrows)* in the molar regions.

open bite.[30] Mouth breathing may be observed in association with a habit of tongue thrusting and an anterior open bite. Marginal and papillary gingivitis is frequently encountered in the maxillary anterior sextant in cases that involve an anterior open bite with mouth breathing. However, the role of mouth breathing as a local causative factor is unclear, because conflicting evidence has been reported.[3,76,77,189]

Restorations that do not conform to the occlusal pattern of the mouth result in occlusal disharmonies that may cause injury to the supporting periodontal tissues. More issues involving deeper initial probing depths, worse prognoses, and greater

mobility have been observed for teeth with occlusal discrepancies as compared with teeth without initial occlusal discrepancies.[68,138] Histologic features of the periodontium for a tooth that has been subjected to traumatic occlusion include: a widened subcrestal periodontal ligament space, a reduction in the collagen content of the oblique and horizontal fibers, an increase in vascularity and leukocyte infiltration, and an increase in the number of osteoclasts on bordering alveolar bone.[15] However, these observations are generally apical and separate from the bacteria-induced inflammation that occurs at the base of the sulcus. On the basis of current human trials, it is still impossible to

Fig. 12.25 Gingival Inflammation and Enlargement Associated With an Orthodontic Appliance and Poor Oral Hygiene.

definitively answer the question—"Does occlusal trauma modify the progression of periodontal attachment loss that is associated with periodontal inflammation?"[175]

Periodontal Complications Associated With Orthodontic Therapy

Orthodontic therapy may affect the periodontium by favoring plaque retention, by directly injuring the gingiva as a result of overextended bands, and by creating excessive forces, unfavorable forces, or both on the tooth and its supporting structures.

Plaque Retention and Composition

Orthodontic appliances tend to retain bacterial plaque and food debris, thereby resulting in gingivitis (Fig. 12.25), and they are capable of modifying the gingival ecosystem. Scanning electron microscopic examination of the orthodontic bracket–tooth junction shows that excess bonding composite around the bracket base creates a critical site for plaque accumulation due to its rough surface texture and the presence of a distinct gap at the composite–enamel interface. A complex community of bacterial plaque may be noted on the excess composite material within 2 to 3 weeks after bonding.[188] An increase in *Prevotella melaninogenica*, *Prevotella intermedia*, and *Actinomyces odontolyticus* and a decrease in the proportion of facultative microorganisms were detected in the gingival sulcus after the placement of orthodontic bands.[39] More recently, *A. actinomycetemcomitans* was found in at least one site in 85% of children who were wearing orthodontic appliances.[142] By contrast, only 15% of unbanded control subjects were positive for *A. actinomycetemcomitans*.

> **KEY FACT**
>
> Orthodontic treatment should not be commenced in the presence of uncontrolled periodontal disease because it will worsen the periodontal condition.

Gingival Trauma and Alveolar Bone Height

Orthodontic treatment is often started soon after the eruption of the permanent teeth, when the junctional epithelium is still adherent to the enamel surface. Orthodontic bands should not be forcefully placed beyond the level of attachment, because this will detach the gingiva from the tooth and result in the apical proliferation of the junctional epithelium with an increased incidence of gingival recession.[145]

> **KEY FACT**
>
> **Adult** patients planning to undergo orthodontic care should undergo pretreatment assessment for their periodontal status and potential risk for root resorption.

The mean alveolar bone loss per patient for adolescents who underwent 2 years of orthodontic care during a 5-year observation period ranged between 0.1 and 0.5 mm.[21] This small magnitude of alveolar bone loss was also noted in the control group and therefore is considered to be of little clinical significance. However, the degree of bone loss during adult orthodontic care may be higher than that observed in adolescents,[112] especially if the periodontal condition is not treated before the initiation of orthodontic therapy. Orthodontic treatment in adults with active periodontitis (evidenced by deep pockets and bleeding on probing) has been shown to accelerate the periodontal disease process.[8,44,211]

Tissue Response to Orthodontic Forces

Orthodontic tooth movement is possible because the periodontal tissues are responsive to externally applied forces.[157,172] Alveolar bone is remodeled by osteoclasts that induce bone resorption in areas of pressure and by osteoblasts that form bone in areas of tension. Although moderate orthodontic forces ordinarily result in bone remodeling and repair, excessive force may produce necrosis of the periodontal ligament and the adjacent alveolar bone.[148-150] Excessive orthodontic forces also increase the risk of apical root resorption.[25,26] The prevalence of severe root resorption (i.e., resorption of more than one-third of the root length) during orthodontic therapy in adolescents has been reported to be 3%.[82] The incidence of moderate to severe root resorption for incisors among adults aged 20 to 45 years has been reported to be 2% before treatment and 24.5% after treatment.[112] Risk factors associated with root resorption during orthodontic treatment include the duration of treatment, the magnitude of the force applied, the direction of the tooth movement, and the continuous versus intermittent application of forces (Fig. 12.26).[147]

> **KEY FACT**
>
> It is important to avoid excessive force and too-rapid tooth movement during orthodontic treatment to prevent injury to the periodontium.

The use of elastics to close a diastema may result in severe attachment loss with possible tooth loss as the elastics migrate apically along the root surface (Fig. 12.27). The surgical exposure of impacted teeth and orthodontic-assisted eruption has the potential to compromise periodontal attachment on adjacent teeth (Fig. 12.28). However, the majority of impacted teeth that are surgically exposed and aided in their eruption by orthodontic treatment subsequently exhibited more than 90% of their attachment as being intact.[71]

Fig. 12.26 (A) Panoramic radiograph illustrating that a limited degree of pretreatment root resorption *(arrows)* existed before orthodontic care. (B) Note that several roots have undergone severe resorption *(arrows)* during 4 years of intermittent orthodontic treatment. (C) The teeth that developed extensive root resorption with accompanying hypermobility have been extracted and replaced with implant-supported crowns.

Fig. 12.27 (A) Maxillary central incisors for which an elastic ligature was used to close a midline diastema. Note the inflamed gingiva and the deep probing depths. (B) Reflection of a full-thickness mucoperiosteal flap reveals elastic ligature *(arrow)* and angular intrabony defects around the central incisors.

It has been reported that the dentoalveolar gingival fibers that are located within the marginal and attached gingiva are stretched when teeth are rotated during orthodontic therapy.[40] The surgical severing or removal of these gingival fibers in combination with a brief period of retention may reduce the incidence of relapse after orthodontic treatment that is intended to realign rotated teeth.[24,125]

Extraction of Impacted Third Molars

Numerous clinical studies have reported that the extraction of impacted third molars often results in the creation of vertical defects distal to the second molars.[9,95,120] This iatrogenic effect is unrelated to flap design,[152] and it appears to occur more often when third molars are extracted from individuals who are more than 25 years old.[9,95,120] Other factors that appear to play a role in the development of lesions on the distal surface of second molars—particularly in those who are more than 25 years old—include the presence of visible plaque, bleeding on probing, root resorption in the contact area between the second and third molars, the presence of a pathologically widened follicle, the inclination of the third molar, and the close proximity of the third molar to the second molar (Fig. 12.29).[95] Other potential iatrogenic adverse consequences of the removal of third molars include permanent paresthesia (i.e., numbness of the lip, tongue,

Fig. 12.28 (A) Radiograph of an impacted maxillary canine that required surgical exposure and orthodontic assistance to erupt. (B) A palatal flap is reflected to reveal bony dehiscence on the maxillary lateral incisor after orthodontic therapy.

Fig. 12.29 Panoramic Radiograph Illustrating a Mesially Impacted Lower Left Third Molar With a Widened Follicle and No Apparent Bone on the Distal Interproximal Surface of the Second Molar. Alternatively, the lower right third molar is vertically impacted and exhibits interproximal bone distal to the second molar and mesial to the third molar.

and cheek), damage to adjacent teeth, mandibular fracture, maxillary tuberosity fracture, displacement of third molars and root tips, oro-antral communications or fistula, and temporomandibular joint complications.[23] Permanent paresthesia occurs at a frequency of approximately 1 of every 100,000 wisdom teeth removed in the United States.[52] The incidence of damage to second molar as a consequence of third molar extraction has been estimated to be 0.3% to 0.4%.[33] Although the incidence of mandibular fracture during or after third molar removal is low (0.003% to 0.005%),[104] it may pose important medicolegal and patient care implications. Iatrogenic displacement of a maxillary third molar into the maxillary sinus[143,209] and displacement of a mandibular third molar into the sublingual, submandibular, pterygomandibular, and lateral pharyngeal spaces[46,209] have been reported with unknown incidence rates.

> **FLASH BACK**
>
> Preoperative use of three-dimensional radiographs in conjunction with extraction of impacted third molars has the potential to minimize the risk of inferior alveolar nerve paresthesia or damage to the adjacent second molar.

For several decades, panoramic radiography has been the standard of choice to assess the state of third molar impaction, including angulation of the tooth, root morphology, root development, related pathology, and, most importantly, the relation between the tooth or roots and the mandibular canal. However, when an overprojection is observed between the impacted third molar and the mandibular canal, or when specific signs suggest a close contact between the third molar and the mandibular canal, CBCT is recommended to be more beneficial in proper treatment planning (Fig. 12.30).[122]

Habits and Self-Inflicted Injuries

Patients may not be aware of their self-inflicted injurious habits that may be important to the initiation and progression of their periodontal disease. Mechanical forms of trauma can stem from the improper use of a toothbrush, the wedging of toothpicks between the teeth, the application of fingernail pressure against the gingiva (Fig. 12.31), pizza burns, and other causes.[20] Sources of chemical irritation include the topical application of caustic medications such as aspirin or cocaine, allergic reactions to toothpaste or chewing gum, the use of chewing tobacco, and concentrated mouthrinses.[176] Accidental and iatrogenic gingival injuries may be caused by a variety of chemical, physical, and thermal sources, yet they are generally self-limited. Iatrogenic injuries are often acute, whereas factitious injuries tend to be more chronic in nature.[156]

> **FLASH BACK**
>
> Sources of self-inflicted injuries include improper use of toothbrushes, wedging toothpicks between teeth, application of fingernail pressure against gingiva, and burns from hot foods. Chemical sources include topical application of caustic medications such as aspirin or cocaine, allergic reaction to toothpaste or chewing gum, use of chewing tobacco, and concentrated mouth rinses.

Fig. 12.30 Segmented Panoramic Images. (A and B) Overprojection between the impacted third molar and the mandibular canal. (C) Signs of close contact between the third molar and the mandibular canal. (D through F) Corresponding core-beam computed tomographic images (axial views) of the impacted third molars reveal the path of the inferior alveolar nerve *(arrows)* (D) lingual to the root, (E) surrounded by three segments of the root, and (F) buccal to the root. (Courtesy Dr. Mansur Ahmad, Minneapolis, MN.)

Fig. 12.31 Gingival Recession on a Maxillary Canine Caused by Self-Inflicted Trauma from the Patient's Fingernail.

Trauma Associated With Oral Jewelry

The use of piercing jewelry in the lip or tongue has become more common among teenagers and young adults (Fig. 12.32A). However, piercings are associated with potential complications including gingival injury or recession[69,99,103,212,216]; damage to teeth, restorations, and fixed porcelain prostheses[47,53,69,103]; increased salivary flow[53,197]; interference with speech, mastication, or deglutition[83,198]; scar tissue formation[197]; and development of metal hypersensitivities.[92]

> **FLASH BACK**
>
> Use of tongue or lip piercing jewelry is associated with localized gingival recession and periodontitis.

Whittle and Lamden[206] surveyed 62 dentists and found that 97% had seen patients with either lip- or tongue-piercing jewelry within the previous 12 months. The incidence of lingual recession with pocket formation (see Fig. 12.32B) and radiographic evidence of bone loss (see Fig. 12.32C) was 50% among subjects with a mean age of 22 years who wore lingual "barbells" for 2 years or longer.[37] Chipped lower anterior teeth were noted in 47% of the patients who wore tongue-piercing jewelry for 4 years or longer. Patients need to be informed of the risks of wearing oral jewelry and cautioned against such practices.

Toothbrush Trauma

Abrasions of the gingiva as well as alterations in tooth structure may result from aggressive toothbrushing in a horizontal or rotary fashion. The deleterious effect of excessively forceful brushing is accentuated when highly abrasive dentifrices are used. The gingival changes that are attributable to toothbrush trauma may be acute or chronic. The acute changes vary with regard to their appearance and duration, from scuffing of the epithelial surface

Fig. 12.33 The Overzealous Use of a Toothbrush Resulted in Denudation of the Gingival Epithelial Surface and Exposure of the Underlying Connective Tissue as a Painful Ulcer.

Fig. 12.32 (A) Tongue pierced with oral jewelry. (B) Probing depth of 8 mm with 10 mm of clinical attachment loss on the lingual surface of the lower central incisor adjacent to the oral jewelry in the pierced tongue. The central incisor was found to be vital. (C) Bone loss associated with a tongue pierced by oral jewelry. (B, Courtesy Dr. Leonidas Batas, Thessaloniki, Greece.)

to denudation of the underlying connective tissue with the formation of a painful gingival ulcer (Fig. 12.33). Diffuse erythema and denudation of the attached gingiva throughout the mouth may be a striking result of overzealous brushing. Signs of acute gingival abrasions are frequently noted when the patient first uses a new brush. Puncture lesions may be produced when heavy pressure is applied to firm bristles that are aligned perpendicular to the surface of the gingiva. A forcibly embedded toothbrush bristle can be retained in the gingiva and cause an acute gingival abscess.

Chronic toothbrush trauma results in gingival recession with denudation of the root surface. Interproximal attachment loss is generally a consequence of bacteria-induced periodontitis, whereas buccal and lingual attachment loss is frequently the result of toothbrush abrasion.[184] The improper use of dental floss may result in lacerations of the interdental papilla.

Chemical Irritation

Acute gingival inflammation may be caused by chemical irritation that results from either sensitivity or nonspecific tissue injury. In allergic inflammatory states, the gingival changes range from simple erythema to painful vesicle formation and ulceration. Severe reactions to ordinarily innocuous mouthwashes, dentifrices, and denture materials are often explainable on this basis.

Acute inflammation with ulceration may be produced by the nonspecific injurious effect of chemicals on the gingival tissues. The indiscriminate use of strong mouthwashes, the topical application of corrosive drugs such as aspirin (Fig. 12.34) or cocaine, and accidental contact with drugs such as phenol or silver nitrate are common examples of chemical exposures that cause irritation of the gingiva. A histologic view of an aspirin-induced chemical burn shows vacuoles with serous exudates and an inflammatory infiltrate in the connective tissue (Fig. 12.35).

Smokeless Tobacco

Snuff and chewing tobacco constitute the two main forms of smokeless tobacco. Snuff is a fine-cut form of tobacco that is available loosely packed or in small sachets. Chewing tobacco is a more coarse-cut tobacco that is available in the form of loose leaves, a solid block, a plug, or a twist of dried leaves. Chewing tobacco is typically placed in the mandibular buccal vestibule for several hours, during which time saliva and dilute tobacco are periodically expectorated.[203] The nicotine uptake of smokeless tobacco is similar to that of smoking cigarettes in that the consumption of a 34-g container of smokeless tobacco is approximately equal to 1.5 packs of cigarettes.[63] Many professional baseball players use chewing tobacco. The perceived benefits of chewing tobacco are those derived from nicotine, including improved mental alertness, diminished reaction time,

Fig. 12.34 Chemical Burn Caused by Aspirin; Note the Sloughing Gingival Tissue and the Resultant Recession.

Fig. 12.36 Oral Leukoplakia in the Vestibule Associated With the Use of Smokeless Tobacco.

Fig. 12.35 Biopsy of an Aspirin-Induced Chemical Burn. Note the intraepithelial vesicles *(V)* and inflammatory infiltrate *(I)* within the underlying connective tissue.

muscle relaxation, and reduced anxiety and appetite.[64,162] A 1990 survey of 1109 professional baseball players in the United States reported that 39% of the players used smokeless tobacco, with 46% of the users exhibiting leukoplakia within the gingiva or the mucosa (Fig. 12.36).[45] Histologic features of oral leukoplakia associated with smokeless tobacco include (1) a chevron-like pattern of hyperkeratosis with focal areas of inflammation and (2) hyperplasia in the basal cell layer (Fig. 12.37). Increased incidences of gingival recession, cervical root abrasion, and root caries have been reported with the use of smokeless tobacco (Fig. 12.38).[139,163,164,193]

The incidence of gingival recession among adolescents who use smokeless tobacco has been reported to be 42%, compared with 17% among nonusers.[35,121,123,127] The Third National Health and Nutrition Examination Survey (NHANES III) investigated the adverse effect of smokeless tobacco on the periodontium and found double the incidence of severe periodontitis (odds ratio, 2.1; 95% confidence interval, 1.2 to 3.7) among 12,932 adults who used smokeless tobacco but who never smoked cigarettes.[48] However, Bergstrom and colleagues found similar incidences of severe periodontitis among both smokeless tobacco users and nonusers.[14] It can be concluded that the use of smokeless tobacco is associated with at least localized gingival recession, clinical attachment loss, leukoplakia, and possibly enhanced susceptibility to severe periodontitis.

Radiation Therapy

Radiation therapy has cytotoxic effects on both normal cells and malignant cells. A typical total dose of radiation for head and neck tumors is in the range of 5000 to 8000 centigray (cGy); 1 cGy is equal to 1 radiation absorbed dose (rad) and equivalent to 50 to 80 Sieverts (Sv).[146] The total dose of radiation is usually given in partial incremental doses, and this is referred to as *fractionation*. Fractionation helps to minimize the adverse effects of radiation while maximizing the death rate for the tumor cells.[50] Fractionated doses are typically administered in the range of 100 to 1000 cGy or 1 to 10 Sv per week.

Radiation treatment induces an obliterative endarteritis that results in soft tissue ischemia and fibrosis; irradiated bone becomes hypovascular and hypoxic.[118] Adverse effects of head and neck radiation therapy include dermatitis and mucositis of the irradiated area as well as muscle fibrosis and trismus, which may restrict access to the oral cavity.[165] The mucositis typically develops 5 to 7 days after radiation therapy is initiated. The severity of the mucositis can be reduced by asking the patient to avoid secondary sources of irritation (e.g., smoking, alcohol, spicy foods) to the mucous membrane. The use of a chlorhexidine digluconate mouth rinse may help to reduce the mucositis.[154] However, most chlorhexidine mouth rinses currently available in the United States have a high alcohol content that may act as an astringent, which dehydrates the mucosa and thus intensifies the pain. Saliva production is permanently impaired when salivary glands that are located within the portal of radiation receive 6000 cGy (60 Sv) or more.[119] Xerostomia results in greater plaque accumulation and a reduced buffering capacity of saliva. Effective oral hygiene, professional dental prophylactic cleanings, fluoride applications, and frequent dental examinations are

Fig. 12.37 (A) Histologic features of oral leukoplakia associated with smokeless tobacco. Note the chevron-like pattern of hyperkeratosis with focal areas of inflammation. (B) Hyperplasia in the basal cell layer.

Fig. 12.38 Oral Leukoplakia, Recession, and Clinical Attachment Loss Associated With the Use of Smokeless Tobacco.

essential to control caries and periodontal disease. The use of customized trays appears to be a more effective method for fluoride application compared with the toothbrush.[88]

Among cancer patients who were treated with high-dose unilateral radiation, periodontal attachment loss and tooth loss were reported to be greater on the irradiated site compared with the nonradiated control side of the dentition.[43] Patients who are diagnosed with oral cancer and who require radiation therapy should ideally be assessed for dental needs (i.e., mucositis, xerostomia, faulty restorations, periapical lesion, coronal and cervical decay, and periodontal status) before the initiation of radiation treatment.[67] The treatment and prevention of trismus, oral fungal infections, odontogenic infections, osteoradionecrosis, decay, and periodontal disease are critical to minimize oral morbidity for these patients. Dental and periodontal infections have the potential to be severe risks for patients who have been treated with head and neck radiation. The risk of osteoradionecrosis for oncology patients can be minimized by evaluating their oral status, providing dental care, and allowing time for tissue repair before the commencement of radiotherapy.[90]

Oral conditions that increase the risk of osteoradionecrosis for patients about to undergo radiation therapy for oral malignancies include periodontal probing depths of more than 5 mm, dental plaque score of more than 40%, and alveolar bone loss of more than 60%.[86] Non-restorable teeth and teeth with significant periodontal problems should be extracted before radiation therapy to reduce the risk of postradiotherapy osteoradionecrosis. (See Chapter 36 for more detail regarding the periodontal management of medically compromised patients.)[90]

The risk of osteoradionecrosis must be evaluated before the performance of atraumatic extractions or limited periodontal surgical procedures in previously irradiated sites. Therefore, the dentist may choose to consult with the patient's oncologist before the initiation of dental therapy. A randomized multicenter clinical trial questioned the merit of using hyperbaric oxygen therapy to treat osteoradionecrosis because, at 1 year after treatment, only 19% of test subjects had responded to hyperbaric oxygen therapy, compared with 32% of placebo subjects.[5] The administration of the combination of pentoxifylline with vitamin E as antioxidant therapy currently shows the greatest promise for revascularization and treatment of osteoradionecrosis sites.[38]

CLINICAL CORRELATION

Use of smokeless tobacco has been associated with localized gingival leukoplakia, recession, clinical attachment loss, and increased susceptibility to severe periodontitis.

A Case Scenario is found on the companion website www.expertconsult.com.

REFERENCES

 References for this chapter are found on the companion website.

13

Influence of Systemic Conditions[a]

For expanded discussions on female sex hormones, genetic disorders, and nutritional influences on periodontal disease, as well as online-only content on hyperparathyroidism, anemia, thrombocytopenia, antibody deficiency disorders, and other systemic conditions, please visit the companion website.

CHAPTER OUTLINE

Many systemic diseases, disorders, and conditions have been implicated as risk indicators or risk factors in periodontal disease. Clinical and basic science research over the past several decades has led to an improved understanding of and appreciation for the complexity and pathogenesis of periodontal diseases.[192] Although there is clear evidence for a bacterial etiology and there are specific bacteria (periodontal pathogens) associated with destructive periodontal disease, the presence of these pathogens does not invariably cause disease. Their absence, on the other hand, appears to be consistent with periodontal health. The role of bacteria in disease etiology and pathogenesis is discussed in Chapters 8 and 9.

Perhaps the most significant advance in our understanding of the pathogenesis of periodontitis is that the host response varies among individuals and that an altered, deficient, or exaggerated host immune response to bacterial pathogens may lead to more severe forms of the disease. In other words, the individual host immune response to periodontal pathogens is very important and likely explains many of the differences in disease severity observed from one individual to the next. Furthermore, systemic diseases, disorders, and conditions alter host tissues and physiology, which may impair the host's barrier function and immune defense against periodontal pathogens, thereby creating the opportunity for destructive periodontal disease to progress.

Evidence also suggests that periodontal infections can adversely affect systemic health with manifestations such as coronary heart disease, stroke, diabetes, preterm labor, low-birth-weight delivery, and respiratory disease.[171] The role of periodontal infections on these systemic health conditions is discussed in Chapter 14.

The relationships between periodontal infections and host defense are complex. A number of environmental, physical, and psychosocial factors have the potential to alter periodontal tissues and the host immune response, thereby resulting in more severe periodontal disease expression. It is important to recognize that the systemic diseases, disorders, or conditions themselves do not cause periodontitis; rather, they may predispose, accelerate, or otherwise increase the disease's progression. This chapter discusses important systemic diseases, disorders, and conditions that have the potential to influence periodontal health.

ENDOCRINE DISORDERS AND HORMONAL CHANGES

Endocrine diseases such as diabetes and hormonal fluctuations that are associated with puberty and pregnancy are well-known examples of systemic conditions that adversely affect the condition of the periodontium. Endocrine disturbances and hormone fluctuations affect the periodontal tissues directly, modify the tissue response to local factors, and produce anatomic changes in the gingiva that may favor plaque accumulation and disease progression. This section describes the evidence that supports the relationships among endocrine disorders, hormonal changes, and periodontal disease.

---

[a]Adapted from the following chapter of Newman and Carranza's *Clinical Periodontology*, 13th edition, Chapter 14: Influence of Systemic Conditions, by Perry R. Klokkevold and Brian L. Mealey.

Diabetes Mellitus

Diabetes mellitus is an extremely important disease from a periodontal standpoint. It is a complex metabolic disorder characterized by chronic hyperglycemia. Diminished insulin production, impaired insulin action, or a combination of both result in the inability of glucose to be transported from the bloodstream into the tissues, which in turn results in high blood glucose levels and the excretion of sugar in the urine. Lipid and protein metabolism are altered in diabetes as well. Uncontrolled diabetes (chronic hyperglycemia) is associated with several long-term complications, including microvascular diseases (retinopathy, nephropathy, or neuropathy), macrovascular diseases (cardiovascular and cerebrovascular conditions), increased susceptibility to infections, and poor wound healing. An estimated 25.8 million individuals (both children and adults)—8.3% of the US population—have diabetes.[43] Approximately 7 million of these individuals are unaware that they have the disease.

There are two major types of diabetes, type 1 and type 2, with several less common secondary types. *Type 1 diabetes mellitus*, which was formerly known as *insulin-dependent diabetes mellitus*, is caused by a cell-mediated autoimmune destruction of the insulin-producing beta cells of the islets of Langerhans in the pancreas, which results in insulin deficiency. Type 1 diabetes accounts for 5% to 10% of all cases of diabetes and most often occurs in children and young adults. This type of diabetes results from a lack of insulin production, and it is very unstable and difficult to control. It has a marked tendency toward ketosis and coma, it is not preceded by obesity, and it requires the injection of insulin to be controlled. Patients with type 1 diabetes mellitus present with the symptoms that are traditionally associated with diabetes, including polyphagia, polydipsia, polyuria, and predisposition to infections.

Type 2 diabetes mellitus, which was formerly known as *non–insulin-dependent diabetes mellitus*, is caused by peripheral resistance to insulin action, impaired insulin secretion, and increased glucose production in the liver. The insulin-producing beta cells in the pancreas are not destroyed by cell-mediated autoimmune reaction. It typically begins as insulin resistance, which leads to the reduced pancreas production of insulin as the demand increases. Type 2 diabetes is the most common form of diabetes, and it accounts for 90% to 95% of all diagnosed cases in adults. Individuals are often not aware they have the disease until severe symptoms or complications occur. Type 2 diabetes generally occurs in obese individuals, and it can often be controlled by diet and oral hypoglycemic agents. Ketosis and coma are uncommon. Type 2 diabetes can manifest with the same symptoms as type 1 diabetes but typically in a less severe form.

An additional category of diabetes is *hyperglycemia* secondary to other diseases or conditions. A prime example of this type of hyperglycemia is gestational diabetes associated with pregnancy. *Gestational diabetes* develops in 2% to 10% of all pregnancies but disappears after delivery. Women who have had gestational diabetes are at increased risk of developing type 2 diabetes. Other secondary types of diabetes are those associated with diseases that involve the pancreas and the destruction of the insulin-producing cells. Endocrine diseases (e.g., acromegaly, Cushing syndrome), tumors, pancreatectomy, and drugs or chemicals that cause altered insulin levels are included in this group. Experimentally induced types of diabetes generally belong in this category, rather than in the categories of type 1 or 2 diabetes mellitus.

KEY FACT

Diabetes mellitus is a disease that impacts periodontal health. Uncontrolled diabetes is associated with long term complications including cardiovascular diseases and poor wound healing. It is estimated that 8.3% of the U.S. population have diabetes, yet approximately 7 million of those affected are unaware they have the disease.

Oral Manifestations

Numerous oral changes have been described in patients with diabetes, including cheilosis, mucosal drying and cracking, burning mouth and tongue, diminished salivary flow, and alterations in the flora of the oral cavity, with greater predominance of *Candida albicans*, hemolytic streptococci, and staphylococci.[1,23,103,166] An increased rate of dental caries has also been observed in patients with poorly controlled diabetes.[77,87] It is important to note that these changes are not always present, that they are not specific, and that they are not pathognomonic for diabetes.[169] Furthermore, these changes are less likely to be observed in patients with well-controlled diabetes. Individuals with controlled diabetes have a normal tissue response, a normally developed dentition, a normal defense against infections, and no increase in the incidence of caries.[244]

The influence of diabetes on the periodontium has been thoroughly investigated. Although it is difficult to make definitive conclusions about the specific effects of diabetes on the periodontium, a variety of changes have been described, including a tendency toward an enlarged gingiva, sessile or pedunculated gingival polyps, polypoid gingival proliferations, abscess formation, periodontitis, and loosened teeth (Fig. 13.1).[116] Perhaps the most striking changes in patients with uncontrolled diabetes are the reductions in the defense mechanisms and the increased susceptibility to infections, which lead to destructive periodontal disease. In fact, periodontal disease is considered to be the sixth complication of diabetes.[152] Periodontitis in patients with type 1 diabetes appears to start after the age of 12 years, and it has a fivefold increased prevalence in teenagers.[50] The prevalence of periodontitis has been reported as 9.8% in 13- to 18-year-old patients, and it increases to 39% in those who are 19 years old and older.

The extensive literature on this subject and the overall impression of clinicians indicate that *periodontal disease in patients with diabetes follows no consistent or distinct pattern.* Severe gingival inflammation, deep periodontal pockets, rapid bone loss, and frequent periodontal abscesses often occur in patients with poorly controlled diabetes and poor oral hygiene (Figs. 13.2 and 13.3).[3] Children with type 1 diabetes tend to have more destruction around the first molars and incisors, but this destruction becomes more generalized at older ages.[49] In patients with juvenile diabetes, extensive periodontal destruction often occurs as a consequence of having more severe disease at a younger age.

Fig. 13.1 Periodontal Condition in Patients With Diabetes. (A) Adult with diabetes (blood glucose level >400 mg/dL). Note the gingival inflammation, spontaneous bleeding, and edema. (B) The same patient as shown in A. Improved control of diabetes was noted after 4 days of insulin therapy (blood glucose level <100 mg/dL). The clinical periodontal condition has improved without local therapy. (C) Adult patient with uncontrolled diabetes. Note the enlarged, smooth, erythematous gingival margins and papilla in the anterior area. (D) The same patient as shown in C. This is a lingual view of the right mandibular area. Note the inflamed and swollen tissues in the anterior and premolar areas. (E) Adult patient with uncontrolled diabetes. There is a suppurating abscess on the buccal surface of the maxillary premolars.

Other investigators have reported that the rate of periodontal destruction appears to be similar for those with diabetes and those without diabetes up to the age of 30 years.[93,238] Older patients with diabetes have a greater degree of periodontal destruction, possibly related to more disease destruction over time. Patients who have had overt diabetes for more than 10 years have a greater loss of periodontal support than those with a diabetic history of less than 10 years.[93] This destruction may also be related to the diminished tissue integrity, which continues to deteriorate over time (see Altered Collagen Metabolism).

Although some studies have not found a correlation between the diabetic state and the periodontal condition, the majority of well-controlled studies show a higher prevalence and severity of periodontal disease in individuals with diabetes compared with nondiabetic persons with similar local factors.[15,23,40,52,113,182,184,186,241] Findings include a greater loss of attachment, increased bleeding on probing, and increased tooth mobility. A study of risk indicators for a group of 1426 patients between the ages of 25 and 74 years revealed that individuals with diabetes were twice as likely to exhibit attachment loss as nondiabetic individuals.[110] The lack of consistency across studies is most likely related to the different degrees of diabetic involvement, variations in the level of disease control and the diversity of indices, and patient sampling from one study to another.

Fig. 13.2 A 60-Year-Old Patient With a Long-Term History of Type 2 Diabetes. (A) Anterior retracted view of the patient's dental and periodontal condition. Note the missing posterior teeth, the supererup-tion of the premolars, and the mild generalized gingival inflammation. (B) Periapical radiographs of the remaining teeth. Note the mild generalized bone loss with localized areas of severe bone loss. The failure to replace the posterior teeth adds to the occlusal burden of the remaining dentition. (C) Clinical photograph of the maxillary premolar area presenting with abscess. Notice the diffuse erythema and inflammation surrounding the abscess area. (D) Periapical radiograph of the maxillary premolar showing extensive bone loss associated with abscess.

Studies have suggested that uncontrolled or poorly controlled diabetes is associated with an increased susceptibility to and severity of infections, including periodontitis.[17,215] Adults who are 45 years of age or older with poorly controlled diabetes (i.e., with a glycated hemoglobin level >9%) were 2.9 times more likely to have severe periodontitis than those without diabetes. The likelihood was even greater (4.6 times) among smokers with poorly controlled diabetes.[43] As with other systemic conditions associated with periodontitis, diabetes mellitus does not cause gingivitis or periodontitis, but evidence indicates that it alters the response of the periodontal tissues to local factors, thereby hastening bone loss and delaying postsurgical healing. Frequent periodontal abscesses appear to be an important feature of periodontal disease in patients with diabetes.

Approximately 40% of adult Pima Indians in Arizona have type 2 diabetes. A comparison of individuals with and without diabetes in this Native American tribe showed a clear increase in the prevalence of destructive periodontitis as well as a 15%

increase in edentulousness among patients with diabetes.[227] The risk of developing destructive periodontitis was increased three-fold in these individuals.[74]

Bacterial Pathogens

The glucose content of gingival fluid and blood is higher in individuals with diabetes than in those without diabetes with similar plaque and gingival index scores.[80] The increased glucose in the gingival fluid and blood of patients with diabetes could change the environment of the microflora, thereby inducing qualitative changes in bacteria that may contribute to the severity of periodontal disease observed in those with poorly controlled diabetes.

Patients with type 1 diabetes mellitus and periodontitis have been reported to have a subgingival flora that is composed mainly of *Capnocytophaga*, anaerobic vibrios, and *Actinomyces* species. *Porphyromonas gingivalis*, *Prevotella intermedia*, and *Aggregatibacter actinomycetemcomitans*, which are common in periodontal

Fig. 13.3 Periodontal Abscess in a 28-Year-Old Patient With Poorly Controlled Type 1 Diabetes. (A) The patient presented with pain and abscess a few weeks after scaling and root planing of the area. (B) Radiograph of the mandibular right premolar area demonstrating severe localized destruction of bone in the area of periodontal abscess. (C) Radiograph of the mandibular right premolar area taken 2 months before the presentation of the abscess. Note the presence of calculus and the level of interproximal bone before the abscess occurred.

lesions of individuals without diabetes, are present in low numbers in those with the disease.[112,167] However, other studies have found scarce *Capnocytophaga* and abundant *A. actinomycetemcomitans* and black-pigmented *Bacteroides*, as well as *P. intermedia*, *Prevotella melaninogenica*, and *Campylobacter rectus*.[166,218] Black-pigmented species—especially *P. gingivalis*, *P. intermedia*, and *C. rectus*—are prominent in severe periodontal lesions of Pima Indians with type 2 diabetes.[90,272] Although these results may suggest an altered flora in the periodontal pockets of patients with diabetes, the exact role of these microorganisms has not been determined. To date, there is insufficient evidence to support the role of a specific altered microflora that is responsible for periodontal disease destruction in patients with diabetes.

Polymorphonuclear Leukocyte Function

The increased susceptibility of patients with diabetes to infection has been hypothesized as being caused by polymorphonuclear leukocyte (PMN) deficiencies that result in impaired chemotaxis, defective phagocytosis, or impaired adherence.[170,241] In patients with poorly controlled diabetes, the functions of PMNs, monocytes, and macrophages are impaired.[120] As a result, the primary defense mounted by PMNs against periodontal pathogens is diminished, and bacterial proliferation is more likely. No alteration of immunoglobulin A (IgA), G (IgG), or M (IgM) has been found in patients with diabetes.[208]

Altered Collagen Metabolism

Chronic hyperglycemia impairs collagen structure and function, which may directly impact the integrity of the periodontium.

Decreased collagen synthesis, osteoporosis, and a reduction in alveolar bone height have been demonstrated in diabetic animals.[94,222] Chronic hyperglycemia adversely affects the synthesis, maturation, and maintenance of collagen and extracellular matrix. In the hyperglycemic state, numerous proteins and matrix molecules undergo a nonenzymatic glycosylation, thereby resulting in *accumulated glycation end-products* (AGEs). The formation of AGEs occurs at normal glucose levels as well; however, in hyperglycemic environments, AGE formation is excessive. Many types of molecules are affected, including proteins, lipids, and carbohydrates. Collagen is cross-linked by AGE formation, which makes the collagen less soluble and less likely to be normally repaired or replaced. Cellular migration through cross-linked collagen is impeded, and perhaps more importantly, tissue integrity is impaired as a result of damaged collagen that remains in the tissues for longer periods (i.e., collagen is not renewed at a normal rate).[110] As a result, collagen in the tissues of patients with poorly controlled diabetes is older and more susceptible to pathogenic breakdown (i.e., less resistant to destruction by periodontal infections).

AGEs and receptors for AGEs (RAGEs) play a central role in the classic complications of diabetes,[34] and they may play a significant role in the progression of periodontal disease as well. Poor glycemic control, with the associated increase in AGEs, renders the periodontal tissues more susceptible to destruction.[221] The cumulative effects of altered cellular response to local factors, impaired tissue integrity, and altered collagen metabolism undoubtedly play a significant role in the susceptibility of patients with diabetes to infections and destructive periodontal disease.

CLINICAL CORRELATION

Chronic hyperglycemia impairs collagen structure and function. Chronic hyperglycemia causes proteins and matrix molecules to undergo a nonenzymatic glycosylation, thereby resulting in AGEs. AGEs and RAGEs play a central role in the classic complications of diabetes, and they most likely play a significant role in the progression of periodontal disease as well.

Metabolic Syndrome

Obesity is a global concern with serious health consequences including diabetes mellitus and cardiovascular disease. It is believed that the condition of excess adipose tissue contributes to an increased systemic proinflammatory response in these individuals. *Metabolic syndrome* is a term used to describe a condition of abdominal obesity combined with two or more of the following metabolic disturbances: hypertension, dyslipidemia, and hyperglycemia. Individuals diagnosed with metabolic syndrome are at increased risk for developing type 2 diabetes mellitus[219] and cardiovascular disease.

Recent evidence suggests that obesity, obesity-related characteristics, and metabolic syndrome in particular may be risk indicators for the severity and progression of periodontitis.[10,142,181,263] Previous studies have documented the relationship between obesity and periodontitis, as well as obesity-related characteristics such as body mass index and future progression of periodontal disease.[102]

The association between periodontitis and metabolic syndrome is thought to be the result of systemic oxidative stress and an increased inflammatory response.[142] It may be explained by common risk factors such as obesity and obesity-related habits, including diet, exercise, and poor oral hygiene.[136] Obesity is associated with increased cytokine production as well as T-cell and monocyte/macrophage dysfunction, factors known to contribute to periodontitis. The proinflammatory cytokines interleukin-6 (IL-6) and tumor necrosis factor alpha (TNF-α), which are elevated in obese individuals, are thought to be produced by activated macrophages that have infiltrated adipose tissue.[136] Although these associations are highly suggestive, the specific mechanisms and relationship between metabolic syndrome and periodontitis remain unknown. More well-designed studies are needed to better understand this relationship.

Female Sex Hormones

Gingival alterations during puberty, pregnancy, and menopause are associated with physiologic hormonal changes in the female patient. During puberty and pregnancy, these changes are characterized by nonspecific inflammatory reactions with a predominant vascular component, which leads clinically to a marked hemorrhagic tendency. Oral changes during menopause may include thinning of the oral mucosa, gingival recession, xerostomia, altered taste, and burning mouth.

The changes associated with each phase of the female life cycle from puberty to menopause are briefly addressed in the online materials associated with this book.

See Chapter 37 for a detailed description of these changes, including management considerations for the periodontal manifestations of hormonal changes in the female patient.

HEMATOLOGIC DISORDERS AND IMMUNE DEFICIENCIES

All blood cells play an essential role in the maintenance of a healthy periodontium. White blood cells (WBCs) are involved in inflammatory reactions, and they are responsible for cellular defense against microorganisms as well as for proinflammatory cytokine release. Red blood cells (RBCs) are responsible for gas exchange and nutrient supply to the periodontal tissues and platelets, and they are necessary for normal hemostasis as well as for the recruitment of cells during inflammation and wound healing. Consequently, disorders of any blood cells or blood-forming organs can have a profound effect on the periodontium.

Certain oral changes (e.g., hemorrhage) may suggest the existence of a blood dyscrasia. However, a specific diagnosis requires a complete physical examination and a thorough hematologic study. Comparable oral changes occur in more than one form of blood dyscrasia, and secondary inflammatory changes produce a wide range of variation in the oral signs.

Gingival and periodontal disturbances associated with blood dyscrasias must be viewed in terms of fundamental interrelationships among the oral tissues, the blood cells, and the blood-forming organs rather than in terms of a simple association of dramatic oral changes with hematologic disease. Hemorrhagic tendencies occur when the normal hemostatic mechanisms are disturbed. Abnormal bleeding from the gingiva or other areas of the oral mucosa that is difficult to control is an important clinical sign that suggests a hematologic disorder. Petechiae (Fig. 13.4) and ecchymosis (Fig. 13.5), observed most often in the soft palate area, are signs of an underlying bleeding disorder. It is essential to diagnose the specific etiology to appropriately address any bleeding or immunologic disorder.

Deficiencies in the host immune response may lead to severely destructive periodontal lesions. These deficiencies may be primary (inherited) or secondary (acquired) and may be caused by either immunosuppressive drug therapy or the pathologic destruction of the lymphoid system. Leukemia, Hodgkin disease, lymphomas, and multiple myeloma may result in secondary immunodeficiency disorders. This section discusses common hematologic and

Fig. 13.4 Petechiae Evident on the Soft Palate of a Patient With an Underlying Bleeding Disorder (Thrombocytopenia).

Fig. 13.5 Ecchymosis That is Evident on the Lateral Aspects of the Soft Palate and Tonsillar Pillars of a Patient With Chemotherapy-Induced Thrombocytopenia.

certain immunodeficiency disorders that are not related to the human immunodeficiency virus or acquired immunodeficiency syndrome. See Chapter 28 for a detailed discussion of patients with human immunodeficiency virus infection.

> ## KEY FACT
>
> Clinicians must be aware that certain oral manifestations (e.g., hemorrhage, ecchymosis) can suggest the existence of a systemic disorder. Atypical gingival and periodontal findings should be assessed in terms of the interrelationships among oral tissues, blood cells, and blood-forming organs, rather than in terms of a simple association of dramatic oral changes with hematologic disease. Determining a specific systemic diagnosis requires a complete physical examination and a thorough hematologic study. Patients should be referred to a medical doctor for comprehensive workup.

Leukocyte (Neutrophil) Disorders

Disorders that affect the production or function of leukocytes may result in severe periodontal destruction. PMNs (i.e., neutrophils) in particular play a critical role in bacterial infections, because PMNs are the first line of defense (see Chapter 8). A quantitative deficiency of leukocytes (e.g., neutropenia, agranulocytosis) is typically associated with a more generalized periodontal destruction that affects all teeth.

Neutropenia

Neutropenia is a blood disorder that results in low levels of circulating neutrophils. It is a serious condition that may be caused by diseases, medications, chemicals, infections, idiopathic conditions, or hereditary disorders. It may be chronic or cyclic and severe or benign. It affects as many as one in three patients who are receiving chemotherapy for cancer. An absolute neutrophil count (ANC) of 1000 to 1500 cells/μL is diagnostic for mild neutropenia. An ANC of 500 to 1000 cells/μL is considered moderate neutropenia, and an ANC of <500 cells/μL indicates a severe neutropenia. Infections are sometimes difficult to manage and may be life threatening, particularly with severe neutropenia.

Agranulocytosis

Agranulocytosis is a more severe neutropenia that involves not only neutrophils but also basophils and eosinophils. It is defined as an ANC of <100 cells/μL. It is characterized by a reduction in the number of circulating granulocytes, and it results in severe infections, including ulcerative necrotizing lesions of the oral mucosa, the skin, and the gastrointestinal and genitourinary tracts. Less severe forms of the disease are called *neutropenia* or *granulocytopenia*.

Drug idiosyncrasy is the most common cause of agranulocytosis, but in some cases, its cause cannot be explained. Agranulocytosis has been reported after the administration of drugs such as aminopyrine, barbiturates and their derivatives, benzene ring derivatives, sulfonamides, gold salts, and arsenical agents.[140,157,174,201] It generally occurs as an acute disease. It may be chronic or periodic, with recurring neutropenic cycles (e.g., cyclic neutropenia).[242]

The onset of disease is accompanied by fever, malaise, general weakness, and sore throat. Ulceration in the oral cavity, the oropharynx, and the throat is characteristic. The mucosa exhibits isolated necrotic patches that are black and gray and that are sharply demarcated from the adjacent uninvolved areas.[130,161] The absence of a notable inflammatory reaction caused by a lack of granulocytes is a striking feature. The gingival margin may or may not be involved. Gingival hemorrhage, necrosis, increased salivation, and fetid odor are accompanying clinical features. With cyclic neutropenia, the gingival changes recur with recurrent exacerbation of the disease.[53] The occurrence of generalized aggressive periodontitis has been described in patients with cyclic neutropenia (Fig. 13.6).[225]

Because infection is a common feature of agranulocytosis, the differential diagnosis involves consideration of such conditions as necrotizing ulcerative gingivitis, noma, acute necrotizing inflammation of the tonsils, and diphtheria. Definitive diagnosis depends on the hematologic findings of pronounced leukopenia and the almost complete absence of neutrophils.

Leukemia

Leukemia is an important disease to understand and appreciate because of its seriousness and its periodontal manifestations. The leukemias are malignant neoplasias of WBC precursors that are characterized by the following: (1) diffuse replacement of the bone marrow with proliferating leukemic cells; (2) abnormal numbers and forms of immature WBCs in the circulating blood; and (3) widespread infiltrates in the liver, spleen, lymph nodes, and other body sites.[207]

According to the cell type involved, leukemias are classified as *lymphocytic* or *myelogenous*. A subgroup of the myelogenous leukemias are the *monocytic* leukemias. The term *lymphocytic* indicates that the malignant change occurs in cells that normally form lymphocytes. The term *myelogenous* indicates that the malignant change occurs in cells that normally form RBCs, some types of WBCs, and platelets. According to their evolution, leukemias can be *acute* (which is rapidly fatal), *subacute,* or *chronic.* In acute leukemia, the primitive blast cells released into the peripheral circulation are immature and nonfunctional; in chronic

Fig. 13.6 Aggressive Periodontitis in 10-Year-Old Boy With Cyclic Neutropenia and Agammaglobulinemia. (A) Clinical presentation of the periodontal condition. Note the severe swelling and inflammation of the marginal and papillary gingiva. There is gross migration of teeth caused by a loss of bone support. (B) Panoramic radiograph demonstrating severe bone loss around all permanent teeth that have erupted into the oral cavity.

Fig. 13.7 Spontaneous Bleeding From the Gingival Sulcus in a Patient With Thrombocytopenia. Normal coagulation is evident by the appearance of the large clot that forms in the mouth. However, platelets are inadequate to establish hemostasis at the site of hemorrhage.

Fig. 13.8 Leukemic Infiltration That Causes Localized Gingival Swelling of the Interdental Papillae Between the Maxillary Lateral and Central Incisors. Note the tense induration of the area.

leukemia, the abnormal cells tend to be more mature and to have normal morphologic characteristics and functions when released into the circulation.

All leukemias tend to displace normal components of the bone marrow elements with leukemic cells, thereby resulting in the reduced production of normal RBCs, WBCs, and platelets, which leads to anemia, *leukopenia* (a reduction in the number of *nonmalignant* WBCs), and thrombocytopenia. Anemia results in poor tissue oxygenation, which makes tissues more friable and susceptible to breakdown. A reduction of normal WBCs in the circulation leads to a poor cellular defense and an increased susceptibility to infections. *Thrombocytopenia* leads to bleeding tendency, which can occur in any tissue but which in particular affects the oral cavity, especially the gingival sulcus (Fig. 13.7). Some patients may have normal blood counts, while leukemic cells reside primarily in the bone marrow. This type of disease is called *aleukemic leukemia*.[100]

The Periodontium in Leukemic Patients

Oral and periodontal manifestations of leukemia may include leukemic infiltration, bleeding, oral ulcerations, and infections. The expression of these signs is more common with acute and subacute forms of leukemia than with chronic forms.

Leukemic infiltration. Leukemic cells can infiltrate the gingiva and, less frequently, the alveolar bone. Gingival infiltration often results in *leukemic gingival enlargement* (see Chapter 18).

A study of 1076 adult patients with leukemia showed that 3.6% of the patients with teeth had leukemic gingival proliferative lesions, with the highest incidence seen in patients with acute monocytic leukemia (66.7%), followed by those with acute myelocytic–monocytic leukemia (18.7%) and acute myelocytic leukemia (3.7%).[66] It should be noted, however, that monocytic leukemia is an extremely rare form of the disease. Leukemic gingival enlargement is not found in edentulous patients or in patients with chronic leukemia, suggesting that it represents the accumulation of immature leukemic blast cells in the gingiva adjacent to tooth surfaces with bacterial plaque. Leukemic gingival enlargement consists of a basic infiltration of the gingival corium by leukemic cells that increases the gingival thickness and creates gingival pockets in which bacterial plaque accumulates, thereby initiating a secondary inflammatory lesion that contributes to the enlargement of the gingiva. It may be localized to the interdental papilla area (Fig. 13.8), or it may expand to include the marginal gingiva and partially cover the crowns of the teeth (Fig. 13.9C and D). Clinically, the gingiva appears bluish red and cyanotic, with a rounding and tenseness of the gingival margin. The abnormal accumulation of leukemic cells in the dermal and subcutaneous connective tissue is called *leukemia*

Fig. 13.9 Adult Male With Acute Myelocytic Leukemia. (A) A view of the patient's face. Note the elevated, flat macules and papules (leukemia cutis) on the right cheek. (B) Close-up view of skin lesions. (C) An intraoral view showing pronounced gingival enlargements of the entire gingival margin and interdental papilla areas of both arches. (D) Occlusal view of the maxillary anterior teeth. Note the marked enlargement in both the facial and the palatal aspects. (Courtesy Dr. Spencer Woolfe, Dublin, Ireland.)

cutis, and it forms elevated and flat macules and papules (see Fig. 13.9A and B).[66,207]

Microscopically, the gingiva exhibits a dense, diffuse infiltration of predominantly immature leukocytes in the attached and marginal gingiva. Occasionally, mitotic figures indicative of ectopic hematopoiesis may be seen. The normal connective tissue components of the gingiva are displaced by the leukemic cells (Fig. 13.10). The nature of the cells depends on the type of leukemia. The cellular accumulation is denser in the entire reticular connective tissue layer. In almost all cases, the papillary layer contains comparatively few leukocytes. The blood vessels are distended and contain predominantly leukemic cells, and the RBCs are reduced in number. The epithelium shows a variety of changes, and it may be thinned or hyperplastic. Common findings include degeneration associated with intercellular and intracellular edema and leukocytic infiltration with diminished surface keratinization.

The microscopic picture of the marginal gingiva differs from that of other gingival locations in that it usually exhibits a notable inflammatory component in addition to the leukemic cells. Scattered foci of plasma cells and lymphocytes with edema and degeneration are common findings. The inner aspect of the marginal gingiva is usually ulcerated, and marginal necrosis with pseudomembrane formation may also be seen.

The periodontal ligament and alveolar bone may also be involved in acute and subacute leukemia. The periodontal ligament may be infiltrated with mature and immature leukocytes. The marrow of the alveolar bone exhibits a variety of changes, such as localized areas of necrosis, thrombosis of the blood vessels, infiltration with mature and immature leukocytes, occasional RBCs, and the replacement of the fatty marrow with fibrous tissue.

In leukemic mice, the presence of infiltrate in marrow spaces and the periodontal ligament results in osteoporosis of the alveolar bone with destruction of the supporting bone and disappearance of the periodontal fibers (Fig. 13.11).[32,41]

Bleeding. Gingival hemorrhage is a common finding in leukemic patients (see Fig. 13.7), even in the absence of clinically detectable gingivitis. Bleeding gingiva can be an early sign of

Fig. 13.10 Human Histologic Appearance of Leukemic Infiltrate With Dense Diffuse Infiltration of Predominantly Immature Leukocytes. The normal connective tissue components of the gingiva are displaced by the leukemic cells. The cellular accumulation is denser in the entire reticular connective tissue layer. (Courtesy Dr. Russell Christensen, University of California, Los Angeles, CA.)

Fig. 13.11 Leukemic Infiltrate in Alveolar Bone in a Leukemic Mouse. Note the leukemic infiltrate causing destruction of the bone and a loss of the periodontal ligament.

Fig. 13.12 Large Ulcerations on the Palate of a Patient With Granulocytopenia Secondary to Leukemia. These atypical ulcerations are caused by a herpesvirus opportunistic infection. Notice the smaller, discrete, round ulcerations that have coalesced into the larger lesion.

leukemia. It is caused by the thrombocytopenia that results from the replacement of bone marrow cells with leukemic cells and from the inhibition of normal stem cell function by leukemic cells or their products.[207] This bleeding tendency can also manifest in the skin and throughout the oral mucosa, where petechiae are often found, with or without leukemic infiltrates. A more diffuse submucosal bleeding manifests as ecchymosis (see Fig. 13.5). Oral bleeding has been reported as a presenting sign in 17.7% of patients with acute leukemia and in 4.4% of patients

with chronic leukemia.[156] Bleeding may also be a side effect of the chemotherapeutic agents used to treat leukemia.

Oral ulceration and infection. In patients with leukemia, the response to bacterial plaque or other local irritation is altered. The cellular component of the inflammatory exudate differs both quantitatively and qualitatively from that found in nonleukemic individuals in that there is a pronounced infiltration of immature leukemic cells in addition to the usual inflammatory cells. As a result, the normal inflammatory response may be diminished.

Granulocytopenia (diminished WBC count) results from the displacement of normal bone marrow cells by leukemic cells, which increases the host susceptibility to opportunistic microorganisms and leads to ulcerations and infections. Discrete, punched-out ulcers that penetrate deeply into the submucosa and are covered by a firmly attached white slough can be found on the oral mucosa.[16] These lesions occur in sites of trauma (e.g., the buccal mucosa) in relation to the line of occlusion or on the palate. Patients with a history of herpesvirus infection may develop recurrent herpetic oral ulcers (often in multiple sites) and large atypical forms, especially after chemotherapy is instituted (Fig. 13.12).[106]

A gingival (bacterial) infection in leukemic patients can be the result of an exogenous bacterial infection or an existing bacterial infection (e.g., gingival or periodontal disease). Acute gingivitis and lesions that resemble necrotizing ulcerative gingivitis are more frequent and more severe in patients with terminal cases of acute leukemia (Figs. 13.13 and 13.14).[22] The inflamed gingiva in patients with leukemia differs clinically from that found in nonleukemic individuals. The gingiva is a peculiar bluish red, it is sponge-like and friable, and it bleeds persistently on the slightest provocation or even spontaneously in leukemic patients. This greatly altered and degenerated tissue is extremely susceptible to bacterial infection, which can be so severe as to cause acute gingival necrosis with pseudomembrane formation (Fig. 13.15) or bone exposure (Fig. 13.16). These are secondary oral changes that are superimposed on the oral tissues that have been altered by the blood dyscrasia. They produce associated disturbances that may be a source of considerable difficulty to the patient, such as systemic toxic effects, loss of appetite, nausea, blood

Fig. 13.13 Adult Female With Acute Myelocytic Leukemia. (A) Anterior view of a patient with acute myelocytic leukemia. The interdental papillae are necrotic, with highly inflamed and swollen gingival tissue at the base of the lesions. (B) Palatal view demonstrating extensive necrosis of the interdental and palatal tissues behind the maxillary incisors.

Fig. 13.14 The Same Patient as Shown in Fig. 13.13 **After Chemotherapy That Resulted in the Remission of Her Leukemia.** (A) An anterior view reveals dramatic improvement in gingival health after the remission of leukemia. Note the loss of interdental papillae as well as gingival recession in the anterior areas. (B) A palatal view shows the extensive loss of gingival tissue around the maxillary incisors.

Fig. 13.16 An Opportunistic Bacterial Infection in an Immunosuppressed Patient Caused the Complete Destruction of the Gingiva, Thus Exposing the Underlying Alveolar Bone.

Fig. 13.15 An Opportunistic Bacterial Infection of the Gingiva in a Patient Who Has Been Hospitalized With Leukemia. The gingival tissue is highly inflamed, bleeding, and necrotic, with pseudomembrane formation.

loss from persistent gingival bleeding, and constant gnawing pain. Eliminating or reducing local factors (e.g., bacterial plaque) can minimize the severe oral changes associated with leukemia. In some patients with severe acute leukemia, symptoms may be relieved only by treatment that leads to the remission of the disease.

In those with chronic leukemia, oral changes that suggest a hematologic disturbance are rare. The microscopic changes of

chronic leukemia may consist of replacing the normal fatty marrow of the jaws with islands of mature lymphocytes or lymphocytic infiltration of the marginal gingiva without dramatic clinical manifestations.

The existence of leukemia is sometimes revealed by a gingival biopsy performed to clarify the nature of a troublesome gingival condition. In such cases, the gingival findings must be corroborated by medical examination and hematologic study. In patients with diagnosed leukemia, gingival biopsy may indicate the extent to which leukemic infiltration is responsible for the altered clinical appearance of the gingiva. *Although such findings are of interest, their benefit to the patient is insufficient to warrant routine gingival biopsy studies in patients with leukemia.* Furthermore, it is important to note that the absence of leukemic involvement in a gingival biopsy specimen does not rule out the possibility of leukemia. A gingival biopsy in a patient with chronic leukemia may reveal typical gingival inflammation without any suggestion of a hematologic disturbance.

See the online material for discussion of additional blood dyscrasias and their influence on periodontal health.

GENETIC DISORDERS

Systemic conditions that are associated with or that predispose an individual to periodontal destruction include genetic disorders that result in an inadequate number or reduced function of circulating neutrophils. This underscores the importance of the neutrophil in the protection of the periodontium against infection. Severe periodontitis has been observed in individuals with primary neutrophil disorders such as neutropenia, agranulocytosis, Chédiak–Higashi syndrome, and lazy leukocyte syndrome. In addition, severe periodontitis has been observed in individuals who exhibit secondary neutrophil impairment, such as those with Down syndrome, Papillon-Lefèvre syndrome, and inflammatory bowel disease.

See the online material for this chapter as well as for Chapter 8 for detailed descriptions of the periodontal manifestations of these genetic disorders and syndromes.

STRESS AND PSYCHOSOMATIC DISORDERS

Psychologic conditions, particularly psychosocial stress, have been implicated as risk indicators for periodontal disease.[88] The most notable example is the documented relationship between stress (e.g., experienced by soldiers at war or by students during examinations) and acute necrotizing ulcerative gingivitis (see Chapters 19 and 27). The presence of necrotizing ulcerative gingivitis among soldiers stressed by wartime conditions in the trenches led to one of the early diagnostic terms used to describe this condition: "trench mouth." Despite this well-known association between stress and necrotizing ulcerative gingivitis, confirming the connection between psychologic conditions and other forms of periodontal disease (e.g., chronic periodontitis) has been elusive. These relationships are difficult to elucidate, because, as with many common diseases, the etiology and pathogenesis of periodontal disease is multifactorial, and the role of individual risk factors is difficult to define.

Some studies have failed to recognize a relationship between psychologic conditions and periodontal disease despite specific efforts to identify them. In a study of 80 patients (40 with aggressive periodontitis and 40 with chronic periodontitis), Monteiro da Silva and colleagues failed to find a relationship between psychologic factors and periodontal disease.[180] The researchers were able to identify depression and smoking as marginally significant in the aggressive periodontitis group. Their inability to find a relationship may be attributed to a lack of significant

differences in psychologic characteristics between the two groups in the study. In an earlier study, the same researchers identified depression and loneliness as significant factors associated with aggressive periodontal disease in 50 patients as compared with 50 periodontally healthy individuals and 50 individuals with chronic periodontitis.[179] Another challenge when defining the relationship between psychosocial status and periodontitis is the myriad confounding factors and the difficulty of controlling for them.[68]

Psychosocial Stress, Depression, and Coping

Several clinical studies and a systematic review of the subject have documented a positive relationship between psychosocial stress and chronic forms of periodontal disease.[198] In case-control studies, individuals with stable lifestyles (based on family structure and employment status) and minimal negative life events had less periodontal disease destruction than individuals with less stable lifestyles (e.g., unmarried, unemployed) and more negative life events.[59] It is now becoming apparent that the effect is not simply a matter of the presence or absence of stress; rather, the type of stress and the ability of the individual to cope with stress correlate with destructive periodontal disease.

All individuals experience stress, but these events do not invariably result in destructive periodontitis. The types of stress that lead to periodontal destruction appear to be more chronic or long term and less likely to be controlled by the individual. Life events such as the loss of a loved one (e.g., spouse, family member), a failed relationship, loss of employment, and financial difficulties are examples of stressful life events that are typically not controllable by the individual or not perceived by the individual as being under his or her control, thereby resulting in a feeling of helplessness. The duration of the stressful life event also has an influence on the total impact of the stress-induced disease destruction.

Financial stress is an example of a long-term, constant pressure that may exacerbate periodontal destruction in susceptible individuals. Genco and colleagues[89] found that individuals with high levels of financial stress and poor coping skills had twice as much periodontal disease as those with minimal stress and good coping skills. Psychologic tests were used to identify and weigh the causes of stress (e.g., children, spouse, finances, single life, work) and to measure individual coping skills. Individuals with problem-focused (practical) coping skills fared better than individuals with emotion-focused (avoidance) coping skills with respect to periodontal disease. As part of their analysis, the researchers also found that chronic stress and inadequate coping could lead to changes in daily habits, such as poor oral hygiene, clenching, and grinding, as well as physiologic changes such as decreased saliva flow and suppressed immunity.

When comparing 89 patients with periodontal disease to 63 periodontally healthy individuals, Wimmer and colleagues[264] found that patients with defensive (emotional) coping skills were more likely to refuse responsibility and to downplay their condition. All patients completed a comprehensive stress assessment questionnaire (given in German) to evaluate their coping behavior. Patients with periodontal disease were less likely to use active coping skills (i.e., situation control) and more likely to cope with stress by averting blame (emotional) than were periodontally healthy individuals.

These studies support the concept that one of the most important aspects related to the influence of stress on periodontal disease destruction is the manner in which the individual copes with the stress. Emotional coping methods appear to render the host more susceptible to the destructive effects of periodontal disease than do practical coping methods. Furthermore, emotional coping is more common in situations that must be accepted and among individuals who feel helpless in the situation.

> ### KEY FACT
>
> The effect of psychosocial stress on the manifestation of disease (i.e., periodontitis) is not simply a matter of the presence or absence of stress; rather, the type of stress and the ability of the individual to cope with stress correlate with destructive periodontal disease.

Stress-Induced Immunosuppression

Stress and psychosomatic disorders most likely impact periodontal health via changes in the individual's behavior and through complex interactions among the nervous, endocrine, and immune systems. Individuals under stress may have poorer oral hygiene, they may start or increase the clenching and grinding of their teeth, and they may smoke more frequently. All of these behavioral changes increase their susceptibility to periodontal disease destruction. Likewise, individuals who are under stress may be less likely to seek professional care.

In addition to the many behavioral changes that may influence periodontal disease destruction, psychosocial stress may also impact the disease through alterations in the immune system. The influence of stress on the immune system and systemic health conditions (e.g., cardiovascular disease) is well known. Stress-related immune system changes clearly have the potential to affect the pathogenesis of periodontal disease as well. One possible mechanism involves the production of cortisol. Stress increases cortisol production from the adrenal cortex by stimulating an increase in the release of adrenocorticotropic hormone from the pituitary gland. Increased cortisol suppresses the immune response directly through the suppression of neutrophil activity, immunoglobulin G production, and salivary IgA secretion. All of these immune responses are critical for the normal immunoinflammatory response to periodontal pathogens (see Chapter 8). The resulting stress-induced immunosuppression increases the potential for destruction by periodontal pathogens. Stress may also affect the cellular immune response directly through an increased release of neurotransmitters, including epinephrine, norepinephrine, neurokinin, and substance P, which interact directly with lymphocytes, neutrophils, monocytes, and macrophages via receptors that cause an increase in their tissue-destructive function. Thus, in a manner similar to cortisol production, the stress-induced release of these neurotransmitters results in an upregulated immune response that increases the potential for destruction by the cellular response to periodontal pathogens.

It is important to remember that, although stress may predispose an individual to more destruction from periodontitis, the presence of periodontal pathogens remains as the essential etiologic factor. In other words, stress alone does not cause or lead to periodontitis in the absence of periodontal pathogens.

Influence of Stress on Periodontal Therapy Outcomes

Psychologic conditions such as stress and depression may also influence the outcome of periodontal therapy. In a large-scale retrospective study of 1299 dental records from a health maintenance organization database, 85 individuals with depression had posttherapy outcomes that were less favorable (below median) than the outcomes of individuals without depression.[73] More than half of these records (697) were complete enough for a comprehensive evaluation that included both periodontal diagnosis and psychologic profiles. The authors concluded that depression might have a negative effect on periodontal treatment outcomes.

A study investigating the relationship between psychologic stress and wound repair in patients after routine surgery (in this case, inguinal hernia open incision repair) revealed that stress impairs the inflammatory response and matrix degradation.[31] Forty-seven adults were given a standardized questionnaire to assess their psychologic stress before surgery. Wound fluids were collected during the first 20 hours after surgery to measure inflammatory markers: IL-1, IL-6, and matrix metalloproteinase-9 (MMP-9). Greater psychologic stress was significantly associated with lower levels of IL-1 and MMP-9 as well as with a significantly more painful, poorer, and slower recovery.

Another study compared the psychiatric characteristics of individuals with different outcomes to periodontal therapy.[11] Two groups were compared to evaluate the psychologic characteristics of 11 individuals who were responsive to periodontal treatment compared with 11 individuals who were not responsive to periodontal treatment. The members of the responsive group had more rigid personalities, whereas those in the nonresponsive group had more passive, dependent personalities. Furthermore, the nonresponsive group reported more stressful life events having occurred in their past.

These studies suggest that both stressful life events and the individual's personality and coping skills are factors to consider when assessing the risk of periodontal disease destruction and the potential for successful periodontal therapy. If patients with emotional or defensive coping skills are identified, care should be taken to ensure that they receive information in a manner that does not elicit a defensive reaction.

Psychiatric Influence of Self-Inflicted Injury

Psychosomatic disorders may result in harmful effects to the health of tissues in the oral cavity through the development of habits that are injurious to the periodontium. Neurotic habits such as grinding or clenching the teeth, nibbling on foreign objects (e.g., pencils, pipes), nail biting, and excessive use of tobacco are all potentially injurious to the teeth and the periodontium. Self-inflicted gingival injuries, such as gingival recession, have been described in both children and adults (Fig. 13.17).

Fig. 13.17 Severe Gingival Recession Localized to the Labial Surface of All Mandibular Incisors. This finding was discovered in an uncooperative, institutionalized adult with mental disorders who had been placed under general anesthesia. The patient was known to pace around the home with all four fingers inside his lower lip.

However, these types of self-inflicted, factitious injuries do not appear to be common among psychiatric patients.[217]

NUTRITIONAL INFLUENCES

Some clinicians enthusiastically adhere to the theory in periodontal disease that assigns a key role to nutritional deficiencies and imbalances. Previous research did not support this view, but numerous problems in experimental design and data interpretation could be responsible for making these research findings inadequate.[5,216] The majority of opinions and research findings regarding the effects of nutrition on oral and periodontal tissues point to the following:

1. *There are no nutritional deficiencies that by themselves can cause gingivitis or periodontitis.* However, nutritional deficiencies can affect the condition of the periodontium and thereby may accentuate the deleterious effects of plaque-induced inflammation in susceptible individuals. Theoretically, one may presume that an individual with a nutritional deficiency is less able to defend against a bacterial challenge as compared with a nutritionally competent individual.
2. *There are nutritional deficiencies that produce changes in the oral cavity.* These changes include alterations of the tissues of the lips, oral mucosa, gingiva, and bone. These alterations are considered to be the periodontal and oral manifestations of nutritional disease.

The role of nutrition in periodontal disease may be related to the effect of nutrition on inflammation. A 2009 review of the literature evaluating the effect of nutritional factors on inflammation demonstrated that subtle shifts in nutritional status are associated with the prevalence of periodontitis.[46] More specifically, the authors reported that the results of contemporary animal and human studies have demonstrated the role of specific micronutrients in the modulation of the host's inflammatory response by reducing inflammatory biomarkers, which may in turn be responsible for periodontal destruction. The evidence for the

effect of nutrition on inflammation is significant. Data suggest that diets that contain foods rich in antioxidants are beneficial, whereas foods that contain high levels of refined carbohydrates are detrimental to the inflammatory process.[46]

See the online material for a review of the existing knowledge of the effects of vitamin and protein deficiencies on changes in the periodontium.

MEDICATIONS

Some medications that are prescribed to cure, manage, or prevent diseases may have adverse effects on periodontal tissues, wound healing, or the host immune response. Bisphosphonates are a class of medications widely prescribed for the treatment of osteoporosis and various types of cancer. They are implicated in osteonecrosis of the jaw (ONJ), a serious condition that is characterized by nonhealing and often painful exposure of nonvital and often sequestrating bone in the jaws. Corticosteroids have long been prescribed to suppress the immune system for the control and management of autoimmune disease, during cancer treatment, and as an antirejection medication after organ transplantation. This section discusses the effect of bisphosphonates and corticosteroids on the periodontium. Readers are referred to Chapter 36 for additional information about these and other important medications.

Bisphosphonates

Bisphosphonate medications are primarily used to treat cancer (via intravenous [IV] administration) and osteoporosis (via oral administration). They act by inhibiting osteoclastic activity, which leads to less bone resorption, less bone remodeling, and less bone turnover.[214] The use of bisphosphonates in cancer treatment is aimed at preventing the often lethal imbalance of osteoclastic activity. During the treatment of osteoporosis, the goal is simply to harness osteoclastic activity to minimize or prevent bone loss and, in many cases, to increase bone mass by creating an advantage for osteoblastic activity. The major differences in the use of bisphosphonates for cancer versus osteoporosis are the potency and route of administration of the specific bisphosphonate medication used. Potency is influenced by the chemical properties, as well as by the binding and release pharmacokinetic properties of these agents as they apply to bone. Specifically, the strength of binding and the ease of release of bisphosphonates with hydroxyapatite make these drugs more or less potent.

Bisphosphonates were first synthesized during the 1950s as a substitute for pyrophosphate, a compound used in detergent. The ability of bisphosphonates to increase bone mass was discovered after animal studies that took place in 1966, but the potential advantage of using bisphosphonates in humans with low bone mass was not appreciated until 1984.[255] The US Food and Drug Administration approved the use of alendronate for osteoporosis in 1995.

The chemical structure of bisphosphonate consists of two phosphate groups covalently bonded to a central carbon (Fig. 13.18). In addition to the two phosphate groups, the central carbon also has two side chains, R1 and R2. Both the short R1 side chain and the long R2 side chain influence the chemical

TABLE 13.1 **Current Non-Aminobisphosphonate and Aminobisphosphonate Medications and Common Therapeutic Uses**

Generic Name	Commercial Name	Route of Administration	Therapeutic Use	Nitrogen-Containing R2 Side Chain	Relative Antiresorptive Potency
Etidronate	Didronel	PO	Paget disease	No	1
Tiludronate	Skelid	PO	Paget disease	No	10
Risedronate	Actonel	PO	Osteoporosis, Paget disease	Yes	5000
Ibandronate	Boniva	PO	Osteoporosis	Yes	10,000
Alendronate	Fosamax	PO	Osteoporosis, Paget disease	Yes	1000
Pamidronate	Aredia	IV	Paget disease, cancer	Yes	100
Zoledronate	Zometa	IV	Cancer	Yes	10,000+

IV, Intravenous; *PO,* by mouth.

Pyrophosphate

Generic bisphosphonate

R1 Enhances binding to hydroxyapatite
-C- Enhances chemical stability
R2 Determines antiresorptive potency

Fig. 13.18 Chemical Structure of a Bisphosphonate Molecule. Two phosphate groups are covalently bonded with a central carbon. The carbon also has two side chains, *R1* and *R2.*

properties and pharmacokinetics. The long R2 side chain also influences the mode of action and determines the strength or potency of the medication. Bisphosphonates inhibit osteoclasts by two mechanisms that depend on whether the R2 side chain contains nitrogen. Non-aminobisphosphonates are metabolized by osteoclasts to form an adenosine triphosphate analog that interferes with energy production and causes osteoclast apoptosis. Aminobisphosphonates (i.e., risedronate, zoledronate, ibandronate, and alendronate) are more potent and have multiple effects on osteoclasts, including the following: (1) inactivation of adenosine triphosphate, (2) osteoclast cytoskeletal disruption, (3) impairment of osteoclast recruitment, and (4) induction of osteoblasts to produce osteoclast-inhibiting factor.[189] Bisphosphonates also inhibit bone metabolism via antiangiogenic activity.[35]

Table 13.1 lists some of the common bisphosphonate medications used for osteoporosis and cancer treatment that are currently available in the United States.

There is growing evidence that bisphosphonates also affect soft tissues and that they may contribute to ONJ via inhibition of soft tissue healing.[143] An in vitro study by Kim and colleagues suggested that bisphosphonates may act on oral keratinocytes to impair wound healing by inhibiting epithelial migration and wound closure.[133] Interestingly, the effects of bisphosphonates on oral mucosal cells and bone cells share the common mechanism of interference with products of the mevalonate pathway, which may be more significant to the overall problem than the reported apoptosis effects on osteoclasts. The inhibition of farnesyl pyrophosphate synthase leads to inhibition of the mevalonate pathway end product, geranylgeranyl pyrophosphate (Fig. 13.19). This bisphosphonate-inhibited pathway is required for many essential cellular functions in a variety of tissues. In the case of soft tissues, the bisphosphonate-induced senescence of human oral keratinocytes was found to be mediated, at least in part, by inhibition of the mevalonate pathway. Similarly, Fisher and colleagues reported that bisphosphonates inhibit bone resorption via prevention of protein prenylation in osteoclasts that is caused by the inhibition of farnesyl pyrophosphate synthase, resulting in interference with the production of geranylgeranyl pyrophosphate.

Bisphosphonates have a high affinity for hydroxyapatite. They are rapidly absorbed in bone, especially in areas of high activity, which may help explain why bisphosphonate-induced osteonecrosis is found only in the jaws.[255] The bisphosphonate molecule gets incorporated into bone without being metabolized or modified. During the osteoclastic resorption of bone, the trapped bisphosphonate is released and able to affect osteoclasts again. As a result, the half-life of bisphosphonates in the bone is estimated to be 10 years or longer.

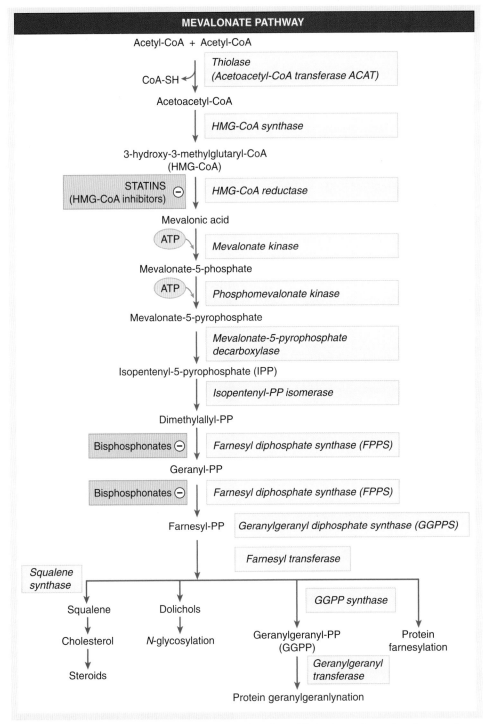

Fig. 13.19 Mevalonate Pathway. Bisphosphonates interfere with the farnesyl pyrophosphate synthase enzyme, which leads to the inhibition of geranylgeranyl pyrophosphate, an important end product for cellular functions.

ONJ associated with bisphosphonates was first described in 2003 by Marx in a report of 36 patients with avascular necrosis of the jaw who had been treated with IV bisphosphonate for malignant tumors.[163] Several case series reporting an association between bisphosphonates and ONJ were published subsequently.[165,212] Various terms have been used to describe this type of ONJ, including *avascular necrosis, bisphosphonate-associated ONJ, bisphosphonate-induced ONJ*, and *bisphosphonate-related ONJ (BRONJ)*.[255] Today, with the widespread recognition of BRONJ, it is important to remember that necrotic bone exposure of the jaw (ONJ) is a condition with multiple possible etiopathogenic factors, including systemic medications, radiation, infection,

Fig. 13.20 Clinical Photograph of Exposed Bone on the Palatal Surface of the Maxilla Adjacent to the Molar Root in a 60-Year-Old Female With Bisphosphonate-Induced Osteonecrosis of the Bone (Maxilla). The bone exposures were noted after about 1 year of treatment with bisphosphonate (Aredia and Zometa). (Courtesy Drs. Eric S. Sung and Evelyn M. Chung, University of California, Los Angeles, CA.)

Fig. 13.21 Clinical Photograph of Exposed Bone on the Lingual Surface of the Posterior Mandible of a 70-Year-Old Male With Bisphosphonate-Induced Osteonecrosis of the Bone (Mandible). The bone exposure was noted after 3 years of bisphosphonate treatment (Aredia and Zometa) for multiple myeloma. (Courtesy Drs. Eric S. Sung and Evelyn M. Chung, University of California, Los Angeles, CA.)

trauma, direct chemical toxicity, and other idiopathic mechanisms; clinicians should carefully consider all factors before making a diagnosis of BRONJ.[8]

The condition of BRONJ has been defined as the exposure and necrosis of portions of the jaw bone in patients who have been exposed to bisphosphonates that has persisted for longer than 8 weeks with no history of radiation therapy to the jaws.[210] The stage of osteonecrosis is used to categorize patients and to make treatment decisions.[2,164,165,210] Stage 0 patients are patients at risk who have been treated with IV or oral bisphosphonates but who have no apparent exposed or necrotic bone. Stage 1 involves exposed or necrotic bone in patients who are asymptomatic with no infection. Stage 2 involves exposed or necrotic bone in patients with pain and clinical evidence of infection. Stage 3 involves exposed or necrotic bone in patients with pain, infection, and one or more of the following: pathologic fracture, extraoral fistula, or osteolysis that extends to the inferior border.

Clinically, BRONJ manifests as exposed alveolar bone that occurs spontaneously or after a traumatic event such as a dental procedure (Figs. 13.20 and 13.21). The sites may be painful, with surrounding soft tissue induration and inflammation. Infection with drainage may be present. Radiographically, lesions appear radiolucent, with sclerosis of the lamina dura, a loss of the lamina dura, or a widening of the periodontal ligament in areas where teeth are present. Histologically, bone appears necrotic, with empty lacunae demonstrating a lack of living osteocytes. In advanced cases, pathologic fracture may be present through the area of exposed or necrotic bone.

The high potency of nitrogen-containing bisphosphonates—especially those administered intravenously for cancer treatment (e.g., zoledronate)—may explain the high incidence of BRONJ in these patients compared with osteoporotic patients taking oral bisphosphonates. The incidence among patients who are being treated for cancer has been reported to range from 2.5% to 5.4%[258] or from 1% to 10%.[35] Estimating the incidence among patients who are taking oral bisphosphonates for osteoporosis is more difficult due to the large number of patients taking this prescription medication and a lack of good reporting or documentation for these patients. Some reports estimate the incidence of BRONJ from oral bisphosphonates to range from 0.007% to 0.04%,[255] whereas other reports suggest a slightly higher incidence that ranges from 0.004% to 0.11%.[231] Clearly, the incidence among patients taking oral bisphosphonates appears to be low.

It has been observed that BRONJ lesions occur most often in areas with dense bone and thin overlying mucosa, such as tori, bony exostoses, and the mylohyoid ridge.[165,211,212] Lesions are found more commonly in the mandible than in the maxilla at a 2:1 ratio.[210] Work by Schaudinn and colleagues suggests that there may be a toxic threshold of accumulated bisphosphonate in the bone that leads to the induction of BRONJ lesions and that measuring or calculating the concentration in bone may be a means of assessing an individual's risk for the development of BRONJ.[220]

In addition to bisphosphonate therapy, other factors are thought to increase individual susceptibility to BRONJ. Potential risk factors that may contribute to BRONJ include systemic corticosteroid therapy, smoking, alcohol, poor oral hygiene, chemotherapy, radiotherapy, diabetes, and hematologic disease.[29] The precipitating factors or trauma-inducing events that lead to BRONJ are reported to include extractions, root canal treatment, periodontal infections, periodontal surgery, and dental implant surgery; however, some cases appear to be idiopathic, with spontaneous exposures.[165] In a retrospective evaluation of patients treated with IV bisphosphonates for metastatic bone cancer from 1996 to 2006, Estilo and colleagues[76] found that the type of cancer, the duration of bisphosphonate therapy, sequential IV bisphosphonate treatment with pamidronate followed by zoledronate, comorbid osteoarthritis, rheumatoid arthritis, and benign hematologic conditions were significantly associated with an increased likelihood of ONJ. In their study, the systemic administration of corticosteroids was not found to be associated with an increased risk of BRONJ.[76]

As stated previously, patients who are being treated for cancer with IV bisphosphonates are at greater risk than patients being treated for osteoporosis with oral bisphosphonates. Dental health care providers should evaluate patients carefully, consider the risks, communicate with medical health care providers, inform patients, and consider treatment options and risks carefully.

> ### KEY FACT
>
> The effects of bisphosphonates on oral hard and soft tissue cells share the common mechanism of interference with products of the mevalonate pathway, which may be more significant to the overall problem than the reported apoptosis effects on osteoclasts. The inhibition of farnesyl pyrophosphate synthase leads to the inhibition of the mevalonate pathway end product, geranylgeranyl pyrophosphate (see Fig. 13.19). This bisphosphonate-inhibited pathway is required for many essential cellular functions in a variety of tissues.

Bisphosphonates and Periodontal Bone Loss

Not surprisingly, the bone-preserving action of bisphosphonates has been studied and advocated for use in the prevention of bone loss from periodontal disease.[243] Several animal studies have shown that bisphosphonates, either applied topically or administered systemically, have the potential to prevent the alveolar bone loss caused by periodontitis.[44,105,173,175,190,229,261] The use of bisphosphonates for bone regeneration has been proposed as well.[243] Although some studies have demonstrated bone preservation with low doses of bisphosphonate, higher doses and longer administration may have a neutral or detrimental effect on bone loss caused by periodontitis.[36,44] In a 2- to 3-year follow-up report of four female patients with periodontitis treated with etidronate (200 mg daily for periods of 2 weeks with 10-week off-drug periods), the potential of this agent to prevent periodontal bone loss was reported.[240] In a 2-year, randomized, placebo-controlled clinical trial of 335 patients treated with alendronate (70 mg once weekly), no significant difference in alveolar bone loss or alveolar bone density was found.[124] Interestingly, alendronate was found to significantly reduce bone loss relative to controls in a subset of this group (i.e., patients with low mandibular bone mineral density [BMD] at baseline), suggesting that the effect may be more perceptible in cases with less bone mass or less bone density. In another clinical trial of 24 patients (12 experimental and 12 control), alendronate was shown to have a significant positive (bone-preserving) effect on bone density in jaws.[71] The BMD of the maxilla and mandible was measured for all patients with the use of dual-energy x-ray absorptiometry (DEXA) at baseline and after 6 months of treatment (10 mg daily for 6 months).

Corticosteroids

In humans, the systemic administration of cortisone and adrenocorticotropic hormone appears to have no effect on the incidence or severity of gingival and periodontal disease. However, renal transplantation patients receiving immunosuppressive therapy (either prednisone or methylprednisone combined with either azathioprine or cyclophosphamide) have significantly less gingival inflammation than control subjects with similar amounts of plaque.[21,129,141,188,247]

Exogenous cortisone may have an adverse effect on bone quality and physiology. The systemic administration of cortisone in experimental animals resulted in the osteoporosis of alveolar bone.[98] There was capillary dilation and engorgement with hemorrhage into the periodontal ligament and gingival connective tissue, degeneration and a reduction in the number of collagen fibers in the periodontal ligament, and increased destruction of the periodontal tissues associated with inflammation.[98]

Stress increases circulating endogenous cortisol levels through stimulation of the adrenal glands (i.e., the hypothalamic–pituitary–adrenal axis). This increased exposure to endogenous cortisol may have adverse effects on the periodontium by diminishing the immune response to periodontal bacteria (see the Psychosocial Stress, Depression, and Coping section).

See the online material for discussion of additional systemic conditions and their influence on periodontal health.

CONCLUSION

Today, we have a better appreciation for the complexity and significance of interrelationships between periodontal infections and host defense. Genetic, environmental, physical, and psychosocial factors have the potential to alter periodontal tissues and the host immune response, thereby resulting in more severe periodontal disease. It is important to recognize that the systemic diseases, disorders, or conditions themselves do not cause periodontitis; rather, they may predispose, accelerate, or otherwise increase disease progression. This chapter reviewed important systemic diseases, disorders, and conditions that influence periodontal health.

A Case Scenario is found on the companion website.

REFERENCES

 References for this chapter are found on the companion website.

14

Impact of Periodontal Infection on Systemic Health[a]

 For online-only content on periodontal disease and pregnancy outcome, periodontal disease and chronic obstructive pulmonary disease, and periodontal disease and acute respiratory infections, please visit the companion website.

CHAPTER OUTLINE

Knowledge of the pathogenesis of periodontal diseases has evolved markedly over the last 50 years.[82] Periodontal disease is an inflammatory disease initiated by bacterial pathogens. Environmental, physical, social, and host stresses may affect and modify disease expression through a multitude of pathways. Certain systemic conditions can affect the initiation and progression of gingivitis and periodontitis (see Chapter 13). Systemic disorders that affect neutrophil, monocyte, macrophage, and lymphocyte function result in the altered production or activity of host inflammatory mediators.[82,125] These alterations may manifest clinically as the early onset of periodontal destruction or as a more rapid rate of destruction than would occur in the absence of such disorders.

Evidence has also shed light on the relationship between systemic health and oral health: the potential effects of inflammatory periodontal diseases on a wide range of organ systems. This field of periodontal medicine addresses the following important questions:

- Can the inflammatory response to bacterial infection of the periodontium have an effect that is remote from the oral cavity?
- Is periodontal infection a risk factor for systemic diseases or conditions that affect human health?

PATHOBIOLOGY OF PERIODONTITIS

Our understanding of the pathogenesis of periodontitis has changed remarkably over the last 30 years.[82,125,131] The nonspecific accumulation of bacterial plaque was once thought to be the cause of periodontal destruction, but it is now recognized that periodontitis is an infectious disease associated with a small number of predominantly gram-negative microorganisms that exist in a subgingival biofilm.[54] Furthermore, the importance of the host in disease initiation and progression is clearly recognized. Although pathogenic bacteria are necessary for periodontal disease, they are not sufficient alone to cause the disease. A susceptible host is also imperative. In a host who has relatively low susceptibility to disease, bacterial pathogens may have no clinical effect. This may be due to a particularly effective host immunoinflammatory response that eliminates pathogenic organisms while minimizing destruction of native tissues. Conversely, in a host with relatively high disease susceptibility, marked destruction of periodontal tissues may result.

> **KEY FACT**
>
> Although pathogenic bacteria are necessary for periodontal disease, bacteria alone are not sufficient to cause disease. A susceptible host is imperative. In a host with relatively low susceptibility, bacterial pathogens may have little or no clinical effect.

Recognizing the importance of host susceptibility opens a door to understanding the differences in the onset, natural history, and progression of periodontitis seen throughout the scientific

[a]Adapted from the following chapter of Newman and Carranza's Clinical Periodontology, 13th edition: Chapter 15: Impact of Periodontal Infection on Systemic Health, by Brian L. Mealey and Perry R. Klokkevold.

literature. Because of differences in host susceptibility, not all individuals are equally vulnerable to the destructive effects of periodontal pathogens and the immunoinflammatory response to those organisms. Thus patients may not necessarily have similar disease expression despite the presence of similar bacteria. Likewise, the response to periodontal treatment may vary depending on the wound-healing capacity and susceptibility of the host to further disease progression. The importance of host susceptibility is evident in the medical literature. For example, respiratory tract pathogens may have a minimal effect on many individuals, but in a susceptible host, such as an elderly patient, these same pathogens may cause life-threatening respiratory tract illnesses.

There are many systemic conditions that can modify the host's susceptibility to periodontitis. For example, patients with immune suppression may not be able to mount an effective host response to subgingival microorganisms, thereby resulting in more rapid and severe periodontal destruction. Conversely, individuals with a significant increase in the production of proinflammatory mediators may respond to periodontal pathogens with an exuberant inflammatory response that results in the destruction of periodontal tissues. Although the potential impact of many systemic disorders on the periodontium is well documented, evidence suggests that periodontal infection may significantly enhance the risk for certain systemic diseases or alter the natural course of systemic conditions.[b] Although more than 50 different systemic conditions have been associated with periodontal diseases, the evidence base is quite large for many of these conditions. For example, conditions in which the influences of periodontal infection are well documented include coronary heart disease (CHD) and CHD-related events such as angina, infarction, atherosclerosis, and other vascular conditions; stroke; diabetes mellitus; preterm labor, low-birth-weight (LBW) delivery, and preeclampsia; and respiratory conditions such as chronic obstructive pulmonary disease (COPD; Box 14.1).[90,110,132] A smaller but growing evidence base supports an association between poor oral health, tooth loss, or periodontitis and conditions such as chronic kidney disease and renal insufficiency[c]; certain forms of cancer[2,45,118,119,161] affecting the liver, pancreas, and colorectal region; rheumatoid arthritis[29,30]; and altered cognitive function, dementia, and Alzheimer disease.[d] This chapter focuses on those conditions with the strongest evidence base, recognizing that ongoing research will further elucidate relationships between inflammatory periodontal diseases and systemic health.

FOCAL INFECTION THEORY REVISITED

Research in the area of periodontal medicine marks a resurgence in the concept of focal infection. In 1900, British physician William Hunter first developed the idea that oral microorganisms were responsible for a wide range of systemic conditions that were not easily recognized as being infectious in nature.[123,174] He claimed that restoration of carious teeth, instead of extraction,

---

> ### BOX 14.1 Organ Systems and Conditions Possibly Influenced by Periodontal Infection
>
> **Cardiovascular and Cerebrovascular Systems**
> Atherosclerosis
> Coronary heart disease
> Angina
> Myocardial infarction
> Cerebrovascular accident (stroke)
> Erectile dysfunction
> Anemia
>
> **Endocrine System**
> Metabolic syndrome
> Diabetes mellitus
>
> **Reproductive System**
> Preterm and low-birth-weight infants
> Preeclampsia
>
> **Respiratory System**
> Chronic obstructive pulmonary disease
> Acute bacterial pneumonia
>
> **Kidney Diseases**
> Renal insufficiency
> Chronic kidney disease
> End-stage kidney disease
>
> **Autoimmune Diseases**
> Rheumatoid arthritis
> Ankylosing spondylitis
>
> **Cognitive Function**
> Dementia
> Alzheimer disease
>
> **Cancers**
> Colorectal
> Pancreatic
> Hepatocellular
> Others

resulted in the trapping of infectious agents under restorations. In addition to caries, pulpal necrosis, and periapical abscesses, Hunter identified gingivitis and periodontitis as foci of infection. He advocated the extraction of teeth with these conditions to eliminate the source of sepsis. Hunter thought that teeth were prone to septic infection primarily because of their structure and their relationship to alveolar bone. He stated that the degree of systemic effect produced by oral sepsis depended on the virulence of the oral infection and the individual's degree of resistance. He also thought that oral organisms had specific actions on different tissues and that these organisms acted by producing toxins, thereby resulting in low-grade "subinfections" that produced systemic effects over prolonged periods. Finally, Hunter thought that the connection between oral sepsis and resulting systemic conditions could be shown via removal of the causative sepsis through tooth extraction and observation of the improvement in systemic health. Because it explained a wide range of disorders

---

[b]References 90, 110, 121, 133, 150, 174.
[c]References 20, 43, 44, 84, 85, 153.
[d]References 75, 76, 90, 155, 158, 160, 179.

for which there was no known explanation at the time, Hunter's theory became widely accepted in Britain and eventually in the United States, leading to the wholesale extraction of teeth.

The focal infection theory fell into disrepute during the 1940s and 1950s, when widespread extraction—often of the entire dentition—failed to reduce or eliminate the systemic conditions to which the supposedly infected dentition had been linked.[174] The theory, while offering a possible explanation for perplexing systemic disorders, had been based on very little (if any) scientific evidence. Hunter and other advocates of the theory were unable to explain how focal oral sepsis produced these systemic maladies. They were also unable to elucidate possible interactive mechanisms between oral and systemic health. Furthermore, the suggested intervention of tooth extraction often had no effect on the systemic conditions for which patients sought relief. However, Hunter's ideas did encourage extensive research in the areas of microbiology and immunology.

FLASH BACK

The focal infection theory fell into disrepute during the 1940s and 1950s, when widespread extraction—often of the entire dentition—failed to reduce or eliminate the systemic conditions. The theory, while offering a possible explanation for perplexing systemic disorders, had been based on very little (if any) scientific evidence.

EVIDENCE-BASED CLINICAL PRACTICE

Many of the precepts of the focal infection theory are being revived today in light of recent research demonstrating links between oral and systemic health. However, as expressed by Newman, for the "hypothesis not to fall into disrepute for a second time, there must be no unsubstantiated attributions, no theories without evidence."[123] Today's era of evidence-based medicine and dentistry provides an excellent environment to examine the possible relationships between oral infection and systemic disorders. To establish a relationship between conditions A and B, different levels of evidence must be examined. All scientific evidence is not given the same weight.[64,114,124] The stronger the evidence, the more likely it is that a true relationship exists between the conditions. Table 14.1 describes these various levels of evidence.

For example, when examining the relationship between elevated cholesterol levels and CHD-related events, the literature might initially consist entirely of *case reports* or similar anecdotal information in which individual patients with recent myocardial infarction (MI) are found to have elevated cholesterol levels. These anecdotal reports suggest a possible relationship between elevated cholesterol and MI, but the evidence is weak. The case reports may lead to *cross-sectional studies*, in which a large subject population is examined to determine whether those individuals who had an MI have higher cholesterol levels than other individuals (control subjects) who did not have an MI. Ideally, these cross-sectional studies are controlled for other potential causes or factors associated with MI, such as age, gender, and smoking history. In other words, the subjects with a previous MI would be retrospectively matched with subjects of similar age, gender,

TABLE 14.1 Evaluation of Evidence

Type of Evidence	Strength of Evidence	Description
Case report	+/–	• Provides relatively weak retrospective anecdotal evidence • May suggest that further study is needed
Cross-sectional study	+	• Compares groups of subjects at a single point in time • Stronger than a case report • Fairly easy to conduct • Relatively inexpensive to conduct
Longitudinal study	++	• Follows groups of subjects over time • Stronger than a cross-sectional study • Studies with a control group much stronger than studies without controls • More difficult and expensive to conduct
Intervention trial	+++	• Examines the effects of some intervention • Studies with a control group (i.e., placebo) much stronger than studies without controls • Strongest form of evidence is the randomized controlled intervention trial • Difficult and expensive to conduct
Systematic review	++++	• Systematically evaluates evidence from multiple studies, especially randomized controlled trials • Uses clearly defined guidelines for the selection of evidence to be included or excluded from the review • Examines for heterogeneity in the overall data to indicate variations in study design, sample populations, and assessment methodologies

and smoking history, and their cholesterol levels would then be examined for similarities or differences. Significantly higher cholesterol levels in subjects with a previous MI compared with those without MI offer stronger evidence than case reports; such evidence further substantiates a possible link between elevated cholesterol and MI.

Even stronger evidence is provided by *longitudinal studies*, in which subject populations are examined over time. For example, a group of subjects might periodically have their cholesterol levels evaluated over several years. If individuals with elevated cholesterol levels have a significantly higher rate of MI over time compared with subjects with normal cholesterol levels, then even stronger evidence is available to substantiate the link between cholesterol and MI. Finally, *intervention trials* may be designed to alter the potentially causative condition and to determine the effect of this change on the resultant condition. For example, patients with elevated cholesterol levels may be divided into two groups: a group that uses a cholesterol-lowering drug or diet and a control group that uses no intervention. These two groups might also be compared with a third group of subjects with normal cholesterol levels. Over time, the rate of MI in each group would be determined. If the group receiving the cholesterol-lowering regimen has a significantly lower rate of MI than the group with continued elevations in cholesterol level, strong evidence of a link between cholesterol and MI is established.

Finally, the highest level of evidence is the *systematic review*. A systematic review is not a standard literature review in which the articles selected for review are based on the desires and search methods chosen by the author, often for convenience. In a systematic review, the topic in question is selected before the review begins. For example, the authors may state the question as follows: "As compared with subjects not taking cholesterol-lowering medications, do subjects taking such medications demonstrate a difference in the rate of myocardial infarction?" A specific search strategy is then determined to reveal as much potential data as possible to answer the stated question. The authors state specifically why research papers were included or excluded from the review. If possible, the data are subjected to meta-analysis, a statistical method that combines the results of multiple studies that address a similar research hypothesis. This provides a more robust evaluation of the overall data than one can glean from individual research articles.

At each level of evidence, it is important to determine whether a biologically plausible link exists between conditions A and B. For example, if case reports, cross-sectional studies, longitudinal studies, and intervention trials all support a link between cholesterol levels and MI, the following questions remain:

- How is cholesterol related to MI?
- What are the mechanisms by which cholesterol affects the cardiovascular system and, thus, increases the risk for MI?

These studies evaluate the mechanisms by which conditions A and B might be linked and provide explanatory data that further substantiate the association between the two conditions.

The focal infection theory, as proposed and defended during the early part of the 20th century, was based on almost no evidence. Only the occasional case report and other anecdotes were available to substantiate the theory. Although explanatory mechanisms were proposed, none were validated with scientific research. This theory predated current concepts of evidence-based clinical practice and led to the unnecessary extraction of millions of teeth. Currently, when reexamining the potential associations between oral infections and systemic conditions, it is important (1) to determine what evidence is available; (2) to determine what evidence is still needed to substantiate the associations; and (3) to validate the possible mechanisms of association. This chapter reviews current knowledge that relates periodontal infection to overall systemic health.

SUBGINGIVAL ENVIRONMENT AS A RESERVOIR FOR BACTERIA

The subgingival microbiota in patients with periodontitis provides a significant and persistent gram-negative bacterial challenge to the host that is met with a potent immunoinflammatory response.[126] These organisms and their products, such as *lipopolysaccharides* (LPSs), have ready access to the periodontal tissues and to the circulation via the sulcular epithelium, which is frequently ulcerated and discontinuous. Even with treatment, complete eradication of these organisms is difficult, and their reemergence is often rapid. The total surface area of pocket epithelium in contact with subgingival bacteria and their products in a patient with generalized moderate periodontitis has been estimated to be approximately the size of the palm of an adult hand, with even larger areas of exposure in cases of more advanced periodontal destruction.[131] Bacteremias are common after mechanical periodontal therapy, and they also occur frequently during normal daily function and oral hygiene procedures.[39,92,109] Just as the periodontal tissues mount an immunoinflammatory response to bacteria and their products, systemic challenges associated with these agents also induce a major vascular response.[35,59,139] This host response may offer explanatory mechanisms for interactions between periodontal infection and a variety of systemic disorders.

KEY FACT

The subgingival microbiota in patients with periodontitis provides a significant and persistent gram-negative bacterial challenge to the host. These organisms and their products, such as LPSs, have access to the periodontal tissues and to the circulation via ulcerations in the sulcular epithelium.

PERIODONTAL DISEASE AND MORTALITY

The ultimate medical outcome measure is mortality. A number of studies suggest that an increased mortality rate from various causes is associated with inflammatory periodontal diseases.[e] The Normative Aging Study examined 2280 healthy men every 3 years for longer than 30 years after baseline clinical, radiographic, laboratory, and electrocardiographic examinations. A subset of this population was examined in the Veterans Affairs Dental Longitudinal Study to determine age-related changes in the oral cavity and identify risk factors for oral disease. Clinical examinations were performed, and alveolar bone level measurements were determined from full-mouth radiographs. The mean percentage of alveolar bone loss and mean probing depth were determined for each subject. From the original sample of 804 dentate, medically healthy subjects, a total of 166 died during the study.[46] Periodontal status at the baseline examination was a significant predictor of mortality independent of other factors such as smoking, alcohol use, cholesterol levels, blood pressure, family history of heart disease, education level, and body mass.

---

eReferences 2, 20, 37, 46, 71, 89, 142.

For those subjects with the most alveolar bone loss (>21% alveolar bone loss at baseline), the risk of dying during the follow-up period was 70% higher than for all other subjects. Interestingly, alveolar bone loss increased the risk of mortality more than smoking (52% increased risk), which is a well-known risk factor for mortality. A later evaluation of these same subjects confirmed a higher incidence of CHD-related events such as MI and unstable angina among men younger than 60 years of age with alveolar bone loss compared with those without bone loss.[37]

In a prospective cohort study of 1400 dentate men from Northern Ireland, subjects were divided into thirds (tertiles) based on average periodontal attachment loss.[89] Those with the highest levels of periodontal attachment loss has a significantly higher risk of death compared with those with the least attachment loss. The mortality rate over a 9-year period was 15.7% in those with the greatest attachment loss and 7.9% in those with the lowest level of periodontal attachment loss. In these studies, periodontitis preceded and increased the risk of mortality. However, this finding only establishes an association; it does not confirm causation. It is possible that periodontal disease reflects other health behaviors not evaluated in this study rather than acting as a specific cause of mortality. In other words, patients with poor periodontal health may also have other risk factors that increase mortality rate (e.g., smoking).

When examining research that suggests oral health status is a possible risk factor for systemic conditions, it is important to recognize when other known risk factors for those systemic conditions have been accounted for in the analysis. Host susceptibility factors that place individuals at risk for periodontitis may also place them at risk for systemic diseases such as cardiovascular disease. In these patients, the association may actually be among the risk factors rather than among the diseases. For example, periodontitis and cardiovascular disease share risk factors such as smoking, age, race, male gender, and stress. Genetic risk factors may also be shared.[83] In the Veterans Affairs Dental Longitudinal Study, smoking was an independent risk factor for mortality. When the data were examined to determine whether periodontal status was a risk factor, smoking status and other known risk factors for mortality were removed from the equation to allow for the independent evaluation of periodontal status. Other studies support an association between poor oral health and an increased risk of mortality.[142] In a prospective longitudinal study of subjects with type 2 diabetes, those with severe periodontitis had 3.2 times the risk of death from ischemic heart disease or kidney disease as subjects without periodontitis or with only slight periodontitis, after adjusting for other risk factors, including age, sex, duration of diabetes, glycemic control, macroalbuminuria, body mass index, serum cholesterol concentration, hypertension, and current smoking.[142]

PERIODONTAL DISEASE, CORONARY HEART DISEASE, AND ATHEROSCLEROSIS

To further explore the association between periodontal disease and CHD or atherosclerosis, investigators have studied specific systemic disorders and medical outcomes to determine their relationship to periodontal status. The proceedings of the first international Workshop on Periodontitis and Systemic Disease held by the American Academy of Periodontology (AAP) and the European Federation of Periodontology (EFP) were published in 2013, a major focus of which was on the relationship between periodontitis and atherosclerotic cardiovascular disease.[32,38,136,147] CHD-related events are a major cause of death. MI has been associated with acute systemic bacterial and viral infections and is sometimes preceded by influenza-like symptoms.[102,159] Is it possible that oral infection is similarly related to MI? Traditional risk factors such as smoking, dyslipidemia, hypertension, and diabetes mellitus do not explain the presence of coronary atherosclerosis in a large number of patients. Localized infection that results in a chronic inflammatory reaction has been suggested as a mechanism underlying CHD in these individuals.[113]

In cross-sectional studies of patients with acute MI or confirmed CHD who were compared with age- and gender-matched control patients, patients with MI had significantly worse dental health (e.g., periodontitis, periapical lesions, caries, pericoronitis) than controls.[70,103,104] This association between poor dental health and MI was independent of known risk factors for heart disease, such as age, cholesterol levels, hypertension, diabetes, and smoking. Because atherosclerosis is a major determinant of CHD-related events, dental health has also been related to coronary atheromatosis. Mattila and colleagues[105] performed oral radiographic examinations and diagnostic coronary angiography on men with known CHD and found a significant correlation between the severity of dental disease and the degree of coronary atheromatosis. This relationship remained significant after accounting for other known risk factors for coronary artery disease. Similarly, Malthaner and colleagues[101] found an increased risk of angiographically defined coronary artery disease in subjects with greater bone loss and attachment loss; however, after adjusting for other known cardiovascular risk factors, the relationship between periodontal status and coronary artery disease was no longer statistically significant. There is evidence that the extent of periodontal disease may be associated with CHD. For example, there may be a greater risk for CHD-related events, such as MI, in subjects who have periodontitis affecting a greater number of teeth in the mouth compared with those who have periodontitis involving fewer teeth.[7]

Cross-sectional studies, thus, suggest a possible link between oral health and CHD; however, such studies cannot determine causality in this relationship. Rather, dental diseases may be indicators of general health practices. For example, periodontal disease and CHD are both related to lifestyle and share numerous risk factors, including smoking, diabetes, and low socioeconomic status. Bacterial infections have significant effects on endothelial cells, blood coagulation, lipid metabolism, and monocytes and macrophages.

Longitudinal studies provide compelling data regarding this relationship. According to a 7-year follow-up study of the patients by Mattila and colleagues, dental disease was significantly related to the incidence of new fatal and nonfatal coronary events as well as overall mortality.[106] In a prospective study of a national sample of adults, subjects with periodontitis had a 25% increased risk for CHD compared with those with no or minimal periodontal disease, after adjusting for other known risk factors.[36]

Among males between the ages 25 and 49 years, periodontitis increased the risk of CHD by 70%. The level of oral hygiene was also associated with heart disease. Patients with poor oral hygiene, as indicated by higher debris and calculus scores, had a twofold increased risk for CHD.

In another large prospective study, 1147 men were followed-up for 18 years.[11] During that time, 207 men (18%) developed CHD. When periodontal status at baseline was related to the presence or absence of CHD-related events during the follow-up period, a significant relationship was found. Subjects with more than 20% mean bone loss had a 50% increased risk of CHD compared with those with less than 20% bone loss. The extent of sites with probing depths greater than 3 mm was strongly related to the incidence of CHD. Subjects with probing depths greater than 3 mm on at least half of their teeth had a twofold increased risk, whereas those with probing depths of greater than 3 mm on all of their teeth had more than a threefold increased risk of CHD. This study and others in which the periodontal condition was known to have preceded the CHD-related events have supported the concept that periodontal disease is a risk factor for CHD, independent of other classic risk factors. Not all studies, however, support this concept; some show little independent effect of periodontal status on the risk for CHD after adjusting for commonly accepted cardiovascular risk factors.[65,66] It is particularly difficult to control for smoking as a confounding variable in these studies, because it is such an important risk factor for both periodontal disease and cardiovascular disease. This confounding influence of smoking makes it difficult to clarify the significance of the relationship between the diseases.

Perhaps the best evidence available comes from systematic reviews of studies examining the relationship between periodontal infection and cardiovascular disease. A systematic review and meta-analysis of data from 15 studies showed a significant 14% to 222% increase in the risk of CHD-related events in patients with periodontal disease as compared with those without periodontal disease.[9] A similar systematic review of longitudinal cohort and case-control studies showed a significant increase in the risk of incident MI, angina, or CHD-related death in subjects with periodontitis in five of the six studies reported.[38] This increased risk was noted mainly in younger subjects (i.e., <65 years old). Janket and colleagues[69] performed a meta-analysis of periodontal disease as a risk factor for future cardiovascular events and found an overall 19% increased risk of such events among individuals with periodontitis. The increase in risk was greater (44%) among people younger than 65 years of age. Although this increased risk is fairly modest, the extensive prevalence of periodontal disease in the population may increase the significance of the risk from a public health perspective. Extensive systematic reviews by Scannapieco and colleagues[143] and by an American Heart Association working group[91] concluded that a moderate degree of evidence exists to support an association between periodontal disease and atherosclerosis, MI, and cardiovascular disease independent of known confounders; however, causality is unclear. The results of the 2103 AAP/EFP Workshop on Periodontitis and Systemic Diseases concluded that "there is consistent and strong epidemiologic evidence that periodontitis

imparts increased risk for future cardiovascular disease," but whereas many studies support multiple biological mechanisms to explain this relationship, "intervention trials to date are not adequate to draw further conclusions."[170] That is, insufficient evidence exists to show that the treatment of periodontal disease has any impact on the risk of heart disease.

> **KEY FACT**
>
> There is consistent and strong epidemiologic evidence that periodontitis imparts increased risk for future cardiovascular disease.

Effects of Periodontal Infection

There are numerous mechanisms—both direct and indirect—through which periodontal infection may affect the onset or progression of atherosclerosis and CHD.[77,136,147] Periodontitis and atherosclerosis both have complex etiologic factors that combine genetic and environmental influences. In addition to smoking, the diseases share many risk factors and have distinct similarities with regard to their basic pathogenic mechanisms.

Ischemic Heart Disease

Ischemic heart disease is associated with the processes of atherogenesis and thrombogenesis (Fig. 14.1). Damage to the vascular endothelium, with a subsequent inflammatory reaction, plays a major role in atherosclerosis and ischemic organ damage.[170] Increased viscosity of blood may promote major ischemic heart disease and cerebrovascular accident (stroke) by increasing the risk of thrombus formation.[99] Fibrinogen is a major factor in

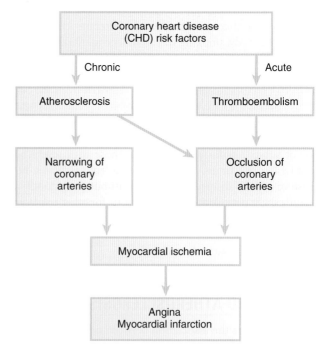

Fig. 14.1 Acute and Chronic Pathways to Ischemic Heart Disease. Coronary heart disease–related events, such as angina and myocardial infarction, may be precipitated by either pathway or both pathways.

Fig. 14.2 Factors That Affect Blood Viscosity in Health. *LDL,* Low-density lipoprotein; *VLDL,* very-low-density lipoprotein.

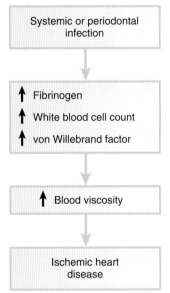

Fig. 14.3 The Effect of Infection on Blood Viscosity. Increased plasma fibrinogen and von Willebrand factor cause hypercoagulability. When they are combined with an increased white blood cell count, the blood viscosity increases, thereby increasing the risk of coronary ischemia.

the promotion of this hypercoagulable state. *Fibrinogen* is the precursor to fibrin, and increased fibrinogen levels increase blood viscosity. Increased plasma fibrinogen is a recognized risk factor for cardiovascular events and peripheral vascular disease (Fig. 14.2).[98] An elevated white blood cell count is also a predictor of heart disease and stroke, and circulating leukocytes may promote the occlusion of blood vessels. Coagulation factor VIII (von Willebrand factor) has likewise been associated with a risk of ischemic heart disease.[137]

Systemic Infections

Systemic infections are known to induce a hypercoagulable state and increase blood viscosity (Fig. 14.3). Fibrinogen levels and white blood cell counts are often increased in patients with periodontal disease.[22,88] Individuals with poor oral health may also have significant elevations in coagulation factor VIII/von Willebrand factor antigen, thereby increasing the risk of thrombus formation. Thus periodontal infection may also promote increased blood viscosity and thrombogenesis, which leads to an increased risk for central and peripheral vascular disease.

Daily Activity

Routine daily activities such as mastication and oral hygiene procedures result in frequent bacteremia with oral organisms.[92] Periodontal disease may predispose the patient to an increased incidence of bacteremia, including the presence of virulent gram-negative organisms associated with periodontitis. There is a greater risk of bacteremia after toothbrushing in patients with higher levels of plaque, calculus, and gingivitis as compared with those with minimal plaque and gingival inflammation.[93] In fact, subjects with generalized gingival bleeding after brushing showed an almost eightfold increase in their incidence of bacteremia as compared with those with minimal gingival bleeding. An estimated 8% of all cases of infective endocarditis are associated with periodontal or dental disease without a preceding dental procedure.[39] The periodontium, when affected by periodontitis, also acts as a reservoir of *endotoxins* (LPSs) from gram-negative organisms. Endotoxins can pass readily into the systemic circulation during normal daily function, thereby inducing damage to the vascular endothelium and precipitating many negative cardiovascular effects. In a study of the incidence of endotoxemia after simple chewing, subjects with periodontitis were four times more likely to have endotoxin present in the bloodstream than subjects without periodontitis. Furthermore, the concentration of endotoxin in the bloodstream was more than fourfold greater in those with periodontitis as compared with healthy subjects.[47]

Thrombogenesis

Platelet aggregation plays a major role in thrombogenesis, and most cases of acute MI are precipitated by thromboembolism. Oral organisms may be involved in coronary thrombogenesis. Platelets selectively bind some strains of *Streptococcus sanguinis,* which is a common component of supragingival plaque, and *Porphyromonas gingivalis,* which is a pathogen closely associated with periodontitis.[60,61] The aggregation of platelets is induced by the *platelet aggregation–associated protein* (PAAP) expressed on some strains of these bacteria.[140] In animal models, intravenous infusion of PAAP-positive bacterial strains resulted in alterations of heart rate, blood pressure, cardiac contractility, and electrocardiogram readings consistent with MI. Platelet accumulation also occurred in the lungs and led to tachypnea. No such changes were seen with the infusion of PAAP-negative strains. PAAP-positive bacteria caused aggregation of circulating platelets, which resulted in the formation of thromboemboli and resultant cardiac and pulmonary changes. Thus periodontitis-associated bacteremia with certain strains of *S. sanguinis* and *P. gingivalis* may promote acute thromboembolic events via interaction with circulating platelets.

Atherosclerosis

Atherosclerosis is a focal thickening of the arterial *intima,* the innermost layer lining the vessel lumen, and the *media,* the thick layer under the intima that consists of smooth muscle, collagen, and elastic fibers (Fig. 14.4).[140] The formation of atherosclerotic plaques is precipitated by damage to vascular endothelium that results in an inflammatory response in which circulating monocytes adhere to the vascular endothelium. Damage to vascular

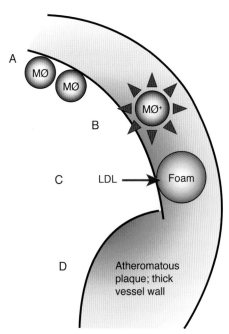

Fig. 14.4 Pathogenesis of Atherosclerosis. (A) Monocytes and macrophages *(MØ)* adhere to the vascular endothelium. (B) Monocytes and macrophages penetrate into the arterial media and produce proinflammatory cytokines and growth factors. (C) The ingestion of oxidized low-density lipoprotein *(LDL)* enlarges monocytes to form foam cells. (D) Smooth muscle proliferation and plaque formation thicken vessel walls and narrow the lumen. *MØ⁺*, Hyperinflammatory monocyte/macrophage phenotype.

endothelium can occur because of the presence of intravascular microorganisms and their products; chemical damage, often resulting from elements of tobacco and other exogenous toxins; and increased shear force along the vascular lining, such as that occurring in hypertension. The adherence of monocytes to the damaged vascular endothelium is mediated by several adhesion molecules on the endothelial cell surface, including intercellular adhesion molecule-1 (ICAM-1), endothelial leukocyte adhesion molecule-1 (ELAM-1), and vascular cell adhesion molecule-1 (VCAM-1).[12,80] These adhesion molecules are upregulated by a number of factors, including bacterial LPSs, prostaglandins, and proinflammatory cytokines. After binding to the endothelial cell lining, monocytes penetrate the endothelium and migrate under the arterial intima. The monocytes ingest circulating low-density lipoprotein in its oxidized state and become engorged, thereby forming the foam cells that are characteristic of atheromatous plaque. After entering the arterial media, monocytes may also transform to macrophages.

A host of proinflammatory cytokines such as interleukin-1 (IL-1), tumor necrosis factor α (TNF-α), and prostaglandin E₂ (PGE₂) are then produced, and they propagate the atheromatous lesion. Mitogenic factors such as fibroblast growth factor and platelet-derived growth factor stimulate smooth muscle and collagen proliferation within the media, thereby thickening the arterial wall.[98] Atheromatous plaque formation and thickening of the vessel wall narrow the lumen and dramatically decrease blood flow through the vessel.[140] Arterial thrombosis often occurs after an atheromatous plaque ruptures. Plaque rupture exposes

circulating blood to arterial collagen and tissue factor from monocytes and macrophages that activate platelets and the coagulation pathway. Platelet and fibrin accumulation forms a thrombus that may occlude the vessel and result in an ischemic event such as angina or MI. The thrombus may separate from the vessel wall and form an embolus, which may also occlude vessels, again leading to an acute event such as MI or cerebral infarction (stroke).

Role of Periodontal Disease in Atherosclerotic Myocardial or Cerebral Ischemia

In animal models, gram-negative bacteria and associated LPSs cause infiltration of inflammatory cells into the arterial wall, proliferation of arterial smooth muscle, and intravascular coagulation. These changes are identical to those seen with naturally occurring atheromatosis. There is strong evidence that periodontal bacteria disseminate from the oral cavity to the systemic vasculature, can be found within distant tissues, and can live within those affected tissues.[136] Furthermore, in animal models, dissemination of periodontal bacteria can induce atherosclerosis in distant vessels. Patients with periodontitis are at increased risk for thickening of the walls of the major coronary arteries.[11] In several studies of atheromas obtained from humans during endarterectomy, more than half of the lesions contained periodontal pathogens, and many atheromas contained multiple different periodontal species.[21,57,181] Periodontal diseases result in chronic systemic exposure to products of these organisms. Low-level bacteremia may initiate host responses that alter coagulability, endothelial and vessel wall integrity, and platelet function, thereby resulting in atherogenic changes and possible thromboembolic events (Fig. 14.5).

> ### CLINICAL CORRELATION
> There is strong evidence that periodontal bacteria disseminate from the oral cavity to the systemic vasculature, can be found within distant tissues, and can live within those affected tissues.

Research has clearly shown a wide variation in host response to bacterial challenge. Some individuals with heavy plaque accumulation and high proportions of pathogenic organisms appear relatively resistant to bone and attachment loss. Others develop extensive periodontal destruction in the presence of small amounts of plaque and low proportions of putative pathogens. Patients with an abnormally exuberant inflammatory response often have a hyperinflammatory monocyte and macrophage phenotype (MØ⁺). Monocytes and macrophages from these individuals secrete significantly increased levels of proinflammatory mediators (e.g., IL-1, TNF-α, PGE₂) in response to bacterial LPSs compared with patients with a normal monocyte and macrophage phenotype. Patients with aggressive periodontitis, refractory periodontitis, and type 1 diabetes mellitus often possess the MØ⁺ phenotype,[13] which appears to be under both genetic and environmental control.

The monocyte and macrophage cell line is intimately involved in the pathogenesis of both periodontal disease and atherosclerosis.

Fig. 14.5 The Influence of Periodontal Infection on Atherosclerosis. Periodontal pathogens and their products result in damage to the vascular endothelium. Monocytes and macrophages enter the vessel wall and produce cytokines that further increase the inflammatory response and propagate the atheromatous lesion. Growth factor production leads to smooth muscle proliferation in the vessel wall. Damaged endothelium also activates platelets, thereby resulting in platelet aggregation and potentiating thromboembolic events. *LPS,* Lipopolysaccharide.

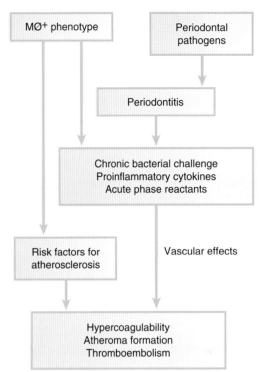

Fig. 14.6 The Cardiovascular and Periodontal Consequences of the Hyperresponsive Monocyte/Macrophage Phenotype *(MØ⁺)*. In combination with other risk factors, the MØ⁺ phenotype predisposes individuals to both atherosclerosis and periodontitis. Bacterial products and inflammatory mediators associated with periodontitis affect vascular endothelium, monocytes and macrophages, platelets, and smooth muscle and may increase blood coagulability. This may further increase atherosclerosis and may result in thromboembolism and ischemic events.

Diet-induced elevations in serum low-density lipoprotein levels upregulate monocyte and macrophage responsiveness to bacterial LPSs. Thus elevated low-density lipoprotein levels, which is a known risk factor for atherosclerosis and CHD, may increase the secretion of destructive and inflammatory cytokines by monocytes and macrophages. This may result not only in the propagation of atheromatous lesions but also in enhanced periodontal destruction in the presence of pathogenic organisms. This is one example of a potential shared mechanism in the pathogenesis of cardiovascular and periodontal diseases. The presence of an MØ⁺ phenotype may place patients at risk for both CHD and periodontitis (Fig. 14.6). Periodontal infections may contribute to atherosclerosis and thromboembolic events by repeatedly challenging the vascular endothelium and arterial wall with bacterial LPSs and proinflammatory cytokines. Vascular monocytes and macrophages in patients with an MØ⁺ phenotype meet this challenge with an abnormally elevated inflammatory response that may directly contribute to atherosclerosis and may precipitate thromboembolic events.[110]

Cardiovascular diseases are increasingly recognized as having a major systemic inflammatory component, further emphasizing possible similarities with inflammatory periodontal diseases.[140] As such, the detection of systemic inflammatory markers plays an increasingly important role in risk assessment for vascular events such as MI and cerebral infarction. Acute-phase proteins

such as *C-reactive protein* (CRP) and fibrinogen are produced in the liver in response to inflammatory or infectious stimuli and act as inflammatory markers.[139] CRP induces monocytes and macrophages to produce tissue factor, which stimulates the coagulation pathway and increases blood coagulability. Increased fibrinogen levels may contribute to this process. CRP also stimulates the complement cascade, further exacerbating inflammation.

Elevations in serum CRP and fibrinogen levels are well-accepted risk factors for cardiovascular disease.[138,139] Research has focused on periodontitis as a potential trigger for systemic inflammation. Serum CRP and fibrinogen levels are often elevated in subjects with periodontitis as compared with subjects without periodontitis.[27,95,176] These acute-phase proteins may act as intermediary steps in the pathway from periodontal infection to cardiovascular disease (see Figs. 14.5 and 14.6). Thus periodontal diseases may have both direct effects on the major blood vessels (e.g., atheroma formation) and indirect effects that stimulate changes in the cardiovascular system (e.g., elevation of systemic inflammatory responses).

Interesting supportive evidence for these mechanisms can be derived from intervention trials in which serum levels of inflammatory mediators and markers are assessed before and after treatment that is aimed at decreasing periodontal inflammation. For example, in subjects with chronic periodontitis, serum levels of IL-6 and CRP are reduced after scaling and root planing.[33] A systematic review and meta-analysis of 25 intervention studies examining periodontitis patients with and without periodontal treatment demonstrated that periodontal treatment was associated with a significant reduction in serum levels of CRP, IL-6, fibrinogen, and TNF-α.[165] Inflammatory periodontal disease (compared with periodontal health) is also associated with altered vascular endothelial function.[34] Altered vascular endothelial function is a major risk factor for acute thrombotic events. After scaling and root planing with a resultant decrease in periodontal inflammation, markers of vascular health improve significantly over time.[34,169] The functional assessment of vascular endothelial function also returns to normal after scaling and root planing.[148,169] These results suggest that periodontal inflammation adversely affects the health of the vascular endothelium, whereas a reduction in inflammation improves endothelial health. Whether these changes directly impact the risk of acute cardiovascular events remains to be determined in prospective controlled clinical intervention trials over long periods; such studies do not currently exist.

Role of Periodontal Disease in Erectile Dysfunction

Erectile dysfunction (ED) is associated with endothelial dysfunction, and elevated levels of oxidative stress and systemic inflammation are common to both periodontal disease and ED. Studies have shown a relationship between ED and periodontitis. In a large case-control study of almost 200,000 subjects in Taiwan, those with ED were significantly more likely to have chronic periodontitis than those without ED, with an overall significant odds ratio of 3.35 after adjusting for confounding variables.[78] Other studies have supported these findings in smaller populations in other countries,[129,152,180] and a systematic review of four studies found a significant association between periodontitis and ED, with an odds ratio of 3.07.[172] An intervention trial was conducted in 120 subjects with ED and chronic periodontitis; 60 subjects received scaling and root planing, and 60 control subjects received no periodontal treatment.[1] Three months later, the treatment group had significant improvement in ED, whereas the control group had no change. These preliminary studies suggest a relationship between periodontitis and ED, but more research is needed to understand the mechanisms of interaction.

PERIODONTAL DISEASE AND STROKE

Ischemic cerebral infarction, or stroke, is often preceded by systemic bacterial or viral infection. In one study, patients with cerebral ischemia were five times more likely to have had a systemic infection within 1 week before the ischemic event than nonischemic control subjects.[52] Recent infection was a significant risk factor for cerebral ischemia; it was independent of other known risk factors such as hypertension, history of a previous stroke, diabetes, smoking, and CHD. Interestingly, the presence of systemic infection before the stroke resulted in significantly greater ischemia and a more severe postischemic neurologic defect than stroke not preceded by infection.[53] Stroke patients with a preceding infection had slightly higher levels of plasma fibrinogen and significantly higher levels of CRP compared with those without infection.

Periodontal Infection Associated With Stroke

Stroke is classified as either hemorrhagic or nonhemorrhagic. Nonhemorrhagic stroke, or ischemic stroke, is usually caused by thromboembolic events and cerebrovascular atherosclerosis, whereas hemorrhagic stroke often results from a vascular bleed such as an aneurysm. Periodontal disease has been associated primarily with an increased risk of nonhemorrhagic stroke. Numerous studies have shown that periodontal disease is associated with an increased risk of stroke. In a case-control study, subjects with severe periodontitis had a 4.3 times higher risk of stroke than subjects with mild or no periodontitis.[51] Severe periodontitis was a risk factor in men but not women, and in those younger but not older than 65 years of age. In a longitudinal study of 1137 dentate men who were followed for a mean of 24 years, subjects with greater than 20% mean radiographic bone loss at baseline were more than three times as likely to have a stroke than subjects with less than 20% bone loss.[74] There was a stronger effect of periodontitis on the risk for stroke among men younger than 65 years of age compared with older subjects. Both large epidemiologic studies and systematic reviews of the evidence have suggested an approximate threefold increased risk of stroke in subjects with periodontitis.[69,177]

As previously discussed, periodontal infection may contribute directly to the pathogenesis of atherosclerosis by providing a persistent bacterial challenge to the arterial endothelium, thereby contributing to the monocyte- and macrophage-driven inflammatory process that results in atheromatosis and narrowing of the vessel lumen. Furthermore, periodontal infection may stimulate a series of indirect systemic effects, such as elevated production of fibrinogen and CRP, which increases the risk of stroke (see Figs. 14.5 and 14.6). Finally, bacteremia with PAAP-positive bacterial strains from supragingival and subgingival plaque can increase platelet aggregation, thereby contributing to thrombus formation and subsequent thromboembolism, which is the leading cause of stroke.[110]

> **CLINICAL CORRELATION**
>
> Periodontal infection may contribute directly to the pathogenesis of atherosclerosis by providing a persistent bacterial challenge to the arterial endothelium, thereby contributing to the monocyte- and macrophage-driven inflammatory process that results in atheromatosis and narrowing of the vessel lumen.

PERIODONTAL DISEASE AND DIABETES MELLITUS

The relationship between diabetes mellitus and periodontal disease has been extensively examined. It is clear from epidemiologic research that diabetes increases the risk for and severity of periodontal diseases.[112] The biological mechanisms through which diabetes influences the periodontium are discussed in Chapter 13. The increased prevalence and severity of periodontitis typically seen in patients with diabetes—especially those with poor metabolic control—has led to the designation of periodontal disease as the "sixth complication" of diabetes.[94] In addition to the five "classic" complications of diabetes, the American Diabetes Association has officially recognized that periodontal disease is common among patients with diabetes, and its Standards of Care include taking a history of current or past dental infections as part of the physician's examination.[4] Since 2009, the American Diabetes Association's Standards of Medical Care in Diabetes have specifically recommended that physicians refer patients with diabetes to a dentist for a comprehensive dental and periodontal examination.[5]

Many studies have examined the effects of diabetes on the periodontium, whereas others have examined the effect of periodontal infection on the control of diabetes.[112] Such studies are difficult to perform because of the influence of ongoing medical management of diabetes during the study. The following questions remain:

- Does the presence or severity of periodontal disease affect the metabolic state of diabetic patients?
- Does periodontal treatment aimed at reducing the bacterial challenge and minimizing inflammation have a measurable effect on glycemic (blood glucose) control?

A review of four studies including more than 22,000 subjects found that the incidence of type 2 diabetes (i.e., new diagnoses) was significantly greater in individuals with periodontal disease than in those without periodontal disease.[15] In a longitudinal study of patients with type 2 diabetes, severe periodontitis was associated with the significant worsening of glycemic control over time.[162] Individuals with severe periodontitis at the baseline examination had a greater incidence of worsening glycemic control over a 2- to 4-year period as compared with those without periodontitis at baseline. In this study, periodontitis was known to have preceded the worsening of glycemic control. Periodontitis has also been associated with the classic complications of diabetes. Diabetic adults with severe periodontitis at baseline had a significantly greater incidence of kidney and macrovascular complications over the subsequent 1 to 11 years than did diabetic adults with only gingivitis or mild periodontitis.[168] This was true despite both groups' having similar glycemic control. One or more cardiovascular complications occurred in 82% of patients with severe periodontitis versus 21% of patients without severe periodontitis. Again, severe periodontitis preceded the onset of clinical diabetic complications in these subjects.

Among patients with diabetes and periodontitis, periodontal therapy may have beneficial effects on glycemic control.[41,112,151,154,164] This may be especially true for patients with relatively poor glycemic control and more advanced periodontal destruction before treatment. A large number of studies, starting as far back as 1960,[175] have examined the impact of periodontal therapy on glycemic control in patients with diabetes. Most of these studies compared scaling and root planing (with or without adjunctive systemic antibiotics) with no periodontal therapy and followed patients for several months to assess changes in glycemic control measured by glycated hemoglobin (HbA1c) values. Others included in the treatment regimen not only scaling and root planing but also extraction of periodontally hopeless teeth and even periodontal surgery. Many of these studies showed a significant improvement in glycemic control, as determined by

reductions in HbA1c values, in the periodontal treatment group compared with the nontreatment group.[55,81,120] Other studies showed minimal change in glycemic control in periodontally treated patients.[3,23,42,157]

When studies of similar treatment regimens demonstrate conflicting results, systematic reviews with meta-analyses of the data are essential to aid the clinician in evaluating the evidence. Numerous systematic reviews and meta-analyses have consistently shown that periodontal therapy is associated with a statistically significant and clinically relevant improvement in glycemic control in patients with diabetes and periodontitis.[41,151,164] However, clinicians must understand that individual patients may or may not have outcomes similar to the average outcome in any given study or systematic review. That is, treatment results vary from patient to patient, and clinicians should not expect the same result in all patients. These studies suggest that periodontal therapy is most likely to result in short-term improvement in glycemia in those patients with diabetes and with severe periodontitis and poor metabolic control who demonstrate marked reduction in periodontal inflammation after treatment. Conversely, individuals with moderately well-controlled diabetes or periodontitis who have less reduction in inflammation may demonstrate no or only minimal changes in glycemic control.

FLASH BACK

Periodontal disease was designated as the "sixth complication" of diabetes because of the increased prevalence and severity of periodontitis typically seen in patients with diabetes, especially those with poor metabolic control.

Most of the studies evaluating the treatment of periodontal disease and its impact on glycemic control have been performed in subjects with type 2 diabetes. However, research suggests that periodontal therapy may have a smaller impact on glycemic control in patients with type 1 diabetes than in those with type 2 disease.[16] In a study of subjects with type 1 and type 2 diabetes with periodontitis, periodontal therapy was associated with a significant improvement in glycemic control overall in those with type 2 diabetes but not in those with type 1 disease, despite improvement in the periodontal condition of both groups.[16]

It is common to observe wide interindividual variability in responses to various medical management approaches in patients with type 1 diabetes. Similarly, wide variability in the impact of periodontal therapy on glycemic control can be expected in the type 1 diabetic population. For example, a study of periodontal therapy in 65 people with type 1 diabetes and chronic periodontitis showed highly variable responses.[167] Although there was an overall improvement in periodontal health after therapy, approximately 35% of subjects had an improvement in glycemic control after treatment, 37% had no significant change, and 28% showed a deterioration of glycemic control. In this study, subjects were divided into those with better baseline glycemic control (i.e., glycated hemoglobin values <8.5%) and those with poorer glycemic control (i.e., glycated hemoglobin values ≥8.5%). Interestingly, twice as many subjects showed improved glycemic control among those whose glycemic control before periodontal treatment was poor compared with those among whom baseline glycemic control was good. Therefore the clinician may anticipate a greater glycemic response to periodontal therapy among those patients with type 1 diabetes whose glycemic control is relatively poor than among those whose glycemic control is already good before periodontal treatment.

Although the routine use of systemic antibiotics for treatment of chronic periodontitis is not justified, patients with poorly controlled diabetes and severe periodontitis may constitute one patient group for whom such therapy is appropriate. Antibiotics remain an adjunct to the necessary mechanical removal of plaque and calculus. The mechanisms by which adjunctive antibiotics may induce positive changes in glycemic control when they are combined with mechanical debridement are unknown at this time. Systemic antibiotics may eliminate residual bacteria after scaling and root planing, thereby further decreasing the bacterial challenge to the host. Tetracyclines are also known to suppress the glycation of proteins and decrease the activity of tissue-degrading enzymes such as matrix metalloproteinases. These changes may contribute to improvements in the metabolic control of diabetes.

Periodontal Infection Associated With Glycemic Control in Diabetes

An understanding of the effects of other infections is useful to delineate the mechanisms by which periodontal infection influences glycemia. It is well known that systemic inflammation plays a major role in insulin sensitivity and glucose dynamics. As discussed previously, periodontal diseases can induce or perpetuate an elevated systemic chronic inflammatory state, which is reflected in increased serum CRP, IL-6, and fibrinogen levels seen in many people with periodontitis.[33,95,163] Inflammation induces insulin resistance, and such resistance often accompanies systemic infections. For example, acute nonperiodontal bacterial and viral infections have been shown to increase insulin resistance and aggravate glycemic control.[141,178] This occurs in individuals either with or without diabetes. Systemic infections increase tissue resistance to insulin through a variety of mechanisms, thereby preventing glucose from entering target cells, causing elevated blood glucose levels, and requiring increased pancreatic insulin production to maintain normoglycemia. Insulin resistance may persist for weeks or even months after the patient has recovered clinically from the illness. In an individual with type 2 diabetes who already has significant insulin resistance, further tissue resistance to insulin as a result of infection may considerably exacerbate poor glycemic control.

It is possible that chronic gram-negative periodontal infections may also result in increased insulin resistance and poor glycemic control.[54,163] In patients with periodontitis, persistent systemic challenge with periodontopathic bacteria and their product results in an upregulation of the immunoinflammatory response, with elevation in serum levels of proinflammatory mediators such as IL-1β, TNF-α, and IL-6, similar to well-recognized systemic infections but on a more persistent, chronic basis (Fig. 14.7). Increased serum levels of several cytokines, including TNF-α and IL-6, are associated with increased insulin resistance. This mechanism would explain the worsening of glycemic control associated with severe periodontitis. Periodontal

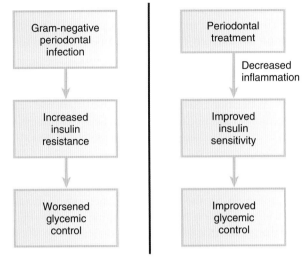

Fig. 14.7 Potential Effects of Periodontal Infection and Periodontal Therapy on Glycemia in Patients With Diabetes.

treatment designed to decrease the bacterial insult and reduce inflammation may result in decreased systemic inflammation, restoring insulin sensitivity over time and thereby resulting in improved metabolic control. The improved glycemic control seen in many studies of periodontal therapy would support such a hypothesis. This mechanism may also explain differences in the glycemic response to periodontal therapy between individuals with type 1 and type 2 diabetes.[16] Because type 2 diabetes is strongly associated with insulin resistance, periodontal therapy that reduces systemic inflammation may improve insulin sensitivity and result in improved glycemic control. Conversely, type 1 diabetes is not strongly associated with insulin resistance, so reduced inflammation after periodontal therapy may not have a major effect on insulin sensitivity in patients with type 1 disease, which would minimize the impact of periodontal treatment in these patients.

PERIODONTAL DISEASE AND ASTHMA

Evidence evaluating the relationship between periodontal disease and asthma is relatively sparse. The largest study has been a case-control study of 220 adults, half with severe asthma and half without asthma.[50] After adjusting for age, smoking habit, education level, and body mass index, people with periodontitis were 4.8 times more likely to have severe asthma than those without periodontitis. Although this study does not demonstrate causation, it suggests a possible link between inflammatory periodontal disease and asthma in adults.

PERIODONTAL MEDICINE IN CLINICAL PRACTICE

The concept of periodontal diseases as localized entities that affect only the teeth and the supporting apparatus is oversimplified. Rather than being confined to the periodontium, inflammatory periodontal diseases may have wide-ranging systemic effects. In most people, these effects are relatively inconsequential, or at least not clinically evident. In susceptible individuals, however, periodontal infection may act as an independent risk factor for systemic disease, and it may be involved in the basic pathogenic mechanisms of these conditions. Furthermore, periodontal infection may exacerbate existing systemic disorders.

Periodontal Disease and Systemic Health

Proper use of the knowledge of potential relationships between periodontal disease and systemic health requires the dental professional to recognize the oral cavity as one of many interrelated organ systems. A palm-sized infection on the leg of a pregnant woman would be of major concern to the patient and her health care provider, given the potential negative consequences of this localized infection on fetal and maternal health. Similarly, a suppurating infection on the foot of a person with diabetes would be cause for immediate evaluation and aggressive treatment, considering the effects of such infections on the metabolic control of diabetes.

Periodontal infection must be viewed in a similar manner. Periodontitis is a gram-negative infection that often results in severe inflammation, and it potentially involves the intravascular dissemination of microorganisms and their products throughout the body. However, periodontitis tends to be a "silent" disease until destruction results in acute oral symptoms. Most patients— and many medical professionals—do not recognize the potential infection that may exist within the oral cavity.

Patient Education

Patient education is a priority. Only 30 years ago, the factors involved in CHD were unclear. At present, however, it would be difficult to find an individual who was unfamiliar with the link between cholesterol and heart disease. This change was precipitated by research that clearly demonstrated the increased risk for heart disease among individuals with high cholesterol levels, followed by intensive education efforts to spread the message from the scientific community to the public at large. It is important to recognize that high cholesterol levels have not been shown to *cause* heart disease in all individuals; rather, they significantly *increase the risk* of disease. Cholesterol has also been demonstrated to have a biologically plausible role in the pathogenesis of CHD.

Similarly, patient education efforts in the realm of periodontal medicine must emphasize the inflammatory nature of periodontal infections, the increased risk for systemic disease associated with the infection, and the biologically plausible role that periodontal infection may play in systemic disease. Few individuals had their cholesterol levels evaluated until knowledge of the link between cholesterol and heart disease became widespread. Likewise, an increased appreciation of the potential effects of periodontal infection on systemic health may result in increased patient demand for periodontal evaluation.

Enhanced community awareness may be derived from newspapers, magazines, and other lay sources. However, the most reliable origin of information should be dental and medical professionals, through daily contact with patients. A pregnant woman usually knows that infections may adversely affect her pregnancy. Individuals with diabetes generally know that infections impair glycemic control. However, many of these patients do not know that occult periodontal infections can have the same effect as more clinically evident infections. The dentist is responsible for diagnosing periodontal infections, providing appropriate treatment, and preventing disease recurrence or progression. Because many medical professionals are unfamiliar with the oral cavity and oral health research, dental professionals must reach out to the medical community to improve patient care through education and communication.[111] Likewise, patients must be educated about disease prevention. Just as patients know that lowering their cholesterol levels may decrease their risk for heart disease, similar knowledge regarding the prevention of periodontal infection should be emphasized. A physician would be remiss if he or she did not provide education about decreasing cholesterol level, losing weight, and ceasing a smoking habit to a patient at risk for CHD. Likewise, controlling the risk factor of periodontal infection requires the dental hygienist to emphasize personal and professional preventive measures that are focused on oral hygiene and regular recall.

CONCLUSIONS

Does periodontal disease *cause* CHD, COPD, or adverse pregnancy outcomes? This question may be answered only by the use of the evidence that is currently available, with the full knowledge that conclusions may change as future evidence dictates. Periodontal disease may increase the risk for many systemic disorders. Biologically plausible mechanisms support the role of periodontal infection in these conditions, but it should not be presented as the cause of such systemic diseases, any more than cholesterol should be said to cause heart disease. Periodontal infection is one of many potential risk factors for a number of systemic conditions. Fortunately, it is a readily modifiable risk factor, unlike age, gender, and genetic influences.

The focal infection theory of the early 20th century was widely and appropriately discredited when treatment based on the theory, which consisted almost solely of tooth extraction, had no effect on the underlying diseases that oral sepsis supposedly caused. Similarly, the clinical utility of our current knowledge base is only now evolving. Future research will further delineate the role of periodontal infection in systemic health. The associations between periodontal infection and conditions such as LBW delivery, diabetes, cardiovascular and cerebrovascular diseases, and respiratory diseases may be further substantiated. Longitudinal studies and intervention trials are needed before any causative role can be assigned.

The field of periodontal medicine offers new insights into the concept of the oral cavity as one system that is interconnected with the whole human body. For many years, the dental profession has recognized the effects of systemic conditions on the oral cavity. Only now, however, are dental professionals beginning to understand more fully the impact of the periodontium on systemic health.

Finally, it is important to appreciate the differences between the science and the art of dental practice as they relate to periodontal medicine. Science is based, in general, on means and standard deviations or standard errors. Thus science may determine that, on average, diabetic patients with periodontal disease have poorer glycemic control than diabetic patients who are periodontally healthy. However, the patient who is sitting in the dental chair at any given time may or may not be a "mean" patient: in other words, she may or may not demonstrate the same relationship that science has determined to exist as an average within the population. She may lie somewhere within or outside the standard deviation. She may have extremely poor glycemic control that is directly related to her extensive periodontal inflammation; she may have average glycemic control; or she may have good glycemic control. The clinical practice of periodontal medicine recognizes that, using an evidence-based approach is key to modern dentistry, each patient is an individual, and he or she may not always fit the average determined by science.

Case Scenarios are found on the companion website.

REFERENCES

References for this chapter are found on the companion website.

Defense Mechanisms of the Gingiva[a]

The gingival tissue is continuously subjected to challenges, influencing the host response type. The epithelial surface, immune response, crevicular fluid, and saliva provide active responses to maintain gingival health. Chapter 4 reviews the role of the epithelium, including its degree of keratinization and its cellular turnover rate. This chapter describes important mechanisms of the gingival response repertoire, including the role of sulcular fluid, junctional epithelium, permeability, sulcular epithelia, sulcular fluid, saliva, and leukocytes.

SULCULAR FLUID

Sulcular fluid, or *gingival crevicular fluid* (GCF), contains an array of biologic mediators, cells, and bacteria. Recognized since the 19th century, its possible role in oral defense was first elucidated by the pioneering work of Waerhaug[110] and Brill and Krasse[14] during the 1950s. The latter investigators applied filter paper to the gingival sulci of dogs that had previously been injected intramuscularly with fluorescein. In this research, within 3 minutes, the fluorescent material was recovered on the paper strips. This reaction indicated the passage of fluid from the bloodstream through the tissues and the exiting of fluid via the gingival sulcus.

In subsequent studies, Brill[11,12] confirmed the presence of GCF in humans and considered it as "transudate." However, others[67,111] demonstrated that GCF is an inflammatory exudate rather than a continuous transudate. In strictly normal gingiva, little or no fluid can be collected.

More recently, interest in the development of tests for the detection or prediction of periodontal disease has resulted in numerous research papers about the components, origin, and function of GCF.[19] Potential markers from crevicular fluid are now used as diagnostic tools for the activity of periodontal diseases and a return to homeostasis, with potential for the evaluation of systemic markers.

Methods of Collection

The most difficult hurdle to overcome when collecting GCF is the scarcity of material that can be obtained from the sulcus. Many collection methods have been tried.[10,13,55,58,69,71,95] These methods include the use of absorbing paper strips, the placement of twisted threads around and into the sulcus, and techniques involving micropipettes and intracrevicular washings. There are limitations to the techniques, including fluid collection, collection time, flow rate, contamination, and reproducibility.

When using the absorbing paper strips to collect GCF, the paper strips are placed within the sulcus (intrasulcular method) or at its entrance (extrasulcular method) (Fig. 15.1). Placement of the filter paper strip in relation to the sulcus or pocket is important. The Brill technique involves inserting it into the pocket until resistance is encountered (see Fig. 15.1A). This method produces some degree of irritation of the sulcular epithelium that by itself can trigger the flow of fluid.

To minimize this irritation, Löe and Holm-Pedersen[67] placed the filter paper strip just at or over the pocket entrance (see Fig. 15.1B to C). In this way, fluid that seeps out is picked up by the strip, but the sulcular epithelium is not in contact with the paper.

Weinstein and colleagues[111] used pre-weighed twisted threads to collect GCF. The threads were placed in the gingival crevice around the tooth, and the amount of fluid collected was estimated by weighing the sample thread.

The use of micropipettes permits the collection of GCF by capillarity. Capillary tubes of standardized length and diameter are placed in the pocket, and their contents are later centrifuged and analyzed.[10,11,13]

Crevicular washings can be used to study GCF from clinically normal gingiva. One method involves the use of an appliance

---

[a]Adapted from the following chapter of Newman and Carranza's Clinical Periodontology, 13th edition: Chapter 16: Defense Mechanisms of the Gingiva, by Marcelo Freire, Jaime Bulkacz, and Fermin A. Carranza.

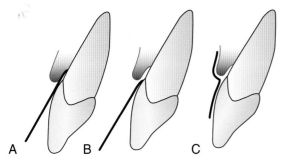

Fig. 15.1 Placement of a Filter Strip in the Gingival Sulcus for the Collection of Fluid. (A) Intrasulcular method. (B and C) Extrasulcular methods.

that consists of a hard acrylic plate that covers the maxilla, with soft borders and a groove that follows the gingival margins; it is connected to four collection tubes. Washings are obtained by rinsing the crevicular areas from one side to the other with the use of a peristaltic pump.[20]

A modification of the previous method involves the use of two injection needles that have been fitted one within the other so that, during sampling, the inside (ejection) needle is at the bottom of the pocket and the outside (collecting) needle is at the gingival margin. The collection needle is drained into a sample tube via continuous suction.[95]

Permeability of Junctional and Sulcular Epithelia

The initial studies by Brill and Krasse[14] involving the use of fluorescein were later confirmed with substances such as India ink[89] and saccharated iron oxide.[20] Substances that have been shown to penetrate the sulcular epithelium include albumin,[88] endotoxin,[87,92] thymidine,[46] histamine,[25] phenytoin,[105] and horseradish peroxidase.[73] These findings indicate permeability to substances with a molecular weight of up to 1000 kD.

Squier and Johnson[104] reviewed the mechanisms of penetration through an intact epithelium. The intercellular movement of molecules and ions along intercellular spaces appears to be a possible mechanism. Substances that take this route do not traverse the cell membranes.

Amount

The amount of GCF collected on a paper strip can be studied in multiple ways. The wetted area can be made more visible by staining with Ninhydrin; it is then measured planimetrically on an enlarged photograph or with a magnifying glass or a microscope.

An electronic method has been devised for measuring the fluid collected on a "blotter" (Periopaper) with the use of an electronic transducer (Periotron, Harco Electronics, Winnipeg, Manitoba, Canada). The wetness of the paper strip affects the flow of an electric current and provides a digital readout. A comparison between the Ninhydrin-staining method and the electronic method performed in vitro revealed no significant differences between the two techniques.[107]

The amount of GCF collected is extremely small. Measurements performed by Cimasoni[20] showed that a strip of paper 1.5-mm wide and inserted 1 mm within the gingival sulcus of a slightly inflamed gingiva absorbs about 0.1 mg of GCF in 3 minutes.

TABLE 15.1	Gingival Crevicular Fluid Diagnostic Tests	
Test Name	**Target**	**References**
Periocheck	Proteinases	Page RC: Host response tests designed for diagnosing periodontal disease. *J Periodontol* 63(4 Suppl):356–366, 1992.
Prognostik	Elastase	http://www.ncbi.nlm.nih.gov/pmc/articles/PMC3118084/
Biolise	Elastase	https://www.ncbi.nlm.nih.gov/pmc/articles/PMC3118084/
MMP dipstick	MMPs	Mäntylä P, Stenman M, Kinane DF, Tikanoja S, Luoto H, Salo T, Sorsa T: Gingival crevicular fluid collagenase-2 (MMP-8) test stick for chair-side monitoring of periodontitis. *J Periodontal Res* 38(4):436–439, 2003.
TOPAS	Bacterial toxins and proteases	http://www.ncbi.nlm.nih.gov/pmc/articles/PMC3118084/
Pocket watch	AST	Mäntylä P, Stenman M, Kinane DF, Tikanoja S, Luoto H, Salo T, Sorsa T: Gingival crevicular fluid collagenase-2 (MMP-8) test stick for chair-side monitoring of periodontitis. *J Periodontal Res* 38:436–439, 2003.

AST, Aspartate aminotransferase; *MMP,* mucous membrane pemphigoid; *TOPAS,* toxic oral pathology assay.

Challacombe[18] used an isotope dilution method to measure the amount of GCF present in a particular space at any given time. His calculations for human volunteers with mean gingival indices of less than 1 showed that the mean GCF volume in the proximal spaces from the molar teeth ranged from 0.43 to 1.56 μL.

Composition

The components of GCF are characterized by individual proteins, metabolites,[67,79,96] specific antibodies, antigens,[33,86] and enzymes of several specificities.[15] The GCF also contains cellular elements.[25,28,113]

Multiple research efforts have attempted to use GCF components to detect or diagnose active disease or to predict which patients are at risk for periodontal disease (Table 15.1).[3] So far, more than 40 compounds found in GCF have been analyzed,[83] but their origin is not known with certainty. These compounds can be derived from the host or produced by bacteria in the gingival crevice, but their source can be difficult to elucidate; examples include β-glucuronidase, which is a lysosomal enzyme, and lactic acid dehydrogenase, which is a cytoplasmic enzyme. The sources of collagenases may be fibroblasts or polymorphonuclear leukocytes (PMNs [neutrophils]),[5,81] or collagenases may be secreted by bacteria.[33] Phospholipases are lysosomal and cytoplasmic enzymes, but they are also produced by microorganisms.[15] The majority of GCF elements detected thus far have been enzymes, but there are nonenzymatic substances as well.

Cellular Elements

Cellular elements found in GCF include bacteria, desquamated epithelial cells, and leukocytes (i.e., PMNs, lymphocytes, and monocytes/macrophages), which migrate through the sulcular epithelium.[25,28]

Electrolytes

Potassium, sodium, and calcium have been studied in the GCF. Most studies have demonstrated a positive correlation of calcium and sodium concentrations with the sodium/potassium ratio seen with inflammation.[52-54] (For more information, see references 51 and 52.)

Organic Compounds

Both carbohydrates and proteins have been investigated as organic compounds within the GCF. Glucose hexosamine and hexuronic acid are two compounds that are found in GCF.[44] Blood glucose levels do not correlate with GCF glucose levels; glucose concentration in GCF is three to four times greater than that in serum.[44] This is interpreted not only as a result of the metabolic activity of adjacent tissues but also as a function of the local microbial flora.

The total protein content of GCF is much less than that of serum.[13,14] No significant correlations have been found between the concentration of proteins in GCF and the severity of gingivitis, pocket depth, or extent of bone loss.[8] Metabolic and bacterial products identified in GCF include lactic acid,[45] urea,[39] hydroxyproline,[85] endotoxins,[101] cytotoxic substances, hydrogen sulfide,[103] and antibacterial factors.[24] Many enzymes have also been identified.

The methodology used to analyze GCF components is as varied as the diversity of those components. Examples include fluorometry to detect metalloproteinases,[25] enzyme-linked immunosorbent assays (ELISAs) to detect enzyme levels and interleukin-1β (IL-1β),[65] radioimmunoassays to detect cyclooxygenase derivatives[80] and procollagen III,[108] high-performance liquid chromatography (HPLC) to detect tinidazole,[62] and direct and indirect immunodot tests to detect acute-phase proteins.[100]

Cellular and Humoral Activity in Gingival Crevicular Fluid

Monitoring periodontal disease is a complicated task, because few noninvasive procedures can follow the initiation and progress of the disease. Analyzing GCF constituents in health and disease may be extremely useful as a result of GCF's simplicity and because GCF can be obtained with noninvasive methods.

The analysis of GCF has identified cell and humoral responses in both healthy individuals and those with periodontal disease.[60] Cellular immune response includes the appearance of cytokines in GCF, but there is no clear evidence of a relationship between cytokines and disease. However, IL-1α and IL-1β are known to increase the binding of PMNs and monocytes/macrophages to endothelial cells, to stimulate the production of prostaglandin E_2 and the release of lysosomal enzymes, and to stimulate bone resorption.[63] Preliminary evidence also indicates the presence of interferon-α in GCF,[60] which may have a protective role in periodontal disease because of its ability to inhibit the bone resorption activity of IL-1β.[41]

Because the amount of fluid recoverable from gingival crevices is small, only the use of very sensitive immunoassays permits the analysis of the specificity of antibodies.[24,26,27] A study comparing antibodies in different crevices with serum antibodies, directed at specific microorganisms, did not provide any conclusive evidence regarding the significance of the presence of antibodies in GCF among individuals with periodontal disease.[60]

Although the role of antibodies in the gingival defense mechanisms is difficult to ascertain, the consensus is that in a patient with periodontal disease, a reduction in antibody response is detrimental, and an antibody response plays a protective role.[59]

Clinical Significance

As an exudate, GCF is a biologic fluid that has potential in diagnostics and disease management.[67] Its presence in clinically normal sulci can be explained, because gingiva that appears clinically normal invariably exhibits inflammation when it is examined microscopically. Commercially available kits for diagnosis are now available (see Table 15.1).

CLINICAL CORRELATION

- Novel diagnostic tools allow evaluations of biomarkers from tissue and oral biofluids.
- Drug delivery targeting oral tissues has optimal absorption and bioavailability.
- Gingival fluid and saliva are biologic fluids that can provide information on human genomics and metagenomics (microbiome, transcriptome, metabolome and proteome).
- Oral immunity is activated through rapid response from innate immune components (fluids, mucosal surfaces, epithelium, cell mediators, molecules, host–bacterial interactions).

The amount of GCF is greater when inflammation is present,[32,98] and is sometimes proportional to the severity of inflammation.[82] GCF production is not increased by trauma from occlusion,[72] but it is increased by the mastication of coarse foods, toothbrushing and gingival massage, ovulation,[65] hormonal contraceptives,[66] prosthetic appliances,[77] and smoking.[74] Other factors that influence the amount of GCF are circadian periodicity and periodontal therapy.

Circadian Periodicity

There is a gradual increase in the amount of GCF from 6 a.m. to 10 p.m., and a decrease thereafter.[9]

Sex Hormones

Female sex hormones increase GCF flow, probably because they enhance vascular permeability.[63] Pregnancy, ovulation,[62] and hormonal contraceptives[64] all increase GCF production.

Mechanical Stimulation

Chewing[11] and vigorous gingival brushing stimulate the flow of GCF. Even minor stimuli represented by intrasulcular placement of paper strips increases the production of fluid.

Smoking

Smoking produces an immediate transient but marked increase in GCF flow but, in the long term, a decrease of salivary and GCF flow.[74]

Periodontal Therapy

There is an increase in GCF production during the healing period after periodontal surgery.[4]

Drugs in Gingival Crevicular Fluid

Drugs that are excreted through the GCF may be used advantageously in periodontal therapy. Bader and Goldhaber[7] demonstrated in dogs that tetracyclines are excreted through the GCF; this finding triggered extensive research that showed a concentration of tetracyclines in GCF as compared with serum.[40] Metronidazole is another antibiotic that has been detected in human GCF[29] (see Chapter 47).

LEUKOCYTES IN THE DENTOGINGIVAL AREA

Leukocytes have been found in clinically healthy gingival sulci in humans and experimental animals. The leukocytes found are predominantly PMNs. They appear in small numbers extravascularly in the connective tissue adjacent to the apical portion of the sulcus; from there, they travel across the epithelium[17,42] to the gingival sulcus, where they are expelled (Figs. 15.2 and 15.3).

Leukocytes are present in sulci even when histologic sections of adjacent tissue are free of inflammatory infiltrate.[91]

Mononuclear cells identified as 58% B lymphocytes, 24% T lymphocytes, and 18% mononuclear phagocytes are present in the sulci. The ratio of T lymphocytes to B lymphocytes was found to be reversed from the normal ratio of about 3:1 found in peripheral blood to about 1:3 in GCF.[113]

Leukocytes are attracted by different plaque bacteria,[50,112] but they can also be found in the dentogingival region of germ-free adult animals.[68,94] Leukocytes were reported in the gingival sulcus in non-mechanically irritated (resting) healthy gingiva, thereby indicating that their migration may be independent of an increase in vascular permeability.[6] The majority of these cells are viable and have phagocytic and killing capacity.[57,84,90] Therefore leukocytes constitute a major protective mechanism against the extension of plaque into the gingival sulcus.

Live and dead leukocytes are found in saliva; this is discussed later in this chapter. The main port of entry of leukocytes into the oral cavity is the gingival sulcus.[97]

SALIVA

Saliva has protective functions and maintains the oral tissues in a physiologic state (Table 15.2). Saliva exerts a major influence on plaque by mechanically cleansing the exposed oral surfaces, buffering acids produced by bacteria, and modulating bacterial activity with immune mediators.[78] Saliva is now considered a main biologic fluid for diagnosis of human health and diseases. Systemic and local disease markers are available through saliva. Available tests allow the individual to measure multi-omics outputs.[22] Functional and static assays are now available as biosensors of health and disease.

Antibacterial Factors

Saliva carries inorganic and organic factors that influence bacteria and their products in the oral environment. Inorganic factors include ions and gases, bicarbonate, sodium, potassium, phosphates, calcium, fluorides, ammonium, and carbon dioxide.

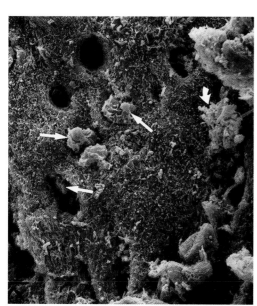

Fig. 15.2 Scanning Electron Microscope View of the Periodontal Pocket Wall. Several leukocytes are emerging *(straight arrows)*, some of which are partially covered by bacteria *(curved arrow)*. Empty holes correspond to tunnels through which leukocytes have emerged.

Fig. 15.3 Scanning Electron Microscope View at Higher Magnification Than Shown in Fig. 15.2. A leukocyte emerging from the pocket wall is covered with bacteria *(small arrows)*. The *large curved arrow* points to a phagosomal vacuole through which bacteria are being engulfed.

TABLE 15.2   Role of Saliva in Oral Health

Function	Salivary Components	Probable Mechanism
Lubrication	Glycoproteins, mucoids	Coating similar to gastric mucin
Physical protection	Glycoproteins, mucoids	Coating similar to gastric mucin
Cleansing	Physical flow	Clearance of debris and bacteria
Buffering	Bicarbonate and phosphate	Antacids
Tooth integrity maintenance	Minerals	Maturation, remineralization
	Glycoprotein pellicle	Mechanical protection
Antibacterial action	Immunoglobulin A	Control of bacterial colonization
	Lysozyme	Breaking of bacterial cell walls
	Lactoperoxidase	Oxidation of susceptible bacteria

Organic factors include lysozyme, lactoferrin, myeloperoxidase, lactoperoxidase, defensins, peptides, and agglutinins such as glycoproteins, mucins, β2-macroglobulins, fibronectins,[108] and antibodies.

Lysozyme is a hydrolytic enzyme that cleaves the linkage between structural components of the glycopeptide muramic acid–containing region of the cell wall of certain bacteria in vitro. Lysozyme works on both gram-negative and gram-positive organisms[47]; its targets include *Veillonella* species and *Actinobacillus actinomycetemcomitans*. It works on the molecular level, protecting the oral cavity and repelling transient bacterial invaders.[49]

The *lactoperoxidase–thiocyanate system* in saliva has been shown to be bactericidal to some strains of *Lactobacillus* and *Streptococcus*[76,93] by preventing the accumulation of lysine and glutamic acid, both of which are essential for bacterial growth. Another antibacterial finding is lactoferrin, which is effective against *Actinobacillus* species.[51]

Myeloperoxidase, an enzyme that is similar to salivary peroxidase, is released by leukocytes; it is bactericidal for *Actinobacillus*,[75] but it has the added effect of inhibiting the attachment of *Actinomyces* strains to hydroxyapatite.[21]

Human α and β-defensins (hBD)-1,-2,-3 are a family of low-molecular-weight antimicrobial peptides. Produced by a number of cells, including neutrophils, they amplify and combat bacterial[1] infections important to homeostasis.

Salivary Antibodies

As with GCF, saliva contains antibodies that are reactive with indigenous oral bacterial species. Although immunoglobulins G (IgG) and M (IgM) are present, the preponderant immunoglobulin found in saliva is *immunoglobulin A* (IgA), whereas IgG is more prevalent in GCF.[106] Major and minor salivary glands contribute all of the secretory IgA and lesser amounts of IgG and IgM. GCF contributes most of the IgG, complement, and PMNs that, in conjunction with IgG or IgM, inactivate or opsonize bacteria.

Salivary antibodies appear to be synthesized locally because they react with bacteria that are indigenous to the mouth, but not with organisms that are characteristic of the intestinal tract.[34,36] Bacteria found in saliva are frequently associated with IgA, and the bacterial deposits on teeth contain both IgA and IgG in quantities that are greater than 1% of their dry weight.[35] It has been shown that IgA antibodies present in parotid saliva can inhibit the attachment of oral *Streptococcus* species to epithelial cells.[30,110] Gibbons and colleagues[34-36] suggested that antibodies in secretions may impair the ability of bacteria to attach to mucosal or dental surfaces.

> ### FLASH BACK
>
> Saliva was known to have protective actions against infection through immunoglobulins only. Now it is clear that enzymes, cytokines, nucleotides, and live cells are part of the host armamentarium.

Enzymes

The *enzymes* that are normally found in saliva are derived from the salivary glands, bacteria, leukocytes, oral tissues, and ingested substances; the major enzyme is parotid amylase. Certain salivary enzymes have been reported in increased concentrations in periodontal disease: hyaluronidase and lipase,[16] β-glucuronidase and chondroitin sulfatase,[38] aspartate aminotransferase and alkaline phosphatase,[109] amino acid decarboxylases,[38] catalase, peroxidase, and collagenase.[56]

Proteolytic enzymes in the saliva are generated by both the host and oral bacteria. These enzymes have been recognized as contributors to the initiation and progression of periodontal disease.[46,70] To combat these enzymes, saliva contains antiproteases that inhibit cysteine proteases such as cathepsins[48] and antileukoproteases that inhibit elastase.[81] Another antiprotease, which has been identified as a tissue inhibitor of matrix metalloproteinase, has been shown to inhibit the activity of collagen-degrading enzymes.[23]

High-molecular-weight mucinous glycoproteins in saliva bind specifically to many plaque-forming bacteria. The glycoprotein–bacteria interactions facilitate bacterial accumulation on the exposed tooth surface.[30,34-36,112] The specificity of these interactions has been demonstrated. The interbacterial matrix of human plaque appears to contain polymers that are similar to salivary glycoproteins and may aid in maintaining the integrity of plaque. In addition, these glycoproteins selectively adsorb to the hydroxyapatite to make up part of the acquired pellicle. Other salivary glycoproteins inhibit the sorption of some bacteria to the tooth surface and to epithelial cells of the oral mucosa. This activity appears to be associated with the glycoproteins that possess blood group reactivity.[2,30,34,36,110] Another effect of mucin is the deletion of bacterial cells from the oral cavity via aggregation with mucin-rich films.

Glycoproteins and a glycolipid that is present on mammalian cell surfaces appear to serve as receptors for the attachment of some viruses and bacteria. Thus the close similarity between the glycoproteins of salivary secretions and the components of the epithelial cell surface suggests that the secretions can competitively inhibit antigen sorption and that they therefore may limit pathologic alterations.

Salivary Buffers and Coagulation Factors

The maintenance of physiologic hydrogen ion concentration (pH) at the mucosal epithelial cell surface and tooth surface is an important function of salivary buffers. The primary effect action of buffers has been investigated with relationship to dental caries. In saliva, the most important buffer is the bicarbonate–carbonic acid system.[69]

Saliva also contains coagulation factors (i.e., factors VIII, IX, and X; plasma thromboplastin antecedent; and Hageman factor) that hasten blood coagulation and protect wounds from bacterial invasion.[61] An active fibrinolytic enzyme may also be present.

Leukocytes

In addition to desquamated epithelial cells, saliva contains all forms of leukocytes, of which the principal cells are PMNs. Whole-blood PMNs are naïve and not activated, whereas the cells found in saliva have interacted with multiple antigens from the microbiome. The number of PMNs varies from person to person at different times of the day, and it is increased in the presence of gingivitis. PMNs reach the oral cavity by migrating through the lining of the gingival sulcus. Living PMNs in saliva are sometimes referred to as *orogranulocytes*, and their rate of migration into the oral cavity is termed the *orogranulocytic migratory rate*. Novel investigation presents the positive correlation between rate of PMN migration and the severity of gingival inflammation, and it is therefore a reliable index for the assessment of gingivitis.[102] In a high-throughput methods, distinct subsets of neutrophils were found in oral mucosa, including naïve, parainflammatory, and proinflammatory cells.[31]

CLINICIAN'S CORNER

What Is the Clinical Importance of Saliva?

Saliva has several important properties, including mechanical, chemical, biologic, and immunologic.[22] Saliva is a viscous, clear, watery fluid secreted from salivary glands, and is a major biologic fluid for diagnosis and "omics" research. Diagnosing local and systemic conditions is possible through salivary markers. Low saliva is a risk factor for caries and periodontal disease. Xerostomia is defined as dry mouth resulting from reduced or absent saliva flow. Xerostomia is a symptom of various medical conditions, and it is a side effect of radiation to the head and neck and a wide variety of medications.

BOX 15.1   Hallmarks of Xerostomia

Features	Healthy	Xerostomia
Flow rate	1–2 mL	<0.1 mg/mL
Sensation	Normal	Dry mouth
Consistency and texture	Resilient and lubricated	Erythematous, sticky

Role in Periodontal Pathology

Saliva modulates plaque initiation, maturation, and metabolism. Salivary flow and composition also influence calculus formation, periodontal disease, and caries. The removal of the salivary glands in experimental animals significantly increases the incidence of dental caries[37] and periodontal disease[43] in addition to delaying wound healing.[99]

In humans, increases of inflammatory gingival conditions, dental caries, rapid tooth destruction, and cervical or cemental caries are associated, at least partially, with decreased salivary gland secretion (xerostomia; Box 15.1). Xerostomia may result from sialolithiasis, sarcoidosis, Sjögren syndrome, Mikulicz disease, irradiation, surgical removal of the salivary glands, and other factors (see Chapters 24 and 35).

FLASH BACK

- Gingival tissue is constantly challenged by external factors.
- Epithelial surface, crevicular fluid, saliva, epithelial surfaces, immune cells, and mediators provide oral immunity.
- Oral diseases, including caries and periodontal diseases, benefit from oral immune components.

A Case Scenario is found on the companion website.

REFERENCES

 References for this chapter are found on the companion website.

Gingival Inflammation[a]

Local innate and specific immunity work to maintain gingival health. Components from the innate immune response include epithelial cells and nonspecific cells within the epithelium, mucins, lysozyme, lactoferrin, lactoperoxidase, and various antimicrobial peptides such as histatins, beta-defensins, and protease inhibitors. Epithelial cells (keratinocytes) are reactive and express a variety of receptors, including Toll-like receptors, and produce a variety of cytokines on activation.

The pathologic changes of gingivitis are initiated by a host response to oral microorganisms attached to the tooth and those in or near the gingival sulcus. These organisms are capable of synthesizing products (e.g., collagenase, hyaluronidase, protease, chondroitin sulfatase, endotoxin) that cause damage to epithelial and connective tissue cells, as well as to intercellular constituents such as collagen, ground substance, and glycocalyx (cell coat). The resultant widening of the spaces between junctional epithelial cells during early gingivitis may permit injurious agents derived from bacteria or bacteria themselves to gain access to the connective tissue.[10,44,48] Microbial products activate cells, including monocytes and macrophages, to produce vasoactive substances such as prostaglandin E2, interferon, tumor necrosis factor, and interleukin-1.[25,38] In addition, interleukin-1β alters the properties of gingival fibroblasts by delaying their death via mechanism-blocking apoptosis. This stabilizes the gingival fibroblast population during inflammation.[54]

Morphologic and functional changes in the gingiva during plaque accumulation have been thoroughly investigated, especially in beagle dogs and humans.[36] A useful framework for the organization and consideration of these data has been devised on the basis of histopathologic, radiographic, and ultrastructural features and biochemical measurements.[37,39] The sequence of events that culminates in clinically apparent gingivitis is categorized as the *initial*, *early*, and *established stages* of disease, with

periodontitis designated as the *advanced stage* (Table 16.1).[38] One stage evolves into the next, with no clear-cut dividing lines.

Despite extensive research, we still cannot definitively distinguish between normal gingival tissue and the initial stage of gingivitis.[36] Most biopsies of clinically normal human gingiva contain inflammatory cells; these consist predominantly of T cells, with very few B cells or plasma cells.[36,49,50] These cells do not create tissue damage, but they appear to be important in the day-to-day host response to bacteria and other substances to which the gingiva is exposed.[36] Under normal conditions, a constant stream of neutrophils is migrating from the vessels of the gingival plexus through the junctional epithelium, to the gingival margin, and into the gingival sulcus and the oral cavity.[43]

STAGE I GINGIVAL INFLAMMATION: THE INITIAL LESION

The first manifestations of gingival inflammation are vascular changes consisting of dilated capillaries and increased blood flow. These initial inflammatory changes occur in response to the microbial activation of resident leukocytes and the subsequent stimulation of endothelial cells. Clinically, this initial response of the gingiva to bacterial plaque (i.e., subclinical gingivitis[26]) is not apparent.

Microscopically, some classic features of acute inflammation can be seen in the connective tissue beneath the junctional epithelium. Changes in blood vessel morphologic features (e.g., widening of small capillaries or venules) and the adherence of neutrophils to vessel walls (margination) occur within 1 week, and sometimes as early as 2 days, after plaque has accumulated (Fig. 16.1).[18,41] The etiopathogenesis of gingival diseases is linked to local or systemic immune response, to innate or adaptive immunity, and to cellular or secretory factors. Leukocytes—mainly polymorphonuclear neutrophils (PMNs)—leave the capillaries by migrating through the walls via diapedesis and emigration (Fig. 16.2).[25,50,51] These can be seen in increased quantities in the connective tissue, the junctional epithelium, and the gingival sulcus (Figs. 16.3 and 16.4).[2,3,24,34,41,45,46] Exudation of fluid from the gingival sulcus[18] and extravascular proteins is present.[20,21]

[a]Adapted from the following chapter of Newman and Carranza's *Clinical Periodontology*, 13th edition, Chapter 17: Gingival Inflammation, by Joseph P. Fiorellini, David M. Kim, Marcelo Freire, Panagiota G. Stathopoulou, and Hector L. Sarmiento.

TABLE 16.1 Stages of Gingivitis

Stage	Time (Days)	Blood Vessels	Junctional and Sulcular Epithelia	Predominant Immune Cells	Collagen	Clinical Findings
I. Initial lesion	2–4	Vascular dilation Vasculitis	Infiltration by PMNs	PMNs	Perivascular loss	Gingival fluid flow
II. Early lesion	4–7	Vascular proliferation	Same as stage I Rete pegs Atrophic areas	Lymphocytes	Increased loss around infiltrate	Erythema Bleeding on probing
III. Established lesion	14–21	Same as stage II, plus blood stasis	Same as stage II but more advanced	Plasma cells	Continued loss	Changes in color, size, texture, and so on

PMNs, Polymorphonuclear leukocytes (neutrophils).

Fig. 16.1 Human Biopsy Sample, Experimental Gingivitis. After 4 days of plaque accumulation, the blood vessels immediately adjacent to the junctional epithelium are distended and contain polymorphonuclear leukocytes (neutrophils) *(PMNs)*. Neutrophils have also migrated between the cells of the junctional epithelium *(JE)*. *OSE,* Oral sulcular epithelium (magnification, ×500). (From Payne WA, Page RC, Ogilvie AL, et al: Histopathologic features of the initial and early stages of experimental gingivitis in man. *J Periodontal Res* 10:51, 1975.)

However, these findings are not accompanied by manifestations of tissue damage that are perceptible at the light microscopic or ultrastructural level; they do not form an infiltrate, and their presence is not considered to indicate pathologic change.[36]

Subtle changes can also be detected in the junctional epithelium and perivascular connective tissue at this early stage. For example, the perivascular connective tissue matrix becomes altered, and there is exudation and deposition of fibrin in the affected area.[36] In addition, lymphocytes soon begin to accumulate (see Fig. 16.2D). The increased migration of leukocytes, and their accumulation within the gingival sulcus, may be correlated with an increased flow of gingival fluid into the sulcus.[4]

The character and intensity of the host response determine whether this *initial lesion* resolves rapidly, with restoration of the tissue to a normal state; alternatively, it may evolve into a chronic inflammatory lesion. If the latter occurs, an infiltrate of macrophages and lymphoid cells appears within a few days.

STAGE II GINGIVAL INFLAMMATION: THE EARLY LESION

The *early lesion* evolves from the *initial lesion* within about 1 week after the beginning of plaque accumulation.[35,41] Clinically, the early lesion may appear as early gingivitis, and it overlaps with and evolves from the initial lesion with no clear-cut dividing line. As time goes on, clinical signs of erythema may appear, mainly because of the proliferation of capillaries and the increased formation of capillary loops between rete pegs or ridges (Fig. 16.5). Bleeding on probing may also be evident.[1] Gingival fluid flow and the numbers of transmigrating leukocytes reach their maximum between 6 and 12 days after the onset of clinical gingivitis.[26]

Microscopic examination of the gingiva reveals leukocyte infiltration in the connective tissue beneath the junctional epithelium, which consists mainly of lymphocytes (75%, with the majority being T cells)[41,47] but also includes some migrating neutrophils as well as macrophages, plasma cells, and mast cells. All of the changes seen in the initial lesion continue to intensify with the early lesion.[15,28,30,35,47] The junctional epithelium becomes densely infiltrated with neutrophils, as does the gingival sulcus, and may begin to show the development of rete pegs or ridges.

The amount of collagen destruction also increases[12,28,47]; 70% of the collagen is destroyed around the cellular infiltrate. The main fiber groups that are affected appear to be the circular and dentogingival fiber assemblies. Alterations in blood vessel morphologic features and vascular bed patterns have also been described.[18,19]

PMNs that have left the blood vessels in response to chemotactic stimuli from plaque components travel to the epithelium and cross the basement lamina; they are found in the epithelium, emerging in the pocket area (see Fig. 16.3). PMNs are attracted to bacteria and engulf them during the process of phagocytosis (Fig. 16.6). PMNs release their lysosomes in association with the ingestion of bacteria.[23] Fibroblasts show cytotoxic alterations,[40] with a decreased capacity for collagen.

Fig. 16.2 Human Biopsy, Experimental Gingivitis. (A) Control biopsy specimen from a patient with good oral hygiene and no detectable plaque accumulation. The junctional epithelium is on the left. The connective tissue *(CT)* shows few cells other than fibroblasts, blood vessels, and a dense background of collagen fibers (magnification, ×500). (B) Biopsy specimen taken after 8 days of plaque accumulation. The connective tissue is infiltrated with inflammatory cells, which displace the collagen fibers. A distended blood vessel *(V)* is seen in the center magnification (i.e., clear spaces around the cellular infiltrate at ×500). (C) After 8 days of plaque accumulation, the connective tissue next to the junctional epithelium at the base of the sulcus shows a mononuclear cell infiltrate and evidence of collagen degeneration (i.e., clear spaces around the cellular infiltrate (magnification, ×500). (D) The inflammatory cell infiltrate at higher magnification (×1250). After 8 days of plaque accumulation, numerous small *(SL)* and medium-sized *(ML)* lymphocytes are seen within the connective tissue. Most of the collagen fibers around these cells have disappeared, presumably as a result of enzymatic digestion. (From Payne WA, Page RC, Ogilvie AL, et al: Histopathologic features of the initial and early stages of experimental gingivitis in man. *J Periodontal Res* 10:51, 1975.)

Meanwhile, on the opposite side of molecular events, collagen degradation is related to matrix metalloproteinases (MMPs). Different MMPs are responsible for extracellular matrix remodeling within 7 days of inflammation, which is directly related to MMP-2 and MMP-9 production and activation.[54]

STAGE III GINGIVAL INFLAMMATION: THE ESTABLISHED LESION

Over time, the *established lesion* evolves. It is characterized by a predominance of plasma cells and B lymphocytes, and it is probably in conjunction with the creation of a small gingival pocket

Fig. 16.3 Scanning Electron Micrograph Showing a Leukocyte Traversing the Vessel Wall to Enter Into the Gingival Connective Tissue.

Fig. 16.4 Early Human Gingivitis Lesion. There is an area of lamina propria subjacent to the crevicular epithelium that shows a capillary with several extravascular lymphocytes and one lymphocyte within the lumen. The specimen also exhibits a considerable loss of perivascular collagen density (magnification, ×2500). (Courtesy Dr. Charles Cobb, Kansas City, Missouri, United States.)

Fig. 16.5 Marginal Gingivitis and Irregular Gingival Contour. Note the rolling at the free gingival margins as well as the shine of the tissue due the loss of stippling.

Fig. 16.6 Scanning Electron Micrograph of a Leukocyte Emerging to the Pocket Wall and Covered With Bacteria and Extracellular Lysosomes. *B,* Bacteria; *EC,* epithelial cells; *L,* lysosomes.

Fig. 16.7 Marginal Supragingival Plaque and Gingivitis.

lined with a pocket epithelium.[46] The B cells that are found in the established lesion are predominantly of the immunoglobulin G1 and G3 subclasses.[36]

With chronic gingivitis, which occurs 2 to 3 weeks after the beginning of plaque accumulation, the blood vessels become engorged and congested, venous return is impaired, and the blood flow becomes sluggish (Fig. 16.7). The result is localized gingival *anoxemia*, which superimposes a somewhat bluish hue on the reddened gingiva.[17] The extravasation of erythrocytes into the connective tissue and the breakdown of hemoglobin into its component pigments can also deepen the color of the chronically inflamed gingiva. The established lesion can be described as moderately to severely inflamed gingiva.

In histologic sections, an intense and chronic inflammatory reaction is observed. Several detailed cytologic studies have

Fig. 16.8 Established Gingivitis in a Human Subject. An area of crevicular epithelium exhibits enlarged intercellular spaces with numerous microvilli and desmosomal junctions. Several lymphocytes, both small and large, are seen migrating through the epithelial layer (magnification, ×3000).

Fig. 16.9 Advanced Gingivitis in a Human Subject. This specimen from the lamina propria exhibits plasma cell degeneration, with abundant cellular debris visible (magnification, ×3000). (Courtesy Dr. Charles Cobb, Kansas City, Missouri, United States.)

been performed on chronically inflamed gingiva.[13-15,40,46,49,53] A key feature that differentiates established lesions is the increased number of plasma cells, which become the preponderant inflammatory cell type. Plasma cells invade the connective tissue not only immediately below the junctional epithelium but also deep into the connective tissue, around the blood vessels, and between the bundles of collagen fibers.[6] The junctional epithelium reveals widened intercellular spaces that are filled with granular cellular debris, including lysosomes derived from disrupted neutrophils, lymphocytes, and monocytes (Fig. 16.8). The lysosomes contain acid hydrolases that can destroy tissue components. The junctional epithelium develops rete pegs or ridges that protrude into the connective tissue, and the basal lamina is destroyed in some areas. In the connective tissue, collagen fibers are destroyed around the infiltrate of intact and disrupted plasma cells, neutrophils, lymphocytes, monocytes, and mast cells (Fig. 16.9).

The predominance of plasma cells is thought to be a primary characteristic of established lesions. However, several studies of human experimental gingivitis have failed to demonstrate plasma cell predominance in the affected connective tissues,[7,8,49] including one study of 6 months' duration.[1] An increase in the proportion of plasma cells was evident with long-standing gingivitis, but the time for development of classic "established lesions" may exceed 6 months.

An inverse relationship appears to exist between the number of intact collagen bundles and the number of inflammatory cells.[51] Collagenolytic activity is increased in inflamed gingival tissue[16] by the enzyme collagenase. Collagenase is normally present in gingival tissues[5]; it is produced by some oral bacteria and by PMNs.

Enzyme histochemistry studies have shown that chronically inflamed gingivae have elevated levels of acid and alkaline phosphatase,[55] β-glucuronidase, β-glucosidase, β-galactosidase, esterases,[29] aminopeptidase,[33,42] and cytochrome oxidase.[9] Neutral mucopolysaccharide levels are decreased,[53] presumably as a result of degradation of the ground substance.

Established lesions of two types appear to exist; some remain stable and do not progress for months or years,[32,33,52] and others seem to become more active and convert to progressively destructive lesions. In addition, established lesions appear to be reversible, in that the sequence of events that occurs in the tissues as a result of successful periodontal therapy seems to be essentially the reverse of the sequence of events observed as gingivitis develops. As the flora reverts from that characteristically associated with destructive lesions to that associated with periodontal health, the percentage of plasma cells decreases greatly and the lymphocyte population increases proportionally.[27,31]

STAGE IV GINGIVAL INFLAMMATION: THE ADVANCED LESION

The extension of the lesion into alveolar bone characterizes the fourth stage, which is known as the *advanced lesion*[40] or *phase of periodontal breakdown.*[26] This phenomenon is described in detail in Chapters 22, 23, and 25.

Microscopically, fibrosis of the gingiva is present and there is widespread manifestation of inflammatory and immunopathologic tissue damage.[36] At the advanced stage, the presence of plasma cells dominates the connective tissue, and neutrophils continue dominating the junctional epithelium.

Patients with experimental gingivitis had significantly more plaque accumulation, higher interleukin-1β levels, and lower interleukin-8 concentrations at 28 days.[11]

Gingivitis will progress to periodontitis only in individuals who are susceptible. Patients who had sites with consistent bleeding (gingival index = 2) had 70% more attachment loss as compared with sites that were not consistently inflamed (gingival index = 0). Teeth with noninflamed sites consistently had a 50-year survival rate of 99.5%, whereas teeth with consistently inflamed gingiva had a 63.4% survival rate over 50 years. On the basis of this longitudinal study of the natural history of periodontitis in a well-maintained male population, persistent gingivitis represents a risk factor for periodontal attachment loss and tooth loss in males.[22] However, whether periodontitis can occur without a precursor of gingivitis is not known at this time.

REFERENCES

 References for this chapter are found on the companion website.

Clinical Features of Gingivitis[a]

Experimental gingivitis studies provided the first empiric evidence that the accumulation of microbial biofilm on clean tooth surfaces results in the development of an inflammatory process in gingival tissue.[42,69] Research also shows that local inflammation persists as long as the microbial biofilm is present adjacent to the gingival tissues and the inflammation resolves after meticulous removal of the biofilm.[69]

The prevalence of gingivitis is evident worldwide. Epidemiologic studies indicate more than 82% of adolescents in the United States have gingivitis and signs of gingival bleeding. A similar or higher prevalence of gingivitis is reported for children and adolescents in other parts of the world.[4] A significant percentage of adults also show signs of gingivitis; more than half of the US adult population is estimated to exhibit gingival bleeding, and other populations have even higher levels of gingival inflammation.[3,5,6,8,66] Plaque remains the primary etiologic factor causing gingivitis, but other factors can affect the development of periodontal disease. Experimental gingivitis studies suggest an important role of the host response in the development and degree of gingival inflammation.[82]

Clinical features of gingivitis can be characterized by any of the following clinical signs: redness and sponginess of the gingival tissue, bleeding on provocation, changes in contour, and the presence of calculus or plaque with no radiographic evidence of crestal bone loss.[10] Histologic examination of inflamed gingival tissue reveals ulcerated epithelium. Inflammatory mediators negatively affect epithelial function as a protective barrier. Repair of this ulcerated epithelium depends on the proliferative or regenerative activity of the epithelial cells, and removal of the etiologic agents that triggered gingival breakdown is essential.

---

[a]Adapted from the following chapter of Newman and Carranza's Clinical Periodontology, 13th edition: Chapter 18: Clinical Features of Gingivitis, by Joseph P. Fiorellini, Hector L. Sarmiento, David M. Kim, and Yu-Cheng Chang.

COURSE AND DURATION

Gingivitis can develop with sudden onset and have a short duration, and it can be painful. A less severe phase of this condition can also occur.

Chronic gingivitis develops slowly and has a long duration. It is painless, unless it is complicated by acute or subacute exacerbations, and it is the type that is most often encountered (Fig. 17.1). Chronic gingivitis is a fluctuating disease in which inflammation persists or resolves and areas of inflammation may change over time.[30,36]

Recurrent gingivitis reappears after having been eliminated by treatment or after disappearing spontaneously.

DESCRIPTION

Localized gingivitis is confined to the gingiva of a single tooth or group of teeth and affects less than 30% of the remaining teeth. *Generalized gingivitis* involves more than 30% of the remaining teeth.

Marginal gingivitis involves the gingival margin, and it can include a portion of the contiguous attached gingiva. *Papillary gingivitis* involves the interdental papillae, and it often extends into the adjacent portion of the gingival margin. Papillae are involved more frequently than the gingival margin, and the earliest signs of gingivitis often occur in the papillae. *Diffuse gingivitis* affects the gingival margin, the attached gingiva, and the interdental papillae. Gingival disease in individual cases is described by combining the preceding terms as follows:

- *Localized marginal gingivitis* is confined to one or more areas of the marginal gingiva (Fig. 17.2).
- *Localized diffuse gingivitis* extends from the margin to the mucobuccal fold in a limited area (Fig. 17.3).
- *Localized papillary gingivitis* is confined to one or more interdental spaces in a limited area (Fig. 17.4).

Fig. 17.1 Chronic Gingivitis. The marginal and interdental gingivae are smooth, edematous, and discolored. Isolated areas of acute response are seen.

Fig. 17.2 Localized Diffuse, Intensely Red Area on the Facial Surface of Tooth #7 and Dark Pink Marginal Changes in the Remaining Anterior Teeth.

Fig. 17.3 Generalized Marginal Gingivitis in the Lower Jaw With Areas of Diffuse Gingivitis.

Fig. 17.4 Generalized Papillary Gingivitis.

Fig. 17.5 Generalized Marginal and Papillary Gingivitis.

Fig. 17.6 Generalized Diffuse Gingivitis Involves the Marginal, Papillary, and Attached Gingivae.

- *Generalized marginal gingivitis* involves the gingival margins in relation greater than 30 % of the teeth. The interdental papillae are usually affected (Fig. 17.5).
- *Generalized diffuse gingivitis* involves the entire gingiva. Because the alveolar mucosa and attached gingiva are affected, the mucogingival junction is sometimes obliterated (Fig. 17.6). Systemic conditions can be involved in the case of generalized diffuse gingivitis and should be evaluated if they are suspected as an etiologic cofactor.

HALLMARKS OF GINGIVITIS		
Feature	**Healthy Gingiva**	**Gingivitis**
Color	Coral pink (or consistent with the degree of melanin pigmentation)	Red
Contour	Knife-edged and scalloped	Rolled with bulbous papillae
Consistency and texture	Firm and resilient with stippling of the attached gingiva	Edematous and with loss of stippling

CLINICAL FINDINGS

A systematic approach is required for the evaluation of the clinical features of gingivitis. The clinician should focus on subtle tissue alterations because they may have diagnostic significance. A systematic clinical approach requires an orderly examination of the gingiva for color, contour, consistency, position, and ease and severity of bleeding and pain. This section discusses these clinical characteristics and the microscopic changes that are responsible for each.

Fig. 17.7 Bleeding on Probing. (A) To explore mild edematous gingivitis, a probe is introduced to the bottom of the gingival sulcus. (B) Bleeding appears after a few seconds.

GINGIVAL BLEEDING ON PROBING

The two earliest signs of gingival inflammation that precede established gingivitis are increased gingival crevicular fluid production and bleeding from the gingival sulcus on gentle probing (Fig. 17.7). Chapter 15 discusses gingival crevicular fluid in detail.

Gingival bleeding varies in severity, duration, and ease of provocation. Bleeding on probing (BOP) is easily detected clinically and, therefore, is of value for early diagnosis and for prevention of more advanced gingivitis. BOP appears earlier than a change in color or other visual signs of inflammation.[36,37,46] The use of bleeding rather than color changes to diagnose early gingival inflammation is advantageous, in that bleeding is a more objective sign that requires less subjective estimation by the examiner.

An estimated 53.2 million (50.3%) US adults who are 30 years of age or older exhibit gingival bleeding.[5] Probing pocket depth measurements by themselves are of limited value in assessing the extent and severity of gingivitis. For example, gingival recession may result in a reduction of probing depth and cause inaccurate assessment of the periodontal status.[7] BOP is widely used by clinicians and epidemiologists to measure disease prevalence and progression, measure outcomes of treatment, and motivate patients to perform necessary home care.[24] See Chapter 7 for several gingival indices that are based on bleeding[2,16,53] and for more information on probing.

Gingival BOP indicates an inflammatory lesion in the epithelium and the connective tissue that exhibit specific histologic differences compared with healthy gingiva.[25] Although gingival BOP may not be a good diagnostic indicator of clinical attachment loss, its absence is an excellent negative predictor of future attachment loss.[34] The absence of gingival BOP is desirable and implies a low risk of future clinical attachment loss. Longitudinal findings revealed that sites with consistent bleeding (gingival index = 2) had 70% more attachment loss than sites that were not inflamed over a 26-year period in 565 male patients. Persistent gingivitis can be considered a risk factor for periodontal attachment loss that may lead to tooth loss.[35]

Numerous studies have shown that current cigarette smoking suppresses the gingival inflammatory response, and smoking was found to exert a strong, chronic, dose-dependent suppressive effect on gingival BOP in the Third National Health and Nutrition Examination Survey (NHANES III).[19] Research has revealed an increase in gingival BOP in patients who quit smoking,[54] and people who are committed to a smoking cessation program should be informed about the possibility of an increase in gingival bleeding associated with smoking cessation.

GINGIVAL BLEEDING CAUSED BY LOCAL FACTORS

Factors that contribute to plaque retention and may lead to gingivitis include anatomic and developmental tooth variations, caries, frenum pull, iatrogenic factors, malpositioned teeth, mouth breathing, overhangs, partial dentures, lack of attached gingiva, and recession. Orthodontic treatment and fixed retainers are associated with increased plaque retention and increased BOP.[38,78]

Chronic and Recurrent Bleeding

The most common cause of abnormal gingival BOP is chronic inflammation.[50] The bleeding is chronic or recurrent, and it is provoked by mechanical trauma (e.g., toothbrushing, toothpicks, food impaction).

In gingival inflammation, histopathologic alterations that result in abnormal gingival bleeding include dilation and engorgement of the capillaries and thinning or ulceration of the sulcular epithelium (Fig. 17.8). Because the capillaries are engorged and closer to the surface and because the thinned, degenerated epithelium is less protective, stimuli that are normally innocuous cause rupture of the capillaries, and gingival bleeding occurs. Sites that bleed on probing have a greater area of inflamed connective tissue (i.e., cell-rich, collagen-poor tissue) than sites that do not bleed. In most cases, the cellular infiltrate of sites that bleed on probing is predominantly lymphocytic, which is a characteristic of Stage II (early) gingivitis.[9,17,25]

Histologic evaluations of animal specimens have revealed that during the early stages of gingivitis, expression of the cytokines (i.e., matrix metalloproteinases [MMPs]) that are responsible for connective tissue breakdown is ubiquitous. Different MMPs play roles in this breakdown at different stages (e.g., a decrease of MMP-14 activity at day 7 of inflammation; immediate increase in MMP-2, especially with fibroblastic stimulation). MMP-9 expression peaked 5 days after gingivitis occurrence, which is also regulated by macrophages and neutrophils. Extracellular matrix remodeling was regulated with MMP-2 and MMP-9 production and activation by the host inflammatory response.[39]

Fig. 17.8 Microscopic View of the Interdental Space in a Human Autopsy Specimen. Note the inflammatory infiltrate and thinned epithelium in the area adjacent to the tooth and the collagenous tissue in the outer half of the section.

CLINICAL CORRELATION

Medications and Gingival Bleeding
- Drugs such as antiplatelet medications (e.g., aspirin) or anticoagulants (e.g., warfarin) that are prescribed for specific medical indications also increase the bleeding tendencies of gingival tissues.
- Women taking oral contraceptives are significantly more prone to gingivitis and, therefore, to gingival bleeding.

The severity of bleeding and the ease of its provocation depend on the intensity of inflammation. After the vessels are damaged and ruptured, interrelated mechanisms induce hemostasis.[73] The vessel walls contract, blood flow diminishes, blood platelets adhere to the edges of the tissue, and a fibrous clot is formed that contracts and results in approximation of the edges of the injured area. Bleeding recurs when the area is irritated.

In cases of moderate or advanced periodontitis, BOP is a sign of active tissue destruction. Acute episodes of gingival bleeding is caused by injury, and can occur spontaneously in patients with gingival disease. Laceration of the gingiva by toothbrush bristles during aggressive toothbrushing or by sharp pieces of hard food can cause gingival bleeding, even in the absence of gingival disease. Gingival burns from hot foods or chemicals increase the ease of gingival bleeding.

Spontaneous bleeding or bleeding on slight provocation can occur with acute necrotizing ulcerative gingivitis. With this condition, engorged blood vessels in the inflamed connective tissue are exposed by ulceration of the necrotic surface epithelium.

GINGIVAL BLEEDING ASSOCIATED WITH SYSTEMIC CHANGES

With some systemic disorders, gingival hemorrhage occurs spontaneously or after irritation (usually generalized), and it is excessive and difficult to control. These hemorrhagic diseases represent a wide variety of conditions that vary with regard to etiologic factors and clinical manifestations. Such conditions have the common feature of a hemostatic mechanism failure that results in abnormal bleeding in the skin, internal organs, and other tissues, including the oral mucosa.[71]

Hemorrhagic disorders in which abnormal gingival bleeding is encountered include vascular abnormalities (e.g., vitamin C deficiency, allergy such as Henoch-Schönlein purpura), platelet disorders[27] (e.g., thrombocytopenic purpura), hypoprothrombinemia (e.g., vitamin K deficiency), other coagulation defects (e.g., hemophilia, leukemia, Christmas disease), deficient platelet thromboplastic factor as a result of uremia,[47] multiple myeloma,[12] and postrubella purpura.[30] The effects of hormonal replacement therapy, oral contraceptives, pregnancy, and the menstrual cycle are also reported to affect gingival bleeding.[43,65,79,80] In women, long-term depression-related stress exposure may increase concentrations of interleukin-6 in gingival crevicular fluid and worsen periodontal conditions, producing elevated levels of gingival inflammation and increased pocket depths.[32]

CLINICAL CORRELATION

Pregnancy Gingivitis
Pregnancy gingivitis affects many pregnant women and is primarily caused by the hormonal imbalances associated with pregnancy. It is characterized by mild to severe gingival inflammation along with pain and, in some cases, significant hyperplasia and bleeding. In most patients, the condition normally resolves by itself after delivery, when the hormonal levels return to normal.

Changes in sex hormones are established as significant modifying factors in gingivitis, especially among adolescents. Several reports show notable effects of fluctuating estrogen and progesterone levels on the periodontium, starting as early as puberty.[1,55] Diabetes is an endocrine condition with a well-characterized effect on gingivitis.[78] In diabetes, marked inflammation affects both epithelial and connective tissues, leading to degeneration of the dermal papilla, an increase in the number of inflammatory cells, the destruction of reticulin fibers, and an accumulation of dense collagen fibers that causes fibrosis.[70]

Several medications are also found to have adverse effects on the gingiva. For example, anticonvulsants, antihypertensive calcium channel blockers, and immunosuppressive drugs cause gingival enlargement (see Chapter 18), which can cause gingival inflammation and bleeding. The American Heart Association has recommended over-the-counter aspirin as a prophylactic and therapeutic agent for cardiovascular disease, and aspirin is often prescribed for other conditions such as rheumatoid arthritis, osteoarthritis, rheumatic fever, and other inflammatory joint diseases.[28] It is important to consider aspirin's effect on bleeding during a routine dental examination to avoid false-positive readings that could result in an inaccurate diagnosis.[67] Chapter 18 discusses periodontal involvement in hematologic disorders.

COLOR CHANGES IN THE GINGIVA

The color of the gingiva is determined by several factors, including the number and size of blood vessels, the epithelial thickness, the quantity of keratinization, and the pigments in the epithelium.

Color Changes With Gingivitis

Change in color is an important clinical sign of gingival disease. The normal gingival color is coral pink or consistent with the degree of skin pigmentation, and is produced by the tissue's vascularity and modified by the overlying epithelial layers. The gingiva becomes red when vascularization increases or the degree of epithelial keratinization is reduced or disappears. The color becomes pale when vascularization is reduced (in association with fibrosis of the corium) or epithelial keratinization increases. Chronic inflammation intensifies the red or bluish red color due to vascular proliferation and a reduction of keratinization. Venous stasis contributes a bluish hue. The gingival color changes with increasing chronicity of the inflammatory process. The changes start in the interdental papillae and gingival margin and then spread to the attached gingiva.

Proper diagnosis and treatment depend on understanding the tissue changes that alter the color of the gingiva at the clinical level. Color changes in acute gingival inflammation differ in both nature and distribution from those in patients with chronic gingivitis. The color changes can be marginal, diffuse, or patchlike, depending on the underlying acute condition. With acute necrotizing ulcerative gingivitis, the involvement is marginal; with herpetic gingivostomatitis, it is diffuse; and with acute reactions to chemical irritation, it is patchlike or diffuse.

CLINICAL CORRELATION

Mouth Breathing and Gingival Inflammation
Gingivitis in the maxillary buccal area of the oral cavity is a common finding in patients who are mouth breathers. The affected gingiva typically appears red, shiny, and edematous, which is thought to be related to the surface dehydration caused by mouth breathing.

Color changes vary with the intensity of inflammation. Initially, there is an increase in erythema. If the condition does not worsen, this is the only color change until the gingiva reverts to normal. With severe acute inflammation, the red color gradually becomes a dull, whitish gray. The gray discoloration produced by tissue necrosis is demarcated from the adjacent gingiva by a thin, sharply defined erythematous zone. Chapter 13 provides detailed descriptions of the clinical and pathologic features of the various forms of acute gingivitis.

Metallic Pigmentation

Heavy metals (i.e., bismuth, arsenic, mercury, lead, and silver) that are absorbed systemically as a result of therapeutic use or occupational or household exposures can discolor the gingiva

Fig. 17.9 Bismuth Gingivitis. Note the linear black discoloration of the gingiva in a patient who is receiving bismuth therapy.

Fig. 17.10 Discoloration of the Gingiva is Caused by Embedded Metal Particles (i.e., Amalgam).

and other areas of the oral mucosa.[45] These changes are rare, but they should be ruled out in suspected cases.

Metals typically produce a black or bluish line in the gingiva that follows the contour of the margin (Fig. 17.9). The pigmentation may also appear as isolated black blotches involving the interdental marginal and attached gingiva. This is different from the tattooing produced by the accidental embedding of amalgam or other metal fragments (Fig. 17.10).[15]

COLOR CHANGES ASSOCIATED WITH SYSTEMIC FACTORS

Many systemic diseases can cause color changes in the oral mucosa, including the gingiva.[22] In general, these abnormal pigmentations are nonspecific, and they should stimulate further diagnostic efforts or referral to the appropriate specialist.[68]

Endogenous oral pigmentation can be caused by melanin, bilirubin, or iron.[45] *Melanin* oral pigmentation (physiologic pigmentation) is normal, and is often found in highly pigmented ethnic groups (see Chapter 17). Diseases that increase melanin pigmentation include the following:

- Addison disease is caused by adrenal dysfunction, and it produces isolated patches of discoloration that vary from bluish black to brown.
- Peutz-Jeghers syndrome produces intestinal polyposis and melanin pigmentation in the oral mucosa and lips.
- Albright syndrome (i.e., polyostotic fibrous dysplasia) and von Recklinghausen disease (i.e., neurofibromatosis) produce areas of oral melanin pigmentation.

The skin and mucous membranes can also be stained by *bile pigments.* Jaundice is best detected by examination of the sclera, but the oral mucosa may also acquire a yellowish color. The deposition of *iron* in hemochromatosis may produce blue-gray pigmentation of the oral mucosa. Several endocrine and metabolic disturbances, including diabetes and pregnancy, can result in color changes. Blood dyscrasias such as anemia, polycythemia, and leukemia also can induce color changes.

Exogenous factors that are capable of producing color changes in the gingiva include atmospheric irritants, such as coal and metal dust, and coloring agents in food and lozenges. Tobacco causes hyperkeratosis of the gingiva, and it can induce a significant increase in melanin pigmentation of the oral mucosa.[56] Localized bluish black areas of pigment are often caused by amalgam implanted in the mucosa (see Fig. 17.10).

The need for aesthetics in dentistry has increased, with a growing demand for a pleasing smile. This has made many individuals more aware of their gingival pigmentation, which may be apparent when smiling and speaking.[20,21] Traditionally, gingival depigmentation has been carried out with the use of nonsurgical and surgical procedures, including chemical, cryosurgical, and electrosurgical techniques. However, those techniques were met with skepticism because of their various degrees of success.

Lasers have been used to ablate cells that produce the melanin pigment; a nonspecific laser beam destroys the epithelial cells, including those at the basal layer. Selective ablation using a laser beam with a wavelength that is specifically absorbed by melanin effectively destroys the pigmented cells without damaging the nonpigmented cells. In both cases, radiation energy is transformed into ablation energy, resulting in cellular rupture and vaporization with minimal heating of the surrounding tissue.[76]

CHANGES IN GINGIVAL CONSISTENCY

Chronic and acute inflammations produce changes in the normal firm and resilient consistency of the gingiva. In patients with chronic gingivitis, destructive (i.e., edematous) and reparative (i.e., fibrotic) changes coexist, and the consistency of the gingiva is determined by their relative predominance (Figs. 17.11 and 17.12). Table 17.1 summarizes the clinical alterations in the consistency of the gingiva and the microscopic changes that produce them.

Calcified Masses in the Gingiva

Calcified microscopic masses may be found in the gingiva.[14,52] They can occur alone or in groups, and they vary with regard to size, location, shape, and structure. Such masses may be calcified material that was removed from the tooth and traumatically displaced into the gingiva during scaling,[52] root remnants, cementum fragments, or cementicles. Chronic inflammation and fibrosis, an occasional foreign body, and giant-cell activity occur in reaction to the masses, which are sometimes enclosed in an osteoid-like matrix. Crystalline foreign bodies have been described in the gingiva, but their origin has not been determined.[60]

TABLE 17.1	Clinical and Histopathologic Changes in Gingival Consistency	
Clinical Changes	**Underlying Microscopic Features**
Chronic Gingivitis	
1. Soggy puffiness that pits on pressure	1. Infiltration by fluid and cells of inflammatory exudate
2. Marked softness and friability, with ready fragmentation on exploration with probe and pinpoint surface areas of redness and desquamation	2. Degeneration of connective tissue and epithelium associated with injurious substances that provoke inflammation and inflammatory exudate; change in the connective tissue–epithelium relationship, with inflamed, engorged connective tissue expanding to within a few epithelial cells of the surface; thinning of epithelium and degeneration associated with edema and leukocyte invasion, separated by areas in which rete pegs are elongated to connective tissue
3. Firm, leathery consistency	3. Fibrosis and epithelial proliferation associated with long-standing chronic inflammation
Acute Gingivitis	
1. Diffuse puffiness and softening	1. Diffuse edema of acute inflammatory origin; fatty infiltration in xanthomatosis
2. Sloughing with grayish, flakelike particles of debris adhering to eroded surface	2. Necrosis with formation of pseudomembrane composed of bacteria, polymorphonuclear leukocytes, and degenerated epithelial cells in fibrinous meshwork
3. Vesicle formation	3. Intercellular and intracellular edema with degeneration of nucleus and cytoplasm and rupture of cell wall

Fig. 17.11 Chronic Gingivitis. Swelling, loss of stippling, and discoloration occur when inflammatory exudate and edema are the predominant microscopic changes. The gingiva is soft and friable and bleeds easily.

Fig. 17.12 Chronic Gingivitis. Firm gingiva is produced when fibrosis predominates in the inflammatory process.

Toothbrushing

Toothbrushing has various effects on the consistency of the gingiva, such as promoting keratinization of the oral epithelium, enhancing capillary gingival circulation, and thickening alveolar bone.[44,49,77] In animal studies, mechanical stimulation by toothbrushing was found to increase the proliferative activity of the junctional basal cells in dog gingiva by 2.5 times compared with the use of a scaler.[31] These findings may indicate that toothbrushing causes an increased turnover rate and desquamation of the junctional epithelial surfaces. This process may repair small breaks in the junctional epithelium and prevent direct access to the underlying tissue by periodontal pathogens.[81]

CHANGES IN GINGIVAL SURFACE TEXTURE

The surface of normal gingiva usually exhibits numerous small depressions and elevations that give the tissue an orange-peel appearance referred to as *stippling*.[13] Stippling is restricted to the attached gingiva and is predominantly localized to the subpapillary area, but it extends to various degrees into the interdental papilla.[61] Although the biologic significance of gingival stippling is not known, some investigators conclude that the loss of stippling is an early sign of gingivitis.[33,61] However, clinicians must take into consideration that its pattern and extent vary in different mouth areas, among patients, and with age.

In patients with chronic inflammation, the gingival surface is smooth and shiny or firm and nodular, depending on whether the dominant changes are exudative or fibrotic. A smooth surface texture is also produced by epithelial atrophy in atrophic gingivitis, and peeling of the surface occurs with chronic desquamative gingivitis. Hyperkeratosis results in a leathery texture, and drug-induced gingival overgrowth produces a nodular surface.

CLINICAL CORRELATION

Stippling and Its Clinical Importance

Healthy, attached gingiva has a pitted orange-peel appearance on its surface. This surface feature, called *stippling*, is an external reflection of the underlying connective tissue projections into the overlying epithelium. Presence of stippling in the attached gingiva is indicative of gingival health, and this surface feature is usually lost when the tissue is edematous.

CHANGES IN GINGIVAL POSITION

Traumatic Lesions

A feature of gingival disease classification is the recognition of nonplaque-induced traumatic gingival lesions as distinct gingival conditions.[11] Traumatic lesions—whether chemical, physical, or thermal—are among the most common lesions in the mouth. Sources of chemical injuries include aspirin, hydrogen peroxide, silver nitrate, phenol, and endodontic materials. Physical injuries can include lip, oral, and tongue piercings, which can result in gingival recession. Thermal injuries can result from hot drinks and foods.

In acute cases, the appearance of slough (i.e., necrotizing epithelium), erosion, or ulceration and accompanying erythema are common features. In chronic cases, permanent gingival defects usually take the form of gingival recession. Typically, the localized nature of the lesions and lack of symptoms readily eliminate them from the differential diagnosis of systemic conditions that may exist with erosive or ulcerative oral lesions.[64]

Gingival Recession

Gingival recession is a common finding. The prevalence, extent, and severity of gingival recession can increase with age, and this condition is more prevalent among males.[5]

Positions of the Gingiva

By clinical definition, recession is exposure of the root surface by an apical shift in the position of the gingiva. To understand recession, it helps to distinguish between the actual and apparent positions of the gingiva. The *actual position* is the level of the coronal end of the epithelial attachment on the tooth, whereas the *apparent position* is the level of the crest of the gingival margin (Fig. 17.13). The severity of recession is determined by the apparent position of the gingiva. However, the actual gingival position is used to determine the clinical attachment loss. For example, in periodontal disease, the inflamed pocket wall covers part of the denuded root; some of the recession is hidden, and some maybe visible. The total amount of clinical attachment loss is the sum of the two.

Recession refers to the location of the gingiva rather than to its condition. Receded gingiva can be inflamed, but it may be normal except for its position (Fig. 17.14). Recession can be localized to one tooth or a group of teeth, or it may be generalized throughout the mouth.

Gingival recession increases with age; the incidence varies from 8% among children to 100% after 50 years of age.[84] This led some investigators to assume that recession might be a physiologic process related to aging. However, no convincing evidence has been presented for a physiologic shift of the gingival attachment.[40] The gradual apical shift most likely results from the

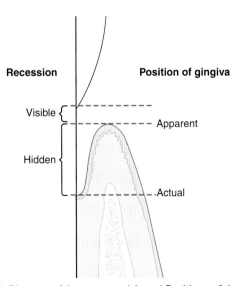

Fig. 17.13 Diagram of Apparent and Actual Positions of the Gingiva and Visible and Hidden Recession.

Fig. 17.14 Degrees of Recession. Recession is slight in teeth #26 and #29 and marked in teeth #27 and #28. The change in gingival contour and the recession, as seen in tooth #28, are referred to as *Stillman clefts.*

cumulative effect of minor pathologic involvement and repeated minor direct trauma to the gingiva. In some populations without access to dental care, however, recession can result from increasing periodontal disease.[29,41]

The following etiologic factors have been implicated in gingival recession: faulty toothbrushing technique (i.e., gingival abrasion), tooth malposition, friction from the soft tissues (i.e., gingival ablation),[72] gingival inflammation, abnormal frenum attachment, and iatrogenic dentistry. Trauma from occlusion has been suggested in the past, but its mechanism of action has never been demonstrated. For example, a deep overbite has been associated with gingival inflammation and recession. Excessive incisal overlap may result in a traumatic injury to the gingiva. Orthodontic movement in a labial direction in monkeys has been shown to result in the loss of marginal bone and connective tissue attachment and in gingival recession.[74]

Standard oral hygiene procedures, including toothbrushing and flossing, frequently lead to transient and minimal gingival injury.[18,62] Although toothbrushing is important for gingival health, faulty technique or brushing with hard bristles can cause significant injury. This type of injury can manifest as lacerations, abrasions, keratosis, or recession, with the facial marginal gingiva being affected most often.[57] In these cases, recession tends to be more frequent and more severe in patients with clinically healthy gingiva, little bacterial plaque, and good oral hygiene.[23,58,59]

CLINICAL CORRELATION

Biologic Width and Gingival Inflammation

Biologic width is the circumferential rim of space around teeth where the junctional epithelium and the underlying connective tissue of the gingiva attach to the teeth. When restoring teeth, if the margins of the restorations violate the biologic width, gingival inflammation ensues. If left untreated, it can lead to bone loss. Crown lengthening is a surgical procedure that is performed clinically (i.e., before restoration delivery) to intentionally create space for the biologic width to reestablish.

Susceptibility to recession is influenced by the position of teeth in the arch,[83] the root-bone angle, and the mesiodistal curvature of the tooth surface.[51] On rotated, tilted, or facially displaced teeth, the bony plate is thinned or reduced in height. Pressure from mastication or moderate toothbrushing damages the unsupported gingiva and produces recession. The effect of

the angle of the root in the bone with recession is often observed in the maxillary molar area. If the lingual inclination of the palatal root is prominent or the buccal roots flare outward, the bone in the cervical area is thinned or shortened, and recession results from repeated trauma of the thin marginal gingiva.

The health of the gingival tissue also depends on properly designed and placed restorative materials. Pressure from a poorly designed partial denture, such as an ill-fitting denture clasp, can cause gingival trauma and recession.[85] Overhanging dental restorations are a contributing factor to gingivitis because of plaque retention. In addition, there is general agreement that placing restorative margins within the biologic width frequently leads to gingival inflammation, clinical attachment loss, and eventually bone loss. Clinically, the violation of biologic width typically manifests as gingival inflammation, deepened periodontal pockets, and gingival recession.

A relationship may exist between smoking and gingival recession (see Chapter 11). The multifactorial mechanisms probably include reduced gingival blood flow and an altered immune response, but current evidence is not conclusive.[26,63]

Clinical Significance

Several aspects of gingival recession make it clinically significant. Exposed root surfaces are susceptible to caries. Abrasion or erosion of the cementum exposed by recession leaves an underlying dentinal surface that can be sensitive. Hyperemia of the pulp and associated symptoms can result from excessive exposure of the root surface.[48] Interproximal recession creates oral hygiene problems and results in plaque accumulation.

CHANGES IN GINGIVAL CONTOUR

Changes in gingival contour are primarily associated with gingival enlargement (see Chapter 18), but changes may also occur with other conditions. Of historical interest are descriptions of indentations of the gingival margin referred to as Stillman clefts (see Fig. 18.14)[75] and McCall festoons. The term *Stillman cleft* has been used to describe a specific type of gingival recession that consists of a narrow, triangular-shaped gingival recession. As the recession progresses apically, the cleft becomes broader, thereby exposing the cementum of the root surface. When the lesion reaches the mucogingival junction, the apical border of oral mucosa is usually inflamed because of the difficulty in maintaining adequate plaque control at this site.

The term *McCall festoon* is used to describe a rolled, thickened band of gingiva that is usually seen adjacent to the cuspids when recession approaches the mucogingival junction. Initially, Stillman clefts and McCall festoons were attributed to traumatic occlusion, and the recommended treatment was occlusal adjustment. However, this association was never proved, and the indentations merely represent peculiar inflammatory changes of the marginal gingiva.[14]

Case Scenarios are found on the companion website.

REFERENCES

 References for this chapter are found on the companion website www.expertconsult.com.

Gingival Enlargement[a,b]

Enlargement of gingiva has many causes and can manifest with various clinical characteristics. A change in the dimensions of gingival tissue is always a pathologic event. Gingival enlargement can be transient and reversible or can be chronic and irreversible. As in other pathologic processes, inflammation of the periodontal tissues typically results in three outcomes: complete resolution of inflammation and restoration of tissue integrity (i.e., homeostasis), destruction of periodontal tissues and loss of attachment (i.e., chronic periodontitis), or fibrosis.

Fibrosis is a component of the defense mechanism against progression of periodontal inflammation. During this process, fibroblasts play a major role by generating excessive amounts of collagen and noncollagenous proteins of the extracellular matrix. Increased matrix deposition is not sufficiently balanced by the enzymatic degradation of the matrix composition (e.g., collagen), resulting in fibrotic changes in soft tissues. Fibrosis of gingival tissues is commonly referred to as *gingival hyperplasia*. In contrast to other tissues in which fibrosis is observed, gingival lesions are usually inflamed due to accumulation of bacteria and reduced oral care. Gingival overgrowth (GO) lesions are unique in their pathogenetic mechanisms.

Pathologic enlargements of gingival tissues were recognized in ancient civilizations and linked to systemic conditions as early as the 18th century. Most common forms of gingival enlargement result from systemic use of various medications. The first scientific report on drug-induced gingival overgrowth (DIGO)

was published in 1939, when the anticonvulsant diphenylhydantoinate was associated with gingival enlargement.[58] Later studies provided significant insights into the complex molecular and cellular mechanisms underlying gingival enlargement. Because many forms of gingival enlargement are associated with systemic factors and conditions, understanding the exact pathogenesis of lesions is essential for designing better approaches to treatment.

This chapter focuses on the clinical, etiologic, and pathologic aspects of gingival enlargement used to develop novel and targeted approaches to therapy. Neoplastic enlargement of gingival tissues associated with benign or malignant oral cancers is not covered in depth because the field of oral pathology has evolved beyond the scope of this chapter and can be found in oral pathology textbooks that provide extensive coverage of oral tumors.

TERMINOLOGY AND CLASSIFICATION

Gingival enlargement and *GO* are used interchangeably with *hyperplasia*, *hypertrophy*, and *fibrosis*. *Hyperplasia* is an increase in the number of cells in tissues that results in increased tissue volume. *Hypertrophy* refers to increased tissue size and volume resulting from increased cell size. Although their pathogenetic mechanisms are different, hyperplasia and hypertrophy usually occur simultaneously when cellular involvement in hyperplasia most likely triggers the overgrowth.

Fibrosis refers to a pathologic process in which disrupted wound healing is associated with defective cell proliferation, cell-to-cell interactions, cell-to-matrix interactions, and matrix deposition and with an impaired immune system response. In this regard, fibrosis is defined as a pathologic lesion, whereas hyperplasia and hypertrophy can be viewed as a pathologic process.

All of these terms refer to different pathogenetic states. In gingival tissues, they are associated with various phases of inflammation. Hyperplastic, hypertrophic, and fibrotic changes are observed during gingival enlargement and cannot be accurately differentiated. This chapter therefore uses *GO* or *gingival enlargement* to refer to all pathologic forms in periodontal tissues.

Classification of GO is based on etiologic factors. The most common form results from systemic use of medications and

---

[a]Adapted from the following chapter of Newman and Carranza's *Clinical Periodontology*, 13th edition: Chapter 19: Gingival Enlargement, by Alpdogan Kantarci, Fermin A. Carranza, Eva Hogan.

[b]Note: In the 2018 Classification of Periodontal and Periimplant Diseases and Conditions, "chronic periodontitis" and "aggressive periodontitis" disease categories are grouped under a single category called "periodontitis" and are further characterized based on a multidimensional staging and grading system. In this chapter, the term "aggressive periodontitis" is still used because the related studies were conducted before the 2018 classification. Readers are referred to Chapter 6 for the detailed discussion on periodontal disease classification.

is called *drug-induced gingival overgrowth*. Three families of drugs can lead to DIGO: anticonvulsants, calcium channel blockers, and immunosuppressants. GO also is associated with severe systemic diseases such as leukemia and with genetic factors. Any form that cannot be classified among these GO forms is known as *idiopathic GO*. GO can also be the result of inflammatory changes due to gingivitis. GO cases are classified as follows:

- Inflammatory enlargement due to chronic gingivitis
- Drug-induced enlargement
- GO associated with systemic conditions
- GO associated with systemic diseases
- Gingival fibromatosis

Enlargement of the gingiva can be indirectly associated with changes in the dimensions of underlying osseous structures. Although not covered in depth in this chapter, neoplastic lesions in the oral cavity can manifest with fibrotic lesions and can appear clinically similar to other forms of GO. Regardless of the cause, all forms of gingival enlargement have distinct pathologic characteristics that should be carefully considered during treatment. It is important to identify the cause and confounding etiologic factors that lead to different forms of GO.

DIAGNOSIS

Because GO is frequently associated with systemic conditions, the general health of the patient and his or her drug use should be carefully managed. GO is one of the most serious pathologies in periodontal medicine, and it requires a meticulous differential diagnosis for selecting a therapeutic approach tailored to the patient's systemic status.

Accurate diagnosis requires a thorough review of the medical history of the patient. Gingival enlargement is distinguished as localized or generalized. Generalized GO can affect marginal gingiva; localized forms are often confined to papillae. Previous classifications also distinguished between diffuse and discrete enlargements, which are sometimes difficult to differentiate. However, these categorizations can be critical for determining the correct cause of the pathology.

In periodontal tissues, indices are important for quantification of the extent and severity of GO. Various indices have been proposed. For example, the degree of gingival enlargement can be scored as follows:

- Grade 0: no signs of gingival enlargement
- Grade I: enlargement confined to interdental papilla
- Grade II: enlargement involves papilla and marginal gingiva
- Grade III: enlargement covers three-fourths or more of the crown

Regardless of the method used for measuring the extent and severity of GO lesions, an accurate assessment is critical for identifying the inflammatory and fibrotic components. Indices should be chosen based on practicality of the data acquired to allow clinicians to select the method of therapy (e.g., gingivectomy and gingivoplasty vs. nonsurgical treatment measures) and plan the maintenance phase.

TYPES OF GINGIVAL ENLARGEMENT

Inflammatory Enlargement of Gingiva Due to Gingivitis

Clinical Manifestations

All changes in gingival tissues manifest with some degree of inflammation. In some cases, gingival enlargement is a direct outcome of gingivitis without any complicating factors or involvement of systemic conditions. When a patient with gingival enlargement is seen, the initial assessment is made by careful visual examination of abnormalities of gingival contours, texture, and color, which are compared with normal standards. Visual inspection is accompanied by a detailed medical history to exclude potential systemic factors and conditions. Dental irregularities, dysfunctional habits, and oral care efficiency are considered in the evaluation, and clinical measurements should be recorded.

Inflammatory GO originates as a slight ballooning of the interdental papilla and marginal gingiva. In the early stages, it produces swelling around the involved teeth, which can increase in size until it covers part of the crowns. Gingival enlargement may be localized or generalized. It progresses slowly and painlessly unless it is complicated by acute infection or trauma (Figs. 18.1 and 18.2). Occasionally, chronic inflammatory GO occurs as a discrete sessile or pedunculated mass that resembles a tumor. It can be interproximal or located on the marginal or attached gingiva. Painful ulceration sometimes occurs in the fold between the mass and the adjacent gingiva.

Fig. 18.1 Chronic Inflammatory Gingival Enlargement Localized to the Anterior Region.

Fig. 18.2 Chronic Inflammatory Gingival Enlargement.

Etiology

Acute inflammatory enlargement of the gingiva is usually caused by a mechanical, chemical, or physical irritation and can be resolved by removal of the irritant. Mouth breathing, impacted food items, and poor oral hygiene are most commonly responsible for acute inflammatory reactions in gingival tissues. Acute lesions are normally localized to marginal or papillary gingiva.

The main etiologic factor for acute inflammatory gingival enlargement is trauma. Traumatic lesions occur when a foreign substance (e.g., toothbrush bristle) is forcefully embedded in the gingiva and complicated by resident microbes. Trauma-induced injuries result in a chronic process characterized by granulation tissue formation and fibrosis.

KEY FACT

The main etiologic factor for acute inflammatory gingival enlargement is trauma. Traumatic lesions occur when a foreign substance (e.g., toothbrush bristle) is forcefully embedded into the gingiva and the situation is complicated by the presence of microbial pathogens. Trauma-induced injuries result in a chronic process characterized by granulation tissue formation and fibrosis. Because nerve tissue does not proliferate, pain is uncommon.

Acute inflammatory enlargement can lead to the formation of gingival abscess. Gingival abscess is a localized, painful, and rapidly expanding lesion (Fig. 18.3). It is typically limited to the marginal gingiva or the interdental papilla. In its early stages, it appears as a red swelling with a smooth, shiny surface. The lesion usually becomes fluctuant and pointed; a surface orifice and a purulent exudate occur in 24 to 48 hours. Adjacent teeth may become sensitive to percussion. The lesion usually ruptures spontaneously. Because of an acute inflammatory process, the gingival abscess consists of a purulent exudate of a diffuse infiltration of polymorphonuclear leukocytes, edematous tissue, and vascularization. The surface epithelium has various degrees of intracellular and extracellular edema, invasion by leukocytes, and sometimes ulceration. The lesion is confined to the gingiva, and it should be distinguished from periodontal abscess.

Chronic inflammatory GO is commonly associated with microbial biofilm. Biofilm can be linked to a lack of proper oral hygiene, orthodontic appliances, faulty restoration margins, misaligned teeth, oral habits, an open bite, or other factors favoring plaque accumulation.

Gingivitis and gingival enlargement are often seen in patients who are mouth breathers. The gingiva appears red and edematous, with a diffuse surface shininess of the exposed area. The maxillary anterior region is commonly involved. In many cases, the altered gingiva is clearly demarcated from the adjacent, unexposed normal gingiva (Fig. 18.4). Irritation from surface dehydration is attributed to mouth breathing. However, comparable changes have not been reproduced by air-drying the gingiva of experimental animals, suggesting that the pathogenesis of mouth breathing–associated gingival changes is far more complex.

Plasma cell gingivitis sometimes manifests as a mild marginal gingival enlargement that extends to the attached gingiva. The gingiva appears red, friable, and sometimes granular and bleeds easily. The lesion is located on the oral aspect of the attached gingiva and is different from plaque-induced gingivitis.

In addition to the acute and chronic forms of gingival enlargements associated with gingivitis, inflammatory lesions can be observed in other forms of GO. Systemic conditions also cause inflammatory changes in gingiva. The distinction should be made very early in treatment planning, and the involvement of drugs, systemic conditions, and neoplastic lesions should be carefully ruled out.

Histopathology

Inflammatory enlargement of the gingiva typically follows the sequence of the inflammatory process. Chronic inflammatory GO lesions show the exudative and proliferative features of chronic inflammation (Fig. 18.5). Lesions that are deep red or bluish red are soft and friable with a smooth, shiny surface and bleed easily. These lesions have a preponderance of inflammatory cells and fluid, along with vascular engorgement, new capillary formation, and associated degenerative changes. Lesions that are relatively firm, resilient, and pink have a greater fibrotic component, with an abundance of fibroblasts and collagen fibers.

In patients with plasma cell gingivitis, the oral epithelium shows spongiosis and infiltration with inflammatory cells. Ultrastructurally, there are signs of damage in the lower spinous layers and the basal layers. The underlying connective tissue contains a dense infiltrate of plasma cells that also extends to the oral epithelium, producing a dissecting type of injury. Associated cheilitis and glossitis have been reported.[89]

Fig. 18.3 Gingival Abscess on the Facial Gingival Surface in the Space Between the Cuspid and the Lateral Incisor, Unrelated to the Gingival Sulcus.

Fig. 18.4 Gingival Enlargement in a Mouth Breather. The lesion is sharply circumscribed in the anterior marginal and papillary areas.

Plasma cell gingivitis is believed to be allergic in origin and possibly a reaction to components of chewing gum, dentifrices, or various dietary items. Cessation of exposure to the allergen brings resolution of the lesion. In rare instances, marked inflammatory gingival enlargements with a predominance of plasma cells can appear; they are associated with aggressive periodontitis.[77] A solitary plasma cell tumor (i.e., plasmocytoma) has been described in the nasopharynx and rarely in the oral mucosa.[10] It is a slow-growing, pedunculated tumor with a pink and smooth surface, and it is composed of normal plasma cells. It is usually benign, but in rare cases it can be an oral manifestation of multiple myeloma, which is a malignant B-cell tumor of the bone marrow.

Treatment

Chronic enlargement of the gingiva due to gingivitis is reversible and can be resolved by removal of the etiologic factors, including the biofilm, and correction of environmental factors. In severe forms of inflammatory enlargement, surgical approaches may be required.

Drug-Induced Overgrowth of Gingiva

Most common forms of DIGO are attributed to the use of anticonvulsants, calcium channel blockers, and immunosuppressants prescribed to patients for serious health concerns. The prevalence of DIGO substantially varies for different medications and among studies. Three drugs associated with DIGO are phenytoin, nifedipine, and cyclosporine. Approximately 20 other medications are linked to DIGO. An estimated 30% to 80% of the patients using these medications are at risk for overgrowth lesions. Genetic factors, drug dosage, and local factors can affect the development and severity of DIGO.[91,101]

DIGO frequently results in impaired oral hygiene, biofilm accumulation, and gingival inflammation. Increased prevalence of gingival infection and inflammation among patients with DIGO poses risk for their general health.[20,24,69] The inciting drugs are being replaced with alternatives, but they remain the drugs of choice in many countries for the treatment of specific conditions. Alternatives have also been linked to DIGO, and GO associated with medication use continues to be a clinical problem in dentistry and medicine.

CLINICAL CORRELATION

Anticonvulsants, calcium channel blockers, and immunosuppressants are prescribed to patients with serious health concerns such as epilepsy, hypertension, and solid organ transplantation, respectively. DIGO is a major dental problem due to impaired oral hygiene, biofilm accumulation, and gingival inflammation, and it poses a risk for the general health of these patients.

DIGO lesions usually develop fast and become chronic over time (Fig. 18.6). The first signs of overgrowth are observed as early as 3 months of drug use as a localized nodular enlargement of the interdental papilla. Because most of the medications associated with DIGO are prescribed for an extended time, the lesions expand and, in some cases, cover the crowns of the teeth. Severe forms of DIGO may result in complete coverage of dental surfaces (Fig. 18.7). Clinically, there are subtle differences in how the lesions manifest depending on the type of medication used. Dental biofilm and bacterial infection frequently lead to inflamed tissues characterized by edema and bleeding (Fig. 18.8). The degree of fibrosis and inflammation depend on the dose, duration, and type of drug; oral hygiene; individual susceptibility, including genetic factors; and environmental influences.[100,102]

Anticonvulsants

Phenytoin (diphenylhydantoinate) is a drug of choice for the treatment of grand mal, temporal lobe, and psychomotor seizures,

Fig. 18.5 Survey Section of Chronic Inflammatory Gingival Enlargement Shows the Inflamed Connective Tissue Core and Strands of Proliferating Epithelium.

Fig. 18.6 Gingival Enlargement Associated With Phenytoin Therapy. (A) Facial view. (B) Occlusal view of the maxillary arch.

Fig. 18.7 Phenytoin-Induced Gingival Enlargement.

Fig. 18.8 Combined Gingival Enlargement Resulted from the Inflammatory Involvement of a Phenytoin-Induced Overgrowth.

and it has been linked to GO for more than 70 years.[67] Other anticonvulsant agents such as phenobarbital and valproic acid have been associated with GO less often than phenytoin.[61,85] The estimated prevalence of phenytoin-induced GO is approximately 50%.[22] Clinical onset occurs as early as 1 month, and increasing severity is seen in 12 to 18 months.[1,14,29]

Phenytoin-induced GO lesions frequently occur on the anterior buccal maxilla and mandible, and the entire dentition can be covered in severe cases.[19,62] Phenytoin-induced GO is characterized by enlargement of interdental papillae and increased thickening of the marginal tissues,[4] causing aesthetic and functional problems, such as malpositioning of teeth, difficulty in speech, and impaired oral hygiene.[80]

Calcium Channel Blockers

Calcium channel blockers are a group of drugs commonly used to treat hypertension, angina pectoris, coronary artery spasm, and cardiac arrhythmia.[67] Benzothiazepine derivatives (e.g., diltiazem), phenylalkylamine derivatives (e.g., verapamil), and dyhydropyridines (e.g., amlopidine, felodipine, isradipine, nicardipine, nifedipine, nitrendipine, oxodipine, nimodipine, nisoldipine) are different types of calcium channel blockers that have been associated with some degree of DIGO.[c]

The first case of GO associated with the calcium channel blocker nifedipine was reported in 1984.[83] Among patients taking the medication, the prevalence of nifedipine-induced GO is highly

variable, ranging from 6% to 83%.[7,35,36,95] Clinically, interdental papillae are affected, and overgrowth is limited to attached and marginal gingiva, which is normally observed on the anterior segments.[90] Nifedipine-induced GO can coexist with periodontitis and attachment loss that is different from other forms of DIGO.

Immunosuppressants

Cyclosporin A has been the immunosuppressant of choice for preventing rejection of solid organ and bone marrow transplants and for treatment of autoimmune conditions.[44] The prevalence of cyclosporin A–induced GO has been reported to be approximately 30%, but it can be much higher, especially for pediatric populations.[57]

The first case of cyclosporin A–induced GO was reported in 1983.[84] Clinically, the lesions are more inflamed and bleed more than other forms of DIGO and are commonly limited to buccal surfaces. Severity of the lesions can be similar to those of phenytoin and nifedipine. They affect the entire dentition and interfere with occlusion, mastication, and speech.[37]

Histopathology. Lesions from different types of DIGO demonstrate significant histologic variations.[102] GO biopsies from patients undergoing treatment with phenytoin show a thick, stratified squamous epithelium with long, thin rete pegs extending deep into the connective tissue.[3,19,33] Fibrosis with minimal inflammatory cell infiltration is a common finding.[101] The histologic characteristics of GO induced by calcium channel blockers is similar to phenytoin-induced lesions, including epithelial thickness, rete peg formation, and excessive matrix accumulation (Fig. 18.9).

Cyclosporin A–induced GO also manifests with a thickened epithelium, rete peg formation, and irregular collagen fibers. However, these lesions are characterized with more inflammatory infiltration and vascularization compared with phenytoin and calcium channel blockers (Fig. 18.10; see Fig. 18.9).[84]

> ### KEY FACT
>
> Different types of DIGO lesions demonstrate a thick, stratified squamous epithelium with long, thin rete pegs extending deep into the connective tissue. Fibrosis is a common finding in patients with phenytoin-induced GO. Histologic characteristics of GO induced by calcium channel blockers are similar to those of phenytoin-induced lesions, including epithelial thickness, rete peg formation, and excessive matrix accumulation. Cyclosporin A–induced GO lesions have more inflammatory infiltration and increased vascularization compared with GO caused by phenytoin or calcium channel blockers.

Pathogenesis of drug-induced gingival overgrowth. The pathogenesis of DIGO is complex. The main mechanism is mediated through defective function of gingival fibroblasts. Because gingival fibroblasts are responsible for the matrix deposition of gingival tissues, extensive research has focused on these key cells and their function. Study findings vary, some pathways have not been validated in humans, and data are limited to in vitro and animal studies, but collectively the findings suggest that DIGO-associated medications affect the extracellular matrix metabolism by decreasing collagenase activity and increasing the production of matrix proteins.

---

[c]References 13, 15, 17, 28, 63, 70, and 92.

Fig. 18.9 Microscopic View of Gingival Enlargement Associated With Phenytoin Therapy. (A) Hyperplasia and acanthosis of the epithelium and densely collagenous connective tissue are seen with evidence of inflammation in the area adjacent to the gingival sulcus. (B) High-power view shows extension of deep rete pegs into the connective tissue.

Fig. 18.10 Microscopic View of Cyclosporine-Associated Gingival Enlargement.

Gingival fibroblasts from phenytoin-induced GO are characterized by elevated levels of collagen synthesis.[45] It has been suggested that fibroblasts may be susceptible to the development of DIGO.[45] Gingival fibroblasts from nifedipine-induced GO lesions have defective collagen production due to decreased levels of collagenase activity, which can result in collagen deposition.[99] Through interference with calcium metabolism, calcium channel blockers decrease calcium levels in gingival fibroblasts and T cells, thereby affecting T-cell proliferation or activation and collagen biosynthesis.[7,99]

Cyclosporin A directly impairs collagen synthesis by gingival fibroblasts,[66] with a concomitant rise in the levels of type I collagen.[88] Cyclosporin A also decreases expression of matrix metalloproteinase-1 (MMP-1) and MMP-3.[12] In addition to collagen, which is the major extracellular matrix component of gingival tissues, noncollagenous matrix is affected by the medications that result in DIGO. Glycosaminoglycan metabolism is impaired in patients with phenytoin-induced GO[32] and in response to cyclosporin A treatment of gingival fibroblasts.[75]

In addition to fibroblast metabolism and function, inflammatory regulation of tissue turnover is a major factor in DIGO pathogenesis. Fibroblast functions such as proliferation, differentiation, and production of extracellular matrix are affected by levels of cytokines and growth factors. GO lesions are characterized by increased levels of interleukin-6 (IL-6), IL-1β, platelet-derived growth factor subunit B (PDGFB), fibroblast growth factor 2 (FGF2), transforming growth factor-β (TGF-β), and connective tissue growth factor (CTGF).[d] Macrophages are the main source of these cytokines.[18,23,30,34,79]

The TGF-β1–CTGF axis is an essential mechanism leading to DIGO. TGF-β1 regulates cell proliferation and differentiation and can activate gene expression for the synthesis of extracellular matrix components, including collagen in cyclosporin A–induced GO.[52,86] TGF-β1 induces CTGF mRNA and protein expression in human gingival fibroblasts; the TGF-β1–CTGF pathway directly regulates fibrosis, gingival fibroblast lysyl oxidase, and collagen generation.[47] CTGF expression is increased in all forms of DIGO, with the highest levels occurring in phenytoin-induced GO, which also has the highest levels of fibrosis.[102]

CTGF expression is not limited to the connective tissue. It also is demonstrated in the gingival epithelium, predominantly in the basal epithelial cells close to the connective tissue border.[54] In vitro studies showed that CTGF could be produced by gingival epithelial cells,[54] illustrating a possible mechanism of fibrosis in gingiva, which may be related to crosstalk between epithelial and connective tissue cells. Studies revealed a unique mechanism for TGF-β1–induced CTGF expression in gingival fibroblasts regulated by prostaglandin E_2, cyclic adenosine monophosphate (cAMP), mitogen-activated protein kinases (MAPKs), and activation of Jun N-terminal kinases (JNKs).[11]

A key event in the pathogenetic mechanism of DIGO is some degree of epithelial-mesenchymal transition induced by medications. Highly fibrotic tissues are characterized by increased epithelial-mesenchymal transition, through which epithelial cells in the gingiva acquire fibroblast function, and the process is regulated by CTGF.[97] The molecular pathways of DIGO have been reviewed elsewhere.[101]

Treatment. DIGO cannot be prevented by conventional approaches, but it can be ameliorated by elimination of local factors, plaque control, and regular periodontal maintenance. The most effective treatment of DIGO is withdrawal or substitution of medications. A case report showed resolution of gingival lesions in 1 to 8 weeks after discontinuing the medication.[56] For example, changing nifedipine to another antihypertensive drug, isradipine, caused regression of gingival enlargement.[103] Tacrolimus, used as an alternative for cyclosporin A, resulted in regression of gingival enlargement.[51] However, most alternatives have also been linked to DIGO in recent years.

In addition to withdrawal or substitution of medication, scaling and root planing (root debridement therapy) have given relief to patients with GO.[96] Nonsurgical treatment can eliminate the inflammatory component of DIGO, which can account for 40% of tissue enlargement.[55]

Because the anterior labial gingiva is frequently affected, surgery is commonly performed to solve aesthetic problems. Surgical elimination of DIGO lesions involves gingivectomy and gingivoplasty.[50] However, the recurrence rate for GO among patients taking cyclosporin A or nifedipine was approximately 40% 18 months after the surgery.[50]

Patients should be given oral hygiene instructions, and removal of calculus should be done as needed during recall visits. New pharmacologic strategies, especially using animal models, are being explored.[5]

CLINICAL CORRELATION

DIGO cannot be prevented, but it can be ameliorated by elimination of local factors, plaque control, and regular periodontal maintenance. The most effective treatment for DIGO is withdrawal or substitution of the medication. Nonsurgical treatment results in elimination of the inflammatory component of DIGO. Surgical elimination of DIGO lesions involves gingivectomy and gingivoplasty. The recurrence rate is high. Maintenance should include oral hygiene instructions, and removal of calculus as needed.

---

[d]References 6, 16, 31, 47, 49, 72, 74, 81, 86, 87, 102, and 104.

Gingival Overgrowth Associated With Systemic Conditions

Changes in systemic conditions can lead to gingival enlargement. The causes and clinical features of GO associated with systemic conditions are diverse and usually manifest with amplification of existing inflammation due to bacterial components. These gingival pathologies are referred as *conditioned enlargements* and include lesions associated with hormonal and nutritional etiologic factors. Gingival inflammation due to microbial factors is a prerequisite that hormonal and nutritional changes modify, and some researchers classify these lesions as gingivitis-associated pathologies. However, pregnancy and puberty are causes for hormonal changes. Nutritional factors are rare but have historically included deficits such as vitamin C deficiency. Likewise, allergic reactions may be linked to GO.

Pregnancy-Associated Gingival Overgrowth

Clinical manifestations. GO is a common pathology in pregnancy. Clinically, it manifests as a single mass or multiple tumor-like masses at the gingival margin. Marginal gingival enlargement during pregnancy results from the aggravation of previous inflammation, and its incidence is reported as 10% to 70%. Sometimes, the lesions are observed as single enlargements, referred to as *pregnancy tumors*. Pregnancy tumors are not neoplasms; they represent an inflammatory response to microbial plaque modified by the patient's condition. It usually appears after the third month of pregnancy, but it may occur earlier. The reported incidence is 1.8% to 5%.[64]

Pregnancy-associated GO manifests with a highly varied clinical picture. Enlargement is usually generalized, but it tends to be more prominent interproximally than on the facial and lingual surfaces. The enlarged gingiva is bright red or magenta, soft, and friable, and it has a smooth, shiny surface. Bleeding occurs spontaneously or on slight provocation. The lesion appears as a discrete, mushroom-like, flattened spherical mass that protrudes from the gingival margin or, more often, from the interproximal space and it is attached by a sessile or pedunculated base (Fig. 18.11). It tends to expand laterally, and pressure from the tongue and the cheek perpetuates its flattened appearance. It is dusky red or magenta; it has a smooth, glistening surface that often exhibits numerous deep red, pinpoint markings.

Fig. 18.11 Localized Gingival Enlargement in a 27-Year-Old Pregnant Patient.

Fig. 18.12 Pyogenic Granuloma. (Courtesy Dr. Silvia Oreamuno, San Jose, Costa Rica.)

Fig. 18.13 Microscopic View of Gingival Enlargement in a Pregnant Patient.

Fig. 18.14 Conditioned Gingival Enlargement During Puberty.

The superficial lesion of pregnancy-associated GO usually does not invade the underlying bone. The mass is usually firm, but it may have various degrees of softness and friability. It is usually painless unless its size and shape foster the accumulation of debris under its margin or interfere with occlusion, in which case painful ulceration may occur. Although the microscopic findings are characteristic of gingival enlargement during pregnancy, they are not pathognomonic.

Pyogenic granuloma is similar in clinical and microscopic appearance to the gingival enlargement seen during pregnancy. This lesion manifests as a tumor-like gingival enlargement that is considered an exaggerated response to minor trauma (Fig. 18.12). The exact nature of the systemic conditioning factor has not been identified. The differential diagnosis is based on the patient's history.[9]

Etiology. Hormonal changes are linked to pathology in periodontal tissues. For example, progesterone and estrogen levels increase 10 to 30 times by the end of the third trimester compared with the menstrual cycle.[2] Although mechanistic evidence is lacking, it is hypothesized that these hormonal changes induce an increased vascular permeability, which leads to gingival edema and an increased inflammatory response to dental plaque. During this process, the impaired vascular response and inflammatory milieu can lead to modification of the subgingival microbiota. Although not specific, an increased presence of *Prevotella intermedia, Prevotella melaninogenica,* and *Porphyromonas gingivalis* has been linked to pregnancy-associated GO in vivo and in vitro,[59,60,82] demonstrating that the lesions have strong infectious associations.

Histopathology. Gingival enlargement in pregnancy, *angiogranuloma,* refers to its strong clinical presentation with vascular changes and fibrotic process. Marginal and tumor-like enlargements consist of a central mass of connective tissue, with numerous diffusely arranged, newly formed, and engorged capillaries lined by cuboid endothelial cells (Fig. 18.13) and of a moderately fibrous stroma with various degrees of edema and chronic inflammatory infiltrate. The stratified squamous epithelium is thickened, with prominent rete pegs and some degree of intracellular and extracellular edema, prominent intercellular bridges, and leukocytic infiltration.

Treatment. Similar to other forms of gingival changes associated with hormonal variations during pregnancy, GO lesions are prevented by adequate oral hygiene. Oral care in pregnant women should be meticulous, and patients should be treated by removal of plaque and calculus. Severe cases may require removal during the second trimester; however, removal of the GO lesions without establishment of an optimal oral hygiene regimen ensures recurrence of gingival enlargement. Although spontaneous reduction in the size of gingival enlargement typically follows the termination of pregnancy, complete elimination of the residual inflammatory lesion and GO requires removal of all plaque deposits, elimination of factors that favor its accumulation, and, in some fibrotic cases, surgical intervention.

Treatment of pyogenic granuloma consists of the removal of the lesions and the elimination of irritating local factors. The recurrence rate of pyogenic granuloma is approximately 15%.

Puberty-Associated Gingival Overgrowth

Clinical manifestations. Enlargement of the gingiva is sometimes seen during puberty and occur in male and female adolescents. Clinically, there is a strong association with plaque accumulation. The lesions are usually marginal and interdental, and they are characterized by prominent bulbous interproximal papillae (Fig. 18.14). Often, only the facial gingivae are enlarged, and the lingual surfaces are relatively unaltered. The mechanical action of the tongue and the excursion of food prevent a heavy accumulation of local irritants on the lingual surface.

Etiology. Gingival enlargement during puberty has all of the clinical features that are associated with chronic inflammatory gingival disease. The degree of enlargement and its tendency to recur in the setting of relatively scant plaque deposits distinguish puberty-associated GO from purely gingivitis-associated lesions, suggesting a profound impact by the hormonal changes. The incidence of puberty-associated GO lesions decline with age,[98] further supporting the role of hormonal changes during puberty.

Studies of the subgingival microbiota of children between the ages of 11 and 14 years and their association with clinical parameters implicated *Capnocytophaga* species in the initiation of pubertal gingivitis.[39,71] Other studies have reported that hormonal changes coincide with an increase in the proportion of *P. intermedia* and *Prevotella nigrescens*.[73,106] However, the etiologic role of the changes in microbiota is not clear. It is not known whether changes in inflammatory conditions predispose to a shift in microbial species.

Histopathology. The microscopic appearance of gingival enlargement during puberty is one of chronic inflammation with prominent edema. It cannot be distinguished from other forms of gingivitis-associated GO lesions.

Treatment. After puberty, enlargement undergoes spontaneous reduction, but it does not disappear completely until the plaque and calculus are removed.

Nutrition-Associated Gingival Overgrowth

Malnutrition has been historically associated with several oral lesions. GO has been observed in cases of chronic vitamin C deficiency in patients with scurvy. These lesions are no longer common, but GO is still considered a part of the classic description of scurvy.

Clinical manifestations. Gingival enlargement with vitamin C deficiency is marginal. The gingiva is bluish red, soft, and friable, and it has a smooth, shiny surface. Hemorrhage that occurs spontaneously or on slight provocation and surface necrosis with pseudomembrane formations are common features.

Etiology. Acute vitamin C deficiency alone does not cause gingival inflammation, but it does cause hemorrhage, collagen degeneration, and edema of the gingival connective tissue. These changes modify the response of the gingiva to plaque to the extent that the normal defensive delimiting reaction is inhibited and the extent of the inflammation is exaggerated, thereby resulting in the massive gingival enlargement seen in patients with scurvy.

Histopathology. In patients with vitamin C deficiency, the gingiva has a chronic inflammatory cellular infiltration with a superficial acute response. There are scattered areas of hemorrhage with engorged capillaries. Marked diffuse edema, collagen degeneration, and a scarcity of collagen fibrils and fibroblasts are striking findings.

Treatment. Nutrition-associated GO lesions are rare. Changes in nutrition accompanied by nonsurgical treatment and good oral hygiene usually result in complete resolution of the pathology. In rare cases, surgical removal is indicated.

Gingival Overgrowth Associated With Systemic Diseases

GO may be linked to various systemic diseases. Although uncommon and occurring with different etiopathogenetic mechanisms,

Fig. 18.15 Leukemia-Associated Gingival Enlargement. (Courtesy Dr. Spencer Wolfe, Dublin, Ireland.)

the GO associated with systemic diseases can be linked to serious issues in clinical management. These lesions should be carefully diagnosed.

Leukemia-Associated Gingival Overgrowth

Clinical manifestations. Leukemic gingival enlargement can be diffuse or marginal and localized or generalized. It can appear as a diffuse enlargement of the gingival mucosa, an oversized extension of the marginal gingiva (Fig. 18.15), or a discrete tumor-like interproximal mass. In patients with leukemic enlargement, the gingiva is bluish red, and it has a shiny surface. The consistency is moderately firm, but there is a tendency toward friability and hemorrhage that occur spontaneously or with slight irritation.

Acute painful necrotizing ulcerative inflammatory involvement can occur in the crevice formed at the junction of the enlarged gingiva and the contiguous tooth surfaces. Patients with leukemia may also have a simple chronic inflammation without the involvement of leukemic cells, and they can have the same clinical and microscopic features seen in patients without the systemic disease. However, most cases have features of simple chronic inflammation and leukemic infiltrate. True leukemic enlargement often occurs with acute leukemia but also occurs in subacute leukemia. It seldom occurs with chronic leukemia.

Histopathology. Gingival enlargements in leukemic patients show various degrees of chronic inflammation. Mature leukocytes are seen along with areas of connective tissue that are infiltrated with a dense mass of immature and proliferating leukocytes, the specific nature of which varies with the type of leukemia. Engorged capillaries, edematous and degenerated connective tissue, and epithelium with various degrees of leukocytic infiltration and edema are found. Isolated surface areas of acute necrotizing inflammation with a pseudomembranous meshwork of fibrin, necrotic epithelial cells, polymorphonuclear leukocytes, and bacteria are often seen.

Wegener Granulomatosis

Clinical manifestations. Wegener granulomatosis is a rare disease that is characterized by acute granulomatous necrotizing lesions of the respiratory tract, including nasal and oral defects. Renal lesions develop, and acute necrotizing vasculitis affects the blood vessels. The initial manifestations of Wegener granulomatosis can involve the orofacial region and include oral mucosal ulceration, gingival enlargement, abnormal tooth mobility, exfoliation of teeth, and a delayed healing response. The granulomatous papillary enlargement is reddish purple and bleeds easily on stimulation (Fig. 18.16).

Etiology. The cause of Wegener granulomatosis is unknown, but the condition is considered an immunologically mediated tissue injury. At one time, the usual outcome for patients with this condition was death from kidney failure within a few months, but more recently the use of immunosuppressive drugs has produced prolonged remissions in more than 90% of patients.

Histopathology. Chronic inflammation involves scattered giant cells, foci of acute inflammation, and microabscesses covered by a thin, acanthotic epithelium. Vascular changes have not been described with gingival enlargement in patients with Wegener granulomatosis, probably because of the small size of the gingival blood vessels.

Sarcoidosis

Clinical manifestations. Sarcoidosis is a granulomatous disease of unknown etiology. It starts in individuals during their 20s or 30s, it predominantly affects blacks, and it can involve almost any organ, including the gingiva, in which a red, smooth, painless enlargement may appear.

Histopathology. Sarcoid granulomas consist of discrete epithelioid cells and multinucleated, foreign body–type giant cells with peripheral mononuclear cells.

Gingival Fibromatosis

Clinical manifestations. Gingival fibromatosis can be hereditary or idiopathic. These lesions are rare and occur in highly fibrotic forms of GO.[38,105] Hereditary gingival fibromatosis is the most common form, and it has been linked to several genetic loci.[e] Idiopathic gingival enlargement is a rare condition of undetermined cause.

The enlargement affects the attached gingiva, the gingival margin, and the interdental papillae. The facial and lingual surfaces of the mandible and maxilla usually are affected, but the involvement may be limited to either jaw. The enlarged gingiva is pink, firm, and almost leathery in consistency, and it has a characteristic minutely pebbled surface (Fig. 18.17). In severe cases, the teeth are almost completely covered, and the enlargement projects into the oral vestibule. The jaws appear distorted because of the bulbous enlargement of the gingiva. Secondary inflammatory changes are common at the gingival margin.

Etiology. The genetic basis of hereditary gingival fibromatosis is well established, with different populations having different genetic loci and specific genes.[f] In some families, gingival enlargement is linked to the impairment of physical development. Other syndromes are sometimes colocalized with gingival fibromatosis.[46,65] Idiopathic forms of gingival fibromatosis have not been linked to specific genes, and the condition is designated as idiopathic.

> ## KEY FACT
>
> The genetic basis of hereditary gingival fibromatosis is well established. In some families, gingival enlargement is linked to impairment of physical development. Other syndromes can coexist with gingival fibromatosis. Idiopathic forms of gingival fibromatosis are not linked to any specific genes.

Although the genes associated with lesions of hereditary forms have been identified, the pathogenetic mechanisms linked to these genetic factors are not fully understood. Enlargement usually begins with the eruption of the primary or secondary dentition, and it may regress after extraction, which suggests that the teeth or the plaque attached to them may be initiating factors. The presence of bacterial plaque is a complicating factor. Gingival enlargement has been described in tuberous sclerosis, which is an inherited condition characterized by the triad of epilepsy, mental deficiency, and cutaneous angiofibromas.

Fig. 18.16 Wegener Granulomatosis Affecting the Gingival Tissue.

[e]References 8, 26, 41, 42, 93, 107, and 108.
[f]References 27, 40, 43, 48, 68, 76, 78, 94, 109, and 110.

Fig. 18.17 Idiopathic Gingival Enlargement. (A) Facial view. (B) Occlusal view of the mandibular arch.

Histopathology. In cases of GO with fibromatosis, the lesions are highly fibrotic, with a bulbous increase in connective tissue that is relatively avascular and consists of densely arranged collagen bundles and numerous fibroblasts. The surface epithelium is thickened and acanthotic, with elongated rete pegs.[21,53,54] Histopathology is similar to phenytoin-induced GO with low levels of inflammatory infiltration. However, collagen bundle formation, dominance, and orientation are distinctive in areas where cellular structures are reduced.[21]

Treatment. Treatment of GO lesions manifesting as gingival fibromatosis requires gingivectomy and gingivoplasty. Clinical management is difficult because of the high recurrence rate, and the severity of lesions usually results in extreme crowding and misalignment of teeth. After removal of the fibromatosis lesions, patients may require orthodontic treatment.[25]

OTHER FORMS OF GINGIVAL ENLARGEMENT

Multiple forms of gingival enlargement have various causes. In addition to the types of GO previously discussed in this chapter, the gingiva can be enlarged due to increases in the size of the underlying osseous and dental tissues. These *false enlargements* usually have no abnormal clinical features except for the massive increase in the size of the area. For example, enlargement of the bone subjacent to the gingival area occurs most often with tori and exostoses, but it can also occur with Paget disease, fibrous dysplasia, cherubism, central giant cell granuloma, ameloblastoma, osteoma, and osteosarcoma.

The gingival tissue can appear normal, or it can have unrelated inflammatory changes. Likewise, during the various stages of eruption, particularly of the primary dentition, the labial gingiva can have a bulbous marginal distortion caused by superimposition of the bulk of the gingiva on the normal prominence of the enamel in the gingival half of the crown. This enlargement is called *developmental enlargement,* and it often persists until the junctional epithelium has migrated from the enamel to the cementoenamel junction.

In a strict sense, developmental gingival enlargements are physiologic, and they usually present no problems for patients. However, when the enlargement is complicated by marginal inflammation, the composite picture gives the impression of extensive gingival enlargement (Fig. 18.18).

Neoplastic formations in gingival tissues can be clinically confused with fibrotic enlargements of gingiva. Oral cancer accounts for less than 3% of all malignant tumors in the body, but it is the 6th most common cancer in males and the 12th most common cancer in females. The gingiva is not a common site of oral malignancy, accounting for only 6% of oral cancers.

Epulis is a generic term that is used to clinically designate all discrete tumors and tumor-like masses of the gingiva. It serves to locate the tumor but does not describe it. Most lesions referred to by this term are inflammatory rather than neoplastic. For example, fibromas arise from the gingival connective tissue or from the periodontal ligament. They are slow-growing, spherical tumors that tend to be firm and nodular but that may be soft and vascular. Fibromas are usually pedunculated. Hard fibromas of the gingiva are rare; most of the lesions that are diagnosed clinically as fibromas are inflammatory enlargements.

Histopathologic review of fibromas demonstrates bundles of well-formed collagen fibers with scattered fibrocytes and various degrees of vascularity. The so-called giant cell fibroma contains multinucleated fibroblasts. In another variant, mineralized tissue (i.e., bone, cementum-like material, and dystrophic calcifications) is found; this type of fibroma is called *peripheral ossifying fibroma.*

Similar to fibromas, papillomas are benign proliferations of surface epithelium that are in many cases associated with human papillomavirus (HPV) infection. Gingival papillomas appear as solitary wartlike or cauliflower-like protuberances (Fig. 18.19). They can be small and discrete, or they can be broad, hard elevations with minutely irregular surfaces. The lesions consist of finger-like projections of stratified squamous epithelium that are often hyperkeratotic, with central cores of fibrovascular connective tissue.

Peripheral giant cell granulomas of the gingiva arise interdentally or from the gingival margin. They occur most frequently on the labial surface, and they can be sessile or pedunculated. They vary in appearance from smooth, regularly outlined masses to irregularly shaped, multilobulated protuberances with surface indentations (Fig. 18.20). Ulceration of the margin is occasionally seen. The lesions are painless, vary in size, and can cover several teeth. They can be firm or spongy, and their color varies from pink to deep red or purplish blue.

Clinically, peripheral giant cell granulomas are not easily differentiated from other forms of gingival enlargement. Microscopic

Fig. 18.18 Developmental Gingival Enlargement.

Fig. 18.19 Papilloma of the Gingiva.

examination is required for definitive diagnosis. The word *peripheral* is needed to differentiate from comparable lesions that originate within the jawbone (i.e., central giant cell granulomas). In some cases, the giant cell granuloma of the gingiva is locally invasive and causes destruction of the underlying bone (Fig. 18.21A). Complete removal leads to uneventful recovery. The lesion has numerous foci of multinuclear giant cells and hemosiderin particles in a connective tissue stroma (see Fig. 18.21B). Areas of chronic inflammation are scattered throughout the lesion, with acute involvement occurring at the surface. The overlying epithelium is usually hyperplastic, with ulceration at the base. Bone destruction occasionally occurs within the lesion (Fig. 18.22).

Gingival cysts of microscopic proportions are common, but they seldom reach a clinically significant size. When they do, they appear as localized enlargements that may involve the marginal and attached gingiva. The cysts occur in the mandibular canine and premolar areas, most often on the lingual surface. They are painless, but with expansion they can cause erosion of the surface of the alveolar bone. The gingival cyst should be differentiated from the lateral periodontal cyst, which arises within the alveolar bone adjacent to the root and which is developmental in origin. Gingival cysts develop from odontogenic epithelium or from surface or sulcular epithelium traumatically implanted in the area. Removal is followed by uneventful recovery.

A gingival cyst cavity is lined by a thin, flattened epithelium with or without localized areas of thickening. Less frequently, the following types of epithelium can be found: unkeratinized stratified squamous epithelium, keratinized stratified squamous epithelium, and parakeratinized epithelium with palisading basal cells.

Squamous cell carcinoma is the most common malignant tumor of the gingiva. It may be *exophytic*, manifesting as an irregular outgrowth, or *ulcerative,* appearing as a flat, erosive lesion. It is often symptom free, going unnoticed until complicated by inflammatory changes that can mask the neoplasm but cause pain; it sometimes becomes evident after tooth extraction. These masses are locally invasive, and they involve the underlying bone and periodontal ligament of adjoining teeth and the adjacent mucosa (Fig. 18.23). Metastasis is usually confined to the region above the clavicle; however, involvement that is more extensive can include the lung, liver, or bone.

Fig. 18.22 Bone Destruction in the Interproximal Space Between the Canine and the Lateral Incisor is Caused by the Extension of a Peripheral Giant Cell Reparative Granuloma of the Gingiva. (Courtesy Dr. Sam Toll.)

Fig. 18.20 Gingival Giant Cell Granuloma.

Fig. 18.21 (A) Microscopic survey of a peripheral giant cell granuloma. (B) High-power microscopic study of the lesion demonstrates the giant cells and the intervening stroma.

Fig. 18.23 Squamous Cell Carcinoma of the Gingiva. (A) Facial view shows extensive verrucous involvement. (B) Palatal view shows mulberry-like tissue emerging between the second premolar and the first molar.

Malignant melanoma is a rare oral tumor that tends to occur in the hard palate and maxillary gingiva of older persons. It is usually darkly pigmented, and it is often preceded by localized pigmentation. It can be flat or nodular, and it is characterized by rapid growth and early metastasis. It arises from melanoblasts in the gingiva, cheek, or palate. Infiltration into the underlying bone and metastasis to cervical and axillary lymph nodes are common.

Fibrosarcoma, lymphosarcoma, and reticulum cell sarcoma of the gingiva are rare; only isolated cases have been described in the literature. Kaposi sarcoma often occurs in the oral cavity, particularly in the palate and the gingiva, of patients with acquired immunodeficiency syndrome. Tumor metastasis to the gingiva occurs infrequently.

The low incidence of oral malignancy should not mislead the clinician. Ulcerations that do not respond to therapy in the usual manner and all gingival tumors and tumor-like lesions must be biopsied and submitted for microscopic diagnosis.

In most clinical cases of GO, the clinical appearance is complicated by inflammation, bleeding, and swelling, which further creates difficulty in identifying the cause and pathologic process. A thorough knowledge of GO and the patient's systemic and oral medical histories are critical for designing the treatment and maintaining outcomes. Because some GO forms are linked to systemic and severe diseases, this approach is also essential for securing the patient's safety before treatment is initiated.

A Case Scenario is found on the companion website.

REFERENCES

 References for this chapter are found on the companion website.

Acute Gingival Infections[a]

NECROTIZING ULCERATIVE GINGIVITIS

Necrotizing ulcerative gingivitis (NUG) is a microbial disease of the gingiva that most often occurs in an impaired host. It manifests with the characteristic clinical signs of necrosis and sloughing of the gingival tissues and may be accompanied by systemic symptoms.

Clinical Features

NUG has historically been identified as an acute disease. However, the term *acute* in this case is used as a clinical descriptor and not a diagnosis, because chronic forms of the disease do not exist. Although the acronym *ANUG* is frequently used, it is a misnomer.[66] A summary of acute periodontal lesions advocated the more simplified term, *necrotizing gingivitis,* rather than *NUG,* but the latter term continues to be used in this chapter.[32] Involvement can be limited to a single tooth or group of teeth, or it can be widespread throughout the mouth (Fig. 19.1).

More advanced forms of necrotizing ulcerative disease can include destruction of the periodontal attachment apparatus, including bone,[46] especially in patients with long-standing disease or severe immunosuppression. When periodontal attachment loss and bone loss occur, the condition is called *necrotizing ulcerative periodontitis* (NUP) (see Chapter 27).

History

NUG is characterized by a sudden onset of symptoms, sometimes occurring after an episode of debilitating disease or acute respiratory tract infection. A change in living habits, protracted work without adequate rest, poor nutrition, tobacco use, poor oral hygiene and psychological stress are common features of the patient's history.

Oral Signs

Characteristic lesions are punched-out, craterlike depressions at the crest of the interdental papillae that subsequently extend to the marginal gingiva and rarely to the attached gingiva and oral mucosa. The surface of the gingival crater is covered by a gray, pseudomembranous slough that is demarcated from the remainder of the gingival mucosa by a pronounced linear erythema (see Fig. 19.1A). In some cases, the lesions are denuded of the surface pseudomembrane, thereby exposing the gingival margin, which is red, shiny, and hemorrhagic. The characteristic lesions can progressively destroy the gingiva and the underlying periodontal tissues (see Fig. 19.1B).

Spontaneous gingival hemorrhage and pronounced bleeding after the slightest stimulation are additional characteristic clinical signs (see Fig. 19.1B and C). Other common signs include a fetid odor and increased salivation.

NUG can occur in otherwise disease-free mouths, or it can be superimposed on chronic gingivitis or periodontitis with periodontal pockets. However, NUG does not usually lead to periodontal pocket formation because the necrotic changes involve the gingival and junctional epithelium; healthy epithelium is needed for periodontal pocket deepening (see Chapter 22). Although the numbers are much less, spirochetes and fusiform bacilli are found on normal edentulous mucosa.[65]

> **KEY FACT**
>
> NUG can be superimposed on chronic periodontitis with pockets, but it does not usually lead to pocket formation because the necrotic changes involve the gingival and junctional epithelium.

Oral Symptoms

The lesions are extremely sensitive to touch, and the patient often complains of a constant radiating, gnawing pain that is intensified by eating spicy or hot foods and chewing. There is a metallic foul taste, and the patient is conscious of an excessive amount of pasty saliva.

Extraoral and Systemic Signs and Symptoms

Patients are usually ambulatory and have a minimum of systemic symptoms. Local lymphadenopathy and a slight elevation in temperature are common features of the mild and moderate stages of the disease. In severe cases, patients can have high fever,

---

[a]Adapted from the following chapter of Newman and Carranza's Clinical Periodontology, 13th edition: Chapter 20: Acute Gingival Infections, by Perry R. Klokkevold and Fermin A. Carranza.

Fig. 19.1 Necrotizing Ulcerative Gingivitis. (A) Typical punched-out papilla between the mandibular canine and lateral incisor is covered by a grayish white pseudomembrane. (B) More advanced case shows the destruction of the papillae, which results in an irregular marginal contour. (C) Typical lesions with spontaneous hemorrhage. (D) Generalized involvement of the papillae and the marginal gingiva with whitish necrotic lesions.

increased pulse rate, leukocytosis, loss of appetite, and general lassitude. Systemic reactions are more severe in children. Insomnia, constipation, gastrointestinal disorders, headache, and mental depression sometimes accompany the condition.

In rare cases, severe sequelae such as gangrenous stomatitis and noma have been described.[3,4,19,36] These patients are almost exclusively encountered in populations in developing countries, especially children with systemic disease or malnutrition.[19,32,66]

Clinical Course

The clinical course varies among individuals. The severity of NUG often diminishes without treatment, leading to a subacute stage with milder clinical symptoms. Some patients experience repeated remissions and exacerbations, and the condition can recur in previously treated patients. If untreated, especially in an immunocompromised host, NUG can lead to progressive destruction of the periodontium and gingival recession accompanied by an increase in the severity of systemic complications.[34,58]

Histopathology

Microscopically, the NUG lesion is a nonspecific acute necrotizing inflammation of the gingival margin that involves the stratified squamous epithelium and the underlying connective tissue. The surface epithelium is destroyed and replaced by a meshwork of fibrin, necrotic epithelial cells, polymorphonuclear leukocytes (PMNs, predominantly neutrophils), and various types of microorganisms (Fig. 19.2). This is the zone that appears clinically as the surface pseudomembrane. At the immediate border of the necrotic pseudomembrane, the epithelium is edematous, and the individual cells exhibit various degrees of hydropic degeneration. PMNs infiltrate the intercellular spaces.

Fig. 19.2 In a survey section of interdental papilla in a patient with necrotizing ulcerative gingivitis, the necrotic tissue forms the gray marginal pseudomembrane *(top)*. Ulceration and the accumulation of leukocytes and fibrin replace normal epithelium *(bottom)*.

The underlying connective tissue is markedly hyperemic, with numerous engorged capillaries and a dense infiltration of PMNs. This acutely inflamed zone appears clinically as the linear erythema beneath the surface pseudomembrane. Numerous plasma cells can appear in the periphery of the infiltrate; this is interpreted as an area of established chronic gingivitis on which the acute lesion became superimposed.[33] The epithelium and connective tissue alterations decrease as the distance from the necrotic gingival margin increases, blending gradually with the uninvolved gingiva.

The microscopic appearance of tissues in a NUG lesion is nonspecific. Comparable changes result from trauma, chemical irritation, or the application of caustic medications.

Relationship of Bacteria and the Necrotizing Ulcerative Gingivitis Lesion

Light and electron microscopy have been used to study the relationship of bacteria and the characteristic lesion of NUG. Light microscopy shows that the exudate on the surface of the necrotic lesion contains microorganisms that morphologically resemble cocci, fusiform bacilli, and spirochetes.[81] The layer between the necrotic and living tissue contains enormous numbers of fusiform bacilli and spirochetes in addition to leukocytes and fibrin. Spirochetes and other bacteria invade the underlying living tissue.[6,14,18,43]

Spirochetes have been found as deep as 300 μm from the surface. Most spirochetes in the deeper zones are morphologically different from cultivated strains of *Treponema microdentium*. They occur in nonnecrotic tissue before other types of bacteria, and they can achieve high intercellular concentrations in the epithelium and connective tissue adjacent to the ulcerated lesion.[42]

Smears from the lesions (Fig. 19.3) show scattered bacteria (predominantly spirochetes and fusiform bacilli), desquamated epithelial cells, and occasional PMNs. Spirochetes and fusiform bacteria are usually seen with other oral spirochetes, vibrios, and filaments.

Diagnosis

Diagnosis is based on clinical findings of gingival pain, ulceration, and bleeding. A bacterial smear is not necessary or diagnostic because the bacterial picture is not appreciably different from that of patients with marginal gingivitis, periodontitis, pericoronitis, or primary herpetic gingivostomatitis.[64] However, bacterial studies are useful for the differential diagnosis of NUG and

specific infections of the oral cavity (e.g., diphtheria, thrush, actinomycosis, streptococcal stomatitis).

The microscopic examination of a biopsy specimen is not sufficiently specific to be diagnostic. It can be used to differentiate NUG from specific infections (e.g., tuberculosis) or from neoplastic disease, but it does not differentiate NUG from other necrotizing conditions of nonspecific origin, such as those produced by trauma or caustic medications.

KEY FACT

A bacterial smear or culture is not necessary or definitive in the diagnosis of NUG because the bacterial microbiota is not appreciably different from that of patients with other common inflammatory conditions (e.g., gingivitis, periodontitis). However, bacterial studies are useful for the differential diagnosis of NUG when specific infections of the oral cavity (e.g., diphtheria, thrush, actinomycosis, streptococcal stomatitis) are suspected.

Differential Diagnosis

NUG should be differentiated from other conditions that resemble it in some respects, such as herpetic gingivostomatitis (Table 19.1), chronic periodontitis, desquamative gingivitis (Table 19.2), streptococcal gingivostomatitis, aphthous stomatitis, gonococcal gingivostomatitis, diphtheritic and syphilitic lesions (Table 19.3), tuberculous gingival lesions, candidiasis, agranulocytosis, dermatoses (e.g., pemphigus, erythema multiforme, lichen planus), and stomatitis venenata (see Chapter 21).

Treatment options for these diseases vary dramatically, and misdiagnosis and improper treatment can exacerbate the condition. In the case of primary herpetic gingivostomatitis, early diagnosis can result in treatment with antiviral drugs that would be ineffective for NUG, whereas the treatment of a case of

Fig. 19.3 A Bacterial Smear Was Obtained from a Lesion in a Patient With Necrotizing Ulcerative Gingivitis. *A,* Spirochete; *B, Bacillus fusiformis; C,* Filamentous organism (i.e., *Actinomyces* or *Leptotrichia*); *D, Streptococcus; E, Vibrio; F, Treponema microdentium.*

TABLE 19.1 Differentiation of Necrotizing Ulcerative Gingivitis and Primary Herpetic Gingivostomatitis

Necrotizing Ulcerative Gingivitis	Primary Herpetic Gingivostomatitis
Caused by interaction between host and bacteria, most often fusospirochetes	Caused by specific viral infection
Necrotizing condition	Diffuse erythema and vesicular eruption
Punched-out gingival margin; pseudomembrane that peels off and leaves raw areas	Vesicles that rupture and leave slightly depressed oval or spherical ulcer
Marginal gingiva affected; other oral tissues rarely affected	Diffuse involvement of gingiva; may include buccal mucosa and lips
Uncommon in children	Occurs more frequently in children
No definite duration	Duration of 7–10 days
No demonstrated immunity	Acute episode results in some degree of immunity
Contagion not demonstrated	Contagion

TABLE 19.2 Differentiation of Necrotizing Ulcerative Gingivitis, Chronic Desquamative Gingivitis, and Chronic Periodontal Disease

Necrotizing Ulcerative Gingivitis	Desquamative Gingivitis	Chronic Destructive Periodontal Disease
Bacterial smears show fusospirochetal complex	Bacterial smears reveal numerous epithelial cells and few bacterial forms	Bacterial smears vary
Marginal gingiva affected	Diffuse involvement of marginal and attached gingivae and other areas of oral mucosa	Marginal gingiva affected
Acute history	Chronic history	Chronic history
Painful	May or may not be painful	Painless if uncomplicated
Pseudomembrane	Patchy desquamation of gingival epithelium	Usually no desquamation, but purulent material may appear from pockets
Papillary and marginal necrotic lesions	Papillae do not undergo necrosis	Papillae do not undergo noticeable necrosis
Affects adults of both genders and occasionally affects children	Affects adults, most often women	Usually found in adults, occasionally found in children
Characteristic fetid odor	No odor	Some odor but not strikingly fetid

TABLE 19.3 Differentiation of Necrotizing Ulcerative Gingivitis, Diphtheria, and Secondary Stage of Syphilis

Necrotizing Ulcerative Gingivitis	Diphtheria	Secondary Stage of Syphilis (Mucous Patch)
Caused by interaction between host and bacteria, typically fusospirochetes	Caused by *Corynebacterium diphtheriae*	Caused by *Treponema pallidum*
Affects marginal gingiva	Rarely affects marginal gingiva	Rarely affects marginal gingiva
Membrane removal easy	Membrane removal difficult	Membrane not detachable
Painful condition	Less painful	Minimal pain
Marginal gingivae affected	Throat, fauces, and tonsils affected	Any part of mouth affected
Serologic findings normal	Serologic findings normal	Serologic findings abnormal[a]
Immunity not conferred	Immunity conferred by an attack	Immunity not conferred
Doubtful contagiousness	Contagious	Only direct contact can communicate disease
Antibiotic therapy relieves symptoms	Antibiotic treatment is effective	Antibiotic therapy has excellent results

[a]Wassermann test, Kahn test, and Venereal Disease Research Laboratories (VDRL) test.

herpes with the debridement required for NUG could exacerbate the herpes.

Streptococcal gingivostomatitis is a rare condition that is characterized by a diffuse erythema of the gingiva and other areas of the oral mucosa.[49] In some cases, it is confined as a marginal erythema with marginal hemorrhage. Necrosis of the gingival margin is not a feature of this disease, and there is no fetid odor. Bacterial smears show a preponderance of streptococcal forms, which were identified as *Streptococcus viridans,* but other studies report findings of group A β-hemolytic streptococci.[44]

Agranulocytosis is characterized by a marked decrease in the number of circulating PMNs, lesions of the throat and other mucous membranes, and ulceration and necrosis of the gingiva that can resemble that of NUG and that occurs most commonly after chemotherapy in cancer patients or in patients with leukemia. The oral condition of patients with agranulocytosis is primarily necrotizing, but it lacks the severe inflammatory reaction seen with NUG. Blood studies can differentiate between NUG and the gingival necrosis associated with agranulocytosis.

Vincent angina is a fusospirochetal infection of the oropharynx and throat that is distinguished from NUG, which affects the marginal gingiva. Patients with Vincent angina have a painful membranous ulceration of the throat, with edema and hyperemic patches breaking down to form ulcers that are covered with pseudomembranous material. The process can extend to the larynx and the middle ear.

NUG in leukemia patients results from the reduced host defense mechanisms that occur with the disease. NUG can be superimposed on the gingival tissue alterations caused by leukemia. The differential diagnosis does not require distinguishing between NUG and leukemic gingival changes; instead, it is determined whether leukemia is a predisposing factor in the mouth of a patient with NUG. For example, if a patient with necrotizing involvement of the gingival margin also has diffuse discoloration and generalized edema of the attached gingiva, the possibility of an underlying systemically induced gingival change should be considered. Leukemia is one of the conditions that would need to be ruled out (see Chapter 13).

NUG in the patient with human immunodeficiency virus (HIV) infection has the same clinical features, although it often follows an extremely destructive course that leads to NUP, with a loss of soft tissue and bone and the formation of bony sequestra (see Chapter 28).[29]

CLINICAL CORRELATION

A serious systemic disease or condition such as leukemia or acquired immunodeficiency that renders the host immunocompromised can be the predisposing causative factor leading to acute gingival disease.

Etiology

Role of Bacteria

Plaut[60] in 1894 and Vincent[83] in 1896 postulated that NUG was caused by specific bacteria: fusiform bacilli and spirochetal organisms. Opinions still differ about whether bacteria are the primary causative factors of NUG. Several observations support this concept, including that spirochetal organisms and fusiform bacilli are always found in patients with the disease along with other organisms. Rosebury and colleagues[64] described a fusospirochetal complex that consists of *T. microdentium*, intermediate spirochetes, vibrios, fusiform bacilli, and filamentous organisms in addition to several *Borrelia* species.

Loesche and colleagues[45] described a predominant constant microbiota and a variable microbiota associated with NUG. The constant microbiota is composed of *Prevotella intermedia* in addition to *Fusobacterium*, *Treponema*, and *Selenomonas* species. The variable microbiota consists of a heterogeneous array of bacterial types.

Treatment with metronidazole results in a significant reduction of *Treponema* species, *P. intermedia*, and *Fusobacterium*, with resolution of the clinical symptoms.[17,45] The antibacterial spectrum of this drug provides evidence for the anaerobic members of the microbiota as etiologic agents. These bacteriologic findings have been supported by immunologic data[10] that demonstrated increased immunoglobulin G and M antibody titers for medium-sized spirochetes and *P. intermedia* in patients with NUG compared with titers in patients with chronic gingivitis and healthy controls.

Role of the Host Response

Regardless of whether specific bacteria are implicated in the cause of NUG, the presence of these organisms without other predisposing factors appears to be insufficient to cause the disease. The fusospirochetal microbiota is frequently found in patients who do not have NUG. Exudates from NUG lesions produce fusospirochetal abscesses rather than typical NUG lesions when the exudates are inoculated subcutaneously into experimental animals.[63]

The role of an impaired host response in NUG has long been recognized. Even in the early descriptions of the disease, NUG was associated with physical and emotional stress[12,66] and decreased resistance to infection. NUG has not been produced experimentally in humans or animals, only by inoculation of bacterial exudates from the lesions. In the animal model, local or systemic immunosuppression with glucocorticoids (e.g., ketoconazole) results in more characteristic lesions of NUG in infected animals. Swenson and Muhler used scillaren B, an amorphous glucoside, which reduced tissue resistance to create oral fusospirochetal infections in dogs.[77,78]

NUG is not usually found in well-nourished individuals with a fully functional immune system, since many of the predisposing factors for NUG are associated with immunosuppression. Cogen and colleagues[11] described depression of host defense mechanisms, particularly in PMN chemotaxis and phagocytosis, in patients with NUG. Host–bacteria interactions are described in Chapter 9.

It is essential for the clinician to determine the predisposing factors that lead to immunodeficiency in patients with NUG to address the continued susceptibility of the patient and to determine whether an underlying systemic disease exists. Immunodeficiency may be related to various levels of nutritional deficiency, fatigue caused by chronic sleep deprivation, other health habits (e.g., alcohol, drug abuse), psychosocial factors, or systemic disease. NUG can be the presenting symptom for patients with immunosuppression related to HIV infection.

Local Predisposing Factors

Preexisting gingivitis, injury to the gingiva, and smoking are important predisposing factors. Although NUG can appear in an otherwise disease-free mouth, it most often occurs superimposed on preexisting chronic gingival disease and periodontal pockets. Deep periodontal pockets and pericoronal flaps are particularly vulnerable areas because they offer a favorable environment for the proliferation of anaerobic fusiform bacilli and spirochetes. Areas of the gingiva that are traumatized by opposing teeth in malocclusion (e.g., palatal surface behind the maxillary incisors, labial gingival surface of the mandibular incisors) can predispose an individual to the development of NUG.

The relationship between NUG and smoking has often been mentioned in the literature. Pindborg[58] reported that 98% of his patients with NUG were smokers and that the increasing frequency of this disease correlates with increasing exposure to tobacco smoke. The effect of smoking on periodontal disease in general has been the subject of numerous studies during the past two decades,[2,23,25,37,40,55] and smoking has been established as a high-risk factor for disease (see Chapter 11).

Systemic Predisposing Factors

NUG is not found in a well-nourished individual with a fully functional immune system. It is therefore important for the clinician to determine the predisposing factors for immunodeficiency. Immunodeficiency can be related to various levels of nutritional deficiency, psychosocial stress, fatigue caused by chronic sleep deficiency, other health habits (e.g., alcoholism, drug abuse), and systemic disease (e.g., diabetes, debilitating infection).

Nutritional deficiency. Necrotizing gingivitis has been produced in animals by giving them nutritionally deficient diets.[8,38,52,79,82] Several researchers found an increase in the fusospirochetal microbiota in the mouths of the experimental animals, but the bacteria were regarded as opportunists that proliferated only when the tissues were altered by the deficiency.

A poor diet has been cited as a predisposing factor for NUG and its sequelae in developing African countries, although the effects appear primarily to diminish the effectiveness of the immune response.[20,21,39] Nutritional deficiencies (e.g., vitamin C, vitamin B_2) accentuate the severity of the pathologic changes induced when the fusospirochetal bacterial complex is injected into animals.[76]

Debilitating disease. Debilitating systemic disease can predispose patients to NUG. Systemic disturbances include chronic diseases (e.g., syphilis, cancer), severe gastrointestinal disorders (e.g., ulcerative colitis), blood dyscrasias (e.g., leukemia, anemia), and acquired immunodeficiency syndrome. Nutritional deficiency that results from debilitating disease can be an additional predisposing factor. Experimentally induced leukopenia in animals can produce ulcerative gangrenous stomatitis.[52,80,81] Ulceronecrotic lesions appear in the gingival margins of hamsters that are exposed to total body irradiation[48]; these lesions can be prevented with systemic antibiotics.[47]

Psychosomatic factors. Psychological factors appear to be important in the cause of NUG. The disease often occurs in association with stressful situations (e.g., induction into the armed forces, academic examinations).[27] Psychological disturbances[28] and increased adrenocortical secretion[71] are common in patients with the disease.

A significant correlation between disease incidence and two personality traits—dominance and abasement—suggests a NUG-prone personality.[24] Data from a study evaluating the relationship between personality traits and stress with gingival inflammation and soft tissue pathology in military recruits found that gingival inflammation correlated significantly with personality traits (e.g., tolerance to change, anxiety).[53]

The mechanisms by which psychologic factors create or predispose an individual to gingival damage have not been established. However, alterations in digital and gingival capillary responses that suggest increased autonomic nervous activity have been demonstrated in patients with NUG.[26]

It can be concluded that opportunistic bacteria are the primary etiologic agents of NUG in patients who demonstrate immunosuppression. Stress, smoking, and preexisting gingivitis are common predisposing factors.

Epidemiology and Prevalence

The prevalence of NUG appears to have been rather low in the United States and Europe before 1914. During World Wars I and II, numerous epidemics broke out among the Allied troops, but German soldiers did not seem to have been similarly affected. Epidemic-like outbreaks have also occurred among civilian populations. A study at a dental clinic in Prague, Czech Republic, reported the incidence of NUG as 0.08% among patients 15 to 19 years old, 0.05% among those 20 to 24 years old, and 0.02% among those 25 to 29 years old.[74]

NUG occurs in individuals of all ages, with the highest incidence reported for patients between the ages of 15 and 30 years.[16,41,74,76] It is not common among children in the United States, Canada, and Europe, but it has been reported in children from low socioeconomic groups in underdeveloped countries.[36] In India, 54%[51] and 58%[59] of patients in two studies were younger than 10 years of age.

In a random school population in Nigeria, NUG occurred in 11.3% of children between the ages of 2 and 6 years.[72] In a Nigerian hospital population, it affected 23% of children who were younger than 10 years of age.[20] Studies of African populations typically report a higher prevalence of necrotizing periodontal disease among young children than in those older than 10 years.[1] NUG has been reported in several members of the same family in low socioeconomic groups. Twenty percent of households with children 2 to 6 years of age in a rural Nigerian city had one or more children with NUG.[72] NUG is more common among children with Down syndrome than among other children with mental deficiencies.[5]

Opinions differ with regard to whether NUG is more common during the winter,[41,56] summer, or fall[72] and whether there is a peak seasonal incidence.[15]

Communicability

NUG often occurs in groups in an epidemic pattern. At one time, NUG was considered contagious and required reporting to the community health department, but it was later concluded not to be communicable.[62,68]

A distinction must be made between communicability and transmissibility when referring to the characteristics of disease. The term *transmissible* denotes a capacity for the maintenance of an infectious agent in successive passages through a susceptible animal host.[62] The term *communicable* signifies a capacity for the maintenance of infection by natural modes of spread, such as direct contact through drinking water, food, and eating utensils; by the airborne route; or by arthropod vectors. A disease that is communicable is described as *contagious*. It has been demonstrated that disease associated with the fusospirochetal bacterial complex is transmissible; however, *it is not communicable or contagious.*

Attempts to spread NUG from human to human have been unsuccessful.[69] King[39] traumatized an area in his own gingiva and introduced debris from a patient with a severe case of NUG. There was no response until he happened to fall ill shortly thereafter. After his illness, he observed the characteristic lesion in the experimental area. It can be inferred with reservation from this experiment that systemic debility is a prerequisite for the contagion of NUG.

Because NUG often occurs among groups that use the same kitchen facilities, it is a common impression that the disease is spread by bacteria on eating utensils. However, the growth of fusospirochetal organisms requires carefully controlled conditions and an anaerobic environment; they do not ordinarily survive on eating utensils.[13,31]

The occurrence of NUG in epidemic-like outbreaks does not necessarily mean that it is contagious. The affected groups may be afflicted by the disease as a result of common predisposing factors rather than because of its spread from person to person. In all likelihood, a predisposed immunocompromised host and the presence of appropriate bacteria are necessary for the production of this disease.

> ### KEY FACT
>
> Although certain bacteria (e.g., fusospirochetal complex) are likely responsible for the lesions observed in NUG, immunocompromise appears to be a necessary predisposing condition for the disease.

PRIMARY HERPETIC GINGIVOSTOMATITIS

Primary herpetic gingivostomatitis is an infection of the oral cavity caused by herpes simplex virus (HSV) type 1.[16,49,50,67] It occurs most often among infants and children who are younger than 6 years of age,[7,67,70] but it is also seen in adolescents and adults.

Fig. 19.4 Herpetic Vesicles Recurred in the Lip. (A) Early stage. (B) Late stage, showing brownish, crusted lesions. (From Sapp JP, Eversole LR, Wysocki GP: *Contemporary oral and maxillofacial pathology*, ed 2, St Louis, 2002, Mosby.)

Fig. 19.5 Recurrent intraoral herpetic vesicles are seen (A) in the palate and (B) in the gingiva. The latter location is rare. (From Sapp JP, Eversole LR, Wysocki GP: *Contemporary oral and maxillofacial pathology*, ed 2, St Louis, 2002, Mosby.)

It occurs with equal frequency in male and female patients. In most individuals, however, the primary infection is asymptomatic.

As part of the primary infection, the virus ascends through the sensory and autonomic nerves, where it persists as latent HSV in neuronal ganglia that innervate the site. In approximately one-third of the world's population, secondary manifestations result from various stimuli, such as sunlight, trauma, fever, and stress. Secondary manifestations include herpes labialis (Fig. 19.4), herpetic stomatitis, herpes genitalis, ocular herpes, and herpetic encephalitis. Secondary herpetic stomatitis can occur on the palate, on the gingiva (Fig. 19.5), or on the mucosa as a result of dental treatment that traumatizes or stimulates the latent virus in the ganglia that innervate the area. It may manifest as pain away from the site of treatment 2 to 4 days later. Careful inspection for characteristic vesicles can be diagnostic (see Fig. 19.4).

Clinical Features

Oral Signs

Primary herpetic gingivostomatitis appears as a diffuse, erythematous, shiny involvement of the gingiva and the adjacent oral mucosa, with various degrees of edema and gingival bleeding. During its initial stage, it is characterized by discrete, spherical, gray vesicles, which can occur on the gingiva, labial and buccal mucosae, soft palate, pharynx, sublingual mucosa, and tongue (Fig. 19.6). After approximately 24 hours, the vesicles rupture and form painful small ulcers with red, elevated, halo-like margins

Fig. 19.6 Primary Herpetic Gingivostomatitis in a 12-Year-Old Boy, Who has Diffuse Erythematous Involvement of the Gingiva and a Spherical, Gray Vesicle in the Lip. (Courtesy Dr. Heddie Sedano, University of \California, Los Angeles, and University of Minnesota.)

and depressed yellowish or grayish white central portions. They occur in widely separated areas or in clusters where confluence occurs (Fig. 19.7).

Occasionally, primary herpetic gingivitis occurs without overt vesiculation. The clinical picture consists of diffuse, erythematous, shiny discoloration and edematous enlargement of the gingivae with a tendency to bleed.

The course of the disease is limited to 7 to 10 days. The diffuse gingival erythema and edema that appear early during the course of the disease persist for several days after the ulcerative lesions

Fig. 19.7 Involvement of the lip (A), gingiva (B), and tongue (C) in primary herpetic gingivostomatitis. (From Sapp JP, Eversole LR, Wysocki GP: *Contemporary oral and maxillofacial pathology,* ed 2, St Louis, 2002, Mosby.)

have healed. Scarring does not occur in the areas of healed ulcerations.

Oral Symptoms

The disease is accompanied by generalized soreness of the oral cavity, which interferes with eating, drinking, and oral hygiene. The ruptured vesicles are the focal sites of pain; they are particularly sensitive to touch, thermal changes, foods such as condiments and fruit juices, and the action of coarse foods. In infants, the disease is marked by irritability and refusal to take food.

Extraoral and Systemic Signs and Symptoms

Cervical lymphadenitis, fever as high as 101°F to 105°F (38°C to 40.6°C), and generalized malaise are common.

History

Primary herpetic gingivostomatitis is the result of an acute infection by HSV. There is an acute onset of symptoms.

Histopathology

The virus targets the epithelial cells called *Tzanck cells,* which show ballooning degeneration that consists of acantholysis, nuclear clearing, and nuclear enlargement. Infected cells fuse to form multinucleated cells, and intercellular edema leads to the formation of intraepithelial vesicles that rupture and develop a secondary inflammatory response with a fibropurulent exudate (Fig. 19.8).[54] Discrete ulcerations that result from the rupture of the vesicles have a central portion of acute inflammation, with various degrees of purulent exudate surrounded by engorged blood vessels.

Diagnosis

It is critical to arrive at a diagnosis as early as possible for a patient with a primary herpetic infection. Treatment with antiviral medications can dramatically alter the course of the disease by reducing symptoms and potentially reducing recurrences. The diagnosis is usually established from the patient's history and the clinical findings. Material can be obtained from the lesions and submitted to the laboratory for confirmatory tests, including virus culture and immunologic tests that involve the use of monoclonal antibodies or deoxyribonucleic acid hybridization

Fig. 19.8 Biopsy Showing Intraepithelial Viral Vesicles that Contain Fluid and Debris, With a Large Number of Viruses and Virally Altered Epithelial Cells (i.e., Tzanck Cells). (Courtesy Dr. Heddie Sedano, University of California, Los Angeles, and University of Minnesota.)

techniques.[7,61] This should not delay treatment if strong clinical evidence exists for primary gingivostomatitis.

Differential Diagnosis

Primary herpetic gingivostomatitis should be differentiated from several conditions. Lesions of recurrent aphthous stomatitis (RAS)[22] range from occasional small (0.5 to 1 cm in diameter), well-defined, round or ovoid, shallow ulcers with a yellowish gray central area surrounded by an erythematous halo, which heal in 7 to 10 days without scarring, to larger (1 to 3 cm in diameter), oval or irregular ulcers, which persist for weeks and heal with scarring (Fig. 19.9). The cause is unknown, although immunopathologic mechanisms appear to play a role.

RAS is a different clinical entity from primary herpetic gingivostomatitis. The ulcerations may look the same for the two conditions, but diffuse erythematous involvement of the gingiva and acute toxic systemic symptoms do not occur with RAS. A history of previous episodes of painful mucosal ulcerations suggests RAS rather than primary HSV.

Information about erythema multiforme, bullous lichen planus, and desquamative gingivitis can be found in Chapter 21.

Fig. 19.9 Aphthous Lesion in the Lip. The depressed gray center is surrounded by an elevated red border. (From Sapp JP, Eversole LR, Wysocki GP: *Contemporary oral and maxillofacial pathology*, ed 2, St Louis, 2002, Mosby.)

Fig. 19.10 Pericoronitis. An inflamed coronal flap covers the disto-occlusal surface of the impacted mandibular third molar. Note the swelling and redness. (From Glickman I, Smulow J: *Periodontal disease: clinical, radiographic and histopathologic features*, Philadelphia, 1974, Saunders.)

Communicability

Primary herpetic gingivostomatitis is contagious.[9,44] Most adults have developed immunity to HSV as a result of infection during childhood, which in most cases is subclinical. For this reason, acute herpetic gingivostomatitis usually occurs in infants and children. Recurrent herpetic gingivostomatitis has been reported,[30] although it is not often clinically significant unless immunity is destroyed by debilitating systemic disease. Studies that have demonstrated HSV in periodontal pockets suggest more recurrence of viral replication than has previously been recognized.[75] Secondary herpetic infection of the skin, such as herpes labialis, does recur.[73]

> **CLINICAL CORRELATION**
>
> Acute herpetic gingivostomatitis usually occurs in infants and children because most adults have developed immunity to herpes simplex virus from childhood exposure, often with mild or no symptoms.

PERICORONITIS

The term *pericoronitis* refers to inflammation of the gingiva in relation to the crown of an incompletely erupted tooth (Fig. 19.10). It occurs most often in the mandibular third molar area. Pericoronitis can be acute, subacute, or chronic.

Clinical Features

The partially erupted or impacted mandibular third molar is the most common site of pericoronitis. The space between the crown of the tooth and the overlying gingival flap (i.e., operculum) is an ideal area for the accumulation of food debris and bacterial growth. Even in patients with no clinical signs or symptoms, the gingival flap is often chronically inflamed and infected, and it has various degrees of ulceration along its inner surface. Acute inflammatory involvement is a constant possibility; it may be exacerbated by trauma, occlusion, or a foreign body trapped underneath the tissue flap (e.g., popcorn husk, nut fragment).

Acute pericoronitis is identified by various degrees of inflammatory involvement of the pericoronal flap and adjacent structures and by systemic complications. The inflammatory fluid and cellular exudate increase the bulk of the flap, which can interfere with complete closure of the jaws. It also can be traumatized by contact with the opposing dentition, thereby aggravating the inflammatory involvement.

The resultant clinical picture is a red, swollen, suppurating lesion that is exquisitely tender, with radiating pains to the ear, throat, and floor of the mouth. The patient is extremely uncomfortable as a result of pain, a foul taste, and an inability to close the jaws. Swelling of the cheek in the region of the angle of the jaw and lymphadenitis are common findings. Trismus may be a presenting complaint. The patient can have systemic complications such as fever, leukocytosis, and malaise.

Complications

Involvement can be localized in the form of a pericoronal abscess. It may spread posteriorly into the oropharyngeal area and medially to the base of the tongue, making it difficult for the patient to swallow. Depending on the severity and extent of the infection, there may be involvement of the submaxillary, posterior cervical, deep cervical, and retropharyngeal lymph nodes.[35,57] Peritonsillar abscess formation, cellulitis, and Ludwig angina are infrequent but potential sequelae of acute pericoronitis.

CONCLUSIONS

Acute gingival diseases are similar in that they typically manifest with painful intraoral or perioral lesions and there is a need for urgent treatment to relieve symptoms. However, each case requires careful assessment and an accurate diagnosis, including identification of risk factors. In many cases, there are systemic risk factors that increase susceptibility to acute gingival disease.

A Case Scenario is found on the companion website.

REFERENCES

 References for this chapter are found on the companion website.

Gingival Disease in Childhood[a]

After reviewing anatomic and physiologic changes in the periodontium and dentition, this chapter describes the gingival changes associated with childhood and adolescence.

PERIODONTIUM OF THE PRIMARY DENTITION

(Periodontal diseases during early periods of life are also discussed in Chapters 13, 25, and 26.)

Anatomic and Physiologic Characteristics

- In the edentulous infant, the gingival tissues have thick gingival mucosa and segmentations that correspond with the primary buds (Fig. 20.1).
- A high labial frenum attachment is a normal finding in almost 85% of infants; it may diminish in size with normal development.[58]
- During the primary dentition stage, the normal gingiva continues to be somewhat different from that found in adults. The tissues are pale pink, but they are pink to a lesser degree than the attached gingiva of adults because the thinness of the keratinized layer allows the underlying vessels in children to be more visible.[42]

Stippling appears at about 3 years of age and has been reported for 56% of children between 3 and 10 years of age, with little differences between maxillary and mandibular arches or between boys and girls throughout childhood (Fig. 20.2).[11]

- The interdental gingiva is broad buccolingually and narrow mesiodistally, which is consistent with the morphology of the primary dentition. Its structure and composition are similar to those of the adult gingiva.
- Gingival sulcular depth is shallower in the primary dentition than in the permanent dentition. Probing depths range from 1 to 2 mm, with increasing depth from anterior to posterior.[8,25,61]
- The attached gingiva varies in width anteroposteriorly, with a range of 3 to 6 mm. On the buccal surfaces, the width decreases from anterior to posterior, with some data indicating a narrowing over the canines (Fig. 20.3). The lingual attached gingiva shows an inverse relationship, with an increase in width from anterior to posterior.[25] The gingival width normally increases with age as children transition from the primary to the permanent dentition.[5,8,15,61] The junctional epithelium is thicker in the primary dentition than in the permanent dentition,[10] which is thought to reduce the permeability of the tissues to bacterial toxins.
- Radiographically, the lamina dura is prominent in the primary dentition, with a wider periodontal space than in the permanent dentition. The marrow spaces of the bone are larger, and the crests of the interdental bony septa are flat, with bony crests within 1 to 2 mm of the cementoenamel junction (Fig. 20.4).[26,54]

PERIODONTAL CHANGES ASSOCIATED WITH NORMAL DEVELOPMENT

Significant changes occur in the periodontium as the dentition changes from the primary to the permanent teeth. Most of the changes are associated with eruption and are physiologic in nature. These changes should be distinguished from gingival disease, which can occur simultaneously.

Tooth Eruption

Before the eruption of a primary or permanent tooth, the gingiva reveals a bulge that is firm and pink or blanched as a result of the underlying tooth crown. An eruption cyst occasionally is evident. This fluctuant mass can be filled with blood, and it usually manifests as a bluish or deep-red enlargement of the gingiva over the erupting tooth (Fig. 20.5A). The most common sites of these cysts are the primary first molars and the permanent

[a]Adapted from the following chapter of Newman and Carranza's Clinical Periodontology, 13th edition: Chapter 21: Gingival Disease in Childhood, by Daniela R. Silva, Clarice S. Law, Donald F. Duperon, and Fermin A. Carranza.

Fig. 20.1 Normal Gingiva of an Edentulous 1-Month-Old Child Shows a High Labial Frenulum and Pink and Healthy Tissues. (Copyright Dr. Daniela Silva. All rights reserved.)

Fig. 20.2 Normal Gingiva of a 4-Year-Old Child Shows Light Stippling and Flattened Interproximal Gingiva in Areas of Physiologic Spacing. (Copyright Dr. Daniela Silva. All rights reserved.)

Fig. 20.3 Normal Gingiva of a 4-Year-Old African American Child Demonstrates the Width of the Attached Gingiva, as Illustrated by the Pigmentation that Occurs Only in the Attached Area. (Copyright Dr. Daniela Silva. All rights reserved.)

Fig. 20.4 Bitewing Radiograph of a 6-Year-Old Child Shows the Flattened Interseptal Bone and Bony Crests Within 1–2 mm of the Cementoenamel Junction. (Copyright Dr. Daniela Silva. All rights reserved.)

BOX 20.1

What are the most common symptoms associated with teething that have been proved or confirmed by scientific studies? They are drooling, irritability, decreased appetite, and gum rubbing.

During the period of active tooth eruption, it is normal for the marginal gingiva that surrounds partially erupted teeth to appear prominent; this is most evident in the maxillary anterior region. The prominence is caused by the height of the contour of the erupting tooth and mild inflammation from mastication. Poor oral hygiene can contribute to the development of significant gingivitis in unprotected gingival areas.

Teething

The effect of primary tooth eruption on infant health has been debated for centuries, but there is little scientific evidence regarding the diagnosis and management of the teething child. The period associated with the eruption of the primary teeth in infants can be difficult and stressful for the child and the parents. The timing of primary incisor eruption (i.e., 5 to 12 months of age) coincides with diminution of the passive humoral immunity conferred by the transfer of maternal antibodies through the placenta and establishment of the child's own immunity.[17,29,60] Pain is a common feature of teething as reported by parents and some health care providers. The tooth does not cause the pain; rather, the follicle, which is a rich source of eicosanoids, cytokines, and growth factors, stimulates a localized inflammatory response.[57,60]

Most medical and dental professionals agree that teething does not cause life-threatening illness, but they disagree about which symptoms are associated with tooth eruption. The studies and systematic reviews of symptoms related to teething most commonly include decreased appetite, biting, drooling, gum rubbing, irritability, sucking, and abnormal temperature.[24,28,29,38,39,46,53,57,60,67,68] However, there is no evidence that any of these symptoms can be diagnostic of teething in a child without excluding the possibility of other systemic diseases.

first molars. Many resolve without treatment, but they can be marsupialized if they are painful or interfere with occlusion (see Fig. 20.5B).[14]

As a tooth erupts, the gingival margin and the sulcus develop. At this point, the margin is rounded, edematous, and reddened.

Fig. 20.5 (A) An eruption cyst is seen at the lower right first primary molar area of a 16-month-old child. With this condition, there is transparent, bluish, blue, or blue-black swelling of the alveolar mucosa over a tooth in eruption. (B) An eruption cyst is located at the lower right first primary molar area of a 16-month-old child. After a small incision of the mucosa, the hemorrhagic content was marsupialized. (Copyright Dr. Daniela Silva. All rights reserved.)

Primary Tooth Exfoliation

As with tooth eruption, the process of tooth exfoliation involves changes in the periodontium. The depth of the gingival sulcus increases as the junctional epithelium migrates down the resorbing root of an exfoliating tooth.[9,10] Microscopically, minor traumatic changes demonstrate compression, ischemia, and hyalinization of the periodontal ligament.[49] Changes in the permeability and integrity of the junctional epithelium can make the exfoliating tooth more susceptible to inflammation.[10]

During the process of exfoliation, teeth can change position, leading to changes in occlusion. Malalignment caused by spacing and changes in skeletal relationships related to erupting teeth can contribute to significant trauma of the periodontal structures. With more severe injury, crushing and necrosis of the periodontal ligament can occur. In most patients, these injuries spontaneously resolve as the teeth exfoliate, erupt, and align through the normal growth and development processes.

Other Developmental Issues
Relation of Periodontal Status to Malocclusion

Data indicate an association between abnormal tooth position and gingivitis.[20] Crowding in the mixed dentition can often make plaque and food removal more difficult, increasing the likelihood of gingivitis. Severe changes include gingival enlargement, discoloration, occasional ulceration, and formation of deep pockets or pseudopockets. Gingival health usually can be restored with orthodontic correction, but failure to align the teeth does not necessarily have an effect on periodontal disease later in life.[20]

Mucogingival Problems

The prevalence of mucogingival problems and recession in children ranges from 1% to 19%, depending on the criteria used to assess the condition.[33] Evidence suggests that some mucogingival problems start during the primary dentition as a consequence of developmental aberrations in eruption and deficiencies in

Fig. 20.6 Erupting Permanent Incisors Have Minimal Attached Gingiva. (Copyright Dr. Daniela Silva. All rights reserved.)

the thickness of the periodontium.[42,43] A high frenum attachment may also be a factor in the development of mucogingival problems if there is excess tension at the marginal tissues.[52,62] During the mixed dentition, recession is most often found on the facial aspect of mandibular permanent incisors due to rotations or labial positioning related to space problems. Although erupting permanent lower incisors often show minimal attached gingiva, gingival width often increases as the teeth erupt and stimulate bone development (Fig. 20.6).[15]

The maxillary canine region is prone to localized gingival recession. Late-erupting canines in a crowded dentition can be displaced buccally, erupting into or near unattached gingiva or mucosa and increasing the risk of insufficient gingival tissue width and recession. Recession can also be associated with an anterior open bite as a result of the labial inclination of the teeth.[36] Orthodontic treatment and realignment may be necessary to protect the integrity of the attached gingiva.

Mucogingival problems can result from factitious habits, such as self-inflicted trauma from a fingernail (Fig. 20.7) or excessive toothbrushing by the parent or the child. Because the width of the attached gingiva increases with age, any of these problems may resolve spontaneously, suggesting a cautious approach to treatment with judicious monitoring instead of immediate surgical intervention.[15,54]

GINGIVAL DISEASES OF CHILDHOOD

Plaque-Induced Gingival Disease

Gingivitis is extremely common among children and adolescents, and it affects up to 70% of children who are more than 7 years old.[16,47] Inflammation is usually limited to the marginal gingiva (Fig. 20.8), with undetectable loss of bone or connective tissue attachment in most cases. Although gingivitis does not always progress to periodontitis, the management of gingival disease in children and adolescents is important, because periodontitis is always preceded by gingivitis.[47]

In children and adults, the primary cause of gingivitis is dental plaque, which is related to poor oral hygiene. The relationship between plaque and the gingival index, however, is weak and remains unclear.[9,37,38,41] Although gingivitis is highly prevalent among children, its severity usually is less intense than that found in adults.[10] Similar oral hygiene conditions produce less severe forms of disease in children compared with adults.[47]

As children age, their tendency to develop gingivitis increases.[10] The prevalence of disease is the lowest during the preschool years and increases throughout childhood, peaking during puberty. However, increases in the degree of gingival inflammation do not fully correlate with the amount of plaque, which suggests the influence of other factors.

Clinical Features

The most prevalent type of gingival disease in childhood is *chronic marginal gingivitis* (see Fig. 20.8). The gingival tissues exhibit changes in color, size, consistency, and surface texture that are similar to those of chronic inflammation in the adult. Red, linear inflammation is accompanied by underlying chronic changes, including swelling, increased vascularization, and hyperplasia. Bleeding and increased pocket depth are not found as often in children as in adults, but they may be observed if severe gingival hypertrophy or hyperplasia occurs.[9,47]

Chronic gingivitis in children is characterized by a loss of collagen in the area around the junctional epithelium and an infiltrate that consists mostly of lymphocytes, with small numbers of polymorphonuclear leukocytes, plasma cells, monocytes, and mast cells. Lesions typically have relatively few plasma cells, and they resemble the early nondestructive, nonprogressive lesions that are seen in adults. Unlike the adult inflammatory response, gingivitis in children is dominated by T lymphocytes, with few B lymphocytes and plasma cells in the infiltrate. This difference may explain why gingivitis in children rarely progresses to periodontitis.[34,35,41,55] Gingival histology in children also demonstrates other unique features that may decrease the tendency to progress to severe gingivitis. The junctional epithelium of the primary dentition tends to be thicker than in the permanent dentition,[10] which is thought to reduce the permeability of the gingival structures to bacterial toxins that initiate the inflammatory response.

Fig. 20.7 Gingival Recession on the Maxillary and Mandibular Left Primary Canine Areas is Caused by Self-Inflicted Trauma from the Patient's Fingernail. (Copyright Dr. Daniela Silva. All rights reserved.)

Fig. 20.8 Plaque-Induced Gingivitis Is Limited to the Marginal Gingiva in a 12-Year-Old Girl. (Copyright Dr. Daniela Silva. All rights reserved.)

BOX 20.2A

What are the main differences between chronic marginal gingivitis in children compared with adults? Children with a nonsignificant medical history have less severe gingival bleeding and very seldom have increased pocket depth, as seen in healthy adults. Gingivitis in children is also different from that in adults because the response is dominated by T lymphocytes, with few B lymphocytes and plasma cells in the infiltrate, and it rarely progresses to periodontitis.

BOX 20.2B

In the category of patients with special needs, children with cystic fibrosis[69] or chronic kidney disease[40] have a higher incidence of calculus deposits, which can be caused by increased calcium and phosphate concentrations in saliva.

Children who are fed exclusively with gastric or nasogastric tubes show significant calculus buildup as a result of a lack of function and increased oral pH (Fig. 20.9).[23]

Fig. 20.9 A 5-Year-Old Boy With a History of Liver Transplantation and Gastric Tube Feeding Has a Generalized Calculus Deposit. (Copyright Dr. Daniela Silva. All rights reserved.)

BOX 20.3

What are the most common drugs that cause gingival enlargement in children, and what conditions do they treat? Cyclosporine is an immunosuppressant drug used by patients who have undergone organ transplantation. Phenytoin is an antiepileptic medication, and calcium channel blockers are used to treat hypertension, abnormal heart rhythms, and Raynaud phenomenon.

Calculus

Calculus deposits are uncommon in infants and toddlers, but they can increase with age. About 9% of 4- to 6-year-old children exhibit calculus deposits. By the age of 7 to 9 years, 18% of children have calculus deposits, and by the age of 10 to 15 years, 33% to 43% have some calculus formation.[69]

Microbiology of Disease

Because the intensity of gingival disease increases as a child develops into adulthood, it is important to understand the microbiology of disease, which is discussed further in Chapter 9. The composition of the oral microflora changes as the child matures.[10] Yang and colleagues[70] analyzed samples of dental plaque in children and reported that 71% of 18- to 48-month-old children were infected with at least one periodontal pathogen. Sixty-eight percent were infected with *Porphyromonas gingivalis*, and 20% had *Tannerella forsythia* (previously called *Bacteroides forsythus*).[70] A moderate correlation was found between *T. forsythia* in children and periodontal disease in their mothers. *T. forsythia* has also been associated with gingival bleeding in children.

In a similar study, 60% of children between the ages of 2 and 18 years had detectable levels of *P. gingivalis* in their plaque, and 75% showed similar levels of *Actinobacillus actinomycetemcomitans*. *P. gingivalis* was most strongly associated with the progression of gingivitis and the onset of periodontitis in otherwise healthy children.[45]

Pediatric gingivitis models have demonstrated increased subgingival levels of *Actinomyces*, *Capnocytophaga*, *Leptotrichia*, and *Selenomonas*[16]—pathogens usually not seen in adult gingivitis—thereby raising interest in their potential role in the cause of childhood gingivitis.

Eruption Gingivitis

Gingivitis associated with tooth eruption is so common that the term *eruption gingivitis* has come into frequent use. Although tooth eruption does not directly cause gingivitis, inflammation associated with plaque accumulation around erupting teeth, perhaps due to discomfort caused by brushing these friable areas, may contribute to gingivitis.[10] The gingiva around erupting teeth can appear reddened because gingival margins have not yet keratinized fully and sulcus development is incomplete.

Exfoliating and severely carious primary teeth often contribute to gingivitis caused by plaque accumulation as a result of pain during brushing or food impaction in areas of cavitation. As a normal part of exfoliation, the junctional epithelium migrates under the resorbing tooth, thereby increasing pocket depth and potentially creating a niche for pathogenic bacteria.[10] The discomfort of chewing on severely infected teeth often leads to unilateral chewing on the unaffected side.

Puberty Gingivitis

The incidence of marginal gingivitis increases as a child matures, peaking when he or she is 9 to 14 years old and then decreasing slightly after puberty.[10] Gingival disease that behaves in such a manner is often referred to as *pubertal* (or *puberty*) *gingivitis*. Chapters 18 and 37 continue the discussion of this condition.

The most frequent manifestation of puberty gingivitis is bleeding and inflammation in interproximal areas. Inflammatory gingival enlargement may also occur in males and females, but it typically subsides after puberty (see Fig. 20.8).[44] The altered gingival response during this developmental stage is thought to be the result of hormonal changes that magnify the vascular and inflammatory response to dental plaque[10,47] and that modify the reactions of dental plaque microbes.[22]

Drug-Induced Gingival Enlargement

Gingival enlargement (see Chapter 18) can result from the use of certain drugs. Cyclosporine, phenytoin, and calcium channel blockers, which are used to treat conditions that are encountered during childhood (e.g., organ transplantation, epilepsy, and cardiac anomalies), increase the prevalence of gingival enlargement (Fig. 20.10). A randomized clinical trial found an interesting and significant decrease in the incidence (21%) of phenytoin-induced gingival hyperplasia in children with epilepsy taking oral folic acid supplementation (0.5 mg/day) compared with the control group (88%).[6] Although complicated by the plaque levels along the gingival margin, this form of gingival disease has features that are not typical of chronic marginal gingivitis.[47]

Gingival Changes Related to Orthodontic Appliances

Gingival enlargement can be related to the presence of fixed orthodontic appliances, which complicate plaque removal (Fig. 20.11). Gingival changes can occur within 1 to 2 months of appliance placement. They usually are transient, and they only rarely produce long-term damage to periodontal tissues.[20] The

Fig. 20.10 (A) A 7-year-old boy with a history of aplastic anemia and cyclosporine-induced gingival hyperplasia. (B) The same patient 1 year after gingivectomy and 6 months after the dosage of cyclosporine was decreased to one-half of the initial dosage. (Copyright Dr. Daniela Silva. All rights reserved.)

Fig. 20.11 Chronic Marginal Gingivitis Was a Result of Orthodontic Therapy and Inadequate Oral Hygiene. (Copyright Dr. Daniela Silva. All rights reserved.)

fact that most orthodontic treatment is provided to individuals during puberty, when they are subject to the inflammatory changes associated with puberty gingivitis, may exacerbate the observed effect.

Mouth Breathing

Mouth breathing and lip incompetence, which are together referred to as an *open mouth posture*, are often associated with increased plaque and gingival inflammation.[20] The area of inflammation is often limited to the gingiva of the maxillary incisors. There is usually a clear line of demarcation where the gingiva is uncovered by the lip.

Non–Plaque-Induced Gingival Lesions

Intraoral soft tissue lesions can be encountered in the pediatric population as they are in the adult population. The six most common pediatric intraoral lesions are primary herpetic gingivostomatitis, recurrent herpes simplex, recurrent aphthous stomatitis, candidiasis, angular cheilitis, and geographic tongue.[47]

Most of these lesions manifest without significant differences between the pediatric and adult populations, but two do have specific pediatric considerations.

Primary Herpetic Gingivostomatitis

Primary herpetic gingivostomatitis is an acute-onset viral infection that occurs early during childhood, with a heightened incidence between the ages of 1 and 3 years (see Chapter 19). Among children with primary herpetic infections, 99% are symptom free or have symptoms that are attributed to teething. The remaining 1% can develop significant gingival inflammation and ulceration of the attached gingiva, tongue, palate, and lips (Fig. 20.12).[28,47]

The most important therapeutic measure is to control the child's hydration with bland, nonacetic fluids. Hospitalization may be necessary in some severe cases.

Candidiasis

Candidiasis results from an overgrowth of *Candida albicans*, usually after a course of antibiotics or as a result of congenital or acquired immunodeficiency. It is far less common in children than in adults, and it rarely occurs in a healthy child.[13]

Localized Juvenile Spongiotic Gingival Hyperplasia

Another condition that appears to be unrelated to plaque accumulation is localized juvenile spongiotic gingival hyperplasia. This condition was identified only recently, and its pathogenesis is not well defined. The lesions are localized patches on the attached gingiva that manifest as bright red, raised overgrowths; they are usually painless and associated with easy bleeding. These lesions are most commonly seen on the anterior labial maxillary and mandibular gingiva.[18] Most of the patients with this condition are between the ages of 8 and 14 years (Fig. 20.13).

PERIODONTAL DISEASES OF CHILDHOOD

Although gingivitis is considered to be almost universal among children who are older than 7 years,[16,47] frank periodontal disease with the loss of periodontal attachment and supporting bone is far less common in the pediatric population than in adults.[16]

Fig. 20.12 (A) Acute herpetic gingivostomatitis in a 5-year-old girl produced spontaneous bleeding. The infection is mostly limited to the attached gingiva, tongue, palate, and lips. (B) In the same patient 1 week later, the attached gingiva demonstrates initial healing. (Courtesy Dr. Thomas K. Barber, University of California, Los Angeles Pediatric Dentistry.)

Fig. 20.13 Localized Juvenile Spongiotic Gingival Hyperplasia is Seen in an 11-Year-Old Girl. The papillary gingiva is red, and the gingival overgrowth is prone to easy bleeding. (Courtesy Dr. Chanel McCreedy. All rights reserved.)

The incidence of disease begins increasing between the ages of 12 and 17 years, but the prevalence of severe attachment loss involving multiple teeth remains low at 0.2% to 0.5%.[16] Of the various manifestations of periodontal disease, chronic periodontitis is more prevalent among adults, and aggressive periodontitis is more common among children and adolescents.[16]

> **CLINICAL INSIGHT** Oral hygiene habits should be imprinted early during life, with instructions about proper technique and directions regarding the frequency of plaque removal procedures. These will form a foundation for a lifetime of dedication to periodontal health. Dental hygienists should be aware of the specific periodontal needs of children with particular abnormalities, such as gingival hyperplasia associated with immunosuppression protocols used with organ transplantation, antiseizure medications, and increased severity of periodontal disease in diabetic children.
>
> Children with physical or developmental disabilities deserve special care to ensure that appropriate preventive techniques are available; techniques may include the use of electric toothbrushes and antibacterial mouth rinses. Chapters 25–27 describe the different types of periodontal disease.

Aggressive Periodontitis

Aggressive periodontitis is addressed in greater detail in Chapter 26. Because of the relatively early onset of disease, which occurs around the time of puberty, former classifications mention the developmental stage: early-onset periodontitis, prepubertal periodontitis, and juvenile periodontitis.[16,47] The currently accepted designation of aggressive periodontitis may be further broken down into two forms: localized and generalized. Localized aggressive periodontitis has been defined as "interproximal attachment loss on at least two permanent first molars and incisors, with attachment loss on no more than two teeth other than first molars and incisors."[16]

In young individuals, localized aggressive periodontitis is more common than the generalized form. Studies consistently show that among different geographic locations and racial groups, aggressive periodontitis is most prevalent in African populations and their descendants, ranging between 1% and 5%. The prevalence in whites residing in Europe is 0.1% to 0.5%, and in North America, the disease affects approximately 0.1% to 0.2% of whites, 0.5% to 1% of Hispanics, and 2.6% of African Americans.[2,15,56] Some studies suggest a higher prevalence among Asian children.[2,48,64] Of relevance to the pediatric population is the finding that the classic clinical presentation of localized aggressive periodontitis may be preceded by signs of bone loss around the teeth during the primary dentition.[16]

The generalized form of aggressive periodontitis, which is defined as a generalized interproximal attachment loss, including at least three teeth that are not first molars and incisors, is rare among children (Fig. 20.14). The onset of this form of periodontitis usually occurs after the initiation of adolescence. Overall prevalence is 0.13% among 14- to 17-year-old children[16]; however, the prevalence is higher among individuals with Down syndrome.[4,15,50] A purported genetic influence in the disease process suggests that any signs of disease in a child with a family history of generalized aggressive periodontitis should be investigated further.

Several studies have suggested the involvement of *A. actinomycetemcomitans*[2,18,32,56,59] and *P. gingivalis*[2] in the pathogenesis of

Fig. 20.14 (A) In an 8-year-old African American girl with aggressive periodontitis, the clinical appearance of the mucosa is similar to normal tissue, but the primary canines and molars have mobility, bleeding on probing, and deep pockets. (B) In an 8-year-old African American girl with aggressive periodontitis, radiographs show advanced bone loss at the primary canine and molar areas. (Copyright Dr. Daniela Silva. All rights reserved.)

aggressive periodontitis, with the former found at higher levels in children with the localized form and the latter found at higher levels in those with the generalized form. Both of these pathogens are rare in healthy children, with a prevalence of 4.8%, but the rate is elevated for children with periodontitis, with a reported prevalence of 20%.[48] One study found a very strong association between localized aggressive periodontitis and the prevalence and abundance of *A. actinomycetemcomitans*. The study authors also observed *A. actinomycetemcomitans* as being very site specific; it was more prevalent and abundant in diseased sites compared with healthy sites in individuals with localized aggressive periodontitis.[56]

Chronic Periodontitis

Chronic periodontitis is far less prevalent in this population than it is in adults.[16]

Similar to the adult version, which is discussed in greater detail in Chapter 25, chronic periodontitis can occur in children in the localized form, in which less than 30% of the dentition is affected, and in the generalized form, in which more than 30% of the dentition is affected.

The microbiology of this disease is discussed in Chapter 9. Studies suggest the familial transmission of certain bacteria associated with chronic periodontitis. Strains such as *T. forsythia*, *Prevotella intermedia*, and *Prevotella nigrescens* are found more often in the children of individuals who harbor these types of bacteria.[66] *Fusobacterium nucleatum* and *P. gingivalis* have been identified at significant levels in children of similarly affected parents.[12,30] Levels of these strains increase with age, suggesting that *P. gingivalis* and *T. forsythia* may serve as early markers during screening for periodontal disease.[12,32,63] Although chronic periodontitis may not be highly prevalent among children, early colonization may underscore the importance of early detection, particularly for those at elevated risk for adult forms of the disease.

GINGIVAL MANIFESTATION OF SYSTEMIC DISEASE IN CHILDREN

Systemic diseases that result in periodontitis occur more frequently in children than in adults.[2] Chapter 13 discusses some of the systemic diseases and disorders that affect periodontal health. However, many diseases are expressed differently in children than in adults and therefore merit special mention.

Acute necrotizing gingivitis is rarely seen, except in cases of primary or secondary immune suppression, Down syndrome, or severe malnutrition.[19,50] The child's breath is fetid, and he or she complains of pain and discomfort when eating (see Chapter 19).

Endocrine Disorders and Hormonal Changes
Diabetes Mellitus
Type 1 or insulin-dependent diabetes mellitus occurs more frequently in children and young adults than type 2 or non–insulin-dependent diabetes mellitus. As with diabetic adults, gingival inflammation and periodontitis are more prevalent in affected children than in unaffected individuals.[47,51] Clinical consequences include premature tooth loss and impaired immune response to the oral flora. The severity of periodontal disease is worse in children with poor metabolic control.

Although destructive changes are rare in healthy children, periodontal destruction can be observed in diabetic children, usually appearing around the time of puberty and becoming progressively worse as children mature into adulthood. Disease prevention and fastidious oral hygiene measures should be highly promoted.[31,32]

Hematologic Disorders and Immune Deficiencies
Leukemias
Leukemia is the most common type of cancer in children. Acute lymphocytic leukemia accounts for most cases among children

Fig. 20.15 In a 12-Year-Old Boy With Acute Lymphoblastic Leukemia, There is Generalized Redness of the Marginal Gingiva With Spontaneous Bleeding. (Copyright Dr. Daniela Silva. All rights reserved.)

who are younger than 7 years. Leukemia must be considered as part of the differential diagnosis for children who present with the hallmark features of acute gingival enlargement, ulceration, bleeding, and infection (Fig. 20.15).[1]

Neutrophil Disorders
Neutrophil disorders impair defenses against infections, making afflicted individuals susceptible to severe periodontal destruction (see Chapter 13). Many neutrophil disorders are genetic, including some forms of neutropenia, such as familial and cyclic neutropenia, Chédiak–Higashi syndrome, leukocyte adhesion deficiency, Papillon–Lefèvre syndrome, and Cohen syndrome.[16,27] The diagnosis of the systemic disorder usually occurs before any signs of periodontal destruction appear.

Because periodontal changes are difficult to reverse in children with neutrophil disorders, disease management includes oral hygiene measures, mechanical debridement, antimicrobial therapy, and supportive care for any resultant tissue destruction or tooth loss. Treatment success is unpredictable because of the impact of systemic disease.[16,27]

Congenital Anomalies
Down syndrome is another congenital condition that is diagnosed before the expression of periodontal disease. People with Down syndrome experience a high prevalence of severe aggressive periodontitis during early adulthood. The disease process likely reflects a host susceptibility that results in an exaggerated immune and inflammatory response rather than a reaction to a specific causative microbe.[3,4,19,27] Studies of people with Down syndrome uncovered defective neutrophil chemotaxis, which can lead to significant tissue loss and the progression of periodontitis.[27]

ORAL MUCOSA IN CHILDHOOD DISEASES

Some childhood diseases, such as rubeola (i.e., rubella or measles), varicella (i.e., chickenpox), diphtheria, and scarlatina (i.e., scarlet fever), cause alterations or lesions of the oral mucosa and the underlying tissues. These diseases are explored in textbooks that discuss oral and pediatric pathology.

THERAPEUTIC CONSIDERATIONS FOR PEDIATRIC PATIENTS

The diagnostic process for pediatric patients follows the general outline described in Chapter 30. Medical and dental histories should be recorded for each child, with parents or legal guardians serving as the primary historians. However, differences between the primary and permanent dentition and aspects related to development warrant some differences in clinical practices that involve the care of children.

Periodontal indices do not need to be recorded during the primary dentition unless a child exhibits signs of aggressive periodontitis or other unusual disease processes. More explicit periodontal assessments should begin during mixed dentition, when children have permanent incisors and first molars. Rather than recording full-mouth probing depths, clinicians can focus on selected teeth. For example, a rudimentary assessment of teeth #3, #8, #14, #19, #24, and #30 has been suggested,[20] with notes made regarding gingival health, bleeding on probing, and degree of calculus. This quick screening usually is sufficient for children up to the age of 11 years. Between the ages 12 to 19 years, when most individuals have a full permanent dentition, clinicians should also record pocket depths of more than 4 mm. By this stage of dental development, full-mouth pocket-depth probing may be warranted on the basis of general indicators of each patient's gingival health or risk of disease.

In-office professional plaque control procedures can vary in accordance with a patient's stage of development. Calculus deposits are uncommon in infants and toddlers. Supragingival plaque removal with the use of simple rubber cup coronal polishing or a toothbrush is usually sufficient during the primary dentition.[20] If calculus deposits are evident, selective supragingival scaling can be performed. As the permanent teeth erupt, the prevalence of calculus deposits increases, often necessitating targeted subgingival scaling in addition to supragingival plaque removal.[20]

Chapter 43 discusses plaque control for periodontal patients. In children, however, the dynamic process of developing manual dexterity affects the ability of a child to perform expected procedures. Each child requires an individualized home care program based on his or her ability to perform the requested activities. For young children, plaque control should be a shared responsibility between children and their parents or caregivers. Instruction in plaque control should be delivered to parents and children in language and terms that both understand.

For children who are younger than 7 years, parents or caregivers should be asked to assist with toothbrushing.[20] Children may be encouraged to take a turn brushing their teeth using a simple scrub technique. However, parents should also take a turn to ensure the proper removal of plaque. By the age of 7 years, children usually possess the manual dexterity to brush their teeth on their own and may require only limited adult supervision.[20] More refined brushing techniques can be introduced during adolescence.

The oral hygiene habits of parents and caregivers have a significant influence on children's oral health behavior. An extensive survey of parents in the United Kingdom found that children and parents place a large emphasis on the cosmetic benefit of toothbrushing. Parents who placed more emphasis on the short-term benefits of toothbrushing were more likely to miss brushing the child's teeth in the evening, but when brushing a child's teeth was habitual, there was a significantly higher chance of brushing twice each day.[64]

Mechanical toothbrushes are effective for plaque removal.[20] The use of these devices can be encouraged as soon as children are able to tolerate the vibrating sensations. Mechanical toothbrushes are especially recommended for physically challenged children and individuals with fixed orthodontic appliances.[47]

Flossing is usually not indicated for children during the primary dentition stage because most children have interdental spacing throughout most of their arches. However, as interdental contacts develop, flossing should be added to the home care routine. Studies have demonstrated a decrease in gingival bleeding and the quantity of microbes associated with periodontal disease when tooth and tongue brushing are combined with flossing.[7,21] Limitations in manual dexterity may necessitate parental assistance with flossing during the mixed dentition stage. Adolescents with sufficient manual dexterity can be expected to floss on their own.[20]

Antimicrobial mouth rinses *for chemical plaque control* are not indicated for very young children because of the risk of ingestion of chemical agents.[20] However, rinses may be indicated for older children who demonstrate the ability to expectorate after rinsing.

CONCLUSIONS

The periodontium of the primary dentition is different from that of the permanent dentition. Normal development can result in changes to the periodontium. Plaque-induced gingivitis is very common in children, although it may be less intense than in adults. With the exception of localized aggressive periodontitis, children rarely show signs of periodontitis. Some systemic disorders that are commonly associated with periodontal disease manifest initially during childhood.

Recommendations regarding home plaque control routines should be individualized according to each patient's periodontal disease status and developmental stage. Because early diagnosis ensures the greatest chance for successful treatment, it is paramount that children receive a periodontal examination as part of their routine dental visits.

Case Scenarios are found on the companion website.

REFERENCES

 References for this chapter are found on the companion website.

21

Desquamative Gingivitis[a]

 For online-only content on miscellaneous conditions that mimic desquamative gingivitis, please visit the companion website.

CHAPTER OUTLINE

CHRONIC DESQUAMATIVE GINGIVITIS

Although the condition was first recognized and reported in 1894,[53] the term *chronic desquamative gingivitis (DG)* was not coined by Prinz[36] until 1932. It describes a reaction characterized by intense erythema, desquamation, and ulceration of the free and attached gingiva (Fig. 21.1).[13,28]

Patients can be asymptomatic, but when symptomatic, their complaints range from a mild burning sensation to intense pain. Approximately 50% of DG cases are localized to the gingiva, although patients can have involvement of the gingiva plus other intraoral and extraoral sites.[15,32]

The cause was initially unclear, with a variety of possibilities suggested. Because most cases were diagnosed in women during the fourth and fifth decades of life (although DG can occur as early as puberty or as late as the seventh or eighth decade), hormonal derangement was suspected. In 1960, McCarthy and colleagues[26] suggested that DG was not a specific disease entity but was instead a *gingival response associated with a variety of conditions*. This concept has been supported by numerous immunopathologic studies.[22,25,34,42,48,54]

The use of clinical and laboratory parameters has revealed that approximately 75% of DG cases have a dermatologic genesis. Lichen planus and cicatricial pemphigoid account for 84% of the DG cases.[23,31] However, many other mucocutaneous autoimmune conditions (e.g., bullous pemphigoid, pemphigus vulgaris, linear immunoglobulin A [IgA] disease, dermatitis herpetiformis, lupus erythematosus, chronic ulcerative stomatitis, dermatomyositis, mixed connective tissue disease) can manifest as DG.[23,46]

Other conditions that must be considered in the differential diagnosis of DG include chronic bacterial, fungal, and viral infections and reactions to medications, mouthwashes, and chewing gum. Although less common, Crohn disease, sarcoidosis, some leukemias, and factitious lesions have also been reported to manifest clinically as DG.[37,46,57]

It is important to ascertain the disease responsible for DG to establish the appropriate therapeutic approach. To achieve this goal, a clinical examination is coupled with a thorough history and routine histologic and immunofluorescence studies.[13,25,49,57] Despite a systematic diagnostic approach, the cause of DG cannot be elucidated in up to one-third of cases.[38]

DIAGNOSIS OF DESQUAMATIVE GINGIVITIS: A SYSTEMATIC APPROACH

SG is a clinical term and not a diagnosis. After the condition is identified, a series of laboratory procedures should be used to arrive at a final diagnosis. The success of any therapeutic approach depends on the establishment of an accurate final diagnosis. The following section describes an overview of the systematic approach used to determine the disease that is triggering DG (Fig. 21.2).

Clinical History

A thorough clinical history is mandatory to begin the assessment of DG.[25,33] Data regarding the symptoms associated with this condition and its historical aspects (e.g., lesion onset, whether it has worsened, habits that exacerbate it) provide the foundation for a thorough examination. Information about previous therapy to alleviate the condition should be documented.

Clinical Examination

The distribution pattern of the lesions (e.g., focal or multifocal, with or without confinement to gingival tissues) provides information that can begin to narrow the differential diagnosis.[6,25] A

[a]Adapted from the following chapter of Newman and Carranza's Clinical Periodontology, 13th edition: Chapter 22: Desquamative Gingivitis, by Alfredo Aguirre, Jose Luis Tapia Vazquez, and Yasmin Mair.

simple clinical maneuver such as the Nikolsky sign offers insight into the plausibility of a vesiculobullous disorder.[29]

CLINICAL CORRELATION

The Nikolsky sign is characterized by blister formation or peeling of skin or mucosa when horizontal tangential pressure is applied to the skin or mucosa in patients with vesiculobullous disorders.

Biopsy

Given the extent and number of lesions that may be present in an individual, an incisional biopsy is the best strategy for beginning

Fig. 21.1 In Chronic Desquamative Gingivitis, Irregular, Conspicuous Erythema Involves the Free and Attached Gingival Tissues.

the microscopic and immunologic evaluation.[6] An important consideration is the selection of the biopsy site (Table 21.1).

Management

The approach depends on the practitioner's experience, the systemic impact of the disease, and the systemic complications of the medications. A detailed consideration of these factors dictates three scenarios.

In the first scenario, the dental practitioner takes direct and exclusive responsibility for the treatment of the patient. This occurs with conditions such as erosive lichen planus, which is responsive to topical steroids (Fig. 21.3).

In the second scenario, the dental practitioner collaborates with another health care provider to evaluate and treat a patient concurrently. The classic example is seen with cicatricial pemphigoid, in which dentists and ophthalmologists work together to provide treatment (Fig. 21.4). Although the dental practitioner addresses the oral lesions, the ophthalmologist monitors the integrity of the ocular conjunctiva.

In the third scenario, the patient is immediately referred to a dermatologist for further evaluation and treatment. This occurs with conditions for which the systemic impact of the disease transcends the boundaries of the oral cavity and results in significant morbidity or mortality. Pemphigus vulgaris is an example of a condition that, after diagnosis by the dentist, requires immediate referral to a dermatologist (Fig. 21.5).

Fig. 21.2 The Diagnostic Approach for Desquamative Gingivitis Includes Hematoxylin and Eosin (H&E) and Direct Immunofluorescence (DIF) Evaluation of Biopsy Specimens.

Fig. 21.3 Algorithm for the Treatment of Lichen Planus.

TABLE 21.1   Diagnostic Findings for Conditions That Can Manifest as Desquamative Gingivitis

Disease	Histopathology	DIRECT IMMUNOFLUORESCENCE		INDIRECT IMMUNOFLUORESCENCE
		Biopsy of Perilesional Mucosa	Biopsy of Uninvolved Mucosa	Serum
Pemphigus	Intraepithelial clefting above the basal cell layer; basal cells have a characteristic tombstone appearance; acantholysis	Intercellular deposits in epithelium; IgG in all cases and C3 in most cases	Same as for perilesional mucosa	Intercellular antibodies (IgG) in ≥90% of cases
Cicatricial pemphigoid	Subepithelial clefting with epithelial separation from the underlying lamina propria, leaving an intact basal layer	Linear deposits of C3 with or without IgG at the basement membrane zone in most cases	Same as for perilesional mucosa	Basement membrane zone antibodies (IgG) in 10% of cases
Bullous pemphigoid	Subepithelial clefting with epithelial separation from the underlying lamina propria, leaving an intact basal layer	Linear deposits of C3 with or without IgG at the basement membrane zone in most cases	Same as for perilesional mucosa	Basement membrane zone in 40%–70% of cases
Epidermolysis bullosa acquisita	Similar to bullous and cicatricial pemphigoid	Linear deposits of IgG and C3 at the basement membrane zone in most cases	Same as for perilesional mucosa	Basement membrane zone antibodies (IgG) in 25% of cases
Lichen planus	Hyperkeratosis, hydropic degeneration of the basal layer, and sawtooth rete pegs; lamina propria exhibits dense, bandlike infiltrate, primarily of T lymphocytes; colloid bodies	Fibrillar deposits of fibrin at the dermal–epidermal junction	Negative	Negative
Chronic ulcerative stomatitis	Similar to erosive lichen planus; hyperkeratosis, acanthosis, basal cell layer liquefaction, subepithelial clefting, and lymphohistiocytic chronic infiltrate in a bandlike configuration	IgG deposits in the nuclei of the basal layer of epithelial cells	Same as for perilesional mucosa	ANA specific for basal cells of stratified squamous epithelium
Linear IgA disease	Similar to erosive lichen planus	Linear deposits of IgA at the basement membrane zone	Same as for perilesional mucosa	IgA basement membrane zone antibodies (IgA) in 30% of cases
Dermatitis herpetiformis	Collection of neutrophils, eosinophils, and fibrin in the connective tissue papillae	IgA deposits in the dermal papillae in 85% of cases	IgA deposits in dermal papillae in 100% of cases	IgA endomysial antibodies in 70% of cases; gliadin antibodies in 30% of cases
Systemic lupus erythematosus	Hyperkeratosis, basal cell degeneration, epithelial atrophy, and perivascular inflammation	IgG or IgM with or without C3 deposits at the dermal–epidermal junction	Same as for perilesional mucosa	ANA in >95% of cases; DNA and ENA antibodies in >50% of cases
Chronic cutaneous erythematosus	Hyperkeratosis, basal cell degeneration, epithelial atrophy, and perivascular inflammation	IgG or IgM with or without C3 deposits at the dermal–epidermal junction	Negative	Usually negative
Subacute lupus erythematosus	Less inflammatory cell infiltrate than systemic and chronic cutaneous forms but with similar microscopic features	IgG or IgM with or without C3 deposits at the dermal-epidermal junction in 60% of cases; granular IgG deposits in basal cell cytoplasm in 30% of cases	Same as for perilesional mucosa	ANA in 60%–90% of cases; Ro (SSA) in 80% of cases; RF in 30% of cases; anti-RNP in 10% of cases

ANA, Antinuclear antibodies; *C3,* complement 3; *DNA,* deoxyribonucleic acid; *ENA,* extractable nuclear antigens; *IgA,* immunoglobulin A; *IgG,* immunoglobulin G; *IgM,* immunoglobulin M; *RF,* rheumatoid factor; *RNP,* ribonucleoprotein; *SSA,* Sjögren syndrome antigen A.
Adapted from Rinaggio J, Neiders ME, Aguirre A, Kumar V: Using immunofluorescence in the diagnosis of chronic ulcerative lesions of the oral mucosa, *Compend Contin Educ Dent* 20:943–944, 947–948, 950 passim, 1999.

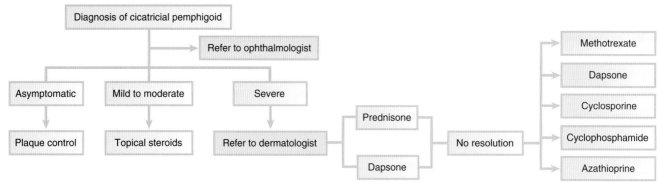

Fig. 21.4 Algorithm for the Treatment of Cicatricial Pemphigoid.

Fig. 21.5 Algorithm for the Treatment of Pemphigus Vulgaris.

When oral treatment is provided, periodic evaluation is needed to monitor the response of the patient to therapy. Initially, the patient should be evaluated at 2 to 4 weeks after beginning treatment to ensure that the condition is under control. Observation should continue until the patient is free of discomfort. Appointments every 3 to 6 months are then appropriate. Medication dosages are usually adjusted during this interval.

Table 21.2 summarizes suggested contemporary therapeutic approaches that can be used to treat selected conditions that can manifest as DG. The dental practitioner plays an important role in the diagnosis and management of DG. The importance of recognizing and properly diagnosing this condition is accentuated by the fact that a serious and life-threatening disease (i.e., squamous cell carcinoma) can mimic DG.[40]

DISEASES THAT CAN MANIFEST AS DESQUAMATIVE GINGIVITIS

Lichen Planus

Lichen planus is a mucocutaneous disorder that classically manifests with bilateral, white striae on the buccal mucosae. The classic reticular subtype is asymptomatic, and no treatment is needed. Atrophic and erosive forms of oral lichen planus are associated with pain and a burning sensation, and topical corticosteroids are the mainstay of treatment. One percent of oral lichen planus cases may develop squamous cell carcinoma.

Pemphigoid

The term *pemphigoid* applies to several cutaneous, immune-mediated, subepithelial bullous diseases that are characterized by a separation of the basement membrane zone, including bullous pemphigoid, mucous membrane pemphigoid (MMP), and pemphigoid (herpes) gestationis.[35,44] Among these conditions, bullous pemphigoid and MMP (i.e., benign MMP or cicatricial pemphigoid) have received considerable attention. Molecular findings for these two diseases indicate that they are separate entities.[44] However, considerable histologic and immunopathologic overlap exists between them, and differentiation may be impossible on the basis of the two criteria.[35]

Mucous Membrane Pemphigoid

MMP (i.e., cicatricial pemphigoid) is a chronic vesiculobullous autoimmune disorder of unknown cause that predominantly affects women during the fifth decade of life. It has rarely been reported in young children.[5,30,44]

KEY FACT

MMP is an autoimmune disorder characterized by ocular and oral lesions. Symblepharon (i.e., scarring resulting in adhesion of the eyelid to the eyeball) is a significant complication of MMP. The diagnosis is made by using hematoxylin and eosin (H&E) and direct immunofluorescence (DIF) studies, and the mainstay of treatment is corticosteroids.

TABLE 21.2 Therapeutic Approaches for Treating Selected Conditions That Manifest as Desquamative Gingivitis

Disease	THERAPY		
	Mild Cases	Recalcitrant Cases	Severe or Refractory Cases
Erosive lichen planus	Delivery of therapeutic agent is enhanced with use of vacuum-formed custom trays **Rx:** Lidex (0.05% fluocinonide) gel **Disp:** One tube (15 g) **Sig:** Apply to affected area pc and hs Monitoring of patient's oral cavity warranted because candidiasis may develop after a few weeks of topical steroid use; concomitant use of antifungal may be necessary **Rx:** Clotrimazole 10-mg troches **Disp:** 90 **Sig:** Dissolve in mouth tid, then expectorate for 30 consecutive days	**Rx:** Protopic (0.1% tacrolimus) ointment **Disp:** One tube (15 g) **Sig:** Apply to affected area bid	Refer to dermatologist for management with systemic corticosteroids
Cicatricial pemphigoid	**Rx:** Lidex (0.05% fluocinonide) gel **Disp:** One tube (15 g) **Sig:** Apply to affected area pc and hs **Rx:** Temovate (0.05% clobetasol propionate) **Disp:** One tube (15 g) **Sig:** Apply to affected area qid		Refer to dermatologist for management with prednisone (20–30 mg/day); concomitant use of azathioprine may be needed; dapsone, sulfonamide, and tetracycline are other alternatives
Pemphigus	Refer to dermatologist for management with prednisone (20–30 mg/day); concomitant use of azathioprine may be needed		
Chronic ulcerative stomatitis	**Rx:** Lidex (0.05% fluocinonide) gel **Disp:** One tube (15 g) **Sig:** Apply to affected area qid **Rx:** Temovate (0.05% clobetasol propionate) **Disp:** One tube (15 g) **Sig:** Apply to affected area qid		

bid, Twice daily; *g,* grams; *hs,* at bedtime; *IU,* international units; *mg,* milligrams; *pc,* after meals; *qid,* four times daily.

Fig. 21.6 A Patient With Pemphigus Vulgaris Has a Large Bulla on the Flexor Surface of the Wrist.

Fig. 21.7 In a Patient With Pemphigus Vulgaris of the Oral Cavity, Multiple and Coalescent Areas of Ulceration Are Covered by Pseudomembranes of Necrotic Epithelium. The patient had large ulcers on the labial mucosa, tongue, and soft palate.

Pemphigus Vulgaris

The pemphigus diseases are a group of autoimmune bullous disorders that produce cutaneous and mucous membranes blisters (Figs. 21.6 and 21.7). Pemphigus vulgaris is the most common of the pemphigus diseases, which also include pemphigus foliaceus, pemphigus vegetans, and pemphigus erythematosus.[41] Pemphigus vulgaris is a potentially lethal chronic condition with a 10% mortality rate and a worldwide annual incidence of 0.1 to 0.5 cases per 100,000 individuals.[3,41,45] A predilection for women, usually after the fourth decade of life, has been observed.[32] However, pemphigus vulgaris has also been reported in unusually young children and even in newborns.[8,41,47,55]

KEY FACT

Pemphigus vulgaris (PV) is a severe autoimmune mucocutaneous disease that warrants immediate referral to a dermatologist or rheumatologist. This condition is potentially lethal if left untreated. Direct and indirect immunofluorescence studies along with H&E staining of biopsy specimens are used to diagnose PV. Systemic steroids are indicated to treat it.

Chronic Ulcerative Stomatitis

Chronic ulcerative stomatitis, which was first reported in 1990,[19] manifests with chronic oral ulcerations and has a predilection for women during the fourth decade of life. The erosions and ulcerations occur predominantly in the oral cavity, with only a few cases exhibiting cutaneous lesions.[7,24,56]

Linear Immunoglobulin A Disease

Linear IgA dermatosis (LAD) is an uncommon mucocutaneous disorder with a predilection for women. The etiopathogenic aspects of LAD are not fully understood, although drug-induced LAD triggered by angiotensin-converting enzyme inhibitors has been reported.[12]

Dermatitis Herpetiformis

Dermatitis herpetiformis is a chronic condition that usually develops in young adults between the ages of 20 and 30 years, and it has a slight predilection for men.[11] Evidence indicates that dermatitis herpetiformis is a cutaneous manifestation of celiac disease. Approximately 25% of patients with celiac disease have dermatitis herpetiformis.

Microscopic examination of the initial lesions of dermatitis herpetiformis reveals focal aggregates of neutrophils and eosinophils among deposits of fibrin at the apices of the dermal pegs.[58]

Subacute Cutaneous Lupus Erythematosus

Patients with subacute cutaneous lupus erythematosus have cutaneous lesions that are similar to those of discoid lupus erythematosus (DLE) but that lack the development of scarring and atrophy.[4] Arthritis and arthralgia, low-grade fever, malaise, and myalgia can occur in up to 50% of patients with subacute cutaneous lupus erythematosus.[4,51]

DRUG-RELATED ERUPTIONS

An increase in the incidence of skin and oral manifestations of hypersensitivity to drugs occurred with the advent of sulfonamides, barbiturates, and various antibiotics. The cutaneous and oral lesions are attributed to the drug acting as an allergen that sensitizes the tissues.

Eruptions in the oral cavity that result from sensitivity to drugs that have been taken orally or parenterally are called *stomatitis medicamentosa*. The local reaction from the use of a medicament in the oral cavity (e.g., stomatitis resulting from topical penicillin use) is referred to as *stomatitis venenata* or *contact stomatitis*. In many cases, skin eruptions accompany the oral lesions.

Most drug eruptions in the oral cavity are multiform. Vesicular and bullous lesions occur most often, but pigmented or nonpigmented macular lesions are also frequently observed. Erosions,

Fig. 21.8 Plasma Cell Gingivitis. The gingiva presents a band of moderate to severe inflammation that is reminiscent of desquamative gingivitis.

which are often followed by deep ulceration with purpuric lesions, can occur. The lesions are seen in different areas of the oral cavity, with the gingiva often being affected.[1,14]

The development of gingival lesions caused by contact allergy to the mercurial compounds in dental amalgam has been documented.[20] Because of financial considerations, biopsy and patch testing may be indicated before the indiscriminate replacement of dental amalgam restorations. Similarly, DG has been reported with the use of tartar control toothpaste. Pyrophosphates and flavoring agents have been identified as the main causative agents of this unusual condition.[10] Oral reactions to cinnamon compounds (i.e., cinnamon oil, cinnamic acid, or cinnamic aldehyde) that are used to mask the taste of pyrophosphates in tartar control toothpaste include an intense erythema of the attached gingival tissues that is characteristic of plasma cell gingivitis (Fig. 21.8).[2,21]

A thorough clinical history usually discloses the source of gingival disturbance. Elimination of the offending agent (i.e., tartar control toothpaste) leads to resolution of the gingival lesions within a week, and challenge with the offending agent leads to recurrence of the oral lesions. If removal of the offending medication is not possible, topical corticosteroids and topical tacrolimus can be used to treat the lesions.[18]

CLINICAL CORRELATION

Diseases That Mimic Desquamative Gingivitis
- Squamous cell carcinoma
- Wegener granulomatosis (strawberry gingivitis)
- Candidiasis
- Graft-versus-host disease
- Crohn disease
- Foreign body gingivitis

Miscellaneous Conditions That Mimic Desquamative Gingivitis

Another group of heterogeneous conditions may masquerade as DG. Factitious lesions, candidiasis, graft-versus-host disease, Wegener granulomatosis, foreign body gingivitis, Kindler syndrome, and squamous cell carcinoma can divert the attention of the clinician and provide a diagnostic challenge.

Factitious lesions are injuries that are consciously and intentionally produced without a clear motive, although guilt, seeking sympathy, or monetary compensation can be the driving forces for this abnormal behavior. Factitious DG has been reported in the literature; it may be difficult to diagnose, and it may become apparent only after extensive and costly laboratory tests fail to reveal the genesis of the lesions.[27]

Candidiasis rarely is limited to the gingival tissues and can simulate DG. Linear gingival erythema is a *Candida*-associated lesion in individuals who are infected with human immunodeficiency virus. It manifests as a ribbon-like red band of the gingival margins and is reminiscent of DG.[43]

Graft-versus-host disease can occur in recipients of allogenic bone marrow transplants. The associated oral lesions occasionally resemble DG (eFig. 21.1).

Wegener granulomatosis is a systemic disease that can manifest with striking alterations that are confined to the gingival tissues. Classically, the gingival tissues exhibit erythema and enlargement, and they are typically described as *strawberry gums* (eFig. 21.2).[9]

Foreign body gingivitis is clinically characterized by red or red and white chronic lesions that can be painful and that are reminiscent of DG. This condition is more common among women approaching the fifth decade of life. Microscopic analysis reveals small (<5 µm in diameter) foreign bodies associated with a chronic inflammatory cell response that can exhibit granulomatous and lichenoid characteristics. Energy-dispersive radiographic microanalysis revealed that most of these foreign bodies originate from dental materials (i.e., abrasives and restorative materials).[16,17]

Kindler syndrome, which involves cutaneous neonatal bullae, poikiloderma, photosensitivity, and acral atrophy, can manifest with oral lesions that are clinically consistent with DG.[39]

A clinical diagnosis of DG requires a series of diagnostic steps before a precise diagnosis can be obtained. The steps include a comprehensive clinical history, clinical-pathologic correlation, microscopic examination (e.g., H&E), and DIF studies.[50] The failure to systematically evaluate a patient with a clinical condition that is consistent with DG can produce poor outcomes. This is particularly true when therapy for a putative DG is established before a biopsy of the lesional tissue is obtained. Every year, we see in our laboratory at least two examples of clinically diagnosed DG for which microscopic and immunofluorescence studies were not performed to rule out the cause of the gingival lesions. The patients were monitored or prescribed topical steroids for several months before the lack of response of the gingival lesions impelled the clinician to obtain a biopsy, which revealed squamous cell carcinoma.[52] Clinicians should be alert to the possibility of squamous cell carcinoma of the gingival tissues with lesions that initially manifest as DG.

A Case Scenario is found on the companion website.

REFERENCES

 References for this chapter are found on the companion website www.expertconsult.com.

22

The Periodontal Pocket and Associated Pathologies[a]

CHAPTER OUTLINE

The periodontal pocket, which is defined as a pathologically deepened gingival sulcus, is one of the most important clinical features of periodontal disease. All types of periodontitis, as outlined in Chapter 6, share histopathologic features, such as tissue changes in the periodontal pocket, mechanisms of tissue destruction, and healing mechanisms. However, they differ with regard to their etiology, natural history, progression, and response to therapy.[30]

POCKET CLASSIFICATION

Deepening of the gingival sulcus may occur as a result of coronal movement (enlargement) of the gingival margin, apical displacement of the gingival attachment, or a combination of the two processes (Fig. 22.1). Pockets can be classified as follows:

- *Gingival pocket* (also called "pseudo-pocket") is formed by gingival enlargement without destruction of the underlying periodontal tissues. The sulcus is deepened because of the increased bulk of the gingiva (Fig. 22.2A).
- *Periodontal pocket* produces destruction of the supporting periodontal tissues, leading to the loosening and exfoliation of the teeth. The remainder of this chapter refers to this type

of pocket. Based on the location of the base of the pocket in relation to the underlying bone, periodontal pockets can be classified into the following types:

- *Suprabony* (*supracrestal* or *supra-alveolar*) occurs when the bottom of the pocket is coronal to the underlying alveolar bone (see Fig. 22.2B).
- *Intrabony* (*infrabony, subcrestal,* or *intraalveolar*) occurs when the bottom of the pocket is apical to the level of the adjacent alveolar bone. With this second type, the lateral pocket wall lies between the tooth surface and the alveolar bone (see Fig. 22.2C).

Pockets can involve one, two, or more tooth surfaces, and they can be of different depths and types on different surfaces of the same tooth and on approximal surfaces of the same interdental space.[28,36] Pockets can also be spiral (i.e., originating on one tooth surface and twisting around the tooth to involve one or more additional surfaces; Fig. 22.3). These types of pockets are most common in furcation areas.

CLINICAL FEATURES

Clinical signs that suggest the presence of periodontal pockets include a bluish red thickened marginal gingiva, a bluish red vertical zone from the gingival margin to the alveolar mucosa, gingival bleeding and suppuration, tooth mobility, diastema formation, and symptoms such as localized pain or pain "deep in the bone." It is important that some pockets have no corresponding visual gingival inflammatory changes. The only reliable method

---

[a]Adapted from the following chapter of Newman and Carranza's *Clinical Periodontology*, 13th edition: Chapter 23: The Periodontal Pocket, by Fermin A. Carranza, Satheesh Elangovan, Paulo M. Camargo.

Fig. 22.1 Illustration of Pocket Formation That Indicates Expansion in Two Directions *(arrows)* from the Normal Gingival Sulcus *(left)* to the Periodontal Pocket *(right)*.

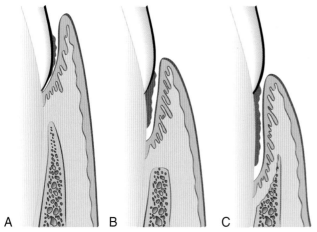

Fig. 22.2 Different Types of Periodontal Pockets. (A) Gingival pocket. There is no destruction of the supporting periodontal tissues. (B) Suprabony pocket. The base of the pocket is coronal to the level of the underlying bone. Bone loss is horizontal. (C) Intrabony pocket. The base of the pocket is apical to the level of the adjacent bone. Bone loss is vertical.

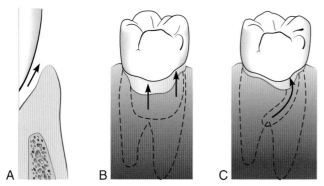

Fig. 22.3 Classification of Pockets According to Involved Tooth Surfaces. (A) Simple pocket. (B) Compound pocket. (C) Complex pocket.

Fig. 22.4 Probing of a Deep Periodontal Pocket. The entire length of the periodontal probe has been inserted to the base of the pocket in the palatal surface of the first premolar.

of locating periodontal pockets and determining their extent is careful periodontal probing of each tooth surface (Fig. 22.4 and Table 22.1). On the basis of depth alone, however, it is sometimes difficult to differentiate between a deep normal sulcus and a shallow periodontal pocket. In such borderline cases, pathologic changes in the gingiva distinguish the two conditions.

For a more detailed discussion of the clinical aspects of periodontal pockets, see Chapter 30.

KEY FACT

Sulcus Versus Periodontal Pocket
Gingival sulcus is the space between the neck of the tooth and the circumferential gingival tissue. Sulcus, when it deepens (as in periodontal disease) due to the apical migration of junctional epithelium, accompanied by attachment loss, it is referred to as a *periodontal pocket*.

PATHOGENESIS

The initial lesion in the development of periodontitis is the inflammation of the gingiva in response to a bacterial challenge. Changes involved in the transition from the normal gingival sulcus to the pathologic periodontal pocket are associated with different proportions of bacterial cells in dental plaque. Healthy gingiva is associated with few microorganisms, mostly coccoid cells and straight rods. Diseased gingiva is associated with increased numbers of spirochetes and motile rods.[38,39,41] However, the microbiota of diseased sites cannot be used as a predictor of future attachment or bone loss, because their presence alone is not sufficient for disease to start or progress.[33]

Pocket formation starts as an inflammatory change in the connective tissue wall of the gingival sulcus. The cellular and fluid inflammatory exudate causes degeneration of the surrounding connective tissue, including the gingival fibers. Just apical to the junctional epithelium, collagen fibers are destroyed,[19,57] and the area is occupied by inflammatory cells and edema (Fig. 22.5).

TABLE 22.1   Correlation of Clinical and Histopathologic Features of the Periodontal Pocket

Clinical Features	Histopathologic Features
1. The gingival wall of the pocket presents various degrees of bluish red discoloration; flaccidity; a smooth, shiny surface; and pitting on pressure.	1. The discoloration is caused by circulatory stagnation; the flaccidity by the destruction of gingival fibers and surrounding tissues; the smooth, shiny surface by atrophy of the epithelium and edema; and the pitting on pressure by edema and degeneration.
2. Less frequently, the gingival wall may be pink and firm.	2. In such cases, fibrotic changes predominate over exudation and degeneration, particularly in relation to the outer surface of the pocket wall. However, despite the external appearance of health, the inner wall of the pocket invariably presents some degeneration and is often ulcerated (see Fig. 22.15).
3. Bleeding is elicited by gently probing the soft-tissue wall of the pocket.	3. Ease of bleeding results from increased vascularity, the thinning and degeneration of the epithelium, and the proximity of engorged vessels to the inner surface.
4. When explored with a probe, the inner aspect of the pocket is generally painful.	4. Pain on tactile stimulation is caused by the ulceration of the inner aspect of the pocket wall.
5. In many cases, pus may be expressed with the application of digital pressure.	5. Pus occurs in pockets with suppurative inflammation of the inner wall.

Fig. 22.5 Interdental Papilla With Suprabony Pockets on Proximal Tooth Surfaces. Note the densely inflamed connective tissue, with the infiltrate extending between the collagen fibers and the proliferating and ulcerated pocket epithelium.

Early concepts assumed that after the initial bacterial attack, periodontal tissue destruction continued to be linked to bacterial action. More recently, it was established that the host's immunoinflammatory response to the initial and persistent bacterial attack unleashes mechanisms that lead to collagen and bone destruction. These mechanisms are related to various cytokines, some of which are produced normally by cells in noninflamed tissue and others by cells that are involved in the inflammatory process, such as polymorphonuclear leukocytes (PMNs), monocytes, and other cells, thereby leading to collagen and bone destruction. This chapter describes the histologic aspects of gingival inflammation and tissue destruction.

KEY FACT

Cytokines are proteins secreted by cells that interact with other cells and eventually lead to a specific cellular response. Cytokines can be proinflammatory or antiinflammatory in nature. Proinflammatory cytokines such as interleukin-1 (IL-1) and tumor necrosis factor-alpha (TNF-α) are implicated strongly in the pathogenesis of periodontal disease progression. Antiinflammatory cytokines such as IL-4 and IL-10 counteract the effects of proinflammatory cytokines.

The two mechanisms associated with collagen loss are as follows: (1) collagenases and other enzymes secreted by various cells in healthy and inflamed tissue, such as fibroblasts,[69] PMNs,[68] and macrophages,[49] become extracellular and destroy collagen (enzymes that degrade collagen and other matrix macromolecules into small peptides are called *matrix metalloproteinases*[70]); and (2) fibroblasts phagocytize collagen fibers by extending cytoplasmic processes to the ligament-cementum interface and degrading the inserted collagen fibrils and the fibrils of the cementum matrix.[19,20]

As a consequence of the loss of collagen, the apical cells of the junctional epithelium proliferate along the root surface and extend finger-like projections that are two or three cells in thickness (Fig. 22.6).

KEY FACT

Matrix Metalloproteinases and Tissue Inhibitors of Metalloproteinases

Matrix metalloproteinases (MMPs) are a group of proteases that play an important role in several biologic processes. Like any protease, they are involved in the degradation of proteins. Specifically, they are important players in extracellular matrix (ECM) degradation and are inhibited by tissue inhibitors of metalloproteinases (TIMPs). The balance between MMPs and TIMPs is critical for the maintenance of ECM remodeling in tissues, including the periodontium.

As a result of inflammation, PMNs invade the coronal end of the junctional epithelium in increasing numbers (Fig. 22.7). The PMNs are not joined to one another or to the epithelial cells by desmosomes. When the relative volume of PMNs reaches approximately 60% or more of the junctional epithelium, the tissue loses cohesiveness and detaches from the tooth surface. Thus the coronal portion of the junctional epithelium detaches from the root as the apical portion migrates, resulting in its apical shift; the oral sulcular epithelium gradually occupies an increasing portion of the sulcus (then a pocket) lining.[59]

Fig. 22.6 Low-Power View of the Base of the Periodontal Pocket and Apical Area. Note the dense inflammatory infiltrate on the area of destroyed collagen fibers and the thin, finger-like extension of epithelium covering the cementum, which has been denuded of fibers.

Fig. 22.7 Base of Periodontal Pocket Showing Extensive Proliferation of Lateral Epithelium Next to Atrophic Areas, Dense Inflammatory Infiltrate, Remnants of Destroyed Collagen Fibers, and the Junctional Epithelium, Which Is Apparently in a Less Altered State Than the Lateral Pocket Epithelium.

Extension of the junctional epithelium along the root requires the presence of healthy epithelial cells. Marked degeneration or necrosis of the junctional epithelium impairs rather than accelerates pocket formation. (This occurs in necrotizing ulcerative gingivitis, which results in an ulcer rather than pocket formation [see Chapter 19].)

Degenerative changes seen in the junctional epithelium at the base of periodontal pockets are usually less severe than those in the epithelium of the lateral pocket wall (see Fig. 22.7). Because the migration of the junctional epithelium requires healthy, viable cells, it is reasonable to assume that the degenerative changes seen in this area occur after the junctional epithelium reaches its position on the cementum.

The degree of leukocyte infiltration of the junctional epithelium is independent of the volume of inflamed connective tissue. This process may occur in gingiva with only slight signs of clinical inflammation.[57]

With continued inflammation, the gingiva increases in bulk, and the crest of the gingival margin extends coronally. The apical cells of the junctional epithelium continue to migrate along the root, and its coronal cells continue to separate from it. The epithelium of the lateral wall of the pocket proliferates to form bulbous, cordlike extensions into the inflamed connective tissue. Leukocytes and edema from the inflamed connective tissue infiltrate the epithelium that lines the pocket, resulting in various degrees of degeneration and necrosis.

The transformation of a gingival sulcus into a periodontal pocket creates an area in which plaque removal becomes impossible, and a feedback mechanism is established. The rationale for pocket reduction is based on the need to eliminate areas of plaque accumulation.

HISTOPATHOLOGY

Changes that occur during the initial stages of gingival inflammation are presented in Chapter 16. After the pocket is formed, several microscopic features are present, which are discussed in this section.

SOFT TISSUE WALL

The connective tissue is edematous and densely infiltrated with plasma cells (approximately 80%), lymphocytes, and a scattering of PMNs.[76] The blood vessels are increased in number, dilated, and engorged, particularly in the subepithelial connective tissue layer.[10] The connective tissue exhibits varying degrees of degeneration. Single or multiple necrotic foci are occasionally present.[48] In addition to exudative and degenerative changes, the connective tissue shows proliferation of the endothelial cells, with newly formed capillaries, fibroblasts, and collagen fibers (see Fig. 22.5).

The junctional epithelium at the base of the pocket is usually much shorter than that of a normal sulcus. Although marked variations are found with regard to the length, width, and condition of the epithelial cells,[58] usually the coronoapical length of the junctional epithelium is reduced to only 50–100 μm.[14] The cells may be well formed and in good condition, or they may exhibit slight to marked degeneration (see Figs. 22.6 and 22.7).

The most severe degenerative changes in the periodontal pocket occur along the lateral wall (Fig. 22.8). The epithelium of the lateral wall of the pocket presents striking proliferative and degenerative changes. Epithelial

Fig. 22.8 View of the Ulcerated Lateral Pocket Wall of a Periodontal Pocket. Note the extension of epithelial cells and the dense accumulation of leukocytes within the epithelium and in the connective tissue.

buds or interlacing cords of epithelial cells project from the lateral wall into the adjacent inflamed connective tissue, and they may extend farther apically than the junctional epithelium (Fig. 22.9A; see also Fig. 22.7). These epithelial projections, as well as the remainder of the lateral epithelium, are densely infiltrated by leukocytes and edema from the inflamed connective tissue. The cells undergo vacuolar degeneration and rupture to form vesicles. Progressive degeneration and necrosis of the epithelium lead to ulceration of the lateral wall, exposure of the underlying inflamed connective tissue, and suppuration. In some cases, acute inflammation is superimposed on the underlying chronic changes.

A comparative study of gingival changes in aggressive and chronic periodontitis revealed more pronounced degenerative changes in the epithelium of aggressive cases with more open intercellular spaces, including microclefts and necrotic areas.[33] The severity of the degenerative changes is not necessarily related to pocket depth. Ulceration of the lateral wall may occur in shallow pockets, and deep pockets are occasionally observed in which the lateral epithelium is relatively intact or shows only slight degeneration. The epithelium at the gingival crest of a periodontal pocket is generally intact and thickened, with prominent rete pegs.

KEY FACTS

Features of Junctional Epithelium
- It acts as a physical barrier against plaque bacteria.
- It is stratified squamous nonkeratinized in nature, which develops by the union of oral epithelium and reduced enamel epithelium during tooth eruption.
- It is attached to the tooth by internal basal lamina and to the connective tissue by external basal lamina.
- It exhibits higher permeability to cells, gingival fluid, and host-defense molecules to flow through.
- It has higher rate of cellular proliferation and turnover.

Fig. 22.9 (A) Lateral wall of a periodontal pocket showing epithelial proliferative and atrophic changes as well as marked inflammatory infiltrate and the destruction of collagen fibers. (B) Slightly apical view of the same patient showing the shortened junctional epithelium.

Fig. 22.10 Scanning Electron Micrograph of a Section of Pocket Wall in Advanced Periodontitis in a Human Specimen Showing Bacterial Penetration Into the Epithelium and Connective Tissue. Scanning electron microscope view of the surface of the pocket wall *(A)*, sectioned epithelium *(B)*, and sectioned connective tissue *(C)*. *Curved arrows* point to areas of bacterial penetration into the epithelium. *Thick white arrows* point to bacterial penetration into the connective tissue through a break in the continuity of the basal lamina. *CF,* Connective tissue fibers; *D,* accumulation of bacteria (rods, cocci, and filaments) on the basal lamina; *F,* filamentous organism on the surface of the epithelium. The *asterisk* points to coccobacillus in the connective tissue.

Bacterial Invasion

Bacterial invasion of the apical and lateral areas of the pocket wall has been described in human chronic periodontitis. Filaments, rods, and coccoid organisms with predominant gram-negative cell walls have been found in intercellular spaces of the epithelium.[24,25] Hillmann and colleagues[33] have reported the presence of *Porphyromonas gingivalis* and *Prevotella intermedia* in the gingiva of aggressive periodontitis cases. *Aggregatibacter actinomycetemcomitans* has also been found in the tissues.[16,44,55]

Bacteria may invade the intercellular space under exfoliating epithelial cells, but they are also found between deeper epithelial cells as well as accumulating on the basement lamina. Some bacteria traverse the basement lamina and invade the subepithelial connective tissue (Figs. 22.10 and 22.11).[56]

The presence of bacteria in the gingival tissues has been interpreted by different investigators as bacterial invasion or as the "passive translocation" of plaque bacteria.[40] This important point has significant clinicopathologic implications and has not yet been clarified.[17,37,41]

Mechanisms of Tissue Destruction

The inflammatory response triggered by bacterial plaque unleashes a complex cascade of events aimed at destroying and removing bacteria, necrotic cells, and deleterious agents. However, this process is nonspecific; in an attempt to restore health, the host's cells (e.g., neutrophils, macrophages, fibroblasts, epithelial cells)

Fig. 22.11 Transmission Electron Micrograph of the Epithelium in the Periodontal Pocket Wall Showing Bacteria in the Intercellular Spaces. *B,* Bacteria; *EC,* epithelial cell; *IS,* intercellular space; *L,* leukocyte about to engulf bacteria. (×8000.)

produce proteinases, cytokines, and prostaglandins that can damage or destroy the tissues.

Chapter 9 describes in detail these aspects of inflammation and the mechanisms of tissue destruction at the molecular level.

Microtopography of the Gingival Wall

Scanning electron microscopy has permitted the description of several areas in the soft tissue (gingival) wall of the periodontal pocket in which different types of activity take place.[52] These areas are irregularly oval or elongated and adjacent to one another, and they measure about 50 to 200 μm. These findings suggest that the pocket wall is constantly changing as a result of the interaction between the host and the bacteria. The following areas have been noted:

1. *Areas of relative quiescence,* showing a relatively flat surface with minor depressions and mounds and occasional shedding of cells (Fig. 22.12A).
2. *Areas of bacterial accumulation,* which appear as depressions on the epithelial surface, with abundant debris and bacterial clumps penetrating into the enlarged intercellular spaces. These bacteria are mainly cocci, rods, and filaments, with a few spirochetes (see Fig. 22.12B).
3. *Areas of emergence of leukocytes,* in which leukocytes appear in the pocket wall through holes located in the intercellular spaces (Fig. 22.13).
4. *Areas of leukocyte-bacteria interaction,* in which numerous leukocytes are present and covered with bacteria in an apparent process of phagocytosis. Bacterial plaque associated with the epithelium is seen either as an organized matrix covered by a fibrin-like material in contact with the surface of cells or as bacteria penetrating into the intercellular spaces (see Fig. 22.12C).

5. *Areas of intense epithelial desquamation,* consisting of semiattached and folded epithelial squames, which are sometimes partially covered with bacteria (see Fig. 22.12D).
6. *Areas of ulceration,* with exposed connective tissue (Fig. 22.14).
7. *Areas of hemorrhage,* with numerous erythrocytes.

The transition from one area to another could result from bacteria accumulating in previously quiescent areas and triggering the emergence of leukocytes and the leukocyte-bacteria interaction. This would lead to intense epithelial desquamation and finally to ulceration and hemorrhage.

Fig. 22.12 Scanning Electron Frontal Micrograph of the Periodontal Pocket Wall. Different areas can be seen in the pocket wall surface. *A,* Area of quiescence. *B,* Bacterial accumulation. *C,* Bacterial-leukocyte interaction. *D,* Intense cellular desquamation. *Arrows* point to emerging leukocytes and holes left by leukocytes in the pocket wall (magnification ×800).

Fig. 22.13 Scanning Electron Micrograph of the Periodontal Pocket Wall, Frontal View, in a Patient With Advanced Periodontitis. Note the desquamating epithelial cells and leukocytes *(white arrows)* emerging onto the pocket space. Scattered bacteria can also be seen *(black arrow)* (magnification ×1500).

Fig. 22.14 Area of Ulceration in the Lateral Wall of a Deep Periodontal Pocket in a Human Specimen (Magnification ×800) *(left).* *A,* Surface of pocket epithelium in a quiescent state. *B,* Area of hemorrhage. Scanning electron microscopy (magnification ×3000) of the square on the left *(right).* Connective tissue fibers and cells can be seen in the bottom of the ulcer.

Periodontal Pockets as Healing Lesions

Periodontal pockets are chronic inflammatory lesions and, thus, are constantly undergoing repair. Complete healing does not occur because of the persistence of the bacterial attack, which continues to stimulate an inflammatory response, thereby causing degeneration of the new tissue elements formed during the continuous effort at repair.

The condition of the soft-tissue wall of the periodontal pocket results from the interplay of the destructive and constructive tissue changes. Their balance determines clinical features such as color, consistency, and surface texture of the pocket wall. If the inflammatory fluid and cellular exudate predominate, the pocket wall is bluish red, soft, spongy, and friable, with a smooth, shiny surface; at the clinical level, this is generally referred to as an *edematous pocket wall.* If there is a relative predominance of newly formed connective tissue cells and fibers, the pocket wall is more firm and pink and clinically referred to as a *fibrotic pocket wall* (see Table 22.1).

Edematous and fibrotic pockets represent opposite extremes of the same pathologic process rather than different disease entities. They are subject to constant modification, depending on the relative predominance of exudative and constructive changes.

Fibrotic pocket walls may be misleading because they do not necessarily reflect what is taking place throughout the pocket wall. The most severe degenerative changes in periodontal tissues occur adjacent to the tooth surface and the subgingival plaque. In some cases, inflammation and ulceration on the inside of the pocket are walled off by fibrous tissue on the outer aspect (Fig. 22.15). Externally the pocket appears pink and fibrotic, despite the inflammatory changes occurring internally.

Pocket Contents

Periodontal pockets contain debris that consists principally of microorganisms and their products (enzymes, endotoxins, and other metabolic products), gingival fluid, food remnants, salivary mucin, desquamated epithelial cells, and leukocytes. Plaque-covered calculus usually projects from the tooth surface (Fig. 22.16). Purulent exudate, if present in the patient, consists of living, degenerated, and necrotic leukocytes; living and dead bacteria; serum; and a scant amount of fibrin.[43] The contents of periodontal pockets, when filtered free of organisms and debris, have been demonstrated to be toxic when injected subcutaneously into experimental animals.[29]

Suppuration (pus) is a common feature of periodontal disease, but it is only a secondary sign. The presence of suppuration or the ease with which it can be expressed from the pocket merely reflects the nature of the inflammatory changes in the pocket wall. It is not an indication of the depth of the pocket or the severity of the destruction of the supporting tissues. Extensive suppuration may occur in shallow pockets, whereas deep pockets may exhibit little or no suppuration. The localized accumulation of suppuration constitutes an abscess, which is discussed later in this chapter.

KEY FACT

Gingival Crevicular Fluid
Gingival crevicular fluid (GCF) is an ultrafiltrate of blood, present in the gingival sulcus space, that contains several molecular components such as bacterial degradation products, host tissue degradation products, and inflammatory mediators. Due to the location and ease of collection, several human clinical studies have been and are currently exploring and validating biomarkers of periodontal disease in GCF. The implant equivalent of GCF is commonly referred to as periimplant sulcular fluid (PISF).

Fig. 22.15 Periodontal Pocket Wall. The inner half is inflamed and ulcerated; the outer half is densely collagenous.

Fig. 22.16 Interdental Papilla With Ulcerated Suprabony Periodontal Pockets on Its Mesial and Distal Aspects. Calculus is present on the approximal tooth surfaces and within the gingiva.

Root Surface Walls

The root surface wall of periodontal pockets often undergoes changes that are significant because they may perpetuate the periodontal infection, cause pain, and complicate periodontal treatment.[11]

> As the pocket deepens, collagen fibers embedded in the cementum are destroyed, and cementum becomes exposed to the oral environment. Collagenous remnants of Sharpey fibers in the cementum undergo degeneration, creating an environment favorable to the penetration of bacteria. Viable bacteria have been found in the roots of 87% of periodontally diseased noncarious teeth.[2,26] Bacterial penetration into the cementum can be found as deep as the cementodentinal junction,[1,18] and it may also enter the dentinal tubules.[27,29] Penetration and the growth of bacteria lead to fragmentation and breakdown of the cementum surface and result in areas of necrotic cementum that are separated from the tooth by masses of bacteria.

Pathologic granules[9] have been observed with light and electron microscopy,[6,7] and they may represent areas of collagen degeneration or areas in which collagen fibrils have not been fully mineralized initially.

In addition, bacterial products (e.g., endotoxins[4,5]) have also been detected in the cementum wall of periodontal pockets. When root fragments from teeth with periodontal disease are placed in tissue culture, they induce irreversible morphologic changes in the cells of the culture. Such changes are not produced by normal roots.[31] Diseased root fragments also prevent the in vitro attachment of human gingival fibroblasts, whereas normal root surfaces allow the cells to attach freely.[3] When placed in the oral mucosa of the patient, diseased root fragments induce an inflammatory response, even if they have been autoclaved.[42]

KEY FACT

Bacterial Endotoxin

Endotoxins are lipopolysaccharide (LPS) in nature and are associated with the cell walls of gram-negative bacteria. LPS is highly immunogenic, which the innate immune system recognizes via Toll-like receptors (TLRs), leading to an immune response. LPS from *P. gingivalis*, a key pathogen in periodontal disease, plays an important role in both triggering and sustaining inflammation in the periodontium.

These changes manifest clinically as softening of the cementum surface; this is usually asymptomatic, but it can be painful when a probe or explorer penetrates the area. They also constitute a possible reservoir for reinfection of the area after treatment. During the course of treatment, these necrotic areas are removed by root planing until a hard, smooth surface is reached. Cementum is very thin in the cervical areas, and scaling and root planing often remove it entirely, exposing the underlying dentin. Sensitivity to cold may result until the pulp tissue forms secondary dentin.

Decalcification and Remineralization of Cementum

Areas of *increased mineralization*[61] are probably a result of an exchange of minerals and organic components at the cementum–saliva interface after exposure to the oral cavity. The mineral content of exposed cementum increases,[60] and the minerals that are increased in diseased root surfaces include calcium,[62] magnesium,[46,62] phosphorus,[46] and fluoride.[46] Microhardness, however, remains unchanged.[51,76] The development of a highly mineralized superficial layer may increase the tooth's resistance to decay.[3]

Areas of demineralization are often related to root caries. Exposure to oral fluid and bacterial plaque results in proteolysis of the embedded remnants of Sharpey fibers; the cementum may be softened, and it may undergo fragmentation and cavitation.[32] Unlike enamel caries, root surface caries tend to progress around rather than into the tooth.[45] Active root caries lesions appear as well-defined yellowish or light-brown areas; they are frequently covered by plaque, and they have a softened or leathery consistency on probing. Inactive lesions are well-defined darker lesions with a smooth surface and a harder consistency on probing.[23]

The dominant microorganism in root surface caries is *Actinomyces viscosus*,[67] although its specific role in the development of the lesion has not been established.[23] Other bacteria, such as *Actinomyces naeslundii*, *Streptococcus mutans*, *Streptococcus salivarius*, *Streptococcus sanguinis*, and *Bacillus cereus*, have been found to produce root caries in animal models. Quirynen and colleagues[50] reported that when plaque levels and pocket depths decrease after periodontal therapy (both nonsurgical and surgical), a shift in oral bacteria occurs, leading to a reduction in periodontal pathogens, an increase in *S. mutans*, and the development of root caries.

A prevalence rate study of root caries among 20- to 64-year-old individuals revealed that 42% had one or more root caries lesions and that these lesions tended to increase with age.[35]

The tooth may not be painful, but exploration of the root surface reveals the presence of a defect, and penetration of the involved area with a probe causes pain. Caries of the root may lead to pulpitis, sensitivity to sweets and thermal changes, or severe pain. Pathologic exposure of the pulp occurs in severe cases. Root caries may be the cause of toothache in patients with periodontal disease and no evidence of coronal decay.

Caries of the cementum requires special attention when the pocket is treated. The necrotic cementum must be removed by scaling and root planing until firm tooth surface is reached, even if this entails extension into the dentin.

Areas of cellular resorption of cementum and dentin are common in roots that are unexposed by periodontal disease.[63] These areas are of no particular significance because they are symptom free, and, as long as the root is covered by the periodontal ligament, they are likely to undergo repair. However, if the root is exposed by progressive pocket formation before repair occurs, these areas appear as isolated cavitations that penetrate into the dentin. These areas can be differentiated from caries of the cementum by their clear-cut outline and hard surface. They may be sources of considerable pain that require the placement of a restoration.

Surface Morphology of Tooth Wall[73]

The following zones can be found in the bottom of a periodontal pocket (Fig. 22.17):

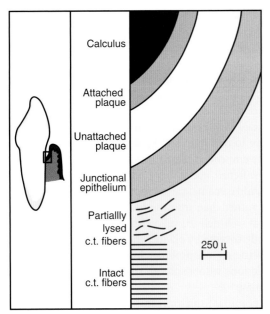

Fig. 22.17 Diagram of the Area at the Bottom of a Pocket. *c.t.,* Connective tissue.

1. *Cementum covered by calculus,* in which all of the changes described in the preceding paragraphs can be found.
2. *Attached plaque,* which covers calculus and extends apically from it to a variable degree (typically 100–500 µm).
3. The zone of *unattached plaque* that surrounds attached plaque and extends apically to it.
4. The zone of *attachment of the junctional epithelium to the tooth.* The extension of this zone, which in normal sulci is more than 500 µm, is usually reduced in periodontal pockets to less than 100 µm.
5. A zone of *semidestroyed connective tissue fibers* may be apical to the junctional epithelium (see the Pathogenesis section earlier in this chapter).[56]

Zones 3, 4, and 5 make up the "plaque-free zone" seen in extracted teeth.[8,12,34,54,73] The total width of the plaque-free zone varies according to the type of tooth (i.e., it is wider in the molars than in the incisors) and the depth of the pocket (i.e., it is narrower in deeper pockets).[53] It is important to remember that the term *plaque-free zone* refers only to attached plaque, because unattached plaque contains a variety of gram-positive and gram-negative morphotypes, including cocci, rods, filaments, fusiforms, and spirochetes. The most apical zone contains predominantly gram-negative rods and cocci.[71]

PERIODONTAL DISEASE ACTIVITY

For many years the loss of attachment produced by periodontal disease was thought to be a slow but continuously progressive phenomenon. More recently, as a result of studies of the specificity of plaque bacteria, the concept of periodontal disease activity has evolved.

According to this concept, periodontal pockets may go through periods of exacerbation and quiescence as a result of

episodic bursts of activity followed by periods of remission. *Periods of quiescence* are characterized by a reduced inflammatory response and little or no loss of bone and connective tissue attachment. A buildup of unattached plaque, with its gram-negative, motile, and anaerobic bacteria (see Chapter 9), starts a *period of exacerbation* during which bone and connective tissue attachment are lost and the pocket deepens. This period may last for days, weeks, or months, and it is eventually followed by a period of remission or quiescence, during which gram-positive bacteria proliferate and a more stable condition is established.

These periods of quiescence and exacerbation are also known as *periods of inactivity* and *periods of activity.* Clinically, active periods show bleeding, either spontaneously or with probing, and greater amounts of gingival exudate. Histologically, the pocket epithelium appears thin and ulcerated, and an infiltrate composed predominantly of plasma cells,[18] PMNs,[49] or both is seen. Bacterial samples from the pocket lumen that are analyzed with darkfield microscopy show high proportions of motile organisms and spirochetes.[41]

Methods to detect periods of activity or inactivity are currently being investigated (see the companion website).

SITE SPECIFICITY

Periodontal destruction most often does not occur in all parts of the mouth at the same time; rather it occurs on a few teeth at a time or even only on some aspects of some teeth at any given time. This is referred to as the *site specificity* of periodontal disease. Sites of periodontal destruction are often found next to sites with little or no destruction. Therefore, the severity of periodontitis increases with the development of new disease sites and with the increased breakdown of existing sites.

PULP CHANGES ASSOCIATED WITH PERIODONTAL POCKETS

The spread of infection from periodontal pockets may cause pathologic changes in the pulp. Such changes may give rise to painful symptoms, or they may adversely affect the response of the pulp to restorative procedures. Involvement of the pulp in periodontal disease occurs through either the apical foramen or the lateral pulp canals after pocket infection reaches them. Atrophic and inflammatory pulpal changes occur in such cases.

RELATIONSHIP OF ATTACHMENT LOSS AND BONE LOSS TO POCKET DEPTH

The severity of the attachment loss in pocket formation is generally but not always correlated with the depth of the pocket. This is because the degree of attachment loss depends on the location of the base of the pocket on the root surface, whereas pocket depth is the distance between the base of the pocket and the crest of the gingival margin. Pockets of the same depth may be associated with different degrees of attachment loss (Fig. 22.18),

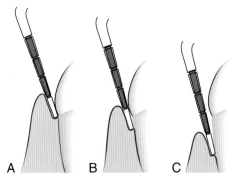

Fig. 22.18 Same Pocket Depth With Different Amounts of Recession.
(A) Gingival pocket with no recession. (B) Periodontal pocket of similar depth as shown in part (A) but with some degree of recession. (C) Pocket depth the same as shown in parts (A) and (B) but with still more recession.

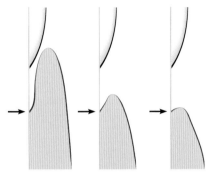

Fig. 22.19 Different Pocket Depths With the Same Amount of Attachment Loss. *Arrows* point to the bottom of the pocket. The distance between the *arrow* and the cementoenamel junction remains the same despite different pocket depths.

and pockets of different depths may be associated with the same amount of attachment loss (Fig. 22.19).

The severity of bone loss is generally but not always correlated with pocket depth. Extensive attachment and bone loss may be associated with shallow pockets if the attachment loss is accompanied by recession of the gingival margin, and slight bone loss can occur with deep pockets.

AREA BETWEEN BASE OF POCKET AND ALVEOLAR BONE

Normally, the distance between the apical end of the junctional epithelium and the alveolar bone is relatively constant. The distance between the apical extent of calculus and the alveolar crest in human periodontal pockets is most constant, having a mean length of 1.97 mm (±33.16%).[66,72]

The distance from attached plaque to bone is never less than 0.5 mm and never more than 2.7 mm.[73-75] These findings suggest that the bone-resorbing activity induced by the bacteria is exerted within these distances. However, the finding of isolated bacteria or clumps of bacteria in the connective tissue[56] and on the bone surface[25] may modify these considerations.

RELATIONSHIP OF POCKET TO BONE

In infrabony pockets, the base of the pocket is apical to the crest of the alveolar bone, and the pocket wall lies between the tooth and the bone. The bone loss is in most cases vertical. Alternatively, in suprabony pockets, the base is coronal to the crest of the alveolar bone, and the pocket wall lies coronal to the bone. The type of bone loss is always horizontal.

This creates some microscopic differences that have some therapeutic importance. They are the relationship of the soft-tissue wall of the pocket to the alveolar bone, the pattern of bone destruction, and the direction of the transseptal fibers of the periodontal ligament (Figs. 22.20 to 22.22).[15]

In suprabony pockets, the alveolar crest gradually attains a more apical position in relation to the tooth, but it retains its general morphology and architecture. The interdental fibers that run over the bone from one tooth to the other maintain their usual horizontal direction. In infrabony pockets, the morphology of the alveolar crest changes completely, with the formation of an angular bony defect. The interdental fibers in this case run over the bone in an oblique direction between the two teeth of the interdental space.[15,75] This may affect the function of the area and also necessitate a modification in treatment techniques (see Chapter 50).[13,15] Table 22.2 summarizes the distinguishing features of suprabony and infrabony pockets. The classification of infrabony pockets is discussed in Chapter 23.

CLINICAL CORRELATION

Pocket Reduction Surgeries
Pocket reduction surgeries are aimed at reducing the probing pocket depths in patients with periodontitis. Depending on the disease presentation, one can take a resective or regenerative approach. Suprabony pockets are primarily treated by resective procedures such as gingivectomy or periodontal flap and osseous surgery, whereas infrabony defects with multiple walls (that are contained) are generally treated using regenerative approaches.

PERIODONTAL ABSCESS

A periodontal abscess is a localized purulent inflammation in the periodontal tissues (Fig. 22.23). It is also known as a *lateral abscess* or a *parietal abscess*. Abscesses that are localized in the gingiva, are caused by injury to the outer surface of the gingiva, and do not involve the supporting structures are called *gingival abscesses*. Gingival abscesses may occur in the presence or absence of a periodontal pocket.

Periodontal abscess formation may occur in the following ways:
1. Extension of infection from a periodontal pocket deep into the supporting periodontal tissues and localization of the suppurative inflammatory process along the lateral aspect of the root.
2. Lateral extension of inflammation from the inner surface of a periodontal pocket into the connective tissue of the pocket wall. Formation of the abscess results when drainage into the pocket space is impaired.

Fig. 22.20 Radiographic and Microscopic Features of Intrabony Pockets. (A) Radiograph of a mandibular canine and premolar area showing angular bone loss mesial to the second premolar. The type of bone loss between the first premolar and the canine is not radiographically apparent. (B) Mesiodistal histologic section of the teeth seen in (A) showing an intrabony pocket mesial to the second premolar as well as suprabony pockets distal to the second premolar and mesial and distal to the first premolar. The mesial suprabony pocket of the first premolar appears to be coronal to a vertical bone loss. (C) Higher-power view of the area between the premolars. Note the angular bone loss and the transseptal fibers that cover the bone. (D) Higher-power view of the area between the premolars stained with Mallory connective tissue stain, clearly showing the direction of transseptal fibers. (E) Higher-power view of the area between the first premolar and the canine. Note the abundant calculus, the dense leukocytic infiltration of the gingiva, and the angulation of the transseptal fibers and bone. The pocket is still suprabony. (F) Mallory stain of a similar area to the one shown in part E. Note the destruction of the gingival fibers caused by inflammation and the angular fibers formed over angular bone loss and less affected by the inflammation. Transseptal fibers extend from the distal surface of the premolar over the crest of the alveolar bone into the intrabony pocket. Note the leukocytic infiltration of the transseptal fibers. (From Glickman I, Smulow J: *Periodontal disease: clinical, radiographic and histopathologic features*, Philadelphia, 1974, Saunders.)

TABLE 22.2 Distinguishing Features of Suprabony and Intrabony Periodontal Pockets

Suprabony Pocket	Intrabony Pocket
1. The base of the pocket is coronal to the level of the alveolar bone.	1. The base of the pocket is apical to the crest of the alveolar bone so that the bone is adjacent to the soft-tissue wall (see Fig. 22.2).
2. The pattern of destruction of the underlying bone is horizontal.	2. The pattern of bone destruction is vertical (angular; see Figs. 22.20 and 22.21).
3. Interproximally, transseptal fibers that are restored during progressive periodontal disease are arranged horizontally in the space between the base of the pocket and the alveolar bone (see Fig. 22.22).	3. Interproximally, transseptal fibers are oblique rather than horizontal. They extend from the cementum beneath the base of the pocket along the alveolar bone and over the crest to the cementum of the adjacent tooth (see Fig. 22.20).
4. On the facial and lingual surfaces, periodontal ligament fibers beneath the pocket follow their normal horizontal-oblique course between the tooth and the bone.	4. On the facial and lingual surfaces, periodontal ligament fibers follow the angular pattern of the adjacent bone. They extend from the cementum beneath the base of the pocket along the alveolar bone and over the crest to join with the outer periosteum.

Fig. 22.21 After Raising a Flap for the Treatment of the Infrabony Pockets, the Vertical Bone Loss Around the Mesial Roots of the Mandibular First and Second Molars Can be Seen.

Fig. 22.24 Microscopic View of a Periodontal Abscess Showing the Dense Accumulation of Polymorphonuclear Leukocytes Covered by Squamous Epithelium.

Fig. 22.22 Two Suprabony Pockets in an Interdental Space. Note the normal horizontal arrangement of the transseptal fibers.

Fig. 22.23 Periodontal Abscess on an Upper Right Central Incisor.

3. Formation in a pocket with a tortuous course around the root. A periodontal abscess may form in the cul-de-sac, the deep end of which is shut off from the surface.

4. Incomplete removal of calculus during treatment of a periodontal pocket. The gingival wall shrinks, thereby occluding the pocket orifice, and a periodontal abscess occurs in the sealed-off portion of the pocket.

5. After trauma to the tooth or with perforation of the lateral wall of the root in endodontic therapy. In these situations, a periodontal abscess may occur in the absence of periodontal disease.

Periodontal abscesses are classified according to location as follows:

1. *Abscess in the supporting periodontal tissues along the lateral aspect of the root.* With this condition, a sinus generally occurs in the bone that extends laterally from the abscess to the external surface.

2. *Abscess in the soft-tissue wall of a deep periodontal pocket.*

Microscopically, an abscess is a localized accumulation of viable and nonviable PMNs within the periodontal pocket wall. The PMNs liberate enzymes that digest the cells and other tissue structures, thereby forming the liquid product known as *pus*, which constitutes the center of the abscess. An acute inflammatory reaction surrounds the purulent area, and the overlying epithelium exhibits intracellular and extracellular edema and the invasion of leukocytes (Fig. 22.24).

The localized acute abscess becomes a chronic abscess when its purulent content drains through a fistula into the outer gingival surface or into the periodontal pocket and the infection that is causing the abscess is not resolved.

The bacterial invasion of tissues has been reported in abscesses; the invading organisms were identified as gram-negative cocci, diplococci, fusiforms, and spirochetes. Invasive fungi were also found and were interpreted as being "opportunistic invaders."[21] Microorganisms that colonize the periodontal abscess have been reported to be primarily gram-negative anaerobic rods.[47]

LATERAL PERIODONTAL CYST

The periodontal cyst, which is also called *lateral periodontal cyst*, is an uncommon lesion that produces localized destruction of the periodontal tissues along a lateral root surface, most often in the mandibular canine–premolar area.[22,65] It is considered to be derived from the rests of Malassez or other proliferating odontogenic rests.[64]

A periodontal cyst is usually asymptomatic, without grossly detectable changes, but it may present as a localized, tender swelling. Radiographically, an interproximal periodontal cyst appears on the side of the root as a radiolucent area bordered by a radiopaque line. Its radiographic appearance cannot be differentiated from that of a periodontal abscess.

Microscopically, the cystic lining may be (1) a loosely arranged, thin, nonkeratinized epithelium, sometimes with thicker proliferating areas, or (2) an odontogenic keratocyst.[22]

A Case Scenario is found on the companion website.

REFERENCES

 References for this chapter are found on the companion website.

Bone Loss and Patterns of Bone Destruction[a]

Periodontitis is an inflammatory condition of the teeth and their supporting structures. The inflammatory process, which occurs as a response to the bacterial biofilm insult, has detrimental effects on the periodontal unit, which results in the destruction of periodontal ligament fibers and bone loss.

The height and density of the alveolar bone are normally maintained by an equilibrium, which is regulated by local and systemic influences, between bone formation and bone resorption.[12,15] When resorption exceeds formation, both bone height and bone density may be reduced (Video 23.1).

Bone loss is a consequence of the inflammatory process observed in periodontitis. The degree of bone loss does not necessarily correlate with the depth of periodontal pockets, the severity of ulceration of the pocket wall, or the presence or absence of suppuration. A reduced but healthy periodontium may exist in areas where bone loss occurred in the past (Fig. 23.1).

BONE DESTRUCTION CAUSED BY THE EXTENSION OF GINGIVAL INFLAMMATION

The most common cause of bone destruction in periodontitis is the extension of inflammation from the marginal gingiva into the supporting periodontal tissues. The migration of the bone surface and the initial bone loss that follows marks the transition from gingivitis to periodontitis.

Periodontitis is always preceded by gingivitis, but not all gingivitis progresses to periodontitis. Some cases of gingivitis never become periodontitis, and other cases go through a brief gingivitis phase and rapidly develop into periodontitis. The factors responsible for the extension of inflammation to the supporting structures, thereby initiating the conversion of gingivitis to periodontitis,

are not clearly understood and are likely to be related to individual susceptibility to the insult presented by the bacterial biofilm or microbiologic changes that occur in the pocket environment and surrounding tissues.

> In periodontitis, the existing bone level is the result of past episodes of bone loss from the disease process, but the changes present in the soft tissue wall of the pocket is the result of the ongoing inflammatory process. The degree of bone loss does not necessarily correlate with the depth of the periodontal pockets, the severity of ulceration of the pocket wall, or the presence or absence of exudate.

As stated previously, the transition from gingivitis to periodontitis is associated with changes in the composition of the bacterial biofilm. In advanced stages of disease, the number of motile organisms and spirochetes increases, whereas the number of coccoid and straight rods decreases.[29] The cellular composition of the infiltrated connective tissue also changes with increasing severity of the lesion (see Chapter 8). Fibroblasts and lymphocytes predominate in Stage 1 gingivitis, whereas the number of plasma cells and blast cells increases gradually as the disease progresses. Seymour and colleagues[54,55] have postulated a stage of "contained" gingivitis, in which T lymphocytes are preponderant; they suggest that, as the lesion becomes a B-lymphocyte lesion, it becomes progressively destructive.

The extension of the inflammatory process into the supporting structures of a tooth may be modified by the pathogenic potential of biofilm and the susceptibility/resistance of the host. The latter includes immunologic activity and other tissue-related mechanisms, such as the degree of fibrosis of the gingiva, probably the width of the attached gingiva, and the reactive fibrogenesis and osteogenesis that occur peripheral to the inflammatory lesion.[48] Some studies suggest that the quality of the host response to a similar bacterial insult varies, resulting in some individuals being more susceptible to the destructive aspects of periodontitis than others.

[a]Adapted from the following chapter of Newman and Carranza's Clinical Periodontology, 13th edition: Chapter 24: Bone Loss and Patterns of Bone Destruction, by Paulo M. Camargo, Henry H. Taikei, Fermin A. Carranza.

Fig. 23.1 (A) An area of inflammation extending from the gingiva into the suprabony area. (B) Extension of inflammation along the blood vessels and between collagen bundles.

Histopathology

Gingival inflammation extends along the collagen fiber bundles and follows the course of the blood vessels through the loosely arranged tissues around them into the alveolar bone (see Fig. 23.1).[63] Although the inflammatory infiltrate is concentrated in the marginal periodontium, the reaction is a much more diffuse one, often reaching the bone and eliciting a response before evidence of crestal resorption or loss of attachment exists.[37] In the upper molar region, inflammation can extend to the maxillary sinus, resulting in thickening of the sinus mucosa.[36]

Interproximally, inflammation spreads to the loose connective tissue around the blood vessels, through the fibers, and then into the bone through vessel channels that perforate the crest of the interdental septum at the center of the crest (Fig. 23.2), toward the side of the crest (Fig. 23.3), or at the angle of the septum. In addition, inflammation may enter the bone through more than one channel. Less frequently, the inflammation spreads from the gingiva directly into the periodontal ligament and from there into the interdental septum (Fig. 23.4).[1]

Facially and lingually, inflammation from the gingiva spreads along the outer periosteal surface of the bone (see Fig. 23.4) and penetrates into the marrow spaces through vessel channels in the outer cortex.

Along its course from the gingiva to the bone, the inflammation destroys the gingival and transeptal fibers, reducing them to disorganized granular fragments interspersed among the inflammatory cells and edema.[41] However, there is a continuous tendency to recreate transeptal fibers across the crest of the interdental septum farther along the root as the bone destruction progresses (Fig. 23.5). As a result, transeptal fibers are present, even in cases of extreme periodontal bone loss. The dense transeptal fibers form a firm covering over the bone that is encountered during

Fig. 23.2 Inflammation That Extends From the Pocket Area *(top)* Between the Collagen Fibers, Which Are Partially Destroyed.

periodontal flap surgery after the superficial granulation tissue is removed.[46]

After inflammation reaches the bone via extension from the gingiva (Fig. 23.6), it spreads into the marrow spaces and replaces the marrow with a leukocytic and fluid exudate, new blood vessels, and proliferating fibroblasts (Fig. 23.7). Multinuclear osteoclasts and mononuclear phagocytes increase in number,

Fig. 23.3 (A) Extension of inflammation into the center of the interdental septum. Inflammation from the gingiva penetrates the transseptal fibers and enters the bone around the blood vessel in the center of the septum. (B) The cortical layer at the top of the septum has been destroyed, and the inflammation penetrates into the marrow spaces.

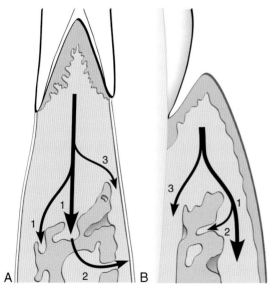

Fig. 23.4 Pathways of Inflammation From the Gingiva Into the Supporting Periodontal Tissues in a Patient With Periodontitis. (A) Interproximally, from the gingiva into the bone *(1)*, from the bone into the periodontal ligament *(2)*, and from the gingiva into the periodontal ligament *(3)*. (B) Facially and lingually, from the gingiva along the outer periosteum *(1)*, from the periosteum into the bone *(2)*, and from the gingiva into the periodontal ligament *(3)*.

Fig. 23.5 Reformation of Transseptal Fibers. A mesiodistal section through the interdental septum shows gingival inflammation and bone loss. Recreated transseptal fibers can be seen above the bone margin, where they have been partially infiltrated by the inflammatory process.

Fig. 23.6 Extension of Inflammation Has Reached the Crestal Bone Surface.

Fig. 23.8 Osteoclasts and Howship Lacunae in the Resorption of Crestal Bone.

Fig. 23.7 Interdental Septum in a Human Autopsy Section. Extensive inflammatory infiltrate has invaded the marrow spaces, entering from both the mesial and distal aspects. Fatty bone marrow has been replaced by inflammatory cells and fibrous marrow.

and the bone surfaces appear to be lined with Howship lacunae (Fig. 23.8).

In the marrow spaces, resorption proceeds from within and causes a thinning of the surrounding bony trabeculae and an enlargement of the marrow spaces; this is followed by the destruction of the bone and a reduction in bone height. Normally, fatty bone marrow is partially or totally replaced by a fibrous type of marrow in the vicinity of the resorption.

Bone destruction in periodontal disease is not a process of bone necrosis.[23] It involves the activity of living cells along viable bone. With the exception of necrotic bone that is visible in distinct pathogenic processes such as necrotizing ulcerative periodontitis and bisphosphonate-related osteonecrosis of the jaws, all bone present in areas with periodontitis is viable, live bone. In periodontitis, bone resorption may be related to the analogy of the bone attempting to run away from the infectious/inflammatory process; this may be seen as a host protection mechanism.

The amount of inflammatory infiltrate correlates with the degree of bone loss but not with the number of osteoclasts. However, the distance from the apical border of the inflammatory infiltrate to the alveolar bone crest correlates with both the number of osteoclasts on the alveolar crest and the total number of osteoclasts.[47] Similar findings have been reported in experimentally induced periodontitis in animals.[28]

Radius of Action

Garant and Cho[10] suggested that locally produced bone resorption factors may need to be present in the proximity of the bone surface to exert their action. Page and Schroeder,[43] on the basis of Waerhaug's measurements made on human autopsy specimens,[60,61] postulated a range of about 1.5 to 2.5 mm in which bacterial biofilm can induce loss of bone. Beyond 2.5 mm, there is little or no effect; interproximal angular defects can appear only in spaces that are wider than 2.5 mm, because narrower spaces would end up with horizontal bone loss. Tal[57] corroborated this concept with measurements in human patients.

Large defects that greatly exceed a distance of 2.5 mm from the tooth surface (as described in aggressive types of periodontitis) may be caused by the presence of bacteria in the tissues.[6,10,50]

Rate of Bone Loss

In a study of Sri Lankan tea laborers with no oral hygiene and no dental care, Löe and colleagues[31] found the rate of bone loss averages about 0.2 mm per year for facial surfaces and about 0.3 mm per year for proximal surfaces when periodontal disease was allowed to progress untreated.

However, the rate of bone loss may vary, depending on the type of disease present. Löe and colleagues[32] also identified the following three subgroups of patients with periodontal disease on the basis of the interproximal loss of attachment and tooth mortality (loss of attachment can be equated with loss of bone, although attachment loss precedes bone loss by about 6 to 8 months[17]):

1. Approximately 8% of persons had a rapid progression of periodontal disease that was characterized by a yearly loss of attachment of 0.1 mm to 1 mm.
2. Approximately 81% of individuals had moderately progressive periodontal disease with a yearly loss of attachment of 0.05 mm to 0.5 mm.
3. The remaining 11% of persons had minimal or no progression of destructive disease with a yearly loss of attachment of 0.05 mm to 0.09 mm.

Periods of Destruction

Periodontal destruction often occurs in an episodic, intermittent manner, with periods of inactivity or quiescence that alternate with destructive periods that result in the loss of collagen and alveolar bone and the deepening of the periodontal pocket.

Periods of destructive activity are associated with subgingival ulceration and an acute inflammatory reaction that results in the rapid loss of alveolar bone[43,52]; it has been hypothesized that this coincides with the conversion of a predominantly T-lymphocyte lesion to one with a predominantly B-lymphocyte–plasma cell infiltrate.[55] Microbiologically, these lesions are associated with an increase in the loose, unattached, motile, gram-negative, anaerobic pocket flora, whereas periods of remission coincide with the formation of a dense, unattached, nonmotile, gram-positive flora with a tendency to mineralize.[39]

It has also been suggested that, in some individuals, the onset of periods of destruction coincide with tissue invasion by one or several bacterial species, and that this is followed by an advanced local host defense that controls the attack.[50]

> The dense network transseptal fiber that is attached interdentally from tooth to tooth is one of the barriers that protects the interdental bone from the inflammatory process. Even after these fibers are initially destroyed, they continually reform and are the fibers found during periodontal flap surgery.

Mechanisms of Bone Destruction

The factors involved in bone destruction in periodontal disease are bacterial and host mediated. The bacterial biofilm products induce the differentiation of bone progenitor cells into osteoclasts and stimulate gingival cells to release mediators that have the same effect.[20,53] Bacterial biofilm products and inflammatory mediators can also act directly on osteoblasts or their progenitors, thereby inhibiting their action and reducing their numbers.

In addition, in patients with rapidly progressing diseases (e.g., aggressive periodontitis), bacterial microcolonies or single bacterial cells have been found between collagen fibers and over the bone surface, suggesting a direct effect.[6,9,53]

Several host factors released by inflammatory cells are capable of inducing bone resorption in vitro, and they play a role in periodontal disease. These include host-produced prostaglandins and their precursors, interleukin-1α, interleukin-β, and tumor necrosis factor α.

Bone Formation in Periodontal Disease

Areas of bone formation are also found immediately adjacent to sites of active bone resorption and along trabecular surfaces at a distance from the inflammation in an apparent effort to reinforce the remaining bone (i.e., buttressing bone formation). This estrogenic response is clearly found in experimentally produced periodontal bone loss in animals.[7] In humans, it is less obvious, but it has been confirmed by histometric[4,5] and histologic studies.[13]

Autopsy specimens from individuals with untreated disease occasionally show areas in which bone resorption has ceased and new bone is being formed on previously eroded bone margins. This confirms the intermittent character of bone resorption in periodontitis, and it is consistent with the varied rates of progression observed clinically in individuals with untreated periodontal disease.

The periods of remission and exacerbation (or inactivity and activity, respectively) appear to coincide with the quiescence or exacerbation of gingival inflammation as manifested by changes in the extent of bleeding, the amount of exudate, and the composition of bacterial biofilm (see Chapters 16 and 17).

The presence of bone formation in response to inflammation, even in those with active periodontal disease, has an effect on the outcome of treatment. The basic aim of periodontal therapy is the elimination of inflammation to inhibit the stimulus for bone resorption and, therefore, to allow the inherent constructive tendencies to predominate.

BONE DESTRUCTION CAUSED BY TRAUMA FROM OCCLUSION

Another cause of periodontal bone destruction is trauma from occlusion, which can occur in the absence or presence of inflammation.

In the absence of inflammation, the changes caused by trauma from occlusion vary from increased compression and tension of the periodontal ligament and increased osteoclasis of alveolar bone to necrosis of the periodontal ligament and bone and the resorption of bone and tooth structure. These changes are reversible in that they can be repaired if the offending forces are removed. However, persistent trauma from occlusion results in funnel-shaped widening of the crestal portion of the periodontal ligament with resorption of the adjacent bone.[30] These changes, which may cause the bony crest to have an angular shape, represent adaptation of the periodontal tissues aimed at "cushioning" increased occlusal forces; however, the modified bone shape may weaken tooth support and cause tooth mobility.

When it is combined with inflammation, trauma from occlusion may aggravate the bone destruction caused by the inflammation[30] and result in many different bone patterns.

BONE DESTRUCTION CAUSED BY SYSTEMIC DISORDERS

Local and systemic factors regulate the physiologic equilibrium of bone. When a generalized tendency toward bone resorption exists, bone loss initiated by local inflammatory processes may be magnified.

This systemic influence on the response of alveolar bone, as envisioned by Glickman[12] during the early 1950s, considers a systemic regulatory influence in all cases of periodontal disease. In addition to the virulence of biofilm bacteria, the nature of the systemic component rather than its presence or absence influences the severity of the periodontal destruction. This concept of a role played by systemic defense mechanisms has been validated by the studies of immune deficiencies and host modulation in severely destructive types of periodontitis.

Interest has increased concerning the possible relationship between periodontal bone loss and osteoporosis.[11] Osteoporosis is a physiologic condition of postmenopausal women that results in the loss of bone mineral content as well as structural bone changes. Periodontitis and osteoporosis share a number of risk factors (e.g., aging, smoking, certain diseases, medications that interfere with healing). Some studies show a relationship between skeletal density and oral bone density; between crestal height and residual ridge resorption; and among osteopenia and periodontitis, tooth mobility, and tooth loss.[18,21,22,51,59]

Periodontal bone loss may also occur with generalized skeletal disturbances (e.g., hyperparathyroidism, leukemia, histiocytosis X) via mechanisms that may be totally unrelated to the more common biofilm-induced, inflammatory periodontal lesion.

> In the absence of inflammation, the localized bone loss caused by trauma from occlusion is reversible (can be repaired) if the offending forces are removed.

FACTORS DETERMINING BONE MORPHOLOGY IN PERIODONTAL DISEASE

Normal Variation in Alveolar Bone

Considerable normal variation exists within the morphologic features of alveolar bone, and this affects the osseous contours produced by periodontal disease. The anatomic features that substantially affect the bone-destructive pattern of periodontal disease include the following:

- Thickness, width, and crestal angulation of the interdental septa
- Thickness of the facial and lingual alveolar plates
- Presence of fenestrations and dehiscences
- Alignment of the teeth
- Root and root trunk anatomy
- Root position within the alveolar process
- Proximity with another tooth surface

For example, angular osseous defects cannot form in thin facial or lingual alveolar plates, which have little or no cancellous bone between the outer and inner cortical layers. In such cases, the entire crest of the plate is destroyed, and the height of the bone is reduced in a horizontal fashion (Fig. 23.9).

Exostoses

Exostoses are outgrowths of bone of varied size and shape. Palatal exostoses have been found in 40% of human skulls.[42] They can occur as small nodules, large nodules, sharp ridges, spikelike projections, or any combination of these examples (Fig. 23.10).[38] Exostoses have been described in rare cases as developing after the placement of free gingival grafts.[42]

> Angular osseous defects—as often seen in the interdental areas of the posterior dentition—cannot form in thin radicular, facial, or lingual alveolar bone. These areas have little or no cancellous bone between the outer and inner cortical layers. In these anatomic areas, the entire crest of the plate is destroyed, and the height of the bone is reduced in a horizontal fashion.

Buttressing Bone Formation

Bone formation sometimes occurs in an attempt to buttress bony trabeculae that are weakened by resorption. When this

Fig. 23.9 (A) Lower incisor with thin labial bone. Bone loss can become vertical only when it reaches thicker bone in apical areas. (B) Upper molars with thin facial bone, where only horizontal bone loss can occur. (C) Upper molar with a thick facial bone that allows for vertical bone loss.

Fig. 23.10 Occlusal (A) and palatal (B) views of exostosis on the first and second molars.

Fig. 23.11 Lipping of Facial Bone. There is a peripheral buttressing bone formation along the external surface of the facial bony plate and at the crest. Note the deformity in the bone produced by the buttressing bone formation and the bulging of the mucosa.

occurs within the jaw, it is termed *central buttressing bone formation.* When it occurs on the external surface, it is referred to as *peripheral buttressing bone formation.*[13] The latter may cause bulging of the bone contour, which sometimes accompanies the production of osseous craters and angular defects (Fig. 23.11).

Food Impaction

Interdental bone defects often occur where the proximal contact is light or absent. Physical pressure and the additional collection of bacteria from food impaction contribute to interproximal resorption and the development of reverse bone architecture. In some cases, the poor proximal relationship may result from a shift in tooth position as a result of extensive bone destruction that precedes food impaction. In patients with this condition, food impaction is a complicating factor rather than the cause of the bone defect.

Rapid Localized Periodontitis[b]

Rapid localized periodontitis usually results in attachment and bone loss around incisors and first molars, particularly in cases where the disease is observed in teenagers. Although such bone loss is usually horizontal in nature around incisors, a vertical or angular pattern of alveolar bone destruction is found around the first molars in aggressive periodontitis. The cause of the

[b]Formerly termed *aggressive localized periodontitis* and historically called *periodontosis.*

localized bone destruction associated with this type of periodontal disease is unknown (see Chapter 26).

BONE DESTRUCTION PATTERNS IN PERIODONTAL DISEASE

Periodontal disease alters the morphologic features of the bone in addition to reducing bone height. An understanding of the nature and pathogenesis of these alterations is essential for effective diagnosis and treatment.[45]

Horizontal Bone Loss

Horizontal bone loss is the most common pattern of bone loss in periodontal disease (Fig. 23.12A and B). The bone is reduced in height, but the bone margin remains approximately perpendicular to the tooth surface. The interdental septa and the facial and lingual plates are affected but not necessarily to an equal degree around the same tooth.

Vertical or Angular Defects

Different types of bone deformities can result from periodontal disease. These usually occur in adults, but they have also been reported in human skulls with deciduous dentitions.[24] Their presence may be suggested on radiographs, but careful probing and surgical exposure of the areas are required to determine their exact conformation and dimensions.

Vertical or angular defects are those that occur in an oblique direction, leaving a hollowed-out trough in the bone alongside the root; the base of the defect is located apical to the surrounding bone (Figs. 23.13A and B and 23.14). In most instances,

Fig. 23.12 Horizontal bone loss in the anterior (A) and posterior (B) areas. Notice the increased distance between the marginal bone and the cementoenamel junction; yet the overall bone contour is scalloped, indicating that bone resorption has affected the buccal and interproximal surfaces to a similar degree.

angular defects have accompanying infrabony periodontal pockets; infrabony pockets, on the other hand, must always have an underlying angular defect.

Goldman and Cohen classified angular defects on the basis of the number of osseous walls.[16] Angular defects may have one, two, or three walls (Figs. 23.15 and 23.16). Continuous defects that involved more than one surface of a tooth, in a shape that is similar to a trough, are called *circumferential defects* (Fig. 23.17). The number of walls in the apical portion of the defect is often greater than that in its occlusal portion, in which case the term *combined osseous defect* is used (Fig. 23.18).

Vertical defects that occur interdentally can generally be seen on the radiograph, although thick, bony plates may sometimes obscure them. Angular defects can also appear on facial and lingual or palatal surfaces, but these defects are more difficult to visualize on radiographs. Surgical exposure is the only sure way to determine the presence and configuration of vertical osseous defects.

Vertical defects increase with age.[40,44,64] Approximately 60% of people with interdental angular defects have only a single defect.[40] Vertical defects detected radiographically have been reported to appear most often on the distal[40] and mesial surfaces.[44] However, three-wall defects are more frequently found on the mesial surfaces of the upper and lower molars.[25]

> The localized angular bone loss in aggressive periodontitis is usually located around the first molars and the incisors. These osseous lesions may be present in teenagers.

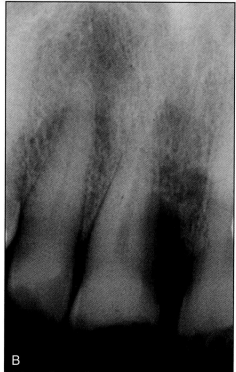

Fig. 23.13 Clinical (A) and radiographic (B) views of a vertical (angular) defect mesial of the upper right central incisor. Note the periodontal probe in a more apical position than the surrounding walls of the bony defect.

Fig. 23.14 Vertical (Angular) Defects Mesial of the First and Second Molars.

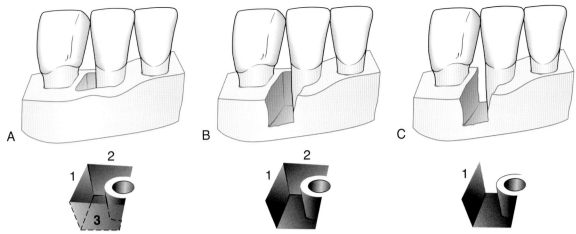

Fig. 23.15 Diagrammatic Representation of One-, Two-, and Three-Walled Vertical Defects on the Right Lateral Incisor. (A) Three bony walls: distal *(1)*, lingual *(2)*, and facial *(3)*. (B) Two-wall defect: distal *(1)* and lingual *(2)*. (C) One-wall defect: distal wall only *(1)*.

Fig. 23.16 Clinical examples of a three-wall defect mesial of the first bicuspid (A), two-wall defect mesial of the lower canine (buccal wall is missing) (B), and one-wall defect mesial of the first molar (buccal and lingual walls are missing) (C).

Fig. 23.17 Circumferential (Troughlike) Defect on the Buccal and Distal Aspects of the First Molar. Notice that the defect extends into the buccal furcation.

Fig. 23.18 Combined Type of Osseous Defect. Because the facial wall is half the height of the distal *(1)* and lingual *(2)* walls, this is an osseous defect with three walls in its apical half and two walls in its occlusal half.

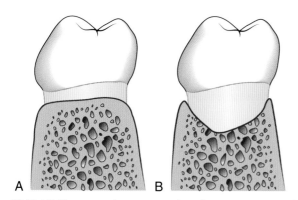

Fig. 23.19 (A) Diagrammatic representation of an osseous crater in a buccolingual section between two lower teeth. *Left,* Normal bone contour. *Right,* Osseous crater. (B) Clinical aspect of an osseous crater between the two bicuspids—notice the buccal and lingual bone walls.

Osseous Craters

Osseous craters are a specific type of two-wall defect; they present as concavities in the crest of the interdental bone that is confined within the facial and lingual walls (Fig. 23.19). Craters have been found to make up about one-third (35.2%) of all defects and about two-thirds (62%) of all mandibular defects; they occur twice as often in posterior segments as in anterior segments.[33,34]

Fig. 23.20 Examples of Positive (Normal) and Negative (Reverse) Osseous Architecture on the Lower Left Posterior Segment. The interproximal bone level in the interdental space between the two bicuspids is more coronal than on the buccal aspect of both teeth, whereas the interproximal bone level in the interdental space between the second bicuspid and the first molar shows the bone level to be apical to the buccal bone.

The heights of the facial and lingual crests of a crater have been found to be identical in 85% of cases, with the remaining 15% being almost equally divided between higher facial crests and higher lingual crests.[49]

The following reasons for the high frequency of interdental craters have been suggested[33,34,49]:

- The interdental area collects biofilm and is difficult to clean.
- The normal flat or even slightly concave buccolingual shape of the interdental septum in the lower molars may favor crater formation.
- Vascular patterns from the gingiva to the center of the crest may provide a pathway for inflammation.

Bulbous Bone Contours

Bulbous bone contours are bony enlargements that are caused by exostoses (see Fig. 23.10), adaptation to function, or buttressing bone formation. They are found more frequently in the maxilla than in the mandible.

Reversed Architecture

Reverse (or negative) alveolar bone architecture is the result of a loss of interdental bone, without a concomitant loss of radicular (buccal or lingual/palatal) bone, thereby reversing the normal (or positive) architecture (Fig. 23.20). Negative architecture is more common in the maxilla of patients with periodontitis.[40]

Ledges

Ledges are plateau-like bone margins that are caused by the resorption of thickened bony plates (Fig. 23.21).

Fig. 23.21 Example of Bone Ledge on the Lingual Aspect of the Bicuspid and Molar.

A

B

Fig. 23.22 Grade II Furcation on the Buccal Aspect of the Lower First Molar. (A) Periodontal probe in place showing a 5-mm pocket. (B) After the flap was elevated, it revealed horizontal bone loss.

Furcation Involvement

The term *furcation involvement* refers to the invasion of the bifurcation and trifurcation of multirooted teeth by periodontitis. The prevalence of furcation-involved molars is not clear.[8,44] Although some reports indicate that the mandibular first molars are the most common sites and that the maxillary premolars are the least common,[26] other studies have found a higher prevalence in the upper molars.[64] The number of furcation involvements increases with age.[26,27]

The denuded furcation may be visible clinically or covered by the wall of the pocket. The extent of the involvement is determined by exploration with a periodontal or Nabers probe (Fig. 23.22A and B).

Furcation involvements have been classified as grades I through IV according to the amount of tissue destruction. Grade I involves incipient bone loss; grade II involves partial bone loss (cul-de-sac); and grade III involves total bone loss with a through-and-through opening of the furcation, but the opening of the furcation is not visible due to the gingiva, which covers the orifice. Grade IV is similar to grade III but includes gingival recession that exposes the furcation to view.

Microscopically, furcation involvement presents no unique pathologic features. It is simply the apical extension of the periodontal pocket along a multirooted tooth. During its early stages, widening of the periodontal space occurs with cellular and fluid inflammatory exudation, and this is followed by epithelial proliferation into the furcation area from an adjoining periodontal pocket. Extension of the inflammation into the bone leads to resorption and a reduction in bone height. The bone-destructive pattern may produce horizontal loss, but angular osseous defects associated with intrabony pockets may also exist (Fig. 23.23). Biofilm, calculus, and bacterial debris occupy the denuded furcation space.

The destructive pattern of a furcation involvement varies in different cases and with the degree of involvement. Bone loss

Fig. 23.23 Different Degrees of Furcation Involvement in a Human Autopsy Specimen. Furcation involvement is found in all three molars, with an advanced lesion in the second molar and an extremely severe lesion in the first molar that is combined with the exposure of the entire mesial root.

Fig. 23.24 Clinical examples of grade I furcation involvement (A) and grade II furcation involvement (B).

around each individual root may be horizontal or angular, and frequently a crater develops in the interradicular area (Fig. 23.24A and B). Probing to determine the presence of these destructive patterns must be done horizontally and vertically around each involved root and in the crater area to establish the depth of the vertical component.

Furcation involvement is a stage of progressive periodontal disease, and it has its same etiology. The difficulty and sometimes the impossibility[2,3] of controlling biofilm in furcations are responsible for the presence of extensive lesions in this area.[62]

The role of trauma from occlusion in the etiology of furcation lesions is controversial. Some assign a key role to trauma, thinking that furcation areas are most sensitive to injury from excessive occlusal forces.[14] Others deny the initiating effect of trauma and consider that inflammation and edema caused by biofilm in the furcation area tend to extrude the tooth, which then becomes traumatized and sensitive.[56,62]

Other factors that may play a role are the presence of enamel projections into the furcation,[35] which occurs in about 13% of multirooted teeth, and the proximity of the furcation to the cementoenamel junction, which occurs in about 75% of cases of furcation involvement.[27]

The presence of accessory pulpal canals in the furcation area may extend pulpal inflammation to the furcation.[19] This possibility should be carefully explored, particularly when mesial and distal bone retains its normal height. Accessory canals that connect the pulp chamber floor to the furcation have been found in 36% of maxillary first molars, 12% of maxillary second molars, 32% of mandibular first molars, and 24% of mandibular second molars.[58]

The diagnosis of furcation involvement is made by clinical examination and careful probing with a specially designed probe (see Chapter 30). Radiographic examination of the area is helpful, but lesions can be obscured by the angulation of the beam and the radiopacity of neighboring structures (see Chapter 31).

For more detailed clinical considerations involved with the diagnosis and treatment of furcation involvement, see Chapters 30 and 31.

CONCLUSION

The understanding of the anatomy, histology, and pattern of bone loss for the diagnosis of and prognosis for periodontal disease is of major importance in determining the therapy that must be rendered. In the final analysis, it is the loss of bone that will determine the retention, maintenance, or loss of the dentition in periodontal disease.

A Case Scenario is found on the companion website.

REFERENCES

 References for this chapter are found on the companion website.

Masticatory System Disorders That Influence the Periodontium[a]

The ability to understand the anatomy and function of the masticatory system and to interpret relevant diagnostic information correctly is a prerequisite to fulfilling comprehensive standards of care.

The masticatory system consists of the:

- temporomandibular joints (TMJs)
- the masticatory muscles
- the teeth in occlusion
- the neurologic and vascular supplies that support all of these structures

Research suggests that masticatory system disorders include many varied conditions with multiple possible contributing factors rather than different manifestations of a single disease or syndrome.[1,34,42]

TEMPOROMANDIBULAR JOINT

Harmonious function of the TMJs results from the coordination of the muscles of mastication by intricate mechanisms of neurologic control. Understanding the dynamics and the relationship of the TMJ to the associated muscles and nerves provides the working knowledge required for effective assessment and diagnosis.

The TMJ is one of the most complex joints in the human body. It is capable of providing both hinging (rotation) and gliding (translation) movements, and it is able to resist incredible forces of mastication. The TMJ is formed by the head of the condyle of the mandible as it fits into the articular fossa of the temporal bone (Fig. 24.1). The body of the mandible effectively connects both condyles so that neither condyle functions independently of the other. Interposed between the head of the condyle and the articular surface of the temporal bone is the articular disc, which consists of dense connective tissue; this results in a compound joint with two joint cavities (Fig. 24.2). The articulating surfaces of the osseous structures are essentially convex in a healthy situation; hence the biconcave configuration of the articular disc compensates for the opposing convexities. The articular surfaces

of the condyles and the temporal bones consist of fibrous connective tissue, which renders them resistant to breakdown and capable of repair. Deep to the superficial connective tissue layer, articular cartilage provides the cellular and structural basis for the response to the functional loading and movement of the TMJs.[34,45,68] The discal ligaments and attachments to the capsule, along with the disc itself, become the means of separating the joint into superior and inferior joint spaces (see Figs. 24.1 and 24.2). Synovial lubrication of the articular surfaces is a function of the production of synovial fluid by endothelial cells along the borders of each joint cavity and at the anterior extent of the retrodiscal tissues.[22,23,34,45,64,65]

MUSCLES AND NERVES OF THE MASTICATORY SYSTEM

The muscles and nerves of the masticatory system are extensively reviewed elsewhere.

CENTRIC RELATION

The mandible is suspended from the cranial base by ligaments and muscles. The understanding of mandibular movement begins with an initial reference point for each condyle, which is usually referred to as *centric relation;* this clinically determined relationship of the mandible to the maxilla occurs when both condyle-disc assemblies are in their most superior position in the maxillary (or glenoid) fossa and against the slope of the articular eminence of the temporal bone.

An individual's susceptibility to masticatory system disorders determines whether that person adapts with minimal consequence or develops dysfunction or degeneration.[15,22,23,45,60]

DYSFUNCTION AND DETERIORATION

The general terms for occlusal parafunction used in this text include *bruxism,* which is the grinding of the teeth, and *clenching,* which is when a person holds the teeth firmly together with significant force. Bruxism is usually confirmed by the observation of excessive tooth wear. The clenching type of parafunction can

---

[a]Adapted from the following chapter of *Newman and Carranza's Clinical Periodontology,* 13th edition: Chapter 26: Masticatory System Disorders That Influence the Periodontium, by Michael J. McDevitt.

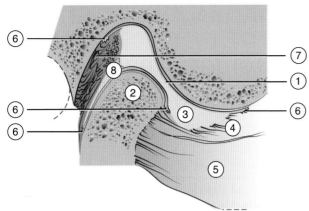

Fig. 24.1 Lateral View of a Cross-Section Through the Temporomandibular Joint. *(1)*, Posterior slope of the articular eminence of the temporal bone; *(2)*, head of the condyle; *(3)*, articular disc (note the biconcave shape); *(4)*, superior lateral pterygoid muscle (note the attachment to both the head of the condyle and the articular disc); *(5)*, inferior lateral pterygoid muscle; *(6)*, synovial tissue; *(7)*, retrodiscal tissue; and *(8)*, discal ligament attachment to the posterior surface of the head of the condyle. (Modified from Dawson PE: *Evaluation, diagnosis, and treatment of occlusal problems*, ed 2, St. Louis, 1989, Mosby.)

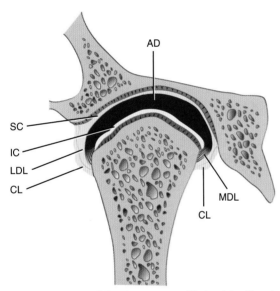

Fig. 24.2 Anterior View of the Temporomandibular Joint Showing the Collateral Ligaments. *AD*, Articular disc; *CL*, capsular ligament; *IC*, inferior joint cavity; *LDL*, lateral discal ligament; *MDL*, medial discal ligament; *SC*, superior joint cavity. (From Okeson JP: *Management of temporomandibular joint disorders and occlusion*, ed 4, St. Louis, 1998, Mosby.)

be distinguished from the grinding of the teeth, and it appears to be more often associated with masticatory system disorders than does bruxism.[18,28,29,33,47,49] Sleep bruxism may include both tooth grinding and clenching, and it appears to occur primarily during Stage 1 and Stage 2 (i.e., non–rapid eye movement) sleep. These episodes often occur in association with short brain and cardiac reactivations called "microarousals." Rhythmic masticatory muscle activity is relatively common among nonbruxers, but the frequency and intensity of the muscle contraction is substantially greater for the sleep bruxer. The central pattern generator of the primate brain stem does not modulate or reduce

BOX 24.1   Differential Diagnosis of Orofacial Pain

Intracranial Pain Disorders[31,32,34,40,44,48]
Neoplasm, aneurysm, abscess, hemorrhage, hematoma, and edema

Primary Headache Disorders (Neurovascular Disorders)[36,41]
Migraine, migraine variants, cluster headache, paroxysmal hemicrania, cranial arteritis, carotidynia, and tension-type headache[2,37,38,45]

Neurogenic Pain Disorders[40,41]
Paroxysmal neuralgias: Trigeminal, glossopharyngeal, nervus intermedius, and superior laryngeal neuralgias[57]
   Continuous pain disorders: Deafferentation pain syndromes (peripheral neuritis, postherpetic neuritis, posttraumatic and postsurgical neuralgia, and neuralgia-inducing cavitational osteonecrosis[9,10])
   Sympathetically maintained pain[12]

Intraoral Pain Disorders
Dental pulp, periodontium, mucogingival tissues, and tongue[7,39,40,67]

Temporomandibular Disorders
Masticatory muscle, temporomandibular joint, and associated structures

Associated Structures[19,20,43,44,45]
Ears, eyes, nose, paranasal sinuses, throat, lymph nodes, salivary glands, and neck

Axis II Mental Disorders
Somatoform disorders
   Pain syndromes of psychogenic origin
   Compiled by the American Academy of Orofacial Pain.

muscle contraction during sleep as it does during waking hours. In addition, the amplification of oral parafunction has been reported in association with a patient's intake of selective serotonin reuptake inhibitors (e.g., Prozac).[5,22,23,45,50,61]

OROFACIAL PAIN

Discomfort associated with masticatory system disorders falls under the larger umbrella of orofacial pain. Pain associated with TMJ dysfunction is most frequently muscular in origin,[22] and it may be amplified by both occlusal parafunction and stress.[30] Although pain itself is a complex entity,[59] a working knowledge of even the uncommon sources of pain perceived in the region of the masticatory system is essential to providing comprehensive diagnosis and treatment.

Sources of dental or periodontal pain should be identified by clinical, radiographic, and historic information. Nondental sources of pain include TMJ structures, muscles, cervical structures, neuropathies, vascular inflammation, all types of headache, sleep disorders, systemic disorders, and psychoimmune neurologic sources.[44] A survey of 45,700 American households revealed that 22% of respondents had experienced some type of orofacial pain during the previous 6 months, thereby establishing a meaningful probability that the periodontal patient's list of symptoms includes pain.[4]

Box 24.1 provides the current list of possible sources of orofacial pain. This list was prepared by the American Academy of Orofacial Pain.[44]

Headache is perceived primarily within the trigeminal nerve pathways, although other cranial and cervical nerves may offer painful sensory input.[34,44,55] Pain that originates in masticatory system structures, which are also innervated by the trigeminal nerve, requires diagnostic differentiation from headache.[56] Headache can present in myriad forms, and it can influence the perception of pain and the diagnosis of the origin of pain.[33,44]

Pain of dental and periodontal origin must be clearly defined and differentiated from heart attack, sinus pain, and myofascial pain.[44,45] Pain that originates in pulpal or periodontal nociceptors can be differentiated with a comprehensive clinical and radiographic evaluation. Orofacial pain that originates in the TMJs or the muscles of mastication can result from neoplasm, macrotrauma, repeated microtrauma, systemic disease, and anatomic predisposition.

Occlusal parafunction, extended dental appointments, metabolic imbalances, and sympathetic nervous system influences have been associated with this painful muscular reaction. An extended period of a limited range of mandibular movement can result in fibrosis of the muscle and related attachments, thereby creating a painless condition called myofibrotic contracture.[44] Chronic myofascial pain temporomandibular disorder (TMD) patients may actually experience significantly greater background masseter muscle activity as a primary basis for their pain rather than sleep bruxism being the dominant influence.[51] Another study suggests that daytime clenching is more likely the primary reason for myofascial pain rather than rhythmic masticatory muscle activity during sleep even when it is in conjunction with sleep bruxism.[54]

Otolaryngologic symptoms associated with masticatory system disorders have been reported and include degrees of deafness, tinnitus, and vertigo.[8,13,16,17, 19,20, 27,35,43,45,46,52,53,66] Trauma and postural stress in the cervical spine can be responsible for both the perception and the origin of pain within the masticatory system.[6,11,34,45]

Sleep-disordered breathing may also play a role in a patient's orofacial pain through various potential mechanisms.[3] Sleep bruxism has been associated with hypoxia and arousals during sleep disruption.[14,25,62,63] Pain tolerance appears to be diminished with sleep deprivation.[58] Oral appliances that have been prescribed for sleep-disordered breathing have the potential to cause at least transient symptoms of temporomandibular disorders as a result of the mandibular advancement that needs to be experienced for them to be effective.[21,24] Oral appliances prescribed for sleep bruxism may represent an additional airway obstruction for the patient with obstructive sleep apnea.[26]

ACKNOWLEDGMENTS

I would like to acknowledge the encouragement and the recommendation of references provided by Dr. Henry Gremillion during the revision of this chapter.

A Case Scenario is found on the companion website.

REFERENCES

 References for this chapter are found on the companion website.

Chronic Periodontitis[a,b]

CHAPTER OUTLINE

Chronic periodontitis is the most prevalent form of periodontitis, and it generally shows the characteristics of a slowly progressing inflammatory disease. Periodontitis belongs to the group of complex inflammatory diseases in humans. In this context, the word *complex* not only describes the fact that there are multiple clinical symptoms that account for the disease but also explains the multiple factors that lead to and influence periodontal inflammation. Chronic periodontitis occurs most frequently in adults. Nonetheless, it may also be diagnosed in children and adolescents when associated with chronic plaque and calculus accumulation. Therefore chronic periodontitis should be understood as age-associated, but not age-dependent, complex chronic inflammation of the periodontal tissues. As described in this chapter, systemic or environmental factors (e.g., diabetes mellitus, smoking) modify the host immune response to the dental biofilm so that the periodontal destruction becomes more progressive. The current classification system suggests that when systemic disease is associated, the ICD[c] code should be used to classify the patients.

Periodontitis is a highly prevalent progressing disease, and it affects approximately 10.5% to 12% of the world's population.[45] Periodontitis has been found to exert adverse effects on systemic health, and in this context, important pathologic interdependencies with, for example, diabetes mellitus have been identified.[10,33,56,74] Also, it is known that systemic inflammatory markers, such as the C-reactive protein (CRP), are elevated in patients with periodontitis.[70,97] In general, chronic periodontitis is considered as a slowly progressing disease, but in the presence of severe systemic conditions or environmental factors, such as smoking, this inflammatory disease progresses more rapidly.

The classic definition described chronic periodontitis as "an infectious disease resulting in inflammation within the supporting tissues of the teeth, progressive attachment loss, and bone loss."[25] The etiopathologic factors that lead to periodontal inflammation and, subsequently, destruction of periodontal tissues have been widely studied, and the interplay between the microbial environment and the individual host immune response has gained attention in the scientific community (discussed later).

Chronic periodontitis represents major clinical and etiologic characteristics such as (1) microbial biofilm formation (dental plaque), (2) periodontal inflammation (gingival swelling, bleeding on probing), and (3) attachment as well as alveolar bone loss.

Besides the local immune response to the dental biofilm, periodontitis may also be associated with a number of systemic disorders and defined syndromes. In most cases, patients with systemic diseases, which lead to impaired host immunity, may also show periodontal destruction. On the other hand, periodontitis is not only limited to the area of the oral cavity but may be associated with severe systemic diseases such as cardiovascular disease, stroke, and diabetes mellitus.[53,71,74,80]

This chapter discusses clinical features that have been described for chronic periodontitis, based on the consensus of the 1999 World Workshop in Periodontics and classified by the 2018 classification sytsem.[9] In addition, the etiology is summarized in categories explaining the known factors (microbiologic, immunologic, genetic, and environmental) involved in the pathology of chronic periodontitis.

CLINICAL FEATURES

General Characteristics

Characteristic clinical findings in patients with untreated chronic periodontitis include the following symptoms (see the case presentation in Figs. 25.1 to 25.6):
- Supragingival and subgingival plaque (and calculus)
- Gingival swelling, redness, and loss of gingival stippling

---

[a]Adapted from the following chapter of *Newman and Carranza's Clinical Periodontology*, 13th edition: Chapter 27: Chronic Periodontitis, by Henrik Dommisch and Moritz Kebschull.

[b]Editorial note:
As we look into the future to anticipate what the role of dental hygienist will be, I think it is essential for them to have direct access at the point of care, in all sorts of practice/treatment environments. It is important to know the immunologic and microbiologic basis of disease, just as it is important to understand the role of genetics. The profession is required to have a "body of evidence" to support their clinical work. The current ADHA strategic plan calls for dental hygienists to "diagnose" and "treat." This book and chapters like this one give them the background to begin to do so.

[c]International Classification of Diseases and Related Health Codes (ICD).

Fig. 25.1 Clinical Features of Generalized Chronic Periodontitis in a 49-Year-Old, Medically Healthy Male Patient Who Presented to the Clinic for the First Time. The patient reported smoking 15 cigarettes per day. Note the abundant dental plaque and calculus deposits, gingival redness and swelling, and alteration of the gingival texture (loss of gingival stippling). The patient noticed multiple recessions. In this case, recessions were the result from loss of clinical attachment and alveolar bone. (A) Right lateral view. (B) Frontal view. (C) Left lateral view. (D) Maxillary view. (E) Mandibular view. (Reprinted from Kebschull M, Dommisch H: Resektive parodontalchirurgie, *Zahnmedizin up-2-date* 525–545, 2012.)

Fig. 25.2 Collage of the Radiographic Periodontal Status (a Total of 11 X-Rays) at the Time of Diagnosis (Compare Figs. 25.1 and 25.3). Generalized horizontal and localized angular, vertical bone loss on the mesial and distal sites of molars was noted. Radiographs present deep subgingival restorations (teeth #2 and #19), overhanging margins of restorations (teeth #14 and #15), carious lesion (tooth #14), and insufficient root canal treatment (tooth #18). (Reprinted from Kebschull M, Dommisch H: Resektive parodontalchirurgie, *Zahnmedizin up-2-date*, 525–545, 2012.)

Fig. 25.3 Documentation of the Periodontal Attachment Level in the Same Patient (See Fig. 25.1) at the Time of the First Visit. The *red line* displays the gingival margin reflecting recessions. Clinical attachment loss is illustrated by the filled *(blue)* area on the root surfaces. The deepest periodontal pocket measured was 9 mm. Class I *(green)* and class II *(yellow)* furcation involvement were documented. Bleeding upon periodontal probing (gingival inflammation) is reflected by *orange dots*. Due to the history of smoking, the bleeding on probing score was relatively low, although the patient presented advanced attachment loss. Tooth mobility is indicated by the *green line* (tooth #19). The *red boxes* indicate probing depths 5 mm or greater. (Reprinted from Kebschull M, Dommisch H: *Resektive parodontalchirurgie, Zahnmedizin up-2-date,* 525–545, 2012.)

Fig. 25.4 Subsequent to the Antiinfective Therapy and Periodontal Reevaluation, Resective Peri-odontal Surgery Was Performed in the Patient Introduced in Figs. 25.1 to 25.3. Surgical method: apically repositioned flap. (A) Intrasulcular incision at buccal sites; notice class I furcation involvement on tooth #14. (B) Paramarginal incision at palatal sites, excision of a distal wedge. (C–D) Sutured using 5-0 Prolene, buccal and palatal view, respectively. (E) Occlusal view after suturing. (F) Occlusal view 1 week post surgery. Tooth #14 received endodontic therapy and crown restoration prior to periodontal surgery. (Reprinted from Kebschull M, Dommisch H: Resektive parodontalchirurgie, *Zahnmedizin up-2-date*, 525–545, 2012.)

- Altered gingival margins (rolled, flattened, cratered papillae, recessions)
- Pocket formation
- Bleeding on probing
- Attachment loss
- Bone loss (angular/vertical or horizontal)
- Root furcation involvement
- Increased tooth mobility

- Change in tooth position
- Tooth loss

Chronic periodontitis can be clinically revealed by means of periodontal screening and recording (PSR), diagnosed by an assessment of the clinical attachment level and the detection of inflammatory changes in the marginal gingiva (see Fig. 25.1). Measurements of periodontal probing pocket depth in combination with the location of the marginal gingiva allow conclusions

Fig. 25.5 Subsequent to the Antiinfective Therapy and Periodontal Reevaluation, Resective Periodontal Surgery Was Performed in the Patient Introduced in Figs. 25.1 to 25.4. Surgical method: apically repositioned flap. (A) Intrasulcular incision at buccal sites; notice class I furcation involvement on tooth #19 and horizontal bone loss in teeth #18 to #20. (B) Sutured using 5-0 Prolene, buccal view. (Reprinted from Kebschull M, Dommisch H: Resektive parodontalchirurgie, *Zahnmedizin up-2-date*, 525–545, 2012.)

regarding the loss of clinical attachment (see Figs. 25.3 and 25.6). Dental radiographs reveal the extent of bone loss indicated by the distance between the cemento-enamel junction and the alveolar bone crest (see Fig. 25.2).

The distinction between aggressive and chronic periodontitis, and the ability to assign a Grade under the current classification system, is sometimes difficult, because the clinical features may be similar at the time of the first examination. At later time points during treatment, aggressive and chronic periodontitis may be differentiated by the rate of disease progression over time, the familial nature of aggressive disease, and the presence of local as well as systemic factors.

Disease Distribution

Chronic periodontitis exhibits a site-specific clinical picture, where attachment and bone loss are not equally distributed throughout the dentition as well as around teeth. Local inflammation, pocket formation, attachment loss, and bone loss are the sequelae of the direct exposure to the subgingival plaque (dental biofilm) and local inflammatory responses. Periodontal pocket formation, attachment, and bone loss may develop on one or more sites of a tooth, while other sites remain at a physiologic attachment level. Due to the site-specific nature and based

on the number of teeth with clinical attachment loss, chronic periodontitis can be classified into the following categories:

- *Localized chronic periodontitis*, meaning that less than 30% of the teeth show attachment and bone loss
- *Generalized chronic periodontitis*, meaning that 30% or more of the teeth show attachment and bone loss
- *Molar-incisor*, as discussed in Chapter 6

During chronic periodontitis, the local inflammatory response may lead to different patterns of bone loss, including vertical (angular) and horizontal bone destruction. Although vertical bone loss is associated with intrabony pocket formation, horizontal bone loss is usually associated with suprabony (supraalveolar) pockets.

Key Differences Between Gingivitis and Chronic Periodontitis

Plaque-Induced Gingivitis	Chronic Periodontitis
Inflammation of the gingiva without attachment/bone loss.	Inflammation of periodontal apparatus with attachment/bone loss.
With optimal oral hygiene, this condition can be resolved completely (reversible).	The attachment loss is irreversible, in spite of successfully controlling the inflammation.
Not all sites with gingivitis progress to periodontitis	All patients with chronic periodontitis must have experienced prior gingivitis
The dental implant counterpart of gingivitis is peri-implant mucositis.	The dental implant counterpart of periodontitis is peri-implantitis.

Disease Severity

With chronic periodontitis, severity and extent of periodontal destruction will occur over time in combination with systemic disorders impairing or enhancing host immune responses. Patients with chronic periodontitis experience a progression in attachment and bone loss as they become older. If untreated, and oral hygiene behaviors remain unchanged, initial chronic periodontitis eventually leads to tooth loss and may negatively impact distant organs by the uncontrolled progression of periodontal inflammation and by the systemic spread of infection. Relative to the degree of attachment and bone loss, disease severity can be described in four stages as initial (Stage I), moderate (Stage II), severe with potential for further tooth loss (Stage III), and severe with potential for loss of dentition (Stage IV). These degrees are defined as follows:

- *Mild chronic periodontitis:* clinical attachment loss of 1 to 2 mm
- *Moderate chronic periodontitis:* clinical attachment loss of 3 to 4 mm
- *Severe chronic periodontitis:* clinical attachment loss of 5 mm or more

Symptoms

Chronic periodontitis is commonly a slowly progressing complex disease without a pain experience. Most patients are unaware

Fig. 25.6 Documentation of the Periodontal Attachment Level in the Same Patient (See Figs. 25.1 to 25.5) After Active Periodontal Therapy Was Completed and the Supportive Periodontal Therapy Was Initiated. *Green dots* denote furcation involvement and white boxes indicate probing depths 3 mm or less, while, 4 mm probing depths are indicated in *orange boxes*. The *red line* displays the gingival margin reflecting recessions after therapy. Clinical attachment loss is illustrated by the filled *(blue)* area on the root surfaces. The deepest periodontal pocket measured was 4 mm. (Reprinted from Kebschull M, Dommisch H: Resektive parodontalchirurgie, *Zahnmedizin up-2-date* 525–5, 2012.)

that they have developed a chronic disease. For the majority of patients, gingival bleeding during oral hygiene procedures or eating may be the first sign of disease occurrence. Areas with advanced periodontal inflammation may present with purulence emanating from the periodontal pocket. As a result of gingival

recession, patients may notice black triangles between teeth or tooth sensitivity in response to temperature changes (cold and heat). In addition, food impaction may occur in the space of interdental triangles, leading to increased discomfort and bad breath. In cases with advanced attachment and bone loss, tooth mobility, tooth movement, fanned out or elongated front teeth, and on rare occasion tooth loss may be reported. In cases with advanced disease progression, areas of localized dull pain or pain sensations radiating to other areas of the mouth or head may occur.

KEY FACT

Site Specificity of Chronic Periodontitis
Not all sites in the mouth are equally prone to chronic periodontitis, and it exhibits site specificity. The progression of the disease occurs in certain sites but not uniformly. Interproximal sites, in general, are more prone to periodontal destruction, compared to buccal/facial sites.

Disease Progression

Chronic periodontitis may develop at any time in life. First clinical signs of inflammation may occur even during adolescence when the oral hygiene is neglected and dental plaque and calculus were allowed to accumulate. In general, the progression rate of chronic periodontitis is slow, so that symptoms of the disease appear around the age of 40 or later in life. Onset and the rate of disease progression, however, may be influenced by a number of modifiable (e.g., smoking, diet) and nonmodifiable (e.g., genetic disorders and risk issues) factors. In this context, patients who develop a metabolic disorder, such as diabetes mellitus, may exhibit a much higher progression rate of chronic periodontitis along with increased alveolar bone loss, periodontal bleeding, and pocketing.[74,96,101] Thus diabetes mellitus and the degree of blood sugar control belong to the most important systemic factors that are directly correlated with periodontal disease.

The progression pattern of chronic periodontitis does not show equal degrees of attachment loss on each affected site over time. Although some sites exhibit more rapid periodontal breakdown over time, the attachment level remains static at other sites in the dentition for longer time periods.[59] Interestingly, disease progression is more rapid at interproximal sites compared to oral or buccal areas of neighboring teeth.[57,60] This phenomenon may be explained by the fact that these interproximal areas become wider along with disease progression, recession development, and the related increased probability of plaque accumulation and food impaction in those areas. Plaque control becomes more difficult, and interproximal furcation areas, interproximal caries, root caries, overhanging restoration margins, and tooth crowding may further promote interproximal attachment loss.

As chronic periodontitis exhibits individual and heterogeneous progression patterns throughout the dentition, three different models have been proposed to describe the rate of disease progression and determine the degree of attachment loss over time[18] as follows[93]:

- The continuous model:
  - Describes slow and continuous disease progression
  - Suggests that sites exhibit a constant progression rate of attachment loss throughout the duration of the disease
- The random or episodic-burst model:
  - Describes the episodic occurrence of short progressive bursts of periodontal destruction followed by periods of stagnation

- Sites, teeth, and the chronology of bursts and stagnation are subject to random effects
- The asynchronous, multiple-burst model:
  - Describes the occurrence of periodontal destruction (bursts) during defined periods, which are asynchronously interrupted by periods of stagnation or remission for individual sites and teeth

Prevalence

Chronic periodontitis is considered to be one of the most common chronic diseases in humans, and the prevalence of the disease increases with age equally in both genders. In general, 40% of patients aged 50 years or older and almost 50% of patients aged 65 years or older show signs of mild-to-moderate periodontal destruction. The prevalence of severe forms of periodontitis also increases with age. From 11% to 30% of patients develop severe periodontitis at the age of 40 years or older (Figs. 25.7 and 25.8).[15,23,29,40,95] The worldwide prevalence for severe chronic periodontitis is estimated at 10.5% to 12% of the world's population.[45]

RISK FACTORS FOR DISEASE

A number of factors influence the etiopathogenesis of chronic periodontitis. The composition of the oral microflora and the amount of dental biofilm (plaque) are major etiologic factors. In this context, the extent of the periodontal destruction depends on the host immune competence as well as genetic predispositions influencing the individual susceptibility to disease. In addition, both systemic diseases and environmental factors interfere with the development and progression of chronic periodontitis. The risk factors described in the following sections (microbiological, local, systemic, immunologic, genetic, environmental, and behavioral) may occur simultaneously, or a selection of factors is present in patients with chronic periodontitis. The degree of the individual risk factor contribution differs among patients, so it is worthwhile not only to identify the risk factors but also to specify the degree of contribution of each risk factor.

The prior history of gingivitis and periodontitis should be considered as general predictors for the development or progression of chronic periodontitis.[57] It is possible that the disease could not be successfully treated in the first place. The reason for an unsuccessful treatment outcome can be as simple as the patient's unwillingness (noncompliant patients) to understand the disease or perform proper oral hygiene. On the other hand, reasons for disease progression can also be more complex when nonmodifiable factors—such as genetic predispositions/syndromes, severe immunologic disorders, other therapies (e.g., organ transplantations) that affect the patient's immune status, lack of dexterity, or other systemic diseases—are present. This highlights the complexity of not only the development but also the progression/reoccurrence of chronic periodontitis. Several risk factors that contribute to the patient's susceptibility to chronic periodontitis are discussed next.

Microbiologic Aspects

Plaque accumulation on tooth and gingival surfaces (dental biofilm formation) at the dentogingival junction is considered

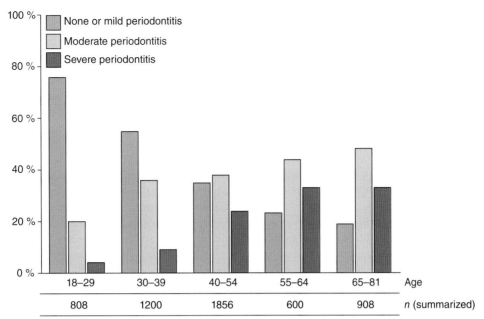

Fig. 25.7 Prevalence for Periodontitis in the United States and Germany (2007–2009). (Data from Genco et al., 2007,[29] and Holtfreter et al., 2009,[40] and reviewed in Demmer & Papapanou, 2010.[15])

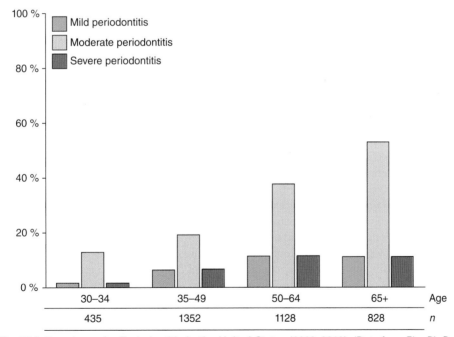

Fig. 25.8 Prevalence for Periodontitis in the United States (2009–2010). (Data from Eke PI, Dye BA, Wei L, et al: Prevalence of periodontitis in adults in the United States: 2009 and 2010, *J Dent Res* 91:914–20, 2012.)

the primary initiating agent in the etiology of gingivitis and chronic periodontitis.[57] As the dental biofilm develops, early signs of an inflammatory reaction occur in the gingival margin (gingivitis) without attachment loss. In general, optimal plaque control leads to the complete resolution of this early gingival inflammation.[63] With neglected oral hygiene, on the other hand, inflammation will progress and eventually result in the loss of attachment

around teeth.[57] Although not all patients with gingivitis develop periodontitis, it is known that all patients with periodontitis experienced prior gingivitis. The occurrence of periodontitis depends on the individual immune response that modifies the onset and progression of the disease.[57,69,71]

Attachment and bone loss are associated with an increase in the proportion of gram-negative organisms in the subgingival biofilm, with specific increases in organisms known to be pathogenic and virulent. *Porphyromonas gingivalis, Tannerella forsythia,* and *Treponema denticola,* otherwise known as the *red complex bacteria,* are frequently associated with ongoing attachment and bone loss in chronic periodontitis.[92] Development and progression of chronic periodontitis may not depend on the presence of one specific bacterium or bacterial complex alone. It is assumed that chronic periodontitis is the sequelae of a multispecies infection with a number of different bacteria that influence the proinflammatory immune response of the host.[47,83] Furthermore, the concept of host–microbial interactions has gained scientific attention. It has been found that increased numbers of periodontal pathogens contribute to the development of a dysbiotic (imbalanced) microbial environment, which is triggered by the inflammatory milieu in the periodontal pocket.[2,37] This concept describes a shift from a symbiotic microbial environment to the development of dysbiosis within the biofilm involving so-called keystone pathogens, such as *P. gingivalis,* as a polymicrobial synergistic effect.[34-36] Periodontal pathogens such as *P. gingivalis* may then invade the periodontal tissue and therewith induce further immune responses with increasing concentrations of proinflammatory mediators that may enhance periodontal breakdown. In addition, a number of periodontal pathogens are capable of producing proteases that directly affect the tissues and host immune responses.[71]

Local Factors

Plaque accumulation and biofilm development are the primary causes of periodontal inflammation and destruction. Therefore factors that facilitate plaque accumulation or prevent plaque removal by oral hygiene procedures can be detrimental to the patient. Plaque-retentive factors are important in the development and progression of chronic periodontitis because they retain microorganisms in proximity to the periodontal tissues, providing an ecologic niche for biofilm maturation. Calculus is considered the most important plaque-retentive factor because of its ability to retain and harbor plaque bacteria on its rough surface as well as inside.[43,90] As a consequence, calculus removal is essential for the maintenance of a healthy periodontium. In addition, the tooth morphology may influence plaque retention. Roots may show grooves or concavities and, in some instances, enamel projections on the surface or furcation entrances. Those morphologic variations may facilitate plaque retention, subgingival calculus formation, and disease progression.[30,41,79] In addition, subgingival and overhanging margins of restorations, carious lesions that extend subgingivally, and furcations exposed by loss of bone promote plaque retention.[51,102]

Common Retentive Local Factors That Contribute to Chronic Periodontitis

- Dental calculus
- Crown margins
- Restoration overhangs
- Furcation involvement
- Deep probing depths
- Anatomic grooves on the roots
- Subgingival caries or resorptive lesions

Systemic Factors

Chronic periodontitis is a complex disease that may not be limited to infection at local sites, but in several instances, periodontitis is also associated with other systemic disorders, such as Haim-Munk syndrome, Papillon-Lefèvre syndrome, Ehlers-Danlos syndrome, Kindler syndrome, and Cohen syndrome. Patients who suffer from diseases that impair host immune responses (e.g., HIV/AIDS) may also show periodontal destruction. Further, it is also known that osteoporosis, severe unbalanced diet, and stress, as well as dermatologic, hematologic, and neoplastic factors, interfere with periodontal inflammatory responses. In addition to defined syndromes, periodontitis is also associated with severe systemic diseases such as diabetes mellitus, cardiovascular disorders, stroke, and lung disorders.[1,10,46,68,71,99,100,103]

Periodontitis is now considered as the sixth most common complication of diabetes mellitus.[28,62] For diabetes mellitus and periodontitis, there is a known interaction during which both diseases mutually correlate to each other.[55] Patients with diabetes mellitus exhibit a higher risk to develop periodontitis, and the periodontal infection/inflammation may negatively interfere with the glycemic control of the diabetic patient.[74] A number of studies showed that prevalence, severity, and prognosis of periodontitis are associated with the incidence of diabetes mellitus. It was found that the average pocket depth as well as the clinical attachment loss was increased in patients with diabetes mellitus (independently from the type of diabetes mellitus).[16,48,74,82] Patients with poor glycemic control tend to experience more severe progression of periodontitis compared with patients with good glycemic control. Regarding the progression of severe periodontitis, no difference was found between patients with good glycemic control and nondiabetic patients.[101] With diabetes mellitus, advanced glycation end products (AGEs) may arise, which lead to the release of free oxygen and proinflammatory mediators (cytokines). AGEs may also promote chemotaxis and adhesion of inflammatory cells to periodontal tissues, and increased apoptosis of fibroblasts and osteoblasts may occur.[32] Furthermore, patients with diabetes mellitus tend to show a higher body mass index, and therefore increased concentrations of adipokines that directly influence inflammatory responses were found.[75] Hyperglycemia per se leads to the release of proinflammatory mediators in the bloodstream, which in turn promote increased glucose concentration.[74] Periodontal therapy may contribute to glycemic control of the diabetic patient. It was shown that the systematic therapy of chronic periodontitis leads to an at least short-term reduction of glycated hemoglobin (HbA1c) of approximately 0.3% up to 0.6%.[7,10,42,58,91] Each therapy regimen that contributes to achieve reduction of glycated hemoglobin may decrease the risk of diabetes-related long-term consequences, such as myocardial infarction, microvascular complications, and many others.[74]

In the context of diabetes mellitus, a number of patients exhibit an increased body weight (obesity), which also correlates with the prevalence and severity of periodontal attachment and bone loss.[67] The negative effect of a high body mass index with regard to the outcome of periodontal therapy was comparable to the negative effect that has been described for smoking.[94]

Immunologic Factors

Chronic periodontitis is a disease induced by bacteria organized in the dental biofilm. Onset, progression, and severity of the disease depend, however, on the individual host immune response.[27,69] Patients may show alterations of peripheral monocytes, which relate to reduced reactivity of lymphocytes or enhanced B-cell response.[69,71] Not only B cells and macrophages, but also periodontal ligament cells, gingival fibroblasts, and epithelial cells synthesize proinflammatory mediators—such as interleukin-1β (IL-1 β), IL-6, IL-8, prostaglandin-E2 (PGE2), tumor-necrosis factor α (TNF-α), and many others—that modify innate and adaptive immune responses at periodontal sites.[12,19-22,49,76]

Proinflammatory mediators regulate synthesis and secretion of matrix-metalloproteinases (MMPs) and receptor-activator-of-NF-κB-ligand (RANKL). In periodontal lesions, MMPs contribute to soft and hard tissue degradation during active inflammatory processes.[27] RANKL binds to its receptor RANK on the cell surface of premature osteoclasts, and therewith it initiates osteoclast differentiation leading to degradation of alveolar bone.[27,49,76] Physiologically, osteoprotegerin (OPG) is an inhibitor of RANKL, and during periodontitis, an imbalance between OPG and RANKL promotes further bone degradation.[27]

In addition, reduced counts in neutrophils (polymorphonuclear neutrophils [PMNs]) influence the degree of periodontal inflammation. Congenital neutropenia (Kostmann syndrome) leads not only to an increased susceptibility to infection in general but also to severe chronic periodontitis. Patients with Kostmann syndrome show reduced levels of antimicrobial peptides, such as the cathelicidin (LL-37) and neutrophil peptides (α defensins), which impair their innate immune response.[8,77] LL-37 is an effective antimicrobial peptide that is synthesized from inactive precursors, and mutations in the cathepsin C gene hinder cleavage, and therewith activation, of LL-37. Those genetic alterations contribute to the severity and progression of chronic periodontitis (Papillon-Lefèvre syndrome, Haim-Munk syndrome).[14,39]

Genetic Factors

Periodontitis is considered to be a complex inflammatory disease influenced by local, systemic, and immunologic factors (discussed earlier). Each factor is, in turn, directly related to individual genetic conditions. Several genetic disorders are known to show periodontal destruction as one of their major symptoms. For example, Papillon-Lefèvre syndrome is a well-known genetic disorder (a defect on chromosome 11) that exhibits not only palmoplantar hyperkeratosis but also severe periodontitis.[24,38,52] Besides Papillon-Lefèvre syndrome, Haim-Munk syndrome, Ehlers-Danlos syndrome, Down syndrome, Kindler syndrome, Cohen syndrome, and congenital neutropenia (Kostmann syndrome) are other genetic disorders that have been related to periodontal disease. These genetic conditions are discussed extensively in Chapter 8.

Periodontal disease has been found in different family members (twins, siblings) and generations of one family. Early twin studies suggested the involvement of genetic susceptibility factors in the etiopathogenesis of periodontitis.[64] In a number of studies, the prevalence of aggressive and chronic periodontitis has been investigated in families with a history of one or more family members with periodontitis. The data from those studies showed variable results with a likelihood for heritability of up to 50%. Variations are mainly due to different study designs as well as the number of evaluated individuals.[3,61,65,84]

Treatment of Chronic Periodontitis

Chronic periodontitis can be treated effectively by a systematic periodontal therapy that includes optimal long-term plaque control, debridement of soft and hard deposits, or surgical pocket reduction (case-dependently either resective osseous surgery or regenerative surgery; see Figs. 25.4 and 25.5). Depending on the individual periodontal risk, each patient should be remotivated, reinstructed, and retreated (if necessary) during a systematic supportive periodontal therapy regimen (revisits every 3, 6, or 12 months; see Fig. 25.6).

In addition, other genetic variations (single nucleotide polymorphisms [SNPs], genetic copy number variations) that have so far not been identified as responsible for certain syndromes may also directly influence innate and adaptive immune responses, as well as the structure of periodontal tissues. The identification of genes that are relevant to the development of periodontitis has led to new scientific concepts and findings. There are at least two different strategies (candidate genes and genome-wide associations) to identify genetic variances in relation to disease. In candidate gene studies, certain already known variances (SNPs) are correlated to a specific phenotype such as periodontitis. Therefore a hypothesis is required in order to choose specific SNPs in relevant genes. The data from those studies showed variable results, making it challenging to draw clear conclusions. In this context, studies on SNPs in the IL-1 gene led to the early conclusion that alterations in sequences of immunologically relevant genes may explain the heritability of periodontitis.[50] Conflicting data in the literature, however, indicate inconclusive knowledge regarding SNPs in the IL-1 gene and their potential role in the heritability and etiopathogenesis of periodontitis.[54] Also, it seems implausible that a single polymorphism in a specific gene sequence can cause a complex inflammatory disease, such as periodontitis, without causing any other symptoms relevant to one's systemic health. Thus genome-wide association studies (GWASs) have become more relevant. Here, a high number of DNA-sequence variances are evaluated at the same time. In contrast to candidate gene studies, no hypotheses are required for GWASs, so that there is no potential bias during analysis. In several GWASs, a number of new genes have been identified to be associated with periodontitis. One of the best-replicated genes is called *ANRIL* (antisense RNA in the lnc locus). *Antisense RNA in the lnc Locus (ANRIL)* is associated not only with periodontitis but also with cardiovascular disease, which underlines potential systemic interactions.[13,86-88] The role of *ANRIL* during the development of periodontitis is subject to ongoing investigations. It is known that it represents a noncoding regulatory RNA, which is involved during the regulation of cell division and in affecting other genes that play a role in the glucose and lipid metabolism (*ADIPOR1, VAMP3, C11ORF10*).[6,17,104] In addition to *ANRIL*, genetic variances (SNPs) in the sequences of the glucosyltransferase-6 domain containing 1 gene (*GLT6D1*), the plasminogen gene *(PLA)*, and the neuropeptide Y gene *(NPY)* have been associated with periodontal disease.[26,85,89] Due to the current technical and scientific progress, it may be expected that more genes will be identified to be associated with periodontitis in the future.

Environmental and Behavioral Factors

In addition to microbial, immunologic, and genetic factors, the development and progression of chronic periodontitis is further influenced by environmental and behavioral factors such as smoking and psychological stress[69,71] Smoking is a major risk factor for the development and progression of generalized chronic periodontitis.[4] Periodontitis is influenced by smoking in a dose-dependent manner. The intake of more than 10 cigarettes per day tremendously increases the risk of disease progression when compared with nonsmokers and former smokers, respectively.[98]

Compared to nonsmokers, the following features are found in smokers[5,44,73,81]:

- Increased periodontal pocket depth with more than 3 mm
- Increased attachment loss
- More recessions
- Increased loss of alveolar bone
- Increased tooth loss
- Fewer signs of gingivitis (less bleeding upon probing)
- A greater incidence of furcation involvement

Due to the consumption of tobacco, reactive oxygen (radicals) is released that chemically irritates periodontal tissues by DNA damage, lipid peroxidation of cell membranes, damage of endothelial cells, and the induction of smooth muscle cell growth.[66]

Psychological factors, such as stress and depression, also negatively influence the progression of chronic periodontitis.[31] Patients with periodontitis often report the experience of family- or work-related stress.[72] Positive correlations between cortisol levels and periodontal indices (plaque index, gingival index), bone loss, and missing teeth were recorded.[18,31,78] In addition, stress as an etiologic factor was even strongly associated with periodontitis when patients were smokers compared with nonsmokers.[11]

Stress and Periodontal Disease: Potential Mechanisms

1. Immunosuppression via cortisol secretion
2. Poor oral hygiene compliance in patients with chronic stress
3. Patients with stress are less likely to seek professional care
4. Patients with stress may smoke more frequently
   Case Scenarios are found on the companion website.

REFERENCES

 References for this chapter are found on the companion website.

Aggressive Periodontitis (Periodontitis Grade C)

OVERVIEW

Periodontitis is the pathologic manifestation of the host response against bacterial challenge that stems from a polymicrobial biofilm at the biofilm–gingival interface.[48] There are several subforms of the disease primarily defined by their clinical phenotype (i.e., the rate of disease progression and other features) rather than their (still partially unknown) etiology. This chapter addresses aggressive periodontitis, a clinically challenging subform of periodontitis featuring rapid loss of periodontal attachment and tooth-supporting bone in otherwise healthy patients. In this chapter, forms of disease characterized by a rapid rate of progression are discussed. As there must be a period of time between initial and subsequent clinical observations in order to characterize the rate of progression, most of the time, patients with moderate to severe stages of disease are discussed. All of the forms of diseases in this chapter are grade C or rapid rate of progression.

CLASSIFICATION AND CLINICAL CHARACTERISTICS

Features

The 1999 International Classification Workshop defined the entity of aggressive periodontitis, Periodontitis Grade C, to be characterized by three primary features (Table 26.1)[37]:

1. *Rapid loss of attachment and tooth-supporting bone.* In aggressive periodontitis, as compared with the more common chronic periodontitis, the loss of attachment progresses significantly faster. To evaluate this rapid course of destruction, the evaluation of clinical or radiographic data from earlier points in time (allowing for making an estimate of the start of disease) is necessary.[49] Note that the age of the patient is not by itself a primary criterion for the diagnosis of aggressive periodontitis. Because earlier clinical records are often not available, many clinicians argue that severe loss of attachment in young patients conceivably must be due to a rapid course of disease progression. This, however, is not generally true—neglect of all oral hygiene in a periodontitis-susceptible individual over a decade will lead to severe attachment loss, even with a slow rate of progression. On the other hand, severe attachment loss in an older individual is not necessarily the result of long-lasting, slowly progressing disease. It is therefore inappropriate to use the age of an individual as a primary diagnostic criterion for the distinction of aggressive and chronic periodontitis. Note that in chronic periodontitis, there are reportedly periods of rapid disease progression that can by themselves be misinterpreted as aggressive periodontitis.

2. *Subject is otherwise healthy (i.e., not with any systemic disease or condition that could be responsible for the present periodontitis).* There are systemic diseases that lead to severely altered host defenses against periodontal pathogens, often resulting in rapid loss of attachment and tooth loss at an early age. This disease is designated "periodontitis as a manifestation of systemic disease" (see Chapter 14). Note that the specific properties or abnormalities of some types of immune cells listed here and reported to be often associated with the diagnosis of aggressive periodontitis do not themselves qualify for the aforementioned diagnosis.

3. *Familiar aggregation.* Familiar aggregation of aggressive periodontitis cases is a feature that can be evaluated by medical/dental history questionnaires and interviewing the patient. It is, however, advisable to verify similar cases in the family, if possible, as many individuals may not be fully aware of their diagnoses, and not a few cases of "bad teeth that run in the family" turn out to be caries related or likely due to chronic periodontitis. In addition, the workshop defined several secondary features that are generally found in aggressive periodontitis cases but that are not universally necessary to diagnose the disease entity:

   a. Inconsistency of the low amounts of present etiologic factors and the observed pronounced tissue destruction.
   b. Strong colonization by *Aggregatibacter actinomycetemcomitans* and (in some populations) *Porphyromonas gingivalis*.
   c. Immunologic differences that do not entail the diagnosis "periodontitis as a manifestation of systemic disease":
      • Hyperresponsive macrophages.
      • Abnormalities of neutrophil function.
   d. Self-limiting disease.

TABLE 26.1 Diagnostic Criteria to Distinguish Chronic and Aggressive Periodontitis

Criterion	Aggressive Periodontitis	Chronic Periodontitis
Rate of progression	Rapid	Slow; rapid episodes possible
Familiar aggregation	Typical	Can be present when families share imperfect oral hygiene habits
Presence of etiologic factors (plaque, calculus, overhanging restorations, etc.)	Often minimal	Often commensurate with observed periodontal destruction
Age	Often in young patients (<35 years) but can be found in all age groups	Often in older patients (>55 years) but can be found in all age groups
Clinical inflammation signs	Sometimes lacking (especially in localized aggressive periodontitis)	Commensurate with etiologic factors

TABLE 26.2 Diagnostic Criteria for Localized and Generalized Aggressive Periodontitis

Criterion	Localized Aggressive Periodontitis	Generalized Aggressive Periodontitis
Age of onset	Circumpubertal	Most often <30 years of age but can occur in older individuals too
Serum antibody response against infecting agents	Robust	Poor
Destruction pattern	Localized attachment loss at incisors and first molars—interproximal attachment loss at ≥2 permanent teeth, one of which is a first molar, and involvement of ≤2 teeth, other than first molars and incisors	Generalized interproximal attachment loss at ≥3 permanent teeth other than first molars and incisors
Additional		Episodic nature of attachment loss

Subgroups

Aggressive periodontitis can be subclassified by extent and distribution into a localized and generalized form. The diagnosis of the subcategory is based on clinical, radiographic, and historical data. These include the age of onset, the involvement of teeth other than first molars and incisors (the first permanent teeth to erupt), and the presence of a systemic antibody response against periodontal pathogens (see Table 26.2).

Generalized Aggressive Periodontitis

Generalized aggressive periodontitis (GAP) is the subgroup of periodontal disease characterized by the highest severity and extent of disease, Stage III and IV, but also by its large heterogeneity. The diagnosis of GAP encompasses the diseases previously classified as *generalized juvenile periodontitis (GJP)* and *rapidly progressive periodontitis (RPP)*.

Two gingival tissue responses can be found in cases of GAP (Figs. 26.1 and 26.2). One is a severe, acutely inflamed tissue, often proliferating, ulcerated, and fiery red. Bleeding may occur spontaneously or with slight stimulation. Suppuration may be an important feature. This tissue response is believed to occur in the destructive stage, in which attachment and bone are actively lost.

In other cases, the gingival tissues may appear pink, free of inflammation, and occasionally with some degree of stippling, although stippling may be absent. However, despite the apparently mild clinical appearance, deep pockets can be demonstrated by probing. Page and Schroeder believed that this tissue response coincides with periods of quiescence in which the bone level remains stationary.[50]

Localized Aggressive Periodontitis

Localized aggressive periodontitis (LAP) is usually found in younger individuals than those affected by GAP (Figs. 26.3 and 26.4). It is characterized by more pronounced systemic antibody titers against periodontal pathogens than found in patients with GAP. This could indicate that in individuals susceptible to disease, but with the ability to enact a robust response against pathogens, the disease might be limited in extent (i.e., LAP), whereas in individuals with a lesser humoral response, the disease would not be limited to the first permanent teeth (i.e., the patient would develop GAP). This would mean that LAP and GAP would merely be phenotypic variations of the same underlying disease. This assumption is backed by several reports that show a sequence of LAP and GAP in the same individuals over time.[9,25,65] On the other hand, several lines of evidence exist that support a claim that LAP constitutes a disease on its own, with dissimilar underlying molecular and cellular mechanisms.

EPIDEMIOLOGY

The question of the prevalence of aggressive periodontitis in different populations is complicated by the fact that the currently used classification[3] is relatively young and not easy to apply in epidemiologic studies. Therefore, many available studies either (1) report on older, previously used entities of periodontitis that showed early onset or rapid progression but are not interchangeable with aggressive periodontitis or (2) report only on periodontitis severity, and not on diagnosis (for detailed reviews, see Albandar[2] and Susin and Albandar[69]). The problem of a lacking

Fig. 26.1 Case Presentation: Generalized Aggressive Periodontitis. Generalized aggressive periodontitis in a 28-year-old white female, nonsmoking patient. (A) Clinical views with minimal amounts of calculus and plaque. (B) Radiographically, bone loss ≥50% was present at all teeth.

universal case definition and changing classification systems for epidemiologic research is critical, because different case definitions for periodontitis in adolescents described differences in prevalence of up to 10-fold.[41]

Case Definition

The diagnosis of aggressive periodontitis in epidemiologic studies is difficult, because all primary criteria for the disease—rapid progression, systemic health, and familiar aggregation—are

difficult to assess reliably in the setting of such a study. The criteria of systemic health and familiar aggregation would require extensive interviews and thorough verification. The rapid progression of disease can consistently be documented only by following a subject longitudinally and performing at least two subsequent examinations within a reasonable time frame or (as noted previously) be extrapolated from older clinical or radiographic records. These, however, are frequently not available and would add extensive bias to the study, as prior providers of oral

Fig. 26.2 Case Presentation: Generalized Aggressive Periodontitis. Severe generalized aggressive periodontitis in a 22-year-old black male patient with a family history of early tooth loss through periodontal disease. (A) Clinical view showing minimal plaque and inflammation. A provisional wire-and-resin splint had been placed by the general-practice dentist to stabilize the teeth. (B) Radiographs showing the severe, generalized nature of the disease with all erupted teeth affected.

care were not calibrated. Radiographic examinations at the time of examination are, in the setting of an epidemiologic study, most often unfeasible.[2]

As a result, to date, methodologically sound epidemiologic studies investigating aggressive periodontitis as defined by the 1999 Workshop and now the 2018 Periodontal Classification are sparse (e.g., the study performed in a population of young Israeli army recruits).[38]

Therefore, to be able to assess the prevalence of aggressive periodontitis in other populations, Demmer and Papapanou[13] proposed to utilize the generally accepted case definition (see Chapter 6) for periodontitis proposed by a working group of the US Centers for Disease Control and Prevention (CDC) and the American Academy of Periodontology[14,51] in combination with the age of the study subject. Specifically, they assessed available studies for the proportion of subjects of ≤25 years of age with moderate or severe periodontitis according to the CDC definition, and the proportion of subjects 26 to 35 years of age with severe periodontitis (CDC definition). Similarly, Susin and Albandar[69] used a combination of diagnostic criteria to identify possible aggressive periodontitis cases in studies not designed following the 1999 classification.

Localized Aggressive, Grade C, Periodontitis

The prevalence of LAP in an Israeli army population aged 18 to 30 years was 4.3%. In this cohort, the presence of LAP was highly correlated with North African origin and current smoking.[38] A study of 830 Moroccan school students aged 12 to 25 years using the modified aggressive periodontitis definition of Albandar et al.[2] reported a prevalence of 4.9% for aggressive periodontitis, with approximately 70% exhibiting strong attachment loss at the molar sites.[31]

In addition to these data, several studies have examined the prevalence of LJP, the predecessor of LAP (however, not exactly interchangeable), from diverse populations. The prevalence of this disease in geographically diverse adolescent populations was estimated at less than 1%. Most reports suggested a low prevalence of about 0.2%.[39] Two independent radiographic studies of 16-year-old adolescents, one in Finland[57] and the other in Switzerland,[33] followed the strict diagnostic criteria delineated by Baer[6] and reported a prevalence rate of 0.1%. A clinical and radiographic study of 7266 English adolescents aged 15 to 19 years also showed a prevalence rate of 0.1%.[56] In the United States, a national survey of adolescents aged 14 to 17 years reported that 0.53% had LJP.[39] Blacks were at much higher risk for LJP, and black male teenagers were 2.9 times more likely to have the disease than black female adolescents. In contrast, white female teenagers were more likely to have LJP than white male adolescents. Several other studies have found the highest prevalence of LJP among black male patients,[9,43,56] followed in descending order by black female, white female, and white male patients.[43]

JCP was reported to affect both male and female individuals and is seen most frequently in the period between puberty and 20 years of age. Some studies have suggested a predilection for female patients, particularly in the youngest age groups,[25] whereas others reported no male-female differences in incidence when studies are designed to correct for ascertainment bias.[22]

Fig. 26.3 Case Presentation: Localized Aggressive Periodontitis. Localized aggressive periodontitis in a 15-year-old black female patient who had a twin with a similar disease. (A) Clinical view showing minimal plaque and inflammation except for localized inflammation on the distal side of the maxillary left central incisor and the mandibular right central incisor. (B) Radiographs showing localized, vertical, angular bone loss associated with the maxillary and mandibular first molars and the mandibular central incisors. The maxillary incisors show no apparent involvement. (C) Surgical appearance of the localized, vertical, angular bony defects affecting the mandibular incisors. Note the wide circumferential nature of the defects and the lack of calculus on the root surfaces.

Generalized Aggressive Periodontitis

Among young Israeli army recruits, 1.8% had GAP.[38] When using extrapolation, as proposed by Demmer and Papapanou, a prevalence of about 1% to a maximum of 15% within the age range was found, depending on the study. Specifically, data from the German Study of Health in Pomerania indicate an extrapolated prevalence within the age group of 13% (≤29 years) and 7% (30 to 39 years), whereas the highest extrapolated prevalence was found in the Eerie County study, with up to 15% of the age group.

Note that, as indicated previously, using prior epidemiologic data for the heterogeneous predecessors of GAP, GJP, and RPP to assess GAP prevalence is not possible because these entities are not interchangeable with GAP. In contrast, LJP, although still different from LAP by definition, can be used as a surrogate for LAP.

Current Understanding

Taken together, these data primarily show that the discrimination of aggressive periodontitis and other forms of periodontitis is not always easy, especially when the patient is seen for only a single examination, as is the case in most epidemiologic studies. The prevalence of aggressive periodontitis of approximately 1% to 15% in subjects of ≤35 years of age, in combination with the severity and tendency for rapid progression of this disease, strongly suggests that all patients in this age group should be screened regularly for the presence of periodontal disease.

PATHOBIOLOGY AND RISK FACTORS

All forms of periodontitis share certain common pathobiologic principles as polymicrobial, biofilm-mediated chronic inflammatory diseases at the biofilm–gingival interface. These principles

Fig. 26.4 Case Presentation: Localized Aggressive Periodontitis. Localized aggressive periodontitis in an 18-year old white female, nonsmoking patient. Familiar aggregation was reported. (A) Clinical view showing recessions at incisors and first molars. (B) Intraoperative view showing massive localized, angular bony defect associated with a first molar. (C) Radiographs showing pronounced localized, angular bone loss. (Courtesy Dr. Hendrik Schulze, Bonn, Germany.)

are addressed in detail in Chapters 7 to 9. Herein, we focus on the biologic reasons for the rapid course of destruction in aggressive periodontitis, including work investigating the specific properties of aggressive periodontitis in periodontal microbiology, immunology, and genetics.

Microbiology

Periodontitis is caused by specific microorganisms in a susceptible host.[53] In the subgingival biofilm, up to 700 bacterial species have been identified,[34] some of which were identified to be causative.[11] Details on the current knowledge on different periodontal microorganisms are summarized in Chapters 8 and 9.

The observed higher rate of disease progression in aggressive versus chronic periodontitis could possibly be partially explained by the presence of specific microorganisms that cause and perpetuate tissue destruction. In addition, the reported familiar aggregation of aggressive periodontitis cases could also be, to a certain point, explained by an infection and within-family transmission of specific microorganisms.

Therefore several studies have sought to identify the specific microbial properties of aggressive periodontitis cases. However, when evaluating generalized and localized aggressive periodontitis as a single entity and solely focusing on a small number of "classic" pathogens, it has been concluded that microbiologic infection patterns could not reliably distinguish between this entity and chronic periodontitis cases.[45]

However, data from a limited number of studies using both classic microbiologic tools and more recent molecular techniques suggest that differences exist in the microbiologic composition between (1) localized aggressive periodontitis and both generalized aggressive and chronic periodontitis and (2) generalized aggressive and chronic periodontitis[17,20,35,54] (for a review, see Armitage[4]).

Specific Bacteria in Localized Aggressive Periodontitis

In LAP, the situation appears to be different. Here, several lines of evidence point to a strong role of specific microorganisms, most notably *A. actinomycetemcomitans*. For decades, this bacterial species has been associated with LAP[7,10,66] and could predict the development of LAP in two longitudinal studies.[18,24] Longitudinal studies are of critical importance for demonstrating a causal relationship, whereas cross-sectional studies can by definition only show correlations that cannot be used to infer causality.

In the first longitudinal study, age-, gender- and race-matched juvenile carriers and noncarriers of *A. actinomycetemcomitans* (serotypes a, b, c equally distributed, no JP2) were followed longitudinally. After 1 year of follow-up, 80% of the carriers, but only 10% of the noncarriers, had developed periodontitis.[18]

In the second, larger longitudinal study, the highly leukotoxic *A. actinomycetemcomitans* (serotype b) strain JP2, which has a 530-bp deletion in its leukotoxin gene operon that leads to a 10- to 20-fold higher production of leukotoxin,[23] was found to be directly related to the occurrence of LAP in children in northern Africa. Specifically, the OR for future attachment loss in carriers of the JP2 strain was 18.0 as compared with 3.0 for carriers of other, non-JP2 strains of *A. actinomycetemcomitans*.[24] Similar findings can be found in West African countries (e.g., Ghana[1]) in contrast to eastern parts of Africa where no studies have reported on JP2 clone strain in patients with periodontitis.[15]

A recent study on the occurrence of JP2 clone strains in patients with aggressive periodontitis shows a high incidence in both LAP and GAP, suggesting that both subclasses could be more related than initially thought.[16]

In addition, it needs to be noted that, as with all entities of periodontitis, LAP is clearly not a monoinfection with *A. actinomycetemcomitans* but features a polymicrobial biofilm. Supporting this notion are reports of confirmed cases of LAP that did not carry *A. actinomycetemcomitans*.[35,46]

Host Response to Bacterial Challenge

The inflammatory host response toward pathogens is generally attributed to be responsible for a larger proportion of the tissue destruction in periodontitis than the invading periodontal pathogens themselves. The rapid progression of aggressive periodontitis implies that, in addition to the aforementioned composition of the subgingival microbiologic flora, specific properties of this inflammatory response render the individuals with aggressive periodontitis both more susceptible to disease and more prone to lose more attachment in a shorter time.

Host Responses Specific to Aggressive Periodontitis

In GAP, one review concluded that "there appears to be no difference between aggressive and chronic periodontitis in terms of their histopathology and immunopathology."[67] Still, it has to be acknowledged that this could mean that no differences exist or rather that "the differences between both disease entities only reflect variations in the degree of severity of susceptibility rather than actual different immune-pathologies."[19]

However, stronger activation of natural killer cells and natural killer T-cells in aggressive periodontitis has been suggested to be causative for the observed more pronounced tissue destruction in aggressive periodontitis.[32,47] A distinction of chronic and aggressive periodontitis based on molecular markers (gingival tissue transcriptional signatures) using machine learning algorithms was possible with excellent sensitivity and specificity. At the same time, this work identified substantial diagnostic imprecision in the current classification.[29]

Abnormalities in Localized Aggressive Periodontitis

Earlier work has suggested that individuals with LAP were characterized by an inherited defect of neutrophil function, leading to a dampened immune response against the microflora inhabiting the periodontal pocket.[74] Specifically, when challenged with periodontal pathogens, the LAP neutrophils were reported to show impaired chemotaxis, phagocytosis, and killing of bacteria. Alternatively, it was also hypothesized that these impaired defense properties were in fact acquired defects caused by prolonged exposure to an inflammatory microenvironment.

Today, the understanding of neutrophil biology is that neutrophils arriving at a site with uncontrolled periodontal inflammation are primed to attack the invading pathogens by releasing lytic enzymes. These enzymes may, on the other hand, accelerate tissue destruction. It is hypothesized that the observed dampened neutrophil function in deep aggressive periodontitis lesions is due to the heavy commitment of primed neutrophils to debridement, so that less potency remains for chemotaxis and defense.[55]

Genetics: Family Studies

A familiar aggregation of aggressive periodontitis cases is a secondary feature of the disease entity (i.e., it is often, but not always, found in aggressive periodontitis). To assess the familiar component of the disease, twin studies were performed[8,42] showing a strong genetic component with likely autosomal dominant inheritance mode and a 70% (African Americans) to 73% (Caucasians) penetrance.[42]

Genetics: Polymorphisms

Accordingly, there has been extensive work on the inherent genetic traits underlying this familiar aggregation.[36,68] First, it was suspected that an inherent susceptibility for periodontitis would likely be due to mutations of the DNA encoding for proteins of inflammatory mediators (candidate gene approach). DNA regions selected based on a priori knowledge of the disease pathobiology were assessed for sequence variations, most often single nucleotide polymorphisms (SNPs). Based on small sample sizes and often suboptimal study design, conceivably leading to false-positive results,[36,63] SNPs within genes encoding for cytokines such as interleukins (e.g., IL-1α, IL-1β, and IL-6) were reported to be associated with aggressive periodontitis. However, with current knowledge, it has to be realized that these findings were possibly spurious or the result of confounding—all of the "classical" candidate gene associations could not be replicated in today's larger and better controlled cohorts.[59] Note that in the case of genetic association studies, meta-analyses are not generally suitable tools to overcome the problems of small, heterogeneous cohorts.

Use of the genome-wide association study (GWAS) has been made possible by technologic advances in the field of high-throughput analysis. Using a GWAS of a large number of aggressive periodontitis cases and controls, a number of common susceptibility loci for myocardial infarction and aggressive periodontitis could be identified and replicated in independent cohorts.[58,60-62]

Taken together, these data indicate that there is evidence for a strong genetic component in aggressive periodontitis. It is very likely that the low number of identified and replicated susceptibility loci for aggressive periodontitis is due to too few samples and issues in study design rather than to a lacking biologic association (for reviews, see Laine et al.[36] and Vaithilingam et al.[73]).

Environmental Factors Affecting Susceptibility

The amount and duration of smoking are important variables that can influence the extent of destruction seen in young adults.[72] Patients with GAP who smoke have more affected teeth and more loss of clinical attachment than nonsmoking patients with GAP.[21] However, smoking may not have the same impact on attachment levels in younger patients with LAP.[64]

Current Developments

Based on the aforementioned still incomplete current understanding of the specific microbiologic, immunologic, and genetic properties of the clinical symptom-based periodontitis entities aggressive and chronic periodontitis, research now focuses on the assessment of whether these entities are in fact sufficiently distinct with respect to their underlying pathobiology to form etiology-based clinical classes. For these analyses, novel unbiased high-throughput methodology such as microarrays and next-generation sequencing are employed.[26-28,30]

THERAPEUTIC CONSIDERATIONS IN AGGRESSIVE PERIODONTITIS PATIENTS

CLINICIAN'S CORNER

Aggressive periodontitis is defined by rapid attachment loss in clinically healthy individuals. There is considerable familiar aggregation. Aggressive periodontitis is most often found in younger individuals but can occur at any age. The entity is subdivided into two categories, localized and generalized aggressive periodontitis.

Localized aggressive periodontitis (LAP) primarily affects first molars and incisor teeth in adolescents with deep pockets and advanced bone loss. It occurs in less than 1% of adolescents. There is a strong, hitherto only partially understood genetic component. In addition, the anaerobic gram-negative bacterium *Aggregatibacter actinomycetemcomitans* in the subgingival plaque biofilm was causally linked to LAP development in adolescents.

Generalized aggressive periodontitis (GAP) usually occurs first in young adults and may be present in some populations in up to 15% of the age group. Smoking may play a role because smokers with GAP have more teeth involved and more advanced pockets than nonsmokers.

Considerations for Antiinfective Therapy of Aggressive Periodontitis

Antiinfective therapy in patients with aggressive periodontitis appears to benefit strongly from the adjunctive use of systemic antibiotics (see Chapter 52).[12]

Considerations for Surgical Therapy of Aggressive Periodontitis

In general, individuals with aggressive periodontitis, especially LAP, have to undergo surgical therapy more often than the average periodontitis patient.[12] This is due to (1) the often much more pronounced loss of attachment with deep periodontal pockets that are challenging to instrument[5,40] and (2) the high prevalence of vertical defects, notably in LAP, that need to be resolved.[52]

Considerations for Supportive Periodontal Therapy of Aggressive Periodontitis Patients

Patients with aggressive periodontitis are understood to have an especially virulent microbiologic burden in combination with alterations in their host defense that render them more prone to rapid attachment loss, even in the absence of seemingly adequate numbers of etiologic factors. This suggests that during the maintenance phase, utmost care needs to be taken to optimize the self-performed oral hygiene in order to minimize the amount of plaque that could eventually lead to a new, rapid loss of attachment. Therefore, many clinicians recommend performing supportive periodontal therapy, including regular assessments of periodontal parameters, at least every 3 months—even in subjects who show particularly high levels of oral hygiene proficiency and independent of the periodontal risk assessment (PRA) tool that appears to be of limited use in aggressive periodontitis.[44]

Considerations for Oral Rehabilitation and Implant Therapy in Aggressive Periodontitis Patients

Dental implants today allow for the routine, predictable, functional, and esthetic replacement of lost teeth. Still, there are concerns about the incidence of peri-implantitis, an inflammatory condition of dental implants with parallels to periodontal disease for which no defined, predictable treatment protocols exist to date. Peri-implantitis risk is linked to a history of periodontal disease in the individual treated with dental implants. Limited data exist that show an even stronger risk for developing the disease in patients with aggressive periodontitis as compared to patients with chronic periodontitis or periodontally healthy controls.[70,71]

Case Scenarios are found on the companion website.

REFERENCES

 References for this chapter are found on the companion website.

Necrotizing Ulcerative Periodontitis[a]

Necrotizing ulcerative periodontitis (NUP) is a necrotizing periodontal disease (NPD) as defined in the most recent 2018 classification system. It is often an extension of necrotizing ulcerative gingivitis (NUG) into the periodontal structures, leading to the loss of periodontal attachment and bone. Alternatively, NUP and NUG may be different diseases. To date, there is little evidence to support the progression of NUG to NUP or to establish a relationship between the two conditions as a single disease entity. However, numerous clinical descriptions and case reports of NUP clearly demonstrate many clinical similarities between them. Until a distinction between NUG and NUP can be proved or disproved, it has been suggested that NUG and NUP be classified together under the broader category of *necrotizing periodontal diseases*, although with differing levels of severity.[1,11,15] Because *ulceration* is secondary to necrosis, the term ulcerative is removed in the newly implemented classification system.[1a,11a]

NUG has been recognized and described in the literature for centuries.[17] The features of NUG are presented in Chapter 19. The lesions of NUG are confined to the gingiva without a loss of periodontal attachment or alveolar bone support; this is the feature that distinguishes NUG from NUP.

CLINICAL FEATURES

Clinical cases of NUP are defined by necrosis and ulceration of the coronal portion of the interdental papillae and gingival margin, with a painful bright-red marginal gingiva that bleeds easily. This is similar to the clinical features of NUG. The distinguishing feature of NUP is the *destructive progression* of the disease, which includes periodontal attachment and bone loss. Deep interdental osseous craters typify the periodontal lesions of NUP (Fig. 27.1). However, "conventional" periodontal pockets with deep probing depth are not found because the ulcerative and necrotizing gingival lesion destroys the marginal epithelium and connective tissue, resulting in gingival recession. Periodontal pockets are formed because the junctional epithelial cells remain viable and can therefore migrate apically to cover areas of lost connective tissue attachment. The necrosis of the junctional epithelium in patients with NUG and NUP creates an ulcer that prevents this epithelial migration, so that a pocket cannot form. Advanced lesions of NUP lead to severe bone loss and tooth mobility, may ultimately leading to tooth loss. In addition to these manifestations, as previously mentioned, patients with NUP may present with oral malodor, fever, malaise, or lymphadenopathy.

> **KEY FACT**
>
> NUP cases are defined by necrosis and ulceration of the coronal portion of the interdental papillae. Gingival margins are bright red and bleed easily. Lesions are painful. The feature that distinguishes NUP from NUG is the destructive progression of NUP, which includes periodontal attachment and bone loss.

MICROSCOPIC FINDINGS

In a study involving the use of transmission electron microscopy and scanning electron microscopy of the microbial plaque overlying the necrotic gingival papillae, Cobb and colleagues[2] demonstrated striking histologic similarities between NUP in HIV-positive patients and previous descriptions of NUG in HIV-negative patients. Microscopic examination revealed a surface biofilm composed of a mixed microbial flora with different morphotypes and a subsurface flora with dense aggregations of spirochetes (i.e., the bacterial zone). Below the bacterial layers were dense aggregations of polymorphonuclear leukocytes (PMNs) (i.e., the neutrophil-rich zone) and necrotic cells (the necrotic zone). The biopsy technique used in this study did not allow for the observation of the deepest layer and thus was not able to identify the spirochetal infiltration zone, which is classically described in NUG lesions. In addition to the NUG-like microscopic features of NUP described in this study, high levels of yeasts and herpes-like viruses were observed. This last finding is most likely indicative of the conditions afforded to

---

[a]Adapted from the following chapter of Newman and Carranza's Clinical Periodontology, 13th edition: Chapter 29: Necrotizing Ulcerative Periodontitis, by Perry R. Klokkevold and Fermin A. Carranza.

Fig. 27.1 Necrotizing Ulcerative Periodontitis in a 45-year-old HIV-Negative White Male Patient.
(A) Buccal view of the maxillary cuspid–bicuspid area. (B) Palatal view of the same area shown in (A).
(C) Buccal view of the mandibular anteriors. Note the deep craters associated with bone loss.

opportunistic microbes in the immunocompromised host (i.e., HIV-positive patients).

PATIENTS WITH HIV/AIDS

Gingival and periodontal lesions with distinctive features are frequently found in patients with HIV infection and AIDS. Many of these lesions are atypical manifestations of inflammatory periodontal diseases that arise during the course of HIV infection and as a result of the patient's concomitant immunocompromised state. Linear gingival erythema, NUG, and NUP are the most common HIV-associated periodontal conditions reported in the literature.[16] Chapter 28 provides detailed descriptions of these and other atypical periodontal diseases that occur in the patient with HIV.

NUP lesions found in patients with HIV or AIDS can present with features similar to those seen in HIV-negative patients. Other complications reported in this population included the progression of the lesions to involve large areas of soft tissue necrosis with the exposure of bone and the sequestration of bone fragments. This type of severe, progressive lesion with extension into the vestibular area and palate is referred to as *necrotizing ulcerative stomatitis*.

CLINICAL CORRELATION

Periodontal attachment and bone loss associated with NUP in an immunocompromised host (i.e., HIV-positive or AIDS) may be extremely rapid. NUP lesions in these patients are likely to be much more destructive and may also be associated with complications that are extremely rare among patients without HIV or AIDS.

ETIOLOGY OF NECROTIZING ULCERATIVE PERIODONTITIS

The etiology of NUP has not been determined, although a mixed fusiform–spirochete bacterial flora appears to play a key role. Because bacterial pathogens are not solely responsible for causing the disease, some predisposing "host" factors may be necessary. Numerous predisposing factors have been attributed to NUG, including poor oral hygiene, preexisting periodontal disease, smoking, viral infections, immunocompromised status, psychosocial stress, and malnutrition. One case report attributed heavy tobacco use as the most significant contributing factor associated with NUP in a 21-year-old who had been smoking (>20 cigarettes per day) and chewing tobacco since the age of 7 years.[20] **Smoking, malnutrition, and high plaque levels all increase the risk of NUG and must be changed to achieve successful treatment.**

Clinicians should check all patients who present with NUP to ascertain their HIV status. NUP can progress rapidly and lead to tooth exfoliation, so treatment should include local debridement, local antiplaque agents, and systemic antibiotics. The early diagnosis and treatment of NUP are crucial, because the osseous defects that occur during the late stages of the disease are extremely difficult to resolve.

Microbial Flora

Assessment of the microbial flora of NUP lesions is almost exclusively limited to studies involving patients with HIV or AIDS, with some conflicting evidence. Murray and colleagues[15] reported that cases of NUP in HIV-positive patients demonstrated significantly greater numbers of the opportunistic fungus *Candida albicans* and a higher prevalence of *Aggregatibacter actinomycetemcomitans*,

Prevotella intermedia, Porphyromonas gingivalis, Fusobacterium nucleatum, and *Campylobacter* species as compared with HIV-negative controls. In addition, they reported a low or variable level of spirochetes, which is inconsistent with the flora associated with NUG. Citing differences in microbial flora, they refuted the notion that the destructive lesions seen in HIV-positive patients were related to NUG lesions; they suggested that the flora of NUP lesions in HIV-positive patients is comparable to that of chronic periodontitis lesions, thus supporting their concept that necrotizing periodontitis in the HIV-positive patient is an aggressive manifestation of chronic periodontitis in the immunocompromised host.

In contrast with these findings, Cobb and colleagues[2] reported that the microbial composition of NUP lesions in HIV-positive patients was very similar to that of NUG lesions, as discussed previously. Researchers used electron microscopy to describe a mixed microbial flora with various morphotypes in 81.3% of specimens. The subsurface microbial flora featured dense aggregations of spirochetes in 87.5% of specimens. The authors also reported opportunistic yeasts and herpes-like viruses in 65.6% and 56.5% of NUP lesions, respectively. The differences between these reports may be explained by the limitations of obtaining viable cultures of spirochetes[15] as compared with the more complete sample assessment with electron microscopic observation of spirochetes.[2]

Spirochetes have the ability to modulate the host's innate and adaptive immune responses and to stimulate host inflammatory reactions,[5] which may reduce the local immune competence and facilitate the development of necrotizing disease.[9] Activated herpesviruses have the capacity to deregulate the host's immune system, which may lead to an increase in the colonization and activity of other pathogenic microorganisms. *Candida albicans* has been reported to produce eicosanoids, leading to the release of proinflammatory mediators, which may facilitate spirochete colonization and invasion and promote the development of NPDs.[8,9]

> **KEY FACT**
>
> Patients with NUP are more likely to be immunocompromised. Although a mixed fusiform–spirochete bacterial infection appears to play a key role in the etiology of NUP, bacterial pathogens are not solely responsible. Predisposing "host" factors appear to be necessary. Factors that have been attributed to NUG include poor oral hygiene, preexisting periodontal disease, smoking, viral infections, immunocompromised status, psychosocial stress, and malnutrition.

Psychologic Stress

Most studies evaluating the role of stress on NPD have involved subjects with NUG[4,12,18,19] and thus have not specifically addressed the role of stress on NUP. Patients with NUG have been found to have had significantly more anxiety, higher depression scores, a greater magnitude of recent stressful events, more overall distress and adjustments related to these events, and more negative life events.[3,10] Although the role of stress in the development of NUP has not been reported specifically, the many similarities between NUG and NUP would suggest that similar relationships to stress may exist.

The mechanisms that predispose an individual with stress to necrotizing ulcerative periodontal diseases have not been established.

MALNUTRITION

Direct evidence of the relationship between malnutrition and NPD is limited to descriptions of necrotizing infections in severely malnourished children. Lesions that resemble NUG but that progress to become *gangrenous stomatitis* or noma have been described in children with severe malnutrition in underdeveloped countries. Jimenez and Baer[14] reported cases of NUG among malnourished children and adolescents between the ages of 2 and 14 years in Colombia. In the advanced stages, NUG lesions extended from the gingiva to other areas of the oral cavity, becoming gangrenous stomatitis (noma) and causing exposure, necrosis, and sequestration of the alveolar bone. Later, Jimenez and colleagues reported that 44 of the 45 cases of necrotizing disease (NUG = 29, NUP = 7, and noma = 9) documented from 1965 to 2000 were from a low socioeconomic group and that malnutrition was associated with nearly all of the necrotizing conditions (29/29 NUG cases, 6/7 NUP cases, and 9/9 noma cases).[13] In a study of socioeconomically deprived Nigerian children with NUG (153 cases), Enwonwu and colleagues confirmed malnutrition by measuring circulating micronutrients.[7] As compared with neighborhood counterparts, the children with NUG and micronutrient deficiencies demonstrated dysregulated cytokine production with a complex interplay of elevated proinflammatory and antiinflammatory mediators.

> **KEY FACT**
>
> A fusiform-spirochete infection along with weakened host immune system seem to play a major role in the pathogenesis of necrotizing ulcerative periodontitis.

A possible explanation is that malnutrition, particularly when extreme, contributes to a diminished host resistance to infection and necrotizing disease. It is well documented that many of the host defenses—including phagocytosis; cell-mediated immunity; and complement, antibody, and cytokine production and function—are impaired in malnourished individuals.[6] The depletion of nutrients to cells and tissues results in immunosuppression and increases disease susceptibility. Therefore it is reasonable to conclude that malnutrition can predispose an individual to opportunistic infections or intensify the severity of existing oral infections.

CONCLUSION

NUP and NUG share many clinical and microbiologic features, but NUP is distinguished by a more severe condition with periodontal attachment and bone loss. Some individuals with NUP have severe, rapidly progressive disease. It appears that an impaired immune response and lowered host resistance to infection are significant factors in the onset and progression of NUP. The best example of an immunocompromised host with a predisposition for NUP is the patient with HIV or AIDS. As with the other infection-related complications of HIV and AIDS, the immuno-compromised status of affected patients renders them vulnerable to opportunistic periodontal infections, including NUP. Several predisposing factors have been identified in cases of NUG that may also play a role in NUP, including smoking, viral infections, psychosocial stress, and malnutrition. Although none of these factors alone is sufficient to cause necrotizing disease, when they occur together with an immunocompromised status, there is a potential to adversely influence the host response or resistance to infection.

A case scenario may be found on the companion website.

REFERENCES

 References for this chapter are found on the companion website.

Pathology and Management of Periodontal Problems in Patients With Human Immunodeficiency Virus Infection[a,b]

For online-only content on pathogenesis, classification and staging, adverse drug effects, and necrotizing ulcerative stomatitis as well as expanded content about the oral and periodontal manifestations of human immunodeficiency virus infection and gingival and periodontal diseases, please visit the companion website.

CHAPTER OUTLINE

Acquired immunodeficiency syndrome (AIDS) is characterized by profound impairment of the immune system. The condition was first reported in 1981, and a viral pathogen, the human immunodeficiency virus (HIV), was identified in 1984.[169] The condition was originally thought to be restricted to male homosexuals. Subsequently it was also identified in male and female heterosexuals and bisexuals who participated in unprotected sexual activities or who inject drugs of abuse (injected drug users, or IDUs).[144] Currently sexual activity and drug abuse remain the primary means of transmission.

HIV has a strong affinity for cells of the immune system, most specifically those that carry the CD4 cell surface receptor molecule. Thus helper T lymphocytes (T4 cells) are most profoundly affected, but monocytes, macrophages, Langerhans cells, and some neuronal and glial brain cells may also be involved.[98] Viral replication occurs continuously in the lymphoreticular tissues of the lymph nodes, spleen, gut-associated lymphoid cells, and macrophages.[215,216]

In 1986, a second type of HIV was isolated in western Africa, and subsequently the two were named HIV-1 and HIV-2. Infection with HIV-2 was first reported in the United States in 1987 in an individual who had migrated from western Africa. The two viruses apparently originated in different simian species. HIV-2 is very similar to HIV-1 but appears to be less virulent and causes AIDS much more slowly. Infection with HIV-2 is rarely identified outside of Africa and countries that have been intimately associated with that area. During subsequent years, various subgroups of the viruses have been identified. HIV-1 consists of three named subgroups: M (main or major), N (new or non-M), and O (outlier). HIV-1 subgroup M is primarily responsible for the worldwide HIV epidemic. There are at least 10 subtypes of HIV-1 M, with subtype B being the most common. It has also been learned that coinfection with varying groups or subgroups can result in circulating recombinant forms of viral strains. There are also eight known HIV-2 subgroups. There is evidence that this growing plethora of viral mutations may play a role in the increasing resistance to antiretroviral therapy. It is known, for example, that HIV-2 possesses a natural resistance to nonnucleoside reverse transcriptase inhibitor antiretroviral drugs, and circulating recombinant forms may also develop resistance to drugs being used for treatment.[99,124,165]

Combined therapeutic regimens consisting of antiretroviral agents and protease-inhibiting drugs have resulted in marked improvement in the health status of HIV-infected individuals and occasionally a reduction in viral plasma bioloads to below detectable levels (i.e., <50 copies/mL), although the infection may still be transmissible.[66,88,91,220] Evidence indicates that the virus is never completely eradicated; rather, it is sequestered at low levels in resting CD4 cells even in individuals with no detectable plasma viral ribonucleic acid (RNA).[39,65] These findings suggest that effective combination drug therapy may be necessary throughout the lives of infected individuals. Long-term control of the infection may be difficult because the antiviral agents that

---

[a]Adapted from the following chapter of Newman and Carranza's Clinical Periodontology, 13th edition: Chapter 28: Pathology and Management of Periodontal Problems in Patients With Human Immunodeficiency Virus Infection, by Terry D. Rees.

[b]Note: In the 2018 classification of periodontal and peri-implant diseases and conditions, "chronic periodontitis" and "aggressive periodontitis" disease categories are grouped under a single category called "periodontitis" and are further characterized based on a multidimensional staging and grading system. In this chapter, the term *aggressive periodontitis* is still used because the related studies were conducted before the 2018 classification. Readers are referred to Chapter 6 for a detailed discussion of periodontal disease classification.

are currently used have many adverse side effects and drug-resistant variant viral strains develop readily.[215] In addition, growing evidence suggests that oral pathogenic microorganisms (including putative periodontal pathogens) may help to induce HIV recrudescence by reactivating latently infected dendritic cells, macrophages, or T cells.[79,96,97]

Oral and Periodontal Manifestations of Human Immunodeficiency Virus Infection

Oral lesions are common in HIV-infected patients, although geographic and environmental variables may exist. Previous reports have indicated that most patients with AIDS have head and neck lesions,[171] whereas oral lesions are common among HIV-positive individuals who do not yet have AIDS.[15,77] Several reports have identified a strong correlation between HIV infection and oral candidiasis, oral hairy leukoplakia, atypical periodontal diseases, oral Kaposi sarcoma, and oral non-Hodgkin lymphoma (NHL).[56,59,117]

Oral lesions less strongly associated with HIV infection include melanotic hyperpigmentation, mycobacterial infections, necrotizing ulcerative stomatitis (NUS), miscellaneous oral ulcerations, and viral infections (e.g., herpes simplex virus [HSV], herpes zoster, and condyloma acuminatum). Lesions that are seen in HIV-infected individuals with undetermined frequency include less common viral infections (e.g., CMV, molluscum contagiosum), recurrent aphthous stomatitis, and bacillary angiomatosis (epithelioid angiomatosis).[56]

The advent of HAART has resulted in a greatly diminished frequency of oral lesions associated with HIV infection and AIDS.[30,138,200]

Oral Candidiasis

Candida, a fungus that is found in the normal oral flora, proliferates on the surface of the oral mucosa under certain conditions. A major factor associated with the overgrowth of *Candida* is diminished host resistance, which is seen in debilitated patients or in those who have received immunosuppressive therapy. The incidence of candidal infection has been demonstrated to increase progressively in relation to diminishing immune competency.[121,122,191] Most oral candidal infections (i.e., 85% to 95%) are associated with *Candida albicans,* but other species of *Candida* may also be involved. At least 11 strains of *Candida* have been identified, and non–*Candida albicans* infections are more common among immunocompromised individuals who are already receiving antifungal therapy for *C. albicans.*[118,182]

Candidiasis is the most common oral lesion associated with HIV disease; it has been found in approximately 90% of patients with AIDS.[149,190] It usually has one of four clinical presentations: pseudomembranous, erythematous, or hyperplastic candidiasis or angular cheilitis.[92,137]

Pseudomembranous candidiasis ("thrush") presents as painless or slightly sensitive yellow-white curd-like lesions that can be readily scraped and separated from the surface of the oral mucosa. This type is most common on the hard and soft palate and the buccal or labial mucosa, but it can occur anywhere in the oral cavity (Fig. 28.1).

Fig. 28.1 Palatal Pseudomembranous Candidiasis.

Fig. 28.2 Palatal Erythematous Candidiasis.

Erythematous candidiasis may be present as a component of the pseudomembranous type, appearing as red patches on the buccal or palatal mucosa, or it may be associated with depapillation of the tongue. If the gingiva is affected, it may be misdiagnosed as desquamative gingivitis (Figs. 28.2 to 28.4). Some evidence suggests that erythematous candidiasis is more common among HIV-positive individuals with CD4+ cell counts between 200 and 500/μL, whereas the pseudomembranous form occurs in patient with CD4+ cell counts of less than 200/μL. Viral load is most often elevated to more than 100,000 copies/mL. However, it should be emphasized that any form of candidiasis can be found in individuals who are only minimally immunocompromised.[139]

Hyperplastic candidiasis is the least common form, and it may be seen in the buccal mucosa and the tongue. It is more resistant to removal than the other types (Figs. 28.5 and 28.6).

In *Candida*-related *angular cheilitis,* the commissures of the lips appear erythematous, with surface crusting and fissuring.

The diagnosis of candidiasis is made by clinical evaluation, culture analysis, or microscopic examination of a tissue sample or smear of material scraped from the lesion (oral cytology), which shows hyphae and yeast forms of the organisms

Fig. 28.3 Gingival Erythematous Candidiasis Suggestive of Desquamative Gingivitis.

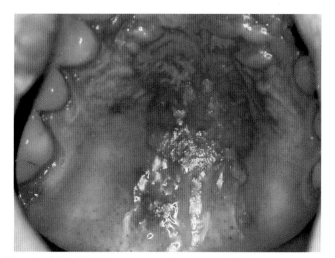

Fig. 28.4 Mixed Erythematous and Pseudomembranous Candidiasis of the Palate.

Fig. 28.5 Mixed Erythematous and Hyperplastic Candidiasis of the Corner of the Mouth.

(Fig. 28.7). When oral candidiasis appears in patients with no apparent predisposing cause, the clinician should be alerted to the possibility of HIV infection.[56] Many patients who are at risk for HIV infection and present with oral candidiasis also have esophageal candidiasis, which is a diagnostic sign of AIDS.[202]

Fig. 28.6 Hyperplastic Candidiasis in the Corner of the Mouth. The lesion persisted despite the use of systemic antifungal drugs.

Oral Hairy Leukoplakia

Oral hairy leukoplakia (OHL) primarily occurs in persons with HIV infection.[83,84] Found on the lateral borders of the tongue, it frequently has a bilateral distribution and may extend to the ventrum. OHL is caused by the Epstein-Barr virus (EBV) and is the only EBV lesion with which viral shedding in saliva is common.[139] The lesion is characterized by an asymptomatic, poorly demarcated keratotic area that ranges in size from a few millimeters to several centimeters (Fig. 28.8A). Often, characteristic vertical striations are present, which impart a corrugated appearance; the surface may also be shaggy and appear hairy when dried. The lesion does not rub off, and it may resemble other keratotic oral lesions.

Microscopically, the OHL lesion shows a hyperparakeratotic surface with projections that often resemble hairs. Beneath the parakeratotic surface, acanthosis and some characteristic "balloon cells" resembling koilocytes are seen (see Fig. 28.8B). It has been demonstrated that these cells contain viral particles of the human herpesvirus group that have been interpreted as EBV.[83,85]

Kaposi Sarcoma and Other Malignancies

Oral malignancies occur more frequently in severely immunocompromised individuals than in the general population. An HIV-positive individual with NHL or Kaposi sarcoma (KS) is categorized as having AIDS (Fig. 28.9). Oral lesions are reported in approximately 4% of individuals with NHL, and the gingiva and palate are common sites. The incidence of oral squamous cell carcinoma may also increase among HIV-infected individuals.[19] KS was a rare disease until the early 1980s. In its classic form, it is found in older men and occasionally in patients who have had organ transplants; it is endemic in parts of Africa. An epidemic form has subsequently been described in HIV-positive individuals, and it is an AIDS-defining condition.[148]

KS is the most common oral malignancy associated with AIDS. This angioproliferative tumor is a rare, multifocal, vascular neoplasm; it was originally described in 1872 as occurring in the skin

Fig. 28.8 **Oral Hairy Leukoplakia on the Left Lateral Border of the Tongue.** (A) Clinical view. (B) Biopsy confirmation of oral hairy leukoplakia. Note the ballooned epithelial cells near the surface of the epithelium.

Fig. 28.7 **Techniques for the Diagnosis of Candidiasis.** (A) Candidal hyphae in a tissue smear after periodic acid–Schiff staining. (B) Culture media specific for *Candida* species. (C) Candidal hyphae in the epithelium of biopsied tissue.

Fig. 28.9 **Non-Hodgkin Lymphoma of the Anterior Mandibular Gingiva.**

of the lower extremities of older men of Mediterranean origin. Today, it is closely associated with homosexual and heterosexual transmission, but it occurs 5 to 10 times more often among MSM than in other groups at high risk for HIV. The causative agent has been identified as human herpesvirus-8 (HHV-8).

Gingival KS lesions may be exacerbated by existing periodontal lesions, or necrotizing periodontal diseases may be superimposed on existing gingival KS. On occasion, the expansion of gingival lesions may result in bone resorption. Increased tooth mobility and loss has also been reported.[146]

Microscopically, KS consists of four components: (1) endothelial cell proliferation with the formation of atypical vascular channels, (2) extravascular hemorrhage with hemosiderin deposition, (3) spindle cell proliferation in association with atypical

vessels, and (4) a mononuclear inflammatory infiltrate consisting mainly of plasma cells (Fig. 28.10).[81]

Non-Hodgkin Lymphoma

Lymphoma represents a heterogeneous malignancy characterized by the proliferation of lymphoid cells. It is broadly classified as Hodgkin disease (14%), or NHL. NHL in individuals with HIV infection is an AIDS-defining condition, and elevated cumulative viremia may be a strong predictor of AIDS-related lymphoma.[222]

Oral lesions usually appear as erythematous, painless enlargements that may become ulcerated as a result of traumatic injury (Fig. 28.11). In some cases, bone involvement occurs, although this is rare in the United States. Lesions commonly affect the

Fig. 28.10 (A) Histologic view of Kaposi sarcoma. This lesion is exophytic and only minimally inflamed (low magnification). (B) Note the sheets of endothelial cells and numerous small blood vessels (high magnification).

Fig. 28.11 Bacillary Angiomatosis Mimicking Kaposi Sarcoma.

gingival, palatal, and alveolar mucosa, and they may mimic dental infections. Diagnosis is based on physical examination, complete blood count with differential, imaging studies, and lymph node and tissue biopsy.[133]

Bacillary (Epithelioid) Angiomatosis

Bacillary (epithelioid) angiomatosis (BA) is an infectious vascular proliferative disease with clinical and histologic features similar to those of KS. BA is caused by facultative intracellular gram-negative mobile bacilli of the genus *Bartonella* and the order Rickettsia (e.g., *Bartonella henselae, Bartonella quintana*).[56,161,177] Cats are the primary host of *B. henselae,* and the infection is usually transmitted to humans by bites, scratches, or fleas (i.e., cat-scratch fever). Humans are the primary reservoir for *B. quintana,* and it is usually transmitted by human lice. BA can occur in immunocompetent persons, but it is most commonly associated with AIDS. Skin lesions are similar to those associated with KS or cat-scratch disease.[45,196] Gingival BA manifests as red, purple, or blue edematous soft-tissue lesions that may cause the destruction of periodontal ligament and bone (see Fig. 28.11).[75]

Oral Hyperpigmentation

An increased incidence of *oral hyperpigmentation* has been described in HIV-infected individuals.[40,105,108,221] Oral pigmented areas often appear as spots or striations on the buccal mucosa, palate, gingiva, or tongue (Fig. 28.12). At present, most reports

Fig. 28.12 Drug-Induced Hyperpigmentation as a Result of Zidovudine Use. (A) Fingernail bed discoloration. (B) Palatal hyperpigmentation in the same patient. (C) Tongue hyperpigmentation in the same patient. Note the similarity between the oral lesions and those caused by adrenal cortex hypofunction (i.e., Addison disease).

describing the oral features of HIV/AIDS or post-HAART HIV/AIDS come from areas of the world where racial pigmentation may be common. In these areas, oral evaluation may often be accomplished by non-dental health care workers. Consequently it is not possible to accurately assess the degree of HIV-related oral hyperpigmentation before or after ART.

In some cases, the pigmentation may relate to the prolonged use of drugs such as zidovudine, ketoconazole, or clofazimine.[221] Zidovudine is also associated with excessive pigmentation of the skin and nails, although similar hyperpigmentation has been reported in some individuals who have never taken zidovudine. On occasion, oral pigmentation may be the result of adrenocorticoid insufficiency induced in an HIV-positive individual by the prolonged use of ketoconazole or by *Pneumocystis jirovecii*, CMV, or other viral infections (see Fig. 28.12).[108]

Atypical Ulcers

Atypical ulcers (nonspecific oral ulcerations) in HIV-infected individuals may have multiple etiologies including neoplasms such as lymphoma, KS, and squamous cell carcinoma. HIV-associated neutropenia may also feature oral ulcerations.

HIV-infected patients have a higher incidence of recurrent herpetic lesions and aphthous stomatitis (Figs. 28.13 and 28.14). Approximately 10% of HIV-infected patients have herpes infection,[153] and multiple episodes are common. The CDC HIV classification system indicates that mucocutaneous herpes that lasts more than 1 month is diagnostic of AIDS in HIV-infected individuals.[32] Aphthae and aphthae-like lesions are common when patients are followed throughout the course of their immunosuppression.[77]

Salivary Gland Disorders and Xerostomia

Salivary gland hypofunction and xerostomia may be most common among HIV-infected men during both the early and advanced stages of HIV infection and immunosuppression. Salivary function does not appear to be affected by HAART despite the fact that some individual antiretroviral medications are reported to induce xerostomia. However, it is clear that xerostomia is a relatively common condition among HIV-infected individuals and that up to 10% of these patients may be affected. Xerostomia appears to become more severe as immunosuppression worsens, and increased candidal carriage is associated with a reduced rate of salivary flow.[100]

Fig. 28.13 Abnormal Herpetic Lesions in Individuals With Human Immunodeficiency Virus. (A) The lip crusting of primary herpetic gingivostomatitis. (B) Ulcerations of the gingiva, the alveolar mucosa, and the vestibule in the same patient. (C) Severe herpes labialis in the commissures of the lip. (D) A close-up view of herpes labialis. Note the fluid-filled vesicles.

Fig. 28.14 Intraoral Aphthous Stomatitis in a Patient With Acquired Immunodeficiency Syndrome. (A) Major aphthous lesion in the left soft palate. (B) Ulcerations of the uvula in the same patient.

Fig. 28.15 Linear Gingival Erythema and Necrotizing Ulcerative Gingivitis in a Patient With Acquired Immunodeficiency Syndrome.

Fig. 28.16 Mild Linear Gingival Erythema. The patient had a T4 count of 9 and a viral load that was too numerous to count.

COMPLICATIONS OF DENTAL TREATMENT

Concerns have been expressed regarding the potential for post-operative complications (e.g., hemorrhage, infection, delayed wound healing) in individuals with HIV or AIDS. Medically compromised patients must be carefully managed in the dental office to avoid undue treatment complications.[48] However, *systematic reviews of the literature indicate that special precautions are usually not necessary based simply on the HIV status of patients when periodontal treatment—involving procedures such as dental prophylaxis, scaling and root planing, periodontal surgery, extractions, and the placement of implants—is being given.* On occasion, the poor overall health status of an individual with AIDS may limit periodontal therapy to conservative minimally invasive procedures, and antibiotic therapy may be required.[10,51,52,74,150] When possible, antibiotics should be avoided in significantly immunocompromised individuals so as to minimize the risk of opportunistic infections (e.g., candidiasis), superinfection, and microorganism drug resistance.[130]

GINGIVAL AND PERIODONTAL DISEASES

Considerable research has focused on the nature and incidence of periodontal diseases in HIV-infected individuals. Some studies suggest that chronic periodontitis ("periodontitis" in the new classification) is more common in this patient population, but others do not. Periodontal diseases are more common among HIV-infected users of injection drugs, but this may relate to poor oral hygiene and a lack of dental care rather than decreased CD4+ cell counts. However, some unusual types of periodontal diseases do seem to occur with greater frequency among HIV-positive individuals.[11,86,107,153,163,199]

Linear Gingival Erythema

A persistent, linear, easily bleeding, erythematous gingivitis has been described in some HIV-positive patients. The intensity of the erythema is disproportionate to the amount of plaque present. There is no ulceration, pocketing, or attachment loss,[206] and the condition does not respond predictably to conventional periodontal therapy. Lesions that are clinically identical to linear gingival erythema (LGE) were observed before the advent of HIV in association with severely immunocompromised individuals or in those with NUG.

LGE may or may not serve as a precursor to rapidly progressive NUP (Figs. 28.15 and 28.16).[76,78] The microflora of LGE may closely mimic that of periodontitis rather than gingivitis. However, *Candida* infection has been implicated as a major etiologic factor, and human herpesviruses have been proposed as possible triggers or cofactors.[7,42,173,192,206] Linear gingivitis lesions may be localized or generalized in nature. The erythematous gingivitis may be limited to marginal tissue, extend into attached gingiva in a punctate or diffuse erythema, or extend into the alveolar mucosa.

Necrotizing Ulcerative Gingivitis

Some reports have described an increased incidence of NUG among HIV-infected individuals, although this has not been substantiated by other studies.[54,77,78,95,175,197]

There is no consensus regarding whether the incidence of NUG increases in HIV-positive patients.[147,150,168,184] However, one study evaluated the HIV status of individuals who presented with necrotizing periodontal diseases, and 69% were found to be HIV seropositive.[185] The treatment of NUG in these patients does not differ from that in HIV-negative individuals (see Chapter 40).

Necrotizing Ulcerative Periodontitis

A necrotizing, ulcerative, rapidly progressive form of periodontitis occurs more frequently among HIV-positive individuals, although such lesions were described long before the onset of the AIDS epidemic. NUP appears to represent an extension of NUG in which the loss of bone and periodontal attachment occurs.[140,184]

NUP is characterized by soft tissue necrosis, rapid periodontal destruction, and interproximal bone loss (Figs. 28.17 to 28.19).[78,156] Lesions may occur anywhere in the dental arches; they are usually localized to a few teeth, although generalized NUP is sometimes present after marked CD4+ cell depletion. Bone is often exposed, which results in necrosis and subsequent sequestration. NUP is severely painful at onset, and immediate treatment is necessary. Occasionally, however, patients undergo spontaneous resolution of the necrotizing lesions, which leave painless, deep, interproximal craters that are difficult to clean and may lead to conventional periodontitis.[76]

Therapy for NUP includes local debridement; scaling and root planing; in-office irrigation with an effective antimicrobial agent such as chlorhexidine gluconate or povidone-iodine (Betadine); and the establishment of meticulous oral hygiene, including the home use of antimicrobial rinses or irrigation.[150,155,176] This therapeutic approach is based on reports that involved only a small number of patients.

In patients with severe NUP, antibiotic therapy may be necessary, but it should be used with caution in HIV-infected patients

Fig. 28.17 Necrotizing Ulcerative Periodontitis. Note the adjacent linear gingival erythema.

Fig. 28.18 Necrotizing Ulcerative Periodontitis in an Otherwise Healthy 19-Year-Old Man Without Human Immunodeficiency Virus. (A) Anterior maxilla. (B) Palatal view.

Fig. 28.19 Early Necrotizing Ulcerative Periodontitis in a Patient With Acquired Immunodeficiency Syndrome. (A) Facial view. (B) Lingual view. (C) Facial view of the complete resolution of necrotizing ulcerative periodontitis after treatment. (D) Lingual view.

to avoid an opportunistic and potentially serious localized candidiasis or even candidal septicemia.[128] If an antibiotic is necessary, metronidazole (250 mg, with two tablets taken immediately and then two tablets taken four times daily for 5 to 7 days) is the drug of choice. The prophylactic prescription of a topical or systemic antifungal agent is prudent if an antibiotic is to be used.

Periodontitis

A number of longitudinal studies and prevalence studies have suggested that HIV-positive individuals are more likely to experience periodontitis than the general population.[11,125,134,164] Most studies, however, do not take into account the level of oral hygiene, the presence of preexisting gingivitis, poor diet, the age of the patient, smoking, other periodontal disease risk factors, the degree of immunodeficiency in the population studied, or whether the individuals in the study are IDUs; these confounding factors cloud the issue.

With proper home care and appropriate periodontal treatment and maintenance, HIV-positive individuals can anticipate reasonably good periodontal health throughout the course of their disease.[102] The median period between initial HIV infection and outright AIDS is approximately 15 years, and the life expectancy of persons living with AIDS has been significantly prolonged with current anti-HIV drug therapy.[20,33]

This indicates that HIV-infected patients are potential candidates for conventional periodontal treatment procedures, including surgery and implant placement. Treatment decisions should be based on the overall health status of the patient, the degree of periodontal involvement, and the motivation and ability of the patient to perform effective oral hygiene (Fig. 28.20).

Clearly, some less common periodontal diseases do occur more frequently in HIV-positive individuals, but these same conditions are also reported among HIV-negative persons. Consequently definitions for these conditions and discussions of their management should not be construed as limiting them to individuals with HIV or AIDS.

PERIODONTAL TREATMENT PROTOCOL

It is imperative that medically compromised patients, including those with HIV or AIDS, be safely and effectively managed in dental practice.[185] Several universal treatment considerations are important to ensure that this goal is achieved.

Fig. 28.20 Periodontal Health in an Individual With Advanced Acquired Immunodeficiency Syndrome.

Health Status

The patient's health status should be determined from the health history, the physical evaluation, and consultation with the patient's physician. Treatment decisions will vary depending on the patient's state of health. For example, delayed wound healing and an increased risk of postoperative infection are possible complicating factors in patients with AIDS, but neither concern should significantly alter treatment planning for an otherwise healthy asymptomatic HIV-infected patient with a normal or near-normal CD4+ count and a low viral bioload.[70,89,117,158]

Infection Control Measures

The clinical management of HIV-infected periodontal patients requires strict adherence to established methods of infection control, which should be based on guidance from the American Dental Association and the CDC. Compliance, especially with standard precautions, will eliminate or minimize risks to both patients and the dental staff.[70,114,210] Immunocompromised patients are potentially at risk for acquiring as well as transmitting infections in the dental office and other health care facilities.[110,129,141]

Goals of Therapy

A thorough oral examination will determine the patient's dental treatment needs. The primary goal of dental therapy should be the restoration and maintenance of oral health, comfort, and function. At the very least, periodontal treatment goals should be directed toward the control of HIV-associated mucosal diseases, such as chronic candidiasis and recurrent oral ulcerations. Acute periodontal and dental infections should be managed, and the patient should receive detailed instructions regarding the performance of effective oral hygiene procedures.[74,93]

Conservative nonsurgical periodontal therapy should be a treatment option for virtually all HIV-positive patients, and the performance of elective surgical periodontal procedures, including implant placement, have been reported.[73,176] NUP or NUS can be severely destructive to periodontal structures, but a history of these conditions does not automatically dictate the extraction of involved teeth unless the patient is unable to maintain effective oral hygiene in the affected areas. Decisions regarding elective periodontal procedures should be made with the informed consent of the patient and after medical consultation when possible.

Maintenance Therapy

It is imperative for the patient to maintain meticulous personal oral hygiene. In addition, periodontal maintenance recall visits should be conducted at short intervals (i.e., every 2 to 3 months), and any progressive periodontal disease should be treated vigorously.[219]

As mentioned previously, systemic antibiotic therapy should be administered with caution. Blood and other medical laboratory tests may be required to monitor the patient's overall health status, and close consultation and coordination with the patient's physician is necessary.

Psychologic Factors

HIV infection of neuronal cells may affect brain function and lead to dementia. This may profoundly influence the responsiveness of affected patients to dental treatment. However, psychologic factors are numerous in virtually all HIV-infected patients even in the absence of neuronal lesions.

Patients may be greatly concerned with the maintenance of medical confidentiality, and such confidentiality must be upheld. Coping with a life-threatening disease may elicit depression, anxiety, and anger in such patients, and this anger may be directed toward the oral health care provider and/or the staff. It is important to display concern and understanding for the patient's situation. Treatment should be provided in a calm, relaxed atmosphere, and stress to the patient must be minimized.[6]

The oral health care team should be prepared to advise and counsel patients regarding their oral health status. Oral health care providers often encounter HIV-infected patients who are unaware of their disease status. Early diagnosis and treatment of HIV infection can have a profound effect on the patient's life expectancy and quality of life, and the oral health care team should be prepared to help patients to obtain testing.[180,187] Any patient with oral lesions that are suggestive of HIV infection should be informed of the findings and, if appropriate, questioned about any previous exposure to HIV. If HIV testing is requested, it must be accompanied by patient counseling; therefore it may be best to obtain such tests through medical referral.

REFERENCES

 References for this chapter are found on the companion website.

Clinical Periodontics

Levels of Clinical Significance[a]

In one study of periodontal tissue regeneration, investigators reported that treatment resulting in a gain of 1.2 mm in clinical attachment level and a reduction of 1 mm in probing pocket depth "may not have a great clinical impact."[5] In another study of a local antimicrobial, the investigators reported that a treatment resulting in a gain of 0.0 mm in clinical attachment level and a reduction of 0.2 mm in probing depth had such clinical significance that it should "be used universally."[27] The American Dental Association (ADA) has defined "a substantial effect" as a mean change in attachment level greater than 0.6 mm.[23] These examples illustrate that different individuals will reach different decisions regarding what is meant by the term *clinical significance*. As a result, the term *clinically significant* has become more useful to marketers than to clinicians.

The term *clinically significant* could be made more relevant by recognizing (1) the nature of the benefits (tangible/intangible) and (2) the size of the treatment effect (large/small). The presence or absence of these two criteria can be used to classify clinical significance into four levels. Before doing so, this chapter describes each classification term.

TANGIBLE VERSUS INTANGIBLE BENEFITS

Controversies remain as to whether outcomes tested in clinical trials designed for drug approval are tangible to the patient.[7,28] Some will argue that the clinical significance of a treatment should depend exclusively on whether the benefits identified are tangible or intangible to the patient who undergoes the procedure.

Tangible benefits are treatment outcomes that reflect how a patient feels, functions, or survives. The word *tangible* is defined

as "capable of being precisely identified or realized by the mind." Examples of tangible benefits could include improved oral health–related quality of life,[13,14] a decrease in self-reported symptoms (e.g., bleeding) after brushing, prevention of tooth loss, or elimination of a painful periodontal abscess. These examples of treatment benefits can precisely be identified or realized by the *patient's mind*—that is, they are tangible. Tangible benefits can also be referred to as "clinically relevant" or "clinically meaningful" benefits.

> **KEY FACT**
>
> The issues with surrogate endpoints were recognized when the first randomized controlled trial in periodontics was published.[4] Almost half a century later, these issues remain largely unaddressed.

Intangible benefits cannot be realized or perceived by the patient's mind. Changes in probing attachment level as a result of scaling, changes in enamel mineralization level as a result of fluoride application, and changes in the size of a periapical radiolucency as a result of root canal treatment are examples of changes that the patient's mind cannot identify or realize; thus they are described as intangible treatment benefits. Intangible treatment benefits can often be measured objectively by the clinician or by laboratory methods.

The first and most important step in assessing the clinical significance of a treatment is to determine whether the documented treatment benefits are tangible or intangible. This distinction is important because intangible benefits often do not translate into tangible benefits. A medication that lowers elevated blood lipid levels (an intangible benefit) may shorten life span (a tangible patient harm). A treatment that increases bone density (an intangible benefit) can increase fracture risk (a tangible patient harm).[10] A treatment that provides extensive periodontal

[a]Adapted from the following chapter of Newman and Carranza's Clinical Periodontology, 13th edition: Chapter 31: Levels of Clinical Significance, by Philippe P. Huijel.

bone regeneration (an intangible benefit) may lead to tooth loss (a tangible harm).[12] A treatment that has been shown to provide tangible benefits has a higher level of clinical significance than a treatment for which only evidence of intangible benefits exists. The finding that implant-supported dentures improve quality of life[1] has a higher level of clinical significance than the finding that scaling increases levels of probing attachment. The finding that an endodontic treatment reliably eliminates tooth pain has a higher level of clinical significance than the finding that chlorhexidine reduces levels of *Streptococcus mutans*.

> ### KEY FACT
>
> True endpoints are tangible outcome measures. Loss of masticatory efficiency in a patient following tooth loss is an example of a tangible outcome. Surrogate endpoints are intangible to patients; examples include probing depth and changes in clinical attachment level following scaling and root planing.

SIZE OF THE TREATMENT EFFECT

A second important criterion for assessing clinical significance is the size of the treatment effect. This involves a comparison of the success rates of the experimental treatment and the control treatment. It can be a subtraction of the success rates, a division of the success rates, or some other mathematical operation. The size of the treatment effect, regardless of how it is calculated, has long been recognized as an important part of assessing clinical significance. The larger the likelihood of obtaining an expected benefit of a treatment (relative to a control treatment), the more clinically significant the treatment is.

The likelihood of obtaining a treatment benefit (relative to the control) largely determines the methodologic and analytic rigor required to establish treatment effectiveness. At one extreme, in all-or-none situations, reliable evidence may result from observations of a small number of patients. For example, no concurrent controlled trials were conducted to assess the effectiveness of general anesthesia. Determining the effectiveness of treatments that achieve a dramatic and immediate effect is straightforward, and only essential scientific principles (e.g., consistency of observations across different operators) are considered sufficient evidence of treatment effectiveness. Reportedly, the statement, "Gentlemen, this is no humbug," were sufficient to convince an audience that general anesthesia was effective.

> ### KEY FACT
>
> As in medicine, randomized controlled trials conducted in periodontics have primarily focused on surrogate endpoints. Having true endpoints in future randomized controlled trials will enhance the clinical applicability and relevance of their results.

At another extreme, if the likelihood of obtaining an expected treatment benefit is small, substantial rigor in both design and analysis of controlled clinical trials is required. The benefits of mammography screening for the early detection of breast cancer, of one "clot-buster" drug over another after a myocardial event,

and of local antibiotics in the treatment of periodontitis are all so small that large randomized controlled trials are required to provide reliable evidence as to whether small benefits indeed are associated with the treatment.

The likelihood of obtaining a treatment benefit is a determinant of clinical significance; the larger the likelihood, the more confident a patient can feel that a treatment will be successful. Although it is possible to have a clear, unequivocal definition of what constitutes a tangible benefit associated with treatment, it is not possible to have a similar rigorous definition of what can be considered a large likelihood.

> ### CLINICAL CORRELATION
>
> Many periodontal treatments result in small changes in clinical attachment levels or probing depths and consequently lead to questions regarding the clinical significance of periodontal therapy. For instance, one systematic review reported by the ADA indicated that the addition of metronidazole to scaling and root planing provided an additional gain of 0.18 mm in attachment level. The ADA refers to such an effect as a "zero effect."[23] Small to zero treatment effects are common in clinical trials in medicine.

DEFINING FOUR LEVELS OF CLINICAL SIGNIFICANCE

Based on the nature of the benefit (tangible/intangible) and the size of the treatment effect (large/small), four levels of clinical significance can be defined (Table 29.1). In order of decreasing levels of significance, these are numbered from 1 to 4.

Level 1 Clinical Significance

Treatments of clinical significance level 1 are the "magic bullets" or "miracle cures" in which the treatment provides a tangible benefit and a large treatment effect. Examples include the use of vitamin C to treat scurvy, bone marrow transplantation to treat leukemia, and a very low-carbohydrate diet to prevent all forms of dental decay. In all three examples, the benefits of the treatment are tangible and the size of the treatment effect is large.

TABLE 29.1   Definition of Levels of Significance Based on Size and Nature of the Benefit

Clinical Significance		SIZE OF THE BENEFIT	
		Large[c]	Small[d]
Nature of the benefit	Tangible[a]	Level 1	Level 2
	Intangible[b]	Level 3	Level 4

[a]Tangible benefits are outcomes that directly measure how a patient feels, functions, or survives.
[b]Intangible benefits are outcomes that are not perceivable by the patient's mind.
[c]A large benefit is defined as one that can reliably be identified using epidemiologic methodology.
[d]A small benefit is defined as one that requires randomized controlled trials for reliable identification.

Understanding the biologic mechanisms of a treatment is not required to establish that the treatment has level 1 clinical significance. Lemon juice was identified as an effective method to prevent scurvy in 1601, but it was not until the beginning of the 20th century that vitamin C was isolated.[20] The dangers of carbohydrates in dental decay were recognized millennia before potential mechanisms of action were understood. Digitalis was discovered as a treatment for "dropsy" long before physicians became aware of the drug's cardiac effects.[26] Lithium is an effective drug for bipolar disorder, but its mechanism of action remains largely unknown.[22] In contrast, hormone replacement therapy (HRT), for which the biologic mechanisms explaining how the drug provided benefits were supposedly well understood, resulted in more harm than good.[11]

> **KEY FACT**
>
> The size of the anticipated treatment effect has a profound impact on the planning of randomized clinical trials. The smaller the treatment effect, the larger the number of patients who will need to be recruited.

Treatments of level 1 clinical significance are not always immediately accepted or widely used. After the observations of Captain James Lancaster on the role of dietary factors in the causation of scurvy, it took British Navy 264 years to come up with a universal preventive policy for this condition.[3] The lack of appreciation of the clinical significance of this level 1 treatment was unfortunate.

It is estimated that 5000 lives a year were needlessly lost from scurvy during this period: that is a total of nearly 800,000 individuals. In the 200 years from 1600 to 1800, nearly a million men died of an easily preventable disease. There are in the whole of human history few more notable examples of official indifference and stupidity producing such disastrous consequences.[19]

Although here it is easy, in retrospect, to determine level 1 clinical significance, it may be difficult to recognize at the time the problem was first noticed.

Level 2 Clinical Significance

Treatments of level 2 clinical significance are those that have demonstrated a tangible benefit but for which the likelihood of obtaining the benefit from treatment is small. As the size of the benefit of one therapy over another decreases, randomized controlled trials (RCTs), large in size and rigorous in execution and analysis, are required to provide unequivocal evidence that the treatment provides tangible patient benefits. Examples of such treatments include the advantages of tissue plasminogen activator (t-PA) over streptokinase[25] and the benefits of penciclovir in the treatment of herpetic lesions.[11]

Determining the clinical relevance of treatments of level 2 clinical significance is an individual choice in which issues such as cost and side effects often play a more important role. For example, the administration of antibiotics to 25 individuals could prevent 1 person from experiencing early implant loss.[6] Is a 4% increased survival probability of dental implants worth the potential side effects of antibiotics? Different individuals, different governments, and different health insurance companies may decide differently on this important question.

> **KEY FACT**
>
> In evidence-based medicine, an all-or-none situation is defined as one of the following two scenarios: (1) either all patients experienced an adverse tangible outcome before the treatment became available but some do not experience it, or (2) some patients experienced the tangible adverse outcome before the treatment became available but none now experience it. All-or-none situations reflect the highest level of evidence.[16]

Level 3 Clinical Significance

Treatments of level 3 clinical significance are the magic bullets or miracle cures in the surrogate world, where the beneficial but intangible effects seem so convincing that the implementation of RCTs may appear to be unethical. Examples of such treatments include highly active antiretroviral therapy (HAART) in patients with acquired immunodeficiency syndrome (AIDS),[15] imatinib (Gleevec) in the treatment of chronic myeloid leukemia,[26] and chlorhexidine varnish in the prevention of caries.[21] In periodontics, examples of treatments of level 3 clinical significance could include complete restoration of periodontal attachment and bone around teeth that had shown extensive destruction of the periodontal apparatus and reconstruction of voluminous amounts of bone on an atrophic mandible for the purpose of placing dental implants.

With a treatment that has the label "level 3 clinical significance," there is always uncertainty as to whether the intangible benefits translate into real, tangible patient benefits. For instance, grafting the periodontal defect with autogenous bone indeed resulted in regenerating prodigious amounts of bone, but about 50% of the teeth were lost due to root resorption.[12] Nonetheless, the larger the effect size observed on the surrogate, the more likely the surrogate benefit translates into a real, tangible patient benefit.[8]

However, assuming that large, intangible treatment benefits invariably translate into tangible benefits remains dangerous, no matter how large the effect on the surrogate endpoint. A 40% chlorhexidine varnish used for the prevention of caries was reported to result in a 99.9% reduction in counts of *Streptococcus mutans* in all 20 subjects treated, and the counts stayed below detectable levels for at least 4 weeks in 9 of the subjects. In contrast, the placebo varnish sealant led to only a 32% reduction of *S. mutans*, and none of the 20 subjects had *S. mutans* below detectable levels for 4 weeks.[16] Based on these data, it was reported that "Chlorzoin will wipe out dental decay much like smallpox." A subsequent RCT in 1240 children at high risk for caries did not translate into a reduction of large cavities in the teeth: the 10% chlorhexidine varnish (Chlorzoin) group had 6.8 D3 lesions (standard deviation, 6.2), and the placebo group had 6.4 D3 lesions (standard deviation, 6.4); in other words, the placebo group had fewer lesions.[24] It has become clear since then that most forms of chlorhexidine are contraindicated in the treatment of caries.[9] A large treatment effect on a surrogate in this instance did not translate into a tangible benefit.

Level 4 Clinical Significance

Treatments of level 4 clinical significance are those that have reliable evidence on small, intangible treatment benefits. Because the treatment effects are small, epidemiologic studies are incapable of identifying treatments of level 4 clinical significance. In other words, rigorously conducted RCTs are necessary to reliably identify a small surrogate benefit. Examples of treatments of level 4 clinical significance include those that cause a small decrease in lipid level, a small drop in blood pressure, or a small decrease in pocket depth. A large leap of faith is often required to jump from the observation that small changes in surrogate endpoints translate into real tangible benefits.

Clofibrate, used to lower lipid levels, is an example of a drug of level 4 clinical significance. Clofibrate reduced mean cholesterol levels from 324 to 224 mg and mean triglyceride levels from 271 to 125 (which can be argued are "not so small" mean changes).[2] Clofibrate was once the most widely prescribed lipid-lowering agent in the United States, but uncertainty remained as to whether it actually provided a tangible patient benefit. Advertisements that appeared widely in medical journals accurately reflected the clinical uncertainty surrounding use of this drug. A textbox within the advertisements stated, "It has not been established whether the drug-induced lowering of serum cholesterol or lipid levels has a detrimental, beneficial, or no effect on the mortality and the morbidity due to atherosclerosis or coronary heart disease. Several years will be required before current investigations will yield an answer to this question." A subsequent World Health Organization (WHO) cooperative trial on clofibrate revealed the wisdom of this disclaimer. The trial outcome showed that clofibrate resulted in excess mortality of 47%, providing yet another example of a misleading surrogate.[18]

Treatments of level 4 clinical significance may cause more harm than good.[17] This observation has significant consequences in periodontics, because approved periodontal therapies are commonly of level 4 clinical significance, and information on their long-term safety and lack of harm is minimal.

SUMMARY

Two important determinants of clinical significance are the nature of the benefit (tangible vs intangible) and the likelihood of obtaining the benefit (as compared with the control treatment). These two characteristics can be used to define four hierarchical levels of clinical significance. Treatments that provide a tangible patient benefit (levels 1 and 2) are of greater value and should correspond to a higher level of clinical significance than treatments with evidence of only intangible benefits (levels 3 and 4). Similarly, treatments with a large likelihood of clinical improvement (levels 1 and 3) are clinically more significant than treatments with a small likelihood of clinical improvement (levels 2 and 4). These four hierarchical levels of clinical significance may help clinicians and patients to communicate more effectively regarding the value of a treatment.

REFERENCES

 References for this chapter are found on the companion website.

30

Periodontal Examination and Diagnosis[a]

 For online-only content on periodontal probing, periodontal charting, clinical indices, periodontal pockets, and periodontal, gingival, and periapical abscesses, please visit the companion website.

CHAPTER OUTLINE

Proper diagnosis is essential to intelligent treatment. Periodontal diagnosis should first determine whether disease is present. It should then identify the disease and its severity and extent. Finally, it should provide an understanding of the underlying pathologic processes and their causes. Part 3 of this book provides detailed descriptions of the different diseases that can affect the periodontium.

The periodontal diagnosis is determined after careful analysis of the case history and evaluation of the clinical signs and symptoms as well as the results of various diagnostic procedures (e.g., probing, mobility assessment, radiographs, blood tests, and biopsies).

The interest should be in the patient who has the disease and not simply the disease itself. Diagnosis must therefore include a general evaluation of the patient and a consideration of the oral cavity.

Diagnostic procedures must be systematic and organized for specific purposes. It is not enough to assemble facts. Findings must be pieced together so that they provide a meaningful explanation of the patient's periodontal problem. The following is a recommended sequence of procedures for the diagnosis of periodontal diseases.

OVERALL APPRAISAL OF THE PATIENT

From the first meeting, the clinician should attempt an overall appraisal of the patient. This includes consideration of the patient's mental and emotional status, temperament, attitude,

and physiologic age, as well as individual preferences toward care, and important aspects of life context that will impact treatment decisions.

HEALTH HISTORY

Most of the health history is obtained at the first visit, and it can be supplemented by pertinent questioning at subsequent visits. The health history can be obtained verbally by questioning the patient and recording his or her responses in the patient chart or by means of a questionnaire that the patient completes prior to the appointment. Fig. 30.1 shows the health history form recommended by the American Dental Association; however, if the health history is obtained on a form, it is important to follow up with an interview to review the form with patient.

The importance of the health history should be clearly explained, because patients often omit information that they feel does not relate to their dental problems. The patient should be made aware of the following: (1) the possible impact of certain systemic diseases, conditions, behavioral factors, and medications on periodontal disease, its treatment, and treatment outcomes; (2) the presence of conditions that may require special precautions or modifications of the treatment procedure (see Chapter 36); and (3) the possibility that oral infections may have a powerful influence on the occurrence, severity and management of a variety of systemic diseases and conditions (see Chapter 14).

The health history should include reference to the following:
1. The date of the last physical exam and the frequency of physical exams and physician visits. If the patient is under the care of a physician, the nature and duration of the problem and its therapy should be discussed. The name, address, and telephone number of the physician should be recorded, because direct interprofessional collaboration may be necessary.

---

[a]Adapted from the following chapter of Newman and Carranza's Clinical Periodontology, 13th edition: Chapter 32: Periodontal Examination and Diagnosis, by Jonathan H. Do, Henry H. Takei, and Fermin A. Carranza. Updated by Peter Loomer, DDS, PhD.

Health History Form

ADA.
American Dental Association
www.ada.org

E-mail: _____ Today's Date: _____

As required by law, our office adheres to written policies and procedures to protect the privacy of information about you that we create, receive or maintain. Your answers are for our records only and will be kept confidential subject to applicable laws. Please note that you will be asked some questions about your responses to this questionnaire and there may be additional questions concerning your health. This information is vital to allow us to provide appropriate care for you. This office does not use this information to discriminate.

Name: _____
Last   First   Middle

Home Phone: *Include area code* ( )
Business/Cell Phone: *Include area code* ( )

Address: _____
Mailing address

City: _____ State: _____ Zip: _____

Occupation: _____

Height: ___ Weight: ___ Date of birth: ___ Sex: M   F

SS# or Patient ID: _____   Emergency Contact: _____   Relationship: _____   Home Phone: ( )   Cell Phone: ( )
Include area codes

If you are completing this form for another person, what is your relationship to that person?

Your Name _____   Relationship _____

Do you have any of the following diseases or problems: (Check DK if you Don't Know the answer to the question)   Yes No DK

Active tuberculosis.. ☐ ☐ ☐
Persistent cough greater than a 3 week duration .... ☐ ☐ ☐
Cough that produces blood.. ☐ ☐ ☐
Been exposed to anyone with tuberculosis.. ☐ ☐ ☐

If you answer yes to any of the 4 items above, please stop and return this form to the receptionist.

Dental Information *For the following questions, please mark (X) your responses to the following questions.*

	Yes	No	DK		Yes	No	DK
Do your gums bleed when you brush or floss?	☐	☐	☐	Do you have earaches or neck pains?	☐	☐	☐
Are your teeth sensitive to cold, hot, sweets or pressure?	☐	☐	☐	Do you have any clicking, popping or discomfort in the jaw?	☐	☐	☐
Does food or floss catch between your teeth?	☐	☐	☐	Do you brux or grind your teeth?	☐	☐	☐
Is your mouth dry?	☐	☐	☐	Do you have sores or ulcers in your mouth?	☐	☐	☐
Have you had any periodontal (gum) treatments?	☐	☐	☐	Do you wear dentures or partials?	☐	☐	☐
Have you ever had orthodontic (braces) treatment?	☐	☐	☐	Do you participate in active recreational activities?	☐	☐	☐
Have you had any problems associated with previous dental treatment?	☐	☐	☐	Have you ever had a serious injury to your head or mouth?	☐	☐	☐
Is your home water supply fluoridated?	☐	☐	☐	Date of your last dental exam:			
Do you drink bottled or filtered water?	☐	☐	☐	What was done at that time?			
If yes, how often? Circle one: DAILY / WEEKLY / OCCASIONALLY							
Are you currently experiencing dental pain or discomfort?	☐	☐	☐	Date of last dental x-rays:			

What is the reason for your dental visit today?

How do you feel about your smile?

Medical Information *Please mark (X) your response to indicate if you have or have not had any of the following diseases or problems.*

	Yes	No	DK		Yes	No	DK
Are you now under the care of a physician?	☐	☐	☐	Have you had a serious illness, operation or been hospitalized in the past 5 years?	☐	☐	☐
Physician Name: ___ Phone: *Include area code* ( )				If yes, what was the illness or problem?			
Address/City/State/Zip:				Are you taking or have you recently taken any prescription or over the counter medicine(s)?	☐	☐	☐
Are you in good health?	☐	☐	☐	If so, please list all, including vitamins, natural or herbal preparations and/or diet supplements:			
Has there been any change in your general health within the past year?	☐	☐	☐	_____			
If yes, what condition is being treated?				_____			
Date of last physical exam:				_____			

© 2007 American Dental Association
Form S500

Fig. 30.1 Medical History Form From the American Dental Association. (Copyright American Dental Association. Reprinted with permission.)

Medical Information
Please mark (X) your response to indicate if you have or have not had any of the following diseases or problems.

(Check DK if you Don't Know the answer to the question)	Yes	No	DK
Do you wear contact lenses?	☐	☐	☐

Joint Replacement. Have you had an orthopedic total joint (hip, knee, elbow, finger) replacement? ☐ ☐ ☐
Date: _____ If yes, have you had any complications? _____

Are you taking or scheduled to begin taking either of the medications, alendronate (Fosamax®) or risedronate (Actonel®) for osteoporosis or Paget's disease? ☐ ☐ ☐

Since 2001, were you treated or are you presently scheduled to begin treatment with the intravenous bisphosphonates (Aredia® or Zometa®) for bone pain, hypercalcemia or skeletal complications resulting from Paget's disease, multiple myeloma or metastatic cancer? ☐ ☐ ☐
Date Treatment began: _____

	Yes	No	DK
Do you use controlled substances (drugs)?	☐	☐	☐
Do you use tobacco (smoking, snuff, chew, bidis)?	☐	☐	☐

If so, how interested are you in stopping?
(Circle one) VERY / SOMEWHAT / NOT INTERESTED

	Yes	No	DK
Do you drink alcoholic beverages?	☐	☐	☐

If yes, how much alcohol did you drink in the last 24 hours? _____
If yes, how much do you typically drink In a week? _____

WOMEN ONLY Are you:

	Yes	No	DK
Pregnant?	☐	☐	☐
Number of weeks: _____			
Taking birth control pills or hormonal replacement?	☐	☐	☐
Nursing?	☐	☐	☐

Allergies - Are you allergic to or have you had a reaction to:
To all **yes** responses, specify type of reaction.

	Yes	No	DK
Local anesthetics _____	☐	☐	☐
Aspirin _____	☐	☐	☐
Penicillin or other antibiotics _____	☐	☐	☐
Barbiturates, sedatives, or sleeping pills _____	☐	☐	☐
Sulfa drugs _____	☐	☐	☐
Codeine or other narcotics _____	☐	☐	☐

	Yes	No	DK
Metals _____	☐	☐	☐
Latex (rubber) _____	☐	☐	☐
Iodine _____	☐	☐	☐
Hay fever/seasonal _____	☐	☐	☐
Animals _____	☐	☐	☐
Food _____	☐	☐	☐
Other _____	☐	☐	☐

Please mark (X) your response to indicate if you have or have not had any of the following diseases or problems.

	Yes	No	DK		Yes	No	DK		Yes	No	DK
Artificial (prosthetic) heart valve	☐	☐	☐	Autoimmune disease	☐	☐	☐	Hepatitis, jaundice or			
Previous infective endocarditis	☐	☐	☐	Rheumatoid arthritis	☐	☐	☐	liver disease	☐	☐	☐
Damaged valves in transplanted heart	☐	☐	☐	Systemic lupus erythematosus.	☐	☐	☐	Epilepsy	☐	☐	☐
Congenital heart disease (CHD)				Asthma	☐	☐	☐	Fainting spells or seizures	☐	☐	☐
Unrepaired, cyanotic CHD	☐	☐	☐	Bronchitis	☐	☐	☐	Neurological disorders	☐	☐	☐
Repaired (completely) in last 6 months	☐	☐	☐	Emphysema	☐	☐	☐	If yes, specify: _____			
Repaired CHD with residual defects	☐	☐	☐	Sinus trouble	☐	☐	☐	Sleep disorder	☐	☐	☐
				Tuberculosis	☐	☐	☐	Mental health disorders	☐	☐	☐
Except for the conditions listed above, antibiotic prophylaxis is no longer recommended for any other form of CHD.				Cancer/Chemotherapy/				Specify: _____			
				Radiation Treatment	☐	☐	☐	Recurrent infections	☐	☐	☐

	Yes	No	DK		Yes	No	DK		Yes	No	DK		Yes	No	DK
Cardiovascular disease.	☐	☐	☐	Mitral valve prolapse	☐	☐	☐	Chest pain upon exertion	☐	☐	☐	Type of infection: _____			
Angina	☐	☐	☐	Pacemaker	☐	☐	☐	Chronic pain	☐	☐	☐	Kidney problems	☐	☐	☐
Arteriosclerosis	☐	☐	☐	Rheumatic fever	☐	☐	☐	Diabetes Type I or II	☐	☐	☐	Night sweats	☐	☐	☐
Congestive heart failure	☐	☐	☐	Rheumatic heart disease	☐	☐	☐	Eating disorder	☐	☐	☐	Osteoporosis	☐	☐	☐
Damaged heart valves	☐	☐	☐	Abnormal bleeding	☐	☐	☐	Malnutrition	☐	☐	☐	Persistent swollen glands			
Heart attack	☐	☐	☐	Anemia	☐	☐	☐	Gastrointestinal disease	☐	☐	☐	in neck	☐	☐	☐
Heart murmur	☐	☐	☐	Blood transfusion	☐	☐	☐	G.E. Reflux/persistent				Severe headaches/			
Low blood pressure	☐	☐	☐	If yes, date: _____				heartburn	☐	☐	☐	migraines	☐	☐	☐
High blood pressure	☐	☐	☐	Hemophilia	☐	☐	☐	Ulcers	☐	☐	☐	Severe or rapid weight loss	☐	☐	☐
Other congenital heart				AIDS or HIV infection	☐	☐	☐	Thyroid problems	☐	☐	☐	Sexually transmitted disease	☐	☐	☐
defects	☐	☐	☐	Arthritis	☐	☐	☐	Stroke	☐	☐	☐	Excessive urination	☐	☐	☐
								Glaucoma	☐	☐	☐				

	Yes	No	DK
Has a physician or previous dentist recommended that you take antibiotics prior to your dental treatment?	☐	☐	☐

Name of physician or dentist making recommendation: _____ | Phone: _____

	Yes	No	DK
Do you have any disease, condition, or problem not listed above that you think I should know about?	☐	☐	☐
Please explain:

NOTE: Both doctor and patient are encouraged to discuss any and all relevant patient health issues prior to treatment.
I certify that I have read and understand the above and that the information given on this form is accurate. I understand the importance of a truthful health history and that my dentist and his/her staff will rely on this information for treating me. I acknowledge that my questions, if any, about inquiries set forth above have been answered to my satisfaction. I will not hold my dentist, or any other member of his/her staff, responsible for any action they take or do not take because of errors or omissions that I may have made in the completion of this form.

Signature of Patient/Legal Guardian: _____ | Date: _____

FOR COMPLETION BY DENTIST
Comments: _____
_____
_____
_____

Fig. 30.1, cont'd

2. Details regarding hospitalizations and operations, including the diagnosis, the type of operation, and any untoward events (e.g., anesthetic, hemorrhagic, or infectious complications) should be obtained.

3. All medical problems (e.g., cardiovascular, hematologic, endocrine), including infectious diseases, sexually transmitted infections, high-risk behavior for human immunodeficiency virus infection, and possible occupational disease, should be inquired.

4. Abnormal bleeding tendencies, such as nosebleeds, prolonged bleeding from minor cuts, spontaneous ecchymosis, a tendency toward excessive bruising, and excessive menstrual bleeding, should be cited. These symptoms should be correlated with the medications that the patient is taking.

5. Information is needed for females regarding the onset of puberty, menopause, menstrual disorders, hysterectomy, pregnancies, and miscarriages.

6. A list of all medications being taken and whether they were prescribed or obtained over the counter should be included. All of the possible effects of these medications should be carefully analyzed to determine their effect, if any, on the oral tissues and also to avoid administering medications that would interact adversely with them. Special inquiry should be made regarding the dosage and duration of therapy with anticoagulants and corticosteroids. Patients who are taking any of the family of drugs called bisphosphonates (e.g., Actonel, Fosamax, Boniva, Aredia, and Zometa), which are often prescribed for osteoporosis, should be cautioned about possible problems related to osteonecrosis of the jaw after undergoing any form of oral surgery involving bone.

7. The patient's allergy history should be taken, including that related to hay fever, asthma, sensitivity to foods, sensitivity to drugs (e.g., aspirin, codeine, barbiturates, sulfonamides, antibiotics, procaine, and laxatives), and sensitivity to dental materials (e.g., latex, eugenol, nickel, and acrylic resins).

8. A family history should be taken, including that of bleeding disorders, cardiovascular disease, diabetes, or periodontal diseases.

9. Detailed information on current and history of alcohol, recreational drugs, and tobacco use, and desire to quit should be elicited.

As part of the overall patient appraisal, baseline vitals—at minimum, blood pressure—should be obtained. For patients who are on medications such as bisphosphonates, anticoagulants, or antiplatelets, or patients who do not know the control of their systemic disease, such as diabetes, hypertension, or immunodeficiency, a medical consultation is required before any treatment can be rendered.

DENTAL HISTORY

Chief Complaint and Current Illness

Some patients may be unaware of any problems. However, many may report bleeding gums, loose teeth, spreading of the teeth with the appearance of spaces where none existed before, foul taste in the mouth, or an itchy feeling in the gums that is relieved by digging with a toothpick. There may also be pain of varied types

and duration, including constant, dull, gnawing pain; dull pain after eating; deep radiating pain in the jaws; acute throbbing pain; sensitivity when chewing; sensitivity to hot and cold; burning sensation in the gums; or extreme sensitivity to inhaled air.

The dental history should include reference to the following:

1. Visits to the dentist should be listed, including their frequency, the date of the most recent visit, the nature of the treatment, and dental prophylaxis, periodontal maintenance, or scaling and root planing by a dentist or hygienist, including the frequency of cleaning and date of the most recent cleaning.

2. The patient's oral hygiene regimen should be described, including toothbrushing frequency, time of day, method, type of toothbrush, and interval when brushes are replaced. Other methods for mouth care, such as mouthrinses, interdental brushes, dental floss, water irrigation, and other devices should also be listed. Whether or not the patient is using a toothpaste with or without fluoride should also be noted.

3. Any orthodontic treatment, including its duration, the approximate date of termination, and use of any retainers, should be noted.

4. If the patient is experiencing pain in the teeth or in the gingiva, the manner in which the pain is provoked, its nature and duration, and the manner in which it is relieved should be described.

5. Note the presence of any gingival bleeding, including when it first occurred; whether it occurs spontaneously, on brushing or eating, at night, or with regular periodicity; whether it is associated with the menstrual period or other specific factors; and its duration of the bleeding and the manner by which it is stopped.

6. A bad taste in the mouth and areas of food impaction should be mentioned.

7. Assess whether the patient's teeth feel "loose" or insecure, if he or she has any difficulty chewing, and whether there is any tooth mobility.

8. Note the patient's general dental habits, such as grinding or clenching of the teeth during the day or at night. Do the teeth or jaw muscles feel "sore" in the morning? Are there other habits to address, such as tobacco smoking or chewing, nail biting, or biting on foreign objects?

9. Discuss the patient's history of previous periodontal problems, including the nature of the condition and, if it was previously treated, the type of treatment received (surgical or nonsurgical), and the approximate period of termination. If, in the opinion of the patient, the present problem is a recurrence of previous disease, what does he or she think caused it?

10. Note whether the patient wears a removable prosthesis. Does the prosthesis enhance or is it a detriment to the existing dentition or the surrounding soft tissues?

11. Does the patient have implants to replace any missing teeth?

> **KEY FACTS**
>
> Periodontal examination and diagnosis must include obtaining a thorough health and dental history.

Fig. 30.2 **Initial Set of Intra-Oral Photographs.** (A) Right lateral view. (B) Frontal view. (C) Left lateral view. (D) Maxillary view. (E) Mandibular view. (From Kebschull M, Dommisch H: Resektive parodontalchirurgie. *Zahnmedizin* up-2-date. 525–545, 2012.)

PHOTOGRAPHIC DOCUMENTATION

An important part of periodontal examination and diagnosis is the documentation of clinical findings. Digital photographic documentation is important and useful for record-keeping, education of both the clinician and the patient, communication with referrals and colleagues, and planning and treatment of high-aesthetic-demand cases. Photographs can provide details that a clinician may not otherwise remember and allow the clinician to evaluate the mouth after the patient leaves and to monitor changes in the tissue over time. If possible, at the beginning of the clinical examination, a set of intraoral photos (Fig. 30.2) should be taken before the tissue is probed and manipulated to obtain an undisturbed baseline of the patient's mouth with gingiva and biofilm intact. These initial photos, when presented to the patient on a large-screen monitor, can be extremely powerful in educating and helping the patient to understand the conditions of his or her mouth; the presence and location of biofilm, inflammation, and any tissue abnormality; and the need for improvement in oral hygiene or treatment.

KEY FACTS

Initial photographs should be taken before the tissue is probed and manipulated to obtain an undisturbed baseline of the patient's mouth with gingiva and biofilm intact.

CLINICAL EXAMINATION

Examination of Extraoral Structures

Clinical examination should begin with an evaluation of the extraoral structures for abnormalities. The temporomandibular joints should be assessed for pain, crepitus, clicking, and range of motion. The muscles of mastication should be palpated for pain and tenderness.

Because periodontal, periapical, and other oral diseases may result in lymph node changes, the dental hygienist should routinely examine and evaluate the lymph nodes of the head and neck. Lymph nodes can become enlarged or indurated as a result of an infectious episode, malignant metastases, or residual fibrotic changes.

Inflammatory nodes become enlarged, palpable, tender, and fairly immobile. The overlying skin may be red and warm. Patients are often aware of the presence of "swollen glands." Primary herpetic gingivostomatitis, necrotizing ulcerative gingivitis, and acute periodontal abscesses may produce lymph node enlargement. After successful therapy, lymph nodes return to normal in a matter of days to weeks.

Examination of the Oral Cavity

The entire oral cavity should be carefully examined, beginning with oral hygiene. The cleanliness of the oral cavity is appraised in terms of the extent of accumulated food debris, biofilm, calculus, and tooth surface stains, as well as biofilm coating of the dorsum of the tongue (Fig. 30.3). Oral malodor, which is also termed *fetor ex ore*, *fetor oris*, or *halitosis*, is a foul or offensive

Fig. 30.3 A biofilm coating of the dorsum surface of the tongue (A) can be a source of oral malodor. When the tongue is heavily coated, the biofilm may need to be scraped off with a spatula (B and C).

odor that emanates from the oral cavity. When present, mouth odors may be of diagnostic significance, and their origin may be either oral or extraoral (remote).[63] Chapter 44 discusses in detail the problems related to oral malodor.

The lips, the floor of the mouth, the tongue, the palate, the vestibule, and the oropharyngeal region should be evaluated for abnormalities and pathologies. The oral mucosa in the lateral and apical areas of the tooth may be palpated for tenderness to detect periapical and periodontal abscesses.

Although not all findings are related to periodontal problems, the dentist should detect all pathologic changes that are present in the mouth and, if necessary, make the appropriate dental or medical referral.

Examination of the Periodontium

The periodontal examination should be systematic and should not immediately begin with insertion of the periodontal probe into the gingival crevice, which can be uncomfortable and traumatic for a patient and may induce bleeding that may make visualization of inflammatory changes in the soft tissue challenging. Periodontal disease occurs as a result of biofilm accumulating on the tooth surface and the adjacent tissue responding to it. Therefore, the periodontal examination should begin with a thorough and careful visual evaluation of the gingival margin to assess biofilm and calculus accumulation as well as inflammatory changes in the soft tissue (Fig. 30.4). Once a thorough visual periodontal assessment has been completed, the gingiva, the gingival crevice, and the subgingival tooth surface are carefully probed. Thorough probing of the gingival crevice and the surrounding tissue provides a wealth of valuable information beyond probing depth and bleeding on probing that is essential to the diagnosis and treatment of periodontal disease.

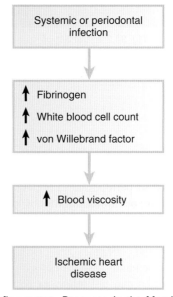

Fig. 30.4 The Inflammatory Response in the Marginal Gingiva Is a Result of Biofilm Accumulation on the Tooth Surface Along the Gingival Margin.

Visual Periodontal Examination

Visual examination begins with drying the tissue and taking a survey of biofilm and calculus accumulation to assess oral hygiene as well as clinical signs of inflammation (erythema, edema, etc.) and recession to assess the presence and severity of disease.

Visual Examination of Biofilm and Calculus

There are many methods available for assessing biofilm and calculus accumulation.[19] The presence of biofilm and supragingival calculus can be observed directly. Biofilm frequently accumulates in concavities along the gingival margins and in embrasure spaces, especially in difficult-to-reach places, such as the distal surface of the distal-most tooth in the quadrant and the lingual surfaces of the mandibular molars. Supragingival calculus commonly

KEY FACTS

Examination of the periodontium consists of two parts: visual examination and tactile examination.

accumulates on the lingual surfaces of the mandibular anterior teeth and the buccal surfaces of the maxillary molars due to the presence of the respective Wharton and Stensen salivary ducts and ineffective biofilm removal. The amount and location of biofilm and supragingival calculus may provide insights into the effectiveness of the patient's biofilm control as well as possible inflammatory changes in the tissue. Biofilm on the buccal and facial surfaces of teeth closest to the midline are most accessible for removal. The presence of biofilm in these areas may suggest inadequate oral hygiene (see Fig. 30.4). The absence of biofilm may not necessarily indicate that the patient practices good oral hygiene at home or that the disease is absent, as many patients, out of courtesy, brush their teeth thoroughly before seeing a dental professional. The presence or absence of biofilm should be correlated to the presence and severity or absence of gingival inflammation.

The presence of subgingival calculus may not be easily detected. Sometimes shallow subgingival calculus may be visible along the gingival margin or through the soft tissue if the soft tissue is thin (Fig. 30.5). Most of the time, subgingival calculus will need to be detected by careful probing of the root surface. The presence of inflammatory changes in the soft tissue may provide clues to the location of the subgingival calculus.

Although radiographs may sometimes reveal heavy calculus deposits interproximally and even on the facial and lingual surfaces, they cannot be relied on for thorough detection of calculus.

Visual Examination of the Gingiva

The gingiva is the keratinized collar of masticatory mucosa around the teeth. It extends from the gingival margin to the mucogingival junction. On the palate, where the mucogingival junction is absent, the gingiva extends apically from the mucogingival junction and merges seamlessly with the mucosa of the hard palate.

The width of the gingiva is the distance from the mucogingival junction to the gingival margin. The mucogingival junction can be determined by stretching the lip and cheek or by placing a probe horizontally in the vestibule and rolling to the mucosa coronally. The mucogingival junction is where the mucosa stops rolling or moving. It is common for teeth to be surrounded by gingiva. However, there may be sites where keratinized tissue is absent and the gingival margin is lined by nonkeratinized mucosa.

Evaluation of the gingiva requires the tissue to be dried before accurate observations can be made. The presence of saliva can obscure details. Once the gingiva is thoroughly dried with gauze, it is evaluated and assessed for inflammatory changes. Subtle inflammatory changes in the marginal gingiva may be best detected by comparing the marginal gingiva to the gingival tissue 2 or 3 mm away from the gingival margin, where the tissue is likely to be healthy. Inflammatory changes at each site are correlated with the presence and severity of biofilm and calculus. If biofilm and supragingival calculus are insignificant, inflammatory changes may suggest the presence of subgingival calculus or other contributing factors.

The appearance of the soft tissue adjacent to a tooth may vary from patient to patient, and from tooth to tooth within the same patient, depending on the location and the anatomy of the area. Generally, healthy gingiva is coral pink or salmon pink in color. The gingival contour consists of sharp, thin, knife-edge margins with scalloped gingival architecture and sharp papillae. The surface texture of healthy gingiva is matte and stippled. The presence of stippling can vary between individuals and sites within the same individual. The absence of stippling does not necessarily imply inflammatory changes in the tissue.

In the presence of inflammatory periodontal disease, the color of the gingiva may be erythematous or cyanotic. Instead of having knife-edge margins and sharp papillae gingival contours, inflamed gingiva may have rolled margins and bulbous papillae. The surface texture in the presence of inflammation may be smooth and shiny, and the gingiva may appear swollen and edematous. Table 30.1 summarizes clinical findings of healthy and inflamed gingiva. Chapter 17 further discusses the clinical features of gingival inflammation.

In individuals with physiologic pigmentation, the gingiva may be pigmented and dark in color. Even so, if healthy, it should exhibit the other features associated with gingival health. Likewise, in the presence of inflammation and disease, it should exhibit many of the characteristics of gingival inflammation (Fig. 30.6).

Fig. 30.5 Subgingival Calculus Can Be Visible on the Tooth Surface Along the Gingival Margin. Its presence is associated with inflammatory changes in the tissue.

Fig. 30.6 The Gingival Inflammation With Papillary and Marginal Erythema Is Associated With Plaque and Calculus.

TABLE 30.1 Clinical Findings of Healthy and Inflamed Gingiva

Gingiva: Healthy	Gingiva: Inflammation
• Color: coral pink or salmon pink	• Color: erythematous, cyanotic
• Consistency: firm/tight, well adapted	• Consistency: edematous, spongy, loosely adapted
• Contour: scalloped, sharp papillae, knife-edge margin	• Contour: bulbous, swollen papillae, rolled margin
• Surface texture: matte, stippled	• Surface texture: smooth, shiny
• Marginal bleeding: absent or slight	• Marginal bleeding: moderate or severe
• Probing depth: 2–3 mm	• Probing depth: >3 mm
• Tissue resistance: present to probe penetration	• Tissue resistance: minimal to probe penetration
• Bleeding on probing: absent or slight	• Bleeding on probing: moderate to severe
• Pain on probing: absent or slight	• Pain: moderate to severe

Fig. 30.7 First Premolar in the Mandibular Left Quadrant Exhibit Gingival Recession and Minimal Keratinized Tissue.

KEY FACTS

Periodontal examination begins with the visual evaluation of the gingival margin for the presence of tooth surface biofilm deposits and inflammatory changes in the gingiva.

Gingival Recession

The location of the gingival margin around teeth should be evaluated and recorded, especially when recession is present. In the absence of attachment loss, the gingival margin is located coronal to the cementoenamel junction (CEJ). The exact location of the gingiva with respect to the CEJ is difficult to ascertain, as the detection of a subgingival cementoenamel can be challenging. When the CEJ is supragingival, recession is the distance from the CEJ to the gingival margin. The presence of recession indicates that attachment loss has occurred, but not necessarily that inflammation is present. At sites with recession, the amount of recession should be recorded, and the presence of biofilm and calculus, the inflammatory changes in the gingiva, and the width of the keratinized tissue should be carefully evaluated (Fig. 30.7).

TACTILE PERIODONTAL EXAMINATION

Tactile periodontal examination begins with the evaluation of the consistency of the gingiva and its adaptation to the tooth as well as the presence of marginal bleeding and suppuration. The gingival crevice is then probed to evaluate the subgingival environment. The tooth surface is carefully probed for aberrations, concavities, furcation, and subgingival calculus. The response of the gingival tissue to probing is appraised in terms of resistance to probe penetration, depth of probe penetration, bleeding on probing, and pain on probing.

Tactile Examination of the Marginal Gingiva

The marginal gingiva is palpated with a periodontal probe to assess its consistency and adaptation to the tooth. Healthy gingiva is firm, resilient, and well adapted to the tooth due to the presence of dense collagen fiber bundles in the lamina propria of the gingiva. When inflamed, the gingiva is edematous, spongy, and loosely adapted to the tooth surface due to the degradation of collagen and the influx of cells and fluid into the lamina propria (Fig. 30.8). In cases of chronic inflammation and in smokers, the gingival tissue may be fibrotic.

Fig. 30.8 The Severely Inflamed Gingiva Is Loosely Adapted to the Tooth.

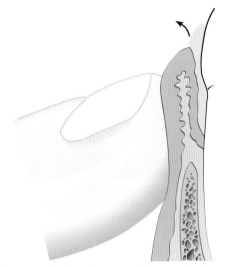

Fig. 30.9 Purulent Exudate Expressed From a Periodontal Pocket by Digital Pressure.

Marginal Bleeding

Marginal bleeding is associated with inflammatory changes in the marginal gingiva. Marginal bleeding can be evaluated by running an instrument such as a probe or rubber tip along the gingival margin. Under pressure, healthy gingival tissue will blanch and not bleed, whereas in the presence of gingival inflammation, marginal bleeding may be observed. The ease and severity of marginal bleeding are correlated with the severity of gingival inflammation.

Suppuration

Palpation of the marginal gingiva with a probe, or digitally by placing the ball of the index finger on the gingiva apical to the margin and pushing coronally toward the gingival margin (Fig. 30.9), may squeeze a white-yellowish exudate from the gingival crevice. The presence of an abundance of neutrophils in the gingival fluid transforms it into a purulent exudate.[5] Suppuration does not occur in all periodontal pockets, but pressure often reveals it in pockets where its presence is not suspected. Several studies[10,11,15,31] have evaluated the association between suppuration

and the progression of periodontitis and have reported that this sign is present in a very low percentage of diseased sites (i.e., 3% to 5%).[5] Therefore, absence of suppuration does not indicate absence of disease.

Tactile Examination of the Gingival Crevice

The probe is inserted into the gingival crevice vertically with the tip of the probe touching and sliding down along the tooth surface to the bottom of the crevice. The probe is "walked" circumferentially around each surface of each tooth to detect the areas of deepest penetration. As the probe tip slides down along the tooth surface, attention is paid to the tactile feel of the gingival tissue and the tooth surface. Healthy gingival tissue will feel tight and resist probe penetration. The tightness of the tissue will increase and the probe will come to a stop. In fact, it is the adhesion of the junctional epithelium to the tooth surface that stops probe penetration in healthy tissue. If the gingival tissue is severely inflamed, the probe may not have any resistance at all as it "falls" to the depth of the gingival crevice.

As the probe tip slides along the tooth surface, if there is no irregularity or subgingival calculus, the tooth surface will feel smooth. If the tooth surface feels rough or if the probe tip stops on a hard surface, its path may be impeded by the presence of subgingival calculus. The probe may need to be moved axially away from the tooth to navigate around the calculus in order for it to penetrate to depth. The presence of subgingival calculus is usually associated with inflammatory changes in the gingival tissue (see Fig. 30.5), the absence of gingival tightness, and the presence of bleeding on probing.

KEY FACTS

When probing, the probe tip should be in contact with the tooth surface as it slides down along the tooth surface to get to the bottom of the gingival crevice. This allows for detection of tooth surface irregularities, furcation invasion, and subgingival calculus.

Additionally, attention should be directed to detecting the presence of periodontal defects, interdental craters, root surface concavities, and furcation invasion. Periodontal defects tend to be associated with deep probing depths and gingival inflammation. To detect an *interdental crater*, the probe should be placed obliquely from both the facial and lingual surfaces to explore the deepest point of the pocket located beneath the contact point. The root surface should be carefully explored and probed to detect concavities and *furcation invasion*. The use of specially designed probes (e.g., Nabers probes) allows for an easier and more accurate exploration of the horizontal component of furcation lesions.

Tactile detection of inflammatory changes in the soft tissue is just as valuable as, if not more valuable than, measuring probing depth and evaluating bleeding on probing. The detection of inflammatory changes in the tissue, subgingival concavities, furcation invasion, and subgingival calculus via probing is instrumental in accurate diagnosis, prognosis, and treatment.

KEY FACTS

Thorough probing of the gingival crevice and the surrounding tissue provides a wealth of valuable information beyond probing depth and bleeding on probing that is essential to the diagnosis and treatment of periodontal disease.

Probing Around Implants

Because implants are susceptible to biofilm-induced inflammatory diseases, probing around them becomes part of the examination and diagnosis. A traditional periodontal probe may be used under light force (e.g., 0.25 N) without damaging the peri-implant mucosal seal.[18] Peri-implant evaluation and probing of implants are further discussed in Chapter 59.

When Not to Probe

Thorough probing of the periodontal pocket and accurate probing depth measurement before, during, and after treatment are essential for diagnosing and monitoring periodontal disease. In the presence of severe gingival inflammation (see Figs. 30.5 and 30.12), accurate probing depth measurement is difficult to obtain without anesthesia due to the pain and discomfort inflicted on the patient with insertion of the periodontal probe into the inflamed periodontal pocket. Therefore, when periodontal disease is overt and obvious clinically and radiographically, thorough probing of the periodontal pocket and accurate probing depth measurement should only occur once the tissue is anesthetized. In cases that require scaling and root planing with anesthesia, accurate probing depth measurement should be delayed until the scaling and root planing appointment. After anesthesia has been administered and before root instrumentation occurs, the periodontal pocket should be thoroughly probed for subgingival calculus, root surface concavities, furcation invasions, and probing pocket depths. Furthermore, in moderate and advanced cases, probing depths will change dramatically with improvement in biofilm control and scaling and root planing (Fig. 30.10). As such, obtaining accurate probing depths at the reevaluation following nonsurgical therapy is much more important than obtaining accurate probing depth at the pretreatment periodontal examination.

Fig. 30.10 (A) Clinical presentation before scaling and root planing. (B) After 4 weeks, oral hygiene instructions and scaling and root planing have improved this patient's periodontal status.

KEY FACTS

In the presence of overt and obvious periodontal disease, it may be best to delay accurate probing depth measurement until the scaling and root planing appointment, when the tissue is anesthetized.

Probing Depth

There are two different pocket depths: (1) the biologic or histologic depth and (2) the clinical or probing depth (Fig. 30.11).[29]

Biologic depth is the distance between the gingival margin and the base of the gingival crevice (i.e., the coronal end of the junctional epithelium). This can be measured only in carefully prepared and adequately oriented histologic sections.

Probing depth is the distance from the gingival margin to the bottom of the probeable crevice (i.e., where the probe tip stops). Probes that are currently used are described in Chapter 45.

Probe penetration can vary depending on the force of introduction, the shape and size of the probe tip, the direction of penetration, the resistance of the tissues, the convexity of the crown, and the degree of tissue inflammation.[5] Probing depth

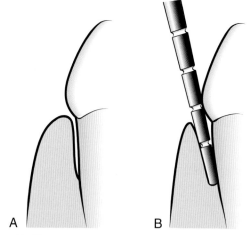

Fig. 30.11 (A) The biologic or histologic pocket depth is the actual distance between the gingival margin and the attached tissues (i.e., the bottom of the pocket). (B) The probing or clinical pocket depth is the depth of probe penetration.

is generally ≤3 mm in gingival health and >3 mm in the presence of gingival inflammation. Several studies have been done to determine the depth of penetration of a probe in a sulcus or pocket. Armitage and colleagues[8] used beagle dogs to evaluate the penetration of a probe with the use of a standardized force

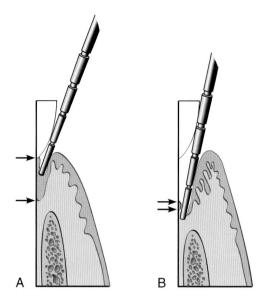

Fig. 30.12 (A) In a normal sulcus, the probe penetrates about one-third to half the length of the junctional epithelium *(between arrows)*. (B) In an inflamed periodontal pocket, the probe penetrates beyond the apical end of the junctional epithelium *(between arrows)*.

of 25 g. They reported that in healthy gingiva, the probe penetrated the junctional epithelium to about two-thirds of its length; in gingivitis cases, it stopped 0.1 mm short of its apical end; and in cases of periodontitis, the probe tip consistently went past the most apical cells of the junctional epithelium (Fig. 30.12).

In human periodontal pockets, the probe tip penetrates to the most coronal intact fibers of the connective tissue attachment.[38,72] The depth of penetration of the probe in the connective tissue apical to the junctional epithelium in a periodontal pocket is about 0.3 mm.[38,66,72] This is important when evaluating differences in probing depth before and after treatment, because the reduction in probe penetration may be a result of reduced inflammatory response rather than a gain in attachment.[37,40]

Probing depth may change from time to time, even in patients with untreated periodontal disease, as a result of changes in the position of the gingival margin. Therefore it may be unrelated to the existing attachment of the tooth.

KEY FACTS

The biologic/histologic pocket depth is always shallower than the clinical/probing pocket depth.

Bleeding on Probing

The insertion of a probe to the bottom of the pocket elicits bleeding if the gingiva is inflamed and if the pocket epithelium is atrophic or ulcerated. Noninflamed sites rarely bleed. In most cases, bleeding on probing is an earlier sign of inflammation than gingival color changes (see Chapter 17).[45] However, color changes may be present without bleeding on probing.[26] Depending on the severity of inflammation, bleeding can vary from a tenuous red

line along the gingival sulcus to profuse bleeding.[1] If periodontal treatment is successful, bleeding on probing will cease.[3]

To test for bleeding after probing, the probe is carefully introduced to the bottom of the pocket and gently moved laterally along the pocket wall. Sometimes bleeding appears immediately after the removal of the probe; other times it may be delayed for a few seconds. Therefore the dental hygienist should recheck for bleeding 30 to 60 seconds after probing.

As a single test, bleeding on probing is not a good predictor of progressive attachment loss; however, its absence is an excellent predictor of periodontal stability.[5] When bleeding is present in multiple sites of advanced disease, bleeding on probing is a good indicator of progressive attachment loss.[5,22] Armitage analyzed the literature on this subject up to 1996; he performed a meta-analysis of the various papers and concluded that the presence of bleeding on probing in a "treated and maintained patient population" is an important risk predictor for increased loss of attachment.[5]

KEY FACTS

In healthy nonsmokers, absence of bleeding on probing is an excellent predictor of periodontal stability.

Pain on Probing

Pain is a cardinal sign of inflammation. Gingival inflammation and periodontal disease in general are painless. However, periodontal probing of the gingival crevice can elicit pain in the gingival tissue. The presence of pain suggests that the gingival tissue is inflamed, and the level of pain is usually related to the severity of gingival inflammation. Unless gingival inflammation is generalized and severe, patients will not feel the same level of pain at every site. Probing of healthy sites will not produce pain, and probing of sites with inflammation will produce pain. Sites that do not exhibit bleeding or obvious clinical signs of inflammation can exhibit pain on probing. Although the dental hygienist cannot directly measure pain on probing, it is useful to make the patient aware that pain indicates inflammation and to ask the patient to pay attention to its presence.

Attachment Loss

Attachment loss is the apical migration of the dentogingival junction—the periodontal attachment apparatus—as a result of the inflammatory response. The dentogingival junction consists of the epithelial attachment and the connective tissue attachment. The dimension of the dentogingival junction is called the *biologic width* and averages 2.04 mm.[21] In healthy conditions, without attachment loss, the connective tissue attachment of the dentogingival junction begins coronally at the CEJ, and the epithelial attachment exists coronal to the connective tissue attachment. With attachment loss, the CEJ becomes exposed. *CAL* measures the *amount* of attachment loss that has occurred, with the CEJ as the reference point. CAL is measured as the distance from the CEJ to the bottom of the probeable crevice.

When the *gingival margin is located on the anatomic crown*, CAL is determined by subtracting the distance from the gingival margin to the CEJ from the probing depth. If both are the same, CAL is zero.

When the gingival margin coincides with the CEJ, CAL is equal to probing depth.

When the gingival margin is located apical to the CEJ, CAL is greater than probing depth. Therefore CAL, or the distance between the CEJ and the bottom of the probeable crevice, is the sum of gingival recession and probing depth. Drawing the gingival margin on the chart where probing depths are entered helps to clarify this important point.[70]

CAL is automatically calculated in many dental practice management software programs as the sum of probing depth and recession. This calculation is accurate only when both probing depth and recession are entered into the software correctly. However, when recession is not entered, many software programs assume the CEJ is at the level of the gingival margin and equate CAL to probing depth. This is not necessarily correct, as many clinicians do not enter a value for recession when the CEJ is subgingival and not visible. As such, automatically calculated CAL values must be scrutinized before they are used to help make a diagnosis.

Attachment Level

Attachment level describes the location *where* the dentogingival junction begins coronally on a tooth. For example, the attachment level of a tooth can be on the coronal third of the root or the apical third of the root. *Clinical attachment level* measures the distance between the attachment level and a reference point on a tooth, such as the CEJ. For example, the attachment level is 3 mm apical to the CEJ. Changes in the attachment level can be the result of a gain or a loss of attachment, and they can provide a better indication of the degree of periodontal destruction or gain. *Shallow pockets attached at the level of the apical third of the root connote more severe destruction than deep pockets attached at the coronal third of the root* (see Chapter 22).

KEY FACTS

CAL measures *how much* attachment loss has occurred using the CEJ as the reference point. Clinical attachment level measures the distance between *where* the periodontal attachment apparatus begins coronally on a tooth and a fixed reference point.

Attached Gingiva

It is important to establish the relationship between the bottom of the pocket and the mucogingival junction, especially at sites with gingival recession and narrow gingival width (see Fig. 30.7). The width of the attached gingiva is the distance between the mucogingival junction and the projection on the external surface of the bottom of the gingival sulcus or the periodontal pocket. It should not be confused with the width of the gingiva, because the latter also includes the marginal gingiva (Fig. 30.13).

The width of the attached gingiva is determined by subtracting the sulcus or pocket depth from the total width of the gingiva (i.e., the gingival margin to the mucogingival line). The amount

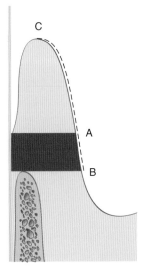

Fig. 30.13 The shaded area shows the attached gingiva, which extends between the projection on the external surface of the bottom of the pocket (A) and the mucogingival junction (B). The keratinized gingiva may extend from the mucogingival junction (B) to the gingival margin (C).

of attached gingiva is generally considered to be insufficient when the stretching of the lip or cheek induces the movement of the free gingival margin.

Other methods that are used to determine the amount of attached gingiva include pushing the adjacent mucosa coronally with a dull instrument and painting the mucosa with Schiller's potassium iodide solution, which stains keratin.

EXAMINATION OF THE TEETH AND IMPLANTS

The teeth are examined for caries, poor restorations, developmental defects, anomalies of tooth form, wasting, hypersensitivity, and proximal contact relationships. The stability, position, and number of implants and their relationship to the adjacent natural dentition are also examined.

Wasting Disease of the Teeth

Wasting is defined as any gradual loss of tooth substance, which is characterized by the formation of smooth, polished surfaces without regard to the possible mechanism of this loss. The forms of wasting are erosion, abrasion, attrition, and abfraction.[47,65]

Erosion, which is also called *corrosion,* is a sharply defined wedge-shaped depression in the cervical area of the facial tooth surface.[55] The long axis of the eroded area is perpendicular to the vertical axis of the tooth. The surfaces are smooth, hard, and polished. Erosion generally affects a group of teeth. During the early stages, it may be confined to the enamel, but it generally extends to involve the underlying dentin as well as the cementum.

The etiology of erosion is not known. Decalcification by acidic beverages[44] or citrus fruits in combination with the effect of acid salivary secretion is a suggested cause. Sognnaes[71] refers to these lesions as *dentoalveolar ablations* and attributes them to forceful frictional action between the oral soft tissues and the adjacent hard tissues. In patients with erosion, the salivary pH,

Fig. 30.14 The Overzealous Use of a Toothbrush Resulted in Denudation of the Gingival Epithelial Surface and Exposure of the Underlying Connective Tissue as a Painful Ulcer. Note the abrasion, a common non-carious cervical lesion noted on the tooth surface.

Fig. 30.15 Flat, Shiny, Discolored Surfaces Produced by Occlusal Wear.

the buffering capacity, and the calcium and phosphorus content have been reported as normal, and the mucin level is elevated.[43]

Abrasion refers to the loss of tooth substance that is induced by mechanical wear other than that of mastication. Abrasion results in saucer-shaped or wedge-shaped indentations with a smooth, shiny surface (Fig. 30.14). Abrasion starts on exposed cementum surfaces rather than on the enamel, and it extends to involve the dentin of the root. A sharp "ditching" around the CEJ appears to be the result of the softer cemental surface as compared with the much harder enamel surface.

Continued exposure to the abrasive agent in combination with decalcification of the enamel by locally formed acids may result in a loss of enamel followed by a loss of the dentin of the crown.

Toothbrushing[26] with an abrasive dentifrice and the action of clasps are frequently mentioned, but aggressive toothbrushing with an abrasive dentifrice is the most common cause.[34] Tooth position (facial) is also a major factor in the abrasive loss of the root surface. The degree of tooth wear from toothbrushing depends on the abrasive effect of the dentifrice and the angle of brushing.[41,42] Horizontal brushing at right angles to the vertical axis of the teeth results in the severest loss of tooth substance. Occasionally, abrasion of the incisal edges occurs as a result of habits such as holding objects (e.g., bobby pins, tacks) between the teeth.

Attrition is occlusal wear that results from functional contact with opposing teeth. Such physical wear patterns may occur on incisal, occlusal, or approximal tooth surfaces. A certain amount of tooth wear is physiologic, but accelerated wear may occur when abnormal anatomic or unusual functional factors are present.

Occlusal or incisal surfaces worn by attrition are called *facets.* When active tooth grinding occurs, the enamel rods are fractured and become highly reflective to light.[79] Thus shiny, smooth, and curviplanar facets are usually the best indicators of ongoing frictional activity (Fig. 30.15). If dentin is exposed, a yellowish-brown discoloration is frequently present. Facets vary with regard to size and location, depending on whether they are produced by physiologic or abnormal wear.[14,77] At least one significant

wear facet has been reported in 92% of adults,[68] and facet prevalence approaches universality.[11,78] Facets are usually not sensitive to thermal or tactile stimulation.

Facets generally represent functional or parafunctional wear as well as iatrogenic dental treatment through coronoplasty (occlusal adjustment). However, coronoplasty does not appear to contribute to higher ratings of wear.[69] Excessive wear may result in the obliteration of the cusps and the formation of either a flat or cuneiform (cupped-out) occlusal surface. Contrary to earlier thought, attrition in young adults from modern societies is not age related.[17,69] This suggests that a significant amount of attrition, when present in young adults, is unlikely to occur as a result of functional wear,[36] and it is probably the result of bruxing activity.[69] Attrition has been correlated with age when older adults are considered.[9,67]

The angle of the facet on the tooth surface is potentially significant to the periodontium. Horizontal facets tend to direct forces on the vertical axis of the tooth to which the periodontium can adapt most effectively. Angular facets direct occlusal forces laterally and increase the risk of periodontal damage. However, gradual attrition may be compensated for by continuous tooth eruption without alveolar bone growth, and it is characterized by a lack of inflammatory changes on the alveolar bone surfaces.[74]

Another mechanism of tooth wear that has been studied is called *abfraction,* and it results from occlusal loading surfaces causing tooth flexure and mechanical microfractures the cervical area.[28] Mechanical microfractures from abfraction weakens the cervical tooth structure and makes it much more susceptible to loss of tooth structure via abrasion (see Fig. 30.14).

These four mechanisms of tooth wear (corrosion, abrasion, attrition, and abfraction) can combine to increase the degree of tooth wear.

Dental Stains

Dental stains are pigmented deposits on the teeth. They should be carefully examined to determine their origin (see Chapter 12).

Hypersensitivity

Root surfaces exposed by gingival recession may be hypersensitive to thermal changes or tactile stimulation. Patients often direct the clinician to the sensitive areas. These may be located by gentle exploration with a probe or cold air.

Proximal Contact Relations

Open contacts allow for food impaction. The tightness of contacts should be checked by means of clinical observation and with dental floss. Abnormal contact relationships may also initiate occlusal changes, such as a shift in the median line between the central incisors with labial flaring of the maxillary canine, buccal or lingual displacement of the posterior teeth, and an uneven relationship of the marginal ridges. Teeth opposite an edentulous site may supererupt, thereby opening the proximal contacts.

Tooth Mobility

All teeth have a slight degree of physiologic mobility, which varies for different teeth and at different times of the day.[52,56] It is greatest when arising in the morning, and it progressively decreases. The increased mobility in the morning is attributed to slight extrusion of the tooth as a result of limited occlusal contact during sleep. During the waking hours, mobility is reduced by chewing and swallowing forces, which intrude the teeth in the sockets. These 24-hour variations are less marked in persons with a healthy periodontium than in those with occlusal habits such as bruxism and clenching.

Single-rooted teeth have more mobility than multirooted teeth, with incisors having the most mobility. Mobility occurs primarily in a horizontal direction, although some axial mobility occurs to a lesser degree.[54]

Tooth mobility occurs in the following two stages:

1. The initial or intrasocket stage occurs when the tooth moves within the confines of the periodontal ligament. This is associated with viscoelastic distortion of the ligament and the redistribution of the periodontal fluids, interbundle content, and fibers.[35] This initial movement occurs with forces of about 100 lb, and it is on the order of 0.05 mm to 0.10 mm (50 μm to 100 μm).[48]
2. The secondary stage occurs gradually and entails elastic deformation of the alveolar bone in response to increased horizontal forces.[50] When a force of 500 g is applied to the crown, the resulting displacement is about 100 μm to 200 μm for incisors, 50 μm to 90 μm for canines, 8 μm to 10 μm for premolars, and 40 μm to 80 μm for molars.[48]

When a force such as that applied to teeth in occlusion is discontinued, the teeth return to their original position in two stages: the first is an immediate, springlike elastic recoil; the second is a slow, asymptomatic recovery movement. The recovery movement is pulsating, and it is apparently associated with the normal pulsation of the periodontal vessels, which occurs in synchrony with the cardiac cycle.[49]

Many attempts have been made to develop mechanical or electronic devices for the precise measurement of tooth mobility.[49,53,55,68] Although standardization of grading mobility would be helpful for the diagnosis of periodontal disease and for

Fig. 30.16 Tooth Mobility Is Checked With a Metal Instrument and One Finger.

evaluating treatment outcomes, these devices are not widely used. As a general rule, mobility is graded clinically by holding the tooth firmly between the handles of two metallic instruments or with one metallic instrument and one finger (Fig. 30.16). An effort is then made to move it in all directions. Abnormal mobility most often occurs faciolingually. Mobility is scored according to the ease and extent of tooth movement according to the Miller Index[46] as follows:

- Mobility no. 1: first distinguishable sign of movement greater than "normal"
- Mobility no. 2: movement of the crown up to 1 mm in any direction
- Mobility no. 3: movement of the crown more than 1 mm in any direction or vertical depression or rotation of the crown in its socket

Physiologic mobility is movement up to 0.2 mm horizontally and 0.02 mm axially. Mobility beyond the physiologic range is termed *abnormal* or *pathologic*. It is pathologic in that it exceeds the limits of normal mobility values; however, the periodontium is not *necessarily* diseased at the time of examination.

Increased mobility is caused by one or more of the following factors:

1. *Loss of tooth support (bone loss)* can result in mobility. The amount of mobility depends on the severity and distribution of bone loss at individual root surfaces, the length and shape of the roots, and the root size compared with that of the crown.[55] A tooth with short, tapered roots is more likely to loosen than one with normal-size or bulbous roots with the same amount of bone loss. One should carefully evaluate postorthodontic cases for possible apical shortening of the root, which may lead to excessive mobility. Because bone loss usually results from a combination of factors and does not occur as an isolated finding, the severity of tooth mobility does not necessarily correspond to the amount of bone loss.

2. *Trauma from occlusion* (i.e., injury produced by excessive occlusal forces or incurred as a result of abnormal occlusal habits such as bruxism and clenching) is a common cause of tooth mobility. Mobility is also increased by hypofunction. Mobility produced by trauma from occlusion occurs initially as a result of resorption of the cortical layer of bone, which leads to reduced fiber support, and later as an adaptation phenomenon that results in a widened periodontal space.

3. *Extension of inflammation* from the gingiva or the periapex into the periodontal ligament results in changes that increase mobility. The spread of inflammation from an acute periapical abscess may increase tooth mobility in the absence of periodontal disease.

4. *Periodontal surgery* temporarily increases tooth mobility immediately after the intervention and for a short period.[58-61]

5. Tooth mobility is increased during *pregnancy,* and it is sometimes associated with the *menstrual cycle* or the use of *hormonal contraceptives.* This is unrelated to periodontal disease, and it occurs presumably because of physicochemical changes in the periodontal tissues.

6. *Pathologic processes of the jaws* that destroy the alveolar bone or the roots of the teeth can also result in mobility. Osteomyelitis and tumors of the jaws belong in this category.

One study[24] has suggested that pockets around mobile teeth harbor higher proportions of *Campylobacter rectus* and *Peptostreptococcus micros* and possibly *Porphyromonas gingivalis* as compared with nonmobile teeth. This hypothesis requires further verification.

KEY FACTS

The three main etiologic factors of tooth mobility are periodontal inflammation, attachment loss, and occlusal trauma.

Trauma From Occlusion

Trauma from occlusion refers to *tissue injury* produced by occlusal forces rather than to the occlusal forces themselves. The criterion that determines that an occlusion is traumatic is whether it causes damage in the periodontal tissues; therefore the diagnosis of trauma from occlusion is made from the condition of the periodontal tissues. The periodontal findings are then used as a guide for locating the responsible occlusal relationships.

Periodontal findings that suggest the presence of trauma from occlusion include excessive tooth mobility, particularly in teeth that show radiographic evidence of a widened periodontal space; vertical or angular bone destruction; infrabony pockets; and pathologic migration, especially of the anterior teeth. These are discussed in more detail in the following sections.

Pathologic Migration of the Teeth

Alterations in tooth position should be carefully noted, particularly with a view toward identifying abnormal forces, a tongue-thrusting habit, or other habits that may be contributing factors (Fig. 30.17). Premature tooth contacts in the posterior region that deflect the mandible anteriorly contribute to the destruction of the periodontium of the maxillary anterior teeth and to pathologic migration. The loss of posterior teeth can lead to facial "flaring" of the maxillary anterior dentition. This is due to the increased trauma that the mandibular anterior dentition places against the palatal surface of the maxillary anterior dentition. Pathologic migration of the anterior teeth in young persons may be a sign of localized aggressive (juvenile) periodontitis.

Sensitivity to Percussion

Sensitivity to percussion is a feature of acute inflammation of the periodontal ligament. Gentle percussion of a tooth at different angles to the long axis often helps with the localization of the site of inflammatory involvement.

Dentition With the Jaws Closed

Examination of the dentition with the jaws closed can detect conditions such as irregularly aligned teeth, extruded teeth, improper proximal contacts, and areas of food impaction, all of which may favor plaque accumulation.

Excessive *overbite,* which is seen most often in the anterior region, may cause impingement of the teeth on the gingiva and food impaction, followed by gingival inflammation, gingival enlargement, and pocket formation. The real significance of the detrimental effect of an excessive anterior overbite on gingival health is still controversial.[2]

In *open-bite* relationships, abnormal vertical spaces exist between the maxillary and mandibular teeth. The condition

Fig. 30.17 Labial Migration of the Maxillary Central Incisors, Especially The Right Incisor.

occurs most often in the anterior region, although posterior open bite is occasionally seen. Reduced mechanical cleansing by the passage of food may lead to accumulation of plaque and debris, calculus formation, and extrusion of teeth.

With *crossbite*, the normal relationship of the mandibular teeth to the maxillary teeth is reversed, with the maxillary teeth being lingual to the mandibular teeth. Crossbite may be bilateral or unilateral, or may affect only a pair of antagonists. Trauma from occlusion, food impaction, spreading of the mandibular teeth, and associated gingival and periodontal disturbances may be caused by crossbite.

Functional Occlusal Relationships

The examination of functional occlusal relationships is an important part of the diagnostic procedure. Dentitions that appear to be normal when the jaws are closed may present marked functional abnormalities. Systematic procedures for the detection and correction of functional abnormalities are presented in Chapter 48.

RADIOGRAPHIC EXAMINATION

The radiographic survey should consist of a minimum of 14 intraoral films and 4 posterior bitewing films (Fig. 30.18). Panoramic radiographs are a simple and convenient method of obtaining a survey view of the dental arch and the surrounding structures (Fig. 30.19). They are helpful for the detection of developmental anomalies, pathologic lesions of the teeth and jaws, and fractures, as well as dental screening examinations of large groups. They provide an informative overall radiographic picture of the distribution and severity of bone destruction with periodontal disease, but *a complete intraoral series is required for periodontal diagnosis and treatment planning.* Chapter 31 gives a detailed description of radiographic interpretation in periodontics.

LABORATORY AIDS TO CLINICAL DIAGNOSIS

When unusual gingival or periodontal problems are detected that cannot be explained by local causes, the possibility of

Fig. 30.18 A Full-Mouth Intraoral Radiographic Series (17 Periapical Films and 4 Bite-Wing Films) Used as an Adjunct for Periodontal Diagnosis.

Fig. 30.19 Panoramic Radiograph Provides an Overview of the Dental Arch and the Surrounding Structures.

contributing systemic factors must be explored. The signs and symptoms of oral manifestations of systemic disease have to be clearly understood and analyzed and their presence discussed with the patient's physician. Chapter 13 presents discussions of many of these problems, and the reader is also directed to standard texts that discuss medical diagnoses for more detailed descriptions of the necessary tests and their interpretation.

Numerous laboratory tests aid in the diagnosis of systemic diseases that may contribute to periodontal and oral diseases; these tests will also be needed to make treatment decisions when dealing with medically compromised patients (see Chapter 36). Analyses of blood smears, blood cell counts, white blood cell differential counts, and erythrocyte sedimentation rates are used to evaluate the presence of blood dyscrasias and generalized infections. Determinations of coagulation time, bleeding time, clot retraction time, prothrombin time, and capillary fragility as well as bone marrow studies may be required at times. The reader is referred to books about medical diagnoses for consideration of this subject.

PERIODONTAL DIAGNOSIS

Once the patient history has been obtained and clinical, radiographic, and other necessary examinations have been performed, the information acquired is synthesized and interpreted to answer three basic diagnostic questions[6] to derive the periodontal diagnosis:

1. What is the disease?
2. How severe is the disease?
3. What is the extent of the disease?

Diseases that can affect the periodontium are listed in the Classification of Periodontal Diseases and Conditions. Severity of periodontal disease is classified based on a three-tier system: slight, mild, early, or initial; moderate; and severe or advanced.

TABLE 30.2 Diagnosis of Biofilm-Induced Inflammatory Periodontal Diseases

Periodontal Diagnosis	Inflammation	Attachment Loss
Healthy	No	No
Biofilm-induced gingivitis	Yes	No
Chronic periodontitis	Yes	Yes
Healthy with a reduced periodontium/with a history of chronic periodontitis	No	Yes

The extent of the disease is classified as generalized or localized. When localized, the extent can be specified to the quadrant, teeth, and even tooth surfaces.

Biofilm-induced inflammatory periodontal diseases are diagnosed based on the presence of inflammation and attachment loss (Table 30.2). In periodontal health, both inflammation and attachment loss are absent. When only inflammation is present, the diagnosis is biofilm-induced gingivitis. When both inflammation and attachment loss are present, the diagnosis is chronic periodontitis. It is possible that when both inflammation and attachment loss are present, biofilm-induced gingivitis is superimposed over a history of chronic periodontitis. However, it is prudent to diagnose the presence of both inflammation and attachment loss as chronic periodontitis due to the following reasons: progression of chronic periodontitis is sporadic, sites with previous attachment loss are susceptible to further attachment loss, and attachment loss is driven by the inflammatory response. Finally, when inflammation is absent and attachment is present, the diagnosis is healthy with a reduced periodontium or with a history of chronic periodontitis.

KEY FACTS

Diagnosis of biofilm-induced inflammatory periodontal diseases is based on the presence of periodontal inflammation and attachment loss.

Currently, the severity of chronic periodontitis is characterized on a three-tier system based on CAL: slight = 1 or 2 mm CAL, moderate = 3 or 4 mm CAL, and severe ≥5 mm CAL. This system is inadequate for two reasons: (1) chronic periodontitis is diagnosed based on the presence of both inflammation and attachment loss, not attachment loss alone; and (2) the link in the relationship between periodontitis and systemic disease is inflammation, not attachment loss. Therefore an ideal classification system should take into consideration the severity of inflammation as well. Furthermore, for cases with mild attachment loss or where the CEJ is subgingival, an accurate determination of CAL is challenging, as it is difficult to accurately determine the location of the CEJ. As such, the severity of attachment loss may depend on the interpretation of radiographic bone loss. Table 30.3 correlates severity of periodontitis to CAL and the distance from the alveolar crest to the CEJ on radiographs.

KEY FACTS

Severity of periodontitis is characterized based on CAL.

Severity of biofilm-induced gingivitis also can be characterized based on a three-tier system of slight, moderate, and severe. However, this can be subjective.

The extent of chronic periodontitis is delineated based on the 30% threshold. Localized chronic periodontitis is defined as chronic periodontitis with a clear pattern of distribution, such as distal surfaces of second molars or ≤30% of teeth are affected.[4] Generalized chronic periodontitis is defined as periodontitis without a clear pattern of distribution or >30% of teeth are affected.[4] The extent of biofilm-induced gingivitis also can be characterized based on the 30% threshold similar to the extent of chronic periodontitis.

When biofilm-induced gingivitis and chronic periodontitis are present simultaneously, if the extent of both is generalized, the diagnosis is simply generalized chronic periodontitis, as the chronic periodontitis is the more advanced progression of the disease. Furthermore, biofilm-induced gingivitis by definition is inflammation without attachment loss, whereas chronic periodontitis is defined as inflammation with attachment loss. A diagnosis of both generalized biofilm-induced gingivitis and generalized chronic periodontitis is contradictory. Biofilm-induced gingivitis may be diagnosed together with chronic periodontitis if the periodontitis is localized. In this situation, the diagnosis is generalized biofilm-induced gingivitis with localized chronic periodontitis. Similarly, if the extent of mild and moderate chronic periodontitis is >30%, the diagnosis is simply generalized moderate chronic periodontitis, as moderate is the more severe of the two types of disease severity.

ASSESSMENT OF BIOFILM CONTROL AND PATIENT EDUCATION

Patients presenting for periodontal consultations typically expect to find out the problems they have and the treatments they need. By the end of the periodontal consultation, it may not be possible to determine the prognosis and formulate a complete treatment plan, as a careful analysis of the information obtained, more diagnostic information, or consultation with other dental and medical professionals may be required. However, the patient should be educated on the problems in his or her mouth, the need for further diagnostics, and the etiologies and prevention of these problems. Clinical photographs, radiographs, and models may be useful to help the patient to better understand the condition of his or her mouth. The patient may be presented with a preliminary treatment plan that may include emergency and palliative treatments and nonsurgical periodontal therapy to control infections.

Although patient education and biofilm control are part of nonsurgical periodontal therapy and not the focus of this chapter, a preventive approach to oral health care demands behavior modification, which requires time, effort, and repetition. As such, every opportunity should be seized to educate patients and alter their behavior. Patients should be given personalized oral hygiene instructions to control biofilm and to improve their oral health and the conditions of the periodontium. It is not uncommon for patients to report brushing and flossing multiple times daily, while having poorly controlled periodontal disease in their mouths. For that reason, the effectiveness of the patient's biofilm control must be evaluated. The patient should be asked to demonstrate biofilm control (toothbrushing, flossing, etc.) in front of a mirror so that both the patient and the dental hygienist can see his or her oral hygiene techniques. The patient should then be taught proper biofilm control techniques with a demonstration in his or her own mouth in front of a mirror. Detailed biofilm control is presented in Chapter 43.

Ideally, unless emergency treatment is required, patients should be given at least 1 or 2 weeks to improve their oral hygiene, to control biofilm and reduce periodontal inflammation, and to appreciate how they can impact their oral health with meticulous biofilm control before any periodontal treatment is rendered.

CONCLUSION

Periodontal examination and diagnosis begins with obtaining a thorough health and dental history. Although the periodontal examination presented in this chapter is divided into two parts, visual examination and tactile examination, in practice both visual and tactile assessments overlap and occur simultaneously, as do the evaluations of teeth and periodontium. Nevertheless, the examination should begin with an overall survey of biofilm and calculus, clinical signs of inflammation, and other obvious signs of disease to obtain insights into the patient's oral hygiene and disease status. As the examination progresses, it becomes more invasive and more specific information is acquired. Once a detailed patient history has been obtained and a thorough clinical examination has been completed, the information collected is

TABLE 30.3   Clinical and Radiographic Guidelines for Determining Severity of Periodontitis

Severity of Periodontitis	Clinical Attachment Loss (mm)	Distance From Alveolar Crest to CEJ (mm)	Radiographic Findings
Health	0	<2	
Mild	1–2	3–4	
Moderate	3–4	5–6	
Severe	≥5	≥7	

CEJ, Cementoenamel junction.

analyzed and synthesized to arrive at a diagnosis. The periodontal examination is the basis from which the diagnosis, prognosis, and treatment plan are derived and from which treatment is ultimately rendered. Therefore a thorough and accurate periodontal examination is of the utmost importance.

KEY FACTS

Examination → Diagnosis → Prognosis ↔ Treatment
- Diagnosis requires thorough and careful examination.
- Prognosis is based on accurate diagnosis.
- Treatment decisions are based on prognosis.
- Treatment decisions are made to improve prognosis.
- Diagnosis and prognosis will change with treatment.

A Case Scenario is found on the companion website.

REFERENCES

References for this chapter are found on the companion website.

31

Radiographic Aids in the Diagnosis of Periodontal Disease[a]

Radiographs are valuable for the diagnosis of periodontal disease, estimation of severity, determination of prognosis, and evaluation of treatment outcome.[6,14,19] However, *radiographs are an adjunct to the clinical examination, not a substitute for it.* Radiographs demonstrate changes in calcified tissue; they do not reveal current cellular activity, but rather reflect the effects of past cellular experience on the bone and roots.

KEY FACTS

Radiographs provide a static view of the currently available periodontal bone. Radiographic information must be considered as one of the elements of the diagnostic workup in conjunction with clinical and historical findings.

NORMAL INTERDENTAL BONE

The evaluation of bone changes in periodontal disease is based mainly on the appearance of the interdental bone because the relatively dense root structure obscures the facial and lingual bony plates. The interdental bone is normally outlined by a thin radiopaque line adjacent to the periodontal ligament (PDL) and at the alveolar crest, referred to as the *lamina dura* (Fig. 31.1). Because the lamina dura represents the cortical bone lining the tooth socket, the shape and position of the root and changes in the angulation of the x-ray beam produce considerable variations in its appearance.

The width and shape of the interdental bone and the angle of the crest normally vary according to the convexity of the proximal tooth surfaces and the level of the cementoenamel junction (CEJ) of the approximating teeth. The faciolingual diameter of the bone is related to the width of the proximal root surface. The angulation of the crest of the interdental septum is generally parallel to a line between the CEJs of the approximating teeth (see Fig. 31.1). When there is a difference in the level of the CEJs, the crest of the interdental bone appears angulated rather than horizontal.

RADIOGRAPHIC TECHNIQUES

In conventional radiographs, periapical and bitewing projections offer the most diagnostic information and are most commonly used in the evaluation of periodontal disease. To properly and accurately depict periodontal bone status, proper techniques of exposure and processing are required. The bone level, pattern of bone destruction, and width of the PDL space as well as the radiodensity, trabecular pattern, and marginal contour of the interdental bone vary as exposure and development time, type of film, and x-ray angulation are modified.[20] Standardized reproducible techniques are required to obtain reliable radiographs for pretreatment and posttreatment comparisons.

Prichard[15] established the following four criteria to determine adequate angulation of periapical radiographs:
1. The radiograph should show the tips of molar cusps with little or none of the occlusal surface showing.
2. Enamel caps and pulp chambers should be distinct.
3. Interproximal spaces should be open.
4. Proximal contacts should not overlap unless teeth are out of line anatomically.

For periapical radiographs, the long-cone paralleling technique most accurately projects the alveolar bone level (Fig. 31.2). The bisection-of-the-angle technique elongates the projected image, making the bone margin appear closer to the crown; the level of the facial bone is distorted more than that of the lingual. Inappropriate horizontal angulation results in tooth overlap, changes the shape of the interdental bone image, alters the radiographic width of the PDL space and the appearance of the lamina dura, and may distort the extent of furcation involvement (see Fig. 31.2).

Periapical radiographs frequently do not reveal the correct relationship between the alveolar bone and the CEJ.[9] This is particularly true in cases where a shallow palate or floor of the mouth does not allow ideal placement of the periapical film. Bitewing projections offer an alternative method that provides better images of the periodontal bone levels. For bitewing radiographs,

[a]Adapted from the following chapter of Newman and Carranza's Clinical Periodontology, 13th edition: Chapter 33: Radiographic Aids in the Diagnosis of Periodontal Disease, by Sotirios Tetradis, Sanjay M. Mallya, and Henry H. Takei.

the film is placed behind the crowns of the upper and lower teeth parallel to the long axis of the teeth. The x-ray beam is directed through the contact areas of the teeth and perpendicular to the film. Thus the projection geometry of the bitewing films allows the evaluation of the relationship between the interproximal alveolar crest and the CEJ without distortion (Figs. 31.3 and 31.4).[17] If the periodontal bone loss is severe and the bone level cannot be visualized on regular bitewing radiographs, films can be placed vertically to cover a larger area of the jaws (Fig. 31.5). More than two vertical bitewing films might be necessary to cover all of the interproximal spaces in the area of interest. Irrespective of the techniques used, it is important that if no direct benefit is anticipated, it is prudent to avoid taking the radiograph, even if it is a small dose. This is based on the radiation safety principle called ALARA, that stands for "as low as reasonably achievable."

Fig. 31.1 Crest of Interdental Bone Normally Parallel to a Line Drawn Between the Cementoenamel Junction of Adjacent Teeth *(Arrow)*. Note also the radiopaque lamina dura around the roots and interdental bone.

KEY FACTS

Bitewing radiography is the preferred imaging technique to depict interproximal periodontal bone levels in the posterior dentition.

BONE DESTRUCTION IN PERIODONTAL DISEASE

Early destructive changes of bone that do not remove sufficient mineralized tissue cannot be seen on radiographs. Therefore slight radiographic changes of the periodontal tissues suggest that the disease has progressed beyond its earliest stages.[4] The earliest signs of periodontal disease must be detected clinically.

Bone Loss

The radiographic image tends to underestimate the severity of bone loss. The difference between the height of the alveolar crest and the radiographic appearance ranges from 0 to 1.6 mm, mostly accounted for by x-ray angulation.

Amount

Radiographs are an indirect method for determining the amount of bone loss in periodontal disease; they show the amount of remaining bone rather than the amount lost. The amount of bone lost is estimated to be the difference between the physiologic bone level and the height of the remaining bone.

Several investigators have analyzed the distance from the CEJ to the alveolar crest.[8,11,13] Most studies, conducted in adolescents, suggest a distance of 2 mm to reflect normal periodontium; this distance may be greater in older patients.

Fig. 31.2 Comparison of Long-Cone Paralleling and Bisection-of-the-Angle Techniques. (A) Long-cone paralleling technique, radiograph of dried specimen. (B) Long-cone paralleling technique, same specimen as shown in (A). Smooth wire is on the margin of the facial plate and knotted wire is on the lingual plate to show their relative positions. (C) Bisection-of-the-angle technique, same specimen as in (A and B). (D) Bisection-of-the-angle technique, same specimen. Both bone margins are shifted toward the crown, the facial margin (smooth wire) more than the lingual margin (knotted wire), creating the illusion that the lingual bone margin has shifted apically. (Courtesy Dr. Benjamin Patur, Hartford, CT.)

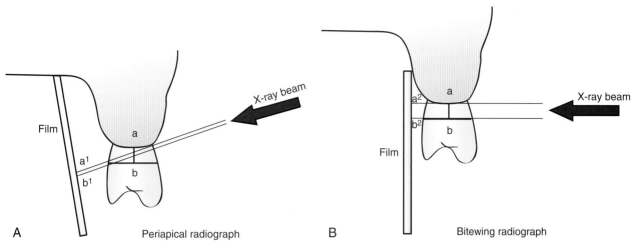

Fig. 31.3 Schematic diagram of periapical (A) and bitewing (B) radiographs. Angulation of the x-ray beam and the film on the periapical radiograph distort the distance between the alveolar crest and the cementoenamel junction (CEJ) (compare a–b vs. a^1–b^1). In contrast, the projection geometry of the bitewing radiograph allows a more accurate depiction (a^2–b^2) of the distance between the alveolar crest and the CEJ (a–b).

Fig. 31.4 Periapical (A) and bitewing (B) radiographs from a full-mouth series of a patient with periodontitis. The periapical film clearly underestimates the amount of bone loss *(white arrows)*. Because of appropriate projection geometry, the height of the alveolar crest is accurately depicted on the bitewing radiograph *(white arrows)*.

Fig. 31.5 Vertical Bitewing Films Can Be Used to Cover a Larger Area of the Alveolar Bone.

Fig. 31.6 Generalized Horizontal Bone Loss.

Distribution

The distribution of bone loss is an important diagnostic sign. It points to the location of destructive local factors in different areas of the mouth and in relation to different surfaces of the same tooth.

Pattern of Bone Destruction

In periodontal disease, the interdental bone undergoes changes that affect the lamina dura, crestal radiodensity, size and shape of the medullary spaces, and height and contour of the bone. The height of interdental bone may be reduced, with the crest perpendicular to the long axis of the adjacent teeth (*horizontal* bone loss, Fig. 31.6). On the other hand, angular or arcuate defects (*angular,* or *vertical,* bone loss, Fig. 31.7) could form.

Fig. 31.7 Angular Bone Loss on First Molar With Involvement of the Furcation.

Fig. 31.8 Angular Bone Loss on Mandibular Molar Partially Obscured by a Dense Mylohyoid Ridge.

Fig. 31.9 Interdental Lesion That Extends to the Facial or Lingual Surfaces in a Troughlike Manner.

Radiographs do not indicate the internal morphology or depth of crater-like defects. Also, radiographs do not reveal the extent of involvement on the facial and lingual surfaces. Bone destruction of facial and lingual surfaces is masked by the dense root structure, and bone destruction on the mesial and distal root surfaces may be partially hidden by superimposed anatomy, such as a dense mylohyoid ridge (Fig. 31.8). In most cases it can be assumed that bone loss seen interdentally continues in either the facial or lingual aspect, creating a troughlike lesion.

Dense cortical facial and lingual plates of interdental bone obscure destruction of the intervening cancellous bone. Thus a deep, crater-like defect between the facial and lingual plates might not be depicted on conventional radiographs. To record destruction of the interproximal cancellous bone radiographically, the cortical bone must be involved. A reduction of only 0.5 to 1 mm in the thickness of the cortical plate is sufficient to permit radiographic visualization of the destruction of the inner cancellous trabeculae.

Interdental bone loss may continue facially or lingually to form a troughlike defect that could be difficult to appreciate radiographically. These lesions may terminate on the radicular surface or may communicate with the adjacent interdental area to form one continuous lesion (Fig. 31.9).

Fig. 31.10 shows two adjacent interdental lesions connecting on the radicular surface to form one interconnecting osseous lesion. Along with clinical probing of these lesions, the use of a radiopaque pointer placed in these radicular defects will demonstrate the extent of the bone loss.

Periodontal bone loss should be differentiated from normal anatomy or anatomic variants that can resemble disease. For example, nutrient canals in the alveolar bone can appear as linear and circular radiolucent areas (Fig. 31.11). These canals can be seen more frequently in the anterior mandible, although they can be present throughout the alveolar ridge.

Finally, it should be emphasized that radiographs can only assess the amount of periodontal bone that is present and deduce the extent of bone loss. However, it is sometimes necessary to determine whether the reduced bone level is the result of periodontal disease that is no longer destructive (usually after treatment and proper maintenance) or whether destructive periodontal disease is present. Differentiation between treated versus active periodontal disease can only be achieved clinically. Radiographically detectable changes in the normal cortical outline of the interdental bone are corroborating evidence of destructive periodontal disease.

RADIOGRAPHIC APPEARANCE OF PERIODONTAL DISEASE

Periodontitis

Radiographic changes in periodontitis follow the pathophysiology of periodontal tissue destruction and include the following:

1. *Fuzziness and disruption of lamina dura* crestal cortication continuity is the earliest radiographic change in periodontitis (Fig. 31.12A and B) and results from bone resorption activated by extension of gingival inflammation into the periodontal bone. Depiction of these early changes depends greatly on the radiographic technique as well as on anatomic variations (thickness and density of interdental bone, position of adjoining teeth). No correlation has been found between crestal lamina dura in radiographs and the presence or absence of clinical inflammation, bleeding on probing, periodontal pockets, or loss of attachment.[16] Therefore it can be concluded that the presence of an intact crestal lamina dura may be an indicator of periodontal health, whereas its absence lacks diagnostic relevance.[1,3]

2. Continued periodontal bone loss and widening of the periodontal space results in a wedge-shaped radiolucency at the mesial or distal aspect of the crest (see Fig. 31.12B). The apex of the area is pointed in the direction of the root.

A

B

C

D

Fig. 31.10 (A) Interdental mesial and distal lesions. (B) Facial or lingual outlines of the actual lesion. (C) Occlusal view of the lesion. (D) Radiograph of mesial and facial lesions.

Fig. 31.11 Prominent Nutrient Canals in the Mandible.

3. Subsequently the destructive process extends across the alveolar crest, thus reducing the height of the interdental bone. As increased osteoclastic activity results in increased bone resorption along the endosteal margins of the medullary spaces, the remaining interdental bone can appear partially eroded (see Fig. 31.12C).

4. The height of the interdental septum is progressively reduced by the extension of inflammation and the resorption of bone (see Fig. 31.12D).

5. A radiopaque horizontal line can frequently be observed across the roots of a tooth. This opaque line demarcates the portion

of the root where the labial or lingual bony plate has been partially or completely destroyed from the remaining bone-supported portion (Fig. 31.13).

> ### KEY FACTS
>
> The earliest changes of periodontal disease often do not manifest on radiographs. Even when radiographic changes are evident, radiographic examination may underestimate the extent of bone loss. Thus assessment of periodontal bone level should be based on combined clinical-radiographic evaluation.

Interdental Craters

Interdental craters are seen as irregular areas of reduced density on the alveolar bone crests. Craters are generally not sharply demarcated but gradually blend with the rest of the bone. Conventional radiographs do not accurately depict the morphology or depth of interdental craters, which sometimes appear as vertical defects.

Furcation Involvement

Definitive diagnosis of furcation involvement is made by clinical examination, which includes careful probing with a specially designed probe (e.g., Nabers). Radiographs are helpful, but root superimposition, caused by anatomic variations or improper technique, can obscure radiographic representation of furcation involvement. As a general rule, bone loss is greater than it appears in the radiograph. A tooth may present marked bifurcation involvement in one film (Fig. 31.14A), but it can appear to

Fig. 31.12 Radiographic Changes in Periodontitis. (A) Normal appearance of interdental bone. (B) Fuzziness and a break in the continuity of the lamina dura at the crest of the bone distal to the central incisor *(left)*. There are wedge-shaped radiolucent areas at the crest of the other interdental bone. (C) Radiolucent projections from the crest into the interdental bone indicate extension of destructive processes. (D) Severe bone loss.

Fig. 31.13 Horizontal Lines Across the Roots of the Central Incisors *(Arrows)*. The area of the roots below the horizontal lines is partially or completely denuded of the facial and lingual bony plates.

Fig. 31.14 (A) Furcation involvement indicated by triangular radiolucency in the bifurcation area of mandibular first molar. The second molar presents only a slight thickening of the periodontal space in the bifurcation area. (B) Same area as in (A) with different angulation. The triangular radiolucency in the bifurcation of the first molar is obliterated, and involvement of the second molar bifurcation is apparent.

be uninvolved in another (see Fig. 31.14B). Radiographs should be taken at different angles to reduce the risk of missing furcation involvement.

A large, clearly defined radiolucency in the furcation area is easy to identify (see Fig. 31.14A), but less clearly defined radiographic changes are often overlooked. To assist in the radiographic detection of furcation involvement, the following diagnostic criteria are suggested:

1. The slightest radiographic change in the furcation area should be investigated clinically, especially if there is bone loss on adjacent roots (Fig. 31.15).

Fig. 31.15 Early Furcation Involvement Suggested by Fuzziness in the Bifurcation of the Mandibular First Molar, Particularly When Associated With Bone Loss on the Roots.

Fig. 31.16 Furcation Involvement of Mandibular First and Second Molars Indicated by Thickening of the Periodontal Space in the Furcation Area. The furcation of the third molar is also involved, but the thickening of the periodontal space is partially obscured by the external oblique line.

2. Diminished radiodensity in the furcation area in which outlines of bony trabeculae are visible suggests furcation involvement (Fig. 31.16).
3. Whenever there is marked bone loss in relation to a single molar root, it may be assumed that furcation is also involved (Fig. 31.17).

Periodontal Abscess

The typical radiographic appearance of a periodontal abscess is a discrete area of radiolucency along the lateral aspect of the root (Figs. 31.18 and 31.19). However, the radiographic picture is often not characteristic (Fig. 31.20). This can be due to the following:

1. *The stage of the lesion.* In the early stages an acute periodontal abscess is extremely painful but presents no radiographic changes.
2. *The extent of bone destruction and the morphologic changes of the bone.*
3. *The location of the abscess.* Lesions in the soft tissue wall of a periodontal pocket are less likely to produce radiographic changes than those deep in the supporting tissues. Abscesses on the facial or lingual surface are obscured by the radiopacity of the root; interproximal lesions are more likely to be visualized radiographically.

Fig. 31.17 Furcation Involvement of the First Molar Partially Obscured by the Radiopaque Lingual Root. The horizontal line across the distobuccal root demarcates the apical portion *(arrow)*, which is covered by bone, from the remainder of the root, where the bone has been destroyed.

Fig. 31.18 Radiolucent Area on Lateral Aspect of Root With Chronic Periodontal Abscess.

Therefore radiographs alone cannot provide a final diagnosis of a periodontal abscess but must be accompanied by careful clinical examination.

Clinical Probing

Regenerative and resective flap designs and incisions require prior knowledge of the underlying osseous topography. Careful probing of these pocket areas after scaling and root planing often requires local anesthesia and definitive radiographic evaluation of the osseous lesions. Radiographs taken with periodontal probes, gutta-percha points, or other indicators (e.g., Hirschfeld pointers) placed into the anesthetized pocket show the true extent of the bone lesion. As indicated previously, the attachment level on the radicular surface or interdental lesions with thick facial or lingual bone cannot be visualized in the radiograph. The use of radiopaque indicators is an efficient and necessary diagnostic aid (Fig. 31.21).

Localized Aggressive Periodontitis

Localized aggressive (formerly "localized juvenile") periodontitis, now termed "periodontitis with molar-incisor distribution," is characterized by the following:

Fig. 31.19 Typical Radiographic Appearance of Periodontal Abscess on Right Central Incisor.

1. Initially, there is bone loss in the maxillary and mandibular incisor or first molar areas, usually bilaterally, resulting in a vertical, arclike destructive pattern (Fig. 31.22).
2. As the disease progresses, loss of alveolar bone may become generalized but remains less pronounced in the premolar areas.

Trauma From Occlusion

Trauma from occlusion can produce radiographically detectable changes in the thickness of the lamina dura, morphology of the alveolar crest, width of the PDL space, and density of the surrounding cancellous bone.[5]

Traumatic lesions manifest more clearly in faciolingual aspects because mesiodistally, the tooth has added stability provided by the contact areas with adjacent teeth. Therefore slight variations in the proximal surfaces may indicate greater changes in the facial and lingual aspects. *The radiographic changes listed next are not pathognomonic for trauma from occlusion and must be interpreted in combination with clinical findings,* particularly tooth mobility, presence of wear facets, pocket depth, and analysis of occlusal contacts and habits.

The *injury phase* of trauma from occlusion produces a loss of the lamina dura that may be noted in apices, furcations, and marginal areas. This loss of lamina dura results in widening of the PDL space (Fig. 31.23). The *repair phase* of trauma from occlusion results in an attempt to strengthen the periodontal structures to better support the increased loads. Radiographically, this is manifested by a widening of the PDL space, which may be generalized or localized.

Although microscopic measurements have determined normal variations in the width of the PDL space along the root surface, these are generally not detected radiographically. Thus, when seen on radiographs, variations in the width of the PDL space suggest that the tooth is being subjected to increased forces. Successful attempts to reinforce the periodontal structures by widening the PDL space can be accompanied by increased width

Fig. 31.20 Chronic Periodontal Abscess. (A) Periodontal abscess *(arrow)* in the left maxillary first premolar area. (B) Extensive bone destruction on the mesial surface of the first premolar. Gutta-percha point traces to the root apex.

Fig. 31.21 (A) Radiograph of maxillary cuspid. This view does not show facial bone loss. (B) Radiograph of same maxillary cuspid as in (A), with gutta-percha points placed in the facial pocket to indicate bone loss.

Fig. 31.22 Localized Aggressive Periodontitis. The accentuated bone destruction in the anterior and first molar areas is considered to be characteristic of this disease.

Fig. 31.23 Widened Periodontal Space Caused by Trauma From Occlusion. Note the increased density of the surrounding bone caused by new bone formation in response to increased occlusal forces.

of the lamina dura and sometimes by condensation of the perialveolar cancellous bone.

More advanced traumatic lesions may result in deep angular bone loss, which, when combined with marginal inflammation, may lead to intrabony pocket formation. In terminal stages, these lesions extend around the root apex, producing a wide, radiolucent periapical image (cavernous lesions).

Root resorption may also result from excessive forces on the periodontium, particularly those caused by orthodontic appliances. Although trauma from occlusion produces many areas of root resorption, these areas are usually of a magnitude insufficient to be detected radiographically.

DIGITAL INTRAORAL RADIOGRAPHY

Advances in digital imaging technology have driven rapid growth of digital intraoral radiography as a convenient alternative to conventional film-based radiography.[10,12,14,23] These technologies have been integrated into patient management systems, enabling dental offices to maintain fully electronic patient records (Fig. 31.24A). The digital records can be easily shared among dental professionals and other health care providers, enabling telediagnosis and facilitating transmission to third parties for reimbursement.

Digital intraoral radiographic systems use either solid-state detectors or photostimulable phosphor (PSP) plates.[21-23] Systems with solid-state detectors use either charge-coupled devices (CCDs) or complementary metal oxide semiconductor (CMOS) chips as image receptors. These receptors are typically wired and connected to a computer using a universal serial bus (USB) connection. Wireless sensors are also available and require the

use of disposable batteries. With CCD/CMOS-based receptors, images are recorded and displayed on a computer monitor virtually in real time. These sensors are bulkier than film, and the active image-recording area is slightly smaller than that of film. A second technology for intraoral radiography is PSP plates. These receptors are the same size as intraoral radiographic film. Unlike CCD/CMOS receptors, PSP plates do not provide a real-time display of the radiographic image. On interaction with x-ray photons, PSP crystals in the plate store energy, creating a latent radiographic image. The stored energy is then released by stimulating the plate with an appropriate wavelength of light. With PSP systems, the workflow is somewhat similar to that with silver halide emulsion film. Following radiographic exposure, the PSP plate is scanned by a laser beam, converting the latent radiographic image into a digital image.

Following capture, digital radiographic images can be enhanced to augment radiographic diagnosis. The brightness and contrast of the image can be altered to highlight specific anatomic regions depending on the diagnostic task. The images can be magnified to allow closer examination of a specific area of interest. Importantly, a variety of image enhancement filters can be applied—for example, to sharpen images (enhance edges). Some software programs have preprogrammed algorithms that can be applied for specific diagnostic tasks—for example, to enhance interproximal caries, periodontal bone, pulp canals, and so forth (see Fig. 31.24B). However, it is important to recognize that such image manipulations can produce artifacts that may be misinterpreted as disease. Clinicians should be aware of such artifacts produced by digital image manipulation. In addition to the image manipulation features, digital radiographic images facilitate patient education, allow for easy storage and sharing with other health care providers, and can be easily integrated into electronic patient records.

ADVANCED IMAGING MODALITIES

Cone-beam computed tomography (CBCT) has revolutionized the field of oral and maxillofacial imaging. CBCT technology and its use in evaluating the implant patient are discussed in Chapter 76. However, CBCT finds application in almost every diagnostic task of clinical dentistry, including the evaluation of periodontal and periapical structures.[18] CBCT offers many advantages over conventional radiography, including accurate three-dimensional imaging of teeth and supporting structures. Although not recommended for every dental patient, CBCT avoids the problems of geometric superimposition and unpredictable magnification and can provide valuable diagnostic information in periodontal evaluation.

As discussed earlier, periapical and bitewing radiographs provide information mostly for interdental bone. However, a three-wall defect that preserves the buccal or lingual cortices can be difficult to diagnose, and the buccal, lingual, and furcational periodontal bone levels are hard to evaluate in conventional radiographs. When clinical examination raises concerns for such areas, CBCT imaging can add diagnostic value. Indeed, as compared with periapical radiographs, CBCT was able to depict the buccal and lingual/palatal surfaces and offered improved

Fig. 31.24 (A) Image display of a full-mouth radiographic series acquired using complementary metal oxide semiconductor receptors. Specific features of the software program allow for image manipulation, measurements, and annotations. (B) The "perio" image enhancement filter applied to highlight the contrast of alveolar bone. Note the presence of calculus and better depiction of the alveolar crestal bone.

Fig. 31.25 Periapical radiograph (A) and sagittal (B), cross-sectional (C), and axial (D) cone-beam computed tomography (CBCT) sections of the mandibular right second molar. No pathology is detected on the periapical radiograph. However, CBCT images clearly illustrate a deep vertical three-wall defect on the distal surface of the mandibular right second molar *(red arrow)*.

visualization of the morphology of the periodontal defect.[7] Furthermore, for assessment of periodontal bone loss, CBCT performed better than digital radiographs in the detection of early furcational defects, three-wall defects, fenestrations, and dehiscence but not in advanced furcation involvement or one- or two-wall and troughlike defects.[2]

Fig. 31.25 illustrates the diagnostic advantage of CBCT in the evaluation of a three-wall defect in the distal surface of tooth #32. A periapical radiograph (see Fig. 31.25A) presents normal bone height at the mesial and distal surfaces of #32. CBCT sections (see Fig. 31.25A and C) clearly demonstrate a three-wall defect on the distal surface of #32. Note that the buccal and lingual cortical plates are well preserved. For this reason, the periodontal defect is not depicted in the periapical radiograph. Similarly, Fig. 31.26 depicts a vertical defect in the interproximal

area between the two right maxillary premolars extending from the alveolar crest to the apical third of the roots toward the palatal aspect of the alveolar ridge. This defect cannot be appreciated on the periapical radiograph.

KEY FACTS

CBCT imaging provides three-dimensional information and overcomes many of the limitations of conventional two-dimensional radiography. However, CBCT imaging is a higher-dose radiation procedure relative to bitewing radiography and is also more expensive. CBCT imaging for periodontal bone evaluation should be considered only for select cases where two-dimensional information is insufficient for diagnostic or treatment planning needs, and it is not recommended for the routine evaluation of periodontal bone loss.

Fig. 31.26 Periapical radiograph (A) and sagittal (B), cross-sectional (C), and axial (D) cone-beam computed tomography (CBCT) sections of the maxillary premolar region. The periapical radiograph demonstrates horizontal bone loss. The CBCT images reveal the presence of a vertical defect between the premolars that extends from the palatal crest to the apical third of the roots. The extent of bone loss is underestimated on the periapical radiograph.

CONCLUSION

Periapical radiographic examination should be part of every patient's periodontal evaluation and coupled with a detailed recording of pocket depths, gingival margin location, and bleeding on probing. Radiographic evaluation should be updated every 2 years. Periapical radiographs often underestimate the amount of periodontal bone loss, and early changes are usually not detected. Significant interdental bone loss can occur and may not be detectable on periapical radiographs because the density of the intact buccal and lingual or palatal bone plates obscure changes that occur as a result of periodontitis. Comparing periapical radiographs of the same area taken at different times will be reliable only for documenting dramatic changes in bone levels, because variations in angulation of the beam, placement of the film, and development of the image make accurate measurements taken over time difficult and unreliable.

Three-dimensional radiographic techniques with CBCT give a much more accurate picture of periodontal bone loss than two-dimensional radiographs and will be more widely used as this technology becomes available in more clinics.

Case Scenarios are found on the companion website.

REFERENCES

 References for this chapter are found on the companion website.

32

Clinical Risk Assessment[a,b]

 For online-only content on risk indicators, risk markers/predictors, and clinical risk assessment for periodontal disease, please visit the companion website.

DEFINITIONS

Risk assessment is defined by numerous components.[2,33] Disease risk is the probability that an individual will develop a specific disease in a given period. The risk of developing the disease will vary from individual to individual.

Risk factors may be environmental, behavioral, or biologic factors that, when present, increase the likelihood that an individual will develop the disease. Risk factors are identified through longitudinal studies of patients with the disease of interest. Exposure to a risk factor or factors may occur at a single point in time, over multiple separate points in time, or continuously. However, to be identified as a risk factor, the exposure must occur before disease onset. Interventions can often be identified and, when implemented, can help modify risk factors.

The term *risk determinant/background characteristic*, which is sometimes substituted for the term *risk factor*, should be reserved for risk factors that cannot be modified. *Risk indicators* are *probable* or *putative* risk factors that have been identified in cross-sectional studies but not confirmed through longitudinal studies. *Risk predictors/markers*, although associated with increased risk for disease, do not cause the disease. These factors also are identified in cross-sectional and longitudinal studies. Box 32.1 lists elements of these categories of risk for periodontal disease.

CLINICAL CORRELATION

Lack of bleeding on probing does appear to serve as an excellent indicator of periodontal health, but the presence of bleeding on probing alone is not a good predictor of future attachment loss.

RISK FACTORS FOR PERIODONTAL DISEASE

Tobacco Smoking

Tobacco smoking is a well-established risk factor for periodontitis.[2,10] A direct relationship exists between smoking and the prevalence of periodontal disease (see Chapter 11). This association is independent of other factors, such as oral hygiene or age.[20] Studies comparing the response to periodontal therapy in smokers, previous smokers, and nonsmokers have shown that smoking has a negative impact on the response to therapy. However, former smokers respond similarly to nonsmokers.[3] These studies demonstrate the therapeutic impact of intervention strategies on patients who smoke (see Chapter 11).

Diabetes

Diabetes is a clear risk factor for periodontitis.[2] Epidemiologic data demonstrate that the prevalence and severity of periodontitis are significantly higher in patients with type 1 or 2 diabetes mellitus than in those without diabetes and that the level of diabetic control is an important variable in this relationship (see Chapter 13).

Pathogenic Bacteria and Microbial Tooth Deposits

It is well documented that the accumulation of bacterial plaque at the gingival margin results in the development of gingivitis

[a]Adapted from the following chapter of Newman and Carranza's Clinical Periodontology, 13th edition: Chapter 34: Clinical Risk Assessment, by Satheesh Elangovan, Karen F. Novak, M. John Novak.
[b]**Note:** In the 2018 Classification of Periodontal and Peri-Implant Diseases and Conditions, *chronic periodontitis* and *aggressive periodontitis* disease categories are grouped under a single category called *periodontitis* and are further characterized based on a multidimensional staging and grading system. In this chapter, the term *aggressive periodontitis* is still used because the related studies were conducted before the 2018 classification. Readers are referred to Chapter 6 for a detailed discussion of the classification of periodontal disease.

BOX 32.1 **Categories of Risk Elements for Periodontal Disease**

Risk Factors
Tobacco smoking
Diabetes
Pathogenic bacteria and microbial tooth deposits

Risk Determinants/Background Characteristics
Genetic factors
Age
Gender
Socioeconomic status
Stress

Risk Indicators
Human immunodeficiency virus (HIV)/acquired immunodeficiency syndrome (AIDS)
Osteoporosis
Infrequent dental visits

Risk Markers/Predictors
Previous history of periodontal disease
Bleeding on probing

and that the gingivitis can be reversed with the implementation of oral hygiene measures.[27] These studies demonstrate a causal relationship between the accumulation of bacterial plaque and gingival inflammation. However, a causal relationship between *plaque accumulation* and *periodontitis* has been more difficult to establish. Often patients with severe loss of attachment have minimal levels of bacterial plaque on the affected teeth, indicating that the *quantity* of plaque is not of major importance in the disease process. However, although quantity may not indicate risk, there is evidence that the composition, or *quality*, of the complex plaque biofilm is important.

In terms of quality of plaque, three specific bacteria have been identified as etiologic agents for periodontitis: *Aggregatibacter actinomycetemcomitans* (formerly *Actinobacillus actinomycetemcomitans*), *Porphyromonas gingivalis*, and *Tannerella forsythia* (formerly *Bacteroides forsythus*).[12] *P. gingivalis* and *T. forsythia* are often found in chronic periodontitis, whereas *A. actinomycetemcomitans* is often associated with aggressive periodontitis. Cross-sectional and longitudinal studies support the delineation of these three bacteria as risk factors for periodontal disease. Additional evidence that these organisms are causal agents includes the following[17]:

1. Their elimination or suppression impacts the success of therapy.
2. There is a host response to these pathogens.
3. Virulence factors are associated with these pathogens.
4. Inoculation of these bacteria into animal models induces periodontal disease.

Although not completely supported by these criteria for causation, moderate evidence also suggests that *Campylobacter rectus*, *Eubacterium nodatum*, *Fusobacterium nucleatum*, *Prevotella intermedia*, *Prevotella nigrescens*, *Peptostreptococcus micros*, *Streptococcus*

intermedius, and *Treponema denticola* are etiologic factors in periodontitis.[12]

It is becoming clear from investigations that the plaque composition shifts from a more symbiotic microbial community to one that is more dysbiotic (an imbalance in the relative abundance of microbes leading to disease), composed primarily of anaerobes, as we go from periodontal health to periodontal disease. Certain pathogens (termed *keystone pathogens*) such as *P. gingivalis*, play a major role in inducing such a shift, converting commensals into disease-provoking microbes (termed *pathobionts*).[18] Therefore the quantity of plaque present may not be as important as the quality of the plaque in determining risk for periodontitis.

Anatomic factors—such as furcations, root concavities, developmental grooves, cervical enamel projections, enamel pearls, and bifurcation ridges—may predispose the periodontium to disease as a result of their potential to harbor bacterial plaque and present a challenge to the dental hygienist during instrumentation. Similarly, the presence of subgingival and overhanging margins in restorations can result in increased plaque accumulation, inflammation, and bone loss. Although not clearly defined as risk factors for periodontitis, anatomic factors and *restorative factors* that influence plaque accumulation may play a role in disease susceptibility for specific teeth.[7]

The presence of *calculus,* which serves as a reservoir of bacterial plaque, has been suggested as a risk factor for periodontitis. Although the presence of some calculus in healthy individuals receiving routine dental care does not result in a significant loss of attachment, the presence of calculus in other groups of patients, such as those not receiving regular care and those with poorly controlled diabetes, can have a negative impact on periodontal health.[33]

RISK DETERMINANTS/BACKGROUND CHARACTERISTICS FOR PERIODONTAL DISEASE

Genetic Factors

Evidence indicates that genetic factors may explain why some patients develop periodontal disease and others do not. Studies conducted in twins have shown that genetic factors influence clinical measures of gingivitis, probing pocket depth, attachment loss, and interproximal bone height.[29-31] The familial aggregation seen in localized and generalized aggressive periodontitis also indicates genetic involvement in these diseases (see Chapter 8).

Kornman and colleagues[23] demonstrated that alterations (*polymorphisms*) in specific genes encoding inflammatory cytokines such as interleukin-1α (IL-1α) and interleukin-1β (IL-1β) were associated with severe chronic periodontitis in nonsmoking subjects.[23] However, results of other studies have shown a limited association between these altered genes and the presence of periodontitis. Overall, it appears that changes in the IL-1 genes may be only one of several genetic changes involved in the risk for chronic periodontitis. Therefore, although alteration in the IL-1 genes may be a valid marker for periodontitis in defined populations, its usefulness as a genetic marker in the general population may be limited.[22]

Immunologic alterations—such as neutrophil abnormalities,[19] monocytic hyperresponsiveness to lipopolysaccharide stimulation in patients with localized aggressive periodontitis,[40] and alterations in the monocyte/macrophage receptors for the F_c portion of antibody[22,50]—also appear to be under genetic control. In addition, genetics plays a role in regulating the titer of the protective immunoglobulin G2 (IgG2) antibody response to *A. actinomycetemcomitans* in patients with aggressive periodontitis (see Chapter 26).[16]

Age

Both the prevalence and severity of periodontal disease increase with age.[8,10,35] It is possible that degenerative changes related to aging may increase susceptibility to periodontitis. However, it is also possible that the loss of attachment and bone seen in older individuals are the result of prolonged exposure to other risk factors over the course of life, creating a cumulative effect over time. In support of this theory, studies have shown minimal loss of attachment in aging subjects enrolled in preventive programs throughout their lives.[36,37] Therefore it is suggested that periodontal disease is not an inevitable consequence of the aging process and that aging alone does not increase disease susceptibility. However, it remains to be determined whether changes related to the aging process—such as medication intake, decreased immune function, and altered nutritional status—interact with other well-defined risk factors to increase susceptibility to periodontitis.

Evidence of loss of attachment may have more consequences in younger patients. The younger the patient, the longer the time for exposure to causative factors. In addition, aggressive periodontitis in young individuals is often associated with unmodifiable risk factors, such as a genetic predisposition to disease.[10] Therefore young individuals with periodontal disease may be at greater risk for continued disease as they age.

Sex and Gender

Sex and gender play a role in periodontal disease.[2] Surveys conducted in the United States since 1960 demonstrate that males have more loss of attachment than do females.[45,47,48] In addition, males have poorer oral hygiene than do females, as evidenced by their higher levels of plaque and calculus.[1,46,48] Therefore sex and gender differences in the prevalence and severity of periodontitis appear to be related to preventive practices rather than any genetic factor.

Socioeconomic Status

Gingivitis and poor oral hygiene can be related to lower socioeconomic status (SES).[2,45,47] This more likely can be attributed to less dental awareness and fewer dental visits compared with more educated individuals with higher SES. After adjusting for other risk factors, such as smoking and poor oral hygiene, lower SES alone does not result in an increased risk for periodontitis (see Chapter 7).

Stress

The incidence of necrotizing ulcerative gingivitis increases during periods of emotional and physiologic stress, suggesting a link between the two.[11,41] Emotional stress may interfere with normal immune function[6,43] and can result in increased levels of circulating hormones, which can affect the periodontium.[39] Stressful life events, such as bereavement and divorce, appear to lead to a greater prevalence of periodontal disease.[14] Moreover, there appears to be an association between psychosocial factors and risk behaviors such as smoking, poor oral hygiene, and chronic periodontitis.[9] Adult patients with periodontitis who are resistant to therapy are more stressed than those who respond to therapy.[5] Individuals with financial strain, other forms of distress, depression, or inadequate coping mechanisms have more severe loss of attachment.[13] Although epidemiologic data on the relationship between stress and periodontal disease are limited, stress may be a putative risk factor for periodontitis.[10]

CLINICAL CORRELATION

The ultimate goal of performing periodontal risk assessment is to develop a personalized treatment plan for a specific patient, taking into account that patient's periodontal risk profile. Once an at-risk patient has been identified and a diagnosis is made, the treatment plan may be modified accordingly.

CONCLUSION

Risk assessment involves identifying elements that either may predispose patients to developing periodontal disease or may influence the progression of disease that already exists. In either case, these patients may require modification of their prognosis and treatment plan. In addition to an evaluation of the factors contributing to their risk, these patients should be educated concerning their risk; when appropriate, suitable intervention strategies should be implemented.

A Case Scenario is found on the companion website www .expertconsult.com.

REFERENCES

 References for this chapter are found on the companion website.

Determination of Prognosis[a]

DEFINITIONS

A *prognosis* is a prediction of the probable course, duration, and outcome of a disease based on a general knowledge of the pathogenesis of the disease and the presence of risk factors for the disease. It is established after the diagnosis is made and before the treatment plan is established. The prognosis is based on specific information about the disease and the manner in which it can be treated, but it also can be influenced by the clinician's previous experience with treatment outcomes (successes and failures) as they relate to the particular case. It is important to note that determination of prognosis is a dynamic process. As such, the prognosis initially assigned requires reevaluation after completion of all phases of therapy, including periodontal maintenance.

Prognosis is often confused with the term *risk*. Risk generally deals with the likelihood that an individual will develop a disease in a specified period (see Chapter 8). *Risk factors* are characteristics that put an individual at increased risk for developing a disease (see Chapter 7). In contrast, *prognosis* is the prediction of the course or outcome of a disease. *Prognostic factors* are characteristics that predict the outcome once the disease is present. In some cases, risk factors and prognostic factors are the same. For example, patients with diabetes or patients who smoke are more at risk for acquiring periodontal disease, and once they have it, they generally have a worse prognosis.

TYPES OF PROGNOSIS

Although some factors may be more important than others when assigning a prognosis (Box 33.1),[33,34] it will benefit the clinician to consider each factor. Historically, prognosis classification schemes were designed based on studies evaluating tooth mortality.[2,3,24,32,33] One scheme[24,33] assigns the following classifications:

Good prognosis: Control of etiologic factors and adequate periodontal support ensure the tooth will be easy to maintain by the patient and dental hygienist.

Fair prognosis: Approximately 25% attachment loss or grade I furcation invasion (location and depth allow proper maintenance with good patient compliance).

Poor prognosis: 50% attachment loss, grade II furcation invasion (location and depth make maintenance possible but difficult).

Questionable prognosis: >50% attachment loss, poor crown-to-root ratio, poor root form, grade II furcation invasion (location and depth make access difficult) or grade III furcation invasion; mobility no. 2 or no. 3; root proximity.

Hopeless prognosis: Inadequate attachment to maintain health, comfort, and function.

It should be recognized that good, fair, and hopeless prognoses in this classification system can be established with a reasonable degree of accuracy. However, poor and questionable prognoses are likely to change to other categories because they depend on a large number of factors that can interact in an unpredictable number of ways.[8,13,46]

In contrast to schemes based on tooth mortality, Kwok and Caton[24] proposed a scheme based on "the probability of obtaining stability of the periodontal supporting apparatus." This scheme is based on the probability of disease progression as related to local and systemic factors (see Box 33.1). Although some of these factors may affect disease progression more than others, consideration of each factor is important in assigning a prognosis. This scheme is as follows:

Favorable prognosis: Comprehensive periodontal treatment and maintenance will stabilize the status of the tooth. Future loss of periodontal support is unlikely.

Questionable prognosis: Local or systemic factors influencing the periodontal status of the tooth may or may not be controllable. If controlled, the periodontal status can be stabilized with comprehensive periodontal treatment. If not, future periodontal breakdown may occur.

Unfavorable prognosis: Local or systemic factors influencing the periodontal status cannot be controlled. Comprehensive

[a]Adapted from the following chapter of Newman and Carranza's Clinical Periodontology, 13th edition: Chapter 35: Determination of Prognosis, by Jonathan H. Do, Henry H. Takei, and Karen F. Novak.

BOX 33.1 Factors to Consider When Determining a Prognosis

Overall Clinical Factors
Patient age
Disease severity
Biofilm control
Patient compliance

Systemic and Environmental Factors
Smoking
Systemic disease or condition
Genetic factors
Stress

Local Factors
Biofilm and calculus
Subgingival restorations

Anatomic Factors
Short, tapered roots
Cervical enamel projections
Enamel pearls
Bifurcation ridges
Root concavities
Developmental grooves
Root proximity
Furcation invasion
Tooth mobility
Caries
Tooth vitality
Root resorption

Prosthetic and Restorative Factors
Abutment selection

periodontal treatment and maintenance are unlikely to prevent future periodontal breakdown.

Hopeless prognosis: The tooth must be extracted.

Because periodontal stability is assessed on a regular basis using clinical measures, it may be more useful in making treatment decisions and prognosis predictions than in trying to determine the likelihood that the tooth will be lost.

In many of these cases, it may be advisable to establish a *provisional prognosis* until phase I therapy is completed and evaluated. The provisional prognosis allows the clinician to initiate treatment of teeth that have a doubtful outlook in the hope that a favorable response may tip the balance and allow teeth to be retained. The reevaluation phase in the treatment sequence allows the dental hygienist to examine the tissue response to scaling, oral hygiene, and root planing, as well as to the possible use of chemotherapeutic agents where indicated. The patient's compliance with the proposed treatment plan also can be determined.

KEY FACT

A prognosis based on whether periodontal stability can be achieved with periodontal therapy and maintenance is as follows: favorable—likely, questionable—maybe, unfavorable—unlikely.

Overall Versus Individual Tooth Prognosis

Prognosis is divided into overall prognosis and individual tooth prognosis. The *overall prognosis* is concerned with the dentition as a whole. Factors that may influence the overall prognosis include patient age; current severity of disease; systemic factors; genetics; smoking; the presence of biofilm, calculus, and other local factors; patient compliance; and prosthetic possibilities (see Box 33.1). The overall prognosis answers the following questions:

- Should treatment be undertaken?
- Is treatment likely to succeed?
- When prosthetic replacements are needed, are the remaining teeth able to support the added burden of the prosthesis?

The *individual tooth prognosis* is determined after the overall prognosis and is affected by that prognosis.[32] For example, in a patient with a poor overall prognosis, the dentist likely would not attempt to retain a tooth that has a questionable prognosis because of local conditions. Many of the factors listed under local factors and prosthetic and restorative factors in Box 33.1 have a direct effect on the prognosis for individual teeth, in addition to any overall systemic or environmental factors that may be present.

FACTORS IN DETERMINATION OF PROGNOSIS

Overall Clinical Factors

Patient Age

For two patients with comparable levels of remaining connective tissue attachment and alveolar bone, the prognosis is generally better for the older of the two. For the younger patient, the prognosis is not as good because of the shorter time frame in which the periodontal destruction has occurred; the younger patient may have an aggressive type of periodontitis, or disease progression may have increased because of systemic disease or smoking. In addition, although the younger patient would ordinarily be expected to have a greater reparative capacity, the occurrence of so much destruction in a relatively short period would exceed any naturally occurring periodontal repair.

Disease Severity

Studies have demonstrated that a patient's history of previous periodontal disease may be indicative of their susceptibility to future periodontal breakdown (see Chapter 7). Therefore the following variables should be carefully recorded because they are important in determining the patient's past history of periodontal disease: probing pocket depth, level of attachment, amount of bone loss, and type of bony defect. These factors are determined by clinical and radiographic evaluation (see Chapters 30 and 31).

Determining clinical attachment loss reveals the approximate extent of root surface that is devoid of periodontal ligament; the radiographic examination shows the amount of root surface still invested in bone. Probing pocket depth is less important than level of attachment because it is not necessarily related to bone loss. In general, a tooth with deep probing depths and little attachment and bone loss has a better prognosis than one with shallow pockets and severe attachment and bone loss. However, a biofilm in deep pockets is difficult to control and may contribute to disease progression.

Prognosis is adversely affected if the base of the pocket (level of attachment) is close to the root apex. The presence of apical disease as a result of endodontic involvement also worsens the prognosis. However, surprisingly good apical and lateral bone repair can sometimes be obtained by combining endodontic and periodontal therapy.

The prognosis is also related to the height of remaining bone. Assuming bone destruction can be arrested, is there enough bone remaining to support the teeth? The answer is readily apparent in extreme cases—that is, when there is so little bone loss that tooth support is not in jeopardy (Fig. 33.1) or when bone loss is so severe that the remaining bone is obviously insufficient for proper tooth support (Fig. 33.2). Most patients, however, do not fit into these extreme categories. The height of remaining bone is usually somewhere in between, making bone level assessment alone insufficient for determining the overall prognosis.

The type of defect also must be determined. The prognosis for horizontal bone loss depends on the height of the existing bone, because it is unlikely that clinically significant bone height regeneration will be induced by therapy. In the case of angular (vertical), intrabony defects, if the contour of the existing bone and the number of osseous walls are favorable, there is an excellent chance that therapy could regenerate bone to approximately the level of the alveolar crest.[44]

When greater bone loss has occurred on one surface of a tooth, the bone height on the less involved surfaces should be taken into consideration when determining the prognosis. Because of the greater height of bone in relation to other surfaces, the center of rotation of the tooth will be nearer the crown (Fig. 33.3). This results in a more favorable distribution of forces to the periodontium and less tooth mobility.[48]

In dealing with a tooth that has a questionable prognosis, the chances of successful treatment should be weighed against any benefits that would accrue to the adjacent teeth if the tooth under consideration were extracted. Strategic extraction of teeth was first proposed as a means of improving the overall prognosis of adjacent teeth or enhancing the prosthetic treatment plan.[9] It has now been expanded to include the extraction of teeth with a questionable prognosis to enhance the likelihood of partial restoration of the bone supporting of the adjacent teeth (Fig. 33.4A to D) or successful implant placement. With the growing evidence of the long-term success of dental implants, it is proposed that a "watch and wait" approach may allow an area to deteriorate to the point that placing an implant is no longer a viable option. This means that the practitioner should weigh the potential success of one treatment option (extraction and implant placement) versus the other (periodontal therapy and maintenance) carefully when assigning a questionable prognosis to teeth.[19]

> ### KEY FACT
>
> Strategic extraction of teeth with unfavorable or questionable prognoses may improve the prognosis of adjacent teeth, enhance the prosthetic treatment, and increase the success rate of implants replacing the strategically extracted teeth.

Biofilm Control

Bacterial biofilm is the primary etiologic factor associated with periodontal disease (see Chapter 9). Therefore, effective removal of biofilm on a daily basis by the patient is critical to the success

Fig. 33.1 (A) Clinical image of mild chronic periodontitis with 1- to 2-mm clinical attachment loss in 40-year-old female. (B) Radiographic images of the patient.

Fig. 33.2 (A) Clinical image of generalized moderate-to-severe chronic periodontitis with 1- to 7-mm PD and 3- to 4-mm clinical attachment loss in a 31-year-old male. (B) Radiographic images of the patient.

Fig. 33.3 Prognosis for Tooth A Is Better Than for Tooth B, Despite Less Bone on One of the Surfaces of A. Because the center of rotation of tooth A is closer to the crown, the distribution of occlusal forces to the periodontium is more favorable than in B.

of periodontal therapy and the prognosis. The dental hygienist, as part of the oral heath care team plays a critical role in educating, individualizing, and modifying behavior to improve oral health.

Patient Compliance and Cooperation

The prognosis for patients with periodontal disease is critically dependent on the patient's attitude, desire to retain the natural teeth, and willingness and ability to effectively control biofilm.

Without these, treatment cannot succeed. Patients should be educated on the etiology and prevention of dental caries and periodontal diseases, and they must be clearly informed of the important role they must play for treatment to succeed. If a patient is unwilling to perform adequate biofilm control and receive the timely periodic maintenance checkups and treatments that the dental care provider deems necessary, the clinician can refuse to accept the patient for treatment. The oral health care provider should make it clear to the patient and in the patient record that further treatment is needed but will not be performed because of a lack of patient cooperation.

Systemic and Environmental Factors
Smoking

Epidemiologic evidence suggests that smoking may be the most important environmental risk factor impacting the development and progression of periodontal disease (see Chapter 11). Therefore, it should be made clear to patients that a direct relationship exists between smoking and the prevalence and incidence of periodontitis. In addition, patients should be informed that smoking affects not only the severity of periodontal destruction but also the healing potential of the periodontal tissues. As a result, patients who smoke do not respond as well to conventional periodontal therapy as do patients who have never smoked.[42,43] Therefore the prognosis in patients who smoke and have slight to moderate chronic periodontitis is generally questionable. In patients with severe chronic periodontitis, the prognosis may be unfavorable or hopeless.

Fig. 33.4 Extraction of Severely Involved Tooth to Preserve Bone on Adjacent Teeth. (A) Extensive bone destruction around the mandibular first molar. (B) Radiograph made years after extraction of the first molar and replacement by a prosthesis. Note the excellent bone support. (C) Extraction of periodontally involved bicuspid and molar. (D) Implant replacement of both teeth. (Courtesy Dr. S. Angha, University of California, Los Angeles.)

However, it should be emphasized that smoking cessation can affect the treatment outcome and therefore the prognosis.[5,16] As such, for patients who stop smoking, the prognosis can improve to favorable in those with slight to moderate chronic periodontitis and to questionable in those with severe chronic periodontitis.

Systemic Disease or Condition

The patient's systemic background affects the overall prognosis in several ways. For example, evidence from epidemiologic studies clearly demonstrates that the prevalence and severity of chronic periodontitis are significantly higher in patients with poorly controlled diabetes than in those whose diabetes is well controlled or those who do not have diabetes (see Chapter 7). Therefore, patients at risk for diabetes should be identified as early as possible and informed of the relationship between periodontitis and diabetes. Similarly, patients diagnosed with diabetes must be informed of the impact of diabetic control on the development and progression of periodontitis. It follows that the prognosis in these cases depends on patient compliance relative to both medical and dental status. Patients with well-controlled diabetes and slight to moderate periodontitis who comply with their recommended periodontal treatment should have a favorable prognosis. Similarly, in patients with other systemic disorders that could affect disease progression, prognosis improves with correction of the systemic problem.

The prognosis is questionable when surgical periodontal treatment is required but cannot be provided because of the patient's health (see Chapter 36). Incapacitating conditions that limit the patient's performance of oral procedures (e.g., Parkinson disease) also adversely affect the prognosis. Newer "automated" oral hygiene devices, such as electric toothbrushes, may be helpful for these patients and may improve their prognosis (see Chapter 43).

Genetic Factors

Periodontal diseases represent a complex interaction between a microbial challenge and the host's response to that challenge, both of which are influenced by environmental factors such as smoking. In addition to these external factors, evidence also indicates that genetic factors play an important role in determining the nature of the host response.[17] Evidence for this type of genetic influence exists for patients with both chronic and aggressive periodontitis. Genetic polymorphisms in the interleukin-1 (IL-1) genes, resulting in increased production of IL-1β, have been associated with a significant increase in risk for severe, generalized, and chronic periodontitis.[23,36] It has been demonstrated that knowledge of the patient's IL-1 genotype and smoking status can aid the clinician in assigning a prognosis.[35] Genetic factors also appear to influence serum immunoglobulin G2 (IgG2) antibody titers and the expression of FcγRII receptors on neutrophils, both of which may be significant in aggressive periodontitis.[17] Other genetic disorders, such as leukocyte adhesion deficiency (LAD) type 1, can influence neutrophil function, creating an additional risk factor for aggressive periodontitis.[17] Finally, the familial aggregation that is characteristic of aggressive periodontitis indicates that additional, as yet unidentified, genetic factors may be important in one's susceptibility to this form of disease (see Chapter 26).

The influence of genetic factors on prognosis is not simple. Although microbial and environmental factors can be altered through conventional periodontal therapy and patient education, genetic factors currently cannot be altered. However, detection of genetic variations linked to periodontal disease can potentially influence the prognosis in several ways. First, early detection of patients at risk because of genetic factors can lead to early implementation of preventive and treatment measures for these patients. Second, identification of genetic risk factors later in the disease or during the course of treatment can influence treatment recommendations, such as the use of adjunctive antibiotic therapy or increased frequency of maintenance visits. Third, identification of young individuals who have not been evaluated for periodontitis but who are recognized as being at risk because of the familial aggregation seen in aggressive periodontitis can lead to the development of early intervention strategies. In each of these cases, early diagnosis, intervention, and alterations in the treatment regimen may lead to an improved prognosis for the patient.

Stress

Physical and emotional stress, as well as substance abuse, may alter the patient's ability to respond to the periodontal treatment performed (see Chapter 7). These factors must be realistically faced when attempting to establish a prognosis.

Local Factors
Biofilm and Calculus

The microbial challenge presented by bacterial biofilm and calculus is the most important local factor in periodontal diseases. Therefore, in most cases, having a favorable prognosis depends on the ability of the patient and the dental hygienist to remove these etiologic factors (see Chapters 9 and 12).

> ### KEY FACT
> Periodontal prognosis depends on the ability of the patient and dental hygienist to effectively remove bacterial biofilm and resolve inflammation.

Subgingival Restorations

Subgingival margins may contribute to increased biofilm accumulation, increased inflammation, and increased bone loss[4,39,47] when compared with supragingival margins. Furthermore, discrepancies in these margins (e.g., overhangs) can negatively impact the periodontium (see Chapter 12). The size of these discrepancies and duration of their presence are important factors in the amount of destruction that occurs. In general, however, a tooth with a discrepancy in its subgingival margins has a worse prognosis than a tooth with well-contoured supragingival margins.

Anatomic Factors

Anatomic factors that may predispose the periodontium to disease and, therefore, affect the prognosis include short, tapered roots with large crowns, cervical enamel projections (CEPs) and enamel pearls, intermediate bifurcation ridges, root concavities, and developmental grooves. The clinician must also consider root proximity and the location and anatomy of furcations when assigning a prognosis.

Prognosis is less favorable for teeth with short, tapered roots and relatively large crowns (Fig. 33.5). Because of the disproportionate crown-to-root ratio and the reduced root surface available for periodontal support,[20] the periodontium may be more susceptible to injury by occlusal forces.

CEPs are flat, ectopic extensions of enamel that extend beyond the normal contours of the cementoenamel junction.[31] CEPs extend into the furcation of 28.6% of mandibular molars and 17% of maxillary molars.[31] CEPs are most likely to be found on buccal surfaces of maxillary second molars.[15,49] Enamel pearls are larger, round deposits of enamel that can be located in furcations or other areas on the root surface.[38] Enamel pearls are seen less frequently (1.1% to 5.7% of permanent molars; 75% appearing in maxillary third molars[38]) than CEPs. An intermediate bifurcation ridge has been described in 73% of mandibular first molars, crossing from the mesial to the distal root at the midpoint of the furcation.[10] The presence of these enamel projections on the root surface interferes with the attachment apparatus and may prevent regenerative procedures from achieving their maximum potential. Therefore their presence may have a negative effect on the prognosis for an individual tooth.

Scaling with root planing is a fundamental procedure in periodontal therapy. Anatomic factors that decrease the efficiency of this procedure can have a negative impact on the prognosis. Therefore, the morphology of the tooth root is an important consideration when discussing prognosis. *Root concavities* exposed through loss of attachment can vary from shallow flutings to deep depressions. They appear more marked on maxillary first premolars, the mesiobuccal root of the maxillary first molar, both roots of mandibular first molars, and the mandibular incisors[6,7] (Figs. 33.6 and 33.7). Any tooth, however, can have a proximal concavity.[12] Although these concavities increase the attachment area and produce a root shape that may be more resistant to torquing forces, they also create areas that can be difficult for oral health care providers and the patient to clean.

Other anatomic considerations that present accessibility problems are developmental grooves, root proximity, and furcation involvement. The presence of any of these can worsen the prognosis. *Developmental grooves,* which sometimes appear in the maxillary lateral incisors (palatogingival groove[50]; Fig. 33.8) or in the lower incisors, create an accessibility problem.[11,14] They initiate on enamel and can extend a significant distance on the root surface, providing a plaque-retentive area that is difficult to instrument. These palatogingival grooves are found on 5.6% of maxillary lateral incisors and 3.4% of maxillary central incisors.[22] Similarly, *root proximity* can result in interproximal areas that are difficult for the dental hygienist and patient to access.

Fig. 33.5 (A) Clinical image of generalized aggressive severe periodontitis with 3- to 13-mm PD and 7- to 15-mm clinical attachment loss in a 32-year-old male. (B) Radiographic images of the patient.

Fig. 33.6 Root Concavities in Maxillary First Molars Sectioned 2 mm Apical to the Furca. The furcal aspect of the root is concave in 94% of the mesiobuccal *(MB)* roots, 31% of the distobuccal *(DB)* roots, and 17% of the palatal *(P)* roots. The deepest concavity is found in the furcal aspects of the mesiobuccal roots (mean concavity, 0.3 mm). The furcal aspect of the buccal roots diverges toward the palate in 97% of teeth (mean divergence, 22 degrees). (Redrawn from Bower RC: Furcation morphology relative to periodontal treatment–furcation root surface anatomy, *J Periodontol* 50:366, 1979.)

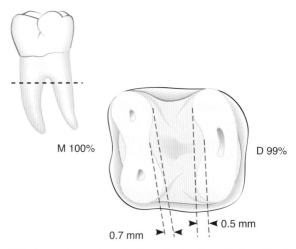

Fig. 33.7 Root Concavities in Mandibular First Molars Sectioned 2 mm Apical to the Furca. Concavity of the furcal aspect was found in 100% of mesial *(M)* roots and 99% of distal *(D)* roots. Deeper concavity was found in the mesial roots (mean concavity, 0.7 mm). (Redrawn from Bower RC: Furcation morphology relative to periodontal treatment–furcation root surface anatomy, *J Periodontol* 50:366, 1979.)

Fig. 33.8 Palatogingival Groove. (A) Probe in place to indicate a deep pocket along the palatogingival groove. (B) Radiograph with a gutta-percha point placed in the pocket. (C) The area is surgically opened. Note the palatogingival groove along the entire palatal portion of the root. (Courtesy Dr. Nadia Chugal, University of California, Los Angeles.)

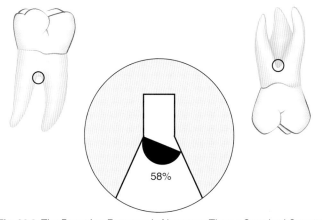

Fig. 33.9 The Furcation Entrance Is Narrower Than a Standard Curette in 58% of First Molars. (Redrawn from Bower RC: Furcation morphology relative to periodontal treatment–furcation root surface anatomy, *J Periodontol* 50:366, 1979.)

Finally, *access to the furcation area* is usually difficult to obtain. In 58% of maxillary and mandibular first molars, the furcation entrance diameter is narrower than the width of conventional periodontal curettes (Fig. 33.9).[7] Maxillary first premolars present the greatest difficulty, therefore, their prognosis is usually unfavorable when the lesion reaches the mesiodistal furcation. Maxillary molars also present some difficulty; sometimes their prognosis can be improved by resecting one of the buccal roots, thereby improving access to the area. When mandibular first molars or buccal furcations of maxillary molars offer good access to the furcation area, the prognosis is usually better.

Tooth Mobility

The principal causes of tooth mobility are loss of alveolar bone, inflammatory changes in the periodontium, and trauma from occlusion. Tooth mobility caused by inflammation and trauma from occlusion may be correctable.[37] However, tooth mobility resulting from loss of alveolar bone is not likely to be corrected. The likelihood of restoring tooth stability is inversely proportional to the extent to which mobility is caused by the loss of supporting alveolar bone.

KEY FACT

Tooth mobility is often used to condemn a tooth to a prognosis of questionable, unfavorable, or hopeless. It must be recognized that, depending on the cause, mobility may be correctable. Eliminating the cause of mobility can stabilize a tooth and improve its prognosis.

Caries, Tooth Vitality, and Root Resorption

For teeth mutilated by extensive caries, the feasibility of adequate restoration and endodontic therapy should be considered before undertaking periodontal treatment. Extensive idiopathic root resorption or root resorption resulting from orthodontic therapy jeopardizes the stability of teeth and adversely affects the response to periodontal treatment. The periodontal prognosis of treated nonvital teeth does not differ from that of vital teeth. New attachment can occur to the cementum of both nonvital and vital teeth.

Prosthetic and Restorative Factors

The overall prognosis requires a general consideration of bone levels (evaluated radiographically) and attachment levels (determined clinically) to establish whether enough teeth can be saved either to provide functional and aesthetic dentition or to serve as abutments for a useful prosthetic replacement of the missing teeth.

At this point, the overall prognosis and individual tooth prognosis overlap because the prognosis for key individual teeth may affect the overall prognosis for prosthetic rehabilitation. For example, saving or losing a key tooth may determine whether other teeth are saved or extracted or whether the prosthesis is fixed or removable (see Fig. 33.4). When few teeth remain, the prosthodontic needs become more important, and sometimes periodontally treatable teeth may have to be extracted if they are not compatible with the design of the prosthesis.

Teeth that serve as abutments are subjected to increased functional demands. More rigid standards are required when evaluating the prognosis of teeth adjacent to edentulous areas. A tooth with a post that has undergone endodontic treatment is more likely to fracture when serving as a distal abutment supporting a distal removable partial denture. Additionally, special oral hygiene measures must be instituted in these areas.

PROGNOSIS OF SPECIFIC PERIODONTAL DISEASES

Many of the criteria used in the diagnosis and classification of the different forms of periodontal disease[1] (see Chapter 6) are also used in developing a prognosis (see Box 33.1). Factors such as patient age, severity of disease, genetic susceptibility, and presence of systemic disease are important criteria in the diagnosis of the condition and in developing a prognosis. These common factors suggest that for any given diagnosis, there should be an expected prognosis under ideal conditions. This section discusses potential prognoses for the various periodontal diseases outlined in Chapter 6.

Prognosis for Patients With Gingival Disease
Biofilm-Induced Gingival Diseases

Gingivitis associated with dental plaque only. Biofilm-induced gingivitis is a reversible disease that occurs when bacterial biofilm accumulates at the gingival margin.[28,30] This disease can occur on a periodontium that has experienced no attachment loss or on a periodontium with nonprogressing attachment loss. In either case, the prognosis is good for patients with gingivitis associated with bacterial biofilm only, provided that all local irritants are eliminated, other local factors contributing to biofilm retention are eliminated, gingival contours conducive to the preservation of health are attained, and the patient cooperates by maintaining good oral hygiene.

Biofilm-induced gingival diseases modified by systemic factors. The inflammatory response to bacterial biofilm at the gingival margin can be influenced by systemic factors, such as endocrine-related changes associated with puberty, menstruation, pregnancy, and diabetes, and the presence of blood dyscrasias. In many cases, the frank signs of gingival inflammation that occur in these patients are seen in the presence of relatively small amounts of bacterial biofilm. Therefore, the long-term prognosis for these patients depends not only on control of bacterial biofilm but also on control or correction of the systemic factors.

Biofilm-induced gingival diseases modified by medications. Gingival diseases associated with medications include drug-influenced *gingival enlargement,* often seen with phenytoin, cyclosporine, and nifedipine and in oral contraceptive–associated gingivitis.

In drug-influenced gingival enlargement, the severity of the lesions is associated with inflammation, which is usually induced by bacterial biofilm. Inflammation may also be induced by repeated trauma (Fig. 33.10). Eliminating the source of inflammation, either trauma or biofilm, can limit the severity of the gingival overgrowth. However, surgical intervention is usually necessary to correct the alterations in gingival contour. Continued use of the drug and persistence of inflammation usually result in recurrence of the enlargement, even after surgical intervention (see Chapter 18). Therefore, the long-term prognosis depends on whether the etiology of the inflammation can be completely eliminated or the patient's systemic problem can be treated with an alternative medication that does not have gingival enlargement as a side effect.

KEY FACT

Inflammation may be induced by biofilm or trauma.

Fig. 33.10 Cyclosporine-associated gingival enlargement. A, Mild involvement located particularly on the papillae between teeth #9 and #10 and teeth #10 and #11. B, Advanced generalized enlargement.

In oral contraceptive–associated gingivitis, frank signs of gingival inflammation can be seen in the presence of relatively little biofilm. Therefore, as seen in biofilm-induced gingival diseases modified by systemic factors, the long-term prognosis in these patients depends not only on the control of bacterial biofilm but also on the likelihood of continued use of oral contraceptives.

Gingival diseases modified by malnutrition. Although malnutrition has been suspected to play a role in the development of gingival diseases, most clinical studies have not shown a relationship between the two. One possible exception is severe vitamin C deficiency. In early experimental vitamin C deficiency, gingival inflammation and bleeding on probing were independent of the biofilm levels present. The prognosis in these patients may depend on the severity and duration of the deficiency and on the likelihood of reversing the deficiency through dietary supplementation.

Non–biofilm-induced gingival lesions. Non–biofilm-induced gingivitis can be seen in patients with a variety of bacterial, fungal, and viral infections.[18] The gingivitis in these patients is not usually attributed to biofilm accumulation and prognosis depends on elimination of the source of the infectious agent. Dermatologic disorders such as lichen planus, pemphigoid, pemphigus vulgaris, erythema multiforme, and lupus erythematosus also can manifest in the oral cavity as atypical gingivitis (see Chapter 21). Prognosis for these patients is linked to management of the associated dermatologic disorder. Finally, allergic, toxic, and foreign-body reactions, as well as mechanical and thermal trauma, can result in gingival lesions. Prognosis for these patients depends on the elimination of the causative agent.

Prognosis for Patients With Periodontitis[b]
Chronic Periodontitis

Chronic periodontitis is a slowly progressive disease associated with well-known local environmental factors.[26] It can present in a localized or generalized form (see Chapter 25). In cases in which the clinical attachment loss and bone loss are not advanced (slight to moderate periodontitis—Stage I or II in the new classification), the prognosis is generally favorable, provided the inflammation can be controlled through good oral hygiene and the removal of local biofilm-retentive factors (see Fig. 33.1). In patients with more severe disease, as evidenced by furcation invasion and tooth mobility, or in patients who are noncompliant with oral hygiene practices, the prognosis may be questionable or unfavorable, and even hopeless.

Aggressive Periodontitis

Aggressive periodontitis can present in a localized or generalized form.[25] Two common features of both forms are (1) rapid

---

[b]In the 2018 Classification of Periodontal and Peri-Implant Diseases and Conditions, "chronic periodontitis" and "aggressive periodontitis" disease categories are grouped under a single category called "periodontitis" and are further characterized based on a multidimensional staging and grading system. In this chapter, the term "aggressive periodontitis" is still used because the related studies were conducted before the 2018 classification. Readers are referred to Chapter 6 for the detailed discussion on periodontal disease classification.

attachment loss and bone destruction in an otherwise clinically healthy patient and (2) a familial aggregation. These patients often present with limited microbial deposits that seem inconsistent with the severity of tissue destruction. However, the deposits that are present often have elevated levels of *Aggregatibacter actinomycetemcomitans* or *Porphyromonas gingivalis*. These patients also may present with phagocyte abnormalities and a hyperresponsive monocyte/macrophage phenotype. These clinical, microbiologic, and immunologic features would suggest that patients diagnosed with aggressive periodontitis (periodontitis grade C with molar incisor pattern) would have an unfavorable prognosis.

However, the clinician should consider additional specific features of the localized form of disease when determining the prognosis (see Fig. 33.5). Localized aggressive periodontitis usually occurs around the age of puberty and is localized to first molars and incisors (periodontitis grade C with molar incisor pattern). The patient often exhibits a strong serum antibody response to the infecting agents, which may contribute to localization of the lesions (see Chapter 26). When diagnosed early, these cases can be treated conservatively with oral hygiene instruction and systemic antibiotic therapy,[41] resulting in a favorable prognosis. When more advanced disease occurs, the prognosis can still be favorable if the lesions are treated with debridement, local and systemic antibiotics, and regenerative therapy.[29,51]

In contrast, although patients with generalized aggressive periodontitis are young (usually under age 30), they present with generalized interproximal attachment loss and a poor antibody response to infecting agents. Secondary contributing factors, such as cigarette smoking, are often present. These factors, coupled with the alterations in host defense seen in many of these patients, may result in a case that does not respond well to conventional periodontal therapy (scaling and root planing, oral hygiene instruction, and surgical intervention). Therefore, these patients often have a questionable or unfavorable prognosis, and the use of systemic antibiotics should be considered to help control the disease (see Chapter 47).

Periodontitis as a Manifestation of Systemic Diseases

Periodontitis as a manifestation of systemic diseases can be divided into the following two categories[21,27]:

1. Periodontitis associated with hematologic disorders such as leukemia and acquired neutropenias
2. Periodontitis associated with genetic disorders such as familial and cyclic neutropenia, Down syndrome, Papillon-Lefèvre syndrome, and hypophosphatasia

Although the primary etiologic factor in periodontal diseases is bacterial plaque, systemic diseases that alter the ability of the host to respond to the microbial challenge may affect the progression of disease and therefore the prognosis for the case. For example, decreased numbers of circulating neutrophils (as in acquired neutropenia) may contribute to widespread destruction of the periodontium. Unless the neutropenia can be corrected, these patients present with a fair to poor prognosis. Similarly, genetic disorders that alter the way the host responds to bacterial plaque (as in LAD syndrome) also can contribute to the development of periodontitis. Because these disorders generally manifest early in life, the impact on the periodontium may be clinically similar to generalized aggressive periodontitis. The prognosis in these cases will be questionable or unfavorable.

Other genetic disorders do not affect the host's ability to combat infections but still affect the development of periodontitis. Examples include (1) hypophosphatasia, in which patients have decreased levels of circulating alkaline phosphatase, severe alveolar bone loss, and premature loss of deciduous and permanent teeth; and (2) Ehlers-Danlos syndrome, a connective tissue disorder, in which patients may present with clinical characteristics of aggressive periodontitis. In both examples the prognosis is questionable or unfavorable.

Necrotizing Periodontal Disease

Necrotizing periodontal disease can be divided into necrotic diseases that affect the gingival tissues exclusively (necrotizing ulcerative gingivitis [NUG]) and necrotic diseases that affect deeper tissues of the periodontium, resulting in a loss of connective tissue attachment and alveolar bone (necrotizing ulcerative periodontitis [NUP]).[40,45] In NUG, the primary predisposing factor is bacterial plaque. However, this disease is usually complicated by the presence of secondary factors such as acute psychologic stress, tobacco smoking, and poor nutrition, all of which contribute to immunosuppression. Therefore, superimposition of these secondary factors on preexisting gingivitis can result in the painful, necrotic lesions characteristic of NUG. With control of both the bacterial plaque and the secondary factors, the prognosis for a patient with NUG is favorable. However, the tissue destruction in these cases is not reversible, and poor control of the secondary factors may make these patients susceptible to recurrence of the disease. With repeated episodes of NUG, the prognosis may worsen to questionable.

The clinical presentation of NUP is similar to that of NUG, except the necrosis extends from the gingiva into the periodontal ligament and alveolar bone. In systemically healthy patients, this progression may have resulted from multiple episodes of NUG, or the necrotizing disease may occur at a site previously affected with periodontitis. In these patients, the prognosis depends on alleviating the biofilm and secondary factors associated with NUG. However, many patients presenting with NUP are immunocompromised by systemic conditions such as human immunodeficiency virus (HIV) infection. In these patients the prognosis depends not only on reducing local and secondary factors but also on dealing with the systemic problem (see Chapter 39).

DETERMINATION AND REASSESSMENT OF PROGNOSIS

Determination of prognosis of a tooth or teeth requires a careful and thorough assessment of the presence of disease and its severity and extent. An accurate prognosis cannot be made without an accurate diagnosis. Once disease has been properly and accurately diagnosed, determining the prognosis can still be difficult, particularly for teeth with disease. Many factors can influence disease progression and the response to therapy, and the specific influence of any one factor is unknown and likely different from one patient to another. In addition, each patient can respond

differently at different times. Moreover, the outcome of therapy significantly depends on the treatment to be rendered, the quality of the treatment, the skills and knowledge of the treating dental hygienist, and patient home care. For these reasons, determining an accurate prognosis can be challenging.

Prognosis of teeth with minimal disease is favorable and by far the easiest to assign with accuracy and precision. As disease develops and severity increases, prognosis becomes progressively harder to assign correctly and accurately, especially for teeth with moderate to advanced disease that have a questionable or unfavorable prognosis. Once disease progresses to a point that teeth are no longer functional or treatable, the prognosis is again easy to determine. These teeth are assigned a hopeless prognosis and the treatment is extraction. However, the treatability of a tooth can be easily skewed by the skills and expertise of the treating clinician, or lack thereof. It is also easier for a clinician to make a diagnosis, determine a prognosis, and create a treatment plan that aligns with his or her expertise. For example, a prosthodontist may assign mandibular incisors with moderate attachment loss and mobility no. 2 a hopeless prognosis and develop a treatment plan that involves replacement of these teeth with a removable partial denture or dental implants. However, with the proper periodontal treatment and effective patient biofilm control, the health and function of these mandibular anterior teeth may be restored and maintained for many years.

It is not always possible to accurately determine the prognosis prior to initiating periodontal treatment. During the periodontal examination, due to the lack of anesthesia, it may not be possible to accurately and carefully probe a tooth to determine the true extent of bone loss and severity of disease. During scaling and root planing under anesthesia, it is possible to probe to the depth of the periodontal pocket. However, the anatomy of the osseous defect may not be determined until a periodontal flap has been elevated and all the granulation tissue removed. As such, the prognosis may change as more specific diagnostic information is discovered.

Prognosis may also change and improve with periodontal treatment or disease progression. During therapy, the patient's motivation and commitment, acknowledged as critical in all forms of periodontal therapy, can be determined, as well as the host response and the healing capacity of the patient. Clearly, enhancing the host response to a microbial biofilm challenge will significantly and positively influence the periodontal prognosis. Likewise, an *inability* to enhance the host response will negatively influence the prognosis. Either outcome, however, will allow the clinician to determine a more accurate prognosis.

A frank reduction in probing depth and inflammation after therapy indicates a favorable response to treatment and may suggest a better prognosis than previously assumed. If the inflammatory changes cannot be controlled or reduced by therapy, the overall prognosis may be unfavorable. In these patients, the prognosis can be directly related to the severity of inflammation. Given two patients with comparable bone destruction, the prognosis may be better for the patient with the greater degree of inflammation because a larger component of that patient's bone destruction may be attributable to local etiologic factors. In addition, therapy allows the dental hygienist an opportunity to work with the patient and the patient's physician to control systemic and environmental factors such as diabetes and smoking, which may have a positive effect on prognosis if adequately controlled.

The progression of periodontitis generally occurs in an episodic manner, with alternating periods of quiescence and shorter destructive stages (see Chapter 22). No methods are available at present to accurately determine whether a given lesion is in a stage of remission or exacerbation. Advanced lesions, if active, may progress rapidly to a hopeless stage, whereas similar lesions in a quiescent stage may be maintainable for long periods. Stable lesions in a patient in periodontal maintenance may also break down and advance due to changes in biofilm control, stress level, or systemic health. For these reasons, prognosis along with diagnosis must be carefully evaluated and reassessed throughout the course of treatment and over time during supportive maintenance therapy.

> **KEY FACT**
>
> Due to the dynamic nature of patients and periodontal disease, prognosis must be reevaluated during all phases of treatment.

CONCLUSION

The periodontal prognosis plays a pivotal role in therapy, as treatment decisions are made based on prognosis and to improve prognosis. Teeth with a hopeless diagnosis are extracted, whereas teeth with more favorable prognoses are treated, with the intent of restoring health and stability and ultimately improving the prognosis. A hopeless prognosis is perhaps the easiest prognosis to assign, because hopeless teeth usually have overt and severe disease. The hopeless prognosis is also perhaps the easiest to be erroneously assigned, due to clinical bias or lack of training and expertise. Therefore, the hopeless prognosis must be assigned with caution, as the consequences are irreversible. It must also be recognized that patients and diseases are dynamic. As such, a prognosis will change and must be reevaluated over time.

> **KEY FACT**
>
> *Examination → Diagnosis → Prognosis ↔ Treatment*
> - Diagnosis requires thorough and careful examination.
> - Prognosis is based on accurate diagnosis.
> - Treatment decisions are based on prognosis.
> - Treatment decisions are made to improve prognosis.
> - Diagnosis and prognosis will change with treatment.

REFERENCES

 References for this chapter are found on the companion website.

34

Treatment Planning and the Rationale for Periodontal Treatment[a]

After the diagnosis and prognosis are established, treatment is planned. The plan should encompass immediate, intermediate, and long-term goals.

The *immediate goals* are the elimination of all infectious and inflammatory processes that cause periodontal and other oral problems that may hinder the patient's general health. Basically, the immediate goals are to bring the oral cavity to a state of health. This requires patient education on infectious oral diseases and disease prevention, oral hygiene instructions, periodontal procedures, endodontics, caries control, oral surgery, and treatment of oral mucous membrane pathologies. Referral to other dental and medical specialties may be necessary.

From a periodontal viewpoint, the immediate goals are important because they consist of the elimination of gingival inflammation and the correction of conditions that cause and perpetuate it. These include not only elimination of root surface accretions but also pocket reduction and the establishment of good gingival contours and mucogingival relationships conducive to periodontal health. Extraction of hopeless teeth, restoration of carious lesions, and correction of poor existing restorations may be necessary.

The *intermediate goals* are the reconstruction of a healthy dentition that not only fulfills all functional and aesthetic requirements but lasts many years. Restoration of health, function, aesthetics, and longevity involves endodontic, orthodontic, periodontal, and prosthodontic considerations, as well as the age, health, and desires of the patient. The financial impact of restoring the dentition to health, function, aesthetics, and longevity requires careful consideration and understanding by the patient. The intermediate goals may be quickly achieved or require treatments over months or even years, depending on the complexity of the case, the therapy involved, and the financial status of the patient.

The *long-term goal* is maintenance of health through prevention and professional maintenance therapy. Once the long-term goal is set, both the patient and the clinician work toward it from the very first visit. Once active disease is controlled, all infectious and inflammatory processes are eliminated, and health

has been attained, health should be maintainable for the rest of the patient's life. Maintenance of health requires patient education on disease prevention and oral hygiene at the onset of treatment, meticulous daily home care by the patient, and patient adherence to professional recall maintenance.

> ### KEY FACT
> Maintenance of health depends on disease prevention, meticulous daily patient home care, and patient adherence to professional recall maintenance at a regular intervals.

The treatment plan is the blueprint for case management. It includes all procedures required for the establishment and maintenance of oral health and involves decisions regarding the following:

- Emergency treatment (pain, acute infections)
- Removal of nonfunctional and diseased teeth, and possibly strategic extraction of healthy teeth to facilitate the prosthetic reconstruction of the patient
- Treatment of periodontal diseases (surgical or nonsurgical, regenerative or resective)
- Endodontic therapy (necessary and intentional)
- Caries removal and placement of temporary and final restorations
- Occlusal adjustment and orthodontic therapy
- Replacement of missing teeth with removable or fixed dental prostheses or dental implants
- Aesthetic demands
- Sequence of therapy

Treatment decisions are made with the diagnosis and prognosis of the individual teeth and the overall dentition in mind. The prognosis is established based on the diagnosis. Treatment decisions are made based on the prognosis and to improve the prognosis. As such, *diagnosis and prognosis will change with treatment.*

Unforeseen developments during treatment may necessitate modification of the initial treatment plan. However, except for emergencies, no therapy should be initiated until a treatment plan has been established.

---

[a]Adapted from the following chapter of Newman and Carranza's Clinical Periodontology, 13th edition: Chapter 36: The Treatment Plan, by Jonathan H. Do, Henry H. Takei, and Fermin A. Carranza.

KEY FACT

Prognosis is established based on diagnosis. Treatment decisions are made based on prognosis and to improve prognosis. Diagnosis and prognosis will change with treatment.

OVERALL TREATMENT PLAN

The aim of the treatment plan is total treatment—that is, the coordination of all the immediate, intermediate, and long-term goals for the purpose of creating a well-functioning dentition in a healthy periodontal environment. The periodontal treatment encompasses different areas of therapeutic objectives for each patient according to their needs. It is based on the diagnosis, prognosis, disease severity, risk factors, and other factors outlined in previous chapters.

Extracting or Preserving a Tooth

Periodontal treatment requires long-range planning. Its value to the patient is measured by the years of healthy functioning of the entire dentition and not by the number of teeth retained at the time of treatment. Treatment is directed at establishing and maintaining the health of the periodontium throughout the mouth rather than attempting spectacular efforts to "save every tooth."

Implant replacement of missing teeth has become a predictable course of therapy. Therefore attempts to save questionable teeth may jeopardize adjacent teeth and lead to the loss of bone needed for future implant therapy. Teeth on the borderline of a hopeless prognosis do not contribute to the overall usefulness of the dentition. Such teeth become sources of recurrent problems for the patient and detract from the value of the greater service rendered by the establishment of periodontal health in the remainder of the oral cavity.

Removal, retention, or temporary (interim) retention of one or more teeth is an important part of the overall treatment plan. A tooth is indicated for extraction under the following conditions:
- It is so mobile that function becomes painful.
- It can cause acute abscesses during therapy.
- There is no use for it in the overall treatment plan.

In some cases a tooth can be retained temporarily, postponing the decision to extract until after treatment is completed. A tooth in this category is retained under the following conditions:
- It maintains posterior stops; the tooth can be removed after treatment, when it is replaced by an implant or another type of prosthesis.
- It maintains posterior stops and may be functional after implant placement in adjacent areas. When the implant is restored, these teeth can be extracted.
- In the anterior aesthetic zone, a tooth can be retained during periodontal therapy and removed when treatment is completed and a permanent restorative procedure can be performed. The retention of this tooth should not jeopardize the adjacent teeth. This approach avoids the need for temporary appliances during therapy.
- Extraction of hopeless teeth can also be performed during periodontal surgery of the adjacent teeth. This approach

reduces the number of appointments needed for surgery in the same area.

In the formulation of the treatment plan, in addition to the proper function of the dentition, aesthetic considerations play an important role. Different patients value aesthetics differently, according to their age, gender, profession, and social status. The clinician should carefully evaluate and consider a final aesthetic outcome of treatment that will be acceptable to the patient without jeopardizing the basic need of attaining health.

With the predictable use of implants, questionable teeth should be carefully evaluated as to whether their removal and replacement with an implant may be a better and more satisfactory course of therapy.

In complex cases, interdisciplinary consultation with other specialty areas is necessary before a final plan can be made. The opinions of orthodontists and prosthodontists are especially important for the final decision in these patients.

Occlusal evaluation and therapy may be necessary during treatment, which may necessitate planning for occlusal adjustment, orthodontics, and splinting (see Chapter 48). The correction of bruxism and other occlusal habits may also be necessary.

Systemic conditions should be carefully evaluated because they may require special precautions during the course of periodontal treatment. The tissue response to treatment procedures may be affected, or the preservation of periodontal health may be threatened after treatment is completed. The patient's physician should always be consulted when the patient presents with medical and systemic problems that may affect the periodontal therapy.

Supportive periodontal care (periodontal maintenance) is also of paramount importance for case maintenance. Such care entails all procedures for maintaining periodontal health. It consists of instruction in oral hygiene, removal of hard and soft deposits, recall evaluation and additional necessary therapies at regular intervals, according to the patient's needs.

SEQUENCE OF THERAPY

The periodontal treatment sequence is presented in Box 34.1, and a nonsurgical periodontal treatment decision tree is presented in Fig. 34.1. Periodontal therapy is an inseparable part of dental therapy, and all treatments must be well coordinated.

Although the phases of treatment are numbered, the recommended sequence does not follow the numbers (Fig. 34.2). Phase I, or the *nonsurgical phase,* is directed to the elimination of the etiologic factors of dental, gingival, and periodontal diseases. When successful, this phase stops the progression of dental and periodontal disease.

Immediately after completion of phase I therapy, immediately followed by reevaluation (if needed), the patient should be placed on the *maintenance phase* (phase IV) to preserve the results obtained and prevent any further deterioration and recurrence of disease. While on the maintenance phase, with its periodic evaluation, the patient enters into the *surgical phase* (phase II) and the *restorative phase* (phase III) of treatment (Fig. 34.3). These phases include periodontal surgery to treat and improve the condition of the periodontal and surrounding tissues. This

BOX 34.1 Periodontal Treatment Sequence

Periodontal Evaluation

Comprehensive periodontal examination

Diagnosis and prognosis

Patient education

- Clinical findings and disease status
- Disease pathogenesis and prevention
- Personalized oral hygiene instruction

Reduction of systemic and environmental risk factors

- Physician consultation
- Smoking cessation

Careful monitoring of blood glucose level and hemoglobin A_{1c} in patients with diabetes

Periodontal treatment plan

- Oral hygiene assessment and education
- Nonsurgical therapy
- Periodontal reevaluation
- Periodontal maintenance

Nonsurgical Therapy

Oral hygiene assessment and education[a]

Infection control

- Nonsurgical periodontal therapy
  - Supragingival and subgingival scaling and root planning (root débridement)
- Extraction of hopeless teeth

Reduction of local risk factors

- Removal or reshaping of overhangs and overcontoured restorations
- Restoration of carious lesions
- Restoration of open contacts

Periodontal Reevaluation

Inquiry of new concerns or problems

Inquiry of changes in patient's medical and oral health status

Oral hygiene assessment and education[a]

Comprehensive periodontal examination

Assessment of outcome of nonsurgical therapy

Determination of required additional nonsurgical and adjunctive therapy

Surgical Therapy

Adjunct to nonsurgical therapy

Should only occur once patient demonstrates proficient biofilm control

Objectives:

- Primary: Access for root instrumentation
- Secondary: Pocket reduction through soft tissue resection, osseous resection, or periodontal regeneration

Periodontal access surgery

- Resective
- Regenerative

Extraction of hopeless teeth

Periodontal plastic surgery

- Mucogingival surgery
- Aesthetic crown lengthening

Preprosthetic surgery

- Prosthetic crown lengthening
- Implant site preparation and implant placement

Periodontal Maintenance Therapy

Inquiry of new concerns or problems

Inquiry of changes in patient's medical and oral health status

Oral hygiene assessment and education[a]

Comprehensive periodontal examination

Professional maintenance care

- Supragingival and subgingival biofilm and calculus removal
- Selective scaling and root planing (root débridement)

Assessment of recall interval and plan for next visit

[a]Patient oral hygiene is critical to the overall short-term and long-term treatment outcome. Therefore oral hygiene must be repeatedly assessed and reinforced at each treatment and maintenance appointment.

Fig. 34.1 Periodontal Treatment Decision Tree.

may include regeneration of the gingiva and bone for function and aesthetics, placement of implants, and restorative therapy.

> ### KEY FACT
>
> Periodontal reevaluation is typically performed 4–8 weeks after nonsurgical periodontal therapy (in the form of scaling and root planing). Revaluation exam allows dental hygienists to assess changes in periodontal parameters such as probing depths and make appropriate treatment recommendations.

EXPLAINING THE TREATMENT PLAN TO THE PATIENT

The following discussion includes suggestions for explaining the treatment plan to the patient.

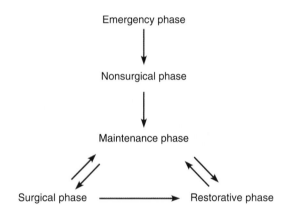

Fig. 34.2 Preferred Sequence of Therapy.

Be specific. Tell your patient, "You have gingivitis" or "You have periodontitis," then explain exactly what the condition is.

Avoid vague statements. Do not use statements such as "You have trouble with your gums" or "Your gums bleed a little." The patient may not understand the significance of such statements and may disregard them.

Begin your discussion on a positive note. Talk about the teeth that can be retained and the long-term service they can be expected to render. Do not begin your discussion with the statement "The following teeth have to be extracted." This creates a negative impression, which adds to the erroneous attitude of hopelessness the patient may already have regarding their mouth. Make it clear that every effort will be made to retain as many teeth as possible, but do not dwell on the patient's loose teeth. Emphasize that the important purpose of the treatment is to prevent the other teeth from becoming as severely diseased as the loose teeth.

Present the entire treatment plan as a unit. Avoid creating the impression that treatment consists of separate procedures, some or all of which may be selected by the patient. Make it clear that dental restorations and prostheses contribute as much to the health of the gingiva as the elimination of inflammation and periodontal pockets. Do not speak in terms of "having the gums treated and then taking care of the necessary restorations later" as if these were unrelated treatments.

Patients often seek guidance from the dental hygienist with questions such as the following:

- "Are my teeth worth treating?"
- "Would you have them treated if you had my problem?"
- "Why don't I just go along the way I am until the teeth really bother me and then have them all extracted?"

Explain that "doing nothing" or holding onto hopelessly diseased teeth as long as possible is inadvisable for the following reasons:

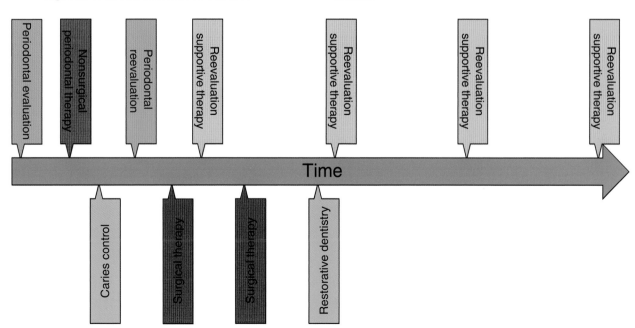

Fig. 34.3 Sample Treatment Timeline. Following nonsurgical periodontal therapy, the patient is placed on periodontal maintenance at regular intervals. Surgical and restorative treatments are scheduled between periodontal recalls.

1. Periodontal disease is a microbial infection, and research has clearly shown it to be an important risk factor for severe life-threatening conditions such as stroke, cardiovascular disease, pulmonary disease, and diabetes, as well as premature low-birth-weight babies in women of childbearing age. Correcting the periodontal condition eliminates a serious potential risk of systemic disease, which in some cases ranks as high on the danger list as smoking.

2. It is not feasible to place restorations or fixed bridges on teeth with untreated periodontal disease because the usefulness of the restoration is limited by the uncertain condition of the supporting periodontal structures.

3. Failure to eliminate periodontal disease not only results in the loss of teeth already severely involved but also shortens the life span of other teeth. With proper treatment, these teeth can serve as the foundation for a healthy, functioning dentition.

Therefore the dental hygienist should make it clear to the patient that if the periodontal condition is treatable, the best results are obtained by prompt treatment. If the condition is not treatable, the teeth should be extracted.

It is the dental professional's responsibility to advise the patient of the importance of periodontal treatment. However, if treatment is to be successful, the patient must be sufficiently interested in retaining his or her natural teeth and committed to changes in oral hygiene self-care. Individuals who are not particularly perturbed by the thought of losing their teeth are generally not good candidates for periodontal treatment.

CONCLUSION

The ultimate goal for every patient is to bring their mouth to a state of health and maintain it long term. This begins with educating the patient on his or her oral problems and the etiologies, treatment, and prevention of these problems. A properly formulated treatment plan is paramount to achieving this goal. A treatment plan is a plan for therapy formulated only after a thorough examination is completed, diagnosis and prognosis have been determined, and the needs and desires of the patient have been taken into consideration. It must be recognized that as diagnosis and prognosis will change with treatment, therapeutic needs may also change. As such, the treatment plan must be fluid and flexible (Box 34.2).

BOX 34.2 Examination → Diagnosis → Prognosis ↔ Treatment

- Diagnosis requires thorough and careful examination.
- Prognosis is based on accurate diagnosis.
- Treatment decisions are based on the prognosis.
- Treatment decisions are made to improve the prognosis.
- Diagnosis and prognosis will change with treatment.

35

Electronic Dental Records and Decision Support Systems[a]

Dental practices are using electronic dental records (EDRs) for patient care to a significant and rapidly rising degree.[15] Early on, computers primarily automated administrative and financial functions, but currently they increasingly support documentation of clinical information, digital radiographs, intraoral photos, and oral disease risk assessments. This shift in EDR use is generating vast amounts of patient data that could provide significant benefits to clinicians and researchers. Previously, clinicians could track individual patient outcomes only through paper-based records, and they typically spent considerable time transcribing that information into an electronic form so that they could analyze the data.

Digitization of patient data creates opportunities to dissect and analyze data in ways not possible before. Clinicians are able to track their patients' treatment progress and risks for various diseases at the individual, group, and practice levels. Analyzing electronic data can generate new knowledge in real time. This chapter discusses the current functions available in EDRs; EDR use by dental practices in the United States, Europe, and other locations throughout the world; commonly used EDRs in the United States and Europe; and the drawbacks and advantages of using EDRs in practice. Finally, the chapter explores the decision support systems available in dentistry, focusing specifically on periodontal disease, and closes with a discussion of the future of EDRs.

FUNCTIONALITIES AND COMPONENTS AVAILABLE IN ELECTRONIC DENTAL RECORDS

An EDR typically includes components such as patient registration, medical and medication history, extraoral and intraoral exams, hard and soft tissue charting, treatment planning, patient education, visit documentation, imaging, and scheduling. This section reviews selected examples of these functions.

Patient Registration

The data captured in patient registration include the patient's name, gender, birth date, identification numbers (such as Social Security and driver's license numbers), and address and contact information. Typically, offices with more than one clinician assign a provider. That makes it easy to list all patients for a particular provider.

Registration also includes an unobtrusive but important data field, the chart number that a patient is assigned automatically as soon as the record is saved. This chart number is the identifier that links together all parts of the electronic record for a particular patient; it is a unique identifier with which all information items for one patient are "stamped."

Another feature of an EDR is that most information on the registration screen is stored in separate fields, called "structured data." Structured data fields can be summarized and analyzed on their own or in combination, enabling some of the powerful reporting and analysis functions found in EDRs.

Periodontal Chart

The sample periodontal chart shown in Fig. 35.1 shows not only the pocket depth and clinical attachment loss but also a graphical presentation of periodontal changes over time. This presentation is difficult to achieve using paper-based periodontal charts.

ELECTRONIC DENTAL RECORD USE IN DENTAL PRACTICES

Since the late 1990s, the use of EDRs in dental practices has risen significantly worldwide, especially in the United States.[13,27] Early on, dental practices used computerized systems primarily for administrative functions, such as patient accounting and billing (94%), insurance processing (90.9%), and patient scheduling (83%).[6] Only 37% of dental practices reported using a

---

[a]Adapted from the following chapter of Newman and Carranza's Clinical Periodontology, 13th edition: Chapter 37: Electronic Dental Records and Decision Support Systems, by Thankam P. Thyvalikakath, Corey Stein, and Titus Schleyer.

Fig. 35.1 Screenshot of the Periodontal Chart in Eaglesoft. (Courtesy Patterson Technology.)

computer to maintain patient records at that time. Studies on EDR use in England and Sweden reported similar figures.[10,20,27,29]

More recent studies have pointed to a marked increase in EDR use for clinical documentation.[6,13,15] In 2010, US dental practices used EDRs to acquire and store radiographs (68%), intraoral photos and videos (67%), examination forms (54%), progress notes (54%), and dental charts (50%).[6] Most practices maintained a hybrid system of patient records, with some information spread across paper and the EDR. Compared with 2% in 2006, in 2012 approximately 15% of practices maintained completely paperless records.[1]

Figs. 35.2 to 35.4 illustrate how clinical information is stored in US solo and group practices, as well as in Scandinavian group dental practices.[15] These figures clearly show that more dental practices in Scandinavian countries store clinical information on computers than in the United States. Meanwhile, nearly all dental schools in the United States and Europe use (primarily commercial) EDR systems in some capacity.[7,16] However, few studies exist on how these systems are used in academic settings.

Commonly Used Electronic Dental Records

Four systems currently hold approximately 75% of the market in EDRs in the United States. They are Dentrix Dental Systems (Henry Schein; 37%), EagleSoft (Patterson Dental; 18%), and

SoftDent and PracticeWorks (Carestream; 20%).[6,13,15] Approximately 100 other companies, most of them fairly small, develop and market EDR systems in the United States. Notable among them are the Windows-based MOGO and the web-based Curve Dental and Dental Symphony. Although no general reports on EDRs commonly used in Europe exist, Al Dente (Nordenta, Horning, Denmark), Dental Suite (Plandent, Helsinki), and Opus (Planmeca, Helsinki) appear to dominate in Scandinavian countries.

Barriers to Using Electronic Dental Records

In spite of the rapid adoption of EDRs, several barriers exist to using them effectively for patient care. These include limited functionality, suboptimal usability and a steep learning curve, insufficient operational reliability, and cost and infection control issues.

Limited Functionality for Communication and Collaboration

Dental personnel collaborate extensively during patient care.[9] However, existing EDRs provide limited support for collaboration and communication among dental team members. In addition, breakdowns related to technology interrupt the workflow, cause rework, and increase the number of steps in work processes.[8]

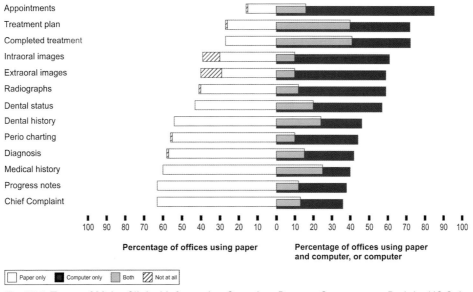

Fig. 35.2 Types of Major Clinical Information Stored on Paper, a Computer, or Both by US Solo Practices. (Reprinted with permission from Schleyer T, Song M, Gilbert G, et al: Electronic dental record use and clinical information management patterns among practitioner-investigators in The Dental Practice-Based Research Network. *J Am Dent Assoc* 144:49–58, 2013.)

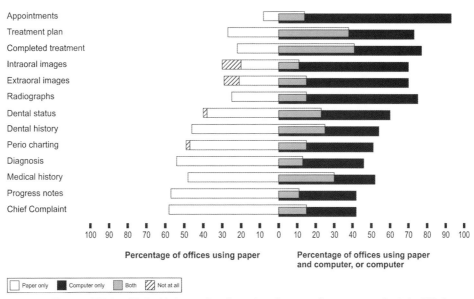

Fig. 35.3 Types of Major Clinical Information Stored on Paper, a Computer, or Both by US Group Practices. (Reprinted with permission from Schleyer T, Song M, Gilbert G, et al: Electronic dental record use and clinical information management patterns among practitioner-investigators in The Dental Practice-Based Research Network. *J Am Dent Assoc* 144:49–58, 2013.)

Suboptimal Usability and Steep Learning Curve

Several studies have reported on the poor usability of existing EDRs.[3,7,13,16,17,29] Two examples of usability problems are the separation of patient information across multiple screens and the frequent mismatch between system design and task flow. As a result, users have to shift their attention from patients to EDRs to navigate through the information and avoid making mistakes. Users believed they spent more time interacting with EDRs than with paper records, resulting in less face time with their patients.

Insufficient Reliability of Electronic Dental Records and Infection Control Issues

System crashes during patient care that lead to loss of patient data and time[13,16] are an example of the insufficient operational reliability of EDRs. Infection control issues are primarily due to the fact that the keyboard and mouse are the primary mechanisms for interacting with a computer. Many practices use auxiliary personnel to control the EDR. Although this workaround is effective, it reduces efficiency and increases the chance of errors.

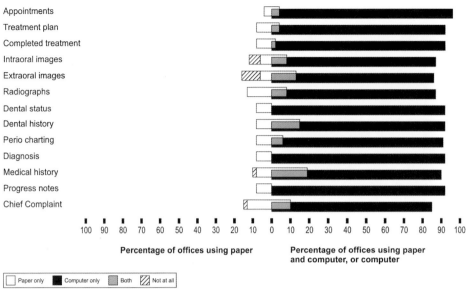

Fig. 35.4 Types of Major Clinical Information Stored on Paper, a Computer, or Both by Scandinavian Groups. (Reprinted with permission from Schleyer T, Song M, Gilbert G, et al: Electronic dental record use and clinical information management patterns among practitioner-investigators in The Dental Practice-Based Research Network. *J Am Dent Assoc* 144:49–58, 2013.)

Challenges to Realizing the Full Potential of Electronic Dental Records

Standards for the Information Content of Electronic Dental Records

As expressed by the adage "dentists and patients forget, but good records remember," complete and comprehensive patient records are essential to support effective decision-making and outcomes research.[28] Currently, no standards exist on what clinical information dental records should or must contain. As more and more dental professionals adopt EDRs to deliver patient care,[15] it is essential that we address the question of what patient information should be documented and how it should be structured.[26] Since the late 1980s, state, national, and international dental organizations have produced many guidelines or standards for essential components of the dental record. Common information categories recommended include personal and demographic information, reason for visit, dental history, medical history, clinical examination information, diagnosis, treatment plan, and informed consent information. However, these recommendations are very general, and dental records vary significantly in the degree to which they meet them.[13] Currently, major work is being pursued toward developing a standard information model for EDRs.[4,26]

Data Representation and Interoperability

Dentistry lacks a standard terminology for documenting and describing dental findings and diagnoses. The World Health Organization's International Classification of Diseases coding system, or ICD, is limited with regard to oral and dental diagnoses. Several terminologies, such as the Systematized Nomenclature of Dentistry (SNODENT)[25] and EZCodes,[21] are being developed and evaluated as standard diagnostic codes for dentistry.

However, standard terminologies alone will not solve the problem of data representation and interoperability. We need to consider how dental data in their totality can be represented on the computer so they can be easily stored, exchanged, and analyzed. Patient records typically consist of free text; numbers; standardized codes; and radiographic, histologic, and clinical images. Although structured data can be represented and analyzed unambiguously, that is not true for free text data and images. Concepts in dental records must be represented to facilitate semantic interoperability and exchange of information across different systems. Ontologies are a powerful way to create computer-based representations that fulfill that goal.[12]

Benefits of Using Electronic Dental Records

In spite of barriers and challenges to using EDRs, tremendous opportunities exist for using them to improve patient care. As mentioned in the introduction, EDRs can provide significant benefits for clinicians and researchers. Using EDRs, clinicians are able to track their patients' treatment progress and risks for various diseases. Other benefits include timely access to patient records, access to patient records regardless of geographic location, simultaneous access to patient records by multiple users, and the ability to generate the best evidence from patient data and built-in decision support systems to reduce errors such as those involving medications and drug-drug interactions. For researchers, digitization creates opportunities to dissect and analyze patient data in ways that were not possible before.[23] Reuse of electronic patient data for dental research is in a nascent stage, but it provides a significant opportunity to help build a "learning health care system." Advantages of using EDR data for research include the ability to conduct studies of significant statistical power due to large sample sizes, obtain well-matched controls, ascertain important potential confounders, identify patients with rare diseases, save study time, collect data in real time, and generate systematic data documentation. We discuss a few of these benefits next.

Risk-Based Decision Support Systems for Periodontal Disease

In periodontology, risk-based decision support systems are the most common type of CDSS. The PreViser Risk Calculator (PRC) (PreViser Corp., Mount Vernon, WA) developed by Page et al.,[19] UniFe developed by Trombelli et al.,[26] and DentoRisk (DentoSystem Scandinavia AB, Stockholm, Sweden) developed by Lindskog et al.[14] are examples of risk assessment tools for periodontal disease. The PRC is a web-based tool developed based on the scientific evidence of the importance of risk factors for periodontal disease. The tool calculates the patient's disease score and risk score based on a mathematical algorithm that assigns relative weights to 11 factors: patient age, smoking history, diagnosis of diabetes, history of periodontal surgery, bleeding on probing, pocket depth, furcation involvement, subgingival restorations, root calculus, vertical bone defects, and radiographic bone loss.[5] The disease score ranges from 0 (no disease) to 100 (severe periodontitis), and the risk score ranges from 1 (lowest) to 5 (highest).

FUTURE OF ELECTRONIC DENTAL RECORDS AND DECISION SUPPORT SYSTEMS IN DENTISTRY

The adoption of EDRs has the potential not just to support clinical care but also to advance research and improve patient outcomes. In addition, EDRs offer the opportunity to move from a reparative to a preventive approach to treating oral diseases.

Many dental diseases, including periodontal disease, are currently being managed using a reparative model, under which dental professionals concentrate on the clinically obvious items that require immediate intervention, focusing less attention on preventing future disease.[18,22] Using this model, the treatment is essentially the same for all patients with identical clinical presentation. EDRs with integrated decision support systems can help with identifying patients at high risk and with providing individualized recommendations. Despite emerging evidence of the validity and clinical utility of these systems for treatment in dentistry and, specifically, periodontology, little evidence suggests that these approaches are adopted broadly in general practice.[11] Leveraging the full functionalities of these systems will require significant work and trained informatics personnel. Dental informatics is an interdisciplinary field that applies computer and information science knowledge and methods to improve information management during clinical care, research, and dental education. Until now, the challenge for dentistry was to transition from paper to EDRs in a very basic fashion. Often, EDRs were designed as close or exact replicas of paper records.

Going forward, this approach will be insufficient. Dentistry now faces the challenge of making sense of electronic data, facilitating clinical care and research, and improving outcomes. It is important that trained dental informaticians, clinicians, educators, and researchers collaborate to accomplish this goal. Dentistry, just like other health care disciplines, is an information-intensive domain. The future success of dentistry depends on how we best use information technology to make sense of data and improve patient care. Informatics holds the key to that success.

REFERENCES

 References for this chapter are found on the companion website.

36

Periodontal Treatment of Medically Compromised Patients[a]

 Content on thyroid and parathyroid disorders, adrenal insufficiency, thrombocytopenic purpuras, nonthrombocytopenic purpuras, blood dyscrasias, renal diseases, liver diseases, and pulmonary diseases can be accessed on the companion website.

CHAPTER OUTLINE

Many patients seeking dental care have significant medical conditions that can alter the course of their oral disease and the therapy provided. Older periodontal patients are more likely to have underlying disease. The therapeutic responsibility of the clinician includes identification of the patient's medical problems to formulate a proper treatment plan. A thorough medical history is paramount.[77] If significant findings are unveiled, consultation with an appropriate physician or referral of the patient is indicated. This will ensure correct management and provide medicolegal coverage for the clinician.

This chapter covers common medical conditions and associated periodontal management. The review of each topic area should be supplemented by consulting other references for more detailed coverage of specific disorders. An understanding these conditions will enable the dental hygienist to treat the total patient, not merely the periodontal reflection of underlying disease.

CARDIOVASCULAR DISEASES

Cardiovascular diseases are the most prevalent category of systemic disease in the United States and many other countries, and they become more common with increasing age.[106] Health histories

should be closely scrutinized for cardiovascular problems, including hypertension, angina pectoris, myocardial infarction (MI), cardiac bypass surgery, cerebrovascular accident (CVA), congestive heart failure (CHF), infective endocarditis (IE), and implanted cardiac pacemakers or automatic cardioverter-defibrillators.

In most cases, the patient's physician should be consulted, especially if stressful or prolonged treatment is anticipated. Short appointments and a calm, relaxing environment will help to minimize stress and maintain hemodynamic stability.

Hypertension

Hypertension, the most common cardiovascular disease, affects more than 50 million American adults, many of whom are undiagnosed.[36] In 2017, the American Heart Association and the American College of Cardiology issued revised guidelines for the evaluation and management of hypertension (Table 36.1).[18,37,45,118]

Compared with previous classification schemes,[41,42] which focused on diastolic blood pressure (BP), the 2017 guidelines[18] emphasize the importance of systolic BP. Systolic BP greater than 130 mm Hg is considered a greater risk factor for cardiovascular disease. Systolic BPs between 120 and 129 mm Hg or diastolic BPs less than or equal to 80 mm Hg are classified as elevated. BP is not considered a disease category or diagnosis; it is instead a term used to describe a condition and identify individuals who are at high risk for hypertension.

The 2017 guidelines classify hypertension into three categories, versus the two under the previous classification schemes *Stage 1 hypertension* is defined as a systolic BP of 130 to 139 mm Hg

[a]Adapted from the following chapter of Newman and Carranza's Clinical Periodontology, 13th edition: Chapter 39: Periodontal Treatment of Medically Compromised Patients, by Perry R. Klokkevold, Brian L. Mealey, and Joan Otomo-Corgel.

TABLE 36.1 Classification of Adult Blood Pressure

Blood Pressure	Systolic		Diastolic
Normal	<120	and	<80
Elevated	120–129	and	<80
Stage 1 hypertension Monitor each visit—advise on risks	130–139	or	80–89
Stage 2 hypertension[a]	≥140	or	≥90
Hypertensive urgency; immediate medical consult	>180	or	>120

[a]risk of providing emergency dental care must outweigh risk of possible hypertensive complications.[18,38,47]

From Whelton, et al: 2017 ACC/AHA/AAPA/ABC/ACPM/AGS/APhA/ASH/ASPC/NMA/PCNA Guideline for the Prevention, Detection, Evaluation, and Management of High Blood Pressure in Adults: A Report of the American College of Cardiology/American Heart Association Task Force on Clinical Practice Guidelines. *J Am Coll Cardiol* 15;71(19):e127–e248, 2018.

or diastolic pressure of 80 to 89 mm Hg. *Stage 2 hypertension* is defined as a systolic pressure greater than 140 mm Hg or diastolic pressure greater than 90 mm Hg. Hypertensive urgency is defined as a systolic pressure greater than 180 mm Hg or a diastolic pressure greater than 120 mm Hg. For a reading within the category of hypertensive urgency, immediate medical consultation is advised.

Hypertension is not diagnosed from a single elevated BP recording. Rather, classification is based on the value of two or more BP readings taken at two or more appointments. The higher systolic or diastolic pressure determines the patient's classification. Patients with hypertension enter dental practices every day, and hypertension is particularly common among the older population. Evidence from the Framingham Heart Study revealed that people with normal BP at age 55 still have a 90% risk of becoming hypertensive later in life.[108]

Hypertension is divided into primary and secondary types. *Primary* (i.e., essential) *hypertension* occurs when no underlying pathologic abnormality can be found to explain the disease. Approximately 95% of hypertensive patients have primary hypertension. The remaining 5% have *secondary hypertension,* in which an underlying cause can be found and is often treated. Conditions responsible for secondary hypertension include renal disease, endocrinologic changes, and neurogenic disorders.

In early hypertension, the patient may be asymptomatic. If not identified, diagnosed, and treated, hypertension can persist and increase in severity, leading eventually to coronary artery disease, angina, MI, CHF, CVA, or kidney failure.[53] The dental office can play a vital role in the detection of hypertension and maintenance care of the patient with hypertensive disease. The first dental office visit should include two BP readings spaced at least 10 minutes apart, which are averaged and used as a baseline. Before the clinician refers a patient to a physician because of elevated BP, readings should be taken at a minimum of two appointments unless the measurements are extremely high (i.e., systolic pressure >180 mm Hg or diastolic pressure >120 mm Hg).

The periodontal recall system is an ideal method for hypertension detection and monitoring. Almost three of every four adult patients with hypertension in the United States do not control their BP well enough to attain the goal of systolic pressure less than 130 mm Hg and diastolic pressure less than 80 mm Hg.[14] Lack of compliance with antihypertensive therapy is the primary reason for this failure. Dental care providers can help to achieve greater success in managing hypertension by taking BP readings at each periodontal recall visit.

Periodontal procedures should not be performed until accurate BP measurements and histories have been taken to identify patients with significant hypertensive disease. The time of day should be recorded because BP varies significantly throughout the day.[70]

Dental treatment for hypertensive patients is safe as long as stress is minimized.[53,59] If a patient is receiving antihypertensive therapy, consultation with the physician may be warranted regarding the individual's current medical status, medications, periodontal treatment plan, and patient care. Many physicians are not knowledgeable about the specific details of dental or periodontal procedures. The dental clinician must inform the physician regarding the estimated degree of stress, length of the procedures, and complexity of the individualized treatment plan. Morning dental appointments were once suggested for hypertensive patients, but evidence indicates that BP usually increases around awakening and peaks at midmorning.[10,70,97] Because lower BP levels occur in the afternoon, afternoon dental appointments may be preferred.

No routine periodontal treatment should be delivered to a patient who is hypertensive and not under medical management. For patients with systolic BP greater than 180 mm Hg or diastolic BP greater than 120 mm Hg, treatment should be limited to emergency care until hypertension is controlled. When treating hypertensive patients, the dental hygienist should not use a local anesthetic containing an epinephrine concentration greater than 1 : 100,000 or a vasopressor to control local bleeding. Local anesthesia without epinephrine can be used for short procedures (<30 minutes). In a patient with hypertensive disease, however, it is important to minimize pain by providing profound local anesthesia to avoid an increase in endogenous epinephrine secretion.[53,59]

The benefits of the small doses of epinephrine used in dentistry far outweigh the potential for hemodynamic compromise. The smallest possible dose of epinephrine should be used, and aspiration before injection of local anesthetics is critical. Intraligamentary injection is usually contraindicated because hemodynamic changes are similar to intravascular injection.[96] If the hypertensive patient exhibits anxiety, use of conscious sedation in conjunction with periodontal procedures may be warranted.[104]

β-adrenergic receptor antagonists (i.e., β blockers) are typically used to treat hypertension (Table 36.2). The β blockers are *cardioselective*, blocking only β1 cardiac receptors (i.e., β1 receptors), or *nonselective*, blocking both β1 cardiac receptors and β2 peripheral receptors (i.e., β2 receptors). Epinephrine, an α-adrenergic and β-adrenergic agonist, increases heart rate through direct stimulation of cardiac β1 receptors. Epinephrine also stimulates α-adrenergic receptors, producing vasoconstriction

TABLE 36.2 Nonselective and Selective β-Adrenergic Receptor Antagonists

Generic Name	Trade Name
Nonselective β-Blockers	
Carvedilol	Coreg
Carteolol hydrochloride	Cartrol
Nadolol	Corgard
Penbutolol sulfate	Levatol
Pindolol	Visken
Propranolol hydrochloride	Inderal; Inderal LA
Timolol maleate	Blocadren
Selective β-Blockers	
Acebutolol hydrochloride	Sectral
Atenolol	Tenormin
Betaxolol hydrochloride	Kerlone
Bisoprolol fumarate	Zebeta
Metoprolol tartrate	Lopressor
Metoprolol succinate	Toprol-XL

Fig. 36.1 As Seen on a Coronary Angiogram, Atherosclerosis Can Result in Narrowing of the Coronary Arteries, Producing Signs and Symptoms of Ischemic Heart Disease.

of arteries, and β2 receptors, causing vasodilation of skeletal muscle arterioles.

Administration of local anesthetics containing epinephrine to patients taking nonselective β blockers (e.g., propranolol, nadolol) can elevate BP.[121] Epinephrine-induced α-adrenergic stimulation results in vasoconstriction and increased BP. Because the patient's nonselective medication has blocked the β2 receptors, epinephrine cannot stimulate the normal compensatory β2 receptor–induced vasodilation. This can result in dramatically increased BP, followed by reflex bradycardia mediated by the vagus nerve and carotid baroreceptors. The end result is a patient with severe hypertension and bradycardia, producing a dangerous decrease in vascular perfusion and possibly causing death. Because of this potential complication, epinephrine-containing local anesthetics should be used cautiously and only in very small amounts in patients taking nonselective β blockers, with careful monitoring of vital signs.[53,121]

The dental hygienist should be aware of the many side effects of antihypertensive medications. *Postural hypotension* is common and can be minimized by slow positional changes in the dental chair.[53] *Depression* is a side effect of which many patients are unaware. Nausea, sedation, oral dryness, lichenoid drug reactions, and gingival overgrowth are associated with certain classes of antihypertensive agents.[59]

CLINICAL CORRELATION

Hypertension, the most common cardiovascular disease, affects more than 50 million American adults, many of whom are undiagnosed. Almost three of every four adults with hypertension do not control their blood pressure well enough. The dental office can play a vital role in the detection of undiagnosed hypertension and the compliance of patients being treated for hypertension. Blood pressure should be taken at the initial visit and at each recall visit and anytime local anesthesia is planned.

Ischemic Heart Disease

Ischemic heart disease (Fig. 36.1) includes disorders such as angina pectoris and myocardial infarction (MI). Angina pectoris occurs when myocardial oxygen demand exceeds supply, resulting in temporary myocardial ischemia.[37] Patients with a history of unstable angina pectoris (i.e., angina that occurs irregularly or on multiple occasions without predisposing factors) should be treated only for emergencies and then in consultation with their physician. Patients with stable angina (i.e., angina that occurs infrequently, is associated with exertion or stress, and is easily controlled with medication and rest) can undergo elective dental procedures. Because stress often induces an acute anginal attack, stress reduction is important. Profound local anesthesia is vital, and conscious sedation may be indicated for anxious patients.[104] Supplemental oxygen delivered by nasal cannula can help to prevent intraoperative anginal attacks.

Patients who manage acute anginal attacks with nitroglycerin are instructed to bring their medication to dental appointments. Nitroglycerin should also be kept in the office medical emergency kit. The patient's nitroglycerin should be readily accessible on the dental tray in case it should be needed during treatment. Because the shelf life of nitroglycerin is relatively short, the expiration date of the patient's nitroglycerin and that of the nitroglycerin in the office's medical emergency kit should be noted.

Patients with angina may be taking longer-acting forms of nitroglycerin (e.g., tablet, patch), β blockers, or calcium channel blockers (also used for treating hypertension) for prevention of angina. Restrictions on the use of local anesthetics containing epinephrine are similar to those for the patient with hypertension. Intraosseous injection with epinephrine-containing local anesthetics using special systems (e.g., Stabident, Fairfax Dental) should be done cautiously in patients with ischemic heart disease because it results in transient increases in heart rate and myocardial oxygen demand.[74]

If the patient becomes fatigued or uncomfortable or has a sudden change in heart rhythm or rate during a periodontal procedure, the procedure should be discontinued as soon as possible. If a patient has an anginal episode in the dental chair, the dental hygienist should do the following:

1. Discontinue the periodontal procedure.
2. Administer 1 tablet (0.3 to 0.6 mg) of nitroglycerin sublingually.
3. Reassure the patient and loosen restrictive garments.
4. Administer oxygen with the patient in a reclined position.
5. If the signs and symptoms cease within 3 minutes, complete the periodontal procedure if possible, making sure that the patient is comfortable. Terminate the procedure at the earliest convenient time.
6. If the anginal signs and symptoms do not resolve with this treatment within 5 minutes, administer another dose of nitroglycerin, monitor the patient's vital signs, call the patient's physician, and be ready to accompany the patient to the emergency department.
7. A third nitroglycerin tablet can be given 5 minutes after the second. Chest pain that is not relieved by three tablets of nitroglycerin indicates likely MI. The patient should be transported to the nearest emergency medical facility immediately.

Nitroglycerin lingual spray formulations have been popular in hospital pharmacies because of their increased shelf life compared with nitroglycerin tablets.[69] The lingual spray can provide greater and more rapid vasodilation with a longer duration of action.[25,82] The convenience and advantages of a nitroglycerin lingual spray are appealing, but the accuracy of dose delivery has been questioned and warrants additional studies before the spray can be recommended to replace the known tablet regimen.[69]

MI is the other category of ischemic heart disease encountered in dental practice. Dental treatment is usually deferred for at least 3 months[5] after MI because the peak mortality rate occurs during this time.[30] After 3 months, MI patients can usually be treated using techniques similar to those for stable angina patients.

Cardiac (aortocoronary) bypass, femoral artery bypass, angioplasty, and endarterectomy have become common surgical procedures in patients with ischemic heart disease. If one of these procedures was performed recently, the physician should be consulted before elective dental therapy to determine the degree of heart damage or arterial occlusive disease, the stability of the patient's condition, and the potential for infective endocarditis (IE) or graft rejection,

Congestive Heart Failure

CHF is a condition in which the pump function of the heart is unable to supply sufficient amounts of oxygenated blood to meet the body's needs.[30] CHF usually begins with left ventricular failure caused by a disproportion between the hemodynamic load and the capacity to handle that load. CHF can be caused by a chronic increase in workload (as in hypertension or aortic, mitral, pulmonary, or tricuspid valvular disease), direct damage to the myocardium (as in MI or rheumatic fever), or an increase in

the body's oxygen requirements (as in anemia, thyrotoxicosis, or pregnancy).

Patients with poorly controlled or untreated CHF are not candidates for elective dental procedures. These individuals are at risk for sudden death, usually from ventricular arrhythmias.[29] For patients with treated CHF, the clinician should consult with the patient's physician regarding the severity of CHF, the underlying cause, and current medical management. Medical management of CHF can include the use of calcium channel blockers, direct vasodilators, diuretics, angiotensin-converting enzyme (ACE) inhibitors, α-receptor blockers, or cardiotonic agents such as digoxin.[27,44] Each medication has potential side effects that can affect periodontal therapy. Because of orthopnea (i.e., inability to breathe unless in an upright position) in some CHF patients, the dental chair should be adjusted to a comfortable level for the patient rather than placed in a supine position. Short appointments, stress reduction with profound local anesthesia, and possibly conscious sedation and use of supplemental oxygen should be considered.[30,53]

Cardiac Pacemakers and Implantable Cardioverter-Defibrillators

Cardiac arrhythmias are most often treated with medications, but some are also treated with implantable pacemakers or automatic cardioverter-defibrillators.[29,53,76] Pacemakers are usually implanted in the chest wall and enter the heart transvenously. Automatic cardioverter-defibrillators are more often implanted subcutaneously near the umbilicus and have electrodes passing into the heart transvenously or directly attached to the epicardium. Consultation with the patient's physician allows determination of the underlying cardiac status, the type of pacemaker or automatic cardioverter-defibrillator in use, and any precautionary measures to be taken.

Automatic cardioverter-defibrillators activate without warning when certain arrhythmias occur. This can endanger the patient during dental treatment because activation often causes sudden patient movement. Stabilization of the operating field during periodontal treatment with bite blocks or other devices can prevent unexpected trauma.

Infective Endocarditis

IE is a disease in which microorganisms colonize damaged endocardium or heart valves.[32] Although the incidence of IE is low, it is a serious disease with a poor prognosis despite modern therapy. The term *infective endocarditis* is preferred to the previous term *bacterial endocarditis* because the disease can also be caused by fungi and viruses. The organisms most often encountered in IE are α-hemolytic streptococci (e.g., *Streptococcus viridans*). However, nonstreptococcal organisms often found in the periodontal pocket have been increasingly implicated, including *Eikenella corrodens, Aggregatibacter actinomycetemcomitans, Capnocytophaga,* and *Lactobacillus* species.[8]

IE has been divided into acute and subacute forms. The acute form involves virulent organisms, usually nonhemolytic streptococci and strains of staphylococci, which invade normal cardiac tissue, produce septic emboli, and cause infections that run a rapid, usually fatal course. The subacute form results from colony formation on damaged endocardium or heart valves by low-grade pathogenic organisms. The classic example is rheumatic carditis from rheumatic fever.

After the American Heart Association (AHA) publication on prevention of IE in 1997,[22] many questioned the efficacy of antimicrobial prophylaxis to prevent IE in patients who undergo dental or other procedures and have suggested that the AHA guidelines should be revised.[26,99] Members of the Rheumatic Fever, Endocarditis, and Kawasaki Disease Committee of the AHA Council on Cardiovascular Disease in the Young and a national and international group of experts on IE extensively reviewed data published on the prevention of IE. The committee concluded that only an extremely small number of IE cases can be prevented by antibiotic prophylaxis for dental procedures (even if such therapy were 100% effective). The guidelines were then changed and published in a 2008 report.[119] The new guidelines advise that IE prophylaxis should be recommended only for cardiac conditions with the highest risk of adverse outcome from IE (Box 36.1). For these patients, antibiotic prophylaxis is recommended for all dental procedures that involve manipulation of the gingival or periapical tissues or perforation of the oral mucosa. Antibiotic prophylaxis is not indicated for individuals solely on the basis of an increased lifetime risk of contracting IE.

The practice of periodontics is intimately concerned with the prevention of IE. However, bacteremia may occur even in the absence of dental procedures, especially in individuals with poor oral hygiene and significant periodontal inflammation. IE is much more likely to result from frequent exposure to random bacteremias associated with daily activities than to be caused by a dental procedure.[119] Prevention of periodontal inflammation is paramount. The AHA states that patients who are at risk for IE should "establish and maintain the best possible oral health to reduce potential sources of bacterial seeding." To provide adequate preventive measures for IE, the dental hygienist's major concern should be to reduce the microbial population in the oral cavity to minimize soft tissue inflammation and bacteremia.

> **KEY FACT**
>
> The updated AHA guidelines on the prevention of IE were published in a 2008 report. They recommend that prophylaxis should be provided only for cardiac conditions with the highest risk of adverse outcomes from IE (see Box 36.1).

Preventive measures to reduce the risk of IE consist of the following:

1. *Define the susceptible patient.* A careful medical history can disclose a susceptible patient. Health questioning should cover the history in all categories of risk. If any doubt exists, the patient's physician should be consulted.
2. *Provide oral hygiene instruction.* Oral hygiene should be practiced with methods that improve gingival health. In patients with significant gingival inflammation, oral hygiene should initially be limited to gentle procedures (i.e., oral rinses and gentle toothbrushing with a soft brush) to minimize bleeding. As gingival health improves, more aggressive oral hygiene can be initiated. Oral irrigators are usually not recommended because their use can induce bacteremia.[64] Susceptible patients should be encouraged to maintain the highest level of oral hygiene after soft tissue inflammation is controlled.
3. *Recommended antibiotic prophylactic regimens should be practiced with all high-risk patients during periodontal treatment* (Table 36.3). If any doubt regarding susceptibility exists, the patient's physician should be consulted. In patients who have been receiving continuous oral penicillin for secondary prevention of rheumatic fever, penicillin-resistant α-hemolytic streptococci are occasionally found in the oral cavity. An alternate regimen is recommended instead. If the periodontal patient is taking a systemic antibiotic as part of periodontal therapy, changes in the IE prophylaxis regimen may be indicated. For example, a patient taking a penicillin agent after regenerative therapy can be placed on azithromycin before the next periodontal procedure. Patients with early-onset forms of periodontitis often have high levels of *A. actinomycetemcomitans* in the subgingival plaque. This organism has been associated with IE and is often resistant to penicillins. In patients with aggressive periodontitis who should be given prophylaxis, Slots and colleagues[95] suggested using tetracycline (250 mg four times daily for 14 days) to eliminate or reduce *A. actinomycetemcomitans*, followed by the conventional prophylaxis protocol at the time of dental treatment.
4. *Periodontal treatment should be designed for susceptible patients to accommodate their degree of periodontal involvement.* The nature of periodontal therapy enhances the problems related to the prophylaxis of subacute IE. Patients are often faced with long-term therapy, healing periods that extend beyond a 1-day antibiotic regimen, multiple visits, and procedures that easily elicit gingival bleeding.

> **BOX 36.1 Cardiac Conditions Associated With the Highest Risk of Adverse Outcome From Infective Endocarditis for Which Prophylaxis With Dental Procedures Is Recommended**[a]
>
> Previous history of infective endocarditis
> Prosthetic cardiac valves or prosthetic material used for cardiac valve repair
> Congenital heart disease (CHD), with the following conditions:
> - Unrepaired cyanotic CHD, including palliative shunts and conduits
> - Completely repaired congenital heart defect with prosthetic material or device, whether placed by surgery or catheter intervention, during the first 6 months after the procedure
> - Repaired CHD with residual defects at or adjacent to the site of a prosthetic patch or prosthetic device (which inhibits endothelialization)
>
> Cardiac transplantation recipients who develop cardiac valvulopathy
>
> [a]American Heart Association recommendations.[119]
> From Wilson W, Taubert KA, Gewitz M, et al: Prevention of infective endocarditis: guidelines from the American Heart Association Rheumatic Fever, Endocarditis, and Kawasaki Disease Committee, Council on Cardiovascular Disease in the Young, and the Council on Clinical Cardiology, Council on Cardiovascular Surgery and Anesthesia, and the Quality of Care and Outcomes Research Interdisciplinary Working Group. *Circulation* 116:1736–1754, 2007.

TABLE 36.3   Recommended Antibiotic Prophylaxis Regimens for Periodontal Procedures in Adults at Risk for Infective Endocarditis

Regimen	Antibiotic	Dosage[a]
Standard oral regimen	Amoxicillin	2.0 g 30–60 min before procedure
Alternate regimen for patients allergic to amoxicillin or penicillin	Clindamycin	600 mg 30–60 min before procedure
	Azithromycin or clarithromycin or	500 mg 30–60 min before procedure
	Cephalexin or cefadroxil[b]	2.0 g 30–60 min before procedure
Regimen for patients unable to take oral medications	Ampicillin	2.0 g intramuscularly or intravenously within 30 min before procedure
Regimen for patients unable to take oral medications and allergic to penicillin	Clindamycin	600 mg intravenously within 30 min before procedure (must be diluted and injected slowly)
	or Cefazolin[b]	1.0 g intramuscularly or intravenously within 30 min before procedure

[a]Adult dosages are listed. Children's dosages are lower.
[b]Cephalosporins should not be used in patients with immediate-type hypersensitivity reactions to penicillins (e.g., urticaria, angioedema, anaphylaxis).

The following guidelines can aid in the development of periodontal treatment plans for patients susceptible to IE:

- Periodontal disease is an infection with potentially wide-ranging systemic effects. For patients at risk for IE, every effort should be made to eliminate this infection. Teeth with severe periodontitis and a poor prognosis may require extraction. Teeth with less severe involvement in a motivated patient should be retained, treated, and maintained closely.
- All periodontal treatment procedures (including probing) require antibiotic prophylaxis; gentle oral hygiene methods are excluded. Pretreatment chlorhexidine rinses are recommended before all procedures, including periodontal probing, because these oral rinses significantly reduce the bacteria on mucosal surfaces.[22]
- To reduce the number of visits required and thereby minimize the risk of developing resistant bacteria, numerous procedures can be accomplished at each appointment depending on the patient's needs and ability to tolerate dental treatment.[53]
- When possible, at least 7 days between appointments (preferably 10 to 14 days) should be allowed. If this is not possible, an alternative antibiotic regimen for appointments within a 7-day period can be selected.
- Evidence does not support or refute a need to place patients at risk for IE on extended antibiotic regimens after treatment.[53] Patients who have had periodontal surgery are not usually placed on antibiotics for the first week of healing unless there

are specific indications to do so. If patients are placed on these regimens, the dosages are inadequate to prevent endocarditis during ensuing appointments. The standard prophylactic antibiotic dose is still needed. For example, if a patient was placed on 250 mg of amoxicillin three times a day for 10 days after periodontal surgery and was to return to the office for more treatment on the seventh day, the patient would require a full 2.0-g dose of amoxicillin before that treatment. Alternatively, clindamycin or azithromycin could be used at the second appointment.

- Regular recall appointments, with an emphasis on oral hygiene reinforcement and maintenance of periodontal health, are extremely important for patients susceptible to IE.

Cerebrovascular Accident

A CVA (i.e., stroke) results from ischemic changes (e.g., cerebral thrombosis caused by an embolus) or hemorrhagic phenomena. Hypertension and atherosclerosis are predisposing factors for CVA and should alert the dental hygienist to evaluate the patient's medical history carefully for the possibility of early cerebrovascular insufficiency and to be aware of the symptoms of this disease. A physician's referral should precede periodontal therapy if the signs and symptoms of early cerebrovascular insufficiency are evident.

To prevent a repeat stroke, active infections should be treated aggressively, because even a minor infection can alter blood coagulation and trigger thrombus formation and ensuing cerebral infarction. The dental hygienist should counsel the patient about the importance of thorough oral hygiene.[78] Poststroke weakness of the facial area or paralysis of extremities can make oral hygiene procedures extremely difficult.[63] The dental hygienist may have to modify the oral hygiene instruments for ease of use, perhaps in consultation with an occupational therapist. Long-term chlorhexidine rinses greatly aid in plaque control.

Dental clinicians should treat post-CVA patients with the following guidelines in mind:

1. No periodontal therapy (except for an emergency) should be performed for 3 months after a CVA because of the high risk of recurrence during this period.
2. After 3 months, periodontal therapy can be performed during short appointments with an emphasis on minimizing stress. Profound local anesthesia should be obtained, using the minimal effective dose of local anesthetic agents. Concentrations of epinephrine greater than 1:100,000 are contraindicated.
3. Light conscious sedation (i.e., inhalation, oral, or parenteral) can be used for anxious patients. Supplemental oxygen is indicated to maintain thorough cerebral oxygenation.
4. Stroke patients are frequently placed on oral anticoagulants. Previously, it was thought that for procedures entailing significant bleeding, such as periodontal surgery or tooth extraction, the anticoagulant regimen might require adjustment, depending on the level of anticoagulation at which the patient is being maintained. However, evidence regarding the risks of altering anticoagulation therapy suggests that it may be prudent to provide treatment without changing it (see "Anticoagulant Medications," further on). Any changes

in anticoagulant therapy regimens for a stroke patient should be done in consultation with the patient's physician.
5. BP should be monitored carefully. Recurrence rates for CVAs are high, as are rates of associated functional deficits.

ENDOCRINE DISORDERS

Diabetes

The patient with diabetes requires special precautions before periodontal therapy. Type 1 diabetes was formerly known as insulin-dependent diabetes, and type 2 diabetes was referred to as non–insulin-dependent diabetes.[55] During the past decade, the medical management of diabetes has changed significantly in an effort to minimize the debilitating complications associated with this disease.[101,107] Blood glucose (i.e., glycemia) levels are more tightly managed through diet, oral agents, and insulin therapy.[54]

If the dental hygienist detects intraoral signs of undiagnosed or poorly controlled diabetes, a thorough history is indicated.[73] The classic signs of diabetes include *polydipsia* (i.e., excessive thirst), *polyuria* (i.e., excessive urination), and *polyphagia* (i.e., excessive hunger, often with unexplained concurrent weight loss). If the patient has any of these signs or symptoms or the dental hygienist suspects diabetes, further investigation with laboratory studies and physician consultation are indicated. Periodontal therapy has limited success in the setting of undiagnosed or poorly controlled diabetes.

If a patient is suspected of having undiagnosed diabetes, the following procedures should be performed:
1. Consult the patient's physician.
2. Analyze laboratory tests (Box 36.2), including fasting blood glucose and casual glucose test results.[4]
3. Rule out acute orofacial infection or severe dental infection; if present, provide emergency care immediately.
4. Establish the best possible oral health through nonsurgical debridement of plaque and calculus. Institute oral hygiene instruction. Limit more advanced care until the diagnosis has been established and good glycemic control obtained.

If a patient is known to have diabetes, it is critical that the level of glycemic control be established before initiating periodontal treatment. The fasting glucose and casual glucose tests provide snapshots of the blood glucose concentration at the time the blood was drawn; these tests reveal nothing about long-term glycemic control. The primary test used to assess glycemic control in a known diabetic individual is the glycated hemoglobin (Hb) assay (Box 36.3). Two tests are available, the HbA1 and HbA1c assays; the HbA1c is used more often.[54] This assay has been shown by a large international study to provide an accurate measure of the average blood glucose concentrations over the preceding 2 to 3 months.[61] Fig. 36.2 is a simplified graphic representation of the data from that study depicting the average blood glucose concentrations for HbA1c values.

The therapeutic goal for many patients is to achieve and maintain an HbA1c below 8%. Patients with relatively well-controlled diabetes (HbA1c <8%) usually respond to therapy similarly to nondiabetic individuals.[19,100,117] Poorly controlled patients (HbA1c >10%) often have a poor response to treatment, with more postoperative complications and less favorable

---

BOX 36.2 Diagnostic Criteria for Diabetes Mellitus

Diabetes mellitus can be diagnosed by any one of the following laboratory methods. Initial results using any method must be confirmed on a subsequent day.

1. A fasting plasma glucose level of 126 mg/dL (7.0 mmol/L) or greater. *Fasting* is defined as no caloric intake for at least 8 hours. The normal fasting glucose level is 70–100 mg/dL.
2. A 2-hour postprandial glucose level of 200 mg/dL (11.1 mmol/L) or greater during an oral glucose tolerance test. The test should be performed using a glucose load containing the equivalent of 75 g anhydrous glucose dissolved in water. The normal 2-hour postprandial glucose level is below 140 mg/dL.
3. A glycated hemoglobin (HbA1c) value of 6.5% (48 mmol/L) or greater. The test should be performed in a laboratory using a method that is certified by the National Glycohemoglobin Standardization Program (NGSP) and standardized according to the Diabetes Control and Complications Trial (DCCT) assay.[a]
4. A random plasma glucose level of 200 mg/dL (11.1 mmol/L) or greater for a patient with classic symptoms of hyperglycemia or hyperglycemic crisis, which include polyuria, polydipsia, and unexplained weight loss. Blood for casual glucose testing can be drawn without regard to the time since the last meal.

[a]In the absence of unequivocal hyperglycemia, results should be confirmed by repeat testing.
Data from American Diabetes Association: 2. Classification and diagnosis of diabetes. *Diabetes Care* 40(Suppl. 1):S11–S24, 2017.

BOX 36.3 Laboratory Evaluation of Diabetes Control by Glycated Hemoglobin Assay Values

Normal	4%–6%
Good diabetes control	<7%
Moderate diabetes control	7%–8%
Action suggested to improve diabetes control	>8%

Data from American Diabetes Association: 2. Classification and diagnosis of diabetes. *Diabetes Care* 40(Suppl. 1):S11–S24, 2017.

---

long-term results[57,100] (see Fig. 13.3 in Chapter 13). Improvements in HBA1c values after periodontal therapy may provide an indication of the potential response.

As discussed in Chapter 13, periodontal infection can worsen glycemic control and should be managed aggressively. Patients with diabetes and periodontitis should receive oral hygiene instructions, mechanical debridement to remove local factors, and regular maintenance. When possible, an HbA1c of less than 10% should be established before surgical treatment is performed. Systemic antibiotics are not needed routinely, although evidence indicates that tetracycline antibiotics in combination with scaling and root planing may positively influence glycemic control. If the patient has poor glycemic control and surgery is absolutely needed, prophylactic antibiotics can be given; penicillins are most often used for this purpose. Frequent reevaluation after active therapy is needed to assess the treatment response and prevent the recurrence of periodontitis.

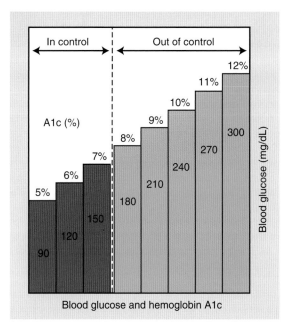

Fig. 36.2 Graphic Representation of Glycated Hemoglobin (HbA1c) Values That Correspond to Estimated Average Blood Glucose Levels.

BOX 36.4   Signs and Symptoms of Hypoglycemia

Shakiness or tremors
Confusion
Agitation and anxiety
Sweating
Tachycardia
Dizziness
Feeling of impending doom
Unconsciousness
Seizures

Almost all patients with diabetes use a glucometer for blood glucose self-monitoring. These devices use capillary blood from a fingerstick to provide blood glucose readings in seconds. Diabetic patients should be asked whether they have a glucometer and how often they use it. Because these devices provide instantaneous assessment of blood glucose, they are highly beneficial in the dental office environment. The following guidelines should be observed:

1. Many dental offices now have glucometers for blood glucose monitoring. If your office does not have a monitor, patients should be asked to bring their glucometers to the dental office at each appointment.
2. Patients should check their blood glucose before any long procedure to obtain a baseline level. Patients with a blood glucose level at or below the lower end of normal before the procedure may become hypoglycemic intraoperatively. It is advisable to have the patient consume some carbohydrate before starting treatment. For example, if a 2-hour procedure is planned and the pretreatment glucose level is 70 mg/dL (i.e., lower end of the normal range), the provision 4 ounces of juice preoperatively may help to prevent hypoglycemia during treatment. If the pretreatment glucose level is excessively high, the dental hygienist should determine whether the patient's glycemic control has recently been poor. This can be done with thorough patient questioning and by determining the most recent HbA1c values. If glycemic control has been poor over the preceding few months, the procedure may have to be postponed until better glycemic control has been established. If glycemic control has been good and the current high glucometer reading is a fairly isolated event, the surgical procedure can proceed.
3. If the procedure lasts several hours, it is often beneficial to check the glucose level during this period to make sure that the patient does not become hypoglycemic.
4. After the procedure, the blood glucose can be checked again to assess fluctuations over time.
5. Any time the patient feels the symptoms of hypoglycemia, the blood glucose level should be checked immediately. This may prevent the onset of severe hypoglycemia, a medical emergency.

The most common dental office complication seen in patients with diabetes who are taking insulin is a symptomatic low blood glucose level (i.e., hypoglycemia) (Box 36.4). Hypoglycemia is also associated with the use of numerous oral agents (Table 36.4). In patients receiving conscious sedation, the warning signs of an impending hypoglycemic episode may be masked, making the patient's glucometer one of the best diagnostic aids. Hypoglycemia does not usually occur until the blood glucose level falls below 60 mg/dL. However, in patients with poor glycemic control who have prolonged hyperglycemia (i.e., high blood glucose levels), a rapid drop in glucose can precipitate signs and symptoms of hypoglycemia at levels well above 60 mg/dL.

As medical management of diabetes has intensified over the past decade, the incidence of severe hypoglycemia has risen.[102] The dental hygienist should question diabetic patients about past episodes of hypoglycemia. Hypoglycemia is more common in patients with better glycemic control. When dental treatment is being planned, it is best to schedule appointments before or after periods of peak insulin activity. This requires knowledge of the pharmacodynamics of the drugs being taken by the diabetic patient. Patients taking insulin are at greatest risk, followed by those taking sulfonylurea agents. Metformin and thiazolidinediones usually do not cause hypoglycemia (see Table 36.4).

Insulins are classified as rapid-acting, short-acting, intermediate-acting, or long-acting agents (Table 36.5). The categories vary in onset, peak, and duration of activity. It is important that the dental hygienist establish exactly which insulin the diabetic patient is taking, the amount, the number of times per day, and the time of the last dose. Periodontal treatment can often be timed to avoid peak insulin activity. Many patients with diabetes take multiple injections each day, in which case it can be difficult or impossible to avoid peak insulin activity. Checking the pretreatment glucose with the patient's glucometer, checking again during a long procedure, and checking again at the end of the procedure will provide a better understanding of the patient's insulin pharmacodynamics and can help to prevent hypoglycemia.

TABLE 36.4 Oral Agents Used for the Management of Diabetes

Agent	Action	Risk of Hypoglycemia[a]
Sulfonylureas (first generation): Chlorpropamide Tolbutamide Tolazamide	Stimulate pancreatic insulin secretion	++
Sulfonylureas (second generation): Glyburide Glipizide	Stimulate pancreatic insulin secretion	+++
Sulfonylureas (third generation): Glimepiride	Stimulate pancreatic insulin secretion	+
Meglitinides: Repaglinide Nateglinide	Stimulate rapid pancreatic insulin secretion (different mechanism from sulfonylureas)	+
Biguanides: Metformin	Block production of glucose by liver; improve tissue sensitivity to insulin	–
Thiazolidinediones: Rosiglitazone Pioglitazone	Improve tissue sensitivity to insulin	–
α-Glucosidase inhibitors: Acarbose Miglitol	Slow absorption of some carbohydrates from gut, decreasing postprandial peaks in glycemia	–
Dipeptidyl peptidase-4 (DPP-4) inhibitors: Sitagliptin Saxagliptin	Inhibit the enzyme DPP-4; enable the pancreas to produce more insulin but only after food ingestion	–
Combination agents	Combine two different oral agents into single drug	Risk depends on which drugs are combined.

[a]Hypoglycemia risk: +++, high; ++, moderate; +, low; –, none.

If hypoglycemia occurs during dental treatment, therapy should be immediately terminated. If a glucometer is available, the blood glucose level should be checked. Treatment guidelines are as follows[54]:

1. Provide approximately 15 g of oral carbohydrate to the patient as
   - 4 to 6 ounces of juice or soda
   - 3 or 4 teaspoons of table sugar
   or
   - Hard candy with 15 g of sugar
2. If the patient is unable to take food or drink by mouth or if he or she is sedated,
   - Give 25 to 30 mL of 50% dextrose intravenously, which provides 12.5 to 15.0 g of dextrose, or
   - Give 1 mg of glucagon intravenously (i.e., glucagon results in rapid release of stored glucose from the liver)
   or
   - Give 1 mg of glucagon intramuscularly or subcutaneously (if no intravenous access).

Emergencies resulting from hyperglycemia are rare in the dental office; they usually take days to weeks to develop. However, the glucometer may be used to rule out hyperglycemic emergencies such as diabetic ketoacidosis, a life-threatening event.

KEY FACT

The most common dental office complication seen in diabetic patients taking insulin is a symptomatic low blood glucose level, or hypoglycemia. It does not usually occur until blood glucose level falls below 60 mg/dL. However, in patients with poor glycemic control who have prolonged hyperglycemia, a rapid drop in glucose can precipitate signs and symptoms of hypoglycemia at higher levels. Dental hygienists must recognize the signs of hypoglycemia and be prepared to manage it. Hypoglycemia is more common in individuals with well-controlled glucose levels.

Consultation with the patient's physician is prudent and allows both practitioners to review the proposed treatment plan and determine whether modifications are needed. When periodontal surgery is indicated, it is usually best to limit the size of the surgical field so that the patient will be comfortable enough to resume a normal diet immediately.

TABLE 36.5 Types of Insulin

Type	Classification	ACTIVITY		
		Onset	Peak	Duration
Lispro (Humalog), aspart (Novolog), glulisine (Apidra)	Rapid acting	15 min	30–90 min	<5 h
Regular R or Novolin R, Velosulin (used in insulin pump)	Short acting	30–60 min	2–3 h 1–2 h	3–6 h 2–3 h
NPH (N), Humulin N, Novolin N	Intermediate acting	2–4 h	4–12 h	14–18 h
Insulin determir (Levemir)	Long acting	1–2 h	Relatively flat (fairly even over 24 h)	Up to 24 h
Glargine (Lantus)	Long acting	6–8 h	There is no peak	20–24+ h

HEMORRHAGIC DISORDERS

Patients with a history of bleeding problems caused by disease or drugs are managed to minimize the risks of hemorrhage. Identification of these patients through the health history, clinical examination, and clinical laboratory tests is paramount. Health questioning should cover (1) the history of bleeding after previous surgery or trauma, (2) past and current drug history, (3) history of bleeding problems among relatives, and (4) illnesses associated with potential bleeding problems.

Clinical examination can detect jaundice, ecchymosis, spider telangiectasia, hemarthrosis, petechiae, hemorrhagic vesicles, spontaneous gingival bleeding, and gingival hyperplasia. Laboratory tests include methods to measure the hemostatic, coagulation, or lytic phase of the clotting mechanism, depending on clues regarding which phase is involved (Table 36.6). These tests include bleeding time, tourniquet test, complete blood cell count, prothrombin time (PT), partial thromboplastin time (PTT), and coagulation time. Bleeding disorders are classified as coagulation disorders, thrombocytopenic purpuras, or nonthrombocytopenic purpuras.

Coagulation Disorders

The main inherited coagulation disorders include hemophilia A, hemophilia B, and von Willebrand disease[73,84] (Table 36.7). *Hemophilia A* results in a deficiency of coagulation factor VIII, and the clinical severity of the disorder depends on the level of factor VIII remaining.[65] Patients with severe hemophilia who have less than 1% of normal factor VIII levels can have severe bleeding on the slightest provocation, whereas those with more moderate hemophilia (i.e., 1% to 5% of factor VIII) have less frequent spontaneous hemorrhage but still bleed with minimal trauma.[53] Patients with mild hemophilia (i.e., 6% to 30% of factor VIII) rarely bleed spontaneously but may still hemorrhage after severe trauma or during surgical procedures.

The dental hygienist should consult the patient's physician before dental treatment to determine the risk of bleeding and treatment modifications required. To prevent surgical hemorrhage, a factor VIII level of at least 30% is needed.[53,65] Parenteral 1-deamino-8-D-arginine vasopressin (DDAVP; desmopressin) can be used to raise factor VIII levels two- to threefold in patients with mild or moderate hemophilia. DDAVP has the significant

TABLE 36.6 Laboratory Tests for Bleeding Disorders

HEMOSTATIC TESTS			
Vascular	**Platelet**	**Coagulation**	**Lysis**
1. Tourniquet test *N:* 10 petechiae *Abn:* >10 petechiae	1. Platelet count *N:* 150,000–300,000/mm³ *Abn:* Thrombocytopenia occurs at <100,000/mm³; clinical bleeding occurs at <80,000/mm³; spontaneous bleeding occurs at <20,000/mm³	1. PT measures extrinsic and common pathways: factors I, II, V, VII, and X. *N:* 11–14 s (depending on laboratory) measured against control PT reported as international normalized ratio (INR): *N:* INR = 1.0 *Abn:* INR >1.5	1. Euglobin clot lysis time *N:* <90 min *Abn:* >90 min
2. Bleeding time *N:* 1–6 min *Abn:* >6 min	2. Bleeding time 3. Clot retraction 4. Complete blood cell count	2. PTT measures intrinsic and common pathways: factors III, IX, XI, and low levels of factors I, II, V, X, and XII. *N:* 25–40 s (depending on laboratory) measured against control *Abn:* >1.5 times normal 3. Clotting (coagulation) time *N:* 30–40 min *Abn:* >1 h	
Associations With Clinical Disease			
Vascular (capillary) wall defect	Thrombocytopenia		Increase in fibrinolytic activity
Rule Out:	**Rule Out:**	**All Three Tests:**	
Thrombocytopenia Purpuras Telangiectasia Aspirin or NSAID therapy Leukemia Renal dialysis	Vascular wall defect Acute or chronic leukemia Aplastic anemia Liver disease Renal dialysis	Liver disease Warfarin therapy Aspirin or NSAID therapy Malabsorption syndrome or long-term antibiotic therapy (lack of vitamin K metabolism) PT: factor VII deficiency PTT: hemophilia Renal dialysis	

Abn, Abnormal; *N,* normal; *NSAID,* nonsteroidal antiinflammatory drug; *PT,* prothrombin time; *PTT,* partial thromboplastin time.

TABLE 36.7 Inherited Coagulation Disorders

Type	Prolonged	Normal	Treatment
Hemophilia A	PTT	PT Bleeding time	DDAVP factor VIII concentrate or cryoprecipitate Fresh frozen plasma Fresh whole blood ε-Aminocaproic acid (Amicar) Tranexamic acid
Hemophilia B	PTT	PT Bleeding time	Purified prothrombin complex concentrate Factor IX concentrates Fresh-frozen plasma
Von Willebrand disease	Bleeding time PTT Variable factor VIII deficiency	PT Platelet count	DDAVP factor VIII concentrate or cryoprecipitate

DDAVP, 1-Deamino-8-D-arginine vasopressin (desmopressin); *PT,* prothrombin time; *PTT,* partial thromboplastin time.

advantage of avoiding the risk of viral disease transmission from factor VIII infusion and is considered the drug of choice in responsive patients. Most patients with moderate or severe hemophilia require the infusion of factor VIII concentrate before surgical procedures. Before 1985, the risk of viral disease transmission from these infusions was high. Since then, virally safe, highly purified monoclonal antibody or recombinant DNA factor VIII products have come into widespread use.

Hemophilia B (i.e., Christmas disease) results in a deficiency of factor IX. The severity of the disorder depends on the relative amount of existing factor IX. Surgical therapy requires a factor IX level of 30% to 50%, which is usually achieved by the administration of purified prothrombin complex concentrate or factor IX concentrate.[65]

Von Willebrand disease results from a deficiency of von Willebrand factor, which mediates the adhesion of platelets to the injured vessel walls and is required for primary hemostasis. Von Willebrand factor also carries the coagulant portion of factor VIII in the plasma. The disorder has three major subtypes with a wide range of clinical severity. Many cases of von Willebrand disease go undiagnosed, and bleeding during dental treatment may be the first sign of the underlying disease. More severe forms require preoperative factor VIII concentrate or the infusion of cryoprecipitate. Patients with milder forms respond favorably to the administration of DDAVP before periodontal surgery or tooth extraction.[65,66]

Periodontal treatment can be performed in patients with these coagulation disorders provided that appropriate precautions are taken. Probing, routine periodontal maintenance, and prophylaxis can usually be done without medical modification. More invasive treatment—such as local block anesthesia, root planing (root debridement), or surgery—dictates prior physician consultation.

Not all coagulation disorders are hereditary. Liver disease affects all phases of blood clotting because most coagulation factors are synthesized and removed by the liver. Patients who have long abused alcohol and those with chronic hepatitis often demonstrate inadequate coagulation. Coagulation can be impaired by vitamin K deficiency, often caused by malabsorption syndromes, or by prolonged antibiotic administration, which alters the intestinal microflora that produces vitamin K. The planning of dental treatment for patients with liver disease should include the following:

1. Physician consultation
2. Laboratory evaluations: PT, bleeding time, platelet count, and PTT (for patients in later stages of liver disease)
3. Conservative nonsurgical periodontal therapy whenever possible
4. Possible hospitalization when surgery is required
   - International normalized ratio (INR; PT) should be less than 2.0; for simple surgical procedures, an INR of less than 2.5 is usually safe.[38]
   - Platelet count should be more than 80,000/mm^3.

KEY FACT

Periodontal treatment can be performed in patients with coagulation disorders provided that appropriate precautions are taken. Probing, scaling, and prophylaxis can usually be done without medical modification. However, more invasive treatment—such as local block anesthesia, root planing, or surgery—should be considered only after consultation with a physician.

Anticoagulant Medications

The most common cause of abnormal coagulation may be drug therapy. Patients with a prosthetic heart valve or a history of MI, CVA, or thromboembolism are frequently placed on anticoagulant therapy using coumarin derivatives such as dicumarol and warfarin.[38,49] These drugs are vitamin K antagonists that decrease the production of vitamin K–dependent coagulation factors II, VII, IX, and X. The effectiveness of anticoagulation therapy is monitored by a PT laboratory test. The recommended level of therapeutic anticoagulation for most patients is an INR of 2.0 to 3.0, with prosthetic heart valve patients usually in the range of 2.5 to 3.5.[38] Traditional recommendations for periodontal treatment are as follows:

1. Consult the patient's physician to determine the nature of the underlying medical problem and the degree of required anticoagulation.
2. The procedure planned determines the acceptable INR. Infiltration anesthesia, scaling, and root planing can be done safely in patients with an INR of less than 3.0. Block anesthesia, minor periodontal surgery, and simple extractions usually require an INR of less than 2.0 to 2.5. Complex surgery or multiple extractions may require an INR of less than 1.5 to 2.0.
3. The physician must be consulted about any changes (i.e., discontinuing or reducing) in anticoagulant dosage until the desired INR is achieved. The dental professional must inform the physician what degree of intraoperative and postoperative bleeding is usually expected with the planned procedure. If the INR is higher than the level at which significant bleeding is likely to accompany a particular procedure, the physician

may elect to change anticoagulant therapy. Often the anticoagulant is discontinued for 2 to 3 days before periodontal treatment (i.e., the clearance half-life of warfarin is 36 to 42 hours), and the INR is checked on the day of therapy. If the INR is within the acceptable target range, the procedure is done and the anticoagulant resumed immediately after treatment.

4. Careful technique and complete wound closure are paramount. For all procedures, the application of pressure can minimize hemorrhage. The use of oxidized cellulose, microfibrillar collagen, topical thrombin, and tranexamic acid should be considered for persistent bleeding.

Discontinuing anticoagulant therapy before dental surgery was common in the past. However, many physicians no longer recommend discontinuing anticoagulation for many procedures because it poses significant risks for patient health.[40,86] Evidence related to the risks of altering anticoagulant therapy and the lack of evidence for bleeding complications suggest that treating patients without reducing or discontinuing medications may be more prudent. Details of anticoagulant or antiplatelet therapy are discussed in the next section.

Heparin is typically used for short-term anticoagulation and is given intravenously, usually in a hospital environment. It is a powerful anticoagulant with a duration of action of 4 to 8 hours. Periodontal treatment is rarely required while a patient is taking heparin.

Antiplatelet Medications

Aspirin interferes with normal platelet aggregation and can result in prolonged bleeding. Because it binds irreversibly to platelets, the effects of aspirin last at least 4 to 7 days. Aspirin is typically used in small doses of 325 mg or less per day, which normally does not alter bleeding time. Patients taking low doses of aspirin daily usually do not have to discontinue aspirin therapy before periodontal procedures.[86] However, higher doses can increase bleeding time and predispose the patient to postoperative bleeding.[53] For patients taking more than 325 mg of aspirin per day, it may have to be discontinued 7 to 10 days before surgical therapy that could result in significant bleeding; this should be done in consultation with the physician.

Nonsteroidal antiinflammatory drugs (NSAIDs) such as ibuprofen also inhibit platelet function. Because NSAIDs bind reversibly, the effect is transitory, lasting only a short time after the last drug dose. The bleeding time is used when questions arise about the potential effect of aspirin or NSAIDs. Aspirin should not be prescribed for patients who are receiving anticoagulant therapy or who have an illness involving the tendency to bleed.

KEY FACT

Discontinuing anticoagulant therapy before an oral surgical procedure was common in the past. Numerous clinicians no longer recommend discontinuing anticoagulation for many procedures because it can pose significant risks to the patient's health. Evidence related to the such risks and the lack of evidence for bleeding complications in these patients suggests that treating them without discontinuing medications may be more prudent.

Leukemia

Altered periodontal treatment for patients with leukemia is based on their enhanced susceptibility to infections, their bleeding tendency, and the effects of chemotherapy.[53] The treatment plan for leukemia patients is as follows:

1. Refer the patient for medical evaluation and treatment. Close cooperation with the physician is required.
2. Before chemotherapy, a complete periodontal treatment plan should be developed, again with a physician (discussed in the previous discussion).
   - Monitor hematologic laboratory values daily: bleeding time, coagulation time, PT, and platelet count.
   - Administer antibiotic coverage before periodontal treatment because infection is a major concern.
   - If systemic conditions allow, extract all hopeless or potentially infectious teeth at least 10 days before the initiation of chemotherapy.
   - Periodontal debridement (i.e., scaling and root planing) should be performed and thorough oral hygiene instructions given if the patient's condition allows. After oral hygiene procedures, twice-daily rinsing with 0.12% chlorhexidine gluconate is recommended. It is important to recognize the potential for bleeding caused by thrombocytopenia. Use pressure and topical hemostatic agents as indicated.
3. During the acute phases of leukemia, patients should receive only emergency periodontal care. Any potential source of infection must be eliminated to prevent systemic dissemination. Antibiotic therapy is frequently the treatment of choice, combined with nonsurgical or surgical debridement as indicated.
4. Oral ulcerations and mucositis are treated palliatively with agents such as viscous lidocaine. Systemic antibiotics may be indicated to prevent secondary infection.
5. Oral candidiasis is common in leukemic patients and can be treated with nystatin suspension (400,000 to 600,000 U/mL four times daily) or clotrimazole vaginal suppositories (10 mg four or five times daily).[56]
6. For patients with chronic leukemia and those in remission, scaling and root planing can be performed without complication, but periodontal surgery should be avoided if possible. Platelet count and bleeding time should be measured on the day of the procedure. If either is low, postpone the appointment and refer the patient to a physician.

MEDICATIONS AND CANCER THERAPIES

Some medications prescribed to cure, manage, or prevent diseases have effects on periodontal tissues, wound healing, or the host immune response that sometimes require modification of treatment. Bisphosphonates, anticoagulation medications, antiplatelet medications, steroids, chemotherapy, and radiation therapy are briefly addressed in this chapter; additional information and advice can be found in other sources.

Bisphosphonates

Bisphosphonate medications are primarily used to treat cancer (i.e., intravenous administration) and osteoporosis (i.e., oral administration). They act by inhibiting osteoclastic activity, which leads to less bone resorption, remodeling, and turnover.[79] Bisphosphonates are used in cancer treatment to prevent the often lethal imbalance of osteoclastic activity. In the treatment of osteoporosis, the goal is to harness osteoclastic activity to minimize or prevent bone loss. The major difference between these applications is the potency and route of administration. Potency is influenced by the chemical properties and pharmacokinetics of these agents in bone. Chapter 13 describes the chemical structure, activity, and role of bisphosphonates in the development of bisphosphonate-related osteonecrosis of the jaw (BRONJ).

Clinically, BRONJ manifests as exposed alveolar bone occurring spontaneously or after a dental procedure. Individuals treated with high-potency, nitrogen-containing bisphosphonates, especially those administered intravenously for cancer treatment (e.g., zoledronate), appear to be at greater risk for BRONJ than those taking oral bisphosphonates for the prevention and treatment of osteoporosis. In patients undergoing cancer treatment, the incidence ranges from 2.5% to 5.4%.[114] It is more difficult to estimate the incidence for patients taking oral bisphosphonates for osteoporosis, but it appears to range from 0.007% to 0.04%.[111] Even if this is an underestimation of the actual risk for individuals taking oral bisphosphonates, the incidence appears to be low. The risk for individuals treated with oral bisphosphonates for a period of less than 3 years appears to be minimal or none.[50] Regular use of oral bisphosphonates for a period greater than 3 years suggests a risk profile that increases with time and length of use.[50]

As with many multifactorial diseases and conditions, it is likely that factors in addition to bisphosphonate therapy contribute to the individual risk of BRONJ. Potential risk factors include systemic corticosteroid therapy, smoking, alcohol, poor oral hygiene, chemotherapy, radiotherapy, diabetes, and hematologic disease.[25] Reported factors for BRONJ include extractions, root canal treatment, periodontal infections, periodontal surgery, and dental implant surgery.[52] Periodontal disease and treatment (especially surgery) poses a risk for patients treated with bisphosphonates. The bacteria-induced inflammatory process of periodontitis that causes bone resorption can lead to bone necrosis. Likewise, periodontal treatment can cause bone necrosis in the setting of bisphosphonates. Caution is warranted in the treatment of all patients being treated with bisphosphonates.

Health care providers must evaluate patients carefully, communicate with other medical health care providers, inform patients, and consider treatment options and risk. A careful intraoral examination is prudent for all patients being treated with intravenous or oral bisphosphonate therapy to determine whether bone exposure exists and to assess local conditions that may predispose them to BRONJ. A thorough medical history should be reviewed, evaluated, and annotated with details about bisphosphonate treatment, including medication type, dose, route of administration, and duration. Comorbidities, such as previous and current medications, treatments, and existing disease or pathology, should be considered. Radiographs should be carefully evaluated for signs of bisphosphonate toxicity.

Marx suggested that a laboratory blood test for the serum C-terminal telopeptide fragment of type I collagen (CTX) could be used to assess an individual's risk of developing BRONJ.[50] Marx reported that lower CTX values were associated with greater risk (eTable 36.2). It is important to recognize that these values are based on the retrospective evaluation of patients with osteonecrosis of the jaw and that prospective studies to validate these findings have not been done. The CTX laboratory test is a measure of the specific C-terminal fragment of type I collagen cleaved by osteoclasts and indicates bone resorption activity. However, its use as a measure of the risk for BRONJ is controversial and not confirmed by prospective studies.

Optimal periodontal and oral health should be achieved and maintained for all patients. For individuals treated with intravenous bisphosphonates, invasive treatments—such as extractions, periodontal surgery, implant surgery, and bone augmentation procedures—should be avoided. Risks must be considered before treating individuals with a history of taking oral bisphosphonates for longer than 3 years. This area of research will continue to evolve as the pathophysiology becomes better understood. Providers are encouraged to consult other sources for updates on this important topic.

KEY FACT

Bisphosphonate therapy and one or more comorbidity factors contribute to the individual risk of bisphosphonate-related osteonecrosis of the jaw (BRONJ). Potential risk factors include systemic corticosteroid therapy, smoking, alcohol, poor oral hygiene, chemotherapy, radiotherapy, diabetes, and hematologic disease.

Anticoagulant or Antiplatelet Therapy

Many patients with a variety of conditions are placed on anticoagulant or antiplatelet medications to prevent thrombosis (i.e., blood clotting) or thromboembolism. Patients at risk who may be on anticoagulant or antiplatelet therapy include those with heart valve replacements, heart rhythm disorders, congenital heart defects, or a history or risk of MI, stroke, or deep vein thrombosis. These medications, although effective in reducing the risk of thrombosis, may increase the risk for bleeding complications, especially in patients undergoing surgical procedures.

The traditional approach to patients on anticoagulant or antiplatelet therapy was to discontinue therapy about 3 to 5 days (antiplatelet therapy) or 7 to 10 days (anticoagulant therapy) before a planned surgical procedure. Evidence and theories about the care of patients on anticoagulant or antiplatelet therapy suggest that treating them (e.g., with periodontal surgery or extractions) without altering their anticoagulant or antiplatelet medications is safe and does not lead to intraoperative or postoperative bleeding complications. The increased risk of morbidity and mortality for those discontinuing the anticoagulant or antiplatelet therapy may be significant.

Controlled clinical studies have demonstrated that intraoperative bleeding is not likely to be a problem with simple extractions or periodontal surgery if antiplatelet therapy (e.g., aspirin) is continued.[6,48] In these studies, there were no episodes of uncontrolled bleeding, all bleeding was controlled with local measures, and there were no cases of postoperative bleeding problems. Conversely, the risk of stopping antiplatelet therapy may be serious. In a retrospective evaluation of 52 patients undergoing cataract surgery, 1 in 10 whose antiplatelet therapy was stopped or reduced suffered a stroke.[81]

Clinical studies of patients on anticoagulant therapy undergoing extractions and other oral surgical procedures have demonstrated minimal bleeding problems when therapy is continued.[12,15,112,113,123] In a review of the literature, Wahl and colleagues[113] reported that only 12 (<1.3%) of 950 patients receiving continuous anticoagulant therapy required more than local measures to control hemorrhage after 2400 minor oral surgical procedures. Most of the 950 patients had anticoagulation levels that were well above currently recommended therapeutic levels. Only three patients (<0.31%) had anticoagulation levels within or below currently recommended therapeutic levels. In contrast, 5 (0.95%) of 526 patients who experienced 575 interruptions of continuous anticoagulant therapy suffered serious embolic complications; 4 patients died.

In a prospective study of 131 patients undergoing 511 extractions, those whose oral anticoagulant therapy was reduced 72 hours before surgery to achieve an INR of 1.5 to 2.0 (target, 1.8) had postoperative bleeding that warranted subsequent local intervention in 10 (15.1%) of 66 patients.[80] Postoperative bleeding occurred in only 6 (9.2%) of 65 patients in the group that continued the regular dosage of oral anticoagulant therapy (mean INR, 2.9).

These studies suggest that the risk of serious morbidity associated with discontinuing anticoagulant or antiplatelet therapy should be avoided and that the risk of bleeding while maintaining this therapy is minimal.

Corticosteroids

Approximately 5% of the adults in the United States habitually take corticosteroids for the treatment of various conditions, potentially putting them at risk for secondary adrenal insufficiency.[46] Patients who habitually use corticosteroids have an increased likelihood of developing hypertension, osteoporosis, and peptic ulcer disease. Care should be taken to minimize the risk of adverse outcomes in these patients. BP should be monitored, and medications that might exacerbate peptic ulceration (e.g., NSAIDs) should be avoided.

Stressful events—such as trauma, illness, surgery, emotional upset, or athletic events—normally increase circulating endogenous cortisol levels by stimulating the HPA axis. Pain appears to increase the requirement for cortisol release.[72] There is concern that the normal release of cortisol in response to a stressful event such as a dental procedure may be impaired in patients exposed to habitual corticosteroid use. The concern is about whether these patients require perioperative supplementation for dental procedures. Historically, recommendations were based on the type, amount, and duration of corticosteroid use. However, current thinking about the need for perioperative corticosteroid supplementation has been adjusted.

Studies investigating the stress response to minor general and oral surgical procedures concluded that significant increases in cortisol were usually not seen until 1 to 5 hours after surgery and appeared to be associated more with postoperative pain and the loss of local anesthesia than with the preoperative and intraoperative stress of the procedure.[7,90,91] Administration of adequate analgesics in the postoperative period can diminish the release (requirement) of cortisol.[7]

Most individuals with adrenal insufficiency can receive routine dental treatment without the need for supplemental glucocorticosteroids.[13,46] Patients taking corticosteroids usually have enough exogenous and endogenous cortisol to handle routine dental procedures if the usual dose is taken within 2 hours of the planned procedure. For most patients, supplemental corticosteroid administration is not required when uncomplicated minor surgical procedures, including periodontal surgery, are performed with local anesthesia with or without sedation.[46] Topical corticosteroids usually have minimal HPA effect, and steroid supplementation is not required for these patients.

Individuals at risk for adrenal crisis who require supplementation include those undergoing lengthy major surgical procedures, those expected to have significant blood loss, and those who have extremely low adrenal function. Low adrenal function can be identified with an ACTH stimulation test. For these individuals, consultation with the physician and steroid supplementation are indicated.

Immunosuppression and Chemotherapy

Immunosuppressed patients have an impaired host defense as a result of an underlying immunodeficiency or use of drugs (primarily related to organ transplantation or cancer chemotherapy).[57,87] Because chemotherapy is often cytotoxic to bone marrow, destruction of platelets and red and white blood cells results in thrombocytopenia, anemia, and leukopenia. Immunosuppressed individuals are at greatly increased risk for infection, and even minor periodontal infections can become life threatening if immunosuppression is severe.[71,73] Bacterial, viral, and fungal infections can manifest intraorally. Patients undergoing bone marrow transplantation require special attention because they receive extremely high-dose chemotherapy and are particularly susceptible to dissemination of oral infections.

Treatment should be directed toward prevention of oral complications that can be life-threatening. The greatest potential for infection occurs during periods of extreme immunosuppression; treatment should be conservative and palliative. It is always preferable to evaluate the patient before initiation of chemotherapy.[57,87] Teeth with a poor prognosis should be extracted, with thorough debridement of remaining teeth to minimize the microbial load. The dental hygienist must teach and emphasize the importance of good oral hygiene. Antimicrobial rinses, such as chlorhexidine, are recommended, especially for patients with chemotherapy-induced mucositis, to prevent secondary infection.

Chemotherapy is usually performed in cycles, with each cycle lasting several days, followed by intervening periods of myelosuppression and recovery. If periodontal therapy is needed during chemotherapy, it is best done the day *before* chemotherapy is given, when white blood cell counts are relatively high. Coordination with the oncologist is critical. Dental treatment should be done when the white blood cell count is above 2000/mm³, with an absolute granulocyte count of 1000 to 1500/mm³.[53]

Radiation Therapy

The use of radiotherapy, alone or in conjunction with surgical resection, is common in the treatment of head and neck tumors. The side effects of ionizing radiation include dramatic perioral changes of significant concern to dental health personnel.[37,56,88] The extent and severity of mucositis, dermatitis, xerostomia, dysphagia, gustatory alteration, radiation caries (Fig. 36.3), vascular changes, trismus, temporomandibular joint degeneration, and periodontal changes depend on the type of radiation used, field of irradiation, number of ports, type of tissue in the field, and dosage.

Patients scheduled to receive head and neck radiation therapy require dental consultation *at the earliest possible time* to reduce the morbidity of known perioral side effects.[85] Preirradiation treatment depends on the patient's prognosis, compliance, and residual dentition in addition to the field, ports, dose, and immediacy of radiotherapy. The initial visit should include panoramic and intraoral radiographs, a clinical dental examination, a periodontal evaluation, and a physician consultation. The physician should be asked about the amount of radiation to be administered, extent and location of the lesion, nature of surgical procedures already performed or to be performed, number of radiation ports, exact fields to be irradiated, mode of radiation therapy, and patient's prognosis (i.e., likelihood of metastasis). Preirradiation treatment should commence immediately after the physician consultation. The first decision should involve possible extractions because radiation can cause side effects that interfere with healing.

For head and neck squamous cell carcinomas, the radiation dose is usually 5000 to 7000 cGy (1 cGy = 1 rad) delivered in a fractionated method (150 to 200 cGy/day over a 6- to 7-week course).[11,56] This is considered full-course radiation treatment, and the degree of perioral side effects depends on which tissues are irradiated (i.e., the radiation fields). If the radiation is administered to the salivary gland tissues, xerostomia will ensue. The parotid is the most radiosensitive of the salivary glands; saliva may become extremely viscous or nonexistent, depending on the dose delivered to the particular gland. Xerostomia causes a decrease in the normal salivary cleansing mechanisms, buffering capacity of saliva, and pH of oral fluids.[56] Oral bacterial populations shift to a preponderance of cariogenic forms (e.g., *Streptococcus mutans*, *Actinomyces* spp., *Lactobacillus* spp.). Radiation-induced caries may progress rapidly, and they primarily affect smooth tooth surfaces (see Fig. 36.3).

High-dose radiation therapy results in hypovascularity of irradiated tissues, with a reduction in wound-healing capacity.[63,109,110] Most severe among the resulting oral complications is osteoradionecrosis (ORN). Decreased vascularity renders the bone less capable of resolving trauma or infection. These events can cause severe destruction of bone. The risk of ORN continues for the remainder of the patient's life and does not decrease with time.[51]

Periodontal disease can be a precipitating factor in ORN.[16,31] Tooth extraction after radiation treatment involves a high risk of developing ORN, and surgical flap procedures are usually discouraged after radiation therapy. For these reasons, it is important that the dental hygienist address the patient's periodontal disease *before* radiation begins when possible. Teeth that are nonrestorable or severely periodontally diseased should be extracted, ideally at least 2 weeks before radiation therapy.[56] Extractions should be performed in a manner that allows primary closure. Mucoperiosteal flaps should be gently elevated; teeth should be extracted in segments; alveolectomy should be performed, allowing no rough bony spicules to remain; and primary closure should be provided without tension. It is not necessary to extract teeth that can be retained with conservative restorative,

Fig. 36.3 (A) In a clinical view of a patient with radiation caries, notice how the caries primarily affected the smooth tooth surfaces, especially cervical areas and cusp tips. (B) Radiographs of anterior teeth of 52-year-old man with postradiation caries. The patient received a dose of 6000 cGy for radiation treatment of the posterior mandible and base of the tongue for squamous cell carcinoma. Radiation caries developed within 1 year after radiation treatment, affecting the cervical areas and incisal edges of the anterior teeth. (A, courtesy Dr. Eric Sung, Hospital Dentistry, University of California Los Angeles.)

endodontic, or periodontal therapy. However, prudence dictates extraction of questionable teeth because periodontal treatment after irradiation may be limited to nonsurgical forms of therapy. Flap surgery or extraction of teeth after radiation can lead to ORN. Management of ORN is often difficult and costly, involving progressively more aggressive treatment if bone does not respond to conservative therapy. Costly hyperbaric oxygen therapy is frequently required for complete resolution.

During radiation therapy, patients should receive weekly prophylaxis, oral hygiene instruction, and professionally applied fluoride treatments, unless mucositis prevents treatment. Patients should be instructed to brush daily with a 0.4% stannous or 1.0% sodium fluoride gel. Custom gel trays allow optimal fluoride application.[109] All remaining teeth should receive thorough debridement (i.e., scaling and root planing).

Postirradiation follow-up consists of palliative treatment given as indicated. Viscous lidocaine can be prescribed for painful mucositis, and salivary substitutes can be given for xerostomia. Daily topical fluoride application and oral hygiene are the best means of preventing radiation caries over time. A long-term, 3-month recall interval is ideal.

PROSTHETIC JOINT REPLACEMENT

The main treatment consideration for patients with prosthetic joint replacement is the potential need for antibiotic prophylaxis before periodontal therapy (eTable 36.3). No scientific evidence indicates that prophylactic antibiotics prevent late prosthetic joint infections, which can occur from transient bacteremia induced by dental treatment.[23,53,89] Although dental-induced bacteremia can theoretically cause prosthetic joint infection, scant reports demonstrate dental treatment as a source of joint infection, and none actually documents a cause-and-effect relationship.[19,77,105]

Reports from the American Dental Association (ADA), American Academy of Orthopedic Surgeons (AAOS), American Academy of Oral Medicine (AAOM), and British Society for Antimicrobial Chemotherapy (BSAC) agree that routine antibiotic prophylaxis before dental treatment is not indicated for most patients with prosthetic joint replacement.[1,2,21,28,103] However, antibiotic prophylaxis is indicated for almost all patients with previous prosthetic joint infections, immunosuppression, rheumatoid arthritis, systemic lupus erythematosus, type 1 diabetes, hemophilia, and malnourishment.[1] Some investigators consider patients with severe periodontal disease or other potential dental infections to be at high risk, and antibiotic prophylaxis may be indicated for them before dental treatment.[62,103]

Between 2009 and 2014, after much controversy and debate among experts, there was a complete shift toward recommending prophylactic antibiotics before dental treatment for life for all patients with prosthetic joint replacements. After further review of the evidence and consensus among experts, new recommendations were published that did not recommend prophylactic antibiotics for dental procedures in patients with prosthetic joint replacement to prevent prosthetic joint infection. A historical description of the changes that were implemented from 2009 to 2012 can be found online (www.ada.org/en/member-center/oral-health-topics/antibiotic-prophylaxis).

Current advice for patients with orthopedic joint replacement stresses the importance of maintaining good dental health and hygiene and seeking prompt attention and treatment for oral infections when they occur. Dental procedures have not been associated with an increased risk of prosthetic joint infection, and the use of prophylactic antibiotics before dental procedures does not reduce the risk of infection.[9,94,122] Given the lack of evidence to support the need for prophylactic antibiotics, the AAOM, ADA, AAOS, and BSAC advise against universal use of antibiotic prophylaxis before dental procedures for the prevention of prosthetic joint infections.

In 2013, the ADA in conjunction with the AAOS published a joint guideline on the prevention of orthopedic implant infections in patients undergoing dental procedures. The publication stated that there was no convincing evidence to support the routine use of prophylactic antibiotics for patients with prosthetic joints.[116] In 2015, the ADA Council on Scientific Affairs published a clinical practice guideline to clearly state the findings of the 2013 ADA/AAOS joint guideline. The clinical practice guideline states that prophylactic antibiotics are not recommended before dental procedures for patients with prosthetic joint implants to prevent prosthetic joint infections.[98]

KEY FACT

In 2015, the American Dental Association (ADA) Council on Scientific Affairs published a clinical practice guideline to clearly state the findings published in the 2013 ADA and American Association of Orthopedic Surgeons (AAOS) joint guideline. The clinical practice guideline states that, to prevent prosthetic joint infections, prophylactic antibiotics are *not* recommended before dental procedures for patients with prosthetic joint implants.

 A Case Scenario is found on the companion website.

REFERENCES

 References for this chapter are found on the companion website www.expertconsult.com.

37

Periodontal Therapy in the Female Patient[a]

 Content on menopause can be accessed on the companion website.

Throughout a woman's life, hormonal changes occur that may affect therapeutic decision making in periodontics. Historically, therapies have been gender biased. Research has provided a keener appreciation of the unique systemic influences on oral, periodontal, and implant tissues. Oral health care professionals now have greater awareness of and can better deal with hormonal influences associated with the reproductive process. Periodontal and oral tissue responses can be altered, creating diagnostic and therapeutic dilemmas. The dental hygienist should recognize, customize, and appropriately alter periodontal therapy according to the individual woman's needs based on her stage of life.

Sex steroids exert profound biologic effects on immune function and bone metabolism.[136] Estrogen can significantly affect the periodontium, including the maturation of gingival epithelium, osteoblastic differentiation of periodontal ligament cells, and bone formation.[135]

This chapter reviews phases of the female reproductive cycle from puberty through menopause. Periodontal manifestations, systemic effects, and clinical management are addressed.

PUBERTY

On average, puberty occurs between the ages of 11 and 14 in most women. The production of sex hormones (i.e., estrogen and progesterone) increases and then remains relatively constant during the remainder of the reproductive phase. The prevalence of gingivitis increases without an increase in the amount of plaque. Gram-negative anaerobes, especially *Prevotella intermedia*, have been associated with puberty gingivitis. Kornman and Loesche[69] postulated that this anaerobic organism may use ovarian hormones as a substitute for vitamin K as a growth factor. Levels of black-pigmented *Bacteroides*, especially *P. intermedia* (formerly known as *Bacteroides intermedius*), are thought to increase with

increased levels of gonadotropic hormones in puberty. *Capnocytophaga* species also increase in incidence and proportion. These organisms have been implicated in the increased bleeding tendency observed during puberty.

Studies of pubertal gingivitis indicate proportionally elevated numbers of motile rods, spirochetes, and *P. intermedia*.[48,96] Statistically significant increases in gingival inflammation and the proportions of *P. intermedia* and *Prevotella nigrescens* have been seen in pubertal gingivitis.[100] A study of 11- to 17-year-old adolescents found higher levels of *Actinobacillus actinomycetemcomitans* and *Fusobacterium nucleatum*, which were associated with bleeding indices, probing depth, and attachment loss.[83]

During puberty, periodontal tissues can have an exaggerated response to local factors. A hyperplastic reaction of the gingiva can occur in areas where food debris, materia alba, plaque, and calculus are deposited. The inflamed tissues become erythematous, lobulated, and retractable. Bleeding can easily occur with mechanical debridement of the gingival tissues. Histologically, the appearance is consistent with inflammatory hyperplasia.

During the reproductive years, women tend to have a more vigorous immune response, including higher immunoglobulin concentrations, stronger primary and secondary responses, increased resistance to the induction of immunologic tolerance, and a greater ability to reject tumors and homografts.[134] Allergy, sensitivity, and asthma occur more often in young males, but after puberty, women become more susceptible than their male counterparts.

> ### KEY FACT
>
> Sex steroids exert profound biologic effects on immune function and bone metabolism. Estrogen can have a significant impact on the periodontium, including the maturation of gingival epithelium, osteoblastic differentiation of periodontal ligament cells, and bone formation. During puberty, periodontal tissues can have an exaggerated response to local factors. A hyperplastic reaction of the gingiva can occur. Inflamed tissues become erythematous, lobulated, and retractable; they also bleed easily. Histologically, the appearance is consistent with inflammatory hyperplasia.

---

[a]Adapted from the following chapter of Newman and Carranza's Clinical Periodontology, 13th edition: Chapter 41: Periodontal Therapy in the Female Patient, by Joan Otomo-Corgel.

Management

During puberty, education of the parent or caregiver is a part of successful periodontal therapy. Preventive care, including a vigorous program of oral hygiene, is also vital.[6] Milder cases of gingivitis respond well to scaling, with frequent oral hygiene reinforcement. Severe cases of gingivitis may require microbial culturing, antimicrobial mouthwashes and local site delivery, or antibiotic therapy. Periodontal maintenance appointments may have to become more frequent when periodontal instability is identified.

The dental hygienist should recognize the periodontal manifestations and intraoral lesions associated with systemic diseases (e.g., diabetes).[24,106] Thorough review of the patient's medical history and medical referral should occur when deemed necessary. The clinician should be aware of the effects of chronic regurgitation of gastric contents on intraoral tissues; this age group is susceptible to eating disorders such as bulimia and anorexia nervosa.[16] *Perimolysis* (i.e., smooth erosion of enamel and dentin), typically on the lingual surfaces of maxillary anterior teeth, varies with the duration and frequency of the behavior.[18] Enlargement of the parotid glands (occasionally sublingual glands) has been estimated to occur in 10% to 50% of patients who binge and purge.[88] A diminished salivary flow rate may be identified, which can increase oral mucous membrane sensitivity, gingival erythema, and caries susceptibility.

MENSES

Periodontal Manifestations

During the reproductive years, the ovarian cycle is controlled by the anterior pituitary gland. The gonadotropin follicle-stimulating hormone (FSH) and luteinizing hormone (LH) are produced by the anterior pituitary gland. The secretion of gonadotropins also depends on the hypothalamus. Ongoing changes in the concentration of the gonadotropins and ovarian hormones occur during the monthly menstrual cycle (Fig. 37.1). Under the influence of FSH and LH, estrogen and progesterone are steroid hormones produced by the ovaries during the menstrual cycle. During the reproductive cycle, the purpose of estrogen and progesterone is to prepare the uterus for implantation of an egg.

The monthly reproductive cycle has two phases. The first is referred to as the *follicular phase.* Levels of FSH are elevated, and estradiol (E2), the major form of estrogen, is synthesized by the developing follicle and peaks approximately 2 days before ovulation. Estrogen stimulates the egg to move down the fallopian tubes (i.e., ovulation) and stimulates proliferation of the stroma cells, blood vessels, and glands of the endometrium.

In the second, or *luteal phase,* the developing corpus luteum synthesizes estradiol and progesterone. Estrogen peaks at 0.2 ng/mL and progesterone at 10.0 ng/mL to complete the rebuilding of the endometrium for implantation of a fertilized egg. If the egg is not fertilized, the corpus luteum involutes, ovarian hormone levels drop, and menstruation ensues. It has been postulated that ovarian hormones increase inflammation in gingival tissues and exaggerate the response to local irritants. Gingival inflammation seems to be aggravated by an imbalance or increase in sex hormones.[56] Menstrual cycle irregularity is a risk indicator for periodontal disease before menopause.[49] Numerous in vitro and in vivo studies have demonstrated that sex hormones affect and modify the actions of cells of the immune system.

Evidence suggests that the interaction between estrogen and cells of the immune system can have nonimmune regulatory effects.[8,23] Possible mechanisms have been suggested for the increase in hormonal gingival interaction in the menstrual cycle.

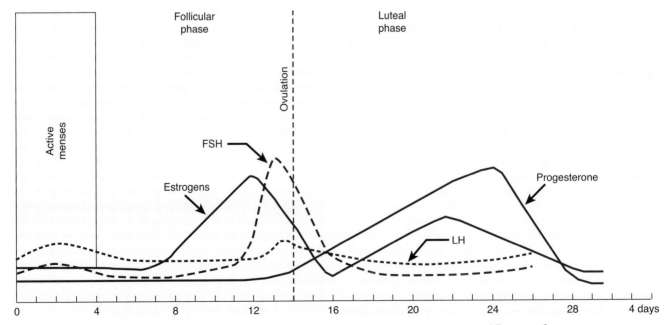

Fig. 37.1 Female Menstrual Cycle, Showing the Peak Levels of Progesterone and Estrogen Compared With Follicle-Stimulating Hormone *(FSH)* and Luteinizing Hormone *(LH).*

Tumor necrosis factor alpha (TNF-α), which fluctuates during the menstrual cycle,[14] elevated prostaglandin E_2 (PGE_2) synthesis,[93] and angiogenetic factors, endothelial growth factors, and receptors may be modulated by progesterone and estrogen, contributing to increases in gingival inflammation during certain stages of the menstrual cycle.[65]

Progesterone has been associated with increased permeability of the microvasculature, altering the rate and pattern of collagen production in the gingiva,[84] increasing folate metabolism,[111,148] and altering the immune response. During menses, progesterone increases from the second week, peaks at approximately 10 days, and dramatically drops before menstruation (based on a 28-day cycle; individual cycles vary). Progesterone plays a role in stimulating the production of prostaglandins that mediate the body's response to inflammation. PGE_2 is one of the major secretory products of monocytes, and the level is increased in inflamed gingiva. Miyagi and colleagues[92] found that the chemotaxis of polymorphonuclear leukocytes (PMNs) was enhanced by progesterone but reduced by estradiol. Testosterone did not have a measurable effect on PMN chemotaxis. The researchers suggested that the altered PMN chemotaxis associated with gingival inflammation might be caused by the effects of sex hormones. Physiologic, experimental, and clinical data confirm differences in immune responses between the two sexes.[157]

Gingival tissues have been reported to be more edematous during menses and erythematous before the onset of menses in some women. One study reported higher gingival indices during ovulation and before menstruation despite reported increases in oral symptoms during menses.[85] An increase of gingival exudate has been observed during the menstrual period and is sometimes associated with a minor increase in tooth mobility.[44] The incidence of postextraction osteitis is also higher during the initiation of menses. No significant hematologic laboratory findings accompany this other than a slightly reduced platelet count and a slight increase in clotting time.

When the progesterone level is highest (during the luteal phase of the cycle), intraoral recurrent aphthous ulcers,[36] herpes labialis lesions, and candidal infections occur in some women in a cyclic pattern. Because the esophageal sphincter is relaxed by progesterone, women may be more susceptible to gastroesophageal reflux disease (GERD) during this time of the cycle. Symptoms of GERD include heartburn, regurgitation, and chest pain; when reflux is severe, some patients develop unexplained coughing, hoarseness, sore throat, gingivitis, or asthma.[126]

Management

During the peak level of progesterone (about 7 to 10 days before menstruation), premenstrual syndrome (PMS) may also occur. There appears to be no significant difference in estrogen and progesterone levels between women with PMS and those without PMS. However, women with PMS seem to have lower levels of certain neurotransmitters such as enkephalins, endorphins, γ-aminobutyric acid (GABA), and serotonin. Depression, irritability, mood swings, and difficulty with memory and concentration are symptoms of neurotransmitter reduction. Patients are more sensitive and less tolerant of procedures, have a heightened gag reflex, and can have an exaggerated response to pain.

Increased gingival bleeding and tenderness associated with the menstrual cycle require closer periodontal monitoring. Periodontal maintenance should be titrated to the individual patient's need; if problematic, 3- to 4-month intervals should be recommended. An antimicrobial oral rinse before cyclic inflammation may be indicated. Emphasis should be placed on oral hygiene. For the patient with a history of excessive postoperative hemorrhage or menstrual flow, the scheduling surgical visits after cyclic menstruation is prudent. Anemia is common, and appropriate consultation with a physician as well as laboratory tests when indicated should be pursued.

During PMS, many women exhibit physical symptoms that include fatigue, cravings for sweet and salty foods, abdominal bloating, swollen hands or feet, headaches, breast tenderness, nausea, and gastrointestinal upset. GERD may make it more uncomfortable for the patient to lie fully supine, especially after a meal, due to a more sensitive gag reflex. The clinician should be aware that nonsteroidal antiinflammatory drugs (NSAIDs), infection, and acidic foods exacerbate GERD. Patients with GERD may take over-the-counter antacids, H_2-receptor antagonists (e.g., cimetidine, famotidine, nizatidine, ranitidine), prokinetic agents (e.g., cisapride, metoclopramide), or proton pump inhibitors (e.g., lansoprazole, omeprazole, pantoprazole, rabeprazole).[127] These medications interact with some antibiotics and antifungals, and a review of their pharmacology is necessary. Fluoride rinses and trays, frequent periodontal debridement, and avoidance of mouthwashes with high alcohol content can reduce the associated gingival and caries sequelae.

PMS is often treated with antidepressants. Selective serotonin reuptake inhibitors (SSRIs) are usually the first-line choice because they have fewer side effects than other antidepressants, do not require blood monitoring, and are safe if overdosed. Women with PMS taking the SSRI fluoxetine had a 70% response rate. Fluoxetine was ranked the fifth most dispensed prescription (i.e., new and refills) in the United States in 1998, but sales slowed when the patent was lifted. Overall, however, SSRIs ranked second in total dollar sales in the 2000s. Sertraline was ranked twelfth and is the drug of choice for the treatment of PMS.[165]

The dental hygienist should be aware that patients taking fluoxetine have increased side effects with highly protein-bound drugs (e.g., aspirin) and that the half-life of diazepam and other central nervous system (CNS) depressants is increased. Other common SSRIs are fluvoxamine, paroxetine, and citalopram. Other prescribed antidepressants include selective serotonin-norepinephrine reuptake inhibitors (SNRIs), tricyclics, trazodone, mirtazapine, nefazodone, and maprotiline.

> ### KEY FACT
>
> Increased gingival bleeding and tenderness associated with the menstrual cycle require close periodontal monitoring. Periodontal maintenance should be adjusted to the individual patient's needs. If problematic, 3- to 4-month recall intervals should be recommended.

The PMS patient may be difficult to treat because of her emotional and physiologic sensitivity. The clinician should treat the gingival and oral mucosal tissues gently. Gauze pads or cotton rolls should be moistened with a lubricant, chlorhexidine rinse, or water before they are placed in the patients prone to develop aphthous or herpetic lesions. Careful retraction of the oral mucosa, cheeks, and lips is also necessary. Because the hypoglycemic threshold is elevated in PMS patients, the clinician should advise them to have a light snack before their appointments. Among menstruating women, 70% have PMS symptoms but only 5% meet the strict diagnostic criteria.

PREGNANCY

Periodontal Manifestations

The link between pregnancy and periodontal inflammation has been known for many years. In 1778, Vermeeren discussed "toothpains" in pregnancy. In 1818, Pitcarin[118] described gingival hyperplasia in pregnancy. Despite awareness regarding pregnancy and its effect on periodontal disease, only recently has evidence indicated an inverse relationship with systemic health. Research confirms that periodontal disease alters the patient's systemic health and adversely affects the well-being of the fetus by elevating the risk for preterm low-birth-weight (PLBW) infants.

In 1877, Pinard[117] recorded the first case of pregnancy gingivitis. Only recently has periodontal research begun to focus on causative mechanisms. Pregnancy gingivitis is extremely common, occurring in 30% to 100% of pregnant women.[51,74,79,131] It is characterized by erythema, edema, hyperplasia, and increased bleeding. Histologically, the description is the same as for gingivitis. However, the etiologic factors are different despite clinical and histologic similarities. Cases range from mild to severe inflammation (Fig. 37.2), which can progress to severe hyperplasia, pain, and bleeding (Figs. 37.3 and 37.4).

Other growths that resemble pregnancy granulomas must be ruled out, such as central giant cell granulomas or underlying systemic diseases. Periodontal status before pregnancy may influence the progression or severity as the circulating hormones fluctuate. The anterior region of the mouth is affected more often, and interproximal sites tend to be most involved.[28] Increased tissue edema can lead to increased pocket depths and may be associated with transient tooth mobility.[120] Anterior site inflammation can be exacerbated by increased mouth breathing, primarily in the third trimester, from pregnancy rhinitis. The gingiva

is the most common site involved (approximately 70% of cases), followed by the tongue and lips, buccal mucosa, and palate.[131] An increase in attachment loss can represent active periodontal infection accelerated by pregnancy.[75]

Pyogenic granulomas (i.e., pregnancy tumors or pregnancy epulis) occur in 0.2% to 9.6% of pregnancies. They are clinically and histologically indistinguishable from pyogenic granulomas occurring in nonpregnant women or in males. Pyogenic granulomas appear most often during the second or third month of pregnancy. Clinically, they bleed easily and become hyperplastic and nodular. When excised, the lesions usually do not leave a large defect. They may be sessile or pedunculated and ulcerated, ranging in color from purplish red to deep blue, depending on the vascularity of the lesion and degree of venous stasis.[11] The lesion classically occurs in an area of gingivitis and is associated

Fig. 37.2 Moderate Form of Pregnancy Gingivitis.

Fig. 37.3 Pyogenic Granuloma of Pregnancy (i.e., Pregnancy Tumor).

Fig. 37.4 Severe Pregnancy Gingivitis With Hyperplasia Can Occur in Patients With Poorly Controlled Non–Insulin-Dependent Diabetes Mellitus. (A) Moderate gingival enlargement. (B) Severe gingival enlargement.

with poor oral hygiene and calculus. Alveolar bone loss is usually not associated with pyogenic granulomas of pregnancy.

Role of Pregnancy Hormones
Subgingival Plaque Composition

Epidemiologic studies indicate a relationship between the level of home care and the severity of gingival inflammation. It appears that the association between signs of gingival inflammation and the amount of plaque is greater after parturition than during pregnancy. An alteration in the compositions of subgingival plaque occurs during pregnancy. Kornman and Loesche[70] found that during the second trimester, gingivitis and gingival bleeding increased without an increase in plaque levels. Bacterial anaerobic/aerobic ratios increased in addition to proportions of *Bacteroides melaninogenicus* and *P. intermedia* (2.2% to 10.1%). The study authors suggested that estradiol or progesterone could substitute for menadione (vitamin K) as an essential growth factor for *P. intermedia* but not *Porphyromonas gingivalis* or *Eikenella corrodens.* There was also an increase in *P. gingivalis* during the 21st through 27th weeks of gestation, but this was not statistically significant. The relative increase in the numbers of *P. intermedia* may be a more sensitive indicator of an altered systemic hormonal situation than clinical parameters of gingivitis.[139]

One study concluded that subgingival levels of bacteria associated with periodontitis did not change. Counts of *P. gingivalis* and *Tannerella forsythia* were higher and associated with bleeding on probing at week 12.[2] Bacterial challenge to the gingival tissues, quantitatively (plaque scores) and qualitatively (*P. gingivalis*), appears to affect the level of gingival inflammation observed during pregnancy.[19]

Periodontal Disease and Preterm Low-Birth-Weight Infants

Although most studies support a causal relationship regarding the hypothesis that periodontitis during pregnancy poses an increased risk of adverse pregnancy outcomes, there are conflicting results. Variations in study results may stem from confounding factors, effect modifiers, populations studied, timing of intervention or evaluation, and severity of periodontal disease based on different definitions.

Several systematic reviews indicate that periodontal disease[133,152,160,161] adversely affects pregnancy outcomes. Intervention trials have shown a positive effect with periodontal therapy and reduction of adverse pregnancy outcomes,[60,81,82,105,146] but three large multicenter trials in the United States did not support these results.[90,102,140] Studies indicate that routine nonsurgical periodontal therapy after the first trimester is not associated with adverse pregnancy outcomes.[90]

Initially, Offenbacher and colleagues[104] provided evidence that untreated periodontal disease in pregnant women could be a significant risk factor for preterm (<37 weeks' gestation) low-birth-weight (<2500 g) infants. The relationship between genitourinary tract infection and PLBW infants is well documented in human and animal studies. Periodontal researchers, suspecting periodontal disease as another source of infection, found that otherwise low-risk women of PLBW infants had significantly more periodontal attachment loss than control women having normal-weight infants at birth.

Current opinion is that the correlation of periodontal disease with PLBW birth may result from infection and is mediated indirectly, principally by the translocation of bacterial products such as endotoxin (i.e., lipopolysaccharide [LPS]) and the action of maternally produced inflammatory mediators.[39] Jared and coworkers[58] found that fetal exposure to oral pathogens in utero increased the risk of neonatal intensive care unit admission and extended length of stay. Concentrations of biologically active molecules, such as PGE_2 and TNF-α, which are usually involved in normal parturition, are raised to artificially high levels by the infection process, which can foster premature labor.[4]

Gram-negative bacteria in periodontal diseases may permit their selective overgrowth or invasion within the genitourinary tract. Han and associates[50] documented hematogenous spread of oral bacteria to the amnion, and Madianos and colleagues[86] showed that oral bacteria crossed the placental barrier and triggered an immune response by the fetus.

Gingival crevicular fluid (GCF) levels of PGE_2 were positively associated with intraamniotic PGE_2 levels ($P = .018$), suggesting that gram-negative periodontal infection presents a systemic challenge sufficient to initiate the onset of premature labor as a source of LPS or through stimulation of secondary inflammatory mediators such as PGE_2 and interleukin-1 beta (IL-1β).[25] Offenbacher and coworkers[103] suggested a dose–response relationship for increasing GCF PGE_2 as a marker of current periodontal disease activity and decreasing birth weight.

Four organisms associated with mature plaque and progressing periodontitis—*T. forsythia*, *P. gingivalis*, *A. actinomycetemcomitans*, and *Treponema denticola*—were detected at higher levels in women who had given birth to PLBW infants compared with normal-birth-weight controls. Despite research supporting the association of periodontal disease and PLBW infants,[26,27] more studies with improved methodology are needed to assess the validity of the association.

KEY FACT

Current opinion suggests a possible association between periodontal disease and PLBW infants. Adverse pregnancy events can result from an infection that is mediated by one of two major pathways: (1) directly by oral microorganisms or (2) indirectly, principally by the translocation of bacterial products such as endotoxin (i.e., lipopolysaccharide) and the action of maternally produced inflammatory mediators.

Preeclampsia

A systematic review of preeclampsia and periodontitis indicated an increased risk during pregnancy. Preeclampsia is a life-threatening condition in late pregnancy that is characterized by high blood pressure and excess protein in the urine. High levels of C-reactive protein are also associated with preeclampsia in this population.[129,137,151]

Maternal Immunoresponse

The maternal immune system is thought to be suppressed during pregnancy, a response that may allow the fetus to survive as an allograft. Documentation of immunosuppressive factors in the sera of pregnant women shows a marked increase in monocytes (which in large numbers inhibit in vitro proliferative responses to mitogens, allogenic cells, and soluble antigen)[150] and pregnancy-specific β_1-glycoproteins, which contribute to diminished lymphocyte responsiveness to mitogens and antigens.[12] The ratio of peripheral helper T cells to suppressor T cells (CD4/CD8) decreases throughout pregnancy.[121]

The changes in maternal immunoresponsiveness suggest an increased susceptibility to developing gingival inflammation. In one study, the gingival index was higher, but percentages of T3 (CD3), T4 (CD4), and B cells appeared to decrease in peripheral blood and gingival tissues during pregnancy compared with a control group.[1] Other studies report decreased PMN (i.e., neutrophil) chemotaxis, depression of cell-mediated immunity, phagocytosis, and decreased T-cell response with elevated ovarian hormone levels, especially progesterone.[119] Decreased in vitro responses of peripheral blood lymphocytes to several mitogens and to a preparation of *P. intermedia* have been reported.[13,80,109] Evidence suggests a decrease in the absolute numbers of CD4+ cells in peripheral blood during pregnancy compared with postpartum.[94,102]

Lapp and colleagues[73] suggested that high levels of progesterone during pregnancy affect the development of localized inflammation by downregulation of IL-6 production, rendering the gingiva less efficient at resisting the inflammatory challenges produced by bacteria. Another study indicated that live preterm birth was associated with decreased levels of immunoglobulin G (IgG) antibody to periodontal pathogens in women with periodontitis when assessed during the second trimester, but this was not associated with birth outcomes.[30]

Ovarian hormone stimulates the production of prostaglandins, particularly PGE$_1$ and PGE$_2$, which are potent mediators of the inflammatory response. With the prostaglandin acting as an immunosuppressant, gingival inflammation can increase when the mediator level is high.[33,107] Kinnby and coworkers[66] found that high progesterone levels during pregnancy influenced plasminogen activator inhibitor type 2 (PAI-2) and disturbed the balance of the fibrinolytic system. Because PAI-2 is an important inhibitor of tissue proteolysis, this research implies that components of the fibrinolytic system may be involved in the development of pregnancy gingivitis.

During pregnancy, sex hormone levels rise dramatically (Box 37.1). Progesterone reaches levels of 100 ng/mL, 10 times the peak luteal phase of menses. Estradiol in the plasma may reach levels 30 times higher than during the reproductive cycle. In early pregnancy and during the normal ovarian cycle, the corpus luteum is the major source of estrogen and progesterone. During pregnancy, the placenta begins to produce estrogens and progesterone.

Estrogen regulates cellular proliferation, differentiation, and keratinization, whereas progesterone influences the permeability of the microvasculature,[76,77] alters the rate and pattern of collagen production, and increases the metabolic breakdown of folate (necessary for tissue maintenance).[163] High concentrations of sex hormones in gingival tissues, saliva, serum, and GCF also can exaggerate the response.

> ### BOX 37.1 Causes of Gingival Responses to Elevated Estrogen and Progesterone During Pregnancy
>
> **Subgingival Plaque Composition**
> - Increase in anaerobic/aerobic ratio
> - Higher concentrations of *Prevotella intermedia* (i.e., substitutes sex hormone for vitamin K growth factor)
> - Higher concentrations of *Bacteroides melaninogenicus*
> - Higher concentrations of *Porphyromonas gingivalis*
>
> **Maternal Immunoresponse**
> - Depression of cell-mediated immunity
> - Decrease in neutrophil chemotaxis
> - Depression of antibody and T-cell responses
> - Decrease in ratio of peripheral helper T cells to suppressor-cytotoxic T cells (i.e., CD4/CD8 ratio)
> - Cytotoxicity directed against macrophages and B cells can diminish immunoresponsiveness
> - Decrease in absolute numbers of CD3+, CD4+, and CD19+ cells in peripheral blood during pregnancy versus postpartum
> - Stimulation of prostaglandin production
>
> **Sex Hormone Concentration**
> *Estrogen*
> - Increases cellular proliferation in blood vessels (e.g., in the endometrium)
> - Decreases keratinization while increasing epithelial glycogen
> - Specific receptors are found in gingival tissues
>
> *Progesterone*
> - Increases vascular dilation and increases permeability, resulting in edema and accumulation of inflammatory cells
> - Increases proliferation of newly formed capillaries in gingival tissues (i.e., increased bleeding tendency)
> - Alters rate and pattern of collagen production
> - Increases metabolic breakdown of folate (i.e., folate deficiency can inhibit tissue repair)
> - Specific receptors are found in gingival tissues
> - Decreases plasminogen activator inhibitor type 2, increasing tissue proteolysis
>
> *Estrogen and Progesterone*
> - Affect ground substance of connective tissue by increasing fluidity
> - Concentrations increase in saliva and fluid, with increased concentrations in serum

Regulation of most cellular processes by hormones occurs through the interaction of these products with intracellular receptors. The resulting effects depend on the concentration of unbound hormone diffused through the cell membrane. Vittek and associates[154] demonstrated specific estrogen and progesterone receptors in gingival tissues, providing direct biochemical evidence that this tissue functions as a target organ for sex hormones. Muramatsu and Takaesu[98] found increasing concentrations of sex hormones in saliva from the first month and peaking in the ninth month of gestation, along with increasing percentages of *P. intermedia*. Probing depth, number of gingival sites with bleeding, and redness increased until 1 month after delivery. Evidence indicates that the concentration of sex hormone in GCF provides a growth medium for periodontal pathogens.

Other Oral Manifestations of Pregnancy

Perimolysis (i.e., acid erosion of teeth) can occur if morning sickness or esophageal reflux is severe and involves repeated vomiting of the gastric contents. Severe reflux can cause scarring of the esophageal sphincter, and the patient may become more susceptible to GERD later in life.

Xerostomia is a frequent complaint among pregnant women. One study found this persistent dryness in 44% of pregnant participants.[31]

A rare finding in pregnancy is *ptyalism* (i.e., sialorrhea). Excessive secretion of saliva usually begins at 2 to 3 weeks' gestation and may abate at the end of the first trimester. The cause of ptyalism has not been identified, but it may result from the inability of a nauseated gravid women to swallow normal amounts of saliva rather than from a true increase in saliva production.[22]

Because pregnancy places the woman in an immunocompromised state, the dental hygienist must be aware of a patient's total health. Gestational diabetes, leukemia, and other medical conditions may appear during pregnancy.

Clinical Management

A thorough medical history is an imperative component of the periodontal examination, especially for the pregnant patient. Because of immunologic alterations, increased blood volume (i.e., ruling out mitral valve prolapse and heart murmurs), and fetal interactions, the dental hygienist must diligently and consistently monitor the patient's medical and periodontal stability. Medical history discussion should include pregnancy complications, previous miscarriages, and recent history of cramping, spotting, or pernicious vomiting. The patient's obstetrician should be contacted to discuss her medical status, periodontal or dental needs, and the proposed treatment plan.

Establishing a healthy oral environment and maintaining optimal oral hygiene are primary objectives for the pregnant patient. A preventive periodontal program consisting of nutritional counseling and rigorous plaque control measures in the dental office and at home should be reinforced. Women of reproductive age, especially those trying to conceive, should be informed of the possible impact of inflammation on the unborn.

Plaque Control

The increased tendency for gingival inflammation to arise during pregnancy should be clearly explained to the patient so that acceptable oral hygiene techniques may be taught, reinforced, and monitored throughout the term. Scaling, polishing, and root planing can be performed whenever necessary during pregnancy. Some practitioners avoid the use of high-alcohol-content antimicrobial rinses for pregnant women and prefer to use non–alcohol-based rinses.

Prenatal Fluoride

The prescription of prenatal fluoride supplements has been an area of controversy. Although two studies have claimed beneficial results,[40,41] others suggest that the clinical efficacy of such supplements is uncertain and that the mechanism by which they might impart cariostasis is unclear.[3] The American Dental Association (ADA) does not recommend the use of prenatal fluoride because its efficacy has not been demonstrated. The American Academy of Pediatric Dentistry also supports this position. The American Academy of Pediatrics has no stated position on prescribing prenatal fluorides.

Treatment

Elective Dental Treatment

Other than good plaque control, it is prudent to avoid elective dental care if possible during the first trimester and the last half of the third trimester. The first trimester is the period of organogenesis, when the fetus is highly susceptible to environmental influences. In the last half of the third trimester, a hazard of premature delivery exists because the uterus is very sensitive to external stimuli. Prolonged chair time may have to be avoided because the woman may be uncomfortable in a supine position.

Supine hypotensive syndrome may occur. In a supine position, the great vessels, particularly the inferior vena cava, are compressed by the gravid uterus. By interfering with venous return, this compression causes maternal hypotension, decreased cardiac output, and eventual loss of consciousness. Supine hypotensive syndrome can usually be reversed by turning the patient on her left side, which removes pressure on the vena cava and allows blood to return from the lower extremities and pelvic area. A preventive 6-in soft wedge (i.e., rolled towel) should be placed on the patient's right side when she is reclined for clinical treatment.

Early in the second trimester is the safest period for providing routine dental care. The emphasis at this time is on controlling active disease and eliminating potential problems that can arise in late pregnancy. Major elective oral or periodontal surgery may be postponed until after delivery. Pregnancy tumors that are painful, interfere with mastication, or continue to bleed or suppurate after mechanical debridement may require excision and biopsy before delivery.

It is hypothesized that when the inflammatory cascade is activated during pregnancy, interventions targeting this pathway may be ineffective in reducing the rate of preterm birth. Treatment during pregnancy may be too late; it is possible that treatment before pregnancy (in nulliparous women) or in the period between pregnancies (for multiparous women, especially those with a history of preterm birth) may yield more promising results.[42]

The American Academy of Periodontology (www.perio.org) developed a position statement regarding the need to provide proper periodontal therapy for pregnant patients (Fig. 37.5). Because of research indicating a possible impact on the fetus, acute infection, abscesses, or other potential disseminating sources of sepsis may warrant prompt intervention irrespective of the stage of pregnancy.[5] A consensus report of a Joint European Workshop of Periodontology and an American Academy of Periodontology Workshop stated that "although periodontal therapy has been shown to be safe and leads to improved periodontal conditions in pregnant women, case-related periodontal therapy, without systemic antibiotics does not reduce overall rates of preterm birth and low birth weight."[132]

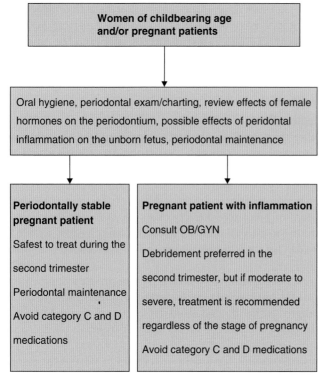

Fig. 37.5 Treatment Algorithm for the Pregnant Patient.

BOX 37.2 US Food and Drug Administration Drug Classification System Based on Potential to Cause Birth Defects

A: Controlled studies enrolling women fail to demonstrate a risk to the fetus in the first trimester (there is no evidence of risk in later trimesters), and the possibility of fetal harm appears remote.

B: Animal reproduction studies have not demonstrated a fetal risk, but there are no controlled studies in pregnant women; or animal reproduction studies have shown an adverse effect (other than decreased fertility) that was not confirmed in controlled studies in women in the first trimester (there is no evidence of risk in later trimesters).

C: Studies in animals have revealed adverse effects on the fetus (i.e., teratogenic, embryocidal, or other), and there are no controlled studies in women, or studies in women and animals are not available. Drugs should be given only if the potential benefit justifies the potential risk to the fetus.

D: There is positive evidence of human fetal risk, but the benefits of use in pregnant women may be acceptable despite the risk (e.g., the drug is needed in a life-threatening situation or for a serious disease for which safer drugs cannot be used or are ineffective).

X: Studies in animals or humans have demonstrated fetal abnormalities, or there is evidence of fetal risk based on human experience, or both, and the risk of using the drug in pregnant women clearly outweighs any possible benefit. The drug is contraindicated in women who are or may become pregnant.

CLINICAL CORRELATION

It is prudent to avoid elective dental care during the first trimester and the last half of the third trimester. The first trimester is the period of organogenesis, and the fetus is highly susceptible to environmental influences. During the last half of the third trimester, the fetus is vulnerable to premature delivery. The uterus is very sensitive to external stimuli. Early in the second trimester is the safest period for providing routine dental care.

Dental Radiographs

The safety of dental radiography during pregnancy has been well established provided that items such as high-speed film, filtration, collimation, and lead aprons are used. However, it is most desirable not to have any irradiation during pregnancy, especially during the first trimester, because the developing fetus is particularly susceptible to radiation damage.[78] When radiographs are needed for diagnosis, the most important aid for the patient is the protective lead apron. Studies have shown that when an apron is used during contemporary dental radiography, gonadal and fetal radiation is virtually unmeasurable.[10]

Even with the obvious safety of dental radiography, x-ray films should be taken selectively during pregnancy and only when necessary and appropriate to aid in diagnosis and treatment. In most cases, only bitewing, panoramic, or selected periapical films are indicated.

Medications

Medication therapy for the pregnant patient is controversial due to effects on the fetus by diffusion across the placenta. Prescriptions should be used only for the duration absolutely essential for the

pregnant patient's well-being and only after careful consideration of potential side effects. The classification system established by the US Food and Drug Administration (FDA) in 1979 to rate fetal risk levels associated with many prescriptions provides safety guidelines (Box 37.2). The prudent practitioner should consult references, such as Briggs and colleagues' *Drugs in Pregnancy and Lactation*[17] and Olin's *Drug Facts and Comparisons*,[108] for information on the FDA pregnancy risk factors associated with prescription medication.

Ideally, no medication should be administered during pregnancy, especially the first trimester.[78] However, it is sometimes impossible to adhere to this rule. Fortunately, most common medications in dental practice can be given during pregnancy with relative safety, although there are a few important exceptions. Tables 37.1 to 37.3 provide guidelines for anesthetic and analgesic, antibiotic, and sedative-hypnotic drugs, respectively.[122,149]

Antibiotics are often needed in periodontal therapy. The effect of a particular medication on the fetus depends on the type of antimicrobial, dosage, trimester, and duration of the course of therapy.[110] Research regarding subgingival irrigation and local site delivery in relation to the developing fetus is inadequate.

Breastfeeding

Medications may enter breast milk and be transferred to the nursing infant, on whom exposure could have adverse effects (Tables 37.4 and 37.5). Unfortunately there is little conclusive information about drug dosage and effects through breast milk; however, retrospective clinical studies and empiric observations coupled with known pharmacologic pathways allow recommendations to be made.[78] The amount of medication excreted in

TABLE 37.1 Local Anesthetic and Analgesic Administration During Pregnancy

Drug	FDA Category	During Pregnancy
Local Anesthetics[a]		
Lidocaine	B	Yes
Mepivacaine	C	Use with caution; consult physician
Prilocaine	B	Yes
Bupivacaine	C	Use with caution; consult physician
Etidocaine	B	Yes
Procaine	C	Use with caution; consult physician
Articaine	B	Yes; no blocks
Analgesics		
Aspirin	C/D, third trimester	Caution; avoid in third trimester
Acetaminophen	B	Yes
Ibuprofen	B/D, third trimester	Use with caution; avoid in third trimester
Codeine[b]	C	Use with caution; consult physician
Hydrocodone[b]	B	Use with caution; consult physician
Oxycodone[b]	B	Use with caution; consult physician
Propoxyphene	C	Use with caution; consult physician

[a]Can use vasoconstrictors if necessary.
[b]Avoid prolonged use.
FDA, U.S. Food and Drug Administration.

TABLE 37.2 Antibiotic Administration During Pregnancy

Drugs	FDA Category	During Pregnancy	Risks
Penicillins	B	Yes	Diarrhea
Erythromycin	B	Yes; avoid estolate form	Intrahepatic jaundice in mother
Clindamycin	B	Yes, with caution	Drug concentrated in fetal bone, spleen, lung, and liver
Cephalosporins	B	Yes	Limited information
Tetracycline	D	Avoid	Depression of bone growth, enamel hypoplasia, gray-brown tooth discoloration
Ciprofloxacin	C	Avoid	Possible developing cartilage erosion
Metronidazole	B	Avoid; controversial	Theoretic carcinogenic data in animals
Gentamicin	C	Caution; consult physician	Limited information
Ototoxicity			
Vancomycin	C	Caution; consult physician	Limited information
Clarithromycin	D	Avoid; use only if potential benefit justifies risk to fetus	Limited information Adverse effects on pregnancy, outcome and embryo and fetal development in animals

FDA, US Food and Drug Administration.

TABLE 37.3 Sedative-Hypnotic Drug Administration During Pregnancy

Drugs	FDA Category	During Pregnancy
Benzodiazepines	D	Avoid
Barbiturates	D	Avoid
Nitrous oxide	Not assigned	Avoid in first trimester; otherwise use with caution; consult physician

FDA, US Food and Drug Administration.

breast milk is usually not more than 1% to 2% of the maternal dose; therefore it is highly unlikely that most medications have any pharmacologic significance for the infant.[159]

Prescribed medication should be taken just after breastfeeding; then nursing should be avoided for 4 hours or more if possible[78,141] to decrease the drug concentration in breast milk.

ORAL CONTRACEPTIVES

Women may have responses to oral contraceptives (OCs) similar to those seen in pregnant patients. Mullally and associates found that current users of OCs had poorer periodontal health.[97] An exaggerated response to local irritants occurs in gingival tissues. Inflammation ranges from mild edema and erythema to severe inflammation with hemorrhagic or hyperplasic gingival tissues. It has been reported that more exudate is present in the inflamed gingival tissues of OC users than in those of pregnant women.[138,164]

Investigators have suggested several mechanisms for the heightened response in gingival tissues. Kalkwarf[63] reported that the response might be caused by an altered microvasculature, increased gingival permeability, and increased synthesis of prostaglandin. Levels of PGE, a potent mediator of inflammation,[34] appear to rise significantly with increasing levels of sex hormones. Jensen and colleagues[62] found dramatic microbial changes in pregnant and OC groups compared with a nonpregnant group. A 16-fold increase in *Bacteroides* species was seen in the OC group versus the nonpregnant group, despite no statistically significant clinical differences in gingival index or GCF flow. The study authors found that the increased female sex hormones substituting for the naphthoquinone requirement of certain *Bacteroides* species was most likely responsible for this increase.

OC-associated gingival inflammation may become chronic (versus the acute inflammation of pregnancy) because of the

TABLE 37.4 Local Anesthetic and Analgesic Administration During Breastfeeding

Drug	During Breastfeeding
Local Anesthetics	
Lidocaine	Yes
Mepivacaine	Yes
Prilocaine	Yes
Bupivacaine	Yes
Etidocaine	Yes
Procaine	Yes
Analgesics	
Aspirin	Avoid
Acetaminophen	Yes
Ibuprofen	Yes
Codeine	Yes
Hydrocodone	No data
Oxycodone	Yes
Propoxyphene	Yes

TABLE 37.5 Antibiotic and Sedative-Hypnotic Administration During Breastfeeding

Drugs	During Breastfeeding
Antibiotics[a]	
Penicillins	Yes
Erythromycin	Yes
Clindamycin	Yes, with caution
Cephalosporins	Yes
Tetracycline	Avoid
Ciprofloxacin	Avoid
Metronidazole	Avoid
Gentamicin	Avoid
Vancomycin	Avoid
Sedative-Hypnotics	
Benzodiazepines	Avoid
Barbiturates	Avoid
Nitrous oxide	Yes

[a]Antibiotics carry a risk of diarrhea and sensitization in the mother and infant.

extended periods that women are exposed to elevated levels of estrogen and progesterone.[68,113] Some have reported that the inflammation increases with prolonged use of OCs. Kalkwarf[63] did not find that duration of use made a significant difference, but the brands used resulted in different responses. Further studies are needed to elucidate the effects of dosage, duration, and type of OC on the periodontium. The concentration of female sex hormones in current OCs is significantly less than that of the 1970s while still providing the same level of contraceptive efficacy.

Salivary composition changed notably in patients taking OCs in studies from the 1970s. Decreased concentrations of protein, sialic acid, hexosamine fucose, hydrogen ions, and total electrolytes have been reported. Salivary flow rates were increased in one report[87] and decreased in 30% of subjects in another report.[32]

The dental literature reports that women taking OCs experience a two- to threefold increase in the incidence of localized osteitis after the extraction of mandibular third molars.[143] The higher incidence of osteitis among these patients may be attributed to the effects of OCs (i.e., estrogens) on clotting factors. However, several studies refute these findings.[21] Evidence is inconclusive on osteitis after third molar extraction and OC use. A spotty melanotic pigmentation of the skin may occur with OC use. This suggests a relationship between the use of OCs and the occurrence of gingival melanosis,[53] especially in fair-skinned individuals.

Management

The medical history should include OCs along with other medications. The patient should be informed of the oral and periodontal side effects of OCs and the need for meticulous home care and compliance with periodontal maintenance. Treatment of gingival inflammation exaggerated by OCs should include establishing an oral hygiene program and eliminating local predisposing factors. Periodontal surgery may be indicated if resolution after initial therapy (i.e., scaling and root planing) is inadequate. It may be advisable to perform extraction of teeth (especially third molars) on nonestrogenic days of the OC cycle (i.e., days 23 to 28) to reduce the risk of a postoperative localized osteitis[37]; however, evidence of this association is inconclusive and warrants further investigation.

Although results from animal studies have demonstrated that antibiotic interference adversely affects contraceptive sex hormone levels, several human studies have failed to support such an interaction.[9,38,99,101] This issue is controversial, and antibiotics could render OCs ineffective in preventing pregnancy. In 1991, an ADA report stated that all women of reproductive age should be informed of the possible reduced efficacy of steroid OCs during antibiotic therapy and advised women to use additional forms of contraception during short-term antibiotic therapy.[7] During long-term antibiotic therapy, women should consult their physician about using high-dose OC preparations. Although only research regarding oral manifestations attributed to OCs has been reported in the literature, the same effects presumably occur with the use of contraceptive implants. Similarly, the remote possibility of reduced efficacy of contraceptive implants with concurrent antibiotic use exists, and women can follow the same precautions as with OC use.

CONCLUSIONS

Clinical periodontal therapy requires an understanding of the dental hygienist's role in supporting the total health and well-being of female patients. Dental professionals do not treat localized infections without affecting other systems and the fetus or the breastfed infant. The periodontal and systemic factors of female patients may alter conventional therapy.

The cyclic nature of the female sex hormones often is reflected in the gingival tissues as initial signs and symptoms. Medical histories and discussions should include thoughtful investigation of the individual patient's problems and needs. Questioning should reflect hormonal stability and medications associated with regulation. Patients should be educated regarding the profound effects that sex hormones have on periodontal and oral tissues and the consistent need for home and office removal of local irritants.

Research regarding female issues and medical/periodontal therapy is in process. In the near future, information about the specific management and causes of sex hormone–mediated infections will enhance the dental professional's ability to provide optimal care to their patients.

A Case Scenario is found on the companion website.

REFERENCES

 References for this chapter are found on the companion website.

38

Periodontal Treatment for Older Adults[a]

🌐 Content on demographics, dental and medical assessment, and risk reduction can be accessed on the companion website.

CHAPTER OUTLINE

In the future, older adults are expected to make up a larger proportion of the population than in the past. Population growth among long-lived older adults contributes to this increase worldwide. For dentistry, this means that older adults are retaining more of their natural dentition. Almost 70% of older adults in the United States have natural teeth.[30] However, retention of teeth may result in more teeth at risk for periodontal disease, and the prevalence of periodontal disease can be associated with aging. This association was addressed by Beck[23] at the 1996 World Workshop on Periodontics: "It may be that risk factors do change as people age or at least the relative importance of risk factors change." This chapter focuses on the associations between aging and oral health, with an emphasis on periodontal health.

THE AGING PERIODONTIUM

Normal aging of the periodontium is a result of cellular aging, which is the basis for the intrinsic changes seen in oral tissues over time. The aging process does not affect every tissue in the same way. For example, muscle and nerve tissue undergo minimal renewal, whereas epithelial tissue, which is one of the primary components of the periodontium, always renews itself.

Intrinsic Changes

In epithelium, a progenitor population of cells (i.e., stem cells) in the basal layer provides new cells. The cells of the basal layer are the least differentiated cells of the oral epithelium. A small subpopulation of these cells produces basal cells and retains the proliferative potential of the tissue. A larger subpopulation of these cells (i.e., amplifying cells) produces cells available for subsequent maturation. This maturing population of cells continually undergoes a process of differentiation or maturation.

By definition, the differentiated cell (i.e., epithelial cell) can no longer divide. Conversely, the basal cell remains as part of the progenitor population of cells ready to return to the mitotic cycle and again produce both types of cells. There is a constant source of renewal (Fig. 38.1).

In the aging process, cell renewal takes place at a slower rate and with fewer cells. The effect is to slow down the regenerative processes. As the progenitor cells wear out and die, there are fewer and fewer of these cells to replace the dead ones. This effect is characteristic of the biologic changes that occur with aging.

> **KEY FACT**
>
> With aging, stem cells undergo exhaustion; this affects the regenerative potential of the organism. Reductions in the number of stem cells and in their response to stimuli in their local environment have been documented.

Through the action of gerontogenes or replicative senescence (i.e., the Hayflick limit and telomere shortening), the number of progenitor cells decreases. Hayflick, an American microbiologist, observed that fetal cells (i.e., fibroblasts) displayed a consistently greater growth potential (i.e., approximately 50 cumulative population doublings) than those derived from adult tissues (i.e., 20 to 30 cumulative population doublings). The decreased cellular component has a concomitant effect of decreasing both cellular reserves and protein synthesis. This causes the oral epithelial tissue to become thin, with reduced keratinization.

Stochastic Changes

Stochastic changes occurring in cells also affect tissue (e.g., glycosylation and cross-linking produce morphologic and physiologic changes). Structures become stiffer, with a loss of elasticity and increased mineralization (i.e., fossilization). With a loss of regenerative power, structures become less soluble and more thermally stable. Somatic mutations lead to decreased protein synthesis and structurally altered proteins. Free radicals contribute to the accumulation of waste in the cell.

[a]Adapted from the following chapter of Newman and Carranza's Clinical Periodontology, 13th edition: Chapter 42: Periodontal Therapy in the Female Patient, by Sue S. Spackman and Janet G. Bauer.

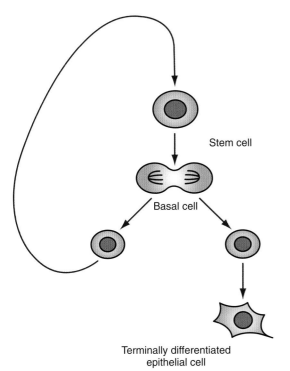

Fig. 38.1 Cell Renewal Cycle in Which the Basal Cell Produces an Epithelial Cell and Then Returns to the Progenitor Cell Population.

Stem cell

Basal cell

Terminally differentiated
epithelial cell

All of these changes decrease the physiologic processes of tissue. Most changes are primarily a result of aging, although some result from physiologic deterioration. For example, loss of elasticity and increased resistance of the tissue can lead to decreased permeability, decreased nutrient flow, and the accumulation of waste in the cell. Vascular peripheral resistance (i.e., decreased blood supply) can decrease cellular function.

Physiologic Changes

In the periodontal ligament, a decrease in the number of collagen fibers leads to a reduction in or loss of tissue elasticity. Decreased vascularity reduces production of mucopolysaccharides.

All of these types of changes are seen in the alveolar bone. With aging, alveolar bone density decreases, bone resorption increases, and vascularity decreases. In contrast, cementum shows cemental thickening.

Functional Changes

With aging, the cells of the oral epithelium and periodontal ligament have reduced mitotic activity, and all cells experience a reduction in metabolic rate. These changes also affect the immune system and periodontium because of the reduced healing capacity and rate. Inflammation develops more rapidly and is more severe. Individuals are highly susceptible to viral and fungal infections because of abnormalities in T-cell function.

Clinical Changes

Compensatory changes that occur during aging or in response to disease manifest clinically as dental or periodontal conditions, such as gingival recession and reductions in bone height. Dental

attrition, a type of tooth wear commonly seen as a normal part of aging, is a compensatory change that acts as a stabilizer between loss of bony support and excessive leveraging from occlusal forces imposed on the teeth.

A reduction in overjet of the teeth manifests as an increase in the edge-to-edge contact of the anterior teeth. Typically, this is related to the approximal wear of the posterior teeth. An increase is seen in the food table area, with loss of sluiceways, and in mesial migration.

Functional changes are associated with a reduced efficiency of mastication. Although effective mastication may remain, efficiency is reduced because of missing teeth, loose teeth, poorly fitting prostheses, or noncompliance of the patient, who may refuse to wear prosthetic appliances.

> ### KEY FACT
>
> **Key Periodontal Changes With Aging**
> - Thinning of oral epithelium and reduced keratinization
> - Reduction or loss of periodontal ligament tissue elasticity
> - Gingival recession
> - Attachment and bone loss
> - Thickening of cementum

PERIODONTAL DISEASES IN OLDER ADULTS

Etiology

Periodontal disease in older adults is usually referred to as *chronic periodontitis*.[45,75] Because periodontitis is a chronic disease, much of the ravage of the disease detected in older adults accumulated over time. The advanced stages of periodontitis are less prevalent than the moderate stages in the older adult population.[27] One theory is that many sites of advanced periodontal disease have resulted in tooth loss earlier in life, suggesting that older age is not a risk factor for periodontal disease.[45,75]

Evidence is limited on whether the risk factors for periodontal disease fluctuate with age.[23] General health status, immune status, diabetes, nutrition, smoking, genetics, medications, mental health status, salivary flow, functional deficits, and finances can modify the relationship between periodontal disease and age.[23,92]

Some frequently prescribed medications for older adults can alter the gingival tissues. *Steroid-induced gingivitis* has been associated with postmenopausal women receiving steroid therapy. *Gingival overgrowth* can be induced by medications such as cyclosporine, calcium channel blockers, and anticonvulsants (e.g., nifedipine, phenytoin) in the setting of poor oral hygiene. Gingival overgrowth further decreases a person's ability to maintain good oral hygiene.[45]

Relation to Systemic Disease

Padilha and colleagues,[65] using data from the Baltimore Longitudinal Study of Aging, reached the conclusion that "the number of teeth is a significant risk indicator for mortality … and that improving oral health and preventing tooth decay may substantially improve the oral status of the population and increase longevity."

A review of the literature by Loesche and Lopatin[57] indicates that poor oral health has been associated with medical conditions such as aspiration pneumonia and cardiovascular disease. In particular, periodontal disease can be associated with coronary heart disease and cerebrovascular accident (CVA). The Surgeon General's Report on Oral Health emphasizes that animal- and population-based studies demonstrate an association between periodontal disease and diabetes, cardiovascular disease, and stroke.[79]

Investigations confirm these associations. For example, a periodontal examination can assist in cardiovascular risk assessment in hypertensive patients. Angeli and coworkers[11] reported an association between periodontal disease and left ventricular mass in patients with untreated essential hypertension. In another investigation, diabetes mellitus type 2 HbA1c levels declined with periodontal therapy in a large study by the US Department of Veterans Affairs in South Carolina.[59]

Pneumonia is a common cause of morbidity and mortality in the older adult. Improvements in oral care have greatly reduced the incidence of pneumonia in elderly nursing home patients. Although the mechanism is under investigation, it is thought that the cough reflex can be improved by reducing the numbers of oropharyngeal microbial pathogens.[85] Expanding on these findings, studies have been conducted on the prevention of ventilator-associated pneumonia. Providing oral therapy for intensive care patients to reduce bacterial colonization in the mouth and teeth can reduce mortality and morbidity rates by 42%.[43]

The presence and extent of periodontal disease may be related to an increased risk of weight loss in older well-functioning adults. This association is independent of smoking and diabetes mellitus. Changes in nutrient intake may be related to periodontal disease and a higher systemic burden of inflammation.[89]

PERIODONTAL TREATMENT PLANNING

Periodontal disease in older adults is not usually a rapidly progressive disease but often manifests as long-standing chronic disease. Because periodontal disease has periods of exacerbation and remission, understanding and documenting periods of active disease compared with quiescent periods is essential to the formulation of the treatment plan and prognosis.[75]

Periodontal disease must be diagnosed regardless of age. The goal of periodontal treatment for all patients is to preserve function and eliminate or prevent the progression of inflammatory disease.[88]

The goal of clinically managing periodontal disease in older adults is based on specific individualized care. The major consideration is improving or maintaining function, with an emphasis on quality-of-life issues. Emphasizing care over cure is the cornerstone of any proposed treatment plan. Prevention, comfort, function, aesthetics, and ease of maintenance are the criteria for successful care of an older adult, particularly a frail or functionally dependent older patient.

Several factors must be considered during treatment planning for older individuals.[75] It is important first to remember that periodontal healing and recurrence of disease are *not* influenced by age.[23] Factors to consider in the older patient are medical and mental health status, medications, functional status, and lifestyle behaviors that influence periodontal treatment, outcome, or progression of disease.[88] Periodontal disease severity, ability to perform oral hygiene procedures, and ability to tolerate treatment should be evaluated during treatment planning. The risks and benefits of surgical and nonsurgical therapy should be considered.[57] The amount of remaining periodontal support or past periodontal destruction, tooth type, number of occlusal contacts, and individual patient preferences are also important.[88]

Dental implants are reliable replacements for missing teeth in older adults[93]; age alone is not a contraindication for implant placement. Risk factors for the success of implants have been investigated. Although aging is a factor in decision making, most failures are associated with smoking, diabetes, head and neck irradiation, and postmenopausal estrogen therapy.[63]

For older adults, a nonsurgical approach is often the first treatment choice. Depending on the nature and extent of periodontal disease, surgical therapy may be indicated. Surgical technique should minimize the amount of additional root exposure. Individuals who respond best to surgical therapy are those who are able to maintain the surgical result. Age alone is not a contraindication to surgery. For individuals who are unable to comply with treatment, have poor oral hygiene, or are medically or mentally compromised or functionally impaired, palliative supportive periodontal care instead of surgical periodontal treatment is often the optimal approach.[57,73]

The US Food and Drug Administration (FDA) approved silver diamine fluoride to reduce sensitivity, and its off-label use can arrest root caries and reduce bacteria on roots, where combined caries and periodontal infections is an issue and traditional dental treatment is not optimal or possible.[48]

A common goal for all older adults is to decrease bacteria through oral hygiene and mechanical debridement. Clinical trials enrolling older adults showed that the development or progression of periodontal disease could be prevented or arrested by controlling plaque. For certain patients, topical antibiotic therapy may complement repeated subgingival instrumentation during supportive care. Oral hygiene maintenance should also focus on root surfaces susceptible to caries.[88] Treatment planning for frail and functionally dependent older adults may be challenging for dental professionals. For this reason, high-quality office-based methods to access evidence-based decision-making programs and accommodating websites were created to help with complicated oral health care issues.[4,74]

Disease Prevention and Maintenance of Periodontal Health in Older Adults

For younger and older people, the most important factors determining a successful outcome of periodontal treatment are plaque control and frequency of professional care. Advanced age does not decrease plaque control,[12] but older adults may have difficulty performing adequate oral hygiene because of compromised health, altered mental status, medications, or altered mobility and dexterity.[88] Older adults may change toothbrushing habits because of disabilities such as hemiplegia due to CVA, visual difficulties, dementia, or arthritis. The newer, lightweight electric-powered toothbrush may be more beneficial than a manual toothbrush for older adults with physical and sensory limitations.

The proportion of people who floss their teeth decreases after 40 years of age.[87] This may be partly caused by impairment of fine motor skills due to disease or injury. Interproximal brushes, shaped wooden toothpicks, and mechanical flossing devices often can be used in place of traditional flossing with satisfactory outcomes.

Multidisciplinary strategies are increasingly becoming part of periodontal health care promotion. Assessments of overall health, functional status, and patient education are fundamental to promoting and maintaining optimal periodontal health. Older adults, their families, and caregivers need to be informed and trained by dental professionals on the appropriate devices, chemotherapeutic agents, and techniques to provide oral self-care and maintain a healthy lifestyle.[39]

The outcomes are instrumental in achieving overall health, oral and periodontal health, self-esteem, nutrition, and quality of life. Barriers to achieving these benefits are access and cost. For older adults who are homebound or institutionalized, these barriers inhibit their achieving and maintaining optimal oral and periodontal health.

Chemotherapeutic Agents
Antiplaque Agents
Patients who are unable to remove plaque adequately due to disease or disability may benefit from antiplaque agents such as chlorhexidine, subantimicrobial tetracycline, or Listerine or its generic counterparts.[61,75,88]

Chlorhexidine is a cationic bisbiguanide that has been used as a broad-spectrum antiseptic in medicine since the 1950s. In Europe, a 0.2% concentration of chlorhexidine has been used for years as a preventive and therapeutic agent.[57,87] Chlorhexidine is bacteriostatic or bactericidal, depending on the dose. Adverse effects of chlorhexidine include an increase in calculus formation, dysgeusia (i.e., altered taste), and permanent staining of teeth.[8] Chlorhexidine is a prescription rinse for short-term use (<6 months); long-term use (>6 months) has not been extensively studied.[87]

The American Dental Association (ADA) Council on Dental Therapeutics[6] has approved chlorhexidine to help prevent and reduce supragingival plaque and gingivitis. Although chlorhexidine has not been studied in older adults, outcomes in younger persons, including those with disabilities, suggest that it is also effective in older adults. Chlorhexidine may be particularly useful for older adults who have difficulty with plaque removal and those who take phenytoin, calcium channel blockers, or cyclosporine and who are at risk for gingival hyperplasia.[75,87]

Subantimicrobial tetracycline (Periostat) is useful in treating moderate to severe chronic periodontitis. The active ingredient in Periostat is doxycycline hyclate. In concert with scaling and root planing, Mohammad and colleagues[61] showed this treatment to be effective in institutionalized older adults. Periostat is contraindicated for patients with an allergy to tetracycline.

Listerine antiseptic and its generic counterparts are approved by the ADA Council on Dental Therapeutics[8] to help prevent and reduce supragingival plaque and gingivitis. The active ingredients in Listerine are methyl salicylate and three essential oils (i.e., eucalyptol, thymol, and menthol). Listerine has been found to be effective in reducing plaque and gingivitis compared with placebo rinses in young healthy adults. It may exacerbate xerostomia because of its high alcohol content, ranging from 21.6% to 26.9%, and it is generally contraindicated in patients under treatment for alcoholism who take disulfiram (Antabuse). Listerine may benefit patients who do not tolerate the taste or staining of chlorhexidine or who prefer OTC medicaments that are less expensive and easier to obtain.[75,87]

Antimicrobial photodynamic therapy (aPDT) is being investigated for the treatment of periodontitis. Using low-powered lasers and cells treated with a drug to make them susceptible to the light, it is possible to kill microorganisms specific to periodontal disease.[34]

Fluoride
Fluoride is an effective caries-preventive agent (see "Periodontal Treatment Planning," earlier). Fluoride's effects are as follows[75,87]:
1. It reduces enamel solubility.
2. It promotes remineralization of early carious lesions.
3. It is bactericidal for bacterial plaque.

Topical fluorides are recommended for the prevention and treatment of dental caries. OTC fluorides include fluoride dentifrices, rinses, and gels that contain concentrations of 230 to 1500 parts per million (ppm) of fluoride ions. Prescription 1.1% neutral sodium fluoride gels are available with a fluoride concentration of 5000 ppm of fluoride ions. Professionally applied fluoride gel, foam, or varnish products have between 9050 and 22,600 ppm of fluoride ions.[8]

Saliva Substitutes
Saliva substitutes, which are intended to match the chemical and physical traits of natural saliva, are available to relieve the symptoms of dry mouth. Their composition varies, but they usually contain salt ions, a flavoring agent, paraben (a preservative), cellulose derivative or animal mucins, and fluoride. The ADA's seal of approval has been granted for some artificial saliva products (e.g., Saliva Substitute, Salivart).[8] Most saliva substitutes can be used as desired by patients and are dispensed in a spray bottle, rinse or swish bottle, or oral swab stick.[8,87] Products such as dry-mouth toothpastes and moisturizing gels are also available. Biotene products such as Oral Balance are marketed to relieve the symptoms of xerostomia.

Patients with dry mouth can benefit from stimulating saliva flow with sugarless candies and sugarless gum. Xylitol chewing gum has been shown to have anticariogenic properties in children. Medicated chewing gum with xylitol and chlorhexidine or xylitol alone has the added benefit of reducing oral plaque and gingivitis in elderly people who live in residential facilities.[9]

Salivary substitutes and stimulants are effective only in the short term. Under investigation is acupuncture-like transcutaneous nerve stimulation (Codetron), a method to treat radiation-induced xerostomia. Unlike traditional acupuncture therapy, Codetron does not use invasive needles to achieve stimulation. This method helps patients produce their own saliva and reduces symptoms of xerostomia for several months. Acupuncture therapy has demonstrated improvements lasting up to 3 years.[95]

CONCLUSIONS

Future oral health care trends will include increased numbers of older adults seeking periodontal therapy. Dental practitioners of the 21st century should be comfortable with providing comprehensive periodontal care for this segment of the population. Aging dental patients have particular oral and general health conditions that dental hygienists should be familiar with detecting, consulting on, and treating. Medical diseases and conditions that occur more often with age may require modification of periodontal preventive tools and the planning and treatment phases of periodontal care.

A Case Scenario is found on the companion website.

REFERENCES

 References for this chapter are found on the companion website.

39

Treatment of Aggressive and Atypical Forms of Periodontitis[a,b]

 For online-only content on periodontitis refractory to treatment, please visit the companion website.

CHAPTER OUTLINE

The majority of patients with common forms of periodontal disease respond predictably well to conventional therapy, including oral hygiene instruction, nonsurgical periodontal debridement, surgery, and supportive periodontal maintenance. However, patients with aggressive forms of periodontitis and some atypical forms of periodontal disease often do not respond as predictably or as favorably to conventional therapy. Fortunately, only a small percentage of patients with periodontal disease are diagnosed with aggressive periodontitis. Patients who are diagnosed with periodontal disease of any type that is *refractory* to treatment present in small numbers as well. Even fewer patients are diagnosed with necrotizing ulcerative periodontitis (NUP). Each of these atypical disease entities poses significant challenges for the clinician, not only because they are infrequently encountered, but also because they may not respond favorably to conventional periodontal therapy.[18,32] Furthermore, the severe loss of periodontal support associated with these cases leaves the dentist faced with uncertainty about treatment outcomes and difficulty in making decisions about whether to save affected teeth or extract them.

AGGRESSIVE PERIODONTITIS

Aggressive periodontitis, by definition, causes rapid destruction of the periodontal attachment apparatus and the supporting alveolar bone (see Chapter 6). The responsiveness of aggressive periodontitis to conventional periodontal treatment is unpredictable,

and the overall prognosis for these patients is poorer than for patients with chronic periodontitis. Because these patients do not respond typically to conventional methods and their disease progresses unusually fast, the logical question is whether there are problems associated with an impaired host immune response that may contribute to such a *different* disease and result in a *limited* response to the usual therapeutic measures. However, in most patients with aggressive periodontitis, numerous attempts to examine immunologic profiles of patients with aggressive periodontitis have failed to identify any specific etiologic factors common to all patients.

The prognosis for patients with aggressive periodontitis depends on (1) whether the disease is generalized or localized, (2) the degree of destruction present at the time of diagnosis, and (3) the ability to control future progression. *Generalized* aggressive periodontitis rarely undergoes spontaneous remission, whereas *localized* forms of the disease have been known to arrest spontaneously.[22] This unexplained curtailment of disease progression has sometimes been referred to as a "burnout" of the disease. It appears that cases of localized aggressive periodontitis often have a limited period of rapid loss of periodontal attachment and alveolar bone, followed by a slower, more chronic phase of disease progression. Overall, patients with generalized aggressive periodontitis tend to have a poorer prognosis because they typically have more teeth affected by the disease and the disease is less likely to go into remission spontaneously compared with localized forms of aggressive periodontitis.

Therapeutic Modalities

Early detection is critically important in the treatment of aggressive periodontitis (generalized or localized), because prevention of further destruction is often more predictable than regeneration of lost supporting tissues. Therefore, at the initial diagnosis, it is helpful to obtain any previously taken radiographs to assess the rate of progression of the disease. Together with future radiographs, this documentation also facilitates the clinician's assessment of treatment success and control of the disease.

Treatment of aggressive periodontitis must be pursued with a logical and regimented approach. Several aspects of treatment

---

[a]Adapted from the following chapter of Newman and Carranza's Clinical Periodontology, 13th edition: Chapter 43: Treatment of Aggressive and Atypical Forms of Periodontitis, by Perry R. Klokkevold.

[b]Note: In the 2018 Classification of Periodontal and Peri-Implant Diseases and Conditions, "chronic periodontitis" and "aggressive periodontitis" disease categories are grouped under a single category called "periodontitis" and are further characterized based on a multidimensional staging and grading system. In this chapter, the term "aggressive periodontitis" is still used because the related studies were conducted before the 2018 classification. Readers are referred to Chapter 6 for the detailed discussion on periodontal disease classification.

must be considered. One of the most important aspects of treatment success is educating the patient about the disease, including the causes and risk factors, and stressing the importance of the patient's role in the success of treatment.[39] Essential therapeutic considerations for the clinician are controlling the infection, arresting disease progression, correcting anatomic defects, replacing missing teeth, and ultimately helping the patient maintain periodontal health with frequent periodontal maintenance care. Educating family members is another important factor, because aggressive periodontitis is known to have familial aggregation. Family members, especially younger siblings of the patient diagnosed with aggressive periodontitis, should be examined for signs of disease, educated about preventive measures, and monitored closely. It cannot be stressed enough that early diagnosis, intervention, and, if possible, prevention of disease is more desirable than attempting to reverse the destruction that results from aggressive periodontitis.

Conventional Periodontal Therapy

Because aggressive periodontitis is primarily of bacterial of origin, initial treatment is comparable to treatment rendered for chronic periodontitis. Conventional periodontal therapy for aggressive periodontitis consists of patient education, oral hygiene improvement, scaling and root planing, and regular (frequent) recall maintenance. It may or may not include periodontal flap surgery.[2] However, the response of aggressive periodontitis to conventional therapy alone may be limited and less predictable. Patients who are diagnosed with aggressive periodontitis at an early stage and are able to enter therapy may have a better outcome than those who are diagnosed at an advanced stage of destruction. In general, the earlier the disease is diagnosed, the more conservative the therapy and the more predictable the outcome.

Teeth with moderate to advanced periodontal attachment loss and bone loss often have a poor prognosis and pose the most difficult challenge. Depending on the condition of the remaining dentition, treatment of these teeth may offer a limited prospect of improvement and may even diminish the overall treatment success. Clearly, some of these teeth should be extracted; however, other teeth may be pivotal to the stability of the dentition, making it desirable to attempt treatment to maintain them. Treatment options for teeth with deep periodontal pockets and bone loss may be nonsurgical or surgical. Surgery may be purely resective, regenerative, or a combination of these approaches.

> ### KEY FACT
>
> Patients who are diagnosed with aggressive periodontitis at an early stage and who are able to enter therapy may have a better outcome than those who are diagnosed at an advanced stage of destruction. In general, the earlier the disease is diagnosed, the more conservative the therapy and the more predictable the outcome. Teeth with advanced periodontal attachment loss and bone destruction often have a poor prognosis and pose the biggest challenge for treatment.

Surgical resective therapy. Resective periodontal surgery can be effective in reducing or eliminating pocket depth in patients

with aggressive periodontitis, but it may be difficult to accomplish if adjacent teeth are unaffected. If a significant height discrepancy exists between the periodontal support of the affected tooth and the adjacent unaffected tooth, the gingival transition (soft tissue following the bone) often results in deep probing pocket depth around the affected tooth that cannot be eliminated. A less-than-ideal outcome must be considered before deciding to treat increased pocket depth surgically.

It is important to realize the limitations of surgical therapy and to appreciate the possible risk that surgical therapy may further compromise teeth that are mobile due to extensive loss of periodontal support. For example, in a patient with severe horizontal bone loss, surgical resective therapy may result in increased tooth mobility that is difficult to manage, and a nonsurgical approach may be preferable. Careful evaluation of the risks versus the benefits of surgery must be performed on a case-by-case basis.

More information on regenerative therapy and online materials for this chapter are found on the companion website.

Antimicrobial Therapy

The presence of periodontal pathogens, specifically *Aggregatibacter actinomycetemcomitans (previously Actinobacillus actinomycetemcomitans)*, has been implicated as the reason that aggressive periodontitis does not respond to conventional therapy alone. These pathogens are known to remain in the tissues after therapy and to reinfect the pocket.[6,45] The use of systemic antibiotics was thought to be necessary to eliminate pathogenic bacteria (especially *A. actinomycetemcomitans*) from the tissues. Indeed, several authors have reported success in the treatment of aggressive periodontitis using antibiotics as adjuncts to standard therapy.[25-27,56]

There is compelling evidence that adjunctive antibiotic treatment frequently results in a more favorable clinical response than mechanical therapy alone.[51] In a systematic review, Herrera and colleagues[17] found that systemic antimicrobials in conjunction with scaling and root planing offered benefits greater than scaling and planing alone in terms of clinical attachment level, probing pocket depth, and reduced risk of additional attachment loss. Patients with deeper, progressive pockets seemed to benefit the most from systemic administration of adjunctive antibiotics. Many different antibiotic types and regimens were reviewed, but because of limitations in comparing data from different studies, definitive recommendations were not possible. In a meta-analysis of the literature (including six randomized clinical trials), Sgolastra and associates[46] found that the systemic use of combined amoxicillin and metronidazole as an adjunct to scaling and root planing for the treatment of generalized aggressive periodontitis resulted in significant clinical attachment gain ($P < .05$) and pocket reduction ($P < .05$) compared with scaling and root planing alone.

Fig. 39.1 shows the results of treatment in a case of aggressive periodontitis treated nonsurgically with scaling and root planing and adjunctive antibiotic therapy. The patient, a 34-year-old Asian man, presented with a complaint of loose teeth and bleeding gums. He requested treatment to save his teeth. Treatment consisted of patient education, including oral hygiene instructions, and nonsurgical therapy with adjunctive antibiotics. All teeth were thoroughly scaled and root planed under local anesthesia over two treatment appointments, and the patient was treated with systemic amoxicillin (500 mg, three times daily for 2 weeks) during the period of treatment. All areas responded favorably, with probing pocket depths decreasing from 3 to 13 mm to 2 to 5 mm. Bleeding on probing diminished from generalized to very few isolated areas. The patient continued on periodontal maintenance with good results for more than 5 years.

More information on the outcomes following treatment of aggressive periodontitis and online materials for this chapter are found on the companion website.

Fig. 39.1 Intraoral Clinical Photographs and Full-Mouth Radiographs Taken Before and After Treatment of Aggressive Periodontitis in a 34-Year-Old Asian Man. (A and B) Intraoral clinical photographs of pretreatment periodontal condition. Notice the gingival edema, inflammation, and bleeding. Probing pocket depths ranged from 3 mm to 13 mm, with generalized bleeding on probing and purulent exudate. (C) Pretreatment full-mouth radiographs demonstrate generalized severe horizontal bone loss. Notice the periapical radiolucency at the apex of the upper left premolar, indicating pulpal disease.

Continued

Fig. 39.1, cont'd (D and E) Intraoral clinical photographs of posttreatment results after 5 years. Treatment included nonsurgical scaling and root planing along with adjunctive systemic antibiotics (amoxicillin). Patient improved his oral hygiene and continued to be seen for professional maintenance every 3 months. Probing pocket depths have been maintained in the range of 2 mm to 5 mm, with only a few localized areas of bleeding on probing. (F) Full-mouth radiographs after 5 years demonstrate no additional bone loss. The endodontically involved maxillary premolar was extracted and replaced with a removable partial denture.

CLINICAL CORRELATION

The use of amoxicillin and metronidazole as an adjunctive therapy to scaling and root planing for the treatment of aggressive periodontitis has been shown to significantly improve clinical attachment gain and pocket depth reduction when compared with scaling and root planing alone. Aggressive periodontitis is a disease with a bacterial etiology.

Microbial testing. Some investigators and clinicians advocate microbial testing to identify the specific periodontal pathogens responsible for disease and selecting an appropriate antibiotic based on sensitivity and resistance. There may be specific cases in which bacterial identification and antibiotic-sensitivity testing is valuable. For example, in some cases of localized aggressive periodontitis, tetracycline-resistant *Actinobacillus* species have been suspected. If an antibiotic susceptibility test determines that tetracycline-resistant species exist in the lesion, the clinician may be advised to consider another antibiotic or an antibiotic combination, such as amoxicillin and metronidazole.[9,40,41]

Local delivery. Local delivery for administration of antibiotics is another approach to the management of localized periodontal infections. The primary advantage of local therapy is that smaller total dosages of topical agents can be delivered inside the pocket, avoiding the side effects of systemic antibacterial agents while increasing the exposure of the target microorganisms to higher concentrations and therefore more therapeutic levels of the medication. Local delivery agents are available in many different forms, including solutions, gels, fibers, and chips (see Chapter 47).[10,11,20]

Full-Mouth Disinfection

Another approach to antimicrobial therapy in the control of infection associated with periodontitis is full-mouth disinfection. The concept, described by Quirynen and coworkers,[41] consists of full-mouth debridement (removal of all plaque and calculus) completed in two appointments within a 24-hour period. In addition to scaling and root planing, the tongue is brushed with chlorhexidine gel (1%) for 1 minute, the mouth is rinsed with chlorhexidine solution (0.2%) for 2 minutes, and periodontal pockets are irrigated with chlorhexidine solution (1%).

Treatment Planning and Restorative Considerations

Successful management of aggressive periodontitis must include tooth replacement as part of the treatment plan. In some advanced cases, the overall treatment success for the patient may be enhanced if severely compromised teeth are extracted. The outcome of treatment for these teeth is limited, and, more importantly, the retention of severely diseased teeth over time may result in additional bone loss and teeth that are further compromised. The risk of further bone loss is an even greater concern now, with the current success and predictability of dental implants and the desire to preserve bone for implant placement. Any additional alveolar bone loss in an area that has already undergone severe bone loss may further compromise residual anatomy and impair the opportunity for tooth replacement with a dental implant. This is especially true for certain areas with poor bone quality or limited bone volume, such as the posterior maxilla. Fortunately, healing of extraction sites is typically uneventful in patients with aggressive periodontitis, and bone augmentation of defect sites is predictable.

In the patient with aggressive periodontitis, the approach to restorative treatment should be chosen based on a single premise: Extract severely compromised teeth early, and plan treatment to accommodate future tooth loss. The teeth with the best prognosis should be identified and considered when planning the restorative treatment. The lower cuspids and first premolars are typically more resistant to loss, probably because of the favorable anatomy (i.e., single roots, no furcations) and easier access for patient oral hygiene. As a rule, an extensive fixed prosthesis should be avoided, and removable partial dentures should be planned in such a way as to allow for the addition of teeth.

When hopeless teeth are extracted, they need to be replaced. The desire to replace missing teeth in a permanent manner without preparation of adjacent teeth for a fixed partial denture has motivated some dentists to attempt transplantation of teeth from one site to another. Transplantation of developing third molars to the sockets of hopeless first molars has been attempted with limited success.[4,24,31] Now, however, the success and predictability of dental implants have obviated the need to transplant teeth to edentulous sites.

Use of Dental Implants

Initially, the use of dental implants was suggested for and implemented in patients with aggressive periodontitis with much caution, because of an unfounded fear of bone and implant loss. However, evidence appears to support the use of dental implants in these patients.[29,33,34,35,55] Therefore, it is possible to consider the use of dental implants in the overall treatment plan for patients with aggressive periodontitis.

CLINICAL CORRELATION

Special consideration must be given to the risk of occlusal overload of implants placed in a periodontally compromised dentition. This is especially true when only one or a few implants are used to replace a limited number of teeth with an implant-supported fixed crown or bridge in a patient with a moderately mobile remaining dentition. The immobility of implants in a dentition that does not have a stable vertical occlusal stop may lead to implant overload.

Periodontal Maintenance

When patients with periodontitis are transferred to maintenance care, their periodontal condition must be stable (i.e., no clinical signs of disease and no periodontal pathogens). Each maintenance visit should consist of a medical history review, an inquiry about any recent periodontal problems, an assessment of risk factors, a comprehensive periodontal and oral examination, thorough root debridement, and prophylaxis, followed by a review of oral hygiene instructions. If oral hygiene is not good, patients may benefit most from a review of oral hygiene instructions and visualization of plaque in their own mouth before debridement and prophylaxis.

Frequent maintenance visits appear to be one of the most important factors in the control of disease and the success of treatment in patients with aggressive periodontitis.[23,49] In a study of 25 individuals with aggressive (early-onset) periodontitis followed with maintenance every 3 to 6 months for 5 years, it was concluded that these patients can be effectively maintained with clinical and microbiologic improvements after active periodontal therapy.[19] High bacterial counts (particularly *Porphyromonas gingivalis* and *Treponema denticola*), the number of acute episodes, the number of teeth lost, smoking, and stress appeared to be significant factors in the small percentage of sites that showed progressive bone loss. In a 5-year follow-up study of 13 patients with aggressive periodontitis treated with comprehensive mechanical, surgical, and antimicrobial therapy and supportive periodontal maintenance every 3 to 4 months, periodontal disease progression was arrested in 95% of the initially affected lesions. Only 2% to 5% experienced discrete episodes of loss of periodontal support.[5]

A supportive periodontal maintenance program aimed at early detection and treatment of sites that begin to lose attachment should be established. The interval between these recall visits is short during the first period after the patient's completion of therapy—usually no longer than 3 months. Acute episodes of gingival inflammation can be detected and managed earlier when the patient is on a frequent monitoring cycle. Monitoring as frequently as every 3 to 4 weeks may be necessary when the disease is thought to be active. If signs of disease activity and progression persist despite therapeutic efforts, frequent visits, and good patient compliance, microbial testing may be indicated. The rate of disease progression may be faster in younger individuals, and therefore the dental hygienist should monitor such patients more frequently. Over time, the recall maintenance interval can be adjusted (more or less often) to suit the patient's level of oral hygiene and control of disease, as determined by each examination.

Close collaboration among members of the treatment team, including the periodontist, general dentist, dental hygienist, and patient's physician, is required for continuity of care and for patient motivation and encouragement. It is important to monitor and observe the patient's overall physical status as well, because weight loss, depression, and malaise have been reported in patients with generalized aggressive periodontitis. Finally, there is a constant need to reinforce patient education about disease etiology and preventive practices (i.e., oral hygiene and control of risk factors).

More information on managing persons with periodontitis refractory to treatment and online materials for this chapter are found on the companion website.

PERIODONTITIS REFRACTORY TO TREATMENT

Although refractory periodontitis is not currently considered a separate disease entity (see Chapter 6), patients who fail to respond to conventional therapy are considered to have periodontitis refractory to treatment. It is possible to characterize any form of periodontal disease (e.g., chronic periodontitis, aggressive periodontitis) as refractory to treatment.

These cases are difficult to manage because the etiology behind their lack of response to therapy is unknown. Initially, because contributing factors may have been overlooked, it is important to evaluate the adequacy of treatment attempts thoroughly and to consider other possible etiologies before concluding that a case truly is refractory. A patient with periodontitis that is refractory to treatment often does not have any distinguishing clinical characteristics on initial examination compared with patients who have periodontitis that responds normally. Therefore the initial treatment would follow conventional therapeutic modalities for periodontitis. After treatment, if the response is not as expected, the dental professional should rule out the following conditions:

1. *Inadequately treated periodontitis.* Most forms of periodontitis can be treated effectively with currently available modalities if they are performed properly. After treatment, if it is determined that the patient has not responded, the dental hygienist must evaluate whether the therapy was adequately performed. Undetected or inaccessible subgingival calculus may be present in one or more areas. Retreatment may be the best way to ensure that therapy was adequately performed. All root surfaces must be meticulously inspected.
2. *Poor plaque control.* Plaque control is essential to the success of periodontal therapy.[36,43,44] Patients must understand the role of bacterial plaque in their disease process, and they must comply with daily oral hygiene instructions. Patient compliance and the adequacy of daily plaque control should be assessed before concluding that a case of periodontitis is refractory to treatment.
3. *Endodontic infection.* The presence of nonperiodontal infections in the area can perpetuate periodontal disease activity and prevent a normal healing response to conventional periodontal therapy. Endodontic infection of teeth in the area should be suspected and ruled out before concluding that a case is refractory to treatment. The clinician should suspect an endodontic etiology, especially in those patients with localized recurrent disease.

A case may be considered *refractory* to treatment only when loss of periodontal attachment and bone continues after well-executed treatment in a patient with good oral hygiene and no other infections or etiologic factors.

Clinicians are in a quandary when presented with a patient who is not responding to periodontal therapy. Therapeutic means must be broad in scope and thorough to ensure that all aspects of the host response are addressed. At a minimum, a frequent and intensive recall maintenance and home care program is necessary. Mechanical debridement with scaling and root planing can reduce total supragingival and subgingival bacterial masses, but major periodontal pathogens may persist. Surgical treatment may aid in providing access for debridement and in elimination of bacterial pathogens.[45] In addition, the morphology of the gingival tissues should be modified to facilitate daily plaque removal by the patient.

Some cases of periodontitis that are refractory to treatment may not respond to a given antibiotic regimen. When this occurs, the clinician should consider a different antimicrobial therapy based on microbial susceptibility analysis. At this point in the therapy, strong consideration should be given to consulting with the patient's physician for evaluation of a possible host immune system deficiency or a metabolic problem such as diabetes.

NECROTIZING ULCERATIVE PERIODONTITIS

NUP is a rare disease, especially in developed countries, and NUP is invariably diagnosed in individuals with a compromised host immune response. The incidence of NUP in specific populations, such as patients who are positive for human immunodeficiency virus (HIV) infection or have acquired immunodeficiency syndrome (AIDS), has been reported to be between 0% and 6%. Most patients diagnosed with NUP have diseases or conditions that impair their host immune response. These patients often have an underlying predisposing systemic factor that renders them susceptible to NUP disease. For this reason, patients presenting with NUP should be treated in consultation with their physician.

CONCLUSIONS

Treatment of aggressive and atypical forms of periodontal disease is challenging for clinicians because these forms are infrequently encountered, can manifest with more severe bone loss, and do not respond as predictably or as favorably to conventional therapy. Fortunately, only a small percentage of patients are diagnosed with these forms of periodontitis. This chapter discussed therapies and rationales for management of these challenging cases.

A Case Scenario is found on the companion website.

REFERENCES

 References for this chapter are found on the companion website.

40

Treatment of Acute Gingival Disease[a]

CHAPTER OUTLINE

The treatment of acute gingival disease entails alleviation of the acute symptoms and elimination of all etiologic factors, including periodontal disease, both chronic and acute, throughout the oral cavity. Treatment is not complete if periodontal pathologic changes or predisposing factors capable of causing them remain. Systemic risk factors that increase susceptibility to these acute gingival diseases also need to be assessed and eliminated or modified if possible.

NECROTIZING ULCERATIVE GINGIVITIS

Necrotizing ulcerative gingivitis (NUG) results from an impaired host response to a potentially pathogenic microflora. Depending on the degree of host compromise or immunosuppression, NUG may occur in a mouth essentially free of other gingival involvement, or it may be superimposed on underlying chronic gingival or periodontal disease. Treatment should include alleviation of the acute symptoms and correction of the underlying chronic gingival or periodontal disease. The former is the simpler part of the treatment; the latter often requires more comprehensive procedures, follow-up, and patient education.

The treatment of NUG consists of (1) alleviation of the acute inflammation by reduction of the microbial load and removal of necrotic tissue, (2) treatment of chronic disease either underlying the acute involvement or elsewhere in the oral cavity, (3) alleviation of generalized symptoms such as fever and malaise, and (4) correction of systemic conditions or factors that contribute to the initiation or progression of gingival changes. Chapter 28 provides further information on the management and treatment of necrotizing ulcerative

periodontitis (NUP) in patients with acquired immunodeficiency syndrome (AIDS).

Treatment of NUG should follow an orderly sequence, according to specific steps, at three clinical visits.

First Visit

At the first visit, the clinician should conduct a comprehensive evaluation of the patient, including a thorough medical history, with special attention to recent illness, living conditions, dietary background, cigarette smoking, type of employment, hours of rest, risk factors for human immunodeficiency virus (HIV) infection, and psychosocial parameters (e.g., stress, depression). The patient is questioned regarding the history of the acute disease, including its onset and duration, as follows:

- Is the disease recurrent?
- Are the recurrences associated with specific factors such as menstruation, particular foods, exhaustion, or mental stress?
- Has there been any previous treatment? When and for how long?

The clinician should also inquire as to the type of treatment received and the patient's impression regarding the effectiveness of previous treatment.

The initial physical examination should include an assessment of general appearance, presence of halitosis, presence of skin lesions, vital signs including temperature, and palpation for the presence of enlarged lymph nodes, especially submaxillary and submental nodes.

The oral cavity is examined for the characteristic NUG lesions distribution and the possible involvement of the oropharyngeal region. Oral hygiene is evaluated, with special attention to the presence of pericoronal flaps, periodontal pockets, and local risk factors (e.g., poorly contoured and ill-fitting restorations, presence and distribution of calculus). Periodontal probing of NUG lesions is likely to be very painful, will not aid in the primary diagnosis, and may need to be deferred until after the acute lesions are resolved.

[a]Adapted from the following chapter of Newman and Carranza's Clinical Periodontology, 13th edition: Chapter 44: Treatment of Acute Gingival Disease, by Perry R. Klokkevold and Fermin A. Carranza.

KEY FACT

The goals of initial therapy for NUG are reduction of the microbial load and removal of necrotic tissue to facilitate the healing process of repair and regeneration so that normal tissue barriers can be reestablished.

The goals of initial therapy are reduction of the microbial load and removal of necrotic tissue to the degree that repair and regeneration of normal tissue barriers can be reestablished. Treatment during the initial visit is confined to the acutely involved areas, which are isolated with cotton rolls and dried. A topical anesthetic is applied, and after 2 or 3 minutes the areas are gently swabbed with a moistened cotton pellet to remove the pseudomembrane and nonattached surface debris. Bleeding may be profuse. Each cotton pellet is used in a small area, then discarded; sweeping motions over large areas with a single pellet are not recommended. After the area is cleansed with warm water, the superficial calculus is removed. Ultrasonic scalers are very useful for this purpose because they do not elicit pain, and the water jet and cavitation aid in lavage of the area.

Subgingival scaling and curettage are contraindicated at this time because these procedures may extend the infection into the deeper tissues and may also cause bacteremia. *Unless an emergency exists, procedures such as extractions or periodontal surgery are postponed until the patient has been symptom-free for 4 weeks, to minimize the likelihood of exacerbating the acute symptoms.*

Antibiotics are effective in the treatment of patients with NUG.[5] Patients with moderate or severe NUG and local lymphadenopathy or other systemic signs or symptoms are placed on an antibiotic regimen of amoxicillin 500 mg orally every 6 hours for 10 days. For amoxicillin-sensitive patients, other antibiotics such as erythromycin (500 mg every 6 hours) or metronidazole (500 mg twice daily for 7 days) are prescribed. Systemic complications should subside in 1 to 3 days. *Antibiotics are not recommended in NUG patients who do not have systemic complications.*

Instructions to the Patient

The patient is discharged with the following instructions:
1. Avoid tobacco, alcohol, and condiments.
2. Rinse with a glassful of an equal mixture of 3% hydrogen peroxide and warm water every 2 hours and/or 0.12% chlorhexidine solution twice daily.
3. Get adequate rest. Pursue usual activities, but avoid excessive physical exertion or prolonged exposure to the sun, as in outdoor activities.
4. Confine toothbrushing to removal of surface debris with either a bland dentifrice or just water and an ultrasoft brush; overzealous brushing and the use of dental floss or interdental cleaners will be painful. Chlorhexidine mouth rinses are also helpful in controlling biofilm throughout the mouth.
5. An analgesic, such as a nonsteroidal antiinflammatory drug (NSAID; e.g., ibuprofen), is appropriate for pain relief.
6. Patients who have systemic complications such as high fever, malaise, anorexia, or general debility are given antibiotics and instructed to get plenty of bed rest and drink lots of fluids.

Patients are asked to report back to the clinician in 1 to 2 days. They should be advised about the extent of total treatment required to resolve the condition and warned that treatment is not complete when pain stops. They should be informed of the presence of chronic gingival or periodontal disease, which must be eliminated to reduce the likelihood of recurrence of the acute symptoms.

A large variety of drugs have been used in the treatment of NUG.[3] Topical drug therapy, however, is only an adjunctive measure; no drug, when used alone, can be considered complete therapy. Systemic antibiotics, when used, also reduce the oral bacterial flora and alleviate the oral symptoms,[12,13] but they are only an adjunct to the complete local treatment that the disease requires. If patients are treated by drugs or systemic antibiotics alone, the acute painful symptoms often reoccur after treatment is discontinued.

Second Visit

At the second visit, 1 or 2 days after the first visit, the patient is evaluated for amelioration of signs and symptoms. The patient's condition is usually improved; the pain is diminished or is no longer present. The gingival margins of the involved areas are erythematous but without a superficial pseudomembrane.

Scaling is performed if necessary and if sensitivity permits. Shrinkage of the gingiva may expose previously covered calculus, which is gently removed. Instructions to the patient are the same as those given previously.

Third Visit

At the next visit, approximately 5 days after the second visit, the patient is evaluated for resolution of symptoms, and a comprehensive plan for management of the patient's periodontal condition is formulated. The patient should be essentially symptom-free at this time. Some erythema may still be present in the involved areas, and the gingiva may be slightly painful on tactile stimulation (Fig. 40.1A and B). The patient is instructed in biofilm control procedures (see Chapter 43), which are essential for the success of the treatment and the maintenance of periodontal health. The patient is further counseled on nutrition, smoking cessation, and other conditions or habits associated with potential recurrence. The hydrogen peroxide rinses are discontinued, but chlorhexidine rinses may be maintained for an additional 2 or 3 weeks. Scaling and root planing is repeated if necessary. Unfortunately, patients often discontinue treatment because the acute condition has subsided; however, this is when comprehensive treatment of the chronic periodontal problem should begin. Patients need to be educated about the importance of comprehensive periodontal treatment and encouraged to complete it.

Appointments should be scheduled for treatment of chronic gingivitis, periodontal pockets, and pericoronal flaps, as well as for elimination of all forms of local risk factors (see Chapter 12). The patient should be reevaluated approximately 4 to 6 weeks after treatment to determine compliance with oral hygiene, health habits, psychosocial factors, the potential need for reconstructive or esthetic surgery, and the interval of subsequent recall visits.

Fig. 40.1 (A) Initial view of the anterior gingival tissues in a 22-year-old white female smoker with acute necrotizing ulcerative gingivitis. (B) Palatal view of the same patient. (C) Facial view of the same patient, 2 days after initial scaling and cessation of smoking. (D) Palatal view of the same patient, 2 days after initial scaling and cessation of smoking. (From Rose LF, Mealey BL, Genco RJ, Cohen DW: *Periodontics: medicine, surgery, and implants*, St. Louis, 2005, Mosby.)

Fig. 40.2 Treatment of Acute Necrotizing Ulcerative Gingivitis. (A) Before treatment. Notice the characteristic interdental lesions. (B) After treatment, showing restoration of healthy gingival contour.

Gingival Changes With Healing

The characteristic lesion of NUG undergoes the following changes during the course of healing in response to treatment:

1. Removal of the surface pseudomembrane exposes underlying red, hemorrhagic, craterlike depressions in the gingiva, indicating inflammation caused by necrosis and microbial infiltration of tissue that has lost the normal barrier function of the epithelium.

2. In the next stage, the bulk and redness of the crater margins are reduced, indicating a reduction in inflammation and reepithelialization, but the surface remains shiny (see Fig. 40.1C and D).

3. This is followed by the early signs of restoration of normal gingival contour and color, indicating reestablishment of the normal barrier function of the epithelium, including keratinization, and further reduction of inflammation.

4. In the final stage, the normal gingival color, consistency, surface texture, and contour may be restored. Portions of the root exposed by the acute disease may be covered by healthy gingiva (Fig. 40.2).

Additional Treatment Considerations
Contouring of Gingiva as an Adjunctive Procedure

Even in cases of severe gingival necrosis, healing often leads to restoration of the normal gingival contour, although normal architecture of the gingiva is only achieved after several weeks or months. However, if there has been loss of interdental bone, if the teeth are irregularly aligned, or if the entire papilla is lost, healing sometimes results in the formation of a shelf-like gingival margin, which favors retention of biofilm and recurrence of gingival inflammation and is an esthetic problem. This can be corrected by an attempt to restore lost tissue through periodontal

Fig. 40.3 Reshaping the Gingiva in the Treatment of Acute Necrotizing Ulcerative Gingivitis. (A) Before treatment. Bulbous gingiva and interdental necrosis are present in the mandibular anterior area. (B) After treatment. Gingival contours are still undesirable. (C) Final result. Physiologic contours are obtained by reshaping the gingiva.

plastic procedures or by reshaping the gingiva surgically (Fig. 40.3). Effective biofilm control by the patient is particularly important to establish and maintain the normal gingival contour in areas of tooth irregularity.

Role of Drugs

A large variety of drugs have been used for topical treatment of NUG. Topical drug therapy is only an adjunctive measure. *No drug, when used alone, can be considered complete treatment.*

Escharotic drugs, such as phenol, silver nitrate, chromic acid, or potassium bichromate, should not be used. They are necrotizing agents that alleviate pain by destroying the nerve endings of the ulcerated gingiva but also destroy young cells that are needed for repair, and delay healing. Repeated use of these agents results in loss of gingival tissue that is not restored when the disease subsides.[4]

> **KEY FACT**
>
> No drug, when used alone, can be considered complete treatment for the resolution of acute gingival disease (e.g., NUG). Local therapy and elimination of risk factors are essential for complete resolution.

Persistent or Recurrent Cases

Adequate local therapy with optimal home care will resolve most cases of NUG. If a case of NUG persists despite therapy or if it recurs, the patient should be reevaluated, with a focus on the following factors:

1. *Reassessment of differential diagnosis to rule out diseases that resemble NUG.* Several diseases and conditions (e.g., desquamative gingivitis) may initially manifest with an appearance similar to that of NUG. A renewed search for skin lesions and other signs or symptoms should be undertaken, with a biopsy if warranted.
2. *Underlying systemic disease causing immunosuppression.* In particular, HIV infection may frequently manifest with symptoms of NUG or NUP. The patient should be reassessed for risk factors and may need counseling about testing for HIV or other suspected underlying systemic diseases (e.g., lymphoproliferative disease). The patient will likely need referral to his or her physician for further evaluation.

3. *Inadequate local therapy.* Too often, treatment is discontinued when the symptoms have subsided, without elimination of the chronic gingival disease and periodontal pockets that remain after the superficial acute condition is relieved. Remaining calculus and other local factors that predispose to gingival inflammation may contribute to recurrence. Recurrent acute involvement in the mandibular anterior area can be associated with persistent pericoronal inflammation arising from partial eruption and pericoronal inflammation of third molars.[9] Anterior involvement is less likely to recur after the third molar situation is corrected.
4. *Inadequate compliance.* Poor biofilm control, heavy use of tobacco, ineffective stress management, and continued malnutrition can also contribute to persistence or recurrence of NUG. The dental hygienist should evaluate the quality and consistency of biofilm control. Further assessment and counseling on tobacco use will also determine the role of tobacco. If the clinician perceives that unresolved psychosocial factors are complicating health, the patient should be referred to an appropriate professional. A reassessment of the patient's nutritional state, with dietary analysis or nutritional testing, may be required.[6,8]

> **CLINICAL CORRELATION**
>
> Acute gingival disease may be a sign of a more serious systemic condition such as HIV infection or another condition that renders the host immunocompromised.

PRIMARY HERPETIC GINGIVOSTOMATITIS

Primary infection with herpes simplex virus (HSV) in the oral cavity results in a condition known as *acute herpetic gingivostomatitis*, which is an oral infection that is often accompanied by systemic signs and symptoms (see Chapter 19). This infection typically occurs in children but can occur in adults as well. It runs a 7- to 10-day course and usually heals without scarring. A recurrent herpetic episode may be precipitated by dental treatment,[14] respiratory infection, sunlight exposure, fever, trauma, exposure to chemicals, or emotional stress in individuals with a history of herpesvirus infection.

Treatment consists of early diagnosis and immediate initiation of antiviral therapy. Historically, therapy for primary herpetic gingivostomatitis consisted of palliative care alone. However, since the development of antiviral therapy, the standard of care now includes the use of antiviral medications. In a randomized, double-blind, placebo-controlled study, Amir and colleagues[1] demonstrated that antiviral therapy with 15 mg/kg of an acyclovir suspension given five times daily for 7 days substantially changed the course of the disease without significant side effects. Acyclovir reduced the duration of symptoms, including fever, from 3 days to 1 day, decreased new extraoral lesions from 5.5 to 0 days, and reduced difficulty with eating from 7 to 4 days. Furthermore, viral shedding stopped at 1 day for the acyclovir group but persisted up to 5 days for the control group. Overall, oral lesions were present for only 4 days in the acyclovir group but persisted for 10 days in the control group. Although no clear clinical evidence indicates that this regimen will reduce recurrences, research data suggest that a greater number of latent virus copies incorporated into ganglia will increase the severity of recurrences.[1]

FLASH BACK

As part of the primary infection, the HSV ascends through the sensory and autonomic nerves, where it persists as latent HSV in neuronal ganglia that innervate the site.

In summary, if primary herpetic gingivostomatitis is diagnosed within 3 days of onset, acyclovir suspension should be prescribed: 15 mg/kg five times daily for 7 days. If diagnosis occurs more than 3 days after onset in an immunocompetent patient, acyclovir therapy may have limited value. All patients, including those who present more than 3 days after disease onset, may receive palliative care, including removal of biofilm and food debris. An NSAID (e.g., ibuprofen) can be given systemically to reduce fever and pain. Patients may either take nutritional supplements or use topical anesthetics (e.g., viscous lidocaine) before eating to aid in proper nutrition during the early phases of acute herpetic gingivostomatitis. Periodontal therapy should be postponed until the acute symptoms subside to avoid the possibility of exacerbation (Fig. 40.4).

Local or systemic application of antibiotics is sometimes advised to prevent opportunistic bacterial or fungal infection of ulcerations, especially in the immunocompromised patient. If the condition does not resolve within 2 weeks, the patient should be referred to a physician for medical consultation.[7] The patient should be informed that herpetic gingivostomatitis is contagious at certain stages, such as when vesicles are present (highest viral titer). All individuals exposed to an infected patient should take precautions. Herpetic infection of a clinician's finger, referred to as *herpetic whitlow*, can occur if a seronegative clinician is exposed and becomes infected with herpesvirus from a patient's herpetic lesions.[10,11]

PERICORONITIS

As described in Chapter 19, pericoronitis refers to inflammation of the excess flap of soft tissue that overlies the crown of an incompletely erupted tooth. It is most frequently associated with mandibular third molars. The treatment of pericoronitis

Fig. 40.4 Treatment of Acute Herpetic Gingivostomatitis. (A) Before treatment. Note diffuse erythema and surface vesicles. (B) Before treatment, palatal view, showing gingival edema and ruptured vesicle on palate. (C) One month after treatment, showing restoration of normal gingival contour and stippling. (D) One month after treatment, palatal view.

depends on several factors, including position and quality of the surrounding tissues, severity of the inflammation, presence and/or risk of systemic complications, and advisability of retaining the involved tooth. All pericoronal flaps, even in the absence of symptoms, should be viewed with suspicion. Strong consideration should be given to removal of any pericoronal flaps that persist as a preventive measure against subsequent acute involvement.

The initial treatment of acute pericoronitis consists of (1) gently flushing the area with warm water to remove debris and exudate and (2) swabbing with antiseptic after the pericoronal flap has been lifted gently away from the tooth with an instrument. The underlying debris is removed, and the area is flushed with warm water. The occlusion is evaluated to determine whether an opposing tooth is contacting the pericoronal flap. It may be necessary to reduce soft tissue surgically and/or adjust the opposing tooth as a palliative measure to alleviate pain. Antibiotics can be prescribed in severe cases and for patients who have clinical evidence of diffuse microbial infiltration of the tissue. If the pericoronal flap is swollen and fluctuant, an incision and drainage procedure may be indicated to establish drainage and relieve pressure.

Once the acute symptoms have subsided, the prognosis of the tooth can be evaluated. The decision is governed by the likelihood that the tooth will continue erupting into a functional position or that impaction and the factors predisposing to pericoronitis will persist. Bone loss on the distal surface of the second molar is a concern when third molars are impacted along the distal surface.[2] The problem is significantly greater if the third molars

are extracted after the roots are formed or when the patient is older (i.e., mid-20s or later). To reduce the risk of bone loss around second molars, partially or completely impacted third molars should be extracted early in their development.

The quality of the soft tissues and the amount of space and vestibular depth are important factors to assess when deciding whether to retain or extract the tooth. If the decision is made to retain the tooth, the pericoronal flap is surgically reduced. It is necessary to reduce and reposition the tissue distal to the coronal aspect of the tooth, as well as remove the pericoronal flap on the occlusal surface. It is critical to leave the patient with a site that is cleansable and maintainable. As always, patient education and appropriate instruction in long-term maintenance of periodontal health is an essential part of successful therapy.

CONCLUSION

The treatment of acute gingival disease requires an accurate assessment and diagnosis of the problem, which includes identification of risk factors. The objective of initial therapy is the alleviation of acute symptoms and elimination of all local and systemic contributing factors. Treatment is not complete if predisposing factors remain. Systemic risk factors that increase susceptibility to acute gingival disease should be eliminated or reduced.

A Case Scenario is found on the companion website.

REFERENCES

 References for this chapter are found on the companion website.

Treatment of Periodontal Abscess[a]

CLASSIFICATION OF ABSCESSES

The periodontal abscess is a localized purulent inflammation of the periodontal tissues.[6,15,18,19] It is classified into three diagnostic groups: gingival abscess, periodontal abscess, and pericoronal abscess. The *gingival abscess* involves the marginal gingival and interdental tissues. The *periodontal abscess* is an infection located contiguous to the periodontal pocket and may result in destruction of the periodontal ligament and alveolar bone. The *pericoronal abscess* is associated with the crown of a partially erupted tooth.[15,18,25]

Periodontal Abscess

Periodontal abscesses are typically found in patients with untreated periodontitis and in association with moderate to deep periodontal pockets.[5,15,18,19,28] Periodontal abscesses often arise as acute exacerbations of preexisting pockets (Fig. 41.1).[6,15,18,19] Primarily related to incomplete calculus removal, periodontal abscesses have been linked to several clinical situations.[8,15-19,27] They have been identified in patients after periodontal surgery,[12]

after preventive maintenance (Fig. 41.2),[7,10,20,24] after systemic antibiotic therapy,[29] and as the result of recurrent disease.[15-17] Conditions in which periodontal abscesses are not related to inflammatory periodontal disease include tooth perforation (endodontic treatment related) or fracture (Fig. 41.3)[1,27] and foreign body impaction.[2,26] Poorly controlled diabetes mellitus has been considered a predisposing factor for periodontal abscess formation (Fig. 41.4).[18,25] Formation of periodontal abscess has been reported as a major cause of tooth loss[12-14,16,17,20-24]; however, with proper treatment followed by consistent preventive periodontal maintenance, teeth with significant bone loss may be retained for many years (see Fig. 41.10).[7]

Gingival Abscess

The gingival abscess is a localized acute inflammatory lesion that may arise from a variety of sources, including microbial plaque infection, trauma, and foreign body impaction.[18,25] Clinical features include a red, smooth, sometimes painful, often fluctuant swelling (Fig. 41.5).[15]

[a]Adapted from the following chapter of Newman and Carranza's Clinical Periodontology, 13th edition: Chapter 45: Treatment of Periodontal Abscess, by Philip R. Melnick and Henry H. Takei.

KEY FACTS

Most periodontal abscesses are due to the incomplete removal of subgingival calculus in a periodontal pocket.

Fig. 41.1 (A) Deep furcation invasions are common locations for the periodontal abscess. (B) Furcation anatomy often prevents the definitive removal of calculus and microbial plaque.

Pericoronal Abscess

The pericoronal abscess results from inflammation of the soft tissue operculum, which covers a partially erupted tooth. This situation is most often observed around the mandibular third molars. As with the gingival abscess, the inflammatory lesion may be caused by the retention of microbial plaque biofilm, food impaction, or trauma.

Acute Versus Chronic Abscess

Abscesses are categorized as acute or chronic. The *acute abscess* is often an exacerbation of a chronic inflammatory periodontal lesion. Influencing factors include increased number and virulence of bacteria combined with lowered tissue resistance and lack of spontaneous drainage.[11,15,28] The drainage may have been prevented by deep, tortuous pocket morphology, debris, or closely adapted pocket epithelium blocking the pocket orifice. Acute abscesses are characterized by painful, red, edematous, smooth, and ovoid swelling of the gingival tissues.[16,17,28] Exudate may be expressed with gentle pressure; the tooth may be percussion sensitive and feel elevated in the socket (Fig. 41.6). Fever and regional lymphadenopathy are occasional findings.[25]

The *chronic abscess* forms after the spreading infection has been controlled by spontaneous drainage, host response, or therapy. Once homeostasis between the host and infection has been reached, the patient may have few or no symptoms.[9]

However, dull pain may be associated with the clinical findings of a periodontal pocket, inflammation, and a fistulous tract.[25]

Box 41.1 compares the signs and symptoms of acute and chronic abscesses.

Periodontal Versus Pulpal Abscess

To determine the cause of an abscess and thus establish a proper treatment plan, it is often necessary to perform a differential diagnosis between periodontal abscess and pulpal abscess (Box 41.2 and Figs. 41.7 and 41.8).[4] Box 41.2 lists the differential diagnosis comparing the signs and symptoms of the two lesions. The correct diagnosis for these two lesions may overlap in some cases, but careful examination and patient questioning are important for an accurate diagnosis, because the therapy for these two lesions is completely different.

SPECIFIC TREATMENT APPROACHES

Treatment of the periodontal abscess includes two phases: resolving the acute lesion, then managing the resulting chronic condition (Box 41.3).[15,18,27]

Acute Abscess

The acute abscess is treated to alleviate symptoms, control the spread of infection, and establish drainage.[15,22] Before treatment, the patient's medical history, dental history, and

Fig. 41.2 Postprophylaxis Periodontal Abscess Resulting From Partial Healing of a Periodontal Pocket Over Residual Calculus.

Fig. 41.4 Localized Periodontal Abscess of a Mandibular Right Canine in a Male Adult With Poorly Controlled Type 2 Diabetes Mellitus. For some patients, periodontal abscess formation may be the first sign of the disease.

Fig. 41.3 (A) Fistula is observed in attached gingiva of a maxillary right canine. (B) Elevated flap shows the cause to be a root fracture.

BOX 41.1   Signs and Symptoms of Periodontal Abscess

Acute Abscess
Mild to severe discomfort
Localized red, ovoid swelling
Periodontal pocket
Mobility
Tooth elevation in socket
Tenderness to percussion or biting
Exudation
Elevated temperature[a]
Regional lymphadenopathy[a]

Chronic Abscess
No pain or dull pain
Localized inflammatory lesion
Slight tooth elevation
Intermittent exudation
Fistulous tract often associated with a deep pocket
Usually without systemic involvement

[a]May indicate the need for systemic antibiotics.
Data from Dahlen G: Microbiology and treatment of dental abscesses and periodontal-endodontic lesions, *Periodontol 2000* 28:206–239, 2002; Meng HX: Periodontal abscess, *Ann Periodontol* 4:79–83, 1999; and Sanz M, Herrera D, van Winkelhoff AJ: The periodontal abscess. In Lindhe J, editor: *Clinical periodontology*, Copenhagen, 2000, Munksgaard.

BOX 41.2   Differential Diagnosis of Periodontal and Pulpal Abscess

Periodontal Abscess
Associated with a preexisting periodontal pocket.
Radiographs show periodontal angular bone loss and furcation radiolucency.
Tests show vital pulp.
Swelling usually includes gingival tissue, with an occasional fistula.
Pain is usually dull and localized.
Sensitivity to percussion may or may not be present.

Pulpal Abscess
The offending tooth may have large restoration.
The tooth may have no periodontal pocket or, if present, it probes as a narrow defect.
Tests show nonvital pulp.
Swelling is often localized to the apex, with a fistulous tract.
Pain is often severe and difficult to localize.
Sensitivity to percussion is noted.

Modified from Corbet EF: Diagnosis of acute periodontal lesions, *Periodontol 2000* 34:204–216, 2004.

Fig. 41.5 Plaque-Associated Gingival Abscess of a Mandibular Right Canine.

Fig. 41.6 Patient Presenting With Acute Abscess Complained of Dull Pain and a Sensation of Tooth Elevation in the Socket. Signs of tissue distention and exudation are evident.

Fig. 41.7 (A) Maxillary right first molar with fistula on the attached gingiva. (B) With local anesthesia, periodontal probe is introduced through the fistula and angled toward the root end. (C) Surgical flap elevation demonstrates failed endodontic therapy and tooth fracture as causing the fistula.

Fig. 41.8 (A) Periodontal abscess of maxillary left first molar. (B) Periodontal probe is used to retract the pocket wall gently.

Fig. 41.9 Gentle Digital Pressure May Be Sufficient to Express Purulent Discharge.

BOX 41.3   Treatment Options for Periodontal Abscess

1. Drainage through pocket retraction or incision
2. Scaling and root planing
3. Periodontal surgery
4. Systemic antibiotics
5. Tooth removal

Modified from Sanz M, Herrera D, van Winkelhoff AJ: The periodontal abscess. In Lindhe J, editor: *Clinical periodontology,* Copenhagen, 2000, Munksgaard.

BOX 41.4   Indications for Antibiotic Therapy in Patients With Acute Abscess

1. Cellulitis (nonlocalized, spreading infection)
2. Deep, inaccessible pocket
3. Fever
4. Regional lymphadenopathy
5. Immunocompromised status

BOX 41.5   Antibiotic Options for Periodontal Infections

Antibiotic of Choice
Amoxicillin, 500 mg
- 1.0-g loading dose, then 500 mg three times a day for 3 days
- Reevaluation after 3 days to determine need for continued or adjusted antibiotic therapy

Penicillin Allergy
Clindamycin
- 600-mg loading dose, then 300 mg four times a day for 3 days

Azithromycin (or Clarithromycin)[a]
- 1.0-g loading dose, then 500 mg four times a day for 3 days

[a]To be used with caution in patients with high baseline cardiovascular risk.
Data from American Academy of Periodontology: Position paper: systemic antibiotics in periodontics. *J Periodontol* 67:1553–1565, 2004.

---

systemic condition are reviewed and evaluated to assist in the diagnosis and determine the need for systemic antibiotics (Boxes 41.4 and 41.5).[3]

Drainage Through the Periodontal Pocket

The peripheral area around the abscess is anesthetized with sufficient anesthetic agents to ensure comfort. The pocket wall is gently retracted with a periodontal probe or curette in an attempt to initiate drainage through the pocket entrance (see Fig. 41.8). Gentle digital pressure and irrigation is used to express the exudate and drain the pocket (Fig. 41.9). If the lesion is minimal and access is uncomplicated, debridement in the form of scaling and root planing may be undertaken at this appointment.

If the lesion is large and drainage cannot be established, root debridement by scaling and root planing or surgical access should be delayed until the major clinical signs have abated.[19,21] In these

patients, use of adjunctive systemic antibiotics[13,14,16,17,19] with a short-term high-dose regimen is recommended (see Box 41.5).[23] Antibiotic therapy alone without subsequent drainage and subgingival scaling is contraindicated.[14]

Drainage Through an External Incision

To drain the abscess, the lesion is dried and isolated with gauze sponges. A topical anesthetic agent is applied, followed by a local anesthetic agent injected peripheral to the lesion. A vertical incision through the most fluctuant center of the abscess is made with a no. 15 surgical blade. The tissue lateral to the incision is separated with a curette or periosteal elevator. The fluctuant matter is expressed, and the wound edges are approximated under light digital pressure with a moist gauze pad.

In abscesses manifesting with severe swelling and inflammation, aggressive mechanical instrumentation should be delayed in favor of antibiotic therapy to avoid damage to healthy contiguous periodontal tissues.[27]

Once bleeding and suppuration have ceased, the patient may be dismissed. For patients who do not need systemic antibiotics, post-treatment instructions include frequent rinsing with warm salt water (1 tbsp/8-oz glass) and periodic application of chlorhexidine gluconate 0.12% oral rinse either by rinsing or applied locally with a cotton-tipped applicator. Reduced physical exertion and increased fluid intake are often recommended for patients showing systemic involvement. Analgesics may be prescribed for comfort. By the following day, the signs and symptoms have usually subsided. If the problem continues and the patient is still uncomfortable, the previously recommended regimen is repeated for an additional 24 hours. This often results in satisfactory healing, and the lesion is then treated as a chronic abscess.[28]

Chronic Abscess

As with a periodontal pocket, the chronic abscess is usually treated with scaling and root planing and, if indicated, surgical therapy.

Surgical treatment is suggested when deep vertical pocket or furcation defects are encountered that are beyond the therapeutic capabilities of nonsurgical instrumentation (Fig. 41.10). Access to subgingival calculus must be achieved in areas of deep pockets. The patient should be advised of the possible postoperative sequelae usually associated with periodontal nonsurgical and surgical procedures. As with the acute abscess, antibiotic therapy may be indicated.[15,19,28]

Gingival Abscess

Treatment of the gingival abscess is aimed at reversal of the acute phase and, when applicable, immediate removal of the cause. To ensure comfort, topical or local anesthesia by infiltration is

---

KEY FACTS

Periodontal abscess due to a deep periodontal pocket often requires a surgical flap to access the subgingival calculus. This also allows the dentist to reduce the pocket at the same surgical appointment.

Fig. 41.10 (A) Chronic periodontal abscess of a maxillary right canine. (B) With local anesthesia, periodontal probe is inserted to determine severity of the lesion. (C) With mesial and distal vertical incisions, a full-thickness flap is elevated, exposing severe bone dehiscence, a subgingival restoration, and root calculus. (D) Root surface has been planed free of calculus, and the restoration has been smoothed. (E) Full-thickness flap has been replaced to its original position and sutured with absorbable sutures. (F) At 3 months, gingival tissues are pink, firm, and well adapted to the tooth, with minimal periodontal probing depth.

administered. When possible, scaling and root planing are completed to establish drainage and remove microbial deposits. In more acute situations, the fluctuant area is incised with a no. 15 scalpel blade, and exudate may be expressed by gentle digital pressure. Any foreign material (e.g., dental floss, impression material) is removed. The area is irrigated with warm water and covered with moist gauze under light pressure.

Once bleeding has stopped, the patient is dismissed with instructions to rinse with warm salt water every 2 hours for the remainder of the day. After 24 hours, the area is reassessed, and if resolution is sufficient, scaling not previously completed is undertaken. If the residual lesion is large or poorly accessible, surgical access may be required.

Pericoronal Abscess

As with other abscesses of the periodontium, treatment of the pericoronal abscess is aimed at management of the acute phase, followed by resolution of the chronic condition. The acute pericoronal abscess is properly anesthetized for comfort, and drainage is established by gently lifting the soft tissue operculum with a curette. If the underlying debris is easily accessible, it may be removed, followed by gentle irrigation with sterile saline. If the patient has regional swelling, lymphadenopathy, or systemic signs, systemic antibiotics may be prescribed.

The patient is dismissed with instructions to rinse with warm salt water every 2 hours, and the area is reassessed after 24 hours. If discomfort was one of the original complaints, appropriate analgesics should be used. Once the acute phase has been controlled, the partially erupted tooth may be definitively treated with either surgical excision of the overlying tissue or removal of the offending tooth.

A Case Scenario is found on the companion website.

REFERENCES

 References for this chapter are found on the companion website.

Phase I Periodontal Therapy[a]

Phase I therapy or cause-related therapy[10] is the first in the chronologic sequence of procedures that constitute periodontal treatment. The objective of phase I therapy is to alter or eliminate the microbial etiology and factors that contribute to gingival and periodontal diseases to the greatest extent possible, thereby halting the progression of disease and returning the dentition to a state of health and comfort.[5] Phase I therapy is referred to by a number of names, including *initial therapy*,[5,10] *nonsurgical periodontal therapy*,[18] and *cause-related therapy*.[10] All terms refer to the procedures performed to treat gingival and periodontal infections up to and including tissue reevaluation, which is the point at which the course of ongoing care is determined.

RATIONALE

Phase I therapy is defined by the evidence-based American Association of Periodontology practice guidelines[5] as the initiation of a comprehensive daily plaque or biofilm control regimen, management of periodontal-systemic interrelationships as needed, and thorough removal of supragingival and subgingival bacterial plaque or biofilm and calculus. Other areas of management include the use of chemotherapeutic agents as necessary and correction of local contributing factors[1-4,6] such as defective restorations and treatment of carious lesions.[7,9,15,16,20] These procedures are a required part of periodontal therapy, regardless of the extent of disease present. In many cases, only phase I therapy is required to restore periodontal health, or it constitutes the preparatory phase for surgical therapy. Figs. 42.1 and 42.2 show

the results of phase I therapy in two patients with chronic periodontitis. Cause-related phase I periodontal therapy has been succinctly stated as the approach *aimed at removal of pathogenic biofilms, toxins, and calculus and the reestablishment of a biologically acceptable root surface.*[10]

Phase I therapy is a critical aspect of periodontal treatment. Data from clinical research indicate that the long-term success of periodontal surgical treatment is dependent on maintaining the plaque or biofilm control results achieved with phase I therapy. In fact, patients who do not have adequate plaque or biofilm control will continue to lose attachment regardless of what surgical procedures are performed.[12] In addition, phase I therapy provides an opportunity for the dental hygienist to evaluate tissue response and provide reinforcement about home care, both of which are crucial to the overall success of treatment.

Based on the knowledge that microbial plaque or biofilm is the major etiologic agent in gingival inflammation, one specific aim of phase I therapy for every patient is *effective daily plaque or biofilm removal* at home. These home care procedures can be complex and time-consuming, and often require changing long-standing habits. Good oral hygiene is easier to accomplish if the tooth surfaces are free of calculus deposits and other irregularities so that they are easily accessible. Management of all contributing local factors is required in phase I therapy. The following list of elements makes up phase I therapy:

1. Patient education and oral hygiene instruction
2. Complete removal of supragingival calculus (see Chapters 45 and 46)
3. Correction or replacement of poorly fitting restorations and other prosthetic devices (see Chapter 52)
4. Restoration or temporization of carious lesions
5. Orthodontic tooth movement (see Chapter 48)
6. Treatment of food impaction areas

[a]Adapted from the following chapter of Newman and Carranza's Clinical Periodontology, 13th edition: Chapter 47: Phase I Periodontal Therapy, by Henry H. Takei.

Fig. 42.1 Results of Phase I Therapy, Severe Chronic Periodontitis. (A) A 45-year-old patient with deep probe depths, bone loss, severe swelling, and redness of the gingival tissues. (B) Results 3 weeks after the completion of phase I therapy. Note that the gingival tissue has returned to a normal contour, with redness and swelling dramatically reduced.

Fig. 42.2 Results of Phase I Therapy, Moderate Chronic Periodontitis. (A) A 52-year-old patient with moderate attachment loss and probe depths in the 4- to 6-mm range. Note that the gingiva appears pink because it is fibrotic. Inflammation is present in the periodontal pockets but disguised by the fibrotic tissue. Bleeding occurs on probing. (B) Lingual view of the patient with more visible inflammation and heavy calculus deposits. (C) and (D) At 18 months after phase I therapy the same areas show significant improvement in gingival health. The patient returned for regular maintenance visits at 4-month intervals.

7. Treatment of occlusal trauma (see Chapter 48)
8. Extraction of hopeless teeth
9. Possible use of antimicrobial agents, including necessary plaque or biofilm sampling and sensitivity testing (see Chapters 9 and 47)

TREATMENT SESSIONS

After careful analysis and diagnosis of the specific periodontal condition present, the dental hygienist must develop a treatment plan that includes all required procedures to treat the periodontal involvement and an estimate of the number of appointments necessary to complete phase I therapy. In most cases, patients require several treatment sessions for complete debridement of the tooth surfaces. All the following conditions are considered when determining the phase I treatment plan[18]:

- General health and tolerance of treatment
- Number of teeth present
- Amount of subgingival calculus
- Probing pocket depths
- Attachment loss
- Furcation involvement
- Alignment of teeth
- Margins of restorations

- Developmental anomalies
- Physical barriers to access the dentition (i.e., limited opening or tendency to gag)
- Patient cooperation and sensitivity to therapy (requiring use of anesthesia or analgesia)

SEQUENCE OF PROCEDURES

Step 1: Plaque or Biofilm Control Instruction

Plaque or biofilm control is an essential component of successful periodontal therapy. Home care instruction should begin at the first treatment appointment and be included in every appointment going forward. Before oral hygiene instruction, the patient must understand the reason that he or she must actively participate in therapy. The explanation of the etiology of the disease must be presented to the patient. Once the patient understands the nature of periodontal disease and the etiology, it will be easier to teach the oral hygiene they must practice. The patient is instructed on the correct technique to remove the plaque or biofilm; this means focusing on applying the bristles at the gingival third of the clinical crowns, where the tooth meets the gingival margin. This technique is sometimes referred to as *targeted oral hygiene* and is synonymous with the Bass technique. Instructions for interdental cleaning with dental floss and interdental brushes is included.[23] The use of the multiple appointment approach to phase I therapy is favored by many dental hygienists because it permits the use of numerous appointments to evaluate, reinforce, and improve the patient's oral hygiene skills. (Chapter 43 details plaque and biofilm control options.)

Step 2: Removal of Supragingival and Subgingival Plaque or Biofilm and Calculus

Calculus is removed using sickles, curettes, ultrasonic instrumentation, or combinations of these devices during one or more appointments. Evidence suggests that the treatment results for chronic periodontitis are similar for all hand and mechanical instruments.[12,13] Most dental hygienists advocate the combination of hand instruments (sickles, curettes) and ultrasonic devices. In the past, it was thought the removal of all cementum was necessary to attain a smooth, glassy, hard surface. The rationale was that cementum became necrotic from penetration of endotoxins from the microbial biofilm and would interfere with healing. Current studies have indicated that endotoxins do not penetrate into the cementum as deeply as once believed and complete removal of the cementum is not necessary, but removal of the plaque or biofilm and calculus is absolutely necessary. In a clinical situation, it is difficult to know whether the removal of some or all of the cementum is achieved.

Laser treatment has also been advocated for periodontal therapy by some clinicians.[8] However, some reviews suggest that further well-designed studies are needed to confirm the outcomes. In addition, gingival curettage, the systematic removal of the soft tissue lining of the pockets, has not been shown to improve the results of treatment. Thorough plaque or biofilm removal and excellent root therapy result in conversion of the soft, edematous, inflamed gingival tissue to a healthier state without removing

this tissue by using intentional soft tissue curettage. Therefore curettage of the soft tissue pocket wall in phase I therapy is no longer advocated.

Photodynamic therapy has also been presented as an adjunct to scaling and root planing. This therapy uses lasers at specific wavelengths to "target microorganisms treated with a photosensitizer." Studies have not found this intervention to be useful as an alternative to scaling and root planing to improve treatment outcomes. Further research is necessary to ascertain the efficacy of this treatment.[12]

Another interesting approach to calculus removal and debridement is full-mouth disinfection. In this technique, full-mouth treatment is performed during one session or multiple sessions within a few days. Disinfectants are used after therapy, with the intention of preventing reinfection of treated sites from untreated sites.[14,17,19,22] This treatment approach is used during phase I therapy by some clinicians, but the results have not been shown to be superior to those of any other phase I therapy.[11,12,21]

Multiple approaches are used to plan and perform nonsurgical phase I therapy. Decisions on how to proceed should be discussed and agreed on by the patient and the dentist/dental hygienist based on the amount of disease present and the patient's tolerance to the therapy.[11] Staged therapy has the advantage of evaluating and reinforcing the oral hygiene status of the patient, but the one- or two-appointment approach can be more efficient in reducing the number of office visits the patient is required to attend.

Step 3: Recontouring Defective Restorations and Crowns

Corrections of restorative defects, which are plaque- or biofilm-retentive areas, are accomplished by smoothing the rough surfaces and removing overhangs from the faulty restorations with burs or hand instruments, or complete replacement of the failing restorations may be necessary. All these steps are important to remove the risk factors that perpetuate the inflammatory process. These procedures can be completed concurrently with other phase I procedures.

Step 4: Management of Carious Lesions

Removal of the carious lesions and placement of either temporary or permanent restorations are indicated in phase I therapy because of the infectious nature of the carious process. Healing of the periodontal tissues is maximized by removing the reservoir of bacteria in these lesions so that they cannot repopulate the microbial plaque.

Step 5: Tissue Reevaluation

After scaling, root planing, and other phase I procedures, the periodontal tissues require approximately 4 weeks to heal. This time allows the connective tissues to heal, and allows for more accurate measurement of probing depths. Patients will also have the opportunity to improve their home care skills to reduce gingival inflammation and adopt new habits that will ensure the success of treatment. At the reevaluation appointment, periodontal pockets are probed, and all related anatomic conditions are carefully evaluated to determine whether further treatment, including periodontal surgery, is indicated. Additional improvement from periodontal surgical procedures can be expected only if phase I therapy results in gingival tissues that are free of significant inflammation and the patient has adopted effective daily plaque or biofilm control procedures.

RESULTS

Scaling and root planing therapy have been studied extensively to evaluate their effects on periodontal disease. Studies have indicated that this treatment is both effective and reliable. Studies ranging from 1 month to 2 years in length demonstrated up to 80% reduction in bleeding on probing and mean probing depth reductions of 2 to 3 mm. Other studies demonstrated that the percentage of periodontal pockets of 4 mm or deeper was reduced by more than 50% and in many cases up to 80%.[9] Figs. 42.1 and 42.2 show examples of the effectiveness of phase I therapy.

Deeper probing depths present the dental hygienist with greatly increased instrumentation challenges due to the complexity of root anatomy and difficulty accessing the root surfaces. Badersten and colleagues[7] reported in the 1980s that residual calculus remained on 44% of the surfaces in deeper pockets. Other studies have confirmed these findings, including studies comparing the use of hand instruments with that of powered scaling instruments.[12]

Additional individual treatments, such as caries control and correction of poorly fitting restorations, clearly help the healing gained by good plaque or biofilm control and debridement by making tooth surfaces accessible to hygiene procedures. Fig. 42.3 demonstrates the effects of an overhanging amalgam restoration

on gingival inflammation in an otherwise healthy periodontium. Maximal healing from phase I treatment is not possible when local conditions retain biofilm and provide reservoirs for repopulation of periodontal pathogens.

HEALING

Healing of the gingival epithelium consists of the formation of a long junctional epithelium rather than new connective tissue attachment to the root surfaces. This long junctional epithelium occurs about 1 week after therapy. Gradual reductions in inflammatory cell population, crevicular fluid flow, and repair of connective tissue result in decreased clinical signs of inflammation, including less redness and swelling. One or two millimeters of recession is apparent at times after treatment as the result of tissue shrinkage.[9] Connective tissue fibers are disrupted and lysed by the disease process and also by the inflammatory reaction to treatment. These tissues require 4 or more weeks to reorganize and heal, and many cases may require several weeks for complete healing.

Transient root sensitivity frequently accompanies the healing process. Although evidence suggests that relatively few teeth become highly sensitive, this problem can be disconcerting to patients. The extent of the sensitivity is diminished with good plaque or biofilm removal, but this may take several weeks to months.[24] Patients should also be warned and educated before the therapy is undertaken regarding the potential outcomes of several changes, such as the teeth appearing longer due to shrinkage of the periodontal tissues and root sensitivity. Knowledge of these

Fig. 42.3 Effects of Overhanging Amalgam Margin on Interproximal Gingiva of Maxillary First Molar in Otherwise Healthy Mouth. (A) Clinical appearance of rough, irregular, and overcontoured amalgam. (B) Gentle probing of interproximal pocket. (C) Extensive bleeding elicited by gentle probing indicating severe inflammation in the area.

changes before therapy will prevent the possibility of patients being overly concerned should they occur. Unexpected and possible uncomfortable consequences of treatment may result in the patient's distrust and loss of motivation to continue therapy.

DECISION TO REFER FOR SPECIALIST TREATMENT

It is fortunate that many periodontally involved cases do not require any further therapy beyond phase I therapy. Therefore, these patients only require routine maintenance therapy and periodic exams at regular recall intervals. However, advanced or complicated cases benefit from specialist care. Heitz-Mayfield and Lang[12] demonstrated that surgical treatment in deep pockets, those greater than 6 mm, resulted in 0.6 mm more probing depth reduction and 0.2 mm more clinical attachment gain than did deep pockets treated with scaling and root planing alone. This study also confirmed that in pockets of 4- to 6-mm probing depth, scaling and root planing resulted in 0.4 mm more attachment gain than surgical procedures, and shallow pockets of 1 to 3 mm had 0.5 mm less attachment loss compared with surgical results.[12] It is critical to be skilled in determining which patients would benefit from specialist care and deciding when a patient should be referred.

The concept of the *critical probing depth* of 5.4 mm is used to assist in making the determination to proceed to surgical intervention. This is the measurement above which therapy will result in clinical attachment gain and below which it will result in clinical attachment loss. This determination was made based on statistical analysis of surgical outcomes data.[12] A similar *5-mm standard* has been commonly used as a guideline for identifying candidates for surgical referral based on the understanding that the typical root length is about 13 mm and the crest of the alveolar bone is at a level approximately 2 mm apical to the bottom of the pocket. When there is 5 mm of clinical attachment loss, the crest of bone is about 7 mm apical to the cementoenamel junction, and therefore, only about half of the bony support for the tooth remains. Periodontal surgery can help improve support for teeth in these cases through pocket reduction and/or regeneration procedures. Fig. 42.4 depicts the relationship of clinical attachment loss to tooth support.

In addition to the 5-mm clinical attachment loss criterion, other factors are considered in the decision to refer to a periodontal specialist:

1. *Extent of the disease and generalized or localized periodontal involvement.* The amount of bone loss, even in localized areas, suggests the need for specialized surgical techniques.
2. *Root length.* Short-rooted teeth are jeopardized to a greater extent by the 5-mm clinical attachment loss criterion than teeth with long roots.
3. *Mobility.* Excessive tooth mobility suggests that contributing factors may be responsible for the mobility. The extent of mobility could mean that the prognosis for the tooth is guarded to poor.
4. *Difficulty of scaling and root planing.* The presence of deep pockets and furcations makes instrumentation difficult, but the results can often be improved with surgical access.

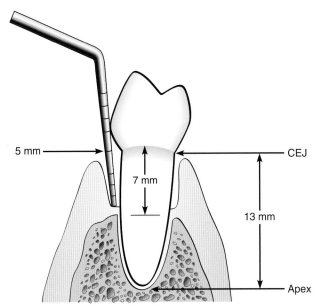

Fig. 42.4 The 5-mm Standard for Referral to a Periodontist Is Based on Root Length, Probing Depth, and Clinical Attachment Loss. The standard serves as a reasonable guideline to analyze the case for referral for specialist care. *CEJ,* Cementoenamel junction. (Redrawn with permission from Armitage G, editor: *Periodontal maintenance therapy,* Berkeley, CA, 1974, Praxis.)

5. *Restorability and importance of particular teeth for reconstruction.* Long-term prognosis of each tooth is important when considering extensive restorative work.
6. *Age of the patient.* Younger patients with extensive attachment loss are more likely to have aggressive forms of disease that require advanced therapy.
7. *Lack of resolution of inflammation after thorough plaque or biofilm removal and excellent scaling and root planing.* If inflammation and progressive deepening of the pocket continue, further therapy will be necessary. Such cases require an understanding of the etiology to determine the best course of treatment.

Every patient is unique, and the decision process for each patient is complex and difficult. The considerations presented in this chapter should provide guidance for understanding the significance of phase I therapy and making referral decisions.

CONCLUSION

The major goal of phase I therapy is to control the factors responsible for periodontal inflammation; this involves educating the patient in the removal of bacterial plaque or biofilm. Phase I therapy also includes scaling, root planing, and other therapies such as caries control, replacement of defective restorations, occlusal therapy, orthodontic tooth movement, and cessation of confounding habits such as tobacco use. Comprehensive reevaluation after phase I therapy is essential to determine treatment options and establish a prognosis. Many patients can attain periodontal disease control with phase I therapy alone and do not require further surgical intervention. For patients who require surgical intervention, phase I therapy is an advantageous element of treatment in that it permits tissue healing, thus improving the surgical management and healing response of the tissues.

Periodontal surgical intervention should be considered for patients with deep pocket depths and those with 5 mm or more of attachment loss after phase I therapy. Periodontal specialists can best provide treatment to preserve the teeth for patients with advanced disease. Moreover, patients who do not demonstrate the ability to control plaque or biofilm on a daily basis effectively are poor candidates for surgery and should be closely monitored on a recall maintenance program unless conditions change.

REFERENCES

 References for this chapter are found on the companion website.

43

Plaque Biofilm Control for the Periodontal Patient[a]

 For online-only content on oral irrigation, caries control, and chemical plaque biofilm control with oral rinses, please visit the companion website.

CHAPTER OUTLINE

Biofilm control, also referred to as periodontal self-care,[32] is an effective way of treating and preventing gingivitis and is an essential part of all procedures involved in the treatment and prevention of periodontal diseases.[50] It is a critical element in the long-term success of all periodontal and dental treatment.[3] In 1965, Löe and colleagues[88] conducted the classic study demonstrating the relationship between microbial plaque biofilm accumulation and the development of experimental gingivitis in humans. Subjects in the study stopped brushing and other plaque biofilm control procedures, thus resulting in the development of gingivitis in every person within 7 to 21 days. The composition of the biofilm bacteria also shifted so that more virulent gram-negative organisms predominated, and these changes were shown to be reversible within 7 days. Good supragingival biofilm control has also been shown to affect the growth and composition of subgingival plaque biofilm so that it favors a healthier microflora and reduces calculus formation.[119] Carefully performed daily home plaque biofilm control, combined with frequent professionally delivered plaque biofilm and calculus removal, reduces the amount of supragingival biofilm, decreases the total number of microorganisms in moderately deep pockets, including furcation areas, and greatly reduces the quantity of periodontal pathogens.[29,60] Reviews of home care procedures in 2011 and 2013 confirmed the positive effects of daily plaque biofilm removal but cautioned that these gains appear to be small, and best results also require professional maintenance care.[32,106]

Microbial biofilm growth occurs within hours, and it must be completely removed at least once every 48 hours in the experimental setting with periodontally healthy subjects to prevent inflammation.[118] The American Dental Association (ADA) recommends that individuals should brush twice per day and use floss or other interdental cleaners once per day to effectively remove microbial plaque biofilms and prevent gingivitis.[3] The ADA recommends twice-daily brushing because most individuals do not adequately remove microbial biofilms at one brushing, and doing it a second time improves the results.

Periodontal lesions are predominantly found in interdental locations, so toothbrushing alone is not sufficient to control gingival and periodontal diseases.[74] It has been demonstrated in healthy subjects that plaque biofilm formation begins on the interproximal surfaces, where the toothbrush does not reach. Masses of biofilm first develop in the molar and premolar areas, followed by the proximal surfaces of the anterior teeth and the facial surfaces of the molars and premolars. Lingual surfaces accumulate the least amount of biofilm. Patients consistently leave more plaque biofilm on the posterior teeth than the anterior teeth, with interproximal surfaces retaining the highest amounts of biofilm. It is in these interproximal areas where periodontal infections and carious lesions begin.[118] In addition, periodontal patients tend to have increased susceptibility to disease[121] due to complex defects in gingival architecture and long exposed root surfaces to clean, which compounds the difficulty of practicing thorough hygiene.

[a]Adapted from the following chapter of Newman and Carranza's Clinical Periodontology, 13th edition: Chapter 48: Plaque Biofilm Control for the Periodontal Patient, by Dorothy A. Perry, Henry H. Takei, and Jonathan H. Do.

CLINICAL CORRELATION

Daily biofilm control practices result in improved periodontal and gingival health. Cessation of plaque control practices for 7–21 days results in:
- Accumulation of thick plaque on tooth surfaces
- Reddened gingiva that bleeds easily
- Shift to more virulent gram-negative flora
- Changes that are completely reversed in about 7 days when plaque control practices are resumed

Chemical inhibitors of plaque biofilm and calculus that are incorporated in mouthwashes or dentifrices also play a role in controlling microbial biofilms.[32] Fluoride delivered through toothpastes and mouthrinses are essential for caries control.[38] Many products are available as adjunctive agents to mechanical techniques. These medicaments, as with any drug, should be recommended and prescribed according to individual patient needs based on risk assessment. The interest in supplementing oral hygiene procedures with natural products has increased in our society. However, the evidence base supporting the use of these products is currently lacking valid studies to determine their efficacy.[22]

Daily biofilm control permits patients to assume responsibility for their own oral health every day. Without it, optimal oral health through periodontal treatment cannot be attained or preserved. Elements of biofilm control include mechanical cleaning and chemical adjuncts.

THE TOOTHBRUSH

Toothbrushes vary in size and design, as well as in length, hardness, and arrangement of the bristles (Fig. 43.1).[114] Some toothbrush manufacturers claim superiority of design for such factors as minor modifications of bristle placement, length, and stiffness. However, research does not indicate significant differences in gingivitis scores or bleeding indices, which are important measures of improved gingival health. In fact, at least one study compared four commercially available toothbrushes for total

Fig. 43.1 Manual Toothbrushes. (A) Toothbrushes from the 19th and 20th centuries, one with an ivory handle from about 1890 *(left)*, one with a composition handle from the 1950s *(center)*, and one with a sterling silver handle from the early 20th century *(right)*. The ivory-handled brush belonged to a dental student who used the handle to practice cutting preparations and filling the "preps" with amalgam or gold foil. (B) Various types of toothbrushes are available; note the variations in brush head and handle design. (C) Brush heads, showing various bristle configurations. (Antique brushes courtesy Dean John D.B. Featherstone, University of California, San Francisco School of Dentistry Historical Collection, San Francisco.)

plaque biofilm removal at a single brushing. All four toothbrushes removed biofilm equally, and the investigators concluded that no one design was superior to the others.[25] In addition, systematic review of multiple studies did not identify a superior design.[32]

FLASH BACK

Early toothbrushes were mostly made of hog bristles and were very stiff and hard. Hard-bristled toothbrushes are shown to abrade tooth surfaces and scratch the gingiva. Few remain on the market, but in general, hard-bristled toothbrushes should be avoided.

When recommending a particular toothbrush, ease of use by the patient and the perception that the brush is effective are the important considerations. The effectiveness and potential injury from different types of brushes depend to a great degree on how the brushes are used. Data from in vitro studies of abrasion by different manual toothbrushes suggest that brush designs that permit the bristles to carry a greater amount of toothpaste while brushing contribute to abrasion more than the bristles themselves.[33] It has been shown that several factors contribute to the problem of abrasion: (1) the use of hard toothbrushes, (2) vigorous horizontal brushing, and (3) the use of extremely abrasive dentifrices; all these factors may contribute to and lead to cervical abrasions of teeth and recession of the gingiva.[73]

Toothbrush Design

Toothbrush bristles are grouped in tufts usually arranged in three or four rows. Rounded bristle ends cause fewer scratches on the gingiva than flat-cut bristles with sharp ends (see Fig. 43.1).[28,114] Two types of bristle material are used in toothbrushes: natural bristles from hogs and artificial filaments made of nylon. Both remove microbial plaque biofilm, but nylon bristle brushes predominate in the market. Bristle hardness is proportional to the square of the diameter and inversely proportional to the square of the bristle length.[56] Diameters of common bristles range from 0.007 inch (0.2 mm) for soft brushes to 0.012 inch (0.3 mm) for medium brushes and 0.014 inch (0.4 mm) for hard brushes.[62] Soft-bristle brushes of the type described by Bass[11] have gained wide acceptance (Fig. 43.2). Handle design characteristics are entirely a matter of personal preference.

Softer bristles are more flexible, clean slightly below the gingival margin when used with a sulcular brushing technique,[12] and reach farther apically to the proximal surfaces (see Fig. 43.2).[45] As indicated earlier, the use of hard-bristled toothbrushes is associated with greater gingival recession.[73] However, the manner in which a brush is used and the abrasiveness of the dentifrice affect abrasion to a greater degree than the bristle hardness itself.[92] Bristle hardness does not significantly affect wear on enamel surfaces.[107]

The amount of force used to brush is not critical for effective plaque biofilm removal.[123] Vigorous brushing is not necessary and can lead to gingival recession, wedge-shaped defects in the cervical area of root surfaces,[108] and painful ulceration of the gingiva.[100]

Toothbrushes must also be replaced periodically, although the amount of visible bristle wear does not appear to affect plaque biofilm removal for up to 9 weeks.[27] Most clinicians recommend that toothbrushes be replaced every 3 to 4 months.

Fig. 43.2 (A) Toothbrushes of different bristle design and configuration. (B) The brush on the *far left* in (A) is the most appropriate of the four brushes displayed for biofilm removal.

KEY FACTS

When recommending toothbrushes, keep these general recommendations in mind:
- Soft nylon bristle toothbrushes clean effectively when used properly and tend not to traumatize the gingiva or root surfaces.
- Toothbrushes become worn due to wear and should be replaced every 3–4 months.
- If patients perceive a benefit from a particular design of toothbrush, they should use it as long as it is not too stiff and hard.

POWERED TOOTHBRUSHES

Electrically powered toothbrushes designed to mimic back-and-forth brushing techniques were invented in 1939. Subsequent models featured circular or elliptical motions, and some had combinations of motions. Currently, powered toothbrushes have oscillating and rotating motions (Fig. 43.3), and some brushes use low-frequency acoustic energy to enhance cleaning ability. Powered toothbrushes rely primarily on mechanical contact between the bristles and the teeth to remove plaque biofilm. The addition of low-frequency acoustic energy generates dynamic fluid movement and provides cleaning slightly away from the bristle tips.[43] The vibrations have also been shown to interfere with bacterial adherence to oral surfaces. Neither the sonic

Fig. 43.3 Powered Toothbrush Designs Offer Options in Head Shape and Size.

Fig. 43.4 Vigorous Toothbrushing With an Abrasive Dentifrice Can Result in Trauma to the Gingiva and Wearing Away of the Tooth Surfaces, Especially Root Surfaces, and Can Contribute to Gingival Recession.

vibration nor the mechanical motion of powered toothbrushes has been shown to affect bacterial cell viability.[90] Hydrodynamic shear forces created by these brushes disrupt biofilm a short distance from the bristle tips, thus explaining the additional interproximal biofilm removal.[66]

Typically, comparison studies of powered toothbrushes, manual toothbrushes, and other powered devices demonstrate slightly improved plaque biofilm removal for the device of interest in short-term clinical trials.[94,105] Patients' acceptance of powered toothbrushes is favorable. One study reported that 88.9% of patients introduced to a powered toothbrush would continue to use it.[125] However, patients have been reported to discontinue the use of the powered toothbrushes after 5 or 6 months, presumably when the novelty has worn off. Powered toothbrushes are shown to improve oral health for the following: (1) children and adolescents; (2) people with physical or mental disabilities; (3) hospitalized patients, including older adults who require the assistance of caregivers for hygiene; and (4) patients with fixed orthodontic appliances. Powered brushes are not shown to provide benefits routinely for patients with rheumatoid arthritis, children who are motivated, or patients with chronic periodontitis.[59]

KEY FACTS

When recommending powered toothbrushes, keep in mind that:
- Powered toothbrushes with oscillating and rotating motions remove plaque biofilm and reduce gingival bleeding slightly better than manual toothbrushes.
- Patients who want to use powered toothbrushes should be encouraged to do so.
- Patients need to be instructed in the proper use of powered devices.
- Patients who lack dexterity, children, and caregivers may particularly benefit from using powered toothbrushes.

DENTIFRICES

Dentifrices aid in cleaning and polishing tooth surfaces. They are mostly in the form of pastes, although powders and gels are also available. The contents of dentifrices are abrasives (e.g., silicon oxides, aluminum oxides, and granular polyvinyl chlorides), water, humectants, soap or detergent, flavoring and sweetening agents, therapeutic agents (e.g., fluoride, pyrophosphates, coloring agents, and preservatives).[57,117] Abrasives are insoluble inorganic salts that enhance the abrasive action of toothbrushing as much as 40 times and make up 20% to 40% of most dentifrices.[92] Tooth powders are much more abrasive than pastes and contain about 95% abrasive materials. The abrasive quality of dentifrices affects enamel slightly and is a much greater concern for patients with exposed root surfaces. Dentin is abraded 25 times faster and cementum is abraded at 35 times the rate of enamel. Therefore, root surfaces with exposed dentin and cementum are easily abraded, leading to notching and tooth sensitivity.[117] It can be concluded that oral hygiene procedures that use abrasive toothpaste are the main cause of hard tissue damage, and it is possible that gingival lesions can also be produced (Fig. 43.4).[100,107] Dentifrices are very useful for delivering therapeutic agents to the teeth and gingiva. The successful caries-preventive effect of *fluoride* incorporated in dentifrices has been proven without question.[116] Fluoride ion must be available in the amount of 1000 to 1100 parts per million (ppm) to achieve caries-reduction effects. Toothpaste products tested by the ADA that have fluoride ion available in the appropriate amount carry the ADA seal of approval to provide for caries control.[5]

"Calculus control" toothpastes, also referred to as "tartar control" toothpastes, contain *pyrophosphates* and have been shown to reduce the deposition of new calculus on teeth as it forms. These ingredients interfere with crystal formation in calculus but do not affect the fluoride ion in the paste or increase tooth sensitivity. Dentifrice with pyrophosphates has been shown to reduce the formation of new supragingival calculus by 30% or more.[69,91,129] Pyrophosphate-containing toothpastes do not affect subgingival calculus formation or gingival inflammation. The inhibitory effect reduces the deposition of new supragingival calculus but does not affect existing calculus deposits. To achieve the greatest effect from calculus control toothpaste, the teeth must be cleaned and completely free of supragingival calculus when adding these products to the daily home care regimen.

KEY FACTS

Considering dentifrices, keep in mind that:
- Dentifrices increase the effectiveness of brushing.
- Products containing fluoride and antimicrobial agents provide additional benefits for controlling caries and gingivitis.
- Patients who form significant amounts of supragingival calculus benefit from the use of a calculus control dentifrice, but remember that calculus formation is directly related to plaque biofilm accumulation.

TOOTHBRUSHING METHODS

Many methods for brushing the teeth have been described and promoted as being efficient and effective. These methods can be categorized primarily according to the pattern of motion when brushing and are primarily of historic interest, as follows[67]:

Roll: Roll[2] or modified Stillman technique[63]
Vibratory: Stillman,[115] Charters,[21] and Bass[12] techniques
Circular: Fones technique[42]
Vertical: Leonard technique[81]
Horizontal: Scrub technique[102]

Patients with periodontal disease are most frequently taught a sulcular brushing technique using a vibratory motion to improve access to the gingival margin areas. It is important for patients to understand that plaque biofilm removal at the dentogingival junction is necessary to prevent caries as well as periodontal disease. This emphasis to clean the area of the dentogingival junction is referred to as *target hygiene* (Takei H: Personal communication, 2009). The method most often recommended is the *Bass technique* because it emphasizes the placement of the bristles at this most important area. Sulcular placement of the bristles and adapting the bristle tips to the gingival margin to reach the supragingival plaque biofilm and accessing some of the subgingival biofilm may be the most important aspects of target hygiene. A controlled vibrating motion is used to dislodge microbial plaque biofilm and avoid trauma. The brush is systematically placed on all the teeth in both arches. Figs. 43.5 and 43.6 illustrate this brushing technique. Patients must understand why, where, and how to practice meaningful plaque biofilm removal properly at the target area to prevent oral diseases.

Bass Technique

1. Place the head of a soft brush parallel to the occlusal plane, with the brush head covering three to four teeth. This hygiene procedure begins at the most distal tooth in the arch and systematically proceeds mesially.[11]
2. Place the bristles at the gingival margin, pointing at a 45-degree angle to the long axis of the teeth.
3. Exert gentle vibratory pressure using short, back-and-forth motions without dislodging the tips of the bristles. This motion forces the bristle ends into the gingival sulcus area (see Fig. 43.5), as well as partly into the interproximal embrasures. The pressure should be firm enough to blanch the gingiva.

Brushing With Powered Toothbrushes

The various mechanical motions built into powered toothbrushes means they do not require special techniques. The patient should

Fig. 43.5 Bass Method. (A) Place the toothbrush so that the bristles are angled approximately 45 degrees from the tooth surfaces. (B) Start at the most distal tooth in the arch, and use a vibrating back-and-forth motion to brush.

Fig. 43.6 Bass Method. (A) Proper positioning of the brush in the mouth aims the bristle tips toward the gingival margin. (B) Diagram shows the ideal placement, which permits slight subgingival penetration of the bristle tips.

Fig. 43.7 Positioning the Powered Toothbrush Head and Bristle Tips so That They Reach the Gingival Margin Is Critical to Achieving the Most Effective Cleaning Results. (A) Straight-head placement. (B) Round-head placement.

place the brush head next to the teeth at the gingival margin, similar to the position with the manual brush (45° to the gingival margin). This is the target hygiene area, and it proceeds systematically around the arch.[122] As indicated earlier, it is the routine brushing method described for manual brushing, except it is with the powered toothbrush (Fig. 43.7).

KEY FACTS

When recommending toothbrushing techniques, remember what research has taught us:
- Targeted hygiene[119] focuses brushing efforts on the critical cervical and interproximal areas of teeth.
- Brushing with either a manual or powered toothbrush requires a systematic routine to be effective.[94]
- Patients will modify any technique to their needs, so emphasize brushing all the surfaces of the teeth effectively.

INTERDENTAL CLEANING AIDS

Any toothbrush, regardless of the brushing method used, does not completely remove interdental plaque biofilms. This is true

for all patients, even for periodontal patients with wide-open embrasures.[47,110] Daily interdental plaque biofilm removal is crucial to augment the effects of toothbrushing because most dental and periodontal diseases originate in interproximal areas.[1]

Tissue destruction associated with periodontal disease often leaves large, open spaces between teeth and exposed root surfaces with anatomic concavities and furcations. These defects also occur after resective periodontal surgery. The best example of an anatomic root concavity is the mesial root surface of the maxillary first bicuspid. With attachment loss, the concavity located on this mesial surface is exposed where plaque biofilm will accumulate. These areas shelter plaque biofilm and are difficult for patients to clean with the toothbrush alone.[74] In addition, dental floss does not reach these concave surfaces (see Fig. 43.16). Patients should understand that the purpose of interdental cleaning is to remove microbial plaque biofilm, not just food that has wedged between two approximating teeth. Many instruments are available for interproximal cleaning, and they should be recommended based on the size of the interdental spaces, the presence of furcations, root surface concavities, tooth alignment, and the presence of orthodontic appliances or other fixed prostheses. Moreover, ease of use and patient cooperation are important considerations. Common aids for interdental hygiene are dental floss, interdental brushes, rubber tips, and wooden or plastic tips.

Dental Floss

Dental floss is the most widely recommended tool for removing biofilm from proximal tooth surfaces.[46] Floss is made from nylon filaments or plastic monofilaments, and it comes in waxed, unwaxed, thick, thin, and flavored varieties. Clinical research has demonstrated no significant differences in the ability of the various types of floss to remove dental plaque biofilm; they all work equally well.[40,61,71,72] Waxed dental floss was thought to leave a waxy film on proximal surfaces, thus contributing to biofilm accumulation and gingivitis. It has been shown, however, that wax is not deposited on tooth surfaces,[101] and improvement in gingival health is unrelated to the type of floss used.[40] Factors influencing the choice of dental floss include the tightness of tooth contacts, the roughness of proximal surfaces, and the patient's manual dexterity, not the superiority of any one product. Recommendations of floss type should be based on ease of use and personal preference. As indicated previously, the limitations of dental floss must also be explained to the patient, and alternative methods must be demonstrated.

Fig. 43.8 Dental Floss Should Be Held Securely in the Fingers or Tied in a Loop.

Fig. 43.9 Dental Floss Technique. The floss is slipped between the contact areas of the teeth (in this case, teeth #7 and #8) and wrapped around the proximal surface, and removes plaque by using several up-and-down strokes. The process must be repeated for the distal surface of tooth #8.

FLASH BACK

Recommended by Bass in the 1930s, and popularized in the 1960s, unwaxed floss is still recommended as being superior to waxed versions. The rationale was that it does not leave a waxy film that would cause more plaque deposition on the interproximal surfaces of the teeth. No evidence supports this. Given that waxed floss is easier for most people to use, patients should floss with whatever type they like. The important thing is that they adopt the flossing habit!

Technique for the Use of Dental Floss

The floss must contact the proximal surface from line angle to line angle to clean effectively. It must also clean the entire proximal surface, including accessible subgingival areas. Flossing technique requires the following:

1. Start with a piece of floss long enough to grasp securely; 12 to 18 inches is usually sufficient. It may be wrapped around the fingers, or the ends may be tied together in a loop.
2. Stretch the floss tightly between the thumb and forefinger (Fig. 43.8) or between both forefingers, and pass it gently through each contact area with a firm back-and-forth motion. Do not snap the floss past the contact area, because this may injure the interdental gingiva. In fact, zealous snapping of floss through contact areas creates proximal grooves in the gingiva.
3. Once the floss is apical to the contact area between the teeth, wrap the floss around the proximal surface of one tooth and slip it under the marginal gingiva. Move the floss firmly along the tooth up to the contact area and gently down into the sulcus again, repeating this up-and-down stroke two or three times (Fig. 43.9). Then move the floss across the interdental gingiva, and repeat the procedure on the proximal surface of the adjacent tooth.

4. Continue through the whole dentition, including the distal surface of the last tooth in each quadrant. When the working portion of the floss shreds or becomes contaminated, move the floss to a fresh portion.

Flossing can be facilitated by using a *floss holder* (Fig. 43.10A). Floss holders are helpful for patients lacking manual dexterity and for caregivers assisting patients in cleaning their teeth. A floss holder should be rigid enough to keep the floss taut when penetrating tight contact areas, and it should be simple to string the floss onto the holder. The disadvantage of these floss holders is that using them tends to be time-consuming because they must be rethreaded frequently when the floss shreds.

Disposable single-use floss holders with prethreaded floss are also available. Short-term clinical studies suggested that plaque biofilm reduction and improvement in gingivitis scores are similar for patients using disposable floss devices and patients who hold the floss with their fingers (see Fig. 43.10B).[19,115]

Powered flossing devices are also available (Fig. 43.11). These devices have been shown to be safe and effective, but they are no better at plaque biofilm removal than holding the floss with the fingers.[26,51]

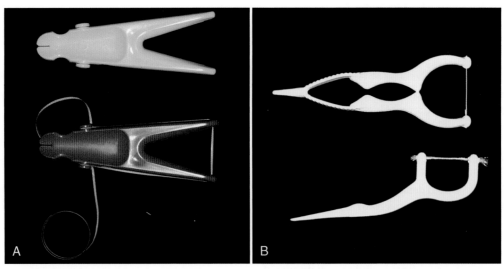

Fig. 43.10 Floss Holders Can Simplify the Manipulation of Dental Floss. (A) Reusable floss tools require stringing the floss around a series of knobs and grooves to secure it. (B) Disposable floss tools have prestrung floss and are easy to use, but the floss may shred and break, requiring several tools to complete flossing the teeth.

Fig. 43.11 Powered Flossing Devices Can Be Easier for Some Patients to Use Than Handheld Floss. The tip is inserted into the proximal space, and a bristle or wand comes out of the tip and moves in a circular motion when the device is turned on *(left)*. Alternately, the device moves the prestrung floss in short motions to provide interproximal cleaning *(right)*.

Establishing a lifelong habit of flossing the teeth is difficult to achieve for both patients and dental professionals, regardless of whether one uses a tool or flosses with fingers. In fact, it is thought that the daily use of dental floss by patients is inconsistent. Investigators reported that only about 8% of young teenagers in Great Britain flossed daily,[89] with similar percentages reported for other countries.[74] It has been suggested that motivational interviewing and instructional techniques are helpful in encouraging this habit.[44] No information is available regarding long-term flossing habits comparing the various instruments used to floss with flossing with one's fingers. However, these instruments may be useful to help individuals begin flossing or to make flossing possible for patients who have limited dexterity.

KEY FACTS

The benefits to gingival health of interproximal cleaning are undisputed.
- Dental floss is a simple and readily available tool to clean where the toothbrush cannot reach. The thorough removal of plaque biofilm from the interdental tooth surfaces is the most important hygiene step in the treatment of periodontal disease.
- Flossing tools work as well as flossing using one's fingers.
- The flossing habit is difficult to establish and requires positive reinforcement during dental visits.

Interdental Brushes

Probably the most effective plaque biofilm removal method for interdental areas, where the papilla does not completely fill the space, is the use of interdental brushes. As indicated earlier, the concave root surfaces, such as the mesial aspect of the maxillary first bicuspid and furcation areas, are usually not cleaned efficiently with dental floss. A comparison study of dental floss and interdental brushes used by patients with moderate to severe periodontal disease indicated that the interproximal brushes removed a greater amount of interproximal plaque biofilm and that the subjects found it easier to use these brushes than dental floss. However, no difference was found when probe depth reductions or bleeding indices were compared.[23] Therefore, interproximal cleaning aids such as dental floss and interdental brushes are excellent for proximal cleaning of teeth when interdental spaces permit their access.[74]

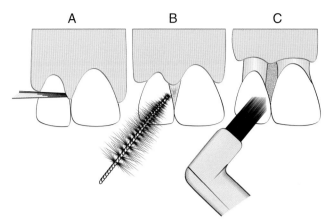

Fig. 43.12 Interproximal Embrasure Spaces Vary Greatly in Patients With Periodontal Disease. (A) In general, embrasures with no gingival recession are adequately cleaned using dental floss. (B) Larger spaces with exposed root surfaces require the use of an interproximal brush. (C) Single-tufted brushes clean efficiently in interproximal spaces with no papillae.

Fig. 43.13 (A) and (B) Interproximal cleaning devices include wooden tips, (C to F) interproximal brushes, and (G) rubber-tip stimulators.

Embrasure spaces vary greatly in size and shape. Fig. 43.12 provides a representation of the size and anatomy of three types of embrasures and the interdental cleaning instrument most often recommended for each. As a general rule, the larger the spaces, the larger the instruments needed to clean them properly.

Technique

An interdental brush of any style is inserted through the interproximal spaces and moved back and forth between the teeth with short strokes. The diameter of the brush should be slightly larger than the gingival embrasures to be cleaned. This size permits the bristles to exert pressure on both proximal tooth surfaces by working their way into concavities on the roots. The brush bristles must also reach the interdental gingival margin.

Single-tufted brushes provide access to furcation areas, or isolated areas of deep recession, and are effective on the lingual surfaces of mandibular molars and premolars. These areas are often missed when using a toothbrush and floss.

Other Interdental Cleaning Devices: Rubber Tips, Wooden Toothpicks, and Tufted Brushes

Other interdental cleaning devices are available for removing microbial plaque biofilm from between the teeth (Fig. 43.13). Rubber tips with angled shanks, tapered wooden toothpicks that are round or triangular in cross-section, and single-tufted brushes are all helpful in attaining interdental hygiene. Many interdental devices have handles and contoured shanks for convenient manipulation around the teeth and in posterior areas. Clinical research has indicated that these devices are all effective for both lingual and facial tooth surfaces, as well as for proximal surfaces.[74,110]

Wooden toothpicks are used with or without a handle (see Fig. 43.13A and B). Access is easier from the buccal surfaces for tips without handles but is limited primarily to the anterior and bicuspid areas. Wooden toothpicks on handles improve access

to all areas and are shown to be as effective as dental floss in reducing plaque biofilm and bleeding scores in subjects with gingivitis.[83] Triangular wooden tips are also available; this design is most useful in the anterior areas when used from the buccal surfaces of the teeth.

Rubber tips are conical and are mounted on handles or the ends of toothbrushes. They are reusable and can be easily adapted to all proximal surfaces in the mouth. The rubber tips that are mounted on handles with a curved shank are excellent not only for cleaning the interdental spaces but also for demonstrating to the patient the location of the plaque biofilm during oral hygiene instruction. For hygiene purposes, the rubber tip should be placed into the embrasure space, resting on the gingiva, and used in a circular motion. It can be applied to interproximal spaces and other defects throughout the mouth and is easily adaptable to lingual surfaces. Plastic tips that resemble wooden or rubber tips are also available and are used in the same way.

Technique

Toothpicks are common devices and readily available in most homes. They can be used around all surfaces of the teeth when attached to commercially available handles (see Fig. 43.13B). Once mounted on the handle, the toothpick is broken off so that it is only 5 or 6 mm long. The tip of the toothpick is used to trace along the gingival margin and into the proximal areas from both the facial and lingual surface of each tooth (Fig. 43.14). Toothpicks mounted on handles are efficient for cleaning along the gingival margin,[46] can penetrate periodontal pockets and furcations, and permit patients to target their hygiene efforts at the gingival margin (Takei H: Personal communication, 2009).

Soft triangular wooden picks or plastic picks are placed in the interdental space with the base of the triangle resting on the gingiva and the sides in contact with the proximal tooth surfaces (Fig. 43.15). The pick is then moved in and out of the embrasure several times to remove the biofilm. The disadvantage of triangular wooden or plastic tips is that they do not reach into the posterior areas or on the lingual surfaces.

Fig. 43.14 Wooden Toothpick. (A) The tip is a common wooden toothpick held in a handle and broken off. It is used to clean subgingivally and reach into periodontal pockets. (B) The tip can also be used to clean along the gingival margins of the teeth and reach under the gingiva.

Fig. 43.15 Triangular Wooden Tips Are Also Popular With Patients. The tip is inserted between the teeth, with the triangular portion resting on the gingival papilla. The tip is moved in and out to remove plaque; however, it is very difficult to use on posterior teeth and from the lingual aspect of all teeth.

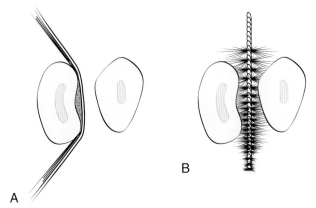

Fig. 43.16 Cleaning of Concave or Irregular Proximal Tooth Surfaces. (A) Dental floss may be less effective than (B) an interdental brush on long root surfaces with concavities.

KEY FACTS

Periodontal patients often have to clean large interdental spaces, so it is extremely important to find an interdental device that is easy to manipulate and that the patient will use regularly.
- Patients may need to try several of the many devices available before finding one that satisfies their needs.
- In general, the largest brush or device that fits into a space will clean most efficiently (Fig. 43.16).

GINGIVAL MASSAGE

Massaging the gingiva with a toothbrush or an interdental cleaning device produces epithelial thickening, increased keratinization, and increased mitotic activity in the epithelium and connective tissue.[17,20,49] The increased keratinization occurs only on the gingiva facing the oral cavity (oral epithelium), but not on the areas more vulnerable to microbial attack, which are the sulcular epithelium and the interdental areas where the gingival col is present. Epithelial thickening, increased keratinization, and blood circulation are shown to be beneficial for restoring gingival health.[48] Improved gingival health associated with interdental

stimulation is the result of inadvertent microbial plaque biofilm removal rather than the effects of gingival massage. No clinical evidence indicates that massaging the gingiva is essential or necessary to attain gingival health.

DISCLOSING AGENTS

Disclosing agents are solutions or wafers that stain bacterial biofilm on the surfaces of the teeth, tongue, and gingiva. Wafers are crushed and rinsed in the mouth for a few seconds before they are expectorated. They can be used as educational and motivational tools to improve the efficiency of plaque biofilm control procedures (eFig. 43.2).[7] Solutions are applied to the teeth as concentrates on cotton swabs or diluted as rinses. They usually produce staining of plaque biofilm, gingiva, tongue, lips, and fingers. Either form, rinses or wafers, can be used for plaque biofilm control instruction in the office and dispensed for home use to help periodontal patients evaluate the effectiveness of their oral hygiene routine.

FREQUENCY OF PLAQUE BIOFILM REMOVAL

In the controlled and supervised environment of clinical research, where well-trained individuals remove all visible plaque biofilm, gingival health can be maintained by one thorough cleaning with brush, floss, and toothpicks every 24 to 48 hours.[29,67,74,77] However, this is not true with most patients. The average daily home care routine lasts less than 2 minutes and removes only 40% of plaque biofilm.[31] It has been reported that improved plaque biofilm removal and therefore improved periodontal health are associated with increasing the frequency of brushing to twice per day.[67,95] Cleaning three or more times per day does not appear to improve periodontal conditions further. Clinical experience has also indicated that more important than the number of times the patient practices oral hygiene during a given day is effective target hygiene, meaning thorough plaque biofilm removal at the proper location. One could be cleaning several times a day, but if the target areas are missed, plaque biofilm will persist in these critical areas.

PATIENT MOTIVATION AND EDUCATION

In periodontal therapy, plaque biofilm control has two important purposes: to minimize gingival inflammation and to prevent the recurrence or progression of periodontal diseases and caries. Daily mechanical removal of plaque biofilm by the patient, including the use of appropriate antimicrobial agents, is the only practical means for improving oral health on a long-term basis. The process requires interest and compliance on the part of the patient and education and instruction from the dental hygienist, followed by encouragement and reinforcement. Keeping records of patients' performance facilitates this process. eFig. 43.3 provides an example of a plaque biofilm control record that permits comparison over time.

Motivation for Effective Plaque Biofilm Control

Motivating patients to perform effective plaque biofilm control is one of the most critical and difficult elements of long-term success in periodontal therapy. It requires commitment by the patient to change poor daily habits and return for regular visits for maintenance therapy. The scope of this compliance problem is immense. It has been shown that patients will stop using interproximal cleaning aids after a very short time. Heasman and associates[58] followed 100 patients treated for moderate to severe periodontal disease who were taught to use one or more interdental cleaning aids. These investigators found that only 20% of the patients used the aids after 6 months. Of the patients who had started using three devices, one-third had stopped all interdental cleaning at 6 months; the others used one or two of the aids.[65] The situation is not any better when patients' willingness to return for maintenance visits is reviewed. In a study of 1280 patients, most of whom had periodontal surgery in multiple sites after intensive scaling, root planing, and home care instruction, 25% never returned for a follow-up visit and only 40% returned regularly.[96] Wilson and colleagues[127] reported that 67% of periodontal patients were noncompliant with return visits in a 20-year retrospective study in a private periodontal practice.

Adopting new habits and returning for maintenance visits are not impossible tasks. To be successful requires the following: (1) the patient must understand the etiology of the disease and its importance in treatment and maintenance; the patient must also be compliant and receptive and must understand the concepts of pathogenesis, treatment, and prevention of periodontal disease; (2) the patient must be willing to alter harmful habits such as smoking; (3) the patient must be able to adjust personal beliefs and values to eliminate risk factors; motivational interviewing and instruction techniques can assist in achieving these goals[44]; and (4) manual skills must be developed to establish an effective plaque biofilm control regimen. In addition, the patient must understand the dental hygienist's critical role in treating and maintaining periodontal health.[103] If none of these factors can be managed, the long-term success of treatment is not likely.

Education and Scoring Systems

Many patients prefer to believe that treatment is a passive process, so it is incumbent on the dental hygienist to educate and reinforce to each patient their personal role in the long-term success of therapy. Today's health-conscious society presents a great advantage with regard to patient education. Most patients have been exposed to what periodontal disease is through television, newspapers, magazines, and the Internet. They must be willing to spend time and money on the many new products that are available. Examples are better-designed toothbrushes and mouthrinses such as chlorhexidine.

Patients must be informed of the importance of maintenance therapy and periodic assessment in the dental office to prevent recurrence of periodontal diseases and identify problems that may arise. These procedures work best when combined with an individualized oral hygiene regimen practiced daily at home. Therefore, patient education and motivating patients about microbial plaque biofilm control procedures are central to care. Many patients believe that "cleanings" every few months are sufficient for calculus and biofilm removal and disease control. Only the combination of regular maintenance visits and conscientious home care has been shown to reduce gingivitis and loss of supporting periodontal tissues over the long term.[85,121]

Periodontal patients should be shown how periodontal disease has manifested in their mouths through demonstrations of plaque biofilm, the bleeding of inflamed gingiva, and where possible, the example of the periodontal probe inserted into the pockets. In addition, it is of educational value for patients to have their oral cleanliness and periodontal condition recorded periodically.[9] The positive improvements in performance can be used for reinforcement. The plaque biofilm control record and the bleeding points index are simple indices that are useful for patient education and motivation.

Plaque Biofilm Control Record (O'Leary Index)

Have the patient use a disclosing solution or tablet and examine each tooth surface (except occlusal surfaces) for the presence or absence of stained biofilm at the dentogingival junction. Plaque biofilm is recorded on the appropriate box in a diagram for four surfaces on each tooth.[97] After all teeth have been scored, the index number is calculated for the percentage of surfaces with biofilm by dividing the number of surfaces with microbial plaque biofilm by the total number of surfaces scored and then multiplying by 100. A reasonable goal is 10% or fewer surfaces with plaque biofilm. If biofilm is always present in the same areas, provide instructions to improve cleaning procedures in those areas. It is extremely difficult to achieve a perfect score of 0, so patients should be rewarded if that is achieved.

Several frequently used plaque biofilm indices do not require staining of the teeth; one of these is the Plaque Index of Silness and Löe.[112] They are convenient to use and often acceptable to patients, even though they are not as dramatic for patient education.

Bleeding Points Index

The bleeding points index provides an evaluation of gingival inflammation around each tooth.[80] Retract the cheek and place the periodontal probe 1 mm into the sulcus or pocket at the distal aspect of the most posterior tooth in the quadrant on the buccal surface. Carry the probe lightly across the length of the sulcus to the mesial interproximal area on the facial aspect. Continue along all the teeth in the quadrant from the facial aspect. Wait 30 seconds, and record the presence of bleeding on the distal, facial, and mesial surfaces on the chart. Repeat on the lingual-palatal aspect, and record bleeding only for the direct lingual surface, not for the mesial or distal surfaces. This results in four separate scores for each tooth and does not score the mesial and distal surfaces twice. Repeat the steps for each quadrant. The percentage of the number of bleeding surfaces is calculated by dividing the number of surfaces that bled by the total number of tooth surfaces (four per tooth) and multiplying by 100 to obtain a percentage. This index is designed to demonstrate gingival inflammation characterized by bleeding rather than the presence of microbial plaque biofilm. Again, a goal of 10% or fewer bleeding points is good, but 0 is ideal. If a few bleeding points repeatedly occur in the same areas, cleaning procedures for those areas should be reinforced or modified because usually a residual piece of subgingival calculus that was not noted during therapy is the cause of the localized gingival bleeding.

Significance of Plaque Biofilm Scores and Bleeding Scores

Plaque biofilm scores are helpful as indicators of patients' compliance and success with daily home care procedures. However, biofilm levels themselves do not necessarily reflect gingival health or risk of disease progression, even though the location of the plaque biofilm is highly correlated with the presence of gingivitis.[88] Bleeding is a much better predictor of success in controlling inflammation and reducing the chance of disease progression. Although bleeding on probing is not the most specific or sensitive measure of health, it has a strong negative correlation with disease progression. If bleeding is absent at any given site in the mouth, reflecting good plaque biofilm control and disease management, it is unlikely that periodontal disease will progress.[79]

Instruction and Demonstration

Patients can reduce the incidence of plaque biofilm and gingivitis with repeated instruction and encouragement much more effectively than with self-acquired oral hygiene habits.[53,110] However, instruction in how to clean teeth must be more than a cursory chairside demonstration on the use of a toothbrush. It is a painstaking procedure that requires the patient's participation, careful supervision with correction of mistakes, and reinforcement during return visits until the patient achieves the necessary proficiency.[82] Any strategy for introducing plaque biofilm control to the periodontal patient includes several elements. Before receiving hygiene instructions, the patient must understand the nature and etiology of the disease. This aspect is important so the patient can understand why plaque biofilm removal on a daily basis is critical. Patients are aware that they have "brushed their teeth" all their lives, but they still have periodontal disease. Instruction on the technique of hygiene should follow an understanding of the disease. At the first instruction visit, the patient should be given a toothbrush and rubber tip along with a hand mirror to observe the procedure in his or her own mouth. The plaque biofilm can be disclosed to allow the patient to see it in the location where it is found (see eFig. 43.1). Many patients do not wish to use the disclosing agent, because it stains many areas in the mouth where staining is not desired. Polished dental restorations do not take up the stain, but the oral mucosa and lips may retain the stain for several hours. Applying petroleum jelly will keep the disclosing agent off the patient's lips. For these patients, the location and true color of the plaque biofilm can be demonstrated with the rubber tip. Once the plaque biofilm is demonstrated, the dental hygienist can proceed with the hygiene instruction in the patient's mouth.

The rubber tip is used to demonstrate the plaque biofilm located at the gingival margin, which is the target area. The nondisclosed plaque biofilm is almost the same color as the teeth, which impresses and educates the patient about the reason for not recognizing biofilm in the past. Toothbrushing should be demonstrated in the patient's mouth while he or she observes with a hand mirror. The patient then repeats the procedure with the dental hygienist giving assistance, correction, and positive reinforcement. Repeat the demonstration and instruction with dental floss and other interdental cleaning aids according to the patient's needs. Depending on the patient's skill and understanding of the technique, instruction on interdental hygiene may be postponed until the patient is able to manipulate the toothbrush properly. The rubber tip is an excellent instrument to demonstrate plaque biofilm, but it is also used to clean the interdental area. The rubber tip is placed interdentally, and the plaque biofilm is removed with a scooping motion.

Encourage patients to clean the teeth thoroughly at least once a day. Be sure to inform them that home care procedures for a full dentition may take 5 to 10 minutes. For complex periodontal cases, home care procedures may take longer, depending on the dexterity of the patient. The patient should set aside a convenient time and place in the daily schedule to perform the hygiene procedures every day. Subsequent visits should be used to reinforce or modify previous instructions and periodically record the state of gingival health and amount of plaque biofilm.

To introduce an oral hygiene program effectively, the dental hygienist must choose a strategy that will be convincing to the patient while understanding that some strategies do not work. Waiting until the end of the appointment when the patient is sore, exhausted, and possibly anesthetized will not be conducive to learning. Failing to provide positive reinforcement, introducing the patient to unfamiliar instruments, and relying only on pamphlets and printed material to provide education are likely to result in an ineffective educational experience.

KEY FACTS

Strategies that will assist you in educating and motivating your patients include:
- Provide encouragement and positive reinforcement.[120] Threats are not effective.
- Demonstrate how devices work, and allow practice time.
- Provide samples so that patients do not have to stop and buy products on the way home because they will not do it.
- Show and reinforce improvements at subsequent appointments, even if changes are modest.

CONCLUSION

- After thorough patient education regarding the disease and the etiology, the hygiene technique is initiated by demonstrating the procedure in the patient's own mouth. The rubber tip is an excellent instrument to demonstrate plaque biofilm. All patients require regular use of a toothbrush, either manual or electric, at least once per day. The brushing method should emphasize access to the gingival margins (dentogingival junction) of all accessible tooth surfaces. Emphasize the importance of *targeted hygiene* and extending as far onto the proximal surfaces as possible.
- Dental floss should be used in all interdental spaces that are filled with gingiva.
- Interdental aids such as interproximal brushes, rubber tips, wooden tips, or toothpicks should be used in all areas where the toothbrush and floss techniques cannot adequately remove the plaque biofilm. This includes large embrasure spaces and furcation areas, as well as the mesial surface of the maxillary

first bicuspid, which presents a concavity on the root surface near the cementoenamel junction.
- Daily at-home subgingival irrigation and lavage are useful for reduction of inflammation and maintenance for patients with residual deep pockets and those who struggle with mechanical interproximal cleaning devices. The effectiveness of irrigation and lavage is enhanced by the addition of a chlorhexidine or essential oil rinse as an irrigant.
- Caries control requires the daily use of a dentifrice with low-concentration fluoride. Topical oral rinses and gels with higher concentrations of fluoride should be used for patients with a high risk for caries.
- Chemical antimicrobial agents, such as chlorhexidine and essential oils, can be used to disinfect the patient's mouth and control infection. These oral rinses may be continued indefinitely. Staining of teeth and taste alteration are side effects that may limit the patient's acceptance of these products.
- Reinforcement of daily plaque biofilm control practices and routine visits to the dental office for maintenance care are essential for successful microbial plaque biofilm control and the long-term success of therapy.

Successful prevention, treatment, and maintenance in periodontal therapy are based on scientific knowledge of the etiology, risk factors, and host resistance involved in periodontal disease. The importance of the patient's understanding of the etiology and active participation in partnership with the therapist to prevent and treat periodontal disease is well understood in the current understanding of periodontal therapy.

A Case Scenario is found on the companion website.

REFERENCES

 References for this chapter are found on the companion website.

44

Breath Malodor[a]

🌐 For online-only content on extraoral causes of breath malodor and the portable volatile sulfur monitor, as well as expanded discussions on epidemiology and etiology of malodor, fundamentals of malodor detection, diagnosis of malodor including organoleptic rating and gas chromatography, and chlorhexidine use in treating malodor, please go to the companion website.

CHAPTER OUTLINE

SEMANTICS AND CLASSIFICATION

Breath odor can be defined as the subjective perception after smelling someone's breath.[112] Other definitions within the literature include noticeably unpleasant odors exhaled in breathing, any disagreeable odor of breath, regardless of its origin, and "any unpleasant odor eliminating from the oral cavity."[5] It can be pleasant, unpleasant, or even disturbing, if not repulsive. If unpleasant, the terms *breath malodor, halitosis, bad breath,* or *fetor ex ore* can be applied. Breath malodor is a common complaint in the general population. One in four persons are reported to have bad breath at a given time in his/her life.[6] It has a significant socioeconomic impact but unfortunately has been neglected until recently by scientists and dental professionals, and it is still hardly covered in the medical curricula. Halitosis can lead to personal discomfort and social embarrassment.[169] Moreover, halitosis can be indicative of underlying diseases. In general, intraoral conditions, like insufficient dental hygiene, periodontitis, or tongue coating are considered to be the most important cause (85%) for halitosis.[110] Therefore, the dental hygienist, dentist, and periodontologist are the first-line professionals to be confronted with this problem.

Miyazaki et al.[80] suggest three main categories of halitosis: genuine halitosis, pseudo-halitosis, and halitophobia. *Genuine halitosis* is the term that is used when the breath malodor really exists and can be diagnosed organoleptically or by measurement of the responsible compounds. A distinction should be made between physiologic and pathologic halitosis (Fig. 44.1).

Transient disturbing odors caused by food intake (e.g., garlic, onions, and certain spices), smoking, or medications (e.g., metronidazole) do not reveal a health problem and are common examples of physiologic halitosis. The same is true for "morning" bad breath, as habitually experienced on awakening. This malodor is caused by decreased salivary flow and increased putrefaction during the night, and it spontaneously disappears after breakfast or after oral hygiene measures. A persistent breath malodor, by definition, does reflect some pathology (pathologic halitosis). The causes of this condition are discussed later in the chapter. When the origin of pathologic halitosis can be found in the oral cavity, one speaks of *oral malodor.* When an obvious breath malodor cannot be perceived but the patient is convinced that he or she suffers from it, this is called *pseudo-halitosis.* If the patient still believes that bad breath is present after treatment of genuine halitosis or diagnosis of pseudo-halitosis, one considers halitophobia, which is a recognized psychiatric condition.[172] Anyone who complains of halitosis to the dental hygienist, objective or subjective (i.e., self-perceived odor not detectable by others/pseudo-halitosis), should be considered a halitosis patient.[5]

KEY DEFINITIONS FOR THE DIAGNOSIS OF BAD BREATH

Genuine halitosis	Malodor that can be verified objectively
Physiologic halitosis	Malodor that is transient and caused by physiologic factors, such as food intake or smoking
Oral malodor or intraoral halitosis	Obvious malodor originating from the oral cavity
Extraoral halitosis	Bad breath originating from pathologic conditions outside the oral cavity
Pseudo-halitosis	Malodor that cannot be perceived objectively even though the patient complains of its existence. This condition can be improved by oral hygiene instruction and counseling.
Halitophobia	No malodor that can be perceived objectively after treatment of halitosis or pseudo-halitosis even though the patient persists in believing that halitosis exists

[a]Adapted from the following chapter of Newman and Carranza's Clinical Periodontology, 13th edition: Chapter 49: Breath Malodor, by Marc Quirynen, Isabelle Laleman,|Sophie De Geest, Charlotte De Hous, Christel Dekeyser, and Wim Teughels. This chapter was updated by Sarah Hughes.

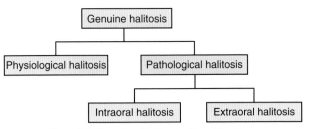

Fig. 44.1 Genuine Halitosis: Classification.

ETIOLOGY

In most patients, breath malodor originates from the oral cavity. Tongue coating is the predominant cause of oral malodor. Furthermore, periodontal diseases (gingivitis and periodontitis) are the second most important causative factors.[b]

A large-scale study including 2000 patients with halitosis complaints showed that for those patients whose bad breath could be objectively detected, the cause was mostly found within the oral cavity (90%). Tongue coating (51%), gingivitis or periodontitis (13%), or a combination (22%) accounted for the majority of the cases.[110] Because a large part of the population has tongue coating or gingivitis/periodontitis, the risk always exists that an intraoral condition is too easily considered as the cause, whereas more important pathologic conditions are overlooked. Indeed, for a minority of patients (4% in the same study), extraoral causes could be identified, including ear, nose, and throat (ENT) disorders, systemic diseases (e.g., diabetes), metabolic or hormonal changes, hepatic or renal insufficiency, bronchial and pulmonary diseases, or gastroenterologic disorders.[29,89,105,110,156]

Intraoral Causes

Tongue coating, poor oral hygiene, gingivitis, and periodontitis are the predominant causative factors.[110,134] In these cases the term *oral malodor* applies. It is the result of the degradation of organic substrates by anaerobic bacteria. During the process of bacterial putrefaction, peptides and proteins present in saliva, food debris, gingival crevicular fluid, interdental plaque, shed epithelial cells, postnasal drip, and blood are hydrolyzed to sulfide-containing and non–sulfide-containing amino acids, which can be further metabolized. The proteolytic degradation of sulfur-containing amino acids (cysteine, cystine, and methionine) by gram-negative bacteria produces sulfur-containing gases such as hydrogen sulfide (H_2S) and methyl mercaptan (CH_3SH).[166]

The most commonly involved bacteria are *Porphyromonas gingivalis, Prevotella intermedia, Prevotella nigrescens, Aggregatibacter actinomycetemcomitans, Campylobacter rectus, Fusobacterium nucleatum, Peptostreptococcus micros, Tannerella forsythia, Eubacterium* spp., and *spirochetes*. A study by Niles and Gaffar[91] made clear that these gram-negative species in particular cause an unpleasant smell by the production of sulfur compounds. However, because of the large microbial diversity found in patients

with halitosis, it is suggested that breath malodor is the result of complex interactions among several bacterial species. One study indicated that some gram-positive microorganisms, such as Streptococcus salivarius, also contribute to oral malodor production by deglycosylating salivary glycoproteins, thus exposing their protein core to further degradation by gram-negative microorganisms.[143] More recently, the presence of Solobacterium moorei, a gram-positive bacterium, has also been linked to oral malodor.[51,52,60]

Thus, for oral malodor, the unpleasant smell of the breath mainly originates from VSCs, especially H_2S, CH_3SH, and (less significantly) dimethyl sulfide ($[CH_3]_2S$), as first discovered by Tonzetich.[153] Other compounds, such as the diamines indole and skatole, the polyamines putrescine and cadaverine, and the carboxylic acids acetic, butyric, and propionic acid, are also formed by proteolytic degradation of non–sulfur-containing amino acids by oral microorganisms.[44]

Tongue and Tongue Coating

The dorsal tongue mucosa, with an area of 25 cm,[103] has a very irregular surface topography.[21,133] The innumerable depressions in the tongue surface are ideal niches for bacterial adhesion and growth, sheltered from cleaning actions.[27,173] Moreover, desquamated cells and food remnants also remain trapped in these retention sites and consequently can be putrefied by the bacteria.[10] A fissured tongue (deep fissures on the dorsum, also called *scrotal tongue* or *lingua plicata*) and a hairy tongue *(lingua villosa)* have an even rougher surface (Fig. 44.2).

Accumulated food remnants intermingled with exfoliated cells and bacteria form a coating on the tongue dorsum. The latter cannot be easily removed because of retention by the irregular surface of the tongue dorsum (see Fig. 44.2). As such, the two factors essential for putrefaction (bacteria and their nutrients) are united. Several investigators have identified the dorsal posterior surface of the tongue as the primary source of oral malodor.[10,20,27,122] Indeed, high correlations have been reported between tongue coating and odor formation.[10,23,81,173]

In both healthy individuals and patients with periodontitis with or without complaints of oral halitosis, a significant positive correlation was found between the presence or amount of tongue coating and levels of VSCs[81,111] and/or organoleptic scores of the mouth odor.[27] In a group of 2000 patients visiting a multidisciplinary halitosis clinic,[110,163] significant correlations were found between organoleptic scores and tongue coating ($R = 0.52$; $P < .001$). In another study,[95] it was also observed that the amount of tongue coating was significantly greater in the halitosis-positive group compared with the halitosis-negative group. Morita and Wang[83] found that the volume of tongue coating and the percentage of sites with bleeding on probing were significantly associated with oral malodor.[83] In 1992, Yaegaki and Sanada[173,174] demonstrated that even in patients with periodontal disease, 60% of the VSCs were produced from the tongue surface.[173,174]

Research has showed that the strongest determinant of the presence of tongue coating is suboptimal oral hygiene. Other influencing factors were periodontal status, presence of a denture, smoking, and dietary habits.[162]

---

[b]References 29, 100, 101, 110, 173, 174.

Fig. 44.2 (A–C) Clinical pictures of heavily coated tongues.

Periodontal Infections

A relationship between periodontitis and oral malodor has been shown. However, periodontally healthy patients can suffer from halitosis, not all patients with gingivitis and/or periodontitis complain about bad breath, and some disagreement exists in the literature over to what extent oral malodor and periodontal disease are related.[10,123,140] Bacteria associated with gingivitis and periodontitis are indeed able to produce VSCs.[c]

Several studies have shown that VSC levels in the mouth correlate positively with the depth of periodontal pockets (the deeper the pocket, the more bacteria, particularly anaerobic species) and that the amount of VSCs in the breath increases with the number, depth, and bleeding tendency of the periodontal pockets.[20,99,110,174] VSCs aggravate the periodontitis process by increasing the permeability of the pocket and mucosal epithelium, therefore exposing the underlying connective tissues of the periodontium to bacterial metabolites. CH_3SH enhances interstitial collagenase production, interleukin-1 production by mononuclear cells, and cathepsin B production, thus further mediating connective tissue breakdown.[72,116] It was shown that human gingival fibroblasts developed an affected cytoskeleton when exposed to CH_3SH.[12,116] Furthermore, the reaction of H_2S with collagen can alter the protein structure, thereby rendering the periodontal ligament and bone collagen more susceptible to destruction by proteases.[90] Investigators have shown, in cases of gingivitis and periodontitis, a decrease in the content of acid-soluble and total collagen in the affected tissues.[132] These findings suggest that increased production of VSCs may accelerate the progression of periodontal disease. Toxic VSCs are able to damage the periodontal tissues and create even more loss of attachment. A mutual reinforcement of the loss of periodontal attachment and production of VSCs occurs, resulting in a vicious cycle.

Some studies, however, have shown that when the presence of tongue coating is taken into account, the correlation between periodontitis and oral malodor is much lower, thus indicating that tongue coating remains a key factor for halitosis. The prevalence of tongue coating is six times higher in patients with periodontitis, and the same bacterial species associated with periodontal disease can also be found in large numbers on the

dorsum of the tongue, particularly when tongue coating is present.[173] The reported association between periodontitis and oral malodor may thus primarily be due to the effects of periodontal disease on tongue coating. It may also explain why other articles did not find a correlation.[10,140]

Other relevant malodorous pathologic manifestations of the periodontium are pericoronitis (the soft tissue "cap" being retentive for microorganisms and debris), major recurrent oral ulcerations, herpetic gingivitis, and necrotizing gingivitis/periodontitis. Microbiologic observations indicate that ulcers infected with gram-negative anaerobes (i.e., *Prevotella* and *Porphyromonas* species) are significantly more malodorous than noninfected ulcers.[11]

CLINICIAN'S CORNER

What is the influence of bad breath in patients with periodontitis?

The increased production of VSCs in people with bad breath may accelerate the progression of periodontal disease. For example, it is known that CH_3SH and H_2S can adversely affect collagen structure and gingival fibroblasts.

Dental Disorders

Possible causes within the dentition are deep carious lesions with food impaction and putrefaction, extraction wounds filled with blood clots, and purulent discharge leading to important putrefaction. Other causes include interdental food impaction in large interdental areas and crowding of teeth favoring food entrapment and accumulation of debris. Acrylic dentures, especially when kept continuously in the mouth at night or not regularly cleaned, can lead to infections (e.g., candidiasis), which produce a typical smell. The denture surface facing the gingiva is porous and retentive for bacteria, yeasts, and debris, which are compounds needed for putrefaction.

Dry Mouth

Saliva has an important cleaning function in the oral cavity. Patients with xerostomia often present with large amounts of plaque on teeth and extensive tongue coating. The increased microbial load and the escape of VSCs when salivary flow is reduced explain the strong breath malodor.[63] Several studies link stress with VSC levels, but it is not clear whether this can simply

---

[c]References 63, 87, 91, 100, 101, 153.

be explained by a reduction of salivary flow.[69,107] Other causes of xerostomia are medication,[82] alcohol abuse,[38] Sjögren syndrome (a common autoimmune rheumatic disease),[76] and diabetes.[164]

Extraoral Causes

For a minority of patients, extraoral causes can be identified, including ENT disorders, systemic disease (e.g., diabetes or kidney disease), metabolic or hormonal changes, hepatic or renal insufficiency, bronchial and pulmonary diseases, or gastroenterologic disorders.[4,7] Moreover, multiple causes may be present at the same time, and over the course of time the etiology may shift.

Extraoral halitosis can be subdivided into two types: non–blood-borne halitosis and blood-borne halitosis.[151] Non–blood-borne halitosis is uncommon, and most information about it comes from case reports. Non–blood-borne halitosis encompasses, for example, throat infections, nasal infections, infections of the respiratory system, lung diseases, and stomach disorders.

Blood-borne halitosis is the result of bad-smelling metabolites that can be formed or absorbed at any place in the body (e.g., the liver, the gut) and transported by the bloodstream to the lungs. Exhalation of these volatiles in the alveolar air then causes halitosis, at least when the concentrations of the bad-smelling metabolites are sufficiently high. The crevicular fluid reflects the circulating molecules in the blood and can thus also play a relevant role, but due to the small amount, probably not a very dominant one.

The extraoral causes are much more difficult to detect, although they can sometimes be recognized by a typical odor. Uncontrolled diabetes mellitus can be associated with a sweet odor of ketones, liver disease can be revealed by a sulfur odor, and kidney failure can be characterized by a fishy odor because of the presence of dimethylamine and trimethylamine.[105]

> **CLINICIAN'S CORNER**
>
> What is the most important cause of halitosis?
>   Tongue coating is the most important cause of halitosis. The innumerable depressions in the tongue surface are ideal niches for bacterial adhesion and growth; additionally, desquamated cells and food remnants also remain trapped in these retention sites. The degradation of organic substrates by anaerobic bacteria results in the production of a range of unpleasant-smelling volatile compounds.

Pseudo-Halitosis or Halitophobia

If a patient presents with complaints but no objective halitosis can be detected, one speaks of pseudo-halitosis or *imaginary breath odor*, which can lead to *halitophobia*.[97] The latter is the case when, even after repeated diagnosis of an absence of bad breath, the patient cannot accept the absence of halitosis. This condition has been associated with obsessive-compulsive disorder and hypochondria. Well-established personality disorder questionnaires (e.g., Symptom Checklist 90) allow the clinician to assess the patient's tendency for illusional breath malodor.[30,31,33] Having a psychologist or psychiatrist at the malodor consultation can be especially helpful for such patients. Because of the complexity of this disorder, a malodor consultation is thus preferably multidisciplinary, combining the knowledge of a periodontologist or dentist/dental hygienist, an ENT specialist, an internist (if necessary), and a psychologist or psychiatrist. In a study of 2000 patients, 16% were diagnosed with pseudo-halitosis or halitophobia.[110]

> **KEY FACT**
>
> Only in a few cases is the cause of bad breath found outside the oral cavity. Thus, dental hygienists play an important role in the diagnosis and treatment of halitosis.

DIAGNOSIS OF MALODOR

Preconsultation Approach

A proper diagnostic approach starts with providing the right information to the patient before the appointment. It is recommended that the patient does not eat garlic, onions, or spices for 2 days before the consultation because they can cause bad breath and body odor that can last from several hours to 2 days.[50] To remove confounding odors, the patient is also instructed to refrain from alcohol, coffee, and smoking during the 12-hour period before the consultation. For the same reason, it is advisable not to use chewing gum, mints, drops, or mouthrinses during the 8 hours preceding the appointment, both for the patient and for the oral malodor judge. The day of the consultation, the use of fragranced shampoo, body lotion, and perfume should also be avoided, so as not to disturb the organoleptic ratings. In most halitosis consultations, the patient is asked not to eat or drink on the morning of the examination. However, if breakfast is consumed, morning bad breath can be excluded.

> **COURSE OF A HALITOSIS CONSULTATION**
> Preconsultation patient information
> Anamnesis—the patient's account of their medical and social history
> Organoleptic examination
> Examination of the breath with portable sulfur monitor
> Oropharyngeal examination
> Explanation of halitosis and instructions for oral hygiene
> If necessary, explanation of additional therapy

The patient should be encouraged to bring a confidant to the consultations who can identify whether the perceived odor is the one previously noticed. Some of these guidelines are crucial not only for the organoleptic evaluation but also for a correct interpretation of the results obtained with certain breath analyzers (see later).

Anamnesis

Each consultation should start with thorough questioning about the breath malodor, eating habits, and medical, dental, and social history. This can be done with a questionnaire that the patient fills out in the waiting room and/or verbally at the beginning of the consultation, depending on the preference of the examiner and the practical possibilities. To start with, the patient should be asked about the frequency of the halitosis (e.g., constantly, every day), the time of appearance during the day (e.g., after meals can indicate a stomach hernia), when the problem first appeared, and whether others have identified the problem (to exclude imaginary breath odor). In addition, the medical history has to be recorded, with an emphasis on medications and systemic diseases of the lungs, liver, kidneys, stomach, and pancreas. Concerning the ENT history, attention should be paid to the presence of nasal obstruction, mouth breathing, postnasal drip, allergy, tonsillitis, dysphagia, and previous ENT encounters. The dental history includes questions assessing the frequency of dental visits, the use of mouthrinses, the presence and maintenance of a dental prosthesis, and the frequency of and instruments used for toothbrushing, interdental cleaning, and tongue brushing and scraping. Finally, the patient is asked about smoking, drinking, and dietary habits.

Examinations

After obtaining a thorough anamnesis, the clinician checks whether an unpleasant odor can be perceived and inspects the mouth to detect possible causes of bad breath. Different ways exist to examine the breath. The easiest and least expensive way is to smell the breath. However, several devices are on the market that mainly detect VSCs.

Organoleptic Rating

Even though devices are available, organoleptic assessment by a judge is still the gold standard in the examination of breath malodor. It is the easiest and most often used method because it gives a reflection of the everyday situation when halitosis is noticed. Moreover, the human nose can smell 10,000 different odors, many more than any device on the market.[50,53] In an organoleptic evaluation, a trained and preferably calibrated "judge" sniffs the expired air and assesses whether it is unpleasant by using an intensity rating.[128] Scoring is normally done according to the intensity scale of Rosenberg, where 0 represents the absence of odor, 1 is barely noticeable odor, 2 is slight malodor, 3 is moderate malodor, 4 is strong malodor, and 5 is severe malodor.[128] In this six-point system, 0 indicates a concentration of odorant below a threshold, 1 to 4 are increasing occupancy of receptor binding sites, and 5 is assumed to be close to saturation.[45,46] To avoid bias, it is advisable that the organoleptic assessment precedes all other measurements.

In an organoleptic assessment, the judge smells a series of air samples (Fig. 44.3), as follows:
1. *Nasal breath odor:* The subject expires through the nose while keeping the mouth closed. When the nasal expiration is

Fig. 44.3 (A) Organoleptic assessment of the oral cavity odor while the patient refrains from breathing. (B) assessment of the oral cavity odor when the patient counts out loud from 1 to 10. (C) A sample of the tongue coating is taken to smell afterward. (D) The nasal odor is rated.

malodorous yet the air expired through the mouth is not, an ENT problem can be suspected.

2. *Oral cavity odor:* The subject opens the mouth and refrains from breathing while the judge places his or her nose close to the mouth opening (approximately 10 cm from the patient's mouth).

3. *Oral cavity odor:* The patient counts from 1 to 10. This reveals the same as described earlier, but favors oral malodor because of drying of the palatal and tongue mucosa.

4. *Tongue coating:* The judge smells a tongue scraping from the posterior part of the tongue, obtained with an odorless plastic spoon or tongue scraper, at a distance of approximately 5 cm from his or her nose. This odor resembles that emanating from the tongue dorsum.

Although the organoleptic assessment is still the gold standard for diagnosis of halitosis, the method also has some important drawbacks. The assessment can, for example, be influenced by several aspects, such as the position of the head, hunger, and the experience of the judge. Odor judges are also supposed to rest their nose for several minutes between tests to avoid habituation. The most important disadvantage of the method, however, is that it clearly has a degree of subjectivity. Researchers are trying to improve the reliability and reproducibility of the organoleptic method.[46] When using a panel of odor judges instead of one judge, the reliability is already considered to increase.[172] Furthermore, the agreement among judges may be improved by standardization of the sense of smell using an odor solution kit for measuring the olfactory response.[178] Training is also considered to reduce odor judges' errors.[85]

Portable Volatile Sulfur Monitor

The Halimeter (Interscan) is an electronic device that detects the presence of VSCs such as H_2S and CH_3SH in breath. The instrument cannot discriminate among the different sulfur compounds. The sensitivity for CH_3SH is five times lower than for H_2S, and the device is almost insensitive to $(CH_3)_2S$.[39] Moreover, ethanol and other compounds can disturb the measurements.

To allow an increase in concentration of VSCs, the patient has to keep his or her mouth closed for 2 to 3 minutes before sampling. The mouth air is aspirated by inserting a drinking straw fixed on the flexible tube of the instrument (Fig. 44.4). The straw is kept inside the mouth, preferably above the posterior part of the tongue dorsum, not touching the oral mucosa or the tongue, while the subject keeps the mouth slightly open and breathes through the nose. The sulfur meter uses a voltammetric sensor that generates a signal when exposed to sulfur-containing gases. Using a recorder or specific software, a graphic presentation can be obtained, called a *haligram* (Fig. 44.5), which gives the response as a function of time. For the most optimal results, the manufacturer recommends performing three measurements and using the average value. Between measurements, it is important

Fig. 44.4 Halimeter.

Fig. 44.5 Haligram. *VSC,* Volatile sulfur compound.

to allow the meter to restabilize before repeating. The monitor needs regular calibration and replacement of the sensor biannually.

The Halimeter is easy to use as a chair-side test and is relatively inexpensive. Patients are usually less embarrassed by this examination than by organoleptic assessment. Moreover the absence of odor in cases of halitophobia can be more convincingly proven than by an organoleptic assessment. Several studies have shown good correlations between the organoleptic measurement and the Halimeter.[126,129] An important drawback of the device is that it detects only sulfur compounds and thus is useful only for intraoral causes of halitosis. The absence of VSCs does not prove that no breath odor is present.

A wide range of threshold limits for halitosis has been proposed. Yaegaki and Sanada[173] recommended a value of 75 ppb as the limit for social acceptance, whereas the Halimeter's manufacturer proposes 150 ppb. Following this recommendation, the sensitivity and specificity of the device for the organoleptic score have been calculated to be 63% and 98%, respectively. Previous studies from our group showed that a reduction in this threshold to 120 ppb improves the sensitivity of the device without detriment to specificity.[163] In patients with oral malodor, VSC concentrations can easily reach 300 to 400 ppb.

Gas Chromatography

A gas chromatograph can analyze air, saliva, or crevicular fluid (Fig. 44.6). About 100 compounds have been isolated from the headspace of saliva and tongue coating, including ketones, alkanes, sulfur-containing compounds, and phenyl compounds.[19] In the expired air of a person, at least 150 compounds can be found.[103,159-161] The most important advantage of the technique is that when coupled with mass spectrometry, it can detect virtually any compound when using adequate materials and conditions. Moreover, it has very high sensitivity and specificity.

Elaborate GC is available only in specialized centers but is especially useful for identifying nonoral causes.[56,102,146,158] It is expensive and requires trained personnel.

A small, portable "gas chromatograph" (OralChroma, Nissha FIS, Inc., Osaka, Japan) has been introduced, which makes this technique available for periodontal clinics (Fig. 44.7). More recently, the second generation of this portable gas chromatograph was introduced: the OralChroma CHM-2. The CHM-2 is a little bit smaller than the first-generation OralChroma, the measurements only take half the time, and it comes with optimized software. Sample collection is done by use of a disposable syringe, which is inserted two-thirds of the way into the oral cavity. The patient must close the mouth for 30 seconds before sample collection, and afterward the sample is injected into the gas chromatograph.

The analysis starts automatically. A software packet, OralChroma Data Manager, collects the data from the OralChroma and graphically displays the sensor responses on a computer screen. After 4 minutes for the OralChroma CHM-2, the process is completed, and the concentrations of the three gases are displayed in either ng/10 mL or ppb (nmol/mol) (Fig. 44.8). The accompanying software packet gives a clear overview of the VSC measurement. However, with the OralChroma CHM-1, sometimes these graphics are not correct because the place of the VSCs is incorrectly assigned in the chromatogram. The latter can be corrected by analyzing the chromatograph.[150,152]

The OralChroma has the capacity to measure the concentration of the three key sulfur compounds (H_2S, CH_3SH, and $[CH_3]_2S$) separately. This can be helpful for a differential diagnosis. A high concentration of CH_3SH compared with H_2S indicates, for example, periodontitis.[174] If only H_2S is increased, a problem with oral hygiene may exist. $(CH_3)_2S$ can indicate an extraoral cause.[149] Just like the Halimeter, the OralChroma cannot detect compounds other than sulfur compounds, and some intraoral and extraoral causes can thus be overlooked. The apparatus needs calibration and the sensor and column need to be replaced every 2 years.[163]

Fig. 44.6 Gas Chromatography Machinery, Including Thermal Desorber *(TD)* to Release Molecules Trapped in Special Collectors, Gas Chromatograph *(GC)* for Separation of Molecules, and Mass Spectrometer *(MS)* for Identification of Molecules.

Fig. 44.7 OralChroma.

Fig. 44.8 Graphic From the OralChroma. The first peak indicates the level of hydrogen sulfide (H_2S), the second the level of methyl mercaptan (CH_3SH), and the third the level of dimethyl sulfide $(CH3)_2S$. 2332.

HALIMETER VERSUS ORALCHROMA

Halimeter	OralChroma
Easy to handle	Easy to handle
Affordable	More expensive
Displays results immediately	Takes 4 min (CHM-2) or 8 min (CHM-1) before measurements are shown
Cannot discriminate among different gases	Can discriminate among hydrogen sulfide, methyl mercaptan, and dimethyl sulfide
Maintenance needed	Maintenance needed

Dark-Field or Phase-Contrast Microscopy

Oral malodor is typically associated with a higher incidence of motile organisms and spirochetes, so shifts in their proportions allow monitoring of therapeutic progress. Another advantage of direct microscopy is that the patient becomes aware of bacteria present in plaque, tongue coating, and saliva. Too often, patients confuse plaque with food remnants.

Oropharyngeal Examination

The oropharyngeal examination includes inspection of deep carious lesions, interdental food impaction, wounds, bleeding of the gums, periodontal pockets, tongue coating, dry mouth, and the tonsils and pharynx (for tonsillitis and pharyngitis).

The tongue coating can be scored with regard to thickness and surface. Several methods have been proposed for thickness; Gross and coworkers in 1975[49] proposed an index ranging from 0 (no coating) to 3 (severe coating). Miyazaki[81] (Fig. 44.9A) assessed tongue-coating status according to area: 0 = none visible, 1 = less than one-third of the tongue dorsum covered, 2 = less than two-thirds, and 3 = more than two-thirds.

Winkel and coworkers[170] considered both the extension and the thickness of the tongue coating. The dorsum of the tongue is divided into six areas, three in the posterior and three in the anterior of the tongue (see Fig. 44.9B). The tongue coating in each sextant is scored as follows: 0 = no coating, 1 = light coating, and 2 = severe coating. A score of 1 is given when the pink color

underneath the coating is still visible; when this is not the case, 2 is given.

Attention should be paid to the morphology of the tongue. For example, the clinician should note whether the tongue looks normal or rough or has a deep sulcus or large papillae vallatae.[170]

Self-Examination

Smelling one's own breath by expiring into the hands in front of the mouth is not relevant because the nose becomes used to the odor,[145] and the smell of the skin and soap used for handwashing may interfere. Moreover, studies have shown that self-assessment of oral malodor is notoriously unreliable, and one should be careful with such information obtained from the patient.[8,32]

CLINICIAN'S CORNER

When one of your patients complains of bad breath and he or she is periodontally healthy but has a thick tongue coating, what can you do?

You give the patient oral hygiene instruction and stress the importance of using a tongue scraper. Optionally, a mouthrinse can be advised, with active ingredients of proven efficacy such as chlorhexidine, cetylpyridinium chloride, or a zinc formulation.

TREATMENT OF ORAL MALODOR

The treatment of oral malodor (with an intraoral origin) should preferably be cause related. Because oral malodor is caused by the metabolic degradation of available proteins to malodorous gases by certain oral microorganisms, the following general treatment strategies can be applied:

- Mechanical reduction of intraoral nutrients (substrates) and microorganisms
- Chemical reduction of oral microbial load
- Rendering malodorous gases nonvolatile
- Masking the malodor

Treatment should be centered on reducing the bacterial load and micronutrients by effective mechanical oral hygiene procedures, including tongue scraping. Periodontal disease should be

Fig. 44.9 (A) Miyazaki tongue coating index. Score 0 = none visible, score 1 = less than one-third of the tongue dorsum covered, score 2 = less than two-thirds, and score 3 = more than two-thirds; here score 2 applies because less than two-thirds of the tongue dorsum is covered. (B) Winkel tongue coating index. Divide the dorsum of the tongue into six areas, (i.e., three in the posterior and three in the anterior part of the tongue). The tongue coating in each sextant is scored as 0 = no coating, 1 = light coating, and 2 = severe coating.

treated and controlled, and as an auxiliary aid, oral rinses containing chlorhexidine and other ingredients may further reduce the oral malodor. If breath malodor persists after these approaches, other sources of the malodor, such as the tonsils, lung disease, gastrointestinal disease, or metabolic abnormalities (e.g., diabetes), should be investigated.

Mechanical Reduction of Intraoral Nutrients and Microorganisms

Because of the extensive accumulation of bacteria on the dorsum of the tongue, tongue cleaning should be emphasized.[17,130,173] Previous investigations demonstrated that tongue cleaning reduces both the amount of coating (and thus bacterial nutrients) and the number of bacteria and thereby improves oral malodor effectively.[27,42,43,49,115] Other reports indicated that the reduction of the microbial load on the tongue after cleaning is negligible and that the reduced malodor probably results from the reduction of bacterial nutrients.[78,109]

Cleaning of the tongue can be done with a normal toothbrush, but preferably with a tongue scraper if a coating is established.[96,98] Tongue cleaning using a tongue scraper reduces halitosis levels by 75% after 1 week.[98] This should be gentle cleaning to prevent soft tissue damage. It is best to clean as far backward as possible; the posterior portion of the tongue has the most coating.[127] Tongue cleaning should be repeated until almost no coating material can be removed.[18] The gagging reflex is often elicited, especially when using brushes[109]; practice helps to prevent this.[16] It can also be helpful to pull the tongue out with a gauze pad. Tongue cleaning has the additional benefit of improving taste sensation.[109,171]

Interdental cleaning and toothbrushing are essential mechanical means of dental plaque control. Both remove residual food particles and organisms that cause putrefaction. Clinical studies have shown that the mechanical action of toothbrushing alone has no appreciable influence on the concentration of VSCs.[147] In a short-term study, Tonzetich[154] showed a short-term effect on bad breath after brushing with a sodium monofluorophosphate toothpaste. However, the effect was half of what was observed when combined with tongue brushing (73% and 30% reduction in VSCs, respectively).[154]

When chronic oral malodor arises as a consequence of periodontitis, professional periodontal therapy is needed.[10,20,99,174] A one-stage full-mouth disinfection, combining scaling and root planing with the application of chlorhexidine, reduced organoleptic malodor levels up to 90% in one study.[111] In another study by the same investigators, initial periodontal therapy had only a weak impact on VSC levels, except when combined with a mouthrinse containing chlorhexidine.[113]

Chewing gum may control bad breath temporarily because it can stimulate salivary flow.[118] The salivary flow itself also has a mechanical cleaning capability. Not surprisingly, therefore, subjects with extremely low salivary flow rate have higher VSC ratings and tongue coating scores than those with normal saliva production.[66] Waler[165] showed that chewing gum without any active ingredient can reduce halitosis modestly.

Chemical Reduction of Oral Microbial Load

Together with toothbrushing, mouth rinsing has become a common oral hygiene practice.[40] Formulations have been modified to carry antimicrobial and oxidizing agents, impacting the process of oral malodor formation. The active ingredients usually include antimicrobial agents such as chlorhexidine, cetylpyridinium chloride (CPC), essential oils, chlorine dioxide (ClO_2), triclosan, amine fluoride and stannous fluoride, hydrogen peroxide (H_2O_2), and baking soda. Some of these agents have only a temporary effect on the total number of microorganisms in the oral cavity.

Chlorhexidine

Chlorhexidine is considered the most effective antiplaque and antigingivitis agent.[1-3,7,58] Its antibacterial action can be explained by disruption of the bacterial cell membrane by the chlorhexidine molecules, thus increasing its permeability and resulting in cell lysis and death.[58,70] Because of its strong antibacterial effects and superior substantivity in the oral cavity, chlorhexidine rinsing provides significant reductions in VSC levels and organoleptic ratings.[14,124,126,157,176]

Unfortunately, as mentioned in some trials, chlorhexidine at a concentration of 0.2% or greater also has some disadvantages, such as increased tooth and tongue staining, unpleasant taste, and some temporary reduction in taste sensation.[34]

Essential Oils

Previous studies evaluated the short-term effect (3 hours) of a well-known, over the counter, oral rinse (which contains essential oils) compared with a placebo rinse.[104] The oral rise was found to be only moderately effective against oral malodor ($\pm$25% reduction vs. 10% for placebo of VSCs after 30 minutes) and caused a sustained reduction in the levels of odorigenic bacteria. Similar VSC reductions were found after rinsing for 4 days.[14]

Chlorine Dioxide

ClO_2 is a powerful oxidizing agent that can eliminate bad breath by oxidation of H_2S, CH_3SH, and the amino acids methionine and cysteine. Studies demonstrated that a single use of a ClO_2–containing oral rinse slightly reduced mouth odor.[36,37]

Two-Phase Oil-Water Rinse

Rosenberg and colleagues[124] designed a two-phase oil-water rinse containing CPC. The efficacy of oil-water-CPC formulations is thought to result from the adhesion of a high proportion of oral microorganisms to the oil droplets that is further enhanced by the CPC. A twice-daily rinse with this product (before bedtime and in the morning) showed reductions in both VSC levels and organoleptic ratings. These reductions were superior to those seen with Listerine and were significantly superior to placebo.[67,124]

Triclosan

Triclosan, a broad-spectrum antibacterial agent, has been found to be effective against most oral bacteria and has good compatibility with other compounds used for oral home care. A pilot study demonstrated that an experimental mouthrinse containing 0.15% triclosan and 0.84% zinc (Zn^{++}) produced a stronger and more prolonged reduction in mouth odor than a well-known over-the-counter oral rinse.[117] The anti-VSC effect of triclosan, however, seems strongly dependent on the solubilizing agents.[175] Flavoring oils or anionic detergents and copolymers are added to increase the oral retention and decrease the rate of release in toothpaste formulations containing triclosan. The effects of these formulations in oral malodor have been illustrated in several studies.[55,92,93,136,137] Significant reduction of breath scores were observed after a single use as well as after a week (28% and >50%, respectively), with a similar effect on VSC levels (57% reduction after 1 week of using the paste).

Amine Fluoride or Stannous Fluoride

The association of amine fluoride with stannous fluoride resulted in encouraging reductions of morning breath odor, even when oral hygiene was insufficient.[108] More recent evidence supporting the use of this rinse has become available. The formulation showed not only short-term but also long-term effects on malodor indicators in patients with obvious malodor.[24]

Stannous fluoride has also been shown to be effective in the management of oral malodor as a component of a dentifrice, reducing both organoleptic scores and VSC levels.[41] A superior short-term and overnight benefit of a stannous-containing dentifrice versus a control dentifrice on morning bad breath was demonstrated in a meta-analysis.[35]

Hydrogen Peroxide

Suarez and colleagues[147] reported that rinsing with 3% H_2O_2 produced impressive reductions ($\pm$90%) in sulfur gases that persisted for 8 hours.

Oxidizing Lozenges

Greenstein and associates[48] reported that sucking a lozenge with oxidizing properties reduced tongue dorsum malodor for 3 hours. This antimalodor effect may be caused by the activity of dehydroascorbic acid, which is generated by peroxide-mediated oxidation of ascorbate in the lozenges.

Baking Soda

Baking soda dentifrices have been shown to confer a significant odor-reducing benefit for up to 3 hours.[13,91] The mechanism by which baking soda produces its inhibition of oral malodor is related to its bactericidal effects.[106]

Conversion of Volatile Sulfur Compounds
Metal Salt Solutions

Metal ions with an affinity for sulfur are efficient in capturing the sulfur-containing gases. Zinc is an ion with two positive charges (Zn^{++}), which will bind to the twice-negatively loaded sulfur radicals and thus reduce the expression of VSCs. The same applies for other metal ions such as stannous, mercury, and copper. Clinically, the VSC inhibitory effect was copper chloride > stannous fluoride > zinc chloride ($CuCl_2 > SnF_2 > ZnCl_2$). In vitro, the inhibitory effect was mercury chloride = copper chloride = cadmium chloride > zinc chloride > stannous fluoride > tin chloride > lead chloride ($HgCl_2 = CuCl_2 = CdCl_2 > ZnCl_2 > SnF_2 > SnCl_2 > PbCl_2$).[177]

Compared with other metal ions, Zn^{++} is relatively nontoxic and noncumulative and gives no visible discoloration. Thus, Zn^{++} has been one of the most-studied ingredients for the control of oral malodor.[165,177] Schmidt and Tarbet[131] reported that a rinse containing zinc chloride was remarkably more effective than a saline rinse (or no treatment) in reducing the levels of both VSCs ($\pm$80% reduction) and organoleptic scores ($\pm$40% reduction) for 3 hours.

As previously noted, an over-the-counter "bad breath" mouthwash containing 0.05% chlorhexidine, 0.05% CPC, and 0.14% zinc lactate has been even more efficient than a 0.2%

chlorhexidine formulation in reducing VSC levels and organoleptic ratings.[114,157] The special effect of this mouthwash may result from the VSC conversion ability of Zn^{++}, besides its antimicrobial action. The combination of Zn^{++} and chlorhexidine seems to act synergistically.[176]

Similar observations have been reported for a chlorhexidine-free mouthrinse. The addition of zinc ions to a basic formulation containing amino fluoride and stannous fluoride caused short- and long-term reduction of oral malodor indicators in volunteers with morning bad breath[167,168] as well as in volunteers with obvious halitosis.[24]

In a study by Hoshi and van Steenberghe,[54] a zinc citrate/triclosan toothpaste applied to the tongue dorsum appeared to control morning breath malodor for 4 hours. If the flavor oil was removed, however, the antimalodor efficacy of the active ingredients decreased. Another clinical study reported up to a 41% reduction in VSC levels after 7 days' use of a dentifrice containing triclosan and a copolymer, but the benefit compared with a placebo was relatively small (17% reduction).[93] Similar reductions were also found in two other more recent studies.[55,92]

Chewing gum can be formulated with antibacterial agents, such as fluoride or chlorhexidine, helping to reduce oral malodor through both mechanical and chemical approaches. Tsunoda and associates[155] investigated the beneficial effect of chewing gum containing tea extracts for its deodorizing mechanism. *Epigallocatechin* is the main deodorizing agent among the tea catechins. The chemical reaction between epigallocatechin and CH_3SH results in a nonvolatile product. Waler[165] compared different concentrations of Zn^{++} in a chewing gum and found that a 2-mg Zn^{++} acetate–containing chewing gum that remained in the mouth for 5 minutes resulted in an immediate reduction in VSC levels of up to 45%, but the long-term effect was not mentioned.

Masking the Malodor

Treatment with rinses, mouth sprays, or lozenges containing volatiles with a pleasant odor has only a short-term effect.[118,119] Typical examples are mint-containing lozenges and the aroma of rinses without antibacterial components.[24]

Another pathway is to increase the solubility of malodorous compounds in the saliva by increasing the secretion of saliva; a larger volume allows the retention of larger volumes of soluble VSCs.[64] The latter can also be achieved by ensuring proper liquid intake or using chewing gum; chewing triggers the periodontal-parotid reflex, at least when the lower (pre)molars are still present.

CONCLUSION

Breath malodor has important socioeconomic consequences and can reveal important diseases. A proper diagnosis and determination of the etiology allow initiation of the proper etiologic treatment. Although tongue coating and (less frequently) periodontitis and gingivitis are by far the most common causes of malodor, the dental hygienist cannot take the risk of overlooking other, more challenging diseases. This can be done with a multidisciplinary consultation or, if this is not feasible, a trial therapy to deal quickly with intraoral causes (e.g., full-mouth one-stage disinfection, including the use of proper mouthrinses, tongue scrapers, and toothpastes). For more detailed information, the reader is encouraged to consult review articles.[47,71,135]

A Case Scenario is found on the companion website.

REFERENCES

 References for this chapter are found on the companion website.

45

Scaling and Root Planing[a]

 For online-only content on general principles of instrumentation, principles of scaling and root planing, and instrument sharpening, please visit the companion website.

CHAPTER OUTLINE

Periodontal instruments are designed for specific purposes, such as calculus removal, biofilm removal, and root planing. On first investigation, the variety of instruments available for similar purposes appear confusing. With experience, however, dental hygienists select a set that fulfills requirements and personal preference.

CLASSIFICATION OF PERIODONTAL INSTRUMENTS

Periodontal instruments are classified according to the purposes they serve, as follows:

1. *Periodontal probes* are used to locate and measure the depth of pockets, as well as determine their pattern on individual tooth surfaces.
2. *Explorers* are used to locate calculus deposits, surface irregularities, overhanging restorations, and caries.
3. *Scaling, root-planing, and curettage instruments* are used for removal of biofilm and calcified deposits from the crown and root of a tooth and removal of altered cementum from the subgingival root surface. Scaling and root planing instruments are classified as follows:
   - *Sickle scalers* are heavy instruments used to remove supragingival calculus.
   - *Curettes* are instruments used for subgingival scaling and root planing.
   - *Hoe, chisel, and file scalers* are used to remove tenacious calculus and altered cementum. Their use is limited compared with that of curettes.
   - *Implant instruments* are plastic or titanium scalers and curettes designed for use on implants and implant restorations.

- *Ultrasonic and sonic instruments* are used for scaling and cleansing tooth surfaces and curetting the soft tissue wall of the periodontal pocket.[42,43,66]
4. *Periodontal endoscopes* are used for deep visualization into subgingival pockets and furcations, thereby allowing the detection of deposits.
5. *Cleansing and polishing instruments*, such as rubber cups, brushes, and dental tape, are used to clean and polish tooth surfaces. Air-powder abrasive systems are also available for supragingival and subgingival cleaning and polishing of tooth, root, and implant surfaces.

The wearing and cutting qualities of some types of steel used in periodontal instruments have been tested,[88,89,157] but specifications vary among manufacturers.[157] Stainless steel is used most often in instrument manufacture. High–carbon content steel instruments are available and are considered by some clinicians to be superior. Newer advanced proprietary manufacturing processes for heat treating and cryogenically tempering stainless steel are producing blades that are sharper and longer lasting than ever before. In addition, other processes produce stainless steel instruments with titanium nitride or other surface coatings. Their cutting edges are sharp when new and hold a sharp edge longer, but wear down during normal use and cannot be resharpened. Each group of instruments has characteristic features; individual therapists often develop variations with which they operate most effectively. Small instruments are recommended to fit into periodontal pockets without injuring the soft tissues.[116,118,119,174]

The parts of each instrument are referred to as the working end, shank, and handle (Fig. 45.1).

Periodontal Probes

Periodontal probes are used to measure the depth of pockets and to determine their configuration. The typical probe is a tapered, rod-like instrument calibrated in millimeters, with a blunt, rounded tip (Fig. 45.2). Several other designs with various millimeter calibrations are available (Fig. 45.3). The World Health

[a]Adapted from the following chapter of Newman and Carranza's Clinical Periodontology, 13th edition: Chapter 50: Scaling and Root Planing, by Anna M. Pattison and Gordon L. Pattison. Material in this chapter was derived from Pattison A, Pattison G, Matsuda S: *Periodontal instrumentation*, ed 3, New York, 2018, Pearson Education.

Fig. 45.1 Parts of a Typical Periodontal Instrument.

Fig. 45.2 Periodontal Probe Is Composed of the Handle, Shank, and Calibrated Working End.

Fig. 45.4 Curved #2 Nabers Probe for Detection of Furcation Areas, With Color-Coded Markings at 3, 6, 9, and 12 mm.

Fig. 45.3 Types of Periodontal Probes. (A) Marquis color-coded probe. Calibrations are in 3-mm sections. (B) University of North Carolina 15 probe, a 15-mm long probe marked at each millimeter and color coded at the 5th, 10th, and 15th millimeters. (C) University of Michigan "O" probe, with Williams markings (at 1, 2, 3, 5, 7, 8, 9, and 10 mm). (D) Michigan "O" probe with markings at 3, 6, and 8 mm. (E) World Health Organization probe, which has a 0.5-mm ball at the tip and markings at 3.5, 8.5, and 11.5 mm and color coding from 3.5 to 5.5 mm.

Fig. 45.5 Five Typical Explorers. (A) #17; (B) #23; (C) EXD 11-12; (D) #3; (E) #3CH pigtail.

Organization probe has millimeter markings and a small, round ball at the tip (see Fig. 45.3E). Ideally, these probes are thin, and the shank is angled to allow easy insertion into the pocket. Many clinicians believe furcation areas can best be evaluated with the curved, blunt Nabers probe (Fig. 45.4).

Explorers

Explorers are used to locate subgingival deposits, surface irregularities, margin discrepancies of restorations, and carious areas, and to check the smoothness of the root surfaces after root planing. Explorers are designed with different shapes and angles, with various uses (Fig. 45.5), as well as limitations (Fig. 45.6). The periodontal probe can also be useful in the detection of subgingival deposits (see Fig. 45.6D).

> **KEY FACT**
>
> Periodontal probes are used to measure the depth of pockets and to determine their configuration.
>
> When measuring a pocket, the probe is inserted with firm, gentle pressure to the epithelial junction at the base of the pocket. The shank should be aligned with the long axis of the tooth surface to be probed. Six measurements are made on each tooth to determine the level of epithelial attachment.

> **KEY FACT**
>
> Explorers are used to locate subgingival deposits, surface irregularities, and carious areas and to check the smoothness of the root surfaces after root planing.

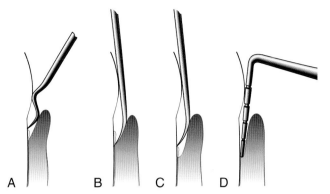

Fig. 45.6 Insertion of Two Types of Explorers and a Periodontal Probe in a Pocket for Calculus Detection. (A) The limitations of the pigtail explorer in a deep pocket. (B) Insertion of the #3 explorer. (C) Limitations of the #3 explorer. (D) Insertion of the periodontal probe.

Fig. 45.8 Basic Characteristics of a Sickle Scaler: Triangular Shape, Double-Cutting Edge, and Pointed Tip.

Fig. 45.7 The Five Basic Scaling Instruments. (A) Curette; (B) sickle; (C) file; (D) chisel; (E) hoe.

Fig. 45.9 Use of a Sickle Scaler for Removal of Supragingival Calculus.

Scaling and Curettage Instruments

Scaling and curettage instruments are illustrated in Fig. 45.7.

Sickle Scalers

Sickle scalers have a flat surface and most have two cutting edges that converge in a sharply pointed tip. The shape of the instrument makes the tip strong so that it will not break off during use (Fig. 45.8). The sickle scaler is used to remove supragingival calculus (Fig. 45.9). Because of the design of this instrument, it is difficult to insert a large sickle blade under the gingiva without damaging the surrounding gingival tissues (Fig. 45.10).

Sickle scalers of the same basic design can be obtained with different blade sizes and shank types to adapt to specific uses. The U15/30 (Fig. 45.11), Ball, and Indiana University sickle scalers are large. Jacquette sickle scalers #1, #2, and #3 have medium-size blades. Curved 204 posterior sickle scalers are available with large, medium, or small blades (Fig. 45.12). The Montana Jack,

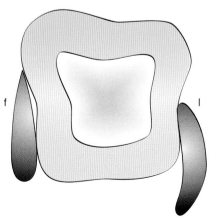

Fig. 45.10 Subgingival Adaptation Around the Root Is Better With the Curette Than With the Sickle. *f*, Facial; *l*, lingual.

Fig. 45.11 Both Ends of a U15/30 Scaler.

Fig. 45.13 The Curette Is the Instrument of Choice for Subgingival Scaling and Root Planing.

Fig. 45.12 Three Different Sizes of 204 Sickle Scalers.

Fig. 45.14 Basic Characteristics of a Curette: Spoon-Shaped Blade and Rounded Tip.

Black Jack, and the Nevi 2, Nevi 3, and Nevi 4 curved posterior sickle scalers are all thin enough to be inserted slightly subgingival for removal of light to moderate ledges of calculus. The selection of these instruments should be based on the area to be scaled. Sickle scalers with straight shanks are designed for use on anterior teeth and premolars. Sickle scalers with contra-angled shanks adapt to posterior teeth.

Curettes

The curette is the instrument of choice for removing deep sub-gingival calculus, root planing, and altered cementum (Fig. 45.13). Each working end has a cutting edge on both sides of the blade and a rounded toe. Curettes are finer than sickle scalers and do not have any sharp points or corners other than the cutting edges of the blade (Fig. 45.14). Therefore curettes can be adapted for and provide good access to deep pockets, with minimal soft tissue trauma (see Fig. 45.10). In cross section, the blade appears semicircular with a convex base. The lateral border of the convex base forms a cutting edge with the face of the semicircular blade. Cutting edges are present on both sides of the blade. Both single- and double-end curettes may be obtained, depending on the preference of the operator.

> **KEY FACT**
>
> The curette is the instrument of choice for removing deep subgingival calculus, root planing, and altered cementum.
>
> As shown in Fig. 45.10, the curved blade and rounded toe of the curette allow the blade to adapt better to the root surface, unlike the straight design and pointed end of a sickle scaler, which can cause tissue laceration and trauma. The two basic types of curettes are universal and area specific.

Universal curettes. Universal curettes have cutting edges that may be inserted in most areas of the dentition by altering and adapting the finger rest, fulcrum, and hand position of the operator. The blade size and the angle and length of the shank may vary, but the face of the blade of every universal curette is at a 90-degree angle (perpendicular) to the lower shank when seen in cross section from the tip (Fig. 45.15A). The blade of the universal curette is curved in one direction from the head of the blade toward the toe. Barnhart curettes #1-2 and #5-6 and Columbia curettes #13-14, #2R-2L, and #4R-4L (Figs. 45.16 and 45.17A) are examples of universal curettes. Other popular universal curettes are Younger-Good #7-8, McCall's #17-18, and Indiana University #17-18 (see Fig. 45.17B).

Area-specific curettes.

Gracey curettes. Gracey curettes are representative of the area-specific curettes, a set of several instruments designed and angled to adapt to specific anatomic areas of the dentition (Fig. 45.18). These curettes and their modifications are probably the best instruments for subgingival scaling and root planing because they provide the best adaptation to complex root anatomy. Gracey

> **KEY FACT**
>
> Universal curettes have cutting edges that may be inserted in most areas of the dentition by altering and adapting the finger rest, fulcrum, and hand position of the operator.

Fig. 45.17 (A) Columbia #4R-4L universal curette. (B) Younger-Good #7-8, McCall's #17-18, and Indiana University #17-18 universal curettes.

Fig. 45.18 Reduced Set of Gracey Curettes. *Left to right,* #5-6, #7-8, #11-12, and #13-14.

Fig. 45.15 Principal Types of Curettes as Seen From the Toe of the Instrument. (A) Universal curette. (B) Gracey curette. Note the offset blade angulation of the Gracey curette.

Fig. 45.16 (A) Double-ended curette for the removal of subgingival calculus. (B) Cross section of the curette blade *(arrow)* against the cemental wall of a deep periodontal pocket. (C) Curette inserted in a pocket with the tip directed apically. (D) Curette in position at the base of a periodontal pocket on the facial surface of a mandibular molar. (E) Curette in position at the base of a pocket on the distal surface of the mandibular molar.

KEY FACT

Gracey curettes are representative of the area-specific curettes, a set of several instruments designed and angled to adapt to specific anatomic areas of the dentition.

Double-ended Gracey curettes are paired in the following manner:

Gracey #1-2 and #3-4: Anterior teeth
Gracey #5-6: Anterior teeth and premolars
Gracey #7-8 and #9-10: Posterior teeth, facial and lingual
Gracey #11-12: Posterior teeth, mesial access (Fig. 45.19)
Gracey #13-14: Posterior teeth, distal access (Fig. 45.20)
Gracey #15-16: Posterior teeth, mesial access
Gracey #17-18: Posterior teeth, distal access

Single-ended Gracey curettes can also be obtained. Although these curettes are designed to be used in specific areas, an experienced operator can adapt each instrument for use in several different areas by altering the position of his or her hand and the position of the patient.

Gracey curettes also differ from universal curettes in that the blade is not at a 90-degree angle to the lower shank. The term *offset blade* is used to describe Gracey curettes because they are angled approximately 70 degrees from the lower shank (see Fig. 45.15B). This unique angulation allows the blade to be inserted in the precise position necessary for subgingival scaling and root planing, provided the lower shank is parallel to the long axis of the tooth surface being scaled.

Fig. 45.19 Gracey #11-12 Curette. For mesial surfaces.

KEY FACT

Gracey curettes also differ from universal curettes in that the blade is not at a 90-degree angle to the lower shank.

Area-specific curettes also have curved blades. Whereas the blade of the universal curette is curved in one direction (Fig. 45.21A), the Gracey blade is curved from shank to toe and also appears to be curved along the side of the cutting edge (see Fig. 45.21B). Table 45.1 lists some of the major differences between Gracey (area-specific) curettes and universal curettes.

Gracey curettes are available with either a "rigid" or "flexible" type of shank. The rigid Gracey has a larger, stronger, and less flexible shank and blade than the standard Gracey. The rigid shank allows the removal of moderate to heavy calculus without using a separate set of heavy scalers, such as sickles and hoes. Although some clinicians prefer the enhanced tactile sensitivity that the flexible shank of the standard Gracey provides, both types of Gracey curettes are suitable for root planing.

More recent additions to the Gracey curette set have been #15-16 and #17-18. The Gracey #15-16 is a modification of the standard #11-12 and is designed for the mesial surfaces of posterior teeth (Fig. 45.22). It consists of a Gracey #11-12 blade combined with the more acutely angled #13-14 shank. When the dental hygienist is using an intraoral finger rest, it is often difficult to position the lower shank of the Gracey #11-12 so that it is parallel to the mesial surfaces of the posterior teeth, especially on the mandibular molars. The newer shank angulation of the Gracey #15-16 allows better adaptation to posterior mesial surfaces from a front position with intraoral rests. If alternative fulcrums, such as extraoral or opposite-arch rests, are used, the Gracey #11-12 works well and the #15-16 is not essential. The Gracey #17-18 is a modification of the #13-14. It has a terminal shank elongated by 3 mm and a more accentuated angulation of the shank to provide complete occlusal clearance and better access to all posterior distal surfaces. The horizontal handle position minimizes interference from opposing arches and allows a more relaxed hand position when scaling distal surfaces. In addition, the blade is 1 mm shorter to allow better adaptation of the blade to distal tooth surfaces.

Fig. 45.20 Gracey #13-14 Curette. For distal surfaces.

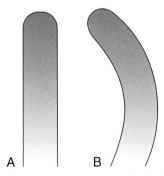

Fig. 45.21 (A) Universal curette as seen with the face of the blade parallel to the floor. Note that the blade is straight. (B) Gracey curette as seen with the face of the blade parallel to the floor. Only the outer convex cutting edge is used.

TABLE 45.1 Comparison of Area-Specific (Gracey) and Universal Curettes

	Gracey Curette	Universal Curette
Area of use	Set of many curettes designed for specific areas and surfaces	One curette designed for all areas and surfaces
Cutting Edge		
Use	One cutting edge used; work with outer edge only	Both cutting edges used; work with either outer or inner edge
Curvature	Blade curves from the shank toward the toe and also appears to curve to the side	Blade curves only from the shank toward the toe, not to the side
Blade angle	Offset blade; face of blade beveled at 60 degrees to shank	Blade not offset; face of blade beveled at 90 degrees to shank

Modified from Pattison G, Pattison A: *Periodontal instrumentation*, ed 2, Norwalk, 1992, Appleton & Lange.

Fig. 45.23 After Five Curettes. Note the extra 3 mm in the terminal shank of After Five curettes compared with standard Gracey curettes. (A) #5-6; (B) #7-8; (C) #11-12; (D) #13-14. (Copyright A. Pattison.)

Fig. 45.24 Comparison of After Five Curette With Standard Gracey Curette. Rigid Gracey #13-14 adapted to the distal surface of the first molar and rigid After Five #13-14 adapted to the distal surface of the second molar. Notice the extralong shank of the After Five curette, which allows deeper insertion and better access. (Copyright A. Pattison.)

KEY FACT

Extended-shank curettes are modifications of the standard Gracey curette design.

Fig. 45.22 Gracey #15-16. New Gracey curette, designed for mesio-posterior surfaces, combines a Gracey #11-12 blade with a Gracey #13-14 shank. (Copyright A. Pattison.)

curettes have one cutting edge on each working end as opposed to two cutting edges on each working end of the universal curette.

Extended-shank curettes. Extended-shank curettes are modifications of the standard Gracey curette design. The terminal shank is 3 mm longer, allowing extension into deeper periodontal pockets of 5 mm or more (Figs. 45.23 and 45.24). Other features of extended shank curettes include a thinned blade for smoother subgingival insertion and reduced tissue distention and a large-diameter, tapered shank. All standard Gracey numbers except for the #9-10 (i.e., #1-2, #3-4, #5-6, #7-8, #11-12, or #13-14) are available in the extended shank. Extended shank curettes are available in flexible or rigid designs. For heavy or tenacious calculus removal, rigid curettes should be used. For light scaling or deplaquing in a periodontal maintenance patient, the thinner flexible curettes will insert subgingivally more easily.

Mini-blade curettes. Mini-blade curettes are modifications of the extended shank curettes. Mini-blade curettes feature blades that are half the length of standard Gracey curettes (Fig. 45.25). The shorter blade allows easier insertion and adaptation in deep, narrow pockets; furcations; developmental grooves; line angles; and deep, tight facial, lingual, or palatal pockets. In any area where root morphology or tight tissue prevents full insertion of the standard Gracey or After Five blade, Mini Five curettes can be used with vertical strokes, with reduced tissue distention and no tissue trauma (Fig. 45.26).

Periodontal maintenance curettes. The most recent Gracey curette innovation is a category called periodontal maintenance Gracey curettes, introduced in November 2015. These instruments are specifically designed for patients with tight tissue, recession, and residual pocket depth following initial periodontal therapy or periodontal surgery. They can also be used on maintenance

Fig. 45.25 Comparison of After Five Curette and Mini Five Curette. The shorter Mini Five blade (half the length) allows increased access and reduced tissue trauma.

Fig. 45.26 Comparison of Standard Rigid Gracey #5-6 With Rigid Mini Five #5-6 on the Palatal Surfaces of the Maxillary Central Incisors. Mini Five curette can be inserted to the base of these tight anterior pockets and used with a straight vertical stroke. The standard Gracey or After Five curette usually cannot be inserted vertically in this area because the blade is too long. (Copyright A. Pattison.)

Fig. 45.27 Micro Mini Five Gracey Curettes. *Left to right,* #1-2, #7-8, #11-12, #13-14. (Copyright A. Pattison.)

| Standard | After Five | Mini Five | Micro Mini Five |

Fig. 45.28 Comparison of Gracey Curette Designs. *Left to right,* Standard #1-2, After Five #1-2, Mini Five #1-2, Micro Mini Five #1-2. (Courtesy Hu-Friedy, Chicago, IL.)

KEY FACT

Mini-blade curettes feature blades that are half the length of standard Gracey curettes. The shorter blade allows easier insertion and adaptation in deep, narrow pockets; furcations; developmental grooves; line angles; and deep, tight facial, lingual, or palatal pockets.

In the past the only solution in most of these areas of difficult access was to use Gracey curettes with a toe-down horizontal stroke. Mini-blade curettes, along with other short-bladed instruments recently introduced, opened a new chapter in the history of root instrumentation by allowing access to areas that previously were extremely difficult or impossible to reach with standard instruments. Mini-blade curettes are available in both flexible and rigid designs. As with the extended shank series, mini-blade curettes are available in all standard Gracey numbers, except the #9-10.

The recently introduced *Micro Mini Five* Gracey curettes (Hu-Friedy) have blades that are 20% thinner and smaller than the mini-blade curettes (Figs. 45.27 and 45.28). These are the smallest of all curettes, and they provide exceptional access and adaptation to tight, deep, or narrow pockets; narrow furcations; developmental depressions; line angles; and deep pockets on facial, lingual, or palatal surfaces. In areas where root morphology or tight, thin tissue prevents easy insertion of other mini-bladed curettes, Micro Mini Five curettes can be used with vertical strokes without causing tissue distention or tissue trauma.

KEY FACT

Micro Mini Five Gracey curettes (Hu-Friedy, Chicago, IL) have blades that are 20% thinner and smaller than the mini-blade curettes. These are the smallest of all curettes, and they provide exceptional access and adaptation to tight, deep, or narrow pockets; narrow furcations; developmental depressions; line angles; and deep pockets on facial, lingual, or palatal surfaces.

Gracey Curvettes comprise another set of four mini-bladed curettes; the Sub-0 and #1-2 are used for anterior teeth and premolars, the #11-12 is used for posterior mesial surfaces, and the #13-14 is used for posterior distal surfaces. The blade length of these instruments is 50% shorter than that of the conventional Gracey curette, and the blade is curved slightly upward (Fig. 45.29). This curvature allows Gracey Curvettes to adapt more closely to the tooth surface than any other curettes, especially on the anterior teeth and on line angles (Fig. 45.30). However, this curvature also carries the risk of gouging or "grooving" into the root surfaces on the proximal surfaces of the posterior teeth when #11-12 or #13-14 is used. Additional features that represent improvements on the standard Gracey curettes are a precision-balanced blade tip in direct alignment with the handle, a blade tip perpendicular to the handle, and a shank closer to parallel with the handle.

Fig. 45.29 Gracey Curvette Blade. This diagram shows the 50% shorter blade of the Gracey Curvette superimposed on the standard Gracey curette blade *(dotted lines)*. Notice the upward curvature of the Curvette blade and blade tip. (Redrawn from Pattison G, Pattison A: *Periodontal instrumentation,* ed 2, Norwalk, 1992, Appleton & Lange.)

Fig. 45.30 Gracey Curvette Sub-0 on the Palatal Surface of a Maxillary Central Incisor. The long shank and short, curved, blunted tip make this a superior instrument for deep anterior pockets. This curette provides excellent blade adaptation to the narrow root curvatures of the maxillary and mandibular anterior teeth. (Copyright A. Pattison.)

Fig. 45.31 Periodontal Maintenance Gracey Curettes (Hu-Friedy) Shorter, Thinner Three-Quarter–Sized Gracey Curettes With Modified Rigid Shanks. *Left to right,* Pattison Gracey Lite #1-2, Pattison Gracey Lite #7-8, Pattison Gracey Lite #11-12, Pattison Gracey Lite #13-14. (Copyright A. Pattison.)

> ### KEY FACT
>
> The most recent Gracey curette innovation is a category called periodontal maintenance Gracey curettes, introduced in November 2015. These instruments are specifically designed for patients with tight tissue, recession, and residual pocket depth following initial periodontal therapy or periodontal surgery.
>
> This newer blade is 1 mm shorter and 20% thinner, and the face of the blade is offset from the terminal shank at 60 degrees as opposed to all other Gracey designs, which are offset at 70 degrees. This slight modification to the blade-to-shank angle and the thinner, narrow blade allow easier insertion and better access to root surfaces with tight tissue and loss of attachment. Working angulation can be achieved without as much tissue distention, thus increasing patient comfort. The three-quarter blade length of this new type of Gracey curette is between the blade lengths of the standard and mini-bladed Gracey curettes. The shorter blade adapts more easily to root anatomy and furcation areas and helps to prevent spanning across root depressions.
>
> The shank length is 2 mm longer than that of the standard Gracey curette, but 1 mm shorter than that of the extended shank Gracey curette. This length enables better access to molar areas with attachment loss but still allows ease of use in the anterior areas where a very long shank is not necessary. The shank angle of the new Gracey #11-12 is between the regular Gracey #11-12 and the Gracey #15-16, and the shank angle of the new Gracey #13-14 is between the regular Gracey #13-14 and the Gracey #17-18. These shank angle modifications were developed to enhance access to the mesial and distal surfaces of the posterior teeth.
>
> The shanks of these newer instruments are rigid so they can withstand firm pressure when removal of residual burnished calculus is necessary. However, they are not designed for moderate or heavy calculus removal. The clinician must be mindful that the instrument blade is at a slightly more closed angle than the traditional Gracey curette, so if more substantial or tenacious calculus is encountered, the clinician must slightly open the blade angulation, or switch to a rigid standard Gracey curette, or use a different manual or ultrasonic instrument.

patients with healthier tight tissue without attachment loss or recession. In both cases, patients require a small, thin blade to allow subgingival insertion with ease (Fig. 45.31).

Langer and Mini-Langer curettes. Langer and Mini-Langer curettes comprise a set of three curettes combining the shank design of standard Gracey #5-6, #11-12, and #13-14 curettes with a universal blade honed at 90 degrees rather than the offset blade of the Gracey curette. This marriage of the Gracey and universal curette designs allows the advantages of the area-specific shank to be combined with the versatility of the universal curette blade. The Langer #5-6 curette adapts to the mesial and distal surfaces of anterior teeth; the Langer #1-2 curette (Gracey #11-12 shank) adapts to the mesial and distal surfaces of mandibular posterior teeth; and the Langer #3-4 curette (Gracey #13-14 shank) adapts to the mesial and distal surfaces of maxillary posterior teeth (Fig. 45.32). These instruments can be adapted to both mesial and distal tooth surfaces without changing instruments. The standard Langer curette shanks are heavier than a finishing Gracey but less rigid than the rigid Gracey. Langer curettes are also available with either rigid or finishing shanks and can be obtained in extended-shank and mini-bladed versions.

Schwartz Periotrievers

Schwartz Periotrievers comprise a set of two double-ended, highly magnetized instruments designed for retrieval of a broken instrument tip from the periodontal pocket (Fig. 45.33). They are indispensable when the clinician has broken a curette tip in a furcation or deep pocket.[148]

Plastic and Titanium Instruments for Implants

Several companies are manufacturing plastic and titanium instruments for use on titanium and other implant abutment

Fig. 45.32 Langer Curettes Combine Gracey-Type Shanks With Universal Curette Blades. *Left to right,* #5-6, #1-2, and #3-4. (Copyright A. Pattison.)

Fig. 45.34 (A) Plastic probe: Colorvue. (B) New Implacare II Barnhart #5-6 cone socket plastic curette tips that screw into an autoclavable stainless steel handle. (Courtesy Hu-Friedy, Chicago, IL.)

Fig. 45.33 Broken Instrument Tip Attached to the Magnetic Tip of a Schwartz Periotriever (Daness Dental Distributors, Nyack, NY). (From Pattison G, Pattison A: *Periodontal instrumentation,* ed 2, Norwalk, 1992, Appleton & Lange.)

Fig. 45.35 New Mini Titanium Implant Scalers (Hu-Friedy, Chicago). *Left to right,* Mini Five Gracey #1-2, Mini Five Gracey #11-12, Langer #1-2, Mini Five Gracey #13-14, 204SD Sickle Scaler.

materials. It is important that plastic or titanium instruments be used to avoid scarring and permanent damage to implants[b] (Figs. 45.34–45.36).

Mini-bladed titanium implant instruments are now available in both universal and Gracey curette designs (see Fig. 45.36B). Although most standard titanium implant instrument blades are large, the newer mini-bladed titanium curettes insert more easily under tight tissue and adapt more easily around implants and implant restorations. They may be used for implant maintenance with careful, light-pressured strokes for biofilm and light calculus removal. Moderate- or heavy-pressured strokes should be avoided to prevent scratching or roughening of implant surfaces. These instruments are not intended for removal of heavy calculus or cement. Such deposits are often found in cases of peri-implantitis with moderate to advanced bone loss and exposure of implant threads. Removal of tenacious deposits requires other forms of instrumentation and surgical treatment of the implant. (See Chapter 58 for information on implant complications.)

---

[b]References 23, 39, 43, 48, 57, 96, 142.

KEY FACT

Several companies are manufacturing plastic and titanium instruments for use on titanium and other implant abutment materials. It is important that plastic or titanium instruments be used to avoid scarring and permanent damage to implants.

Hoe Scalers

Hoe scalers are used for scaling of ledges or rings of calculus (Fig. 45.37). The blade is bent at a 99-degree angle, and the cutting edge is formed by the junction of the flattened terminal surface with the inner aspect of the blade. The cutting edge is beveled at 45 degrees. The blade is slightly bowed so that it can maintain contact at two points on a convex surface. The back of the blade is rounded, and the blade has been reduced to minimal thickness to permit access to the roots without interference from the adjacent tissues.

Fig. 45.36 (A) Micro Mini titanium implant curettes (Paradise Dental Technologies, Missoula, MT). *Left to right,* Gracey #1-2 Micro Mini, Gracey #11-12 Micro Mini, Gracey #13-14 Micro Mini. (B) Mini-bladed titanium implant curettes (LM Instruments, Parainen, Finland): Mini universal curette, Mini Gracey #1-2, Mini Gracey #13-14, Mini Gracey #11-12.

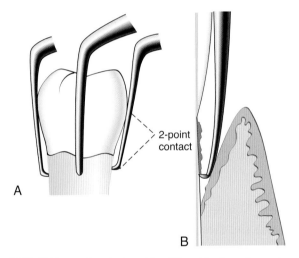

Fig. 45.37 (A) Hoe scalers designed for different tooth surfaces, showing "two-point" contact. (B) Hoe scaler in a periodontal pocket. The back of the blade is rounded for easier access. The instrument contacts the tooth at two points for stability.

Fig. 45.38 (A) Chisel scaler and (B) file scaler.

Hoe scalers are used in the following manner:

1. The blade is inserted into the base of the periodontal pocket so that it makes two-point contact with the tooth (see Fig. 45.37). This stabilizes the instrument and prevents nicking of the root.
2. The instrument is activated with a firm pull stroke toward the crown, with every effort made to preserve the two-point contact with the tooth.

McCall's #3, #4, #5, #6, #7, and #8 comprise a set of six hoe scalers designed to provide access to all tooth surfaces. Each instrument has a different angle between the shank and the handle.

Files

Files have a series of blades on a base (Fig. 45.38). Their primary function is to fracture or crush large deposits of tenacious calculus or burnished sheets of calculus. Files can easily gouge and roughen root surfaces when they are used improperly. Therefore, they are not suitable for fine scaling and root planing. Mini-bladed curettes are currently preferred for fine scaling in areas where files were once used. Files are sometimes used for removing overhanging margins of dental restorations.

KEY FACT

Files have a series of blades on a base. Their primary function is to fracture or crush large deposits of tenacious calculus or burnished sheets of calculus.

Chisel Scalers

The chisel scaler, designed for the proximal surfaces of teeth too closely spaced to permit the use of other scalers, is usually used in the anterior part of the mouth. It is a double-ended instrument with a curved shank at one end and a straight shank at the other (see Fig. 45.38); the blades are slightly curved and have a straight cutting edge beveled at 45 degrees.

The chisel is inserted from the facial surface. The slight curve of the blade makes it possible to stabilize it against the proximal surface, while the cutting edge engages the calculus without nicking the tooth. The instrument is activated with a push motion while the side of the blade is held firmly against the root.

Quétin Furcation Curettes

Quétin furcation curettes are actually hoes with a shallow, half-moon radius that fits into the roof or floor of the furcation. The curvature of the tip also fits into developmental depressions on the inner aspect of the roots. The shanks are slightly curved for better access, and the tips are available in two widths (Fig. 45.39). The BL1 *(buccal-lingual)* and MD1 *(mesial-distal)* instruments are small and fine, with a 0.9-mm blade width. The BL2 and MD2 instruments are larger and wider, with a 1.3-mm blade width.

Fig. 45.39 Quétin Furcation Curettes: BL2 (Larger) and BL1 (Smaller). (Copyright A. Pattison.)

These instruments remove burnished calculus from recessed areas of the furcation where curettes, even mini-bladed curettes, are often too large to gain access. Using mini-bladed Gracey curettes and Gracey Curvettes on the ceiling or floor of the furcation may unintentionally create gouges and grooves. The Quétin instruments, however, are well suited for this area and lessen the likelihood of root damage.

Diamond-Coated Files

Diamond-coated files are unique instruments used for final finishing of root surfaces. These files do not have cutting edges; instead, they are coated with very fine-grit diamond (Fig. 45.40). The most useful diamond files are the buccal-lingual instruments, which are used in furcations and also adapt well to many other root surfaces.

New diamond files are sharply abrasive and should be used with light, even pressure against the root surface to avoid gouging or grooving. When viewing the root surface with the dental endoscope after all tactilely detectable deposits are gone, one can observe small embedded remnants of calculus in the root surface. Diamond files are used similar to an emery board to remove these minute remnants of calculus from the root, to create a surface that is free of all visible accretions. Diamond files can produce a smooth, even, clean, and highly polished root surface.

Diamond files must be used carefully because they can cause overinstrumentation of the root surface. They will remove too much root structure if they are used with excessive force, are poorly adapted to root morphology, or are used too long in one place.

Diamond files are particularly effective when used with the dental endoscope, which reveals residual deposits and directs the clinician to the exact area for instrumentation.

Ultrasonic and Sonic Instruments

Ultrasonic instruments may be used for removing biofilm, scaling, curetting, and removing stain (see Chapter 46).

Fig. 45.40 Diamond Files. (A) #1, #2 and (B) #3, #4. (Brasseler, Savannah, GA.) (C) SDCN 7, SDCM/D 7. (Hu-Friedy, Chicago.) (Copyright A. Pattison.)

Fig. 45.43 Perioscopic Instrumentation Permits Deep Subgingival Visualization in Pockets and Furcations. (Courtesy Perioscopy, Inc., Oakland, CA.)

Fig. 45.41 Perioscopy System, Dental Endoscope. (Courtesy Perioscopy, Inc., Oakland, CA.)

Fig. 45.42 Viewing Periodontal Explorers (Left/Right/Full Viewing) for the Perioscopy System. (Courtesy Perioscopy, Inc., Oakland, CA.)

Dental Endoscope

A dental endoscope has been introduced for use subgingivally in the diagnosis and treatment of periodontal disease (Fig. 45.41). The *Perioscopy* system consists of a 0.99-mm-diameter reusable fiberoptic endoscope over which is fitted a disposable sterile sheath. The fiberoptic endoscope fits onto periodontal probes and ultrasonic instruments that have been designed to accept it (Fig. 45.42). The sheath delivers water irrigation that flushes the pocket while the endoscope is being used, thereby keeping the field clear. The fiberoptic endoscope attaches to a medical-grade charge-coupled device (CCD) video camera and light source that produces an image on a flat-panel monitor for viewing during subgingival exploration and instrumentation. This device allows clear visualization deep into subgingival pockets and furcations (Fig. 45.43). It permits operators to detect the presence and location of subgingival deposits and guides them in the thorough removal of these deposits. Magnification ranges from 24 to 48 times, enabling visualization of even minute deposits of plaque and calculus. Using this device, operators can achieve levels of root debridement and cleanliness that are much more difficult or impossible to produce without it.[160,161,179,180] The Perioscopy system can also be used to evaluate subgingival areas for caries, defective restorations, root fractures, and resorption.

KEY FACT

Using this device, operators can achieve levels of root debridement and cleanliness that are much more difficult or impossible to produce without it. The Perioscopy system can also be used to evaluate subgingival areas for caries, defective restorations, root fractures, and resorption.

Cleansing and Polishing Instruments
Rubber Cups

Rubber cups consist of a rubber shell with or without webbed configurations in the hollow interior (Fig. 45.44). They are used in the handpiece with a special prophylaxis angle. The handpiece, prophylaxis angle, and rubber cup must be sterilized after each patient use, or a disposable plastic prophylaxis angle and rubber cup may be used and then discarded (Fig. 45.45). A good cleansing and polishing paste that contains fluoride should be used and kept moist to minimize frictional heat as the cup revolves. Polishing pastes are available in fine, medium, or coarse grit and are packaged in small, convenient, single-use containers. Aggressive use of the rubber cup with any abrasive may remove the layer of cementum, which is thin in the cervical area.

Dental Tape

Dental tape with polishing paste or polishing strips can be used for polishing proximal surfaces that are inaccessible to other polishing instruments. The tape is passed interproximally while

Fig. 45.44 Metal Prophylaxis Angle With Rubber Cup and Brush.

Fig. 45.45 Disposable Plastic Prophylaxis Angle With Rubber Cup and With Brush.

Fig. 45.46 Cavitron Prophy-Jet Air-Powder Polishing Device. (Courtesy Dentsply International, York, PA.)

Fig. 45.47 Hu-Friedy Ems Air Flow Master Air Polishing Device With Perio and Standard Handpieces and Tips for Both Supragingival and Subgingival Air Polishing. (Courtesy Hu-Friedy, Chicago, IL.)

being kept at a right angle to the long axis of the tooth and is activated with a firm labiolingual motion. Particular care is taken to avoid injury to the gingiva. The area should be cleansed with warm water to remove all remnants of paste.

Air-Powder Polishing

The first specially designed handpiece to deliver an air-powered slurry of warm water and sodium bicarbonate for polishing was introduced in the early 1980s. This device is very effective for removing extrinsic stains and soft deposits (Fig. 45.46). The slurry removes stains rapidly and efficiently by mechanical abrasion and provides warm water for rinsing and lavage. The flow rate of the abrasive cleansing power can be adjusted to increase the amount of powder for heavier stain removal. Currently, many manufacturers produce air-powder polishing systems that use various powder formulas (Fig. 45.47).

The results of studies on the abrasive effect of the air-powder polishing devices using sodium bicarbonate and aluminum trihydroxide on cementum and dentin show that significant tooth substance can be lost.[2,20,117,125] Damage to gingival tissue is transient and insignificant clinically, but amalgam restorations, composite resins, cements, and other nonmetallic materials can be roughened.[13,44,72,94,172] Polishing powders containing glycine or erythritol rather than sodium bicarbonate are commonly used for subgingival biofilm removal from root surfaces.[103,124]

Both supragingival and subgingival air polishing with glycine or erythritol powder are safe and very effective for removal of biofilm from titanium implant surfaces and restorative materials[79,96,136] (Fig. 45.48).

> ### KEY FACT
>
> Both supragingival and subgingival air polishing with glycine or erythritol powder are safe and very effective for removal of biofilm from titanium implant surfaces and restorative materials.
>
> No soft tissue abrasion occurs, and at probing depths of 1 mm to greater than 5 mm, the use of glycine or erythritol powder in an air-polishing device with a subgingival nozzle (Fig. 45.49) is more effective for subgingival biofilm removal than the use of either manual or ultrasonic instruments.[c]

[c]References 14, 46, 47, 63, 64, 102, 109, 126, 128, 129, 149, 175.

Fig. 45.48 Hu-Friedy Ems Air Flow Perio Handy Smaller Air Polishing Device With Subgingival Air Polishing Tip for Glycine or Erythritol Powder Polishing. (Courtesy Hu-Friedy, Chicago, IL.)

Fig. 45.49 Hu-Friedy Ems Perio Flow Tip Disposable Plastic Tip With Millimeter Markings for Subgingival Air Polishing of Implants or Deep Pockets With Glycine or Erythritol Powder. (Courtesy Hu-Friedy, Chicago, IL.)

KEY FACT

The use of glycine or erythritol powder in an air-polishing device with a subgingival nozzle is more effective for subgingival biofilm removal than the use of either manual or ultrasonic instruments.

Patients with a medical history of respiratory illness or hemodialysis are not candidates for the use of the air-powder polishing device.[156,177] Powder containing sodium bicarbonate should not be used on patients with a history of uncontrolled hypertension, sodium-restricted diet, or medication use affecting electrolyte balance.[135] Patients with infectious diseases should not be treated with this device because of the large quantity of aerosol created. A preprocedural rinse with 0.12% chlorhexidine gluconate should be used to minimize the microbial content of the aerosol.[18] High-speed evacuation should also be performed to eliminate as much of the aerosol as possible.[61]

Summary

Various periodontal instruments and devices are specifically designed for examination of the periodontium, removal of calculus and biofilm from tooth and implant surfaces, and root planing.

Important information on techniques for use and sharpening of these instruments is described in detail in the online continuation of this chapter.

A Case Scenario is found on the companion website.

REFERENCES

 References for this chapter are found on the companion website.

46

Sonic and Ultrasonic Instrumentation and Irrigation[a]

CHAPTER OUTLINE

Scaling and root planing are the initial nonsurgical treatments of choice for chronic periodontitis.[22] Practitioners often try to enhance and prolong the outcomes from scaling and root planing. In the office setting, technologic advances and new designs of ultrasonic and sonic power scalers have transformed the role of power-driven oscillating instruments in periodontal therapy.

POWER-DRIVEN INSTRUMENTS: OVERVIEW

Power-driven instruments are everyday mainstays in periodontal therapy and maintenance. They may be used alone or in combination with hand instruments. Evidence indicates that power-driven instruments provide clinical outcomes similar to those derived from hand instruments.[16,17,25,29] Power instrumentation has the potential to make scaling less demanding and more time efficient.[3,25] Potential hazards from using power-driven devices include rough root surfaces, production of bioaerosols, and interference with cardiac pacemakers.[11,24]

CLINICAL CORRELATION

Power instruments are useful tools used alone or in combination with hand instruments. Evidence indicates that power and hand instruments have similar clinical outcomes. Although power instruments can make scaling less demanding, thorough debridement takes time regardless of the type of instrument used.

MECHANISM OF ACTION OF POWER SCALERS

Various physical factors play a role in the mechanism of action of power scalers. These factors include frequency, stroke (power or amplitude), and water flow. In addition to rate of flow, the physiologic effects of water may contribute to the efficacy of power instruments.

Water contributes to three physiologic effects that play a role in the efficacy. These are acoustic streaming, acoustic turbulence, and cavitation. Acoustic streaming is unidirectional fluid flow caused by ultrasound waves. Acoustic turbulence is created when the movement of the tip causes the coolant to accelerate, producing an intensified swirling effect. This turbulence continues until cavitation occurs. Cavitation is the formation of bubbles in water caused by the high turbulence. The bubbles implode and produce shock waves in the liquid, thus creating further shock waves throughout the water.[11,27] In vitro, the combination of acoustic streaming, acoustic turbulence, and cavitation has been shown to disrupt biofilm.[8,28]

TYPE AND BENEFIT OF POWER INSTRUMENTS

Sonic units work at a frequency of 2000 to 6500 cycles per second and use a high- or low-speed air source from the dental unit. Water is delivered via the same tubing used to deliver water to a dental handpiece. Sonic scaler tips are large in diameter and universal in design. A sonic scaler tip travels in an elliptical or orbital stroke pattern. This stroke pattern allows the instrument to be adapted to all tooth surfaces. Box 46.1 outlines the advantages and disadvantages of mechanized instruments compared with manual instruments.

Magnetostrictive ultrasonic devices work in a frequency range of 18,000 to 50,000 cycles per second (Fig. 46.1). Metal stacks that change dimension when electrical energy is applied power the magnetostrictive technology. Vibrations travel from the metal stack to a connecting body that causes the vibration of the working tip. Tips move in an elliptical or orbital stroke pattern. This gives the tip four active working surfaces (Fig. 46.2).

Piezoelectric ultrasonic units work in a frequency range of 18,000 to 50,000 cycles per second (Fig. 46.3). Ceramic disks located in the handpiece power the piezoelectric technology and change in dimension as electric energy is applied. Piezoelectric tips move primarily in a linear pattern, giving the tip two active surfaces (Fig. 46.4). Various insert tip designs and shapes are available for use.

Efficiency

Modified tip designs allow for access in many areas, including furcations. Newer, slimmer designs operate effectively at lower power settings, thus improving patients' comfort. Flat-edged tips

[a]Adapted from the following chapter of Newman and Carranza's Clinical Periodontology, 13th edition: Chapter 51: Sonic and Ultrasonic Instrumentation and Irrigation, by Carol A. Jahn.

BOX 46.1 Advantages and Disadvantages of Mechanized Instruments Compared With Manual Instruments

Advantages
Increased Efficiency
Multiple surfaces of tip are capable of removing deposits
No need to sharpen
Less chance for repetitive stress injuries
Large handpiece size
Reduced lateral pressure
Less tissue distention
Water
Lavage
Irrigation
Acoustic microstreaming

Disadvantages
More Precautions and Limitations
Client comfort (water spraying)
Aerosol production
Temporary hearing shifts
Noise
Less tactile sensation
Reduced visibility

From Darby ML, Walsh MM: *Dental hygiene*, ed 3, St. Louis, 2010, Saunders.

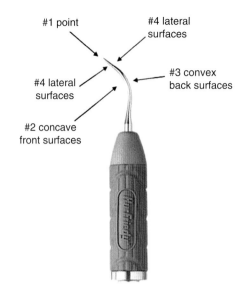

Fig. 46.2 Working Sides of a Magnetostrictive Tip. (Courtesy Hu-Friedy, Chicago, IL.)

#1 point
#4 lateral surfaces
#4 lateral surfaces
#3 convex back surfaces
#2 concave front surfaces

Fig. 46.3 A Piezoelectric Ultrasonic Device. (Courtesy Hu-Friedy, Chicago, IL.)

Fig. 46.1 Magnetostrictive Ultrasonic Device. (Courtesy Dentsply Sirona, York, PA.)

(rectangular in cross section) or bladed designs seem to engage deposits and remove them more efficiently than conical (in cross section) tips.

Tip Designs

Some tips are designed to remove heavy supragingival calculus or debride periodontal pockets definitively. Large-diameter tips are created with a universal design and are indicated for the removal of large, tenacious deposits. A medium to medium-high power setting is generally recommended. Thinner-diameter tips may be site specific in design. The straight-tip design is ideal for use in treating patients with gingivitis and periodontal maintenance patients (Fig. 46.5).[18] The right and left contra-angled instruments allow for greater access and adaptation to root morphology. These inserts are designed to work on a low power setting. A deactivated tip can be used for exploration. The amount of water delivered for lavage can be controlled through the selection of either traditional flow or focused-tip delivery flow. Contra-angled designs and larger ergonomic grips enhance comfort and ergonomics (Figs. 46.6 and 46.7).

Fig. 46.4 Working Sides of a Piezoelectric Tip. (Courtesy Hu-Friedy, Chicago, IL.)

Fig. 46.5 An Ultrasonic Insert With Universal Design. (Courtesy Dentsply Sirona, York, PA.)

Fig. 46.6 Site-Specific Designed Insert. (Courtesy Dentsply Sirona, York, PA.)

CLINICAL OUTCOMES OF POWER-DRIVEN INSTRUMENTS

Numerous clinical outcomes have been evaluated from the use of power-driven instruments. Reviews of the literature have found the effectiveness of subgingival debridement using ultrasonic or sonic scalers to be similar to that achieved with hand instruments.[1,17,25,29]

It is well established that power-driven instruments remove bacterial biofilm and calculus through mechanical action.[6,7,10,20,23] With the advent of newer designs and thinner tips, plaque biofilm removal from root surfaces may be effectively accomplished by power scalers.[18] Power-driven instruments have been shown to be effective in removing calculus, similar to hand instrumentation.[10,20] Ultrasonic instruments, through high-speed action, produce cavitational activity and acoustic microstreaming that some believe may help enhance the disruption of bacteria in subgingival biofilm.

Fig. 46.7 Site-Specific Designed Insert. (Courtesy Dentsply Sirona, York, PA.)

> **KEY FACT**
>
> Power-driven instruments are not just for heavy calculus removal. Depending on tip design and size, they are beneficial for supragingival calculus removal, subgingival debridement, and general plaque biofilm removal.

The primary expected clinical outcomes from scaling and root planing are reductions in bleeding and probing depth and a gain in clinical attachment.[22] Comparing power scalers with hand instruments, both types demonstrate similar outcomes for reductions in bleeding on probing and probing depth and gains in clinical attachment.[4,13,16] Because the opening of a furcation is narrower than with conventional hand instruments, power scalers may be recommended as a means to improve access when scaling this type of defect.[2]

Special Considerations

Power-driven instruments are used with some caution. Due to aerosol production, proper infection control procedures need to be implemented. Considerations are warranted in patients with chronic obstructive or infective respiratory diseases.

Root Surface Roughness

The data is mixed on whether power-driven instruments cause more root surface roughness than hand instruments do.[9,11,12,21] Although it could be assumed that using the device at a higher power may cause more roughness, this has not been proven.[10] It is also not known how much root surface roughness affects the healing process.[11] Power-driven instruments may increase the roughness of resin or glass ionomer restorative materials; therefore, repolishing post scaling is recommended.[5]

Aerosol Production

Power-driven devices produce bioaerosols and splatter, which can contaminate the operator and remain in the air for up to 30 minutes.[26] Good infection control practices can minimize the hazard. Data have shown that preprocedural rinsing with 0.12% chlorhexidine and high-speed evacuation are the most efficient ways to reduce bioaerosols.[15]

> ### KEY FACT
>
> Bioaerosols from power-driven devices can remain in the air for up to 30 minutes. If the operator's face mask becomes damp during the procedure, it should be changed. A face shield may be required. To help minimize bioaerosols, preprocedural rinsing and high-speed evacuation have been shown to be effective.

Cardiac Pacemakers

The use of ultrasonics on patients with cardiac pacemakers is somewhat controversial.[24] Newer models of pacemakers often have bipolar titanium insulation that is believed to make ultrasonic and sonic instruments generally safe for use. An in vivo study supports this; 12 patients underwent continuous electrocardiogram monitoring during piezoelectric ultrasonic scaling and had no abnormal pacemaker functions.[14] Conversely, an in vitro study found that ultrasonic scalers interfered with the activity of dual-system pacemakers.[19] If in doubt, consult with the physician regarding any precautions or warnings from the manufacturer of the product. Box 46.2 outlines the indications, precautions, and contraindications of using mechanized instrumentation.

PRINCIPLES OF INSTRUMENTATION

Ultrasonic technique is different from instrumentation with hand scalers. A pen grasp is used with an ultrasonic scaler, often along with an extraoral fulcrum (Fig. 46.8). The purpose of the extraoral fulcrum is to allow the operator to maintain a light grasp and have easier access physically and visually to the oral cavity. Alternate cross-arch or opposite-arch fulcrums are acceptable alternatives.

> ### CLINICAL CORRELATION
>
> Instrumentation with the ultrasonic device is different from hand instrumentation. A pen grasp with light pressure is preferred, as is using an extraoral fulcrum. Deposits are removed coronally to apically. For deposits in the embrasure area, a horizontal or transverse stroke is recommended.

Light pressure is used with a power instrument. The tip is traveling at a set frequency in a set stroke pattern. Increased clinician pressure on the tip causes decreased clinical efficacy.

Sonic or ultrasonic instrumentation requires removal from the coronal to the apical portion of the deposit. This stroke pattern allows the insert to work at its optimal stroke pattern

> **BOX 46.2 Indications, Precautions, and Contraindications for Use of Mechanized Instruments**
>
> **Indications**
> - Supragingival debridement of dental calculus and extrinsic stains
> - Subgingival debridement of calculus, oral biofilm, root surface constituents, and periodontal pathogens
> - Removal of orthodontic cement
> - Gingival and periodontal conditions and diseases
> - Surgical interventions
> - Margination (reduces amalgam overhangs)
>
> **Precautions**
> - Unshielded pacemakers
> - Infectious diseases: human immunodeficiency virus, hepatitis, tuberculosis (active stages)
> - Demineralized tooth surface
> - Exposed dentin (especially associated with sensitivity)
> - Restorative materials (porcelain, amalgam, gold, composite)
> - Titanium implant abutments unless using special insert (e.g., Quixonic SofTip Prophy Tips)
> - Children (primary teeth)
> - Immunosuppression from disease or chemotherapy
> - Uncontrolled diabetes mellitus
>
> **Contraindications**
> - Chronic pulmonary disease: asthma, emphysema, cystic fibrosis, pneumonia
> - Cardiovascular disease with secondary pulmonary disease
> - Swallowing difficulty (dysphagia)

From Darby ML, Walsh MM: *Dental hygiene,* ed 3, St. Louis, 2010, Saunders.

Fig. 46.8 Pen Grasp of Tip. (Courtesy Hu-Friedy, Chicago, IL.)

and frequency for quick, effective deposit removal. For coronal deposits located in the embrasure area, a horizontal or transverse tip orientation is recommended. A deplaquing stroke should be used when the focus is removal of biofilm and soft debris for the resolution of gingival inflammation. This stroke entails accessing every square millimeter of the tooth surface during ultrasonic deplaquing as a result of the limited lateral dispersion of the lavage subgingivally (Videos 46.1 to 46.7).

CONCLUSION

Power scalers have emerged from being adjuncts for removing heavy supragingival calculus to a tool used for all aspects of scaling: plaque biofilm removal, supragingival scaling, and subgingival scaling. The clinical outcomes achieved are similar to those seen with hand instrumentation. The advantages gained from using power instruments are potentially greater access subgingivally and in furcation areas and increased efficiency in time needed for scaling.

A Case Scenario is found on the companion website.

REFERENCES

 References for this chapter are found on the companion website.

47

Systemic and Local Anti-Infective Therapy for Periodontal Diseases[a,b]

SYSTEMIC ANTIBIOTICS—BACKGROUND AND DEFINITIONS

It has been well established that the various periodontal diseases are caused by bacterial infection. Bacteria begin reattaching to tooth surfaces soon after the teeth have been cleaned and start to form a *biofilm*. Over time, this supragingival plaque biofilm becomes more complex, which leads to a succession of bacteria that are more pathogenic. Bacteria grow in an apical direction and become subgingival. Eventually, as bone is destroyed, a periodontal pocket is formed. In a periodontal pocket, the bacteria form a highly structured and complex biofilm. As this process continues, the bacterial biofilm extends so far subgingivally that the patient cannot reach it during oral hygiene efforts. In addition, this complex biofilm may now offer some protection from the host's immunologic mechanisms in the periodontal pocket as well as from antibiotics used for treatment. It has been suggested that an antibiotic strength that is 500 times greater than the usual therapeutic dose may be needed to be effective against bacteria that have become arranged in biofilms.[54]

CHAPTER HIGHLIGHTS

Systemic Administration of Antibiotics
Tetracyclines
Metronidazole
Penicillins
Cephalosporins
Clindamycin
Ciprofloxacin
Macrolides

It is therefore logical to treat periodontal pockets by mechanically removing local factors (including the calculus that harbors bacteria) and by disrupting the subgingival plaque biofilm itself. Mechanical removal includes manual instrumentation (e.g., scaling and root planing [SRP]) and machine-driven instrumentation (e.g., ultrasonic scalers), and these procedures can be considered "anti-infective therapy." Many chemotherapeutic agents are now available to clinicians who treat periodontal diseases. *Systemic* anti-infective therapy (oral antibiotics) and *local* anti-infective therapy (placing anti-infective agents directly into the periodontal pocket) can reduce the bacterial challenge to the periodontium. It is also possible that systemically administered nonsteroidal antiinflammatory agents may play a role in future adjunctive therapy.[100,147]

Bacteria and their toxic products may cause a loss of attachment and a loss of bone. Ultimately, however, the host's own immunologic response to this bacterial infection can cause even more bone destruction (i.e., indirect bone loss) than that caused by pathogenic bacteria and their by-products. This immunologic response can be influenced by environmental (e.g., tobacco use), acquired (e.g., systemic disease), or genetic risk factors.[125] Chemotherapeutic agents can modulate the host's immune response to bacteria and reduce the host's self-destructive immunologic response to bacterial pathogens, thereby reducing bone loss.[113,116,119] It is also incumbent on health care providers to counsel patients

[a]Adapted from the following chapters of Newman and Carranza's Clinical Periodontology, 13th edition: Chapter 52: Systemic and Local Anti-infective Therapy for Periodontal Diseases, by Sebastian G. Ciancio and Angelo J. Mariotti, and Chapter 53: Locally Delivered, Controlled-Release Antimicrobials, by Richard D. Finkelman, Hector L. Sarmiento, and Alan M. Polson.

[b]In the 2018 Classification of Periodontal and Peri-Implant Diseases and Conditions, "chronic periodontitis" and "aggressive periodontitis" disease categories are grouped under a single category called "periodontitis," and are further characterized based on a multidimensional staging and grading system. In this chapter, the term "aggressive periodontitis" is still used because the related studies were conducted before the 2018 classification. Readers are referred to Chapter 6 for detailed discussion on periodontal disease classification.

about the detrimental effects of systemic factors, including medications, stress, and tobacco use.[54]

This chapter reviews the indications and protocols for optimizing the use of systemically administered anti-infective agents during the treatment of periodontal diseases. It is important to note that there has been significant work with the use of a systematic *evidence-based approach* to evaluate the various anti-infective and host modulation therapies.[153] Meta-analysis of similar research studies has given power to statistical analysis to evaluate anti-infective chemotherapeutic agents for the treatment of periodontal disease. Unfortunately, a standardized research protocol has not yet been implemented. As a result, some studies, although relevant, have not been used in the evidence-based approach because of their study design. Further evidence-based and similar research is needed to define more precise protocols for the use of anti-infective agents to treat various periodontal diseases.

KEY FACT

Bacteriostatic Versus Bactericidal Antibiotics
Pharmacologic agents that prevent the growth of bacteria are bacteriostatic antibiotics, whereas pharmacologic agents that actually kill the bacteria are bactericidal antibiotics. Examples of bacteriostatic antibiotics include tetracycline and clindamycin, and penicillin and metronidazole are good examples of bactericidal antibiotics.

DEFINITIONS

An anti-infective agent is a *chemotherapeutic agent* that acts by reducing the number of bacteria present. An antibiotic is a naturally occurring, semisynthetic, or synthetic type of anti-infective agent that destroys or inhibits the growth of select microorganisms, generally at low concentrations. An antiseptic is a chemical antimicrobial agent that can be applied topically or subgingivally to mucous membranes, wounds, or intact dermal surfaces to destroy microorganisms and inhibit their reproduction or metabolism. In dentistry, antiseptics are widely used as the active ingredient in antiplaque and anti-gingivitis oral rinses and dentifrices. Disinfectants (a subcategory of antiseptics) are antimicrobial agents that are generally applied to inanimate surfaces to destroy microorganisms.[28]

When anti-infective agents are administered orally, many of these agents can be found in the gingival crevicular fluid (GCF). The purpose of a *systemic administration* of antibiotics is to reduce the number of bacteria present in the diseased periodontal pocket; this is often a necessary adjunct for controlling bacterial infection, because bacteria can invade periodontal tissues, thereby making mechanical therapy alone sometimes ineffective.[3,26,27,46,123]

A single chemotherapeutic agent can also have a dual mechanism of action. For example, tetracyclines (especially doxycycline) are chemotherapeutic agents that can reduce collagen and bone destruction via their ability to inhibit the enzyme collagenase. As antibiotic agents, they can also reduce periodontal pathogens in periodontal tissues.[27]

SYSTEMIC ADMINISTRATION OF ANTIBIOTICS

Background and Rationale

The treatment of periodontal diseases is based on their infectious nature (Table 47.1). Ideally, the causative microorganisms should be identified, and the most effective agent should be selected with the use of antibiotic-sensitivity testing. Although this appears simple, the difficulty lies primarily in identifying the specific etiologic microorganisms rather than the microorganisms that are simply associated with various periodontal disorders.[27]

An ideal antibiotic for use in the prevention and treatment of periodontal disease should be specific for periodontal pathogens, allogenic, nontoxic, substantive, not in general use for the treatment of other diseases, and inexpensive.[47] Currently, however, an ideal antibiotic for the treatment of periodontal disease does not exist.[74] Although oral bacteria are susceptible

---

TABLE 47.1 Antibiotics Used to Treat Periodontal Diseases

Category	Agent	Major Features
Penicillin[a]	Amoxicillin	Extended spectrum of antimicrobial activity; excellent oral absorption; used systemically
	Augmentin[b]	Effective against penicillinase-producing microorganisms; used systemically
Tetracyclines	Minocycline	Effective against a broad spectrum of microorganisms; used systemically and applied locally (subgingivally)
	Doxycycline	Effective against a broad spectrum of microorganisms; used systemically and applied locally (subgingivally)
		Chemotherapeutically used in subantimicrobial doses for host modulation (Periostat)
	Tetracycline	Effective against a broad spectrum of microorganisms
Quinolone	Ciprofloxacin	Effective against gram-negative rods; promotes health-associated microflora
Macrolide	Azithromycin	Concentrates at sites of inflammation; used systemically
Lincomycin derivative	Clindamycin	Used in penicillin-allergic patients; effective against anaerobic bacteria; used systemically
Nitroimidazole[c]	Metronidazole	Effective against anaerobic bacteria; used systemically and applied locally (subgingivally) as gel

[a]Indications: localized aggressive periodontitis, generalized aggressive periodontitis, medically related periodontitis, and refractory periodontitis.
[b]Amoxicillin and clavulanate potassium.
[c]Indications: localized aggressive periodontitis, generalized aggressive periodontitis, medically related periodontitis, refractory periodontitis, and necrotizing ulcerative periodontitis.

to many antibiotics, no single antibiotic at the concentrations achieved in body fluids inhibits all putative periodontal pathogens.[150] Indeed, a combination of antibiotics may be necessary to eliminate all putative pathogens from some periodontal pockets (Table 47.2).[111]

As always, the clinician, in concert with the patient, must make the final decision regarding any treatment. Thus the treatment of an individual patient must be based on the patient's clinical status, the nature of the colonizing bacteria, the ability of the agent to reach the site of infection, and the risks and benefits associated with the proposed treatment plan. The clinician is responsible for choosing the correct antimicrobial agent. Some adverse reactions include allergic or anaphylactic reactions, superinfections of opportunistic bacteria, development of resistant bacteria, interactions with other medications, upset stomach, nausea, and vomiting.[4] Most adverse reactions take the form of gastrointestinal upset.[74] Other concerns include the cost of the medication and the patient's willingness and ability to comply with the proposed therapy.

No consensus exists regarding the magnitude of risk for the development of bacterial resistance. The common and indiscriminate use of antibiotics worldwide has contributed to increasing numbers of resistant bacterial strains since the late 1990s, and this trend is likely to continue given the widespread use of antibiotics.[24,42,151] The overuse, misuse, and widespread prophylactic application of anti-infective drugs are some of the factors that have led to the emergence of resistant microorganisms. Increasing levels of resistance of subgingival microflora to antibiotics have been correlated with the increased use of antibiotics in individual countries.[24,146] However, researchers have noted that the subgingival microflora tends to revert to

similar proportions of antibiotic-resistant isolates 3 months after therapy.[44,61]

Tetracyclines

Tetracyclines have been widely used for the treatment of periodontal diseases. They have been frequently used to treat refractory periodontitis, including *localized aggressive periodontitis* (LAP) (see Table 47.1).[73,152] Tetracyclines have the ability to concentrate in the periodontal tissues and inhibit the growth of *Aggregatibacter actinomycetemcomitans*. In addition, tetracyclines exert an anticollagenase effect that can inhibit tissue destruction and may help with bone regeneration.[23,83,149]

Pharmacology

The tetracyclines are a group of antibiotics that are produced naturally from certain species of *Streptomyces* or derived semisynthetically. These antibiotics are bacteriostatic and are effective against rapidly multiplying bacteria. They generally are more effective against gram-positive bacteria than against gram-negative bacteria. Tetracyclines are effective for the treatment of periodontal diseases in part because their concentration in the gingival crevice is 2 to 10 times that found in serum.[2,13,52] This allows a high drug concentration to be delivered into the periodontal pockets. In addition, several studies have demonstrated that tetracyclines at a low GCF concentration (i.e., 2 to 4 μg/mL) are very effective against many periodontal pathogens.[14,15]

Clinical Use

Tetracyclines have been investigated as adjuncts for the treatment of LAP.[73,131] *A. actinomycetemcomitans* is a microorganism that is frequently associated with LAP, and it invades tissue. Therefore the mechanical removal of calculus and plaque from root surfaces may not eliminate this bacterium from the periodontal tissues. Systemic tetracycline can eliminate tissue bacteria and has been shown to arrest bone loss and suppress *A. actinomycetemcomitans* levels in conjunction with SRP.[130] This combination therapy allows for the mechanical removal of root surface deposits and the elimination of pathogenic bacteria from within the tissues.[138] Increased posttreatment bone levels have been noted with the use of this method (Figs. 47.1 to 47.4).

As a result of increased resistance to tetracyclines, metronidazole or amoxicillin with metronidazole has been found to be more effective for the treatment of aggressive periodontitis in children and young adults. Some investigators think that metronidazole in combination with amoxicillin–clavulanic acid is the preferable antibiotic.[148]

Long-term use of low antibacterial doses of tetracyclines has been advocated in the past. One long-term study of patients taking low doses of tetracycline (i.e., 250 mg/day for 2 to 7 years) demonstrated the persistence of deep pockets that did not bleed after probing. These sites contained high proportions of tetracycline-resistant gram-negative rods *(Fusobacterium nucleatum)*. After the antibiotic was discontinued, the flora was characteristic of sites with disease.[74] Therefore it is not advisable to prescribe a long-term regimen of tetracyclines because of the possible development of resistant bacterial strains.[79] Although tetracyclines were often used in the past as anti-infective agents,

TABLE 47.2 Common Antibiotic Regimens Used to Treat Periodontal Diseases[a]		
	Regimen	**Dosage/Duration**
Single Agent		
Amoxicillin	500 mg	Three times daily for 8 days
Azithromycin	500 mg	Once daily for 4–7 days
Ciprofloxacin	500 mg	Twice daily for 8 days
Clindamycin	300 mg	Three times daily 10 days
Doxycycline or minocycline	100 mg to 200 mg	Once daily for 21 days
Metronidazole	500 mg	Three times daily for 8 days
Combination Therapy		
Metronidazole + amoxicillin	250 mg of each	Three times daily for 8 days
Metronidazole + ciprofloxacin	500 mg of each	Twice daily for 8 days

[a]These regimens are prescribed after a review of the patient's medical history, periodontal diagnosis, and antimicrobial testing. Clinicians must consult pharmacology references such as *Mosby's GenRx*[95] or the manufacturer's guidelines for warnings, contraindications, and precautions.
Data from Jorgensen MG, Slots J: Practical antimicrobial periodontal therapy, *Compend Contin Educ Dent* 21:111, 2000.

Fig. 47.1 Panoramic Image of 17-Year-Old African American Male Exhibiting Signs of Localized Aggressive Periodontitis. (Photo courtesy Dr. Sasi Sunkari.)

Fig. 47.2 Image of Anterior Dentition in 17-Year-Old African American Male With Localized Aggressive Periodontitis. (Photo courtesy Dr. Sasi Sunkari.)

especially for LAP and other types of aggressive periodontitis, they are now frequently replaced by more effective combination antibiotics.[74]

Specific Agents

Tetracycline, minocycline, and doxycycline are semisynthetic members of the tetracycline group that have been used in periodontal therapy.

Tetracycline

Treatment with tetracycline hydrochloride requires the administration of 250 mg four times daily. It is inexpensive, but compliance may be reduced by the need to take the medication so frequently. Side effects include gastrointestinal disturbances, photosensitivity, hypersensitivity, increased blood urea nitrogen levels, blood dyscrasias, dizziness, and headache. In addition,

tooth discoloration occurs when this drug is administered to children who are 12 years old or younger.

> **KEY FACT**
>
> **Tetracycline and Tooth Discoloration**
> Tetracycline has the ability to chelate with calcium and therefore gets deposited in mineralized tissues such as bone or teeth during the mineralization process, resulting in yellow to brown discoloration of teeth.

Minocycline

Minocycline is effective against a broad spectrum of microorganisms. In patients with adult periodontitis, it suppresses spirochetes and motile rods as effectively as SRP, with suppression evident up to 3 months after therapy. Minocycline can be given

Fig. 47.3 Preoperative Radiograph of Anterior Mandible in Localized Aggressive Periodontitis Patient. (Photo courtesy Dr. Sasi Sunkari.)

Fig. 47.4 Postoperative Radiograph of Anterior Mandible in Localized Aggressive Periodontitis Patient Treated With a Combination of Antibiotic Therapy, Scaling and Root Planing, and Surgical Intervention. (Photo courtesy Dr. Sasi Sunkari.)

twice daily, thereby facilitating compliance as compared with tetracycline. Although it is associated with less phototoxicity and renal toxicity than tetracycline, minocycline may cause reversible vertigo. Minocycline administered at a dose of 200 mg/day for 1 week results in a reduction of total bacterial counts, complete elimination of spirochetes for up to 2 months, and improvement of all clinical parameters.[28,29]

Side effects are similar to those of tetracycline; however, there is an increased incidence of vertigo. It is the only tetracycline that can permanently discolor erupted teeth and gingival tissue when administered orally.

Doxycycline

Doxycycline has the same spectrum of activity as minocycline and can be equally effective.[27] Because doxycycline can be given only once daily, patients may be more compliant. Compliance is also improved because its absorption from the gastrointestinal tract is only slightly altered by calcium, metal ions, or antacids, as is absorption of other tetracyclines. Side effects are similar to those of tetracycline hydrochloride; however, it is the most photosensitizing agent in the tetracycline category.

The recommended dosage when doxycycline is used as an anti-infective agent is 100 mg twice daily the first day, which is then reduced to 100 mg daily. To reduce gastrointestinal upset, 50 mg can be taken twice daily after the initial dose. When given

as a sub-antimicrobial dose (to inhibit collagenase), 20 mg of doxycycline twice daily is recommended.[23,34]

Metronidazole
Pharmacology

Metronidazole is a nitroimidazole compound that was developed in France to treat protozoal infections. It is bactericidal to anaerobic organisms and is thought to disrupt bacterial DNA synthesis in conditions with a low reduction potential. Metronidazole is not the drug of choice for treating *A. actinomycetemcomitans* infections. However, metronidazole is effective against *A. actinomycetemcomitans* when used in combination with other antibiotics.[111,112] Metronidazole is also effective against anaerobes such as *Porphyromonas gingivalis* and *Prevotella intermedia*.[53]

Clinical Use

Metronidazole has been used clinically to treat acute necrotizing ulcerative gingivitis, chronic periodontitis, and aggressive periodontitis. It has been used as monotherapy and also in combination with root planing and surgery or with other antibiotics. Metronidazole has also been used successfully to treat necrotizing ulcerative gingivitis.[86]

Studies in humans have demonstrated the efficacy of metronidazole for the treatment of periodontitis.[84] A single dose of metronidazole (250 mg orally) appears in both serum and GCF in sufficient quantities to inhibit a wide range of suspected periodontal pathogens. When it is administered systemically (i.e., 750 mg/day to 1000 mg/day for 2 weeks), metronidazole reduces the growth of anaerobic flora, including spirochetes, and it decreases the clinical and histopathologic signs of periodontitis.[84] The most common regimen is 250 mg three times daily for 7 days.[86] Currently, the critical level of spirochetes that is needed to diagnose an anaerobic infection, the appropriate time to give metronidazole, and the ideal dosage or duration of therapy are unknown.[53] As monotherapy (i.e., with no concurrent root planing), metronidazole is inferior and at best only equivalent to root planing. Therefore if it is used, metronidazole should not be administered as monotherapy.

Soder and colleagues[132] demonstrated that metronidazole was more effective than placebo for the management of sites that were unresponsive to root planing. Nevertheless, many patients still had sites that bled with probing, despite metronidazole therapy. The existence of refractory periodontitis as a diagnostic consideration indicates that some patients do not respond to conventional therapy, which may include root planing, surgery, or both.

Studies have suggested that when it is combined with amoxicillin or amoxicillin–clavulanate potassium (Augmentin), metronidazole may be of value for the management of patients with LAP or refractory periodontitis. This is discussed in more detail later in this chapter.

Side Effects

Metronidazole has an Antabuse effect and therefore causes unpleasant symptoms when alcohol is ingested. The response is generally proportional to the amount ingested and can result in severe cramps, nausea, and vomiting. Products that contain alcohol should be avoided during therapy and for at least 1 day after therapy is discontinued. Metronidazole also inhibits warfarin metabolism. Patients who are undergoing anticoagulant therapy should avoid metronidazole, because it prolongs prothrombin time.[86] It also should be avoided in patients who are taking lithium. This drug produces a metallic taste in the mouth, which may affect compliance.

Penicillins
Pharmacology

Penicillins are the drugs of choice for the treatment of many serious infections in humans and are the most widely used antibiotics. Penicillins are natural and semisynthetic derivatives of broth cultures of the *Penicillium* mold. They inhibit bacterial cell wall production and therefore are bactericidal.

Clinical Use

Penicillins other than amoxicillin and amoxicillin–clavulanate potassium (Augmentin)—have not been shown to increase periodontal attachment levels, and their use in periodontal therapy does not appear to be justified.

Side Effects

Penicillins may induce allergic reactions and bacterial resistance.

KEY FACT

Penicillin Allergy
Up to 10% of patients may be allergic to penicillin. Reactions to ingestion of penicillin or its derivatives, such as amoxicillin, in allergic patients can range from skin rash to life-threatening anaphylaxis.

Amoxicillin

Amoxicillin is a semisynthetic penicillin with an extended anti-infective spectrum that includes gram-positive and gram-negative bacteria. It demonstrates excellent absorption after oral administration. Amoxicillin is susceptible to penicillinase, which is a β-lactamase produced by certain bacteria that breaks the penicillin ring structure and thus renders penicillins ineffective.

Amoxicillin may be useful for the management of patients with aggressive periodontitis in both localized and generalized forms. The recommended dosage is 500 mg three times daily for 8 days.[74,75]

Amoxicillin–Clavulanate Potassium

The combination of amoxicillin with clavulanate potassium makes this anti-infective agent resistant to penicillinase enzymes produced by some bacteria. Amoxicillin with clavulanate (Augmentin) may be useful for the management of patients with LAP or refractory periodontitis.[100] Bueno and colleagues[22] reported that Augmentin arrested alveolar bone loss in patients with periodontal disease that was refractory to treatment with other antibiotics, including tetracycline, metronidazole, and clindamycin.

Cephalosporins
Pharmacology

The family of β-lactams known as cephalosporins is similar in action and structure to the penicillins. These drugs are frequently used in medicine, and they are resistant to a number of β-lactamases that are normally active against penicillin.

Clinical Use

Cephalosporins are generally not used to treat dental-related infections. The penicillins are superior to cephalosporins with regard to their range of action against periodontal pathogenic bacteria.

Side Effects

Patients who are allergic to penicillins must be considered to be allergic to all β-lactam products. More specifically, up to 10% of patients who have an allergy to penicillin may also have an adverse reaction to cephalosporins. Rashes, urticaria, fever, and gastrointestinal upset have all been associated with cephalosporins.[151]

Clindamycin
Pharmacology

Clindamycin is effective against anaerobic bacteria and has a strong affinity for osseous tissue.[145] It is effective for situations in which the patient is allergic to penicillin.

Clinical Use

Clindamycin has demonstrated efficacy in patients with periodontitis that is refractory to tetracycline therapy. Walker and colleagues[151] showed that clindamycin helped stabilize refractory patients; the dosage used was 150 mg four times daily for 10 days. Jorgensen and Slots[75] recommend a regimen of 300 mg twice daily for 8 days.

Side Effects

Clindamycin has been associated with pseudomembranous colitis, but the incidence is higher with cephalosporins and ampicillin. When needed, however, clindamycin can be used with caution, but it is not indicated for patients with a history of colitis. Diarrhea or cramping that develops during clindamycin therapy may be indicative of colitis, and it should be discontinued. If symptoms persist, the patient should be referred to an internist.

Ciprofloxacin
Pharmacology

Ciprofloxacin is a quinolone that is active against gram-negative rods, including all facultative and some anaerobic putative periodontal pathogens.[95]

Clinical Use

Because it demonstrates a minimal effect on *Streptococcus* species, which are associated with periodontal health, ciprofloxacin therapy may facilitate the establishment of a microflora that is associated with periodontal health. At present, ciprofloxacin is the only antibiotic in periodontal therapy to which all strains of *A. actinomycetemcomitans* are susceptible. It has also been used in combination with metronidazole.[111]

Side Effects

Nausea, headache, metallic taste in the mouth, and abdominal discomfort have been associated with ciprofloxacin. Quinolones inhibit the metabolism of theophylline, and caffeine and concurrent administration can produce toxicity. Quinolones have also been reported to enhance the effects of warfarin and other anticoagulants.[151]

Macrolides
Pharmacology

Macrolide antibiotics contain a many-membered lactone ring to which one or more deoxy sugars are attached. They inhibit protein synthesis by binding to the 50S ribosomal subunits of sensitive microorganisms. Macrolides can be bacteriostatic or bactericidal, depending on the concentration of the drug and the nature of the microorganism. The macrolide antibiotics used for periodontal treatment include erythromycin, spiramycin, and azithromycin.

Clinical Use

Erythromycin does not concentrate in GCF and is not effective against most putative periodontal pathogens. For these reasons, erythromycin is not recommended as an adjunct to periodontal therapy.

Spiramycin is active against gram-positive organisms; it is excreted in high concentrations in saliva. It is used as an adjunct to periodontal treatment in Canada and Europe but is not available in the United States. Spiramycin has a minimal effect on attachment levels.

Azithromycin is a member of the azalide class of macrolides. It is effective against anaerobes and gram-negative bacilli. After an oral dosage of 500 mg four times daily for 3 days, significant levels of azithromycin can be detected in most tissues for 7 to 10 days.[18,68] The concentration of azithromycin in tissue specimens from periodontal lesions is significantly higher than that of normal gingiva.[89] It has been proposed that azithromycin penetrates fibroblasts and phagocytes in concentrations that are 100 to 200 times greater than that of the extracellular compartment. Azithromycin is actively transported to sites of inflammation by phagocytes, where it is released directly into the sites of inflammation as the phagocytes rupture during phagocytosis.[48] Therapeutic use requires a single dose of 250 mg/day for 5 days after an initial loading dose of 500 mg.[151]

Data have suggested that azithromycin may be an effective adjunctive therapy for increasing attachment levels in patients with aggressive periodontitis[60] as well as for reducing the degree of gingival enlargement.[31] These data must be carefully considered because they were derived from small subject populations. Currently, the literature presents conflicting reports regarding the efficacy of this antibiotic as an adjunct to periodontal therapy. One study concluded that adjunctive azithromycin provides no additional benefit over nonsurgical periodontal treatment for the parameters investigated in patients with severe generalized chronic periodontitis. Furthermore, an additional study reported that there was an increase in cardiovascular deaths among patients who received azithromycin; this increase was most pronounced among patients with a high baseline risk of cardiovascular disease. As a result of this study, the U.S. Food and Drug Administration issued a warning that the drug can alter the electrical activity of the heart, which may lead to a potentially fatal heart rhythm known as *prolonged QT interval.* This rhythm causes the timing of the heart's contractions to become irregular. The warning stated that physicians should use caution when giving the antibiotic to patients who are known to have this condition or who are at risk for cardiovascular problems.

To ascertain the efficacy of azithromycin for the management of periodontal diseases, future studies will need to increase the number of subjects, improve diagnostic methods and tools, and determine the appropriate dose, duration, and frequency of azithromycin therapy.

SERIAL AND COMBINATION ANTIBIOTIC THERAPY
Rationale

Because periodontal infections may contain a wide variety of bacteria, no single antibiotic is effective against all putative pathogens. Indeed, differences exist in the microbial flora associated with the various periodontal disease syndromes.[152] These "mixed" infections can include a variety of aerobic, microaerophilic, and anaerobic bacteria, which may be both gram negative and gram positive. In these cases, it may be necessary to use more than one antibiotic, either serially or in combination.[112] Before combinations of antibiotics are used, however, the periodontal pathogens being treated should be identified and antibiotic-susceptibility testing performed.[154]

Clinical Use

Antibiotics that are bacteriostatic (e.g., tetracycline) generally require rapidly dividing microorganisms to be effective. They do not function well if a bactericidal antibiotic (e.g., amoxicillin) is given concurrently. *When both types of drugs are required, they are best given serially rather than in combination.*

Rams and Slots[112] reviewed combination therapy involving the use of systemic metronidazole along with amoxicillin, amoxicillin–clavulanate (Augmentin), or ciprofloxacin. The metronidazole–amoxicillin and metronidazole–Augmentin combinations provided excellent elimination of many organisms in adults with LAP who had been treated unsuccessfully with tetracyclines and mechanical debridement. These drugs have an additive effect that involves the suppression of *A. actinomycetemcomitans.* Tinoco and colleagues[142] found metronidazole and amoxicillin to be clinically effective for the treatment of LAP, although 50% of patients who were treated with this regimen harbored *A. actinomycetemcomitans* 1 year later. The metronidazole–ciprofloxacin combination is effective against *A. actinomycetemcomitans;* metronidazole targets obligate anaerobes, and ciprofloxacin targets facultative anaerobes. This is a powerful combination against mixed infections. Studies of this drug combination for the treatment of refractory periodontitis have documented marked clinical improvement. This combination may provide a therapeutic benefit by reducing or eliminating pathogenic organisms and a prophylactic benefit by giving rise to a predominantly streptococcal microflora.[111]

Systemic antibiotic therapy in combination with mechanical therapy appears to be valuable for the treatment of recalcitrant periodontal infections and LAP infections that involve *A. actinomycetemcomitans.* Antibiotic treatment should be reserved for specific subsets of periodontal patients who do not respond to conventional therapy. The selection of specific agents should be guided by the results of cultures and sensitivity tests for subgingival plaque microorganisms.

Pharmacologic Implications

Principles of antibiotic therapy for the proper selection of an antibiotic minimally require identification of the causative organism, determination of the antibiotic sensitivity, and an effective method of administration.[67] The use of antibiotics to treat gingival diseases is contraindicated, because this is a local infection that can be easily treated with scaling and appropriate home care by the patient.[140] With regard to destructive periodontal diseases, there are limited data to support the use of systemic antibiotic treatment. Although bacterial infections of the periodontium are considered to be important to initiation of the disease, currently no one microbe or group of microbes has been demonstrated to be the cause of these diseases. It is therefore not surprising that systemic antibiotics have had only a modest effect on the management of periodontal diseases. At this time, systemic antibiotics for the treatment of periodontal diseases have been indicated primarily for adjunctive use in the treatment of aggressive periodontal diseases (Table 47.3).[54,61]

Guidelines for the use of antibiotics in periodontal therapy include the following:

1. The clinical diagnosis and situation dictate the need for possible antibiotic therapy as an adjunct for controlling active periodontal disease (Fig. 47.5). The patient's diagnosis can change over time. For example, a patient who presents with generalized mild chronic periodontitis can return to a diagnosis of periodontal health after initial therapy. However, if the patient has been treated and continues to have active disease, the diagnosis may change to generalized severe chronic periodontitis.

2. Disease activity as measured by continuing attachment loss, purulent exudate, and bleeding on probing[81,82] may be an indication for periodontal intervention and possible microbial analysis through plaque sampling.

TABLE 47.3	Therapeutic Uses of Systemic Antimicrobial Agents for Various Periodontal Diseases	
Disease	**Systemic Antimicrobial Agents**	**Adjunct or Stand-Alone Therapy**
Gingival diseases	Antibiotic use not recommended	Not applicable
Necrotizing ulcerative gingivitis	Antibiotic use not recommended unless there are systemic complications (e.g., fever, swollen lymph nodes)	As an adjunct when necessary
Chronic periodontitis	Limited benefit; antibiotic use not recommended	Not applicable
Aggressive periodontitis	Antibiotic use recommended; for greatest benefit, therapeutic levels of antibiotics should be achieved by the time scaling and root planing are completed (all debridement should be completed within a week); the optimal antibiotic type, dose, frequency, and duration have not been identified	As an adjunct
Necrotizing ulcerative periodontitis	Antibiotic use dependent on the systemic condition of the patient	As an adjunct when necessary
Periodontitis as a manifestation of systemic disease	Antibiotic use dependent on the systemic condition of the patient	As an adjunct when necessary
Periodontal abscess	Antibiotic use not recommended	Not applicable

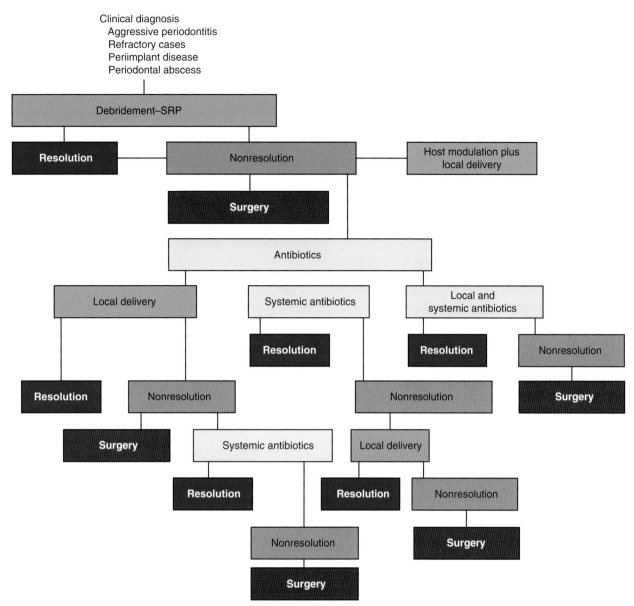

Fig. 47.5 A Decision Tree for the Selection of Antibiotic Therapy. *SRP,* Scaling and root planing.

3. When they are used to treat periodontal disease, antibiotics are selected on the basis of the patient's medical and dental status and current medications,[74] and the results of microbial analysis, if it is performed.

4. Microbiologic plaque sampling may be performed according to the instructions of the reference laboratory. The samples are usually taken at the beginning of an appointment, before instrumentation of the pocket. Supragingival plaque is removed, and an endodontic paper point is inserted subgingivally into the deepest pockets to absorb bacteria in the loosely associated plaque. This endodontic point is placed in reduced transfer fluid or a sterile transfer tube and sent to the laboratory. The laboratory will then send the referring dentist a report that includes the pathogens that are present and any appropriate antibiotic regimen. At this time, there are scant data to suggest that microbial identification from a plaque sample can be used to clinically improve the periodontal condition of the patient.

5. Meta-analyses of randomized clinical trials and quasi-experimental studies have shown that systemic antibiotics can improve attachment levels when they are used as adjuncts to SRP. The same benefits could not be demonstrated when antibiotics were used as a stand-alone therapy.[61]

6. When systemic antibiotics were used as adjuncts to SRP, improvements were observed in the attachment levels of patients with chronic and aggressive periodontitis, although patients with aggressive periodontitis experienced greater benefits.[61] The mean attachment level change depended on the antibiotic used and ranged from 0.09 to 1.10 mm.[61]

7. The identification of which antibiotics were most effective for the treatment of destructive periodontal diseases was limited by the insufficient sizes of the samples found in the

randomized clinical trials used as part of a systematic review.[61] A meta-analysis evaluating eight different antibiotics or antibiotic combinations showed that only tetracycline and metronidazole significantly improved attachment levels when they were used as adjuncts to SRP for patients with destructive periodontal diseases.[61]

8. Debridement of root surfaces, optimal oral hygiene, and frequent periodontal maintenance therapy are important parts of comprehensive periodontal therapy. As mentioned previously, an antibiotic strength that is 500 times greater than the systemic therapeutic dose may be required to be effective against bacteria that have been arranged into biofilm. It is therefore important to disrupt the biofilm physically so that the antibiotic agents can have access to the periodontal pathogens.[54]

9. Although there are adequate data to suggest that systemic antibiotics can be of benefit for the treatment of destructive periodontal diseases, there are limited data available to identify which antibiotics are suitable for which infection; the optimum dosage, frequency, and duration of antibiotic therapy; when the regimen should be introduced during the treatment schedule; the long-term outcomes of antibiotic use; the potential hazards of these agents (e.g., antibiotic resistance, changes in oral microflora)[61]; and the economic ramifications of this type of pharmacologic intervention.

The selection of an antibiotic must be made on the basis of factors other than the empirical decisions made by the clinician. Unfortunately, there is no one best choice of antibiotic at present (i.e., there is no "silver bullet"). Therefore the clinician must integrate the history of the patient's disease, the clinical signs and symptoms, and the results of radiographic examinations and possibly microbiologic sampling to determine the course of periodontal therapy. The clinician must obtain a thorough medical history, including current medications and the possible adverse effects of combining these medicines, before prescribing any antibiotic therapy. The clinician must make the final decision with the patient. Risks and benefits concerning antibiotics as adjuncts to periodontal therapy should be discussed with the patient before antibiotics are used.

LOCALLY DELIVERED ANTIBIOTICS: BACKGROUND AND OBJECTIVES

Chronic periodontitis is a bacterial infection. The focus of most nonsurgical periodontal therapy, including mechanical therapy such as SRP, is to combat infection. Chemical antibacterial strategies include systemic drug delivery, oral rinses or toothpastes, and irrigating devices, but none of these therapies has provided significant clinical benefit in reducing the signs of chronic periodontitis.

In the past few decades, a new strategy has emerged. Several controlled-release delivery systems have been developed to deposit antimicrobials directly into the periodontal pocket and maintain effective concentrations of drug for an extended period. After extensive study, these agents have been declared safe and effective for the treatment of chronic adult periodontitis. In some cases, they are used as monotherapy, and in other cases, they are

administered adjunctively with SRP, which is generally considered by the professional community to be the best approach.

Evidence-based practice, which provides dental treatment based on research, produces optimal care for the greatest number of patients.[96,97] Locally delivered, controlled-release antimicrobials may have the most robust data of any periodontal therapy to support their clinical use. This chapter considers the available clinical data that support the use of these agents for the treatment of chronic periodontitis and provides evidence-based guidance for their use. In this discussion, locally delivered, controlled-release antimicrobials are considered as a drug class rather than individually.

Because appropriate comparative trials have not been performed, there are insufficient data on which to base comparisons of agents or consider differential indications for use. The indications for use of each product are described in their respective full prescribing information. Some commentary is provided regarding these agents and available research for potentially new indications that have not been evaluated by the U.S. Food and Drug Administration (FDA) (Box 47.1).

U.S. Locally Delivered, Controlled-Release Antimicrobials

Three locally delivered, controlled-release antimicrobial products are available for dental use in the United States (Table 47.4): a chlorhexidine-containing chip (PerioChip), a doxycycline gel (Atridox), and minocycline microspheres (Arestin). A fourth product, an ethylene or vinyl acetate copolymer fiber containing the antibiotic tetracycline (Actisite as a 12.7-mg, 9-inch filament), was the first product introduced into the U.S. market in the early 1990s and was the prototypic system. The tetracycline fiber is

---

> **BOX 47.1** **Adjunctive Therapy**
>
> - Adjunctive therapy makes scaling and root planing (SRP) more effective.
> - Because most pockets are quiescent, mean changes are modest when all pockets are included.
> - Significantly more patients show large pocket depth reductions with adjunctive therapy.
> - Clinical responses are evident only after time and with clinical pocket measurements.
> - The greatest clinical benefit is likely to result when adjunctive agents are routinely included as part of SRP procedures and in a long-term periodontal maintenance program.

TABLE 47.4 **Locally Delivered, Controlled-Release Antimicrobials Developed and U.S. Food and Drug Administration Approved for Dental Use in the United States**

Product	Antimicrobial Agent
Actisite[a]	Tetracycline
PerioChip	Chlorhexidine
Arestin	Minocycline
Atridox	Doxycycline

[a]No longer commercially available in the United States.

no longer commercially available in the United States, and its clinical use is not further considered, but it is included because data generated from clinical studies of the product are pertinent to a discussion of the general effects of locally delivered, controlled-release antimicrobials.

Chlorhexidine Chip

The chlorhexidine chip is a small chip (4.0 × 5.0 × 0.35 mm) that contains 2.5 mg of the active ingredient chlorhexidine gluconate in a resorbable, biodegradable matrix of hydrolyzed gelatin that is cross-linked with glutaraldehyde and packaged in individual foil containers (Fig. 47.6A). The chip is stored at 20°C to 25°C (68°F to 77°F), with excursions permitted to 15°C to 30°C (59°F to 86°F). The chlorhexidine chip is placed into the pocket directly from the foil container using a forceps (see Fig. 47.6B).

The chlorhexidine chip is indicated as an adjunct to SRP procedures for the reduction of pocket depth in adults with periodontitis, and it can be used as part of a periodontal maintenance program, which includes good oral hygiene and SRP.[106,134] After placement in the pocket, the chip has been reported to release chlorhexidine into the GCF over 7 to 10 days.[133] Chlorhexidine is active against a broad range of microbes. It disrupts the cell membrane and causes precipitation of the cytoplasm, resulting in cell death. No adverse alterations in the oral microbial flora or overgrowth of opportunistic microorganisms have been observed.[106] The chip is biodegradable and does not require removal, but dental floss should be avoided for 10 days to avoid dislodging it.

Doxycycline Gel

Doxycycline gel is a subgingival, controlled-release delivery product composed of a two-syringe mixing system (Fig. 47.7A). Syringe A contains 450 mg of a bioabsorbable polymeric formulation of 36.7% poly(D,L,-lactide) dissolved in 63.3% N-methyl-2-pyrrolidone. Syringe B contains 50 mg of doxycycline hyclate, equivalent to 42.5 mg of doxycycline. The two syringes are stored at 2°C to 30°C (36°F to 86°F). When mixed, the product is a viscous liquid of 500 mg, which contains 50 mg (10%) of doxycycline hyclate.

Doxycycline gel is indicated for the treatment of chronic adult periodontitis for a gain in clinical attachment, reduction in probing depth, and reduction of bleeding on probing.[11] Doxycycline, a broad-spectrum semisynthetic tetracycline, is bacteriostatic, inhibiting bacterial protein biosynthesis by interfering with transfer RNA (tRNA) and messenger RNA (mRNA) at the ribosome. No overgrowth of opportunistic organisms was observed after use of the doxycycline gel.[11]

Fig. 47.6 Chlorhexidine Gluconate Chip (PerioChip). (A) The chip is packaged in a foil packet *(left)*. The chip is removed from the foil container with a suitable forceps *(right)*. (B) The chip is inserted into the pocket, curved end first *(left)*. After insertion, the chip is pressed apically to the base of the pocket *(right)*. (Reprinted from Wolf HF, Hassell TM: *Color atlas of dental hygiene: periodontology*, ed 1, Stuttgart, Germany, 2006, Thieme, with permission.)

Fig. 47.7 Doxycycline Hyclate Gel (Atridox). (A) Doxycycline gel is packaged as a two-syringe mixing system *(right)*. After mixing the gel, a cannula is attached for injection *(left)*. (B) The two syringes are coupled, and the liquid contents of syringe A are injected into the powder within syringe B; the contents are mixed within the two syringes for 100 cycles (1 cycle/s) and then left within syringe A *(right)*. The mixed solution is injected into the pocket through the cannula attached to syringe A until the pocket is completely filled *(left)*. The pocket contents are covered with a periodontal dressing or a cyanoacrylate dental adhesive. (Reprinted from Wolf HF, Hassell TM: *Color atlas of dental hygiene: periodontology*, ed 1, Stuttgart, Germany, 2006, Thieme, with permission.)

The gel has been reported to release doxycycline in the GCF over 7 days.[139] The doxycycline gel is biodegradable and does not require removal. If not used immediately, the mixed contents in syringe A can be stored in an airtight container at room temperature for a maximum of 3 days. The doxycycline gel is used by injecting the mixed contents of the two syringes directly into the pocket (see Fig. 47.7B). The pocket contents are then covered with a periodontal dressing or a cyanoacrylate dental adhesive.

Minocycline Microspheres

The minocycline microspheres product is a subgingival, controlled-release delivery system containing the antibiotic minocycline hydrochloride incorporated into a bioresorbable poly(glycolide-co-D,L-lactide) polymer in unit-dose cartridges (Fig. 47.8). Each cartridge delivers minocycline hydrochloride equivalent to 1 mg of minocycline free base. Minocycline microspheres are indicated as an adjunct to SRP for the reduction of pocket depth in patients with adult periodontitis and as part of a periodontal maintenance program, which includes good oral hygiene and SRP.[10]

Minocycline belongs to the tetracycline class of antibiotics and has a broad spectrum of activity. Its bacteriostatic, antimicrobial activity results from the inhibition of protein biosynthesis. No overgrowth of opportunistic microorganisms was reported from clinical studies. No changes in the number of minocycline-resistant bacteria, *Candida albicans* or *Staphylococcus aureus*, in the gastrointestinal tract were detected at the end of a 56-day study, although there was a slight increase in the numbers of minocycline-resistant bacteria in periodontal pocket plaque samples after 9 months.[10] The clinical significance of the changes is unknown.

Patients should avoid hard or sticky foods at the treated teeth for 1 week and interproximal cleaning devices for about 10 days. The minocycline microspheres formulation is biodegradable and does not require removal. The cartridges are stored at 20°C to 25°C (68°F to 77°F), with excursions permitted to 15°C to 30°C (59°F to 86°F). Excessive heat should be avoided. The minocycline microspheres are used by injecting the contents of a unit-dose cartridge into the pocket. Neither a periodontal dressing nor an adhesive is needed.

Fig. 47.8 Minocycline Hydrochloride Microspheres (Arestin). Minocycline microspheres are packaged into unit-dose cartridges *(left)*. Microspheres are used by injecting the cartridge contents directly with a syringe into the periodontal pocket *(right)*. (Reprinted from Wolf HF, Hassell TM: *Color atlas of dental hygiene: periodontology*, ed 1, Stuttgart, Germany, 2006, Thieme, with permission.)

Complete details on the use of locally delivered, controlled-release antimicrobials and their safety profiles are available in the full prescribing information for each product.[10,11,106]

Detailed section on non-U.S. locally delivered, controlled-release antimicrobials is available in the online version of this chapter. Online materials for this chapter are found on the companion website.

Rationale for Local Delivery and Controlled Release

Chronic adult periodontitis is a multifactorial disease (Fig. 47.9). The first requirement is a susceptible host, largely due to genetics and not modifiable. Another nonmodifiable risk factor is age. Disease risks that may be modifiable include pathogenic oral plaque microorganisms and behavioral or environmental factors such as tobacco use. Mediating the pathogenesis are host-derived elements, including immune and inflammatory responses that can affect soft and hard tissue metabolism and feed back on the pathogenic flora.

From the most basic perspective, periodontal diseases are bacterial infections; the requirement for bacteria to initiate the periodontal lesion is well recognized. The antibacterial effect of SRP or other mechanical therapy generally results from a reduction of the bacterial load or an alteration of the composition of the bacterial flora at the periodontal site, but the antibacterial effect of mechanical treatment alone is insufficient, providing the rationale for chemically augmenting the mechanical therapy.

Many strategies have been used to deliver antimicrobial agents to the periodontal pocket at effective doses to reduce the bacterial microflora, including systemic administration or local administration by local irrigation of fluid formulations or placement of various gels or ointments. None of these strategies has proved as effective as controlled-release antimicrobials.

A drawback of antimicrobials delivered to the pocket but not in controlled-release formulations results from the dynamics of the GCF. The GCF fills the periodontal pocket space, but the copious flow out of the pocket continuously moves GCF contents to the oral cavity.[49,56] The flow rate can be markedly enhanced in the setting of inflammation. Antimicrobials delivered to the pocket are quickly washed out of the pocket by the GCF, rapidly reducing the concentration of drug locally to sub-antimicrobial

levels (Figs. 47.10 and 47.11). GCF drug concentrations may need to be elevated above usual levels because microorganisms in the pocket can exist within a protective biofilm structure in the periodontal ecosystem[33,135] (for reviews of periodontal microbiology and biofilms, see Palmer,[103] Teughels et al.,[141] or Kuboniwa and Lamont[80]). Bacterial biofilms can be highly resistant to penetration by fluids,[40] emphasizing the critical need for high GCF concentrations of active antimicrobials, which are achievable only with locally delivered, controlled-release agents (see Pharmacokinetics) but not possible with locally delivered antimicrobials not in controlled-release formulations or by systemic routes. Drisko[38] suggested that the high antimicrobial concentrations in the GCF as a result of local delivery could help to reach infected sites within the root or tissue.

Drug concentrations of systemically delivered antimicrobials in the GCF are orders of magnitude less than those achievable with controlled-release local delivery, and they cannot provide equivalent therapy.[124,139] Drug that is transferred from the plasma compartment to the GCF in the periodontal pocket is quickly washed away by the GCF flow (see Fig. 47.10). It was previously thought that systemically delivered tetracyclines markedly concentrated drug in the GCF compared with plasma,[52,105] but the hypothesis was not supported by later studies.[124,139] Some investigators have suggested that systemic therapies, rather than locally delivered agents, should be considered when there are multiple pocket sites for the sake of convenience and to save costs,[55,117] but if high concentrations of an antimicrobial drug are desired in the periodontal pockets, systemic delivery is not the appropriate therapy. Other benefits of locally delivered, controlled-release antimicrobials include decreased systemic, off-target effects and a decreased risk for promoting microbial resistance.

Detailed section on the pharmacokinetics of commonly available locally delivered controlled-release antimicrobials is available in the online version of this chapter. Online materials for this chapter are found on the companion website.

CLINICAL CORRELATION

Controlled-release agents maintain clinically effective intrapocket concentrations of antimicrobial for an extended period of time.

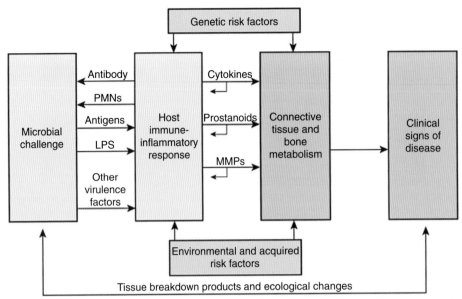

Fig. 47.9 Schematic Representation of the Pathogenesis of Periodontal Diseases and Possible Avenues for Prevention or Treatment. Through several virulence factors such as antigens or lipopolysaccharides *(LPS),* pathogenic microorganisms stimulate a host immune-inflammatory response. Immune elements, including polymorphonuclear leukocytes *(PMNLs)* and antibodies, can inhibit the offending microorganisms, and various cytokines, prostanoids, or enzymes can affect connective tissue and bone metabolism, ultimately resulting in the clinical signs of periodontitis initiation and progression. Genetic factors or environmental/acquired factors can separately affect disease risk. Potential avenues for intervention include scaling and root planing and use of antimicrobial agents to inhibit pocket microorganisms (i.e., affecting the microbial challenge), nonsteroidal or other antiinflammatory agents to inhibit cytokines or prostanoids (i.e., affecting the host immune-inflammatory response), antiresorptive agents (e.g., bisphosphonates) to inhibit osteoclastic bone resorption, and host-modulation therapy (e.g., low-dose oral doxycycline) to inhibit matrix-metalloproteinase *(MMP)* activity (i.e., affecting connective tissue and bone metabolism). (Modified from Page RC, Kornman KS: The pathogenesis of human periodontitis: an introduction, *Periodontology* 2000 14:9–11, 1997.)

LOCAL ADMINISTRATION OF ANTIBIOTICS

Potential Indications

Additional dental indications for locally delivered, controlled-release antimicrobials have not been evaluated by the FDA. Examples include combination adjunctive therapy and adjuncts for surgical therapy or peri-implantitis. Preliminary data for these indications are available and discussed in the following sections.

Combination Adjunctive Therapy

Many local and systemic adjunctive therapies are available with supportive data on their use in patients. None is labeled for use in combination therapy. It seems likely, however, that some practitioners may already be providing off-label combination adjunctive therapy for their patients, even though appropriate data do not exist.

Locally delivered, controlled-release antimicrobials enhance the clinical efficacy of SRP. Similarly, adjunctive systemic therapy with low-dose (20 mg) doxycycline, given orally twice daily as a host-modulating agent (later reported as a once-daily, modified-release formulation[110]) also can enhance the clinical efficacy of SRP.[23,30,109] Reddy and colleague[113] and Ryan and Golub[120] have reviewed matrix metalloproteinase modulation

as a treatment strategy. The question is whether a combination of local antimicrobial and host-modulating adjunctive therapies can provide greater clinical benefit than either adjunctive agent used alone.

In a 6-month clinical trial, combination adjunctive therapies resulted in significantly greater improvements in probing depth and clinical attachment compared with SRP alone.[99] More sites showed a probing depth reduction of 2.0 mm or more, and fewer sites had a residual probing depth 5.0 mm or more.[99] A single case report from this trial was published.[107] Because the appropriate control groups (i.e., SRP plus single adjunctive therapy) were not included in the trial, definitive conclusions regarding increased benefit from combination versus single adjunctive therapy cannot be made. The potential for combined adjunctive therapy to enhance clinical benefit is promising and warrants additional research.

The focus of this chapter is locally delivered, controlled-release antimicrobials. Data support the efficacy of locally delivered, controlled-release antimicrobials,[62] supporting the conclusion that SRP plus adjunctive therapy could be considered a new standard for nonsurgical periodontal therapy. Available data also support the adjunctive efficacy of systemic, low-dose oral doxycycline[23,30,72,110] to an extent that is numerically similar to that reported for locally delivered, controlled-release antimicrobials.

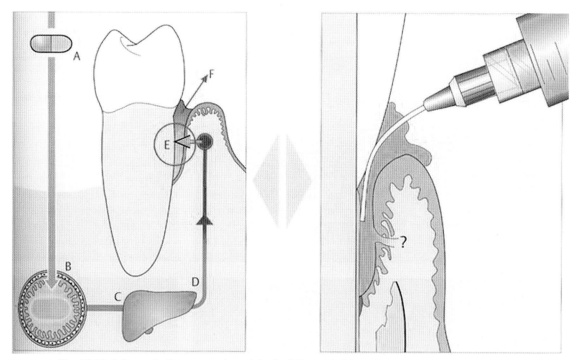

Fig. 47.10 Schematic Representation of the Inability to Achieve Therapeutically Sufficient Concentrations in the Periodontal Pocket for Sufficient Time With Antimicrobials Delivered Systemically or Locally but Not in Controlled-Release Formulations. *Left,* Orally administered drug *(A)* is absorbed in the gastrointestinal tract *(B)*, transported by the portal pathway to the liver *(C)*, and enters the circulatory system *(D)*, from which drug exits the vasculature into the periodontal pocket *(E)*. Drug is quickly eliminated from the pocket into the oral cavity by the copious flow of gingival crevicular fluid (GCF) *(F)*. Locally administered drugs not in controlled-release formulations suffer from the same limitation. *Right,* Locally delivered, controlled-release antimicrobial is administered into the periodontal pocket, where it remains until it degrades, continuously releasing drug into the GCF over time. Antimicrobial drug may be active against plaque bacteria that have invaded the surrounding periodontal tissues. (Reprinted from Wolf HF, Hassell TM: *Color atlas of dental hygiene: periodontology,* ed 1, Stuttgart, Germany, 2006, Thieme, with permission.)

Because appropriate comparative data are not available, comparisons of these therapies is not appropriate, and no conclusion can be reached regarding the most efficacious approach for adjunctive therapy, local or systemic adjunctive therapy or with single or combined agents.

In addition to the possibility of combination adjunctive therapy with a locally delivered agent and host modulatory therapy with low-dose oral doxycycline, Goodson and coworkers[51] reported outcomes from a randomized trial enrolling 231 patients that considered SRP alone and various combinations of SRP, systemic antimicrobials, and surgery using a $2 \times 2 \times 2$ factorial design. Patients were followed for 24 months. Maximal reductions in probing depth and gains in attachment level were observed at 6 months, which were maintained at 24 months in all treatment groups. At 24 months, gains in attachment were increased by systemic antimicrobials (0.50 mm), and probing depth reductions were further augmented by systemic antimicrobials (0.51 mm) and surgical treatment (0.36 mm). Both types of improvements were reduced by smoking.

A detailed section on the application of locally delivered controlled-release antimicrobials in surgical periodontal therapy is available in the online version of this chapter. Online materials for this chapter are found on the companion website.

Surgical Therapy

Pocket sites that do not seem to respond adequately to nonsurgical therapy and evidence residual probing depth with inflammation are often treated with follow-up surgical therapy. A question is whether locally delivered, controlled-release antimicrobials could augment surgical results. This hypothesis was tested in a pilot study by Hellström and coworkers[65] with minocycline microspheres at all pocket sites of 5 mm or more. Sixty patients with at least one nonmolar pocket site with a probing depth of 6 mm or more in each of two quadrants were treated with (1) microspheres at baseline and immediately after each of two surgical procedures at weeks 2 and 3 and again at week 5 or (2) standard surgical therapy. The mean probing depth was reduced in both treatment groups, but the reduction was significantly greater in the test group than in controls at 25 weeks (2.51 ± 0.10 mm vs. 2.18 ± 0.10 mm, $P = .027$). In contrast, the probing depth reduction after SRP with a limited surgical approach using adjunctive minocycline microspheres was not significantly different compared with SRP in a smaller pilot trial.[158]

A specialized periodontal surgical procedure, regenerative surgery, has become a standard procedure in periodontal practice. It had been suggested verbally as early as 1993 (Killoy WJ, personal communication, 2002) and in print in 1998[77,78] that

Subgingival medication concentration

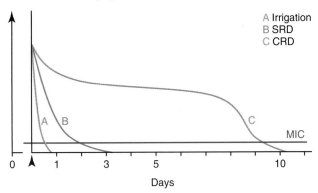

Fig. 47.11 Graph Shows the Release Profile of Locally Delivered, Sustained-Release or Controlled-Release Antimicrobials by Irrigation. Drug concentration in the gingival crevicular fluid (GCF) is diminished rapidly after irrigation *(A)*. Drug concentration can be extended for several days with drug administered in a modified, sustained-release formulation *(B)*. Drug concentration in the GCF can be maintained at therapeutically relevant concentrations for up to 10 days with controlled-release formulations *(C)*. Area under the curve but above the minimal inhibitory concentration *(MIC)* line represents drug concentration in the GCF greater than MIC values. The MIC for subgingival plaque bacteria may be substantially greater than typically reported bacterial MIC values because of the potentially protective effect of a subgingival biofilm formation. *CRD,* Controlled-release delivery; *SRD,* sustained-release delivery; *arrowhead,* administration of locally delivered agent. (Adapted from Wolf HF, Hassell TM: *Color atlas of dental hygiene: periodontology,* ed 1, Stuttgart, Germany, 2006, Thieme, with permission.)

adjunctive locally delivered, controlled-release antimicrobials might improve outcomes after regenerative periodontal surgery. In a pilot trial, the adjunctive use of the chlorhexidine chip with regenerative surgery resulted in more than a 100% greater mean improvement from baseline in bone height and mass 9 months after surgical treatment compared with SRP alone and surgery.[114] Both groups had also received prophylactic systemic antimicrobial treatment before surgery, but the addition of a locally administered antimicrobial resulted in a significant benefit compared with the control arm.

Other reports support the lack of efficacy of systemic antimicrobials[93] and the benefit of locally delivered antimicrobials[157] as adjunctive treatments in the regenerative setting. A microbiologic rationale for the use of locally delivered antimicrobials (i.e., tetracycline fiber) in the regenerative setting was also supported by Sbordone and colleagues.[127] Aichelmann-Reidy and coworkers[1] suggested that regenerative surgical procedures should include an adjunctive, locally delivered, controlled-release antimicrobial agent to provide a more consistent clinical benefit.

These preliminary reports suggested that the adjunctive use of locally delivered, controlled-release antimicrobials can improve clinical outcomes after periodontal surgery in regenerative and nonregenerative settings. These hypotheses require testing in prospective, adequate, and well-controlled trials. None of the three available agents is approved as an adjunct to surgery.

Peri-Implantitis

Similar to periodontitis, peri-implantitis is an inflammatory disease process that is initiated by local microorganisms and which affects the tissues surrounding an implant. An opportunity exists to treat diseased implant sites chemically by targeting the local microflora. There is a potential rationale for the use of locally delivered, controlled-release antimicrobials for the treatment of peri-implantitis. Although the treatment of peri-implantitis is an off-label use, it seems likely that some clinicians have tried local delivery in this setting.

Renvert and coworkers[115] studied 32 patients with at least one implant site with a probing depth of 4 mm or more plus bleeding or exudate on probing. Patients were treated with debridement followed by minocycline microspheres (17 patients, 57 implants) or a chlorhexidine gel formulation (15 patients, 38 implants). Treatments were repeated at 30 and 90 days. Followup examinations were performed at 10 days and 1, 3, 6, 9, and 12 months. There were significant reductions in probing depth compared with chlorhexidine at 1, 3, and 6 months and marked reductions in indicator microorganisms in both treatment groups. The study authors concluded that adjunctive minocycline microspheres could be of value in treating peri-implant lesions.

Buchter and colleagues[21] studied 28 patients with a total of 48 peri-implant defects. Two to 18 weeks before baseline measurements, patients had been treated for peri-implantitis (including scaling with a plastic instrument). Patients then continued to receive this treatment alone or with the additional adjunctive use of the doxycycline gel. At 18 weeks, the test group evidenced a significant reduction in mean probing depth and a significant gain in mean attachment levels compared with controls.

Schar and associates[128] and Bassetti and coworkers[16] studied 40 patients with peri-implantitis who had probing depths of 4 to 6 mm and less than 2 mm of radiographic bone loss that was treated with mechanical debridement and air polishing and adjunctively with local minocycline microspheres or photodynamic therapy for 12 months. A significant decrease in probing depth from baseline values was observed in photodynamic sites up 9 months and in minocycline sites up to 12 months. Decreases in *P. gingivalis* and *Tannerella forsythia* concentrations and in GCF levels of interleukin 1-β (IL-1β) were seen in both groups. There were no significant differences between groups, and no conclusions can be drawn about either therapy compared with mechanical therapy alone because an appropriate control group was not included.

Labels for the available locally delivered, controlled-release antimicrobials do not include an indication for peri-implantitis. Their potential for treating peri-implantitis, however, is an exciting possibility, and one that warrants additional research. Phase III trials are needed to test the hypothesis that locally delivered, controlled-release antimicrobials offer clinical benefit as part of a treatment regimen to manage peri-implantitis.

Tobacco Smoking

Smoking is a well-known risk factor for the development or progression of periodontitis, and it can limit the effectiveness of periodontal therapy.[17,69,76,108] The adjunctive use of locally delivered, controlled-release antimicrobials can enhance the efficacy of SRP in smokers. In a 3-month trial, SRP plus adjunctive doxycycline gel resulted in significantly greater probing depth reduction and clinical attachment gain compared with SRP alone about equally in smokers and nonsmokers.[143] This result was consistent with subset analyses of current smokers, former smokers, and nonsmokers from two 9-month, multicenter trials of doxycycline gel[121] and of smokers versus nonsmokers in studies of minocycline microspheres.[155] Subset analyses of therapy with minocycline microspheres showed that results for smokers were consistent with overall trial results.[102,104]

Consistent results also were seen in a later clinical trial of minocycline microspheres.[57] Beneficial periodontal microbiologic alterations in adjunctively treated sites compared with SRP alone

were reported for doxycycline gel and minocycline microspheres (Fig. 47.12).[57,88,129] A 2-year trial of doxycycline gel with a small number of patients provided further evidence of clinical efficacy.[87]

In a pilot trial to test the use of adjunctive minocycline microspheres in a surgical setting, clinical improvement was seen similarly in smokers and nonsmokers.[65] Adjunctive therapy may lessen the adverse impact of smoking on the periodontium and improve treatment outcomes for patients who smoke. A systematic review of the doxycycline gel and minocycline microspheres found that available data are insufficient to conclude that adjunctive

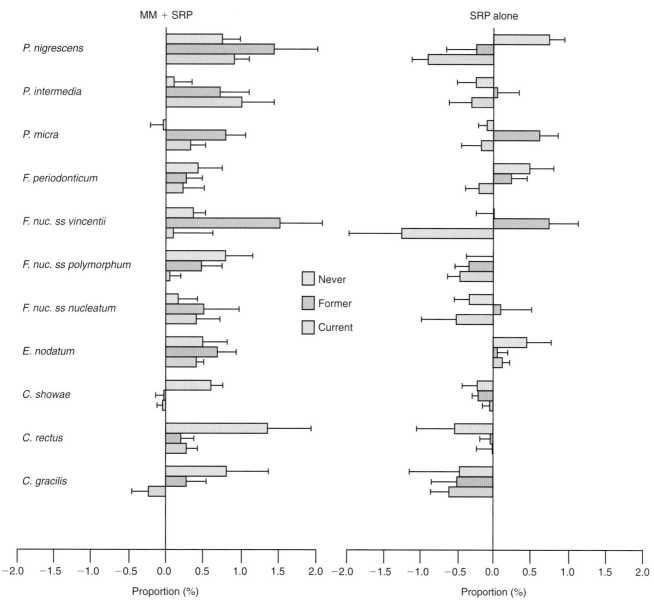

Fig. 47.12 Microbiologic Effects Are Shown After the Adjunctive Administration of Minocycline Microspheres *(Mm)* in Smokers and Nonsmokers. Therapy causes changes in the proportion of orange complex bacteria. Positive changes represent antibacterial effects as reductions in proportions. Negative changes represent proportional increases or proliferation of bacterial groups. *F. nuc.,* *Fusobacterium nucleatum; SRP,* scaling and root planing. (Reprinted from Grossi SG, Goodson JM, Gunsolley JC, et al: Mechanical therapy with adjunctive minocycline microspheres reduces red-complex bacteria in smokers, *J Periodontol* 78:1741, 2007, with permission from the American Academy of Periodontology.)

therapy significantly enhances SRP specifically in smokers, and it recommended additional clinical trials (i.e., adequate and well-controlled trials) to assess outcomes for smokers.[5]

Adverse Effects and Cautions for Use

A complete listing of cautions for use and possible adverse effects as listed on the FDA labels for these locally delivered, controlled-release antimicrobials is beyond the scope of this chapter, but complete details about the use of these products and their safety profiles are available in the full prescribing information.[10,11,106]

Clinicians are cautioned about adverse effects of this class of drugs:

- Potential for hypersensitivity reactions (i.e., not to be used in patients with a known sensitivity to any ingredient)
- Potential for the overgrowth of nonsusceptible microorganisms, including fungi
- Use in pregnancy
- Potential for discoloration during tooth development (i.e., tetracyclines only)
- Use in an acutely abscessed periodontal pocket or in extremely severe periodontal defects with little remaining periodontium
- Use of local mechanical oral hygiene procedures (e.g., toothbrushing, interdental cleaning devices) for approximately 7 to 10 days after administration

The most frequently reported adverse reactions in the clinical trials, without mention of causality, include headache, infection (including upper respiratory tract infection), flu syndrome, pain, tooth disorder and toothache, and various oral signs or symptoms. Toothache was the only adverse reaction that was significantly higher ($P = .042$) in the chlorhexidine chip group compared with placebo.[106]

A detailed section on cost-effectiveness of locally delivered, controlled-release antimicrobials is available in the online version of this chapter. Online materials for this chapter are found on the companion website.

Costs and Outcomes

Locally delivered, controlled-release antimicrobials entail costs. Adjunctive therapy with these products adds cost for the patient in addition to that of SRP, depending on fees charged by the practice. Concerns about the costs and the cost-effectiveness of these agents have proved to be a deterrent to routine clinical use. Although a thorough cost-effectiveness analysis is beyond the scope of this chapter, incorporation of adjunctive therapy into clinical practice warrants some assessment of costs and outcomes.

CASE REPORTS

The indications for the use of locally delivered, controlled-release antimicrobials in clinical practice are detailed in the full prescribing information for each product. Indications include potential use as part of nonsurgical periodontal treatment as adjunctive therapy or monotherapy. Examples of the clinical use of these products as part of nonsurgical periodontal therapy are shown in Figs. 47.13 and 47.14.

CONCLUSIONS

SRP alone are effective for reducing pocket depths, gaining increases in periodontal attachment levels, and decreasing inflammation levels (i.e., bleeding with probing). When systemic

Fig. 47.13 Locally Delivered, Controlled-Release Antimicrobials Can Be Used as Part of Nonsurgical Periodontal Therapy. Evaluation of the patient revealed a pocket depth (PD) of 5+ mm and bleeding on probing (BOP) at tooth #30, mesiolingual (ML) surface. A combination of localized scaling and root planing (SRP) with local delivery of minocycline microspheres was performed for tooth #30. (A) Initial radiograph. (B) PD of 5+ mm with BOP. The patient received localized SRP because this was the only site showing a PD of more than 5 mm. (C) Local delivery is achieved by inserting the syringe before dispensing microspheres into the periodontal pocket. (D) Minocycline microspheres are inserted into the periodontal pocket. (E) At 10 weeks after the procedure, the patient has a 3-mm PD and no BOP at the #30 ML surface. There are no signs of clinical inflammation.

Fig. 47.14 The Patient Had a Pocket Depth (PD) of 6 mm on the Tooth #4 Mesiobuccal (MB) Surface. Therapy included a combination of scaling and root planing (SRP) and local delivery of minocycline microspheres. Follow-up at 12 weeks showed an absence of bleeding on probing (BOP) or other signs of clinical inflammation and a reduced PD. (A) The MB surface of tooth #4 was treated with quadrant SRP in combination with minocycline microspheres. The initial PD at #4 MB was 6 mm. (B) Minocycline microspheres were inserted at tooth #4 MB. (C) Minocycline microspheres were deposited completely at the base of the periodontal pocket. (D) Immediately after application, remnants of the minocycline microspheres can be seen at the level of the free gingival margin. (E) The 12-week postoperative examination revealed a 3-mm PD and no BOP.

antibiotics are used as adjuncts to SRP, the evidence indicates that some systemic antibiotics (e.g., metronidazole, tetracycline) provide additional improvements in attachment levels (0.35 mm for metronidazole; 0.40 mm for tetracycline) when used as adjuncts to SRP.[61] The use of anti-infective chemotherapeutic treatment adjuncts does not result in significant adverse effects for patients.

The decision regarding when to use systemic antimicrobials should be made on the basis of the clinician's consideration of the clinical findings, the patient's medical and dental history,[39,43] the patient's preferences, and the potential benefits of adjunctive therapy with these agents.

Available data support the adjunctive use of locally delivered, controlled-release antimicrobials, which provides significant additional clinical benefit. The evidence supports the idea that adjunctive locally delivered, controlled-release antimicrobials make SRP more effective[62] and have a known safety profile. Based on available data, when these agents are used routinely as adjuncts to SRP as indicated as part of initial periodontal treatment or maintenance therapy, clinicians can expect a significantly greater mean reduction in probing depth compared with SRP alone. SRP plus adjunctive therapy, used in a manner that is consistent

with the approved full prescribing information, could be considered a new standard for nonsurgical periodontal therapy for the management of chronic adult periodontitis.[45]

CLINICAL CORRELATION

SRP plus adjunctive therapy could potentially be considered a new standard for nonsurgical periodontal therapy.

A number of pilot trials have suggested additional indications for adjunctive locally delivered, controlled-release antimicrobials. More research is necessary to test these hypotheses before further clinical comments can be made.

Case Scenarios are found on the companion website.

REFERENCES

 References for this chapter are found on the companion website www.expertconsult.com.

48

Occlusal and Orthodontic Therapy[a]

🌐 For online only content on parafunction, occlusal therapy, preorthodontic osseous surgery, orthodontic treatment of osseous defects, orthodontic treatment of gingival discrepancies, and implant interactions in orthodontics, please visit the companion website.

CHAPTER OUTLINE

Among the numerous local and systemic factors with the potential to influence the progression of periodontitis, the patient's occlusion remains a variable that requires an exact diagnosis. All of the disciplines of dentistry include the comprehensive analysis of occlusal relationships for determination of appropriate care.

The functional demands of the occlusion may fall within or substantially exceed the tolerances and the adaptability of the patient's periodontium and masticatory system. The full range of knowledge and skill needed to analyze all aspects of occlusal anatomy and function is beyond the scope of this chapter, which does present practical guidelines for the assessment and management of the occlusion specific to a patient's unique susceptibility to periodontitis.

PATHOGENESIS

The host-driven inflammatory response of each patient to a pathogenic bacterial biofilm[78] is so specific that the patient is his or her only reference for the interpretation of possible contributing factors to the progressive loss of supporting bone. Destructive events can be episodic and are site specific.

A clinician's diagnostic responsibility includes careful measurement of periodontal structures in the entire circumference of each tooth, accurate documentation, and timely reassessment. Periodontal deterioration that occurs rapidly or that is excessive for a person's age should prompt the clinician to investigate all

variables that can amplify his or her periodontitis. If a local factor such as an occlusal relationship can influence the course of the disease, its analysis must be as precise as any other aspect of the periodontal examination.

EVIDENCE-BASED DECISION-MAKING

In a perfect world, all diagnostic and therapeutic decisions would reflect evidence from multiple prospective clinical trials that have been subject to systematic review. Prospective human investigations of occlusal trauma are considered unethical, and periodontics has conscientiously struggled to reach discipline-wide consensus regarding the interaction of a patient's occlusion with his or her periodontal status.[34] To be clinically applicable, the investigation's methodology must parallel the clinical diagnosis and treatment of an individual with periodontitis.[37]

Historically, data management and statistical credibility and methodology within retrospective studies limited the ability of dedicated researchers to interpret the role of occlusion in an individual's periodontitis experience.[42,76,87] The grouping of data points, especially for large study populations, departs from the site specificity that periodontal diagnosis requires. If occlusal trauma is affecting a tooth, the effect on the periodontium is site specific for only that tooth. Treatment for a patient with periodontitis would never be based on an average of diagnostic references but rather on his or her unique susceptibility, anatomy, occlusion, and history.

[a]Adapted from the following chapters of Newman and Carranza's Clinical Periodontology, 13th edition: Chapter 55: Occlusal Evaluation and Therapy, by Michael J. McDevitt, and Chapter 56: Orthodontics: Interdisciplinary Periodontal and Implant Therapy, by Vincent G. Kokich and Frank Celenza.

KEY FACT

The role of occlusal trauma and its possible influence on the progression of periodontitis is tooth specific.

KEY FACT

Occlusal trauma can amplify (not cause) localized loss of attachment from inflammatory bone damage.

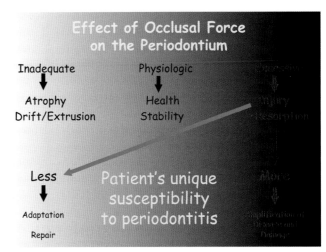

Fig. 48.1 The Degree of Occlusal Force Is Depicted as a Spectrum of White to Black, Representing None to Excessive Force.

In 2001, Nunn and Harrell[70] reported the retrospective findings for a group of patients with periodontitis. The analysis was based on measurement of the loss of attachment of each tooth and the presence or absence of occlusal interferences. This study and a similar investigation[14] confirmed that trauma from occlusion amplified the loss of attachment. Harrell and Nunn[38] also reported that eliminating occlusal interferences had a positive influence on the outcome of treatment when trauma from occlusion was found to be a contributing local factor. The positive influence of occlusal adjustment on the outcome of surgical and nonsurgical periodontal therapies was also reported by Burgett.[19] Evidence supports the possibility that trauma from occlusion can amplify damage to an inflamed periodontium.

Although animal studies do not carry the evidence-based hierarchic weight of ideally structured clinical trials, several newer studies seem to support the potential for excessive occlusal forces to amplify damage from inflammatory periodontitis. In two studies using a periodontitis-induced rat model, occlusal trauma resulted in readily identifiable changes in the periodontal ligament of the experimental group compared with the controls. Greater numbers of osteoclasts, perhaps related to increased receptor activator of nuclear factor κB ligand (RANKL) expression, supported the observation of greater alveolar bone loss in the inflammation plus trauma group. That group also demonstrated increased numbers of immune complexes, which may be a product of the damaged periodontal ligament collagen fibers' greater permeability.[64,93] An in vitro study of human periodontal ligament fibroblasts from healthy individuals and chronic periodontitis patients also supported the observation of significant differences in healthy and diseased periodontal ligament fibroblasts when subjected to compression. Several matrix metalloproteins, interleukin-l6 and interleukin-21, and other inflammation-associated proteins were expressed by the diseased, compressed fibroblasts compared with healthy fibroblasts, suggesting the diseased fibroblasts could produce additional damage to the periodontium of patients with chronic periodontitis.[30]

Interest in occlusion in the discipline of periodontics appears to be increasing, especially with the rapid growth of the replacement of missing teeth with implants. Despite some conflicting reports in the literature, common ground for consensus exists, as shown in Fig. 48.1.

Occlusal force has an effect on the periodontium (see Chapter 24), and that susceptibility to periodontitis is unique to each patient. Occlusal forces occur across a broad spectrum. No or minimal occlusal contact on a tooth results in disuse atrophy of the periodontium, which can result in instability of that tooth. Harmonious occlusal force on a tooth stimulates the physiologic arrangement of the periodontal attachment fibers and osseous architecture and encourages stability. Forces that exceed the tolerance of the periodontium result in resorption of the bone and disruption of the attachment.[44,63,66] In the healthy person, the periodontium around teeth that are subject to excessive occlusal force experiences adaptation and repair or remodeling with no loss of attachment, which often occurs with orthodontics.

For the patient who is losing bone as a result of periodontitis, coupling the ongoing inflammatory disease with excessive occlusal force can amplify destruction and damage to the periodontium of affected teeth.[70] If this conclusion is valid, the dentist has the responsibility to correlate the periodontal status of each tooth with its occlusal responsibilities and possible occlusal excesses.

TERMINOLOGY

The following is a list of key descriptive terms, as used in this chapter, and their common synonyms:

Centric relation: Position of the mandible when both condyle-disc assemblies are in their most superior positions in their respective glenoid fossae and against the slope of the articular eminences of each respective temporal bone.

Disclusion: Separation of certain teeth caused by the guidance provided by other teeth during an excursion. When anterior guidance provides separation of posterior teeth during an excursion, posterior disclusion is achieved.

Excursive movement: Any movement of the mandible away from maximum intercuspation.

Guidance: The pattern of opposing tooth contact during excursive movements of the mandible.

Initial contact in centric relation: The first occlusal contact in the centric relation closure arc.

Interference: Any occlusal contact in the centric relation closure arc or in any excursion that prevents the remaining occlusal surfaces from achieving stable contact or functioning harmoniously or that encourages masticatory system disharmony; also called an *occlusal discrepancy*.

Lateral excursion: Movement of the mandible laterally to the right or to left from maximal intercuspation.

Maximal intercuspation: Position of the mandible when there is maximal interdigitation and occlusal contact between the maxillary and mandibular teeth; also called *centric occlusion* and *intercuspal position.*

Nonworking side: The side of either arch that corresponds with the side of the mandible moving toward the midline during a lateral excursion; also called the *balancing side.*

Protrusion: Movement of the mandible anteriorly from maximal intercuspation.

Retrusion: Movement of the mandible posteriorly relative to a more anterior position.

Working side: The side of either dental arch that corresponds with the side of the mandible moving away from the midline during a lateral excursion.

OCCLUSAL FUNCTION AND DYSFUNCTION

Excellent sources for a comprehensive understanding of dental anatomy and function include textbooks by Ash and Nelson,[8] McNeill,[61] and Dawson.[27,28] Trauma from occlusion is determined by whether the composite of all occlusal forces on a specific tooth exceeds the tolerance or adaptability of its periodontium. Identification of masticatory system disharmonies begins with an appreciation of physiologic norms; this allows the dentist to recognize dysfunctional relationships, which can influence the accuracy of the diagnosis.[28,66,72]

Centric relation is a term used to describe the position of both condyles when they are fully seated in the fossae of their respective temporomandibular joints (TMJs). Rotation of the mandible around an axis through both condyles is called the *centric relation closure arc* (see Chapter 24). This is strictly a skeletal relationship until tooth contact occurs. Maximal intercuspation occurs when opposing teeth make contact, with optimal interdigitation, at the most stable endpoint of mandibular closure. Stability is enhanced by the simultaneous bilateral contact of multiple posterior teeth with occlusal forces in the long axis of most posterior teeth. If the initial tooth contact in the centric relation arc of closure occurs simultaneously with maximal intercuspation, the teeth do not displace the condyles. Conversely, if the teeth are firm and any contact occurs before maximal intercuspation, incline relationships of opposing occlusal surfaces guide the mandible into intercuspal position, thereby requiring one or both condyles to become dislocated from their fossa.[28,70] If the teeth are mobile and contact first in the centric relation closure arc, then *they may move away from opposing teeth rather than cause condylar displacement.*

Cusp–fossa or cusp–marginal ridge relationships of the posterior teeth provide resistance to vertical loading and functional stability for the patient's dentition. When occlusal forces load teeth in their long axis, the periodontium is the most resistant and supportive.[27,28] The anterior teeth can be stable with little occlusal loading in centric occlusion if they are favorably influenced by the oral musculature. If the anterior teeth are in contact in maximal intercuspation, they are coupled.

Movement of the mandible from centric occlusion is called an *excursion.* Movement forward is called a *protrusive excursion,* and movement to either side is called a *lateral excursion.* If the mandible can move posteriorly, it is called *retrusion.* There is evidence that the contact of posterior teeth in excursions can

overload those teeth, which results in negative dental, periodontal, muscular, and TMJ consequences.[1,23,28,72,95-100] The ideal relationship may be a light coupling of the anterior teeth in centric occlusion with immediate separation (i.e., disclusion) of all posterior teeth in all excursions.[97]

During a lateral excursion, posterior teeth that make contact on the same side as the direction of mandibular movement are described as having a working contact. Posterior teeth that make contact on the side opposite the direction of the lateral excursion are described as having a nonworking contact. Although nonworking contacts are classically associated with negative consequences,[100] the analysis of working contacts and the function of anterior teeth are critically important. Contacts that are disruptive to mandibular movement or stressful to individual teeth are called *occlusal interferences* or *discrepancies.* Dentists' ability to analyze the occlusion to identify contacts that can amplify a patient's periodontitis, thereby affecting certain teeth, is strategic to making the correct diagnosis.

Inflammation disrupts the integrity of the attachment apparatus, which results in less resistance to force from opposing teeth. When bone loss has occurred, less root surface area is supported,[5,43] and there are fewer sensory fibers in the periodontal ligament, which limits the protective muscle modulation of the occlusal forces.[80] The dentist must differentiate among inflammation-caused intolerance to occlusal forces, normal forces on teeth with reduced periodontal support, excessive occlusal forces, and well-tolerated forces on teeth affected by periodontitis.

The reader is referred to the online material for more information on the topic of parafunction. Online materials for this chapter are found on the companion website.

PARAFUNCTION

Bruxism can cause occlusal forces on teeth that are susceptible to periodontitis to be increased in intensity or frequency, thereby magnifying the potential amplification of damage.[24,54-55,91] Daytime or awake occlusal parafunction is commonly limited to clenching the teeth during incidents that require a person's focused effort or mental concentration. Patients can be engaged in identification of daytime teeth clenching, as was the case in a study of sleep bruxism and myofascial pain. Awake clenching was reported by 58 of the 60 participants.[81] Selection criteria for a study must be very exacting because self-reports of sleep bruxism by patients is usually unreliable.[79] Patients' identification of their parafunction can help them to understand its importance, and it supports the clinical experience that daytime clenching can be a frequent contributor to a patient's increased susceptibility to bone loss in sites of inflammatory periodontitis.

Nighttime or sleep bruxing of the teeth can take the form of grinding the teeth during various excursions or clenching the teeth. Sleep bruxism is probably an extension of the rhythmic masticatory muscle activity that is also observed in nonbruxers. Why nuclei in the brain stem allow bruxing to occur in some individuals while others are spared is unclear.[24,54-55]

Bruxing is associated with the greater frequency and persistence of TMJ dysfunction, orofacial pain, and possibly periodontal attachment loss.[91] The sensory input of teeth that are subject to bruxism is probably dampened, which may interfere with the diagnosis and treatment.[74] There seems to be limited influence on bruxing tendencies from occlusal interferences.[57] An exception was discovered in a clinical study of 30 bruxers and 30 nonbruxers; there was a significant difference in nonworking interferences in the bruxing population compared with their absence in the nonbruxing group.[83] When these findings are viewed along with those reported by Youdelis and Mann decades ago, the correlation of bruxing and site-specific inflammatory bone damage appears meaningful.[100]

Gerber and Lynd studied selective serotonin reuptake inhibitor–induced movement disorders.[33] They found that selective serotonin reuptake inhibitors such as Prozac encouraged bruxism.

Evidence is emerging that sleep-disordered breathing can influence or be associated with inflammatory diseases such as periodontitis.[18,29,36] Although a causal relationship between obstructive sleep apnea and sleep bruxism has not been firmly established, the reported data and observations support a definite association.[73,88-89] A patient with periodontitis with clinical evidence of occlusal trauma may be experiencing the consequences of sleep-disordered breathing. If an occlusal appliance is being considered to address the periodontal implications of excessive occlusal force experienced by a periodontitis-susceptible patient, compliance may be problematic for a person with sleep-disordered breathing because the appliance can contribute to airway obstruction.[31]

CLINICAL EXAMINATION

Before clinical evaluation, a conversation with the patient can help to provide a more complete diagnosis. With minimal symptoms, a patient may not associate loose teeth or significant dental wear with TMJ dysfunction or orofacial pain with occlusal function or parafunction. The list of questions in Chapter 24 and inquiries specific to the condition of the patient's teeth can help the clinician to open the lines of communication and set the tone for patient education during the clinical examination. Comprehensive evaluation of occlusal anatomy and relationships is accomplished by the analysis of many factors in the clinical setting and by mounted diagnostic casts.

Clinical evaluation of the occlusion is sequenced to support the patient's learning. It should always include a clinical assessment of masticatory system function and identification of disharmonies.

Temporomandibular Disorders Screening and Evaluation

Complete assessment of the masticatory system and identification of temporomandibular disorders are described in Chapter 24 and should be part of a patient's initial comprehensive examination. The temporomandibular disorder screening and clinical evaluation then become part of subsequent examinations.

The patient's range of motion is observed, maximal opening and the lateral and protrusive excursions are measured, and any deviation from the midline during opening and closing is defined. Light finger pressure applied over each TMJ can detect deflection of the tissue while the patient opens and closes the mouth; deflection suggests condyle-disc discoordination. Tenderness

---

BOX 48.1 Temporomandibular Disorder Screening Evaluation

1. Maximal interincisal opening (range, 40–50 mm)
2. Opening or closing pathway
3. Range of lateral and protrusive excursions (7–9 mm)
4. Auscultation for temporomandibular joint sounds
5. Palpation for temporomandibular joint tenderness or tissue displacement
6. Palpation for muscle tenderness
7. Load testing of the patient's temporomandibular joints

---

on palpation can indicate TMJ capsulitis. Listening to the joint with a stethoscope or a Doppler instrument during opening and closing can detect sounds that are consistent with uncoordinated condyle-disc relationships, arthritic changes, and other diagnostic sounds.[28]

Palpation of the muscles of mastication and the related head and neck musculature can reveal muscle tension or spasm related to compensation for occlusal or TMJ disharmonies.[28,72] Load testing of the TMJ is described in Chapter 24. Significant discoveries revealed during the screening examination summarized in Box 48.1 should lead the clinician to complete the comprehensive evaluation.

Testing for the Mobility of Teeth

Two basic methods are used to assess the firmness or looseness of a tooth. Classically, a dental instrument is used to exert pressure in the facial or lingual direction, and the dentist places his or her finger on the opposite side of the tooth to feel and see movement if it occurs (see Chapter 30). Recording a numeric value (range, 0 to 3) for the degree of mobility allows the clinician to track changes that may occur in response to therapy.

The other method is to test for the movement of teeth that are subject to pressure generated by the patient. Fremitus, vibration, or micromovement of a tooth can be felt when patients tap their teeth together. When the patient mimics clenching the teeth and then attempts to move the mandible in excursions, tooth movement can be observed. The patient placing a finger where the clinician felt tooth movement helps the patient to appreciate the looseness of his or her teeth (Fig. 48.2).

If the mobility of the teeth exceeds what is expected on the basis of the loss of support or the level of inflammation observed, trauma from occlusion is included in the diagnosis. The assimilation of all of the occlusal and periodontal diagnostic references can lead the clinician to conclude that even without mobility, there may be evidence of amplified periodontal damage as a result of unfavorable occlusal forces.

KEY FACT

An inflamed periodontium often contributes to the mobility of a tooth.

The reader is referred to the online material for more information on the topics of centric relation assessment, evaluation of excursions, and articulated diagnostic casts. Online materials for this chapter are found on the companion website.

Fig. 48.2 (A) Tactile and visual testing for mobility is done with a dental instrument by the clinician. (B) Tactile and visual testing for mobility is done with the patient clenching and while beginning right lateral excursion by the clinician. (C) The patient feels movement of her tooth when lateral excursion is attempted while the teeth are clenched.

OCCLUSAL THERAPY

Effective nonsurgical therapy usually reduces inflammation within the periodontium and results in some healing of attachment,[65] which often results in mobile teeth becoming more stable. If the clinician concludes that inflammation has been optimally controlled and that occlusal forces on individual teeth still exceed the tolerance of the periodontium, the basis for intervention is established.

The harmonious function of both TMJs and their associated muscles is required for occlusal stability. When there is sufficient evidence of excessive occlusal forces on the patient's teeth or when masticatory system disharmony exists and the patient desires a more stable occlusion, an occlusal appliance is prescribed.

Chapter 24 reviews TMJ anatomy. This can provide a better understanding of the therapy.

> **KEY FACT**
>
> Optimal resolution of inflammation is necessary to accurately interpret tooth mobility.

Occlusal Appliance Therapy

A well-designed and accurately fitted appliance can benefit masticatory system function while encouraging loose teeth in both arches to tighten as the supporting periodontium heals. The bilateral simultaneous contact of all opposing posterior teeth in centric relation, shallow anterior guidance, and the immediate disclusion of all posterior teeth in every excursion are essential elements of maxillary and mandibular occlusal appliances (Figs. 48.3 and 48.4).

Teeth that are opposing an appliance should be loaded as close as possible to their long axis. Maxillary appliances engage a portion of the hard palate, which provides substantial bracing of teeth and resistance to vertical and lateral forces. A horseshoe-shaped maxillary appliance relies on other, possibly compromised teeth to attempt to protect the most mobile teeth. Soft or partial coverage appliances are contraindicated for long-term protection and stabilization.[65] The protective role of occlusal appliances was addressed in the 8-year study by McGuire.[60] Occlusal appliances are not expected to cure bruxism,[59] but they

> **BOX 48.2 Requirements for Occlusal Stability**
>
> 1. Forces on an individual tooth that do not exceed the support and resistance of the tooth's periodontium and that are vertically oriented to the long axis of each tooth as much as possible
> 2. Even and simultaneous contact of all posterior teeth in the centric relation closure or in maximal intercuspation, with minimal difference between the two
> 3. Little or no contact of the anterior teeth in centric occlusion, although such contact is readily available to provide guidance in excursion and to produce posterior disclusion
> 4. Harmonious excursive movement of the mandible within the patient's envelope of function and with complete absence of occlusal interference

are often prescribed for patients with habitual parafunction as a compensating or protective intervention to limit masticatory system disharmony, damage to the teeth, and overstressing of implants.[53]

The reader is referred to the online material for more information on occlusal adjustment. Online materials for this chapter are found on the companion website.

Occlusal Stability for Restorative Dentistry

A stable occlusion is considered a prerequisite for any restorative therapy (Box 48.2). Implants to replace the teeth of a partially dentate patient add to the occlusal considerations. Osseointegration of implants eliminates micromovement, which can allow teeth to accommodate occlusal forces. The extent and timing of occlusal loading and the guidance requirement for each tooth and for each implant must be carefully harmonized (see Chapter 55). This is especially critical if any of the teeth are mobile or the patient bruxes to a significant degree.[92] If bruxism is suspected or the functional forces are considered to be excessive, the occlusal appliance as described may be a valuable application.[53,62]

BENEFITS OF ORTHODONTIC THERAPY

Orthodontic tooth movement may be of substantial benefit to the adult periorestorative patient. Many adults who seek routine

Fig. 48.3 (A) An occlusal appliance is fabricated on accurately mounted diagnostic casts. (B) The entire dental and palatal surface has been carefully relined to promote an optimal stabilizing influence on mobile teeth. (C) There is bilateral, simultaneous contact of the cuspids and all posterior teeth in centric relation, fabricated to enhance axial loading of opposing mandibular teeth. (D) There is smooth, relatively flat anterior guidance with immediate and sustained disclusion of all posterior teeth in protrusion. (E) There is smooth, relatively flat anterior guidance with immediate and sustained disclusion of all posterior teeth in right lateral excursions. (F) There is extreme left lateral excursion with smooth, harmonious transitions across the anterior teeth to maintain the disclusion of all posterior teeth. (G) Marks created by the opposing dentition demonstrate bilateral, simultaneous contact in centric relation and the immediate disclusion of the opposing posterior teeth in all excursions.

restorative dentistry have problems with tooth malposition, which compromises their ability to clean and maintain their dentition. If these individuals also are susceptible to periodontal disease, tooth malposition may be an exacerbating factor that could cause premature loss of specific teeth.

Orthodontic appliances have become smaller, less noticeable, and easier to maintain during orthodontic therapy. Many adults are taking advantage of the opportunity to have their teeth aligned to improve the aesthetics of their smile. Underlying gingival or osseous periodontal defects often can be improved during orthodontic therapy if the orthodontist is aware of the situation and designs the appropriate tooth movement. In addition, implants have become a major part of the treatment plan for many adults with missing teeth. If adjacent teeth have drifted into edentulous spaces, orthodontic therapy is often helpful to provide the ideal amount of space for implants and subsequent

Fig. 48.4 A Mandibular Occlusal Appliance Is Fabricated After Surgery to Provide a Stabilizing Influence for the Incisors in Particular and to Demonstrate Occlusal Attributes Similar to Those of the Maxillary Appliance.

Fig. 48.5 This patient initially had overlapped maxillary central incisors (A), and after initial orthodontic alignment of the teeth, an open gingival embrasure appeared between the centrals (B). Radiography showed that the open embrasure was caused by divergence of the central incisor roots (C). To correct the problem, the central incisor brackets were repositioned (D), and the roots were moved together. This required restoration of the incisal edges after orthodontic therapy (E), because these teeth had worn unevenly before therapy. As the roots were paralleled (F), the tooth contact moved gingivally and the papilla moved incisally, resulting in elimination of the open gingival embrasure.

restorations. This chapter shows the ways in which adjunctive orthodontic therapy can enhance the periodontal health and restorability of teeth and presents the role of implant dentistry in both periodontics and orthodontics.

Orthodontic therapy can provide several benefits to adult periodontal patients. The following seven factors should be considered:

1. Aligning crowded or malpositioned maxillary or mandibular anterior teeth permits adult patients better access to clean all surfaces of their teeth. This could be a tremendous advantage for patients who are susceptible to periodontal disease or do not have the dexterity to maintain oral hygiene.

2. Vertical orthodontic tooth repositioning can improve certain types of osseous defects in periodontal patients. Often, moving the tooth eliminates the need for resective osseous surgery.

3. Orthodontic treatment can improve the aesthetic relationship of the maxillary gingival margins before restorative dentistry. Aligning the gingival margins orthodontically avoids gingival recontouring, which could also entail bone removal and exposure of the roots of the teeth (Fig. 48.5).

Fig. 48.6 Before orthodontic treatment, this patient had significant mesial tipping of the maxillary right first and second molars, causing marginal ridge discrepancies and deep periodontal pockets (A). The tipping produced root proximity between the molars as well as a disruption of the normal gingival anatomy (B). To eliminate the root proximity, the brackets were placed perpendicular to the long axes of the teeth (C). This method of bracket placement facilitated root alignment and elimination of the root proximity, as well as leveling of the marginal ridge discrepancies (D through F).

4. Orthodontic therapy also benefits the patient with a severe fracture of a maxillary anterior tooth that requires forced eruption to permit adequate restoration of the root. Erupting the root allows the crown preparation to have sufficient resistance form and retention for the final restoration.

5. Orthodontic treatment allows open gingival embrasures to be corrected to regain lost papillae. If open gingival embrasures are located in the maxillary anterior region, this can present an aesthetic problem. In most patients, these areas can be corrected with a combination of orthodontic root movement, tooth reshaping, and restoration.

6. Orthodontic treatment could improve adjacent tooth positioning before implant placement or tooth replacement. This is especially true for the patient who has been missing teeth for several years and has drifting and tipping of the adjacent dentition.

7. A common tooth malalignment problem that results in periodontal pockets is the mesially tipped molar. Orthodontic uprighting of tipped molars corrects the deep gingival contours and eliminates or reduces the mesial periodontal pocket (Fig. 48.6).

KEY FACT

Orthodontic therapy can contribute in many ways to help patients with periodontal problems. In selected cases, vertical orthodontic tooth repositioning can improve certain types of osseous defects to eliminate the need for resective periodontal surgery. Many patients have crowded, malaligned, and malpositioned maxillary or mandibular anterior teeth, presenting a difficult biofilm control problem. Aligning the crowded teeth orthodontically will help patients to maintain improved biofilm control. The incorporation of orthodontic therapy in the treatment of these clinical periodontal problems is a great aid to the clinician and the patient.

The reader is referred to the online material for more information on the topic of preorthodontic surgery and orthodontic treatment of osseous defects. Online materials for this chapter are found on the companion website.

KEY FACT

Excellent biofilm control before, during, and after orthodontic therapy is of utmost importance to prevent and control periodontal inflammation. This is especially important during orthodontic therapy because biofilm control is very difficult with the numerous appliances and brackets that are placed on the dentition.

> **KEY FACT**
>
> Furcation problems, especially class III and IV lesions, are challenging to treat and maintain because of the difficulty in attaining access for biofilm control and for scaling and root planing. Hemisection of a furcated molar after endodontic therapy followed by orthodontic separation of the remaining roots is expensive and time consuming and may still have a questionable outcome. With the advent of predictable implant therapy, extraction of such a tooth should be considered.

> **KEY FACT**
>
> Periodontal diagnosis, prognosis, and treatment planning are important in deciding when a tooth is hopeless, because there are orthodontic cases where this knowledge is used to decide when a tooth can be used as a temporary anchor. When a tooth is used for this purpose, the patient is instructed on biofilm control and the tooth is scaled and root planed to eliminate the inflammation. When the tooth is no longer needed for orthodontic anchorage, it can be extracted.

The reader is referred to the online material for more information on the topic of orthodontic treatment of gingival discrepancies. Online materials for this chapter are found on the companion website.

> **KEY FACT**
>
> Orthodontic therapy to assist the periodontal patient with the aesthetic problem of missing interdental papilla is important because it is difficult, and in many cases impossible, to surgically create a missing papilla.

IMPLANT INTERACTIONS IN ORTHODONTICS

Although the interrelationships between the disciplines of orthodontics and implantology might not seem close to the casual observer, in fact they are quite intimate. In addition, the integration of periodontics with orthodontics and implants presents an even more interesting and important combination. Although the conventional orthodontic patient might be quite different in nature from the periodontal patient, there are many useful and interesting interactions between the disciplines that can and should be harnessed for the best treatment outcomes. This is especially true in current treatment planning in which implants are used as anchors to move teeth.

The conventional orthodontic patient might be characterized as an adolescent or young adult, usually with a healthy, although not always complete, dentition. This patient most often does not present with a significant medical or dental history. Conversely, the periodontal patient often does present with a significant and contributory medical history and a long list of dental problems, which often includes restorative considerations. Furthermore, the periodontium will be compromised and in need of treatment, usually preparatory to orthodontic intervention. In addition, there will often be tooth replacement considerations to be sequenced into the therapy. It is in this situation that implant therapy may be part of the treatment scenario. How, then, are

these two divergent patient types to be managed by combining treatment modalities from these three disciplines?

This section delineates some of the interrelationships that can be used for better therapeutic outcomes. When the clinician gains an appreciation for the periodontal apparatus that supports a tooth and applies an understanding of the physiology of tooth movement, one can use the body's reparative and remodeling capacities to effect periodontal alterations as a result of tooth movement. Furthermore, as implant modalities are called upon, a greater demand for accurate tooth position arises. Moreover, as more adult patients are seeking orthodontic and implant treatment, an understanding of the need for and methods of ensuring periodontal health before and during orthodontic and implant care becomes paramount. Consequently, the intimate relationships among these three distinct dental disciplines become apparent in both the treatment planning and treatment execution phases of therapy. We can truly address this topic as *interdisciplinary dentistry*.

The reader is referred to the online material for more information on implant interactions in orthodontics (planning phase, implant anchorage, orthodontic site preparation and orthodontic acceleration). Online materials for this chapter are found on the companion website.

> **KEY FACT**
>
> Implants can be used to facilitate orthodontic mechanotherapy by providing anchorage, and orthodontic treatment can facilitate implant therapy by providing site development. The sequence of therapy is determined by which of these roles are being harnessed. When an implant is used to provide a source of orthodontic anchorage, it should be placed and loaded early in the orthodontic treatment. When orthodontics is being used for site development, the implant placement will follow the orthodontic treatment.

CONCLUSIONS

Confirmation of the appropriateness of occlusal therapy is the product of a thorough evaluation of the patient's occlusion and his or her masticatory system. The sequence of occlusal treatment begins with antiinflammatory therapy and progresses through reversible appliance therapy before any irreversible options are considered. This provides the clinician with the most careful approach to assessing and treating the occlusion of a patient with periodontitis.

There are many benefits to integrating orthodontics and periodontics in the management of adult patients with underlying periodontal defects. The key to treating these patients is communication and proper diagnosis before orthodontic therapy, as well as continued dialog during treatment. Not all periodontal problems are treated in the same way. This chapter provides a framework for the integration of orthodontics to solve periodontal problems.

Significant and fascinating interplays exist between the practices of orthodontics and periodontics, which also includes implantology. Reciprocal relationships can be harnessed through proper sequencing of treatments to enhance outcomes. Utilization of various implants can facilitate orthodontic mechanotherapy, streamline treatment, eliminate compliance dependency, improve predictability, and even introduce new treatment options. Conversely, orthodontic preparation prior to implant placement can yield a more favorable environment through orthodontically induced site development in which both hard and soft tissue can be augmented and remodeled. Furthermore, spatial management of implant sites and neighboring tooth positions is often essential to ideal implant location.

Periodontal treatment preparatory to orthodontic treatment is often required to eliminate inflammation and bolster the investing tooth structures, thereby permitting successful tooth movement without further loss of attachment. Likewise, orthodontic modalities can be used to remodel the hard and soft tissues of the periodontium to benefit various situations, such as defect eradication.

A Case Scenario is found on the companion website.

REFERENCES

 References for this chapter are found on the companion website.

49

Phase II Periodontal Therapy[a]

 For online only content on critical zones in pocket surgery, please visit the companion website.

CHAPTER OUTLINE

Therapy for periodontal disease, which encompasses many techniques and procedures, depends on the disease status and objective of the final outcome. Early problems can be corrected with successful phase I therapy, consisting of biofilm removal by the patient on a daily basis, scaling, and root planing when necessary. Many cases are successfully treated and maintained by phase I therapy.

Many moderate to advanced cases cannot be resolved without surgically gaining access to the root surface for root planing and reducing or eliminating pocket depth to allow the patient to remove biofilm. The surgical phase of therapy is also referred to as phase II therapy. This chapter describes the surgical techniques used for the following purposes:

- Controlling or eliminating periodontal disease
- Correcting anatomic conditions that favor periodontal disease, impair aesthetics, or impede placement of prosthetic appliances
- Placing implants to replace lost teeth and improving the environment for their placement and function

OBJECTIVES OF THE SURGICAL PHASE

The surgical phase of periodontal therapy has the following objectives:

1. To improve the prognosis for teeth and their replacements
2. To improve aesthetics
3. To alter defects of the gingival and mucosal tissues that predispose these areas to disease.

Surgical techniques are used for pocket therapy and for correction of related morphologic problems (i.e., mucogingival

defects). In many cases, therapies are combined to provide one surgical intervention that fulfills both objectives.

Surgical techniques (1) increase access to the root surface, allowing the dentist to remove all irritants; (2) reduce or eliminate pocket depth, making it possible for the patient to maintain the root surfaces free of biofilm; and (3) reshape soft and hard tissues to attain a harmonious topography. Resective or regenerative surgery, or both, is used to reduce pocket depth (Box 49.1) (see Chapter 50).

Three types of techniques are performed on noninflamed tissues and in the absence of periodontal pockets (see Box 49.1):

- *Plastic surgery techniques* are used to create or widen the attached keratinized gingiva by placing grafts of various types.
- *Aesthetic surgery techniques* are used to cover denuded root surfaces resulting from recession and to recreate lost papillae.
- *Preprosthetic techniques* are used to modify the periodontal and neighboring tissues to receive prosthetic replacements. They include crown lengthening, ridge augmentation, and vestibular deepening.

Fig. 49.1 provides a three-tiered classification of the surgical procedures used in periodontics: pocket reduction surgery, periodontal plastic surgery, and preprosthetic surgery. Pocket reduction surgery consists of resective and regenerative procedures, and periodontal plastic surgery includes aesthetic and gingival augmentation (anatomic) procedures. Crown lengthening, ridge preservation/augmentation, and implant procedures are listed under preprosthetic surgery. Periodontal surgical procedures also are available for the placement of dental implants. They include implant placement techniques and a variety of surgical procedures to modify neighboring tissues for the placement of implants. Bone augmentation of the sinus floor or for a narrow edentulous ridge is an example (see Box 49.1).

[a]Adapted from the following chapter of Newman and Carranza's Clinical Periodontology, 13th edition: Chapter 57: Phase II Periodontal Therapy, by Henry H. Takei.

BOX 49.1   Periodontal Surgery

Pocket Reduction Surgery
- Resective (e.g., gingivectomy, apically displaced flap, undisplaced flap with or without osseous resection)
- Regenerative (e.g., flaps with grafts, membranes)

Correction of Anatomic or Morphologic Defects
- Plastic surgery techniques used to widen attached gingiva (e.g., free gingival grafts)
- Esthetic surgery (e.g., root coverage, recreation of gingival papillae)
- Preprosthetic techniques (e.g., crown lengthening, ridge augmentation, vestibular deepening)
- Placement of dental implants, including techniques for site development for implants (e.g., guided bone regeneration, sinus grafts)

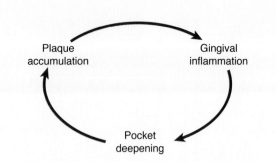

Fig. 49.2 Accumulation of Plaque Leads to Gingival Inflammation and Pocket Deepening, Which Increases the Area of Plaque Accumulation.

Fig. 49.1 Classification of Periodontal Surgery. The surgical procedures accomplished in periodontics are organized as pocket reduction surgery, periodontal plastic surgery, and preprosthetic surgery.

Surgical Pocket Therapy

Surgical pocket therapy can be used to gain access to the diseased root surface to ensure the removal of calculus located subgingivally before surgery and to eliminate or reduce the depth of the periodontal pocket.

Successful periodontal therapy eliminates calculus, plaque or biofilm, and diseased cementum from the tooth surface as much as possible. Numerous investigations have shown that the difficulty of this task increases as the pocket becomes deeper.[2,5] The irregularities and concavities on the root surface also adds to the difficulty of instrumenting the root surfaces.[11,14] Furcations also create problems for scaling and root planing in these areas (see Chapter 45).[4] Most of these problems can be remedied by resecting or displacing the soft-tissue wall of the pocket, which increases the visibility and accessibility of the root surface.[3] The surgical flap technique allows the dentist to overcome these problems of access to the root surface.

Pocket elimination is another important consideration. It consists of reducing the depth of the periodontal pocket to that of a physiologic sulcus to enable cleaning by the patient. By proper case selection, resective and regenerative techniques can be used to accomplish this goal. A pocket makes it impossible for the patient to remove biofilm, which is part of the vicious cycle depicted in Fig. 49.2.

Results of Pocket Therapy

A periodontal pocket can be in an active state or a period of inactivity or quiescence. In an active pocket, underlying bone is being lost (Fig. 49.3, *top left*). It often is diagnosed clinically by bleeding that occurs spontaneously or in response to probing. After phase I therapy, the inflammatory changes in the pocket

Fig. 49.3 Possible Results of Pocket Therapy Are Shown. An active pocket can become inactive and heal by means of a long junctional epithelium. Surgical pocket therapy can result in a healthy sulcus, with or without gain of attachment. Improved gingival attachment promotes restoration of bone height, with re-formation of periodontal ligament fibers and layers of cementum.

wall subside, rendering the pocket inactive and reducing its depth (see Fig. 49.3, *top center*). The extent of this reduction depends on the depth before treatment and the degree to which the depth is the result of the edematous and inflammatory component of the pocket wall (i.e., pseudopocket).

Whether the pocket remains inactive depends on the depth, the individual characteristics of the plaque or biofilm components, and the host response. Recurrence of the initial activity is likely.

Inactive pockets sometimes heal with a long junctional epithelium (see Fig. 49.3, *top right*). This condition can be unstable, and the chance of recurrence and re-formation of the original pocket remains because the epithelial union with the tooth is weak. However, one study in monkeys showed that the long junctional epithelial union could be as resistant to biofilm infection as a true connective tissue attachment.[9]

Several studies reported that inactive pockets could be maintained for long periods with little loss of attachment by means of frequent therapy[6,10,12] and by excellent plaque or biofilm removal by the patient on a daily basis. A more reliable and stable result is obtained by transforming the pocket into a healthy sulcus. The bottom of the healthy sulcus can be located where the bottom of the pocket was localized or coronal to it. In the first case (see Fig. 49.3, *bottom left*), there is no gain of attachment, and the area of the root that was previously the tooth wall of the pocket becomes exposed. Rather than causing recession, periodontal treatment uncovers the recession previously caused by disease.

The healthy sulcus can be located coronal to the bottom of the preexisting pocket (see Fig. 49.3, *bottom center* and *right*). This is conducive to a restored marginal periodontium; the result is a sulcus of normal depth with a gain of attachment. The creation of a healthy sulcus and a restored periodontium entails total restoration of the status that existed before periodontal disease began, which is the ideal result of treatment. The bone regeneration diagram in Fig. 49.3 (*bottom center* and *right)* is for illustrative purpose only because bone regeneration without an osseous wall is seldom achieved.

POCKET ELIMINATION VERSUS POCKET MAINTENANCE

Pocket elimination (i.e., depth reduction to gingival sulcus levels) has traditionally been considered a type of periodontal therapy. It was considered vital because of the need to improve access to root surfaces for the therapist during treatment and for the patient after healing. Prevailing opinion considers deep pockets after therapy to represent a greater risk of disease progression than shallow sites. Individual probing depths are not good predictors of future clinical attachment loss. Conversely, the absence of deep pockets in treated patients is an excellent predictor of a stable periodontium.[5]

Longitudinal studies of different therapeutic modalities over the past 30 years have produced conflicting results,[7,15] probably because of problems created by the split-mouth design. After surgical therapy, pockets that rebound to a shallow or moderate depth can be maintained in a healthy state and without radiographic evidence of advancing bone loss by maintenance visits consisting of scaling and root planing, with oral hygiene reinforcement performed at regular intervals of 3 months or less. In these patients, the residual pocket can be examined with a thin periodontal probe without pain, exudate, or bleeding. This indicates that biofilm has not formed on the subgingival root surfaces.

These findings do not alter the indications and need for periodontal surgery because the results are based on surgical exposure of the root surfaces for thorough elimination of irritants. However, the findings also emphasize the importance of the maintenance phase and close monitoring of the level of attachment and pocket depth along with the other clinical variables (e.g., bleeding, exudation, tooth mobility). *Transformation of the initial deep, active pocket into a shallower, inactive, maintainable pocket requires some form of definitive pocket therapy and constant supervision thereafter.*

Pocket depth is an extremely useful and widely used clinical determination, but it must be evaluated together with the level of attachment and degree of bleeding, exudation, and pain. The most important variable for evaluating whether a pocket is progressing is the *level of attachment,* which is measured in millimeters from the cementum-enamel junction. Apical displacement of the level of attachment places the tooth in jeopardy, not the increase in pocket depth, which may be caused by coronal displacement of the gingival margin.

Pocket depth remains an important clinical variable in making decisions about treatment. Lindhe and colleagues[8] compared the effect of root planing alone or using a modified Widman flap with the resultant level of attachment and in relation to initial pocket depth. They reported that scaling and root-planing procedures induced loss of attachment if performed in pockets shallower than 2.9 mm, whereas gain of attachment occurred in deeper pockets. The modified Widman flap induced loss of attachment if performed in pockets shallower than 4.2 mm but resulted in a greater gain of attachment than root planing in pockets deeper than 4.2 mm. The loss is a true loss of connective tissue attachment, whereas the gain can be considered a false gain because of reduced penetrability of connective tissues apical to the bottom of the pocket after treatment.[9,16]

Probing depths established approximately 6 months after active therapy and healing can be maintained, remain unchanged, or be reduced even further during a maintenance period involving careful reevaluation, plaque or biofilm removal, and root débridement, as necessary every 3 months.[8]

Ramfjord[12] and Rosling[13] and their colleagues reported that a certain pocket depth recurs regardless of the surgical technique used for pocket therapy. *Maintaining this depth without any further loss of attachment becomes the goal.*

REEVALUATION AFTER PHASE I THERAPY

Longitudinal studies found that all patients should be treated initially with scaling, root planing, and plaque or biofilm control and that a final decision on the need for periodontal surgery should be made only after a thorough evaluation of the effects of phase I therapy.[5] Assessment typically is made no less than 1 to 3 months and sometimes as much as 9 months after the completion of phase I therapy.[1] It is customary for reevaluation to be performed 4 to 8 weeks following phase I therapy.[14] Reevaluation of the periodontal condition includes repeat probing of the entire mouth. Calculus, root caries, defective restorations, and signs of persistent inflammation should also be evaluated.

Section on critical zones in pocket surgery is found on the companion Expert Consult website.

INDICATIONS FOR PERIODONTAL SURGERY

The following findings can indicate the need for a surgical phase of therapy:

1. Areas with irregular bony contours, deep craters, and other defects usually require a surgical approach.
2. Pockets around teeth where access to the root surface for complete removal of root irritants is not clinically possible are an indication for surgery. This occurs frequently around molars and premolars.
3. Furcation involvement of grade II or III may require a surgical approach to ensure the removal of irritants around root surfaces. If root resection or hemisection is necessary, surgical intervention will be needed.
4. Intrabony pockets distal to the last molars, which in many cases are complicated by mucogingival problems, often require surgery.
5. Persistent inflammation in areas after past procedures that have moderate to deep pockets may require a surgical approach. These are usually areas where all of the subgingival calculus could not be removed. Cases with shallow pockets and good hygiene but bleeding on probing can be caused by mucogingival problems in areas where there is no keratinized tissue. Trauma to these areas can cause bleeding.

METHODS OF POCKET THERAPY

The methods for pocket therapy can be classified as follows:

1. *New attachment techniques* offer the ideal result because they eliminate pocket depth by reuniting the gingiva with the tooth at a position coronal to the bottom of the preexisting pocket. New attachment involves regeneration of bone, connective tissue, periodontal ligament, and cementum.
2. *Removal of the pocket wall* is the most common method. The wall of the pocket consists of soft tissue and can include bone in the case of intrabony pockets. It can be removed by the following methods:
   - Retraction or shrinkage, where plaque or biofilm removal by the patient and scaling and root planing resolve the inflammatory process, can occur. The gingival tissue shrinks, reducing the pocket depth.
   - Surgical removal of the pocket is done by gingivectomy or the undisplaced flap technique.
   - Apical displacement of the flap is performed with an apically displaced flap.
3. *Removal of the tooth side of the pocket*, which is accomplished by tooth extraction or by partial tooth extraction in the case of furcation involvement (i.e., hemisection or root resection).

Criteria for Selection of the Method of Surgical Therapy

Scientific criteria to establish indications for the use of each technique are difficult to determine. Criteria are based on longitudinal studies that follow a significant number of cases over a number of years, standardization of multiple factors, and long-term clinical experience. Selection of a technique for treating a particular periodontal lesion is based on the following considerations:

1. Characteristics of the pocket: depth, relation to bone, and configuration
2. Accessibility to instrumentation, including furcation involvement
3. Existence of mucogingival problems
4. Response to phase I therapy
5. Patient cooperation, including the ability to perform effective oral hygiene and stop smoking
6. Age and general health of the patient
7. Overall diagnosis of the case: various types of gingival enlargement and stages and grades of periodontitis
8. Aesthetic considerations
9. Previous periodontal treatments

Each variable is analyzed in relation to the pocket therapy techniques available. A specific technique is then selected. The one most likely to successfully solve the problem with the fewest undesirable effects should be selected. Dentists who adhere to one technique to solve all problems do not take advantage of the wide repertoire of techniques that are at their disposal.

Approaches to Specific Pocket Problems

Therapy for Gingival Pockets

Gingival pockets do not have an osseous component (i.e., no attachment loss) and usually have edematous or fibrotic gingival tissue. Two factors are taken into consideration: the character of the pocket wall and the accessibility of the pocket.

The pocket wall can be edematous or fibrotic. *Edematous tissue* shrinks after the elimination of local factors, reducing or totally eliminating pocket depth. Scaling and root planing are the techniques of choice for these cases.

Pockets with a *fibrotic wall* are not appreciably reduced in depth after scaling and root planing. These pockets are eliminated or reduced by surgical therapy. In the past, gingivectomy was frequently used to reduce these pockets. This solved the problem, but in cases of marked gingival enlargement (e.g., severe phenytoin-related enlargement), treatment could leave a large, open wound, and the patient had to endure a painful and prolonged healing process. Currently, a modified flap technique is used, and fewer postoperative problems are associated with primary closure of the wound.

Therapy for Incipient (Stage I) Periodontitis

In patients with slight or incipient periodontitis with minimal attachment and bone loss, the pocket depths are shallow or a moderate depth. In these patients the conservative approach of good oral hygiene, scaling, and root planing when necessary usually suffices to control the disease. Incipient periodontitis that recurs in previously treated sites with good hygiene may require a thorough analysis of the recurrence, which may be caused by remnants of calculus that were missed during previous treatment or other factors such as open margins of a restoration located subgingivally. Occasionally, a surgical approach may be required to correct these problems.

Therapy for Moderate to Severe (Stage II, III, or IV) Periodontitis in the Anterior Areas

Because the maxillary anterior teeth are important aesthetically, techniques that cause the least amount of visual root exposure should be considered. However, each patient has different expectations regarding the final result of therapy. The dentist must explain that the therapy may be a compromise between complete pocket elimination and achieving an aesthetic result that is acceptable to the patient. The patient must be educated before therapy that the result may be some degree of gingival recession and some loss of the interdental papilla.

The anterior dentition has two advantages for using a conservative (nonsurgical) approach: (1) the teeth are all single rooted and easily accessible for subgingival scaling and root planing, and (2) patient compliance and thoroughness in plaque or biofilm control may be easier to attain. *Nonsurgical therapy is therefore the technique of choice for the maxillary anterior dentition.*

In some situations, surgical therapy may be necessary to improve accessibility for root planing, or regenerative therapy may be possible.

When the aesthetic outcome is not the primary consideration and a flap procedure is necessary for root surface access, the *modified Widman flap* can be selected. This technique uses an internal bevel incision approximately 1 to 2 mm from the gingival margin without thinning the flap. This procedure may result in minor recession of the surrounding gingival tissue.

In cases with advanced osseous involvement, bone contouring may be needed despite the resultant root exposure. The technique of choice is the *apically displaced flap with osseous bone contouring.* The dentist must educate the patient before therapy about

the possibility of aesthetic difficulties due to the expected recession of gingival tissue.

Therapy for Moderate to Severe (Stage II, III, or IV) Periodontitis in Posterior Areas

Treatment for the maxillary and mandibular premolars and molars does not entail aesthetic problems but frequently involves difficult access for root therapy. Bone defects occur more often in the posterior area than the anterior, with many areas having deep infrabony lesions and anatomic root problems with concavities, such as the mesial surface of the maxillary first premolar. A difficult problem encountered in the posterior area is the furcation lesion. Because this area can pose insurmountable problems for instrumentation unless a flap is reflected, surgery is frequently indicated.

CONCLUSIONS

Many steps are required to achieve and maintain a healthy periodontal status. After completion of phase I therapy, which consists of patient education, biofilm control, and thorough root therapy, the involved periodontal areas are reevaluated. The necessity of phase II therapy, which is the surgical phase of treatment, depends on the success of the initial phase and the severity of the periodontal condition. Periodontal surgery, which includes plastic, aesthetic, resective, and regenerative procedures, becomes necessary when access for root therapy is required or correction of anatomic or morphologic defects is necessary. Placement of dental implants can be part of this therapy.

REFERENCES

 References for this chapter are found on the companion website.

⊕ For online-only content on the treatment of root sensitivity and hospital periodontal surgery,
please visit the companion website.

CHAPTER OUTLINE

All surgical procedures must be carefully planned. The patient should be adequately prepared medically, psychologically, and practically for all aspects of the intervention. This chapter covers the preparation of the patient and the general considerations that are common to all periodontal surgical techniques. Complications that may occur during or after surgery are also discussed.

Although periodontal surgical procedures are usually performed in the dental office, an online section of this chapter briefly discusses situations that may require hospitalization and treatment using general anesthesia in the operating room. This chapter is concluded with a review of common types of periodontal surgeries and the postoperative management of symptoms resulting from periodontal surgical procedures.

PRINCIPLES OF PERIODONTAL SURGERY

Patient Preparation—Reevaluation After Phase I Therapy

Almost every patient undergoes the so-called initial or preparatory phase of therapy, which consists of thorough scaling and root planing and the removal of all irritants responsible for the periodontal inflammation. When these procedures are executed well and combined with patient education, the results will: (1) eliminate some lesions entirely; (2) render the tissues firm and consistent, thereby allowing for accurate and minimally invasive surgery; and (3) acquaint the patient with the office, the clinician, and the assistants, thereby reducing the patient's apprehension and fear.

[a]Adapted from the following chapters of Newman and Carranza's Clinical Periodontology, 13th edition: Chapter 59: General Principles of Periodontal Surgery, by Perry R. Klokkevold, Henry H. Takei, and Fermin A. Carranza, and Chapter 60: Periodontal Surgical Therapy, by Jonathan H. Do, Henry H. Takei, Michael Whang, and Kitetsu Shin.

> **KEY FACT**
>
> Phase I therapy and reevaluation are important to minimize the necessity for periodontal surgery. When excellent biofilm removal by the patient and scaling and root planing are accomplished, numerous cases may not require surgical therapy, or if it is necessary, the surgical therapy may be minimal.

The reevaluation phase consists of reprobing and reexamining all of the findings that previously indicated the need for the surgical procedure. The persistence of these findings confirms the indication for surgery. The number of surgical procedures, the expected outcome, and the postoperative care necessary are all determined before therapy and are explained to the patient. After all of the important information regarding the surgery is discussed, a final decision is made that incorporates any necessary adjustments to the original plan.

Premedication

For patients who are not medically compromised, the value of administering antibiotics routinely for periodontal surgery has not been clearly demonstrated.[33] However, some studies have reported reduced postoperative complications, including reduced pain and swelling, when antibiotics are given before periodontal surgery and continued for 4 to 7 days after surgery.[3,13,23,37]

The prophylactic use of antibiotics in patients who are otherwise healthy has been advocated for bone-grafting procedures and purported to enhance the chances of new attachment. Although the rationale for such use appears logical, no research evidence is available to support it. In any case, the risks inherent in the administration of antibiotics should be evaluated together with the potential benefits. Additional presurgical medications that may be administered include a nonsteroidal antiinflammatory drug such as ibuprofen (e.g., Motrin) 1 hour before the procedure and an antimicrobial mouthrinse such as 0.12% chlorhexidine gluconate (e.g., Peridex or PerioGard).[50]

Smoking

The deleterious effect of smoking on the healing of periodontal wounds has been amply documented (see Chapter 11).[22,41,57] Patients should be clearly informed of this fact and asked to quit smoking completely or to stop smoking for a minimum of 3 to 4 weeks after the procedure. For patients who are unwilling to follow this advice, an alternate treatment plan that does not include complicated techniques (e.g., regenerative, mucogingival, aesthetic) should be considered.

Informed Consent

The patient should be informed at the initial visit regarding the diagnosis, prognosis, and recommended treatment options including explanations about expected outcomes. The pros and cons of each approach should be discussed, and the patient should be encouraged to ask questions. At the time of surgery, the patient should again be informed both verbally and in writing of the procedure to be performed, including the risks and expected outcomes. Patients should be given the opportunity to ask any additional questions, and once their questions are answered, they should indicate their agreement to undergo the procedure by signing the informed consent form.

Emergency Equipment

The clinician, all assistants, and office personnel should be trained to handle all possible emergencies that may arise. Drugs and equipment for emergency use should be readily available at all times.

The most common emergency is syncope, which is a transient loss of consciousness caused by a reduction in cerebral blood flow. The most common causes of syncope are fear and anxiety. Syncope is usually preceded by a feeling of weakness, and then the patient experiences pallor, sweating, coldness of the extremities, dizziness, and a slowing of the pulse. The patient should be placed in a supine position with the legs elevated; tight clothes should be loosened, and a wide-open airway should be ensured. The administration of oxygen should be started. Unconsciousness may persist for a few minutes. A previous history of syncope during dental appointments should be explored before the treatment is started. If the patient has had other experiences with syncope, every effort should be made to minimize the patient's fear and anxiety, as well as considering the use of oral sedatives. The reader is referred to other texts for a complete analysis of this important topic.[2]

Measures to Prevent Transmission of Infection

Guarding against the danger of transmitting infections to the dental team or to other patients is an important precaution that must be a part of every appointment in the dental office, especially with the threat of acquired immunodeficiency syndrome (AIDS) and hepatitis B virus infection. Universal precautions (e.g., protective attire) and barrier techniques must be incorporated into the surgical protocol of every procedure. These include the use of disposable sterile gloves, surgical masks, and protective eyewear. All surfaces that may be contaminated with blood or saliva and cannot be sterilized (e.g., light handles, unit syringes)

must be covered with sterile aluminum foil or plastic barriers made and approved for office use. Aerosol-producing devices (e.g., ultrasonic scalers) should be used with caution in patients with suspected infections, and their use should be kept to a minimum in all other patients. Special care should be taken when using and disposing of sharp items such as needles and scalpel blades.

Sedation and Anesthesia

Pain control in periodontal surgery is important. Most procedures should be either painless or minimally painful. The patient should be assured of this at the beginning and throughout the procedure. The most reliable means of providing painless surgery is the effective administration of local anesthesia. The area to be treated should be thoroughly anesthetized by means of regional block and local infiltration. Injections directly into the interdental papillae may also be helpful.

Apprehensive and neurotic patients may require special management with antianxiety or sedative–hypnotic agents. Modalities for the administration of these agents include inhalation as well as oral, intramuscular, and intravenous routes. The specific agents and the modality of administration are based on the desired level of sedation, the anticipated length of the procedure, and the overall condition of the patient. Specifically, the patient's medical history and physical and emotional status should be considered when determining the need for sedation, as well as the specific agents and techniques to be used.

Tissue Management

1. *Operate gently and carefully.* In addition to being most considerate to the patient, this is also the most effective way to operate. Tissue manipulation should be precise, deliberate, and gentle. It is essential to be thorough, but traumatic instrumentation must be avoided because it produces excessive tissue injury, causes postoperative discomfort, and delays healing.

2. *Observe the patient at all times.* It is essential to pay careful attention to the patient's reactions. Facial expressions, pallor, and perspiration are distinct signs that may indicate when a patient is experiencing pain, anxiety, or fear. The clinician's responsiveness to these signs can be the difference between success and failure.

3. *Be certain that the instruments are sharp.* Instruments must be sharp to be effective; successful treatment is not possible without sharp instruments. Dull instruments inflict unnecessary trauma as a result of poor cutting and excessive force applied to compensate for their ineffectiveness. A sterile sharpening stone should be available on the operating table at all times.

Scaling and Root Planing

Although scaling and root planing have been performed previously as part of phase I therapy, all exposed root surfaces should be carefully explored and planed as needed during the surgical procedure. In particular, areas of difficult access (e.g., furcations, deep infrabony pockets) often have rough areas or even calculus that was undetected during the preparatory sessions. The assistant who is retracting the tissues and using the aspirator should also check for the presence of calculus and the smoothness of each surface from a different angle.

KEY FACT

The most important objective of periodontal pocket reduction surgery is to gain access to the root surface for scaling and root planing. The exposure of the subgingival root surfaces obtained when the flap is reflected allows not only access for root therapy but also the opportunity to alter the osseous defects that may exist.

Hemostasis

Hemostasis is an important aspect of periodontal surgery because good intraoperative control of bleeding permits accurate visualization of the extent of disease, the pattern of bone destruction, and the anatomy and condition of the root surfaces. It provides the operator with a clear view of the surgical site, which is essential for wound debridement and scaling and root planing. In addition, good hemostasis also prevents excessive loss of blood into the mouth, oropharynx, and stomach.

Periodontal surgery can produce profuse bleeding, especially during the initial incisions and flap reflection. After flap reflection and the removal of granulation tissue, bleeding stops or is considerably reduced. Typically, the control of intraoperative bleeding can be managed with aspiration. Continuous suctioning of the surgical site with an aspirator is indispensable when performing periodontal surgery. The application of pressure to the surgical wound with moist gauze can be a helpful adjunct to control site-specific bleeding. Intraoperative bleeding that is not controlled with these simple methods may indicate a more serious problem and require additional control measures.

For a slow, constant blood flow and for oozing, hemostasis may be achieved with hemostatic agents. Absorbable gelatin sponge (Gelfoam), oxidized cellulose (Oxycel), oxidized regenerated cellulose (Surgicel Absorbable Hemostat), and microfibrillar collagen hemostat (Avitene, CollaCote, CollaTape, CollaPlug) are useful hemostatic agents for the control of bleeding in capillaries, small blood vessels, and deep wounds (Table 50.1).

KEY FACT

Along with the usual procedures to help control hemorrhage during surgery (pressure; irrigation with cold, sterile water; removal of granulation tissue), the use of local anesthesia with epinephrine is also helpful. It is important to remember that this action is effective for a short duration and should not be used toward the end of the surgical procedure. When the patient is dismissed from the appointment and the effect of the vasoconstriction is no longer present, bleeding can occur during the patient's trip home.

Finally, it is imperative to recognize that excessive bleeding may be caused by systemic disorders, including (but not limited to) platelet deficiencies, coagulation defects, medications, and hypertension. As a precaution, all surgical patients should be asked about any current medications that may contribute to bleeding, any family history of bleeding disorders, and hypertension. All patients, regardless of health history, should have their blood pressure evaluated before surgery, and anyone who is diagnosed with hypertension must be advised to see a physician before surgery. Patients with known or suspected bleeding deficiencies or disorders must be carefully evaluated before any surgical procedure. A consultation with the patient's physician is recommended, and laboratory tests should be performed to assess the risk of bleeding. It may be necessary to refer the patient to a hematologist for a comprehensive workup.

Additional information on hemostasis is found on the companion Expert Consult website.

TABLE 50.1 Absorbable Hemostatic Agents

Generic (Brand)	Directions	Adverse Effects	Precautions
Absorbable gelatin sponge (Gelfoam)	May be cut into various sizes and applied to bleeding surfaces	May form nidus for infection or abscess	Should not be overpacked into extraction site or wound—may interfere with healing
Oxidized cellulose (Oxycel)	Most effective when applied to wound dry as opposed to moistened	May cause foreign-body reaction	Extremely friable and difficult to place; should not be used adjacent to bone—impairs bone regeneration; should not be used as a surface dressing—inhibits epithelialization
Oxidized regenerated cellulose (Surgicel Absorbable Hemostat)	May be cut to various shapes and positioned over bleeding sites; thick or excessive amounts should not be used	Encapsulation, cyst formation, and foreign-body reaction possible	Should not be placed in deep wounds—may physically interfere with wound healing and bone formation
Microfibrillar collagen hemostat (Avitene, CollaCote, CollaTape, CollaPlug)	May be cut to shape and applied to bleeding surface	May potentiate abscess formation, hematoma, and wound dehiscence; possible allergic reaction or foreign-body reaction	May interfere with wound healing; placement in extraction sockets has been associated with increased pain
Thrombin (Thrombostat)	May be applied topically to bleeding surface	Allergic reaction can occur in patients with known sensitivity to bovine materials	Must not be injected into tissues or vasculature—can cause severe (and possibly fatal) clotting

KEY FACT

Thrombin is a very effective drug to help coagulate blood and is applied topically. This drug should never be injected into tissues because it can cause serious or even fatal intravascular coagulation. In addition, thrombin is a bovine-derived drug, so caution should be used in the case of patients with a known allergy to bovine products.

HOSPITAL PERIODONTAL SURGERY

For most patients, periodontal surgical procedures are managed well in the dental office with local anesthesia only or with some form of sedation, and are performed in quadrants or sextants, usually at biweekly or longer intervals. However, certain patients and procedures warrant treatment in the hospital operating room with general anesthesia. These include patients who are not well enough to undergo treatment in a dental office and procedures that are more extensive and difficult for patients to endure. Readers are referred to the online material for a discussion of indications and procedures in a hospital setting.

TYPES OF PERIODONTAL SURGERIES

Information on periodontal surgical instruments is found on the companion website.

GINGIVAL SURGERY

Gingival Curettage

The word *curettage* is used in periodontics to describe the scraping of the gingival wall of a periodontal pocket to remove the chronically inflamed tissue. The *excisional new attachment procedure*[38,66,67] is a definitive subgingival curettage procedure that is performed with a knife. Historically, it was thought this tissue hinders healing and new attachment, which necessitate gingival curettage. However, when the root is thoroughly scaled and planed, and the biofilm and calculus are removed, the inflammation in the tissue automatically resolves without tissue curettage. *Therefore, the use of curettage to eliminate the inflamed granulation tissue is unnecessary.* This should not be confused with the elimination of granulation tissue during flap surgery. The reason for the latter is to remove the bleeding tissue that obstructs visualization and prevents the necessary examination of the root surface and the bone. Thus, the removal of granulation tissue during surgery is accomplished for technical rather than biologic reasons. It has been shown that additional curettage does not improve the condition of the periodontal tissues beyond the improvement that results from scaling and root planing alone.

In the anterior maxilla, gingival curettage and root planing apical to the base of the periodontal pocket should be avoided. The removal of the junctional epithelium and the disruption of the connective tissue attachment expose nondiseased cementum. Root planing and the removal of nondiseased cementum may result in attachment loss and gingival recession.

Gingivectomy

The word *gingivectomy* means "excision of the gingiva." By removing the pocket wall, gingivectomy provides visibility and accessibility for complete calculus removal and thorough root planing. This creates a favorable environment for gingival healing and restoration of a physiologic gingival contour.

Although gingivectomy was widely performed in the past, improved understanding of healing and the development of sophisticated flap techniques have relegated it to a lesser role in periodontal surgery. However, it remains an effective form of treatment when indicated (Fig. 50.1).

Gingivectomy may be performed for the following indications[17]:
1. Elimination of suprabony pockets if the pocket wall is fibrous and firm
2. Elimination of gingival enlargements
   Contraindications to gingivectomy include the following:
1. Access to bone required
2. Narrow zone of keratinized tissue
3. Aesthetics
4. Patients with high postoperative risk of bleeding
   The step-by-step technique for gingivectomy is as follows:
Step 1: The periodontal pocket is mapped out on the external gingival surface by inserting a probe to the bottom of the pocket and puncturing the external surface of the gingiva at the depth of probe penetration (see Figs. 50.1C and D; Figs. 50.2 and 50.3).
Step 2: Periodontal knives (e.g., Kirkland) are used for incisions on the facial and lingual surfaces. Orban periodontal knives are used for interdental incisions (see Fig. 50.1E to G). Bard–Parker blades (#12 and #15), and scissors are used as auxiliary instruments. The external bevel incision is started apical to the points marking the course of the pockets,[45,60] and it is directed coronally to a point between the base of the pocket and the crest of the bone. It should be as close as possible to the bone without exposing it to remove the soft tissue coronal to the bone. Exposure of bone is undesirable. If this occurs, healing usually presents minimal complications if the area is adequately covered by the surgical dressing. Either interrupted or continuous incisions may be used. The incision should be beveled at approximately 45 degrees to the tooth surface, and it should re-create the normal festooned pattern of the gingiva. Failure to bevel the incision will leave a broad, fibrous plateau that will delay development of a physiologic contour.
Step 3: Remove the excised pocket wall, irrigate the area, and examine the root surface.
Step 4: Scale and root plane.
Step 5: Cover the area with a surgical dressing (see Fig. 50.1I).

Gingivoplasty

Gingivoplasty is *recontouring the gingiva* in the absence of pockets.[19] It may be accomplished with a periodontal knife, a scalpel, or rotary coarse diamond stones.[40]

Additional information on healing following gingivectomy is found on the companion website.

Fig. 50.1 Results Obtained by Treating a Suprabony Pocket With Gingivectomy. (A and B) Preoperative facial and palatal views. (C) Marking of the depth of the suprabony pocket. (D) The bottoms of the pockets are indicated by pinpoint markings. (E) A beveled palatal incision with an Orban knife. (F) A facial beveled incision with a Bard–Parker #15 blade extends apical to the perforations made by the pocket marker. Note that the beveled incision can also be made with a Kirkland knife. (G) The interdental incision and excision of the pocket wall with a Bard–Parker #12 blade. (H) A completed gingivectomy. (I) The surgical site covered with periodontal dressing. (J) One week after healing. (K and L) Results 22 months after the operation. (Courtesy Dr. Kitetsu Shin, Saitama, Japan.)

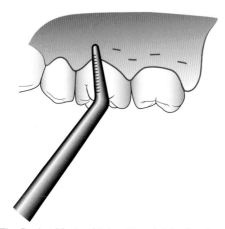

Fig. 50.2 The Pocket Marker Makes Pinpoint Perforations That Indicate Pocket Depth.

Fig. 50.3 Marking the Depth of a Suprabony Pocket. (A) A pocket marker in position. (B) The beveled incision extends apical to the perforation made by the pocket marker.

FLAP SURGERY

Periodontal flaps are used in surgical periodontal therapy to accomplish the following:
1. Access for root instrumentation
2. Gingival resection
3. Osseous resection
4. Periodontal regeneration

To fulfill these purposes, five different flap techniques are used: (1) the modified Widman flap,[44] (2) the undisplaced flap, (3) the apically displaced flap, (4) the papilla preservation flap,[10,56] (5) and the distal terminal molar flap.

The modified Widman flap facilitates root instrumentation. It does not attempt to reduce the pocket depth, but it does eliminate the pocket lining. The objectives of the undisplaced and apically displaced flaps include root surface access and the reduction of probing depth. The choice of which procedure to use depends on two important anatomic landmarks: the transgingival probing depth and the location of the mucogingival junction. These landmarks establish the presence and width of the attached gingiva, which are the basis for the decision. The papilla preservation flap is used when possible in regenerative and aesthetic cases to minimize recession and loss of interdental papillae. The distal terminal molar flap is used for treating pockets and osseous defects on the distal surface of the terminal maxillary and mandibular molars.

Modified Widman Flap

The original Widman[63] flap used two vertical releasing incisions connected by a submarginal scalloped internal bevel incision to demarcate the area of surgery. A full-thickness flap was reflected and the marginal collar of tissue was removed to provide access for root instrumentation and osseous recontouring. In 1974, Ramfjord and Nissle[44] published the "modified Widman flap" (Fig. 50.4), which used only horizontal incisions. This technique offers the possibility of establishing an intimate postoperative adaptation of healthy collagenous connective tissue to tooth surfaces,[6,29,42,44] and it provides access for adequate instrumentation of the root surfaces and immediate closure of the area.

The step-by-step technique for the modified Widman flap is as follows:

Step 1: The first incision (Fig. 50.5A) parallel to the long axis of the tooth is a scalloped internal bevel incision to the alveolar crest starting 0.5 to 1 mm away from the gingival margin (see Fig. 50.4C). The papillae are dissected and thinned to have a thickness similar to that of the remaining flaps.

Step 2: Full-thickness flaps are reflected 2 to 3 mm away from the alveolar crest (see Fig. 50.4D).

Step 3: The second, crevicular incision (see Fig. 50.5B) is made in the gingival crevice to detach the attachment apparatus from the root.

Step 4: The interdental tissue and the gingival collar are detached from the bone with a third incision (Fig. 50.5C; see Fig. 50.4E and F).

Step 5: The gingival collar and granulation tissue are removed with curettes. The root surfaces are scaled and planed (see

Fig. 50.4G and H). Residual periodontal fibers attached to the tooth surface should not be disturbed.

Step 6: Bone architecture is not corrected unless it prevents intimate flap adaptation. Every effort is made to adapt the facial and lingual interdental tissue in such a way that no interdental bone remains exposed at the time of suturing. The flaps may be thinned to allow for close adaptation of the gingiva around the entire circumference of the tooth.

Step 7: The flaps are stabilized with sutures (see Fig. 50.4I and J) and covered with a surgical dressing.

Undisplaced Flap

Currently, the undisplaced flap may be the most frequently performed type of periodontal surgery. For the undisplaced flap, the submarginal scalloped internal bevel incision is initiated at a distance from the tooth that is roughly one-half to two-thirds the interdental transgingival probing depth. This incision can be accomplished only if sufficient attached gingiva remains apical to the incision. Therefore, the two anatomic landmarks, the transgingival interdental probing depth and the mucogingival junction, must be considered to evaluate the amount of attached gingiva that will remain after surgery. The internal bevel incision should be scalloped to create surgical papillae, which are essential to covering the interdental bone (Fig. 50.6). If the tissue is too thick, the flap margin should be thinned with the initial incision. Proper placement of the flap margin at the alveolar crest during closure is important to prevent either recurrence of the pocket or exposure of bone.

The step-by-step technique for the undisplaced flap is as follows:

Step 1: The periodontal probe is inserted into the gingival crevice and penetrates the junctional epithelium and connective tissue down to bone.

Step 2: The mucogingival junction is assessed to determine the amount of keratinized tissue.

Step 3: The initial placement of the submarginal scalloped internal bevel incision is based on the transgingival interdental probing depth and the mucogingival junction (Fig. 50.7). The incision is made parallel to the long axis of the tooth and directed down to the alveolar bone. The angulation of the incision may be altered depending on the thickness of the gingiva, as well as the initial placement of the submarginal scalloped incision, to produce a thin flap margin. The thicker the tissue, the more apically the incision will end (see Fig. 50.7). A short mesial vertical incision may be employed to allow flap release on the palate or to avoid extension of the horizontal incision into the aesthetic area.

Step 4: Full-thickness flaps are reflected 1 mm apical to the mucogingival junction.

Step 5: The crevicular incision is made in the gingival crevice to detach the attachment apparatus from the root.

Step 6: The gingival collar and granulation tissue are removed with curettes. The root surfaces are scaled and planed.

Step 7: Osseous recontouring is performed to eliminate defects and reestablish positive architecture.

Fig. 50.4 Modified Widman Flap Technique. (A) Facial view before surgery. The probing of pockets revealed interproximal depths that ranged from 4 to 8 mm and facial and palatal depths of 2 to 5 mm. (B) Radiographic survey of the area. Note the generalized horizontal bone loss. (C) Facial internal bevel incision. (D) Palatal incision. (E) Elevation of the flap, which left a wedge of tissue attached to its base. (F) Removal of tissue. (G) Tissue removed and ready for scaling and root planing. (H) Scaling and root planing of exposed root surfaces. (I) Continuous, independent sling suture of facial portion of surgery. (J) Continuous, independent sling suture of palatal portion of surgery. (K) Postsurgical result. (Courtesy Dr. Kitetsu Shin, Saitama, Japan.)

Step 8: The flaps are coapted on the alveolar crest with the flap margin well adapted to the roots. The flaps may be trimmed and rescalloped if necessary.

Step 9: The flaps are stabilized with sutures and covered with a surgical dressing.

Apically Displaced Flap

The apically displaced flap is selected for cases that present with a minimal amount (<3 mm) of attached gingiva. For this reason,

the internal bevel incision should be made as close to the tooth as possible (i.e., 0.5 to 1.0 mm). One need not determine where the bottom of the pocket is in relation to the incision for the apically displaced flap, as one would for the undisplaced flap. The flap is placed at the tooth–bone junction by apically displacing the flap. Its final position is not determined by the placement of the first incision.

With some variants, the apically displaced flap can be used for pocket eradication, widening the zone of attached gingiva,

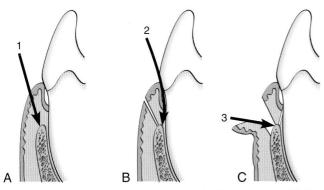

Fig. 50.5 The Three Incisions Necessary for Flap Surgery. (A) First (internal bevel) incision; (B) second (crevicular) incision; and (C) third (interdental) incision.

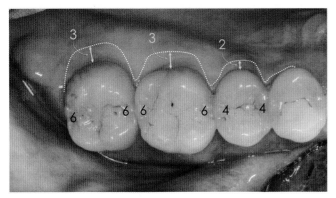

Fig. 50.6 The Submarginal Scalloped Incision Is Placed a Distance of One-Half to Two-Thirds the Transgingival Interdental Probing Depth Away From the Tooth Surface.

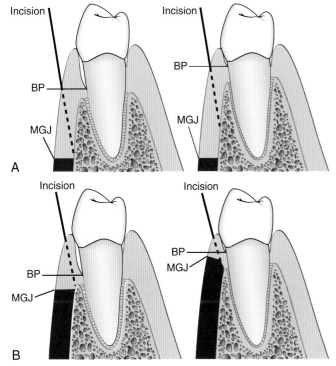

Fig. 50.7 (A and B) The location of two different areas where the internal bevel incision is made in an undisplaced flap. The incision is made at the level of the pocket to discard the tissue coronal to the pocket if remaining attached gingiva is sufficient. *BP,* Bottom of pocket; *MGJ,* mucogingival junction.

or both. Depending on the purpose, the apically displaced flap can be a full-thickness flap or a split-thickness flap. The split-thickness flap requires more precision and finesse, as well as a gingiva that is thick enough to split.

The step-by-step technique for the apically displaced flap is as follows:

Step 1: A marginal scalloped internal bevel incision parallel to the long axis of the tooth is made down to the crest of bone (Fig. 50.8).

Step 2: If used, vertical incisions are made extending beyond the mucogingival junction. It is important that the vertical incisions—and therefore the flap elevation—reach past the mucogingival junction to provide adequate mobility to the flap for its apical displacement.

Step 3: The flap is reflected in full thickness or partial thickness, depending on the thickness of the gingiva and the objective of the surgery.

Step 4: Crevicular and interdental incisions are made, and the marginal collar of tissue is removed.

Step 5: After degranulation, scaling and root planing, and osseous surgery if needed, the flap is displaced apically.

Step 6: If a full-thickness flap was reflected, an independent sling suture positions the flap margin at the alveolar crest, and a surgical dressing can prevent its coronal movement. If a partial-thickness flap was reflected, it can be apically displaced with an independent sling suture, and further stabilized with periosteal sutures. A periodontal dressing can prevent its coronal movement.

After 1 week, dressings and sutures are removed. The area is usually repacked for another week, after which the patient is to brush gently along the gingival margin with a soft brush and interdentally with interdental brushes.

Distal Terminal Molar Flap

The treatment of periodontal pockets on the distal surface of terminal molars is often complicated by the presence of bulbous fibrous tissue over the maxillary tuberosity or prominent retromolar pads in the mandible. Some of these osseous lesions may result from incomplete repair after the extraction of impacted third molars (Fig. 50.9).

Access to these distal areas may be obtained by a single horizontal incision, two converging horizontal incisions, or two parallel incisions extending distally from the distal surface of the terminal molar to the mucogingival junction distal to the tuberosity or the retromolar pad. The distal horizontal incision is connected with the crevicular incision on the distal surface of the terminal molar, which merges mesially with the buccal and lingual or palatal scalloped incisions. If the secondary objective of surgery is regenerative or the buccolingual width of the distal keratinized tissue is limited, a single horizontal incision in keratinized tissue is used. If the secondary objective of surgery is resective and adequate keratinized tissue is present buccolingually, two distal horizontal incisions are placed in keratinized tissue. The two-horizontal incisions technique was described by Robinson[46] and Braden[6] and modified by several other investigators. These techniques are called the *distal wedge* and the *modified distal wedge.*

Fig. 50.8 An Apically Displaced Flap. (A and B) Facial and lingual preoperative views. (C and D) The facial and lingual flaps have been elevated. (E and F) After debridement of the areas. (G and H) The sutures are in place. (I and J) Healing after 1 week. (K) Healing after 2 months. Note the preservation of attached gingiva displaced to a more apical position. (Courtesy Dr. Thomas Han, Los Angeles, CA.)

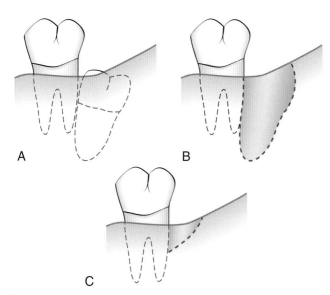

Fig. 50.9 (A) Impaction of a third molar distal to a second molar with little or no interdental bone between the two teeth. (B) Removal of the third molar creates a pocket with little or no bone distal to the second molar. (C) This often leads to a vertical osseous defect distal to the second molar.

The distal wedge technique employs two horizontal incisions that begin at the distal surface of the terminal molar and *converge* distally at the mucogingival junction distal to the tuberosity or the retromolar pad. The modified distal wedge technique employs two *parallel* horizontal incisions that extend distally from the distal surface of the terminal molar and are connected by a transverse incision distal to the mucogingival junction distal to the tuberosity or retromolar pad. The buccolingual distance between the two horizontal incisions in both techniques depends on the transgingival probing depth and the amount of fibrous tissue involved. When the flaps are thinned and the tissue between the two incisions is removed, the two flap edges must approximate each other at a new apical position without overlapping (Fig. 50.10). Generally, the distance between the two parallel incisions is roughly one-half to two-thirds the distal transgingival probing depth; the distance should never be greater than the distance between the buccal and lingual line angles of the tooth.

Maxillary Molars

The treatment of distal pockets in the maxilla is usually less challenging than that in the mandible. The tuberosity presents

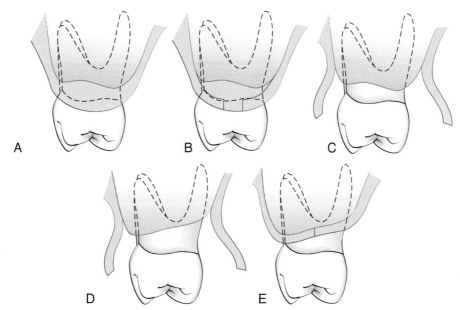

Fig. 50.10 (A) Coronal view from behind a maxillary second molar with an osseous defect. (B) Distal terminal flap surgery employing two horizontal incisions; both buccal and lingual flaps are thinned. (C) Buccal and lingual flaps are elevated, and the "wedge" of tissue is removed. (D) The bone is sloped to the palatal side to eliminate the osseous defect. (E) The flaps are coapted on the bone in the apical position.

Fig. 50.11 (A) Sagittal view of a distal defect on a maxillary second molar. (B) Treatment with a distal wedge results in an acute angle between the tuberosity and the distal surface of the second molar. (C) Treatment with a modified distal wedge results in a wider angle between the tuberosity and the distal surface of the second molar that is more accessible for hygiene.

a greater amount of fibrous attached gingiva than does the retromolar pad. The use of the distal wedge with two converging incisions causes the tissue next to the tooth to be displaced more apically than the tissue away from the tooth. Consequently, healing of a distal wedge in the maxilla results in an acute angle between the distal tooth surface and the tuberosity; it is biofilm-retentive and difficult to clean (Fig. 50.11B). In contrast, the use of the modified distal wedge with two parallel distal incisions allows the soft tissue along the whole length of the distal flap to be evenly displaced apically (see Fig. 50.11C). This is advantageous in the maxilla in maintaining a wide angle between the tooth and the tuberosity that is much easier to clean. Therefore, the modified distal wedge is preferred in the maxilla. The two parallel incisions are usually made at the midline of the tuberosity where the tissue is the thickest, or slightly to the palatal side to maximize buccal keratinized tissue and to provide easier access for flap closure (Fig. 50.12).

> **KEY FACT**
>
> The two parallel distal horizontal incisions in the maxillary tuberosity are advantageous in allowing the soft tissue along the whole length of the distal flap to be evenly displaced. This results in a wide angle between the tooth and the tuberosity that is much easier to clean.

Mandibular Molars

Incisions in the distal mandible differ from those in the tuberosity due to differences in the anatomy of the area. The retromolar pad usually has limited attached gingiva and vestibular depth. The attached gingiva, if present, may not be found directly distal to the molar. The greatest amount may be distolingual or distobuccal, and it may not be over the bony crest. The ascending ramus of the mandible may also create a short or completely eliminate the horizontal area distal to the terminal molar

Fig. 50.12 (A) and (B) Buccal and palatal preoperative views, 6 weeks after completion of scaling and root planing. (C) and (D) Buccal preoperative and postoperative views. In (C), note the ledging on the facial wall of molars and the one-wall defects on both molars. (D) Postoperative view shows the elimination of these defects by osteoplasty on the ledges and ostectomy of the one-wall defects to produce a positive buccal architecture. (E) and (F) Palatal preoperative and postoperative views. In (E), note the pattern of bony loss, which is more severe on the palatal wall. In addition to the facial one-wall defects, an incipient furcation defect is present at the mesial wall of the first molar and a class II furcation is present at the mesial wall of the second molar. (F) Configuration of the defects was such that ostectomy was performed on the palatal roots of both molars to produce a compromise architecture. (G) and (H) Ten-year postoperative views of the buccal and palatal areas showing the pattern of soft tissue adaptation to the surgically produced bony form.

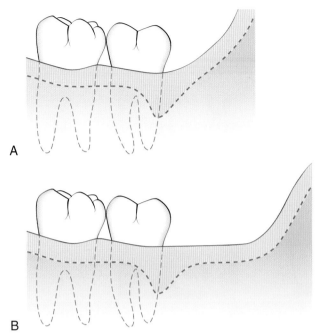

Fig. 50.13 (A) Pocket eradication distal to a mandibular second molar with minimal attached gingiva and a close ascending ramus is anatomically difficult. (B) For surgical procedures distal to a mandibular second molar, abundant attached gingiva and distal space are ideal.

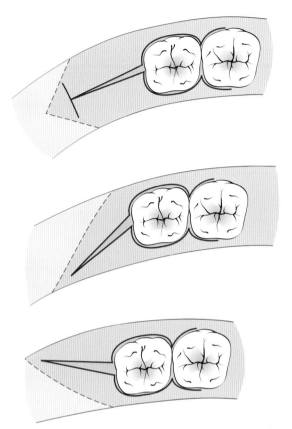

Fig. 50.14 Incision Designs for Surgical Procedures Distal to the Mandibular Second Molar. The incision should follow the areas of greatest attached gingiva and underlying bone.

(Fig. 50.13). The shorter this area, the more difficult it is to treat any deep distal lesion around the terminal molar.

The mandibular retromolar tissue ascends distally to merge with the ascending ramus. This anatomy favors the distal wedge technique in the mandible, although the parallel distal incisions and the single horizontal incision may be used. The two distal incisions should follow the area with the greatest amount of attached gingiva and must be made over bone (Fig. 50.14). Therefore, the incisions could be directed distally or distobuccally, depending on which area has more attached gingiva. Incisions directing distolingually should be avoided due to the potential presence of the lingual nerve.

Papilla Preservation Flap

In current regenerative therapy, bone grafts, membranes, or a combination of these are used with or without other biologics. The flap design should maximize the amount of gingival tissue and papilla retained to cover the material placed in the osseous defect. In the aesthetic area, when surgery is necessary, flap design must minimize recession and loss of interdental papillae. As such, the crevicular incision is the incision of choice for the anterior aesthetic area and regenerative therapy. The interdental papilla is retained with the papilla preservation technique when the interdental space is adequate for reflection of the intact papilla; otherwise, it is split beneath the contact point of the two approximating teeth. The flap is elevated in full thickness without thinning of the flap or the papilla.

The step-by-step technique for the papilla preservation flap (Figs. 50.15 and 50.16) is as follows:

Step 1: A crevicular incision is made around each tooth, with no incisions across the interdental papilla.

Step 2: The preserved papilla can be incorporated into the facial-buccal flap (original papilla preservation technique[56]) or lingual-palatal flap (modified papilla preservation technique[10]). If the preserved papilla is reflected with the facial-buccal flap, the semilunar incision at the base of the papilla is on the lingual-palatal side of the interdental space. If the preserved papilla is reflected with the lingual-palatal flap, the semilunar incision at the base of the papilla is on the facial-buccal side of the interdental space. This semilunar incision dips apically from the line angles of the tooth so that the incision is at least 5 mm from the crest of the papilla.

Step 3: The papilla is then elevated with an Orban knife or curettes and is reflected intact with the flap.

Step 4: The flap is reflected without thinning the tissue.

Additional information on healing following flap surgery is found on the companion website.

Periodontal Dressings (Periodontal Packs)

At completion of the periodontal surgical procedure, clinicians may elect to cover the area with a surgical dressing. In general, dressings have no curative properties but assist healing by protecting the tissue rather than providing "healing factors." The dressing minimizes the likelihood of postoperative infection, facilitates healing by preventing surface trauma during mastication, and protects the patient from pain induced by contact of the wound with food or with the tongue during mastication.

Fig. 50.15 Papilla Preservation Flap. (A) Facial view after sulcular incisions have been made. (B) Straight-line incision in the palatal area about 3 mm from the gingival margins. This incision is then connected to the margins with vertical incisions at the midpart of each tooth. (C) Papillae are reflected with the facial flap. (D) Lingual view after the reflection of the flap. (E) Lingual view after the flap is brought back to its original position. It is then sutured with independent sutures. (F) Facial view after healing. (G) Palatal view after healing. (Courtesy Dr. Thomas Han, Los Angeles, CA.)

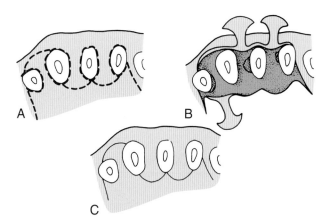

Fig. 50.16 Flap Design for a Papilla Preservation Flap. (A) Incisions for this type of flap are depicted by interrupted lines. The preserved papilla can be incorporated into the facial or the lingual–palatal flap. (B) The reflected flap exposes the underlying bone. Several osseous defects are seen. (C) The flap has been returned to its original position, where it covers all of the interdental spaces.

(For a complete literature review on this subject, see the article by Sachs and colleagues.[48])

Postoperative Instructions

After the dressing is placed, oral and printed postoperative instructions are given before the patient is dismissed from the chair (eBox 50.1).

First Postoperative Week

When the therapy is properly performed, periodontal surgery should present minimal postoperative problems. Patients should be instructed to rinse with 0.12% chlorhexidine gluconate (Peridex, PerioGard) immediately after the surgical procedure and twice daily thereafter until normal biofilm control can be resumed.[45,50,59] The following complications may arise during the first postoperative week, although they are the exception rather than the rule:

1. *Persistent bleeding after surgery.* The dressing is removed, and local anesthesia may be needed before the bleeding areas are located. The bleeding is stopped with pressure, or if necessary, the area may have to be anesthetized and resutured. After the bleeding has been stopped, the area is again re-dressed.

2. *Sensitivity to percussion.* Extension of inflammation into the periodontal ligament may cause sensitivity to percussion. The patient should be questioned regarding the progress of the symptoms. Gradual diminishing discomfort is a favorable sign. The dressing should be removed and the surgical area checked for localized areas of infection or irritation. The area should be irrigated or incised to provide drainage if areas of localized exudate are present. Particles of calculus that may have been overlooked should be removed. Relieving the occlusion can be helpful. Sensitivity to percussion may also be caused by excess dressing, which interferes with the occlusion. Removal of the excess usually corrects the condition.

3. *Swelling.* During the first 2 postoperative days, some patients may report a soft, painless swelling of the cheek in the surgical area. Lymph node enlargement may occur, and the temperature may be slightly elevated. The area of operation itself is usually symptom-free. This type of involvement results from a localized inflammatory reaction to the surgical procedure. It generally subsides by the fourth postoperative day without necessitating the removal of the dressing. If swelling persists, enlarges, or is associated with increased pain, amoxicillin (500 mg) should be taken every 8 hours for 1 week. The patient should also be instructed to apply moist heat intermittently over the area.

4. *Feeling of weakness.* Occasionally, patients report having experienced a "washed-out," weakened feeling for about 24 hours after surgery. This represents a systemic reaction to transient bacteremia induced by the procedure. This reaction can be prevented by premedication with amoxicillin (500 mg) every 8 hours. This protocol should be started 24 hours before the next procedure and continued for 5 days postoperatively.

Removal of the Dressing and Return Visit

When the patient returns in 1 week, the periodontal dressing is removed by inserting a curette along the margin and exerting gentle lateral pressure. Pieces of the dressing retained interproximally and particles adhering to the tooth surfaces are also removed with curettes. Particles of dressing and debris may be enmeshed in the surgical surfaces and should be carefully removed with cotton pliers. The entire area is irrigated with peroxide to remove the superficial debris.

Findings at the Time of Dressing Removal

The following are usual findings when the dressing is removed:
- If *gingivectomy* has been performed, the incised surface is covered with a friable meshwork of new epithelium. This tissue should not be disturbed. If calculus has not been completely removed, red, beadlike protuberances of granulation tissue will persist. The granulation tissue must be removed with a curette to expose the calculus so the root can be planed. Granulation tissue will recur if the residual calculus is not completely removed.
- After a *flap operation*, the areas that correspond to the incisions are epithelialized, but they may bleed readily if irritated. These areas should not be disturbed nor probed.
- The facial and lingual mucosa may be covered with a grayish-yellow or white granular layer of debris that has entered under the dressing. This is easily removed with a moist cotton pellet.

The root surfaces may be sensitive to touch or to thermal change. The patient should be assured that these changes will disappear with time (4 to 6 weeks). The dentition that was beneath the dressing may be stained in a brownish-yellow color that can be removed by polishing at a later date.

- *Fragments of calculus delay healing.* Each root surface should be carefully rechecked visually to be certain that no calculus was missed during surgery. The grooves on the proximal root surfaces and the furcations are areas where calculus is likely to be overlooked.

Redressing

After the dressing is removed, it is usually not necessary to replace it. However, re-dressing for an additional week is advised for the following types of patients: (1) those with a low pain threshold who are particularly uncomfortable when the dressing is removed; (2) those with unusually sensitive root surfaces postsurgically; or (3) those with an open wound where the flap edges have necrosed. Clinical judgment helps when deciding whether to re-dress the area or to leave the initial dressing for a longer period.

> ### KEY FACT
> Periodontal dressings have no curative properties but assist healing by protecting the tissue rather than providing "healing factors." The dressing facilitates healing by preventing surface trauma during mastication and protects the patient from pain induced by contact of the wound with food or with the tongue during mastication.

Tooth Mobility

Tooth mobility usually increases immediately after surgery.[7] This results from edema in the periodontal ligament space from the inflammation that occurs postsurgically. The mobility diminishes to the pretreatment level by the fourth week.[28] The patient should be reassured before surgery that the mobility is temporary.

Mouth Care Between Procedures

Care of the mouth by the patient between the treatments as well as after the surgery is completed is extremely important.[62] These measures should begin after the dressing is removed from the first surgical procedure. The patient has had instructions on oral hygiene before surgical therapy but must be instructed again after surgical therapy. Plaque or biofilm removal post-surgery is different from that of presurgical hygiene because the areas are still healing and uncomfortable.

Vigorous brushing is not feasible during the first week after the dressing is removed. However, the patient is informed that biofilm and food accumulation impair healing and is advised to try to keep the area as clean as possible with the gentle use of a soft toothbrush and light water irrigation. Rinsing with a chlorhexidine mouthwash or applying such a rinse topically with cotton-tipped applicators is indicated for the first few postoperative weeks. Brushing is introduced when the healing of the tissues permits, and the overall hygiene regimen is increased as healing progresses. Patients should be told that (1) some gingival bleeding will occur when the wounded areas are gently cleaned; (2)

this bleeding is normal and will subside as healing progresses; and (3) the bleeding should not deter them from following their oral hygiene regimen.

Management of Postoperative Pain

Periodontal surgery that follows the basic principles outlined here should produce only minimal pain and discomfort.[54] A study of 304 consecutive periodontal surgical interventions revealed that 51.3% of the patients reported minimal or no postoperative pain, and only 4.6% reported severe pain. Of these, only 20.1% took five or more doses of analgesic.[12] The same study indicated that mucogingival procedures result in six times more discomfort and that osseous surgery is three and a half times more uncomfortable than plastic gingival surgery. For the few patients who may have severe pain, the control of pain becomes an important part of patient management.[33]

As indicated earlier, a common source of postoperative pain is overextension of the periodontal dressing onto the soft tissue apical to the mucogingival junction or onto the frena. Overextended dressings cause localized areas of edema that are usually noticed 1 to 2 days after surgery. The removal of excess dressing is followed by resolution in about 24 hours. Extensive and excessively prolonged exposure of bone with poor irrigation during surgery induces greater pain. For most healthy patients, a preoperative dose of ibuprofen (600 to 800 mg) followed by one tablet every 8 hours for 24 to 48 hours is very effective for reducing discomfort after periodontal surgery. Patients are advised to continue taking ibuprofen or acetaminophen thereafter, if needed. If pain persists, acetaminophen plus codeine (Tylenol #3) can be prescribed. Caution should be used when prescribing or dispensing ibuprofen to patients with hypertension that is controlled by medications because it can interfere with the effectiveness of the medication. Patients experiencing severe postoperative pain should be seen on an emergency basis. The area should be anesthetized by infiltration, and the dressing should be removed to allow for the examination of the area in pain. Postoperative pain related to infection is accompanied by localized lymphadenopathy and a slight elevation in temperature.[36] This type of pain should be treated with systemic antibiotics and analgesics.

Management of Postoperative Dentin Hypersensitivity

Dentin or root hypersensitivity is a relatively common problem in periodontal practice. It may occur spontaneously when the root becomes exposed as a result of gingival recession or pocket formation, or it may appear after scaling and root planing and other periodontal surgical procedures. The reader is referred to the online discussion for a detailed discussion of root sensitivity and its management.

Treatment of Sensitive Roots

Root hypersensitivity is a relatively common problem in periodontal practice. It may occur spontaneously when the root becomes exposed as a result of gingival recession or pocket formation, or it may appear after scaling and root planing and other surgical procedures. (See the article by Curro[11] for a literature review of this subject.) This type of sensitivity is manifested as pain that is induced by thermal changes (cold or hot temperature), by citrus fruits or sweets, or by contact with a toothbrush or a dental instrument.

Root sensitivity occurs more frequently in the cervical area of the root, where the cementum is extremely thin. Scaling and root planing procedures remove this thin cementum, thereby inducing the hypersensitivity.

The transmission of stimuli from the surface of the dentin to the nerve endings located in the dental pulp or in the pulpal region of the dentin could result from the odontoblastic process or from a hydrodynamic mechanism (i.e., the displacement of dentinal fluid). The latter process seems more likely and would explain the importance of burnishing desensitizing agents to obturate the dentinal tubule. An important factor for reducing or eliminating hypersensitivity is adequate biofilm control. However, hypersensitivity may prevent biofilm control, and therefore a vicious cycle of escalating hypersensitivity and biofilm accumulation may be created.

The patient should be informed about the possibility of root hypersensitivity before treatment is undertaken. A patient who is educated about any problematic issues before surgery will not complain because he or she is aware and expects the occurrence of the discomfort. The following information on how to cope with the problem should also be given to the patient:

1. Hypersensitivity appears as a result of the exposure of dentin, which is inevitable if calculus, biofilm, and their products, which are buried in the root, are to be removed.
2. Hypersensitivity slowly disappears in a few weeks.
3. An important factor in reducing hypersensitivity is biofilm control.
4. Desensitizing agents do not produce immediate relief and must be used for several days or even weeks to produce results.

Desensitizing Agents

Numerous agents have been proposed to control root hypersensitivity. The clinical evaluation of the many agents proposed is difficult for the following reasons: (1) measuring and comparing pain among patients with different thresholds are difficult, (2) the time table for hypersensitivity before it is completely alleviated is different for each patient, and (3) each desensitizing agent acts differently both in terms of time and the level of relief it offers.

Desensitizing agents can be applied by the patient at home or by the dentist or hygienist in the dental office. The most likely mechanism of action is the reduction of the diameter of the dentinal tubules to limit the displacement of fluid. According to Trowbridge and Silver,[58] this can be attained in the following ways: (1) by the formation of a smear layer produced by burnishing the exposed surface, (2) via the topical application of agents that form insoluble precipitates within the tubules, (3) with the impregnation of tubules with plastic resins, or (4) by sealing the tubules with plastic resins.

Agents used by the patient. The most common agents used by the patient for oral hygiene are dentifrices. Although many dentifrice products contain fluoride, additional active ingredients for desensitization are strontium chloride, potassium nitrate, and sodium citrate. The American Dental Association has approved the following dentifrices for desensitizing purposes: Sensodyne and Thermodent, which contain strontium chloride[5,9,47]; Crest Sensitivity Protection, Denquel, and Promise, which contain potassium nitrate[1,9]; and Protect, which contains sodium citrate. Fluoride rinsing solutions and gels can also be used after the usual biofilm control procedures.[55]

Patients should be aware that several factors must be considered during the treatment of tooth hypersensitivity, including the history and severity of the problem, as well as the physical findings of the tooth or teeth involved. A proper diagnosis is required before any treatment can be initiated so that pathologic causes of pain such as caries, cracked tooth, and other pulpal problems should be ruled out before attempting to treat the hypersensitivity. Desensitizing agents act through the precipitation of crystalline salts on the dentin surface that block dentinal tubules. Patients must be aware that their use will not prove to be effective unless they are used continuously for at least 2 weeks.

Agents used in the dental office. eBox 50.2 lists various office treatments for the desensitization of hypersensitive dentin. These products and treatments aim to decrease hypersensitivity by blocking dentinal tubules with either a crystalline salt precipitation or an applied coating (varnish or bonding agent) on the root surface.[58]

Several agents have been used to precipitate crystalline salts on the dentin surface in an attempt to occlude the dentinal tubules. *Fluoride solutions* and *pastes* historically have been the agents of choice. In addition to their antisensitivity properties, fluoride agents have the advantage of anticaries activity, which is particularly important for patients with a tendency to develop root caries. Certain agents, such as chlorhexidine, decrease the ability of fluoride to bind with calcium on the root surfaces.[1] Thus it is important to advise patients not to rinse or eat for 1 hour after a desensitizing treatment. Currently, potassium oxalate (Protect) and ferric oxalate (Sensodyne Sealant) solutions are the preferred agents, and special applicators have been developed for their use. These agents form insoluble calcium oxalate crystals that occlude the dentinal tubules.[31,34]

The most current method of treatment for hypersensitive dentin is the use of varnishes or bonding agents to occlude dentinal tubules. Newer restorative materials, such as glass-ionomer cements and the dentin bonding agents, are under investigation. These materials are considered for use when the tooth requires recontouring or when difficult cases do not respond to other treatments. Resin primers alone could be promising, but the effects are not permanent, and further investigations are ongoing.[15] Despite some success with decreasing dentin hypersensitivity,

these "dental office" treatments have not been predictable in resolving hypersensitivity, and the success that is achieved is often short-lived. The crystalline salts, varnishes, and other sealants can be washed away over time, and the hypersensitivity may return. Repeated therapy will be necessary to help alleviate the hypersensitivity for these patients.

More recently, attempts have been made to improve the success and longevity of these treatments with the use of lasers. Low-level laser "melting" of the dentin surface appears to seal dentinal tubules without damage to the pulp.[16,25] In a combined treatment modality, the neodymium:yttrium-aluminum-garnet laser has been used to congeal fluoride varnish on root surfaces. This in vitro study demonstrated that the laser-treated fluoride varnish resisted removal by electric toothbrushing, with 90% of tubules remaining blocked. In the control subjects (i.e., those who did not undergo laser treatment), the fluoride varnish was almost completely brushed away.[26] Despite these convincing preliminary results, further research is needed before laser treatment can be considered an effective and predictable means of desensitization.

CONCLUSION

The majority of periodontal surgical procedures can be carried out with the thorough application of local anesthesia. Clinicians have the obligation to ensure a patient-centered approach that includes oral, intravenous, and inhalational sedation in their spectrum of available services for their patients.

The efficient, precise, and minimally traumatic management of tissues is necessary to achieve the most predicable and comfortable result and outcome for the patient. Most patients need oral analgesic support, and they should be given the necessary pain-relieving medications so that an effective level of analgesia is present during the immediate postsurgical period. The use of longer-acting local anesthetic agents (e.g., bupivacaine) and protective periodontal dressings also helps to reduce postsurgical pain.

During the immediate postsurgical weeks, biofilm control and healing are enhanced by the use of antimicrobial mouthrinses such as chlorhexidine. Postsurgical root sensitivity is well controlled by ensuring that biofilm control is optimal, and occasionally desensitizing agents will be needed.

A Case Scenario is found on the companion website.

REFERENCES

 References for this chapter are found on the companion website.

51

Preparation of the Periodontium for Restorative Dentistry[a]

🌐 For online only content on pre-prosthetic surgery, please visit the companion website

CHAPTER OUTLINE

Periodontal health is the *sine qua non*, a prerequisite, of successful comprehensive dentistry.[25] To achieve the long-term therapeutic targets of comfort, good function, treatment predictability, longevity, and ease of restorative and maintenance care, active periodontal infection must be treated and controlled before the initiation of definitive restorative, aesthetic, and implant dentistry. In addition, the residual effects of periodontal disease or anatomic aberrations inconsistent with realizing and maintaining long-term stability must be addressed. This phase of treatment includes techniques performed in anticipation of aesthetic or implant dentistry, such as clinical crown lengthening, covering denuded roots, alveolar ridge preservation or augmentation, and implant site development (Video 51.1).

RATIONALE FOR THERAPY

The many reasons for establishing periodontal health before performing restorative dentistry include the following[52]:

1. Periodontal treatment is undertaken to ensure the establishment of stable gingival margins before tooth preparation. Noninflamed, healthy tissues are less likely to change (e.g., shrink) as a result of subgingival restorative treatment or post-restoration periodontal care.[28,29] In addition, tissues that do not bleed during restorative manipulation allow for a more predictable restorative and aesthetic result.[22,23]

2. Certain periodontal procedures are designed to provide for adequate tooth length for retention, access for tooth preparation, impression making, tooth preparation, and finishing of restorative margins in anticipation of restorative dentistry.[22,47] Failure to complete these procedures before restorative care can add to the complexity of treatment and introduce unnecessary risk for failure.[22]

3. Periodontal therapy should antecede definitive restorative care because the resolution of inflammation may result in the repositioning of teeth[46] or in soft-tissue and mucosal changes.[20,48] Failure to anticipate these changes may interfere with prosthetic designs planned or constructed before periodontal treatment.

4. Traumatic forces placed on teeth with ongoing periodontitis may increase tooth mobility, discomfort, and possibly the rate of attachment loss.[9] Restorations constructed on teeth free of periodontal inflammation, synchronous with a functionally appropriate occlusion, are more compatible with long-term periodontal stability and comfort (see Chapters 17 and 48).

5. Quality, quantity, and topography of the periodontium may play important roles as structural defense factors in maintaining periodontal health. Orthodontic tooth movement and restorations completed without the benefit of periodontal treatment designed for this purpose may be subject to negative changes that complicate construction and future maintenance.[55]

6. Successful aesthetic and implant procedures may be difficult or impossible without the specialized periodontal procedures developed for this purpose.

> ### KEY FACT
> Periodontal treatment is undertaken to ensure the establishment of stable gingival margins before tooth preparation. Non-inflamed, healthy tissues are less likely to change (e.g., shrink) as a result of subgingival restorative treatment or post-restoration periodontal care. In addition, tissues that do not bleed during restorative manipulation allow for a more predictable restorative and aesthetic result.

[a]Adapted from the following chapter of Newman and Carranza's Clinical Periodontology, 13th edition: Chapter 69: Preparation of the Periodontium for Restorative Dentistry, by Philip R. Melnick and Henry H. Takei.

SEQUENCE OF TREATMENT

Treatment sequencing should be based on logical and evidence-based methodologies, taking into account not only the disease state encountered, but also the psychological and aesthetic concerns of the patient. Because periodontal and restorative therapy is situational and specific to each patient, a plan must be adaptable to change depending on the variables encountered during the course of treatment. For example, teeth initially determined to be salvageable may be judged "hopeless," thus altering the established treatment scheme.[20,48]

Generally, the preparation of the periodontium for restorative dentistry can be divided into two phases: (1) control of periodontal inflammation with nonsurgical and surgical approaches and (2) pre-prosthetic periodontal surgery (Box 51.1).

CONTROL OF ACTIVE DISEASE

When the clinician is presented with a patient with different stages of periodontal involvement, this condition is generally treated before one can contemplate any definitive restorative dentistry. This step is the most important part of preparing the periodontium for restorative dentistry. The inflammatory state of the supporting tissues must be eliminated or controlled with biofilm removal, scaling, root planing (root debridement), and, if necessary, periodontal surgery. Please note, if periodontal

> **BOX 51.1   Sequence of Treatment in Preparing Periodontium for Restorative Dentistry**
>
> **Control of Active Disease**
> Emergency treatment
> Extraction of hopeless teeth
> Oral hygiene instructions
> Scaling and root planing
> Reevaluation
> Periodontal surgery
> Adjunctive orthodontic therapy
>
> **Pre-Prosthetic Surgery**
> Management of mucogingival problems
> Preservation of ridge morphology after tooth extraction
> Crown-lengthening procedures
> Alveolar ridge reconstruction

involvement is also coupled with rampant decay, the rampant caries must also be addressed concurrently with periodontal disease. Otherwise, efforts to prepare the periodontium may result in no teeth left to save.

The periodontal therapy is intended to control the active disease (see Chapters 42 to 49). In addition to the removal of biofilm and root surface calculus that are the primary etiologic agents, secondary local factors, such as plaque-retentive overhanging margins and untreated caries, must be addressed.[14,19]

Emergency Treatment

Emergency treatment is undertaken to alleviate symptoms and stabilize acute infection. This includes rampant caries, and endodontic as well as periodontal conditions (see Chapter 41). To the patient, the control of acute pain, especially endodontic, is the most important reason for seeking dental therapy. Therefore, this aspect of therapy must be properly addressed before any other therapy is instituted.

Extraction of Hopeless Teeth

Extraction of hopeless teeth is followed by provisionalization with fixed or removable prosthetics. Retention of hopeless teeth without periodontal treatment may result in bone loss around the adjacent teeth.[32] It is also important to consider the extraction of teeth with a poor prognosis when implant replacement has become a predictable alternative to keeping and attempting periodontal therapy.

Oral Hygiene Measures

As indicated earlier, oral hygiene measures, when properly applied, will reduce plaque biofilm scores and gingival inflammation (see Chapter 43).[30,51] However, in patients with deep periodontal pockets (>5 mm), plaque biofilm control measures alone are insufficient for resolving subgingival infection and inflammation.[5,30] Hygiene alone does not allow the bristles of the brush to reach into the deep pocket area to remove or disturb the plaque biofilm.

Scaling and Root Planing

Scaling and root planing (root debridement) combined with oral hygiene measures have been demonstrated to significantly reduce gingival inflammation and the rate of the progression of periodontitis (see Chapter 45).[3,4,31] This applies even to patients with deep periodontal pockets (Fig. 51.1).[5,15]

Fig. 51.1 Root Planing Has Resolved the Gingival Inflammation of This Patient. Significant improvement in gingival health is observed after root planing (B and C), compared to pretreatment (A).

KEY FACT

When the clinician is presented with a patient with any stage of periodontal involvement, this condition must be treated before one can contemplate any restorative dentistry.

Fig. 51.2 (A) Before treatment. (B) After 4 weeks, oral hygiene instructions and scaling and root planing have improved this patient's periodontal status. However, inflammation associated with pockets deeper than 5 mm suggests a need for periodontal surgery.

Reevaluation

After 4 weeks, the gingival tissues are evaluated to determine oral hygiene adequacy, soft tissue response, and pocket depth changes (see Chapter 42). This permits sufficient time for healing, reduction in inflammation and pocket depths, and gain in clinical attachment levels. However, in deeper pockets (>5 mm), plaque biofilm and calculus removal are often incomplete[2,54] with risk of future breakdown (Fig. 51.2).[8,49] As a result, periodontal surgery to access the root surfaces for instrumentation and to reduce periodontal pocket depths must be considered before restorative care proceeds.

Periodontal Surgery

Periodontal surgery may be required for some patients (see Chapter 50). This should be undertaken with future restorative

and implant dentistry in mind. Some procedures are intended to treat active periodontal disease successfully,[12,37] and others are aimed at preparing the mouth for restorative or prosthetic care.[55] Crown lengthening is an example of such surgery. Both types of surgery are for preparing the periodontium for restorative dentistry.

Adjunctive Orthodontic Therapy

Orthodontic treatment has been shown to be a useful adjunct to periodontal therapy (see Chapter 48).[6,17,18,24,34] It should be undertaken only after active periodontal disease has been controlled. If nonsurgical treatment is sufficient, definitive periodontal pocket therapy may be postponed until after the completion of orthodontic tooth movement. This allows for the advantage of the positive bone changes that orthodontic therapy can provide. However, deep pockets and furcation invasions may require surgical access for root instrumentation in advance of orthodontic tooth movement. Failure to control active periodontitis can result in acute exacerbations and bone loss during tooth movement.[10] As long as the periodontal health is restored, teeth with preexisting bone loss may be moved orthodontically without incurring additional attachment loss.[39,40]

If teeth that are to be orthodontically moved lack keratinized attached gingiva, soft tissue–grafting procedures are often indicated in anticipation of orthodontic therapy. The procedure is necessary to increase the dimension of attached tissue to prevent the possibility of gingival margin recession.[34,55]

KEY FACT

Periodontal surgery is performed for the treatment of active periodontal disease as well as for the pre-prosthetic preparation of the periodontium. Some procedures are intended to treat active disease successfully, and others are aimed at preparing the mouth for restorative or prosthetic care.

CONCLUSION

As described in this and other sections of this textbook, the therapeutic goals of patient comfort, function, aesthetics, predictability, longevity, and ease of restorative and maintenance care are attainable only by a carefully constructed interdisciplinary approach with accurate diagnosis and comprehensive treatment planning serving as the cornerstones. The complex interaction between periodontal therapy and successful restorative dentistry only serves to underscore this premise, and dental hygienists play an important role in establishing a healthy periodontium for these patients with interdisciplinary treatment needs.

Case scenarios are found on the companion website.

REFERENCES

References for this chapter are found on the companion website.

52

Restorative Interrelationships[a]

🌐 For expanded discussions on margin placement, supracrestal attached tissue, and aesthetic tissue management as well as online-only content on special restorative considerations, please visit the companion website.

CHAPTER OUTLINE

Editors' note: An animation (slide show) has been added by the editors as a supplement to the chapter. It was produced by My Dental Hub as a patient education tool and covers the basic elements in a conceptual manner. It is not intended to be a procedural guide for dental professionals.

The relationship between periodontal health and the restoration of teeth is intimate and inseparable. For restorations to survive long term, the periodontium must remain healthy so that the teeth are maintained. For the periodontium to remain healthy, restorations must be critically managed in several areas so that they are in harmony with their surrounding periodontal tissues. To maintain or enhance the patient's aesthetic appearance, the tooth–tissue interface must present a healthy natural appearance, with gingival tissues framing the restored teeth in a harmonious manner. This chapter reviews the key areas of restorative management necessary to optimize periodontal health, with a focus on the aesthetics and function of restorations.

BIOLOGIC CONSIDERATIONS

Margin Placement and Supracrestal Attached Tissue

A dentist is presented with three options for margin placement: supragingival, equigingival (even with the tissue), and subgingival.[50] Supracrestal attached tissue (SAT) was proposed in the most recent classification as the updated terminology for what was previously known as the biologic width. The *supragingival margin* has the least impact on the periodontium. The use of *equigingival margins* (crown margin placement at the level of gingival margin) traditionally was not desirable because they were thought to retain more plaque than supragingival or subgingival margins and therefore resulted in greater gingival inflammation. These concerns are not valid today, not only

because the restoration margins can be aesthetically blended with the tooth, but also because restorations can be finished easily to provide a smooth, polished interface at the gingival margin. From a periodontal viewpoint, both supragingival and equigingival margins are well tolerated. The greatest biologic risk occurs when placing *subgingival margins*.[26] These margins are not as accessible as supragingival or equigingival margins for finishing procedures. In addition, if the margin is placed too far below the gingival tissue crest, it violates the gingival attachment apparatus.

As described in Chapter 4, the dimension of space that the healthy gingival tissues occupy between the base of the sulcus and the underlying alveolar bone is composed of the junctional epithelial attachment and the connective tissue attachment. The combined attachment width is now identified as the *SAT*. Most authors credit Gargiulo, Wentz, and Orban's 1961 study[13] on cadavers with the initial research establishing the dimensions of space required by the gingival tissues. They found that, in the average human, the connective tissue attachment occupies 1.07 mm of space above the crest of the alveolar bone and that the junctional epithelial attachment below the base of the gingival sulcus occupies another 0.97 mm of space above the connective tissue attachment. The combination of these two measurements, averaging approximately 1 mm each, constitutes the SAT (Fig. 52.1). Clinically, this information is applied to diagnose SAT violations when the restoration margin is placed 2 mm or less away from the alveolar bone and the gingival tissues are inflamed with no other etiologic factors evident.

The reader is referred to the online material for more information on periodontal considerations of restoration margins. Online materials for this chapter are found on the companion website.

KEY FACT

Thin gingiva and highly scalloped papilla are more highly prone to recession after normal restorative procedures.

[a]Adapted from the following chapter of Newman and Carranza's Clinical Periodontology, 13th edition: Chapter 70: Restorative Interrelationships, by Frank M. Spear, Todd R. Schoenbaum, and Joseph P. Cooney.

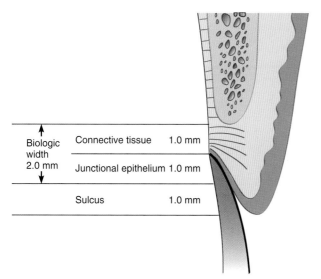

Fig. 52.1 Average Human Supracrestal Attached Tissue (SAT): Connective Tissue Attachment 1 mm in Height; Junctional Epithelial Attachment 1 mm in Height; Sulcus Depth of Approximately 1 mm. The combined connective tissue attachment and junctional epithelial attachment, or SAT, equals 2 mm.

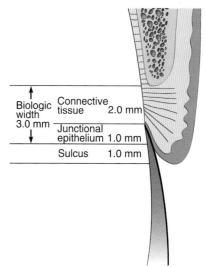

Fig. 52.2 Possible Variations Exist in Supracrestal Attached Tissue (SAT). Connective tissue attachments and junctional epithelial attachments may be variable. In this example, the connective tissue attachment is 2 mm in height, the junctional epithelial attachment 1 mm in height, and the sulcus depth 1 mm, for a combined total tissue height above bone of 4 mm. However, the SAT is 3 mm. This is just one variation that can occur from the average depicted in Fig. 52.1.

Supracrestal Attached Tissue Evaluation

Radiographic interpretation can identify interproximal violations of SAT. However, with the more common locations on the mesiofacial and distofacial line angles of teeth, radiographs are not diagnostic because of tooth superimposition. If a patient experiences tissue discomfort when the restoration margin levels are being assessed with a periodontal probe, it is a good indication that the margin extends into the attachment and that a SAT violation has occurred.

A more positive assessment can be made clinically by measuring the distance between the bone and the restoration margin using a sterile periodontal probe. The probe is pushed through the anesthetized attachment tissues from the sulcus to the underlying bone. If this distance is less than 2 mm at one or more locations, a diagnosis of SAT violation can be confirmed. This assessment is completed circumferentially around the tooth to evaluate the extent of the problem. However, SAT violations can occur in some patients in whom the margins are located more than 2 mm above the alveolar bone level.[14] In 1994, Vacek and colleagues[51] also investigated the SAT phenomenon. Although their average width finding of 2 mm was the same as that previously presented by Gargiulo and associates,[13] they also reported a range of different SATs that were patient specific. They reported SATs as narrow as 0.75 mm in some individuals, whereas others had SATs as tall as 4.3 mm (Fig. 52.2).

This information dictates that specific SAT assessment should be performed for each patient to determine if the patient needs additional SAT, in excess of 2 mm, for restorations to be in harmony with the gingival tissues. The SAT can be identified for the individual patient by probing to the bone level (referred to as "sounding to bone") and subtracting the sulcus depth from the resulting measurement. This measurement must be done on teeth with healthy gingival tissues and should be repeated on more than one tooth to ensure an accurate assessment. The

technique allows the variations in sulcus depths found in individual patients to be assessed and factored into the diagnostic evaluation. The information obtained is then used for definitive diagnosis of SAT violations, the extent of correction needed, and the parameters for placement of future restorations.

Correcting Supracrestal Attached Tissue Violations

SAT violations can be corrected either by surgically removing bone away from proximity to the restoration margin or by orthodontically extruding the tooth and thus moving the margin away from the bone. Surgery is the more rapid of the two treatment options.[40] It is also preferred if the resulting crown lengthening creates a more pleasing tooth length. In these situations, the bone should be moved away from the margin by the measured distance of the ideal SAT for that patient, with an additional 0.5 mm of bone removed as a safety zone.

There is a potential risk of gingival recession after removal of bone.[6] If interproximal bone is removed, there is a high likelihood of papillary recession and the creation of an unaesthetic triangle of space below the interproximal contacts. If the SAT violation is on the interproximal side, or if the violation is across the facial surface and the gingival tissue level is correct, orthodontic extrusion is indicated (Figs. 52.3 to 52.6).[18]

Margin Placement Guidelines

When determining where to place restorative margins relative to the periodontal attachment, it is recommended that the patient's existing sulcular depth be used as a guideline in assessing the SAT requirement for that patient. The base of the sulcus can be viewed as the top of the attachment, and therefore the dentist accounts for variations in attachment height by ensuring that the margin is placed in the sulcus and not in the attachment.[3,24,25,39]

Fig. 52.3 The Left Central Incisor Was Fractured in an Accident 12 Months Ago and Restored at That Time. The patient is unhappy with the appearance of the tissue surrounding the restoration (see Figs. 52.4–52.6).

Fig. 52.4 Radiograph Reveals a Supracrestal Attached Tissue Violation on the Mesial Surface Interproximally. Removal of interproximal bone would create an aesthetic deformity. This patient is better treated with orthodontic extrusion (see Figs. 52.3 and 52.5).

The variations in sulcular probing depth are then used to predict how deep the margin can safely be placed below the gingival crest. With shallow probing depths (1 to 1.5 mm), extending the preparation more than 0.5 mm subgingivally risks violating the attachment. This assumes that the periodontal probe will penetrate into the junctional epithelial attachment in healthy

Fig. 52.5 After Orthodontic Eruption. The tooth has been erupted 3 mm to move the bone and gingiva coronally 3 mm on the left central incisor. It is now possible to reposition the bone surgically to the correct level and position the gingiva to the correct level, reestablishing normal supracrestal attached tissue.

Fig. 52.6 One-Year Recall Photograph After Orthodontic Extrusion, Osseous Surgery, and Placement of a New Restoration for the Patient in Fig. 52.3. Note the excellent tissue health after the reestablishment of supracrestal attached tissue.

gingiva an average of 0.5 mm. With shallow probing depths, future recession is unlikely because the free gingival margin is located close to the top of the attachment. Deeper sulcular probing depths provide more freedom in locating restoration margins farther below the gingival crest. In most circumstances, however, the deeper the gingival sulcus, the greater the risk of gingival recession. Locating the restorative margin deep subgingivally should be avoided, as it increases the difficulty in making an accurate impression, finishing the restoration margins, and increases the likelihood of inflammation and recession.

The reader is referred to the online material for a detailed discussion of the clinical procedures in margin placement. Online materials for this chapter are found on the companion website.

Provisional Restorations

Three critical areas must be effectively managed to produce a favorable biologic response to provisional restorations.[2,53] The marginal fit, crown contour, and surface finish of the interim restorations must be appropriate to maintain the health and position of the gingival tissues during the interval until the final restorations are delivered. Provisional restorations that are poorly adapted at the margins, that are overcontoured or undercontoured, and that have rough or porous surfaces can cause inflammation, overgrowth, or recession of gingival tissues. The outcome can be unpredictable, and unfavorable changes in the tissue architecture can compromise the success of the final restoration.

Marginal Fit

Marginal fit has clearly been implicated in producing an inflammatory response in the periodontium. It has been shown that the level of gingival inflammation can increase corresponding with the level of marginal opening.[11] Margins that are significantly open (several tenths of a millimeter) are capable of harboring large numbers of bacteria and may be responsible for the inflammatory response seen. However, the quality of marginal finish and the margin location relative to the attachment are much more critical to the periodontium than the difference between a 20-μm fit and a 100-μm fit.[26,29,42]

Crown Contour

Restoration contour has been described as extremely important to the maintenance of periodontal health.[17,54] Ideal contour provides access for hygiene, has the fullness to create the desired gingival form, and has a pleasing visual tooth contour in aesthetic areas. Evidence from human and animal studies clearly demonstrates a relationship between overcontouring and gingival inflammation, whereas undercontouring produces no adverse periodontal effect.[31,34] The most frequent cause of overcontoured restorations is inadequate tooth preparation by the dentist, which forces the technician to produce a bulky restoration to provide room for the restorative material. In areas of the mouth in which aesthetic considerations are not critical, a flatter contour is always acceptable.

Subgingival Debris

Leaving debris below the tissue during restorative procedures can create an adverse periodontal response. The cause can be retraction cord, impression material, provisional material, or either temporary or permanent cement.[38] The diagnosis of debris as the cause of gingival inflammation can be confirmed by examining the sulcus surrounding the restoration with an explorer, removing any foreign bodies, and then monitoring the tissue response. It may be necessary to provide tissue anesthesia for patient comfort during the procedure.

Hypersensitivity to Dental Materials

Inflammatory gingival responses have been reported related to the use of nonprecious alloys in dental restorations.[35] Typically, the responses have occurred to alloys containing nickel, although the frequency of these occurrences is controversial.[33] Hypersensitivity responses to precious alloys are extremely rare, and these alloys provide an easy solution to the problems encountered with the nonprecious alloys. Importantly, tissues respond more to the differences in surface roughness of the material than they do to the composition of the material.[1,48] The rougher the surface of the restoration subgingivally, the greater are the plaque accumulation and gingival inflammation. In clinical research, porcelain, highly

polished gold, and highly polished resin all show similar plaque accumulation. Regardless of the restorative material selected, a smooth surface is essential on all materials subgingivally.

AESTHETIC TISSUE MANAGEMENT

Managing Interproximal Embrasures

Current restorative and periodontal therapy must consider a good aesthetic result, especially in the "aesthetic zone." The interproximal papilla is an important part in creating this aesthetic result. The interproximal embrasure created by restorations and the form of the interdental papilla have a unique and intimate relationship.[43,44] The ideal interproximal embrasure should house the gingival papilla without impinging on it and should also extend the interproximal tooth contact to the top of the papilla so that no excess space exists to trap food and to be aesthetically displeasing.

CLINICAL CORRELATION

If you create restorations with no more than 5 mm from the contact to the bone, open gingival embrasures can be avoided. The downside to this approach is that the teeth will look square and blocky. However, some patients can support a 7-mm papilla. Well-made provisional restorations allow accurate determination of actual papilla length.

The clinician most frequently confronts a normal or shallow sulcus with a papilla that appears too short rather than a tall papilla with a deep sulcus. If the embrasure is the ideal width, the papilla assumes a pointed form, has a sulcus of 2.5 to 3 mm, and is healthy. If the embrasure is too narrow, the papilla may grow out to the facial and lingual, form a col, and become inflamed. This information is applied when evaluating an individual papilla with an open embrasure. The papilla in question is compared with the adjacent papillae. If the papillae are all on the same level, and if the other areas do not have open embrasures, the problem is one of gingival embrasure form. If the papilla in the area of concern is apical to the adjacent papillae, however, the clinician should evaluate the interproximal bone levels. If the bone under that papilla is apical to the adjacent bone levels, the problem is caused by bone loss. If the bone is at the same level, the open embrasure is caused by the embrasure form of the teeth and not a periodontal problem with the papilla. The papillae in the anterior maxilla average 4 mm long and are the same heights at the mesial and distal sides of the tooth. Ultimately, deficient papillae and open gingival embrasures are most predictably corrected with restorations to close the space.

The reader is referred to the online material for a brief discussion on the management of open gingival embrasures restoratively and gingival embrasure form for patients with gingival recession. Online materials for this chapter are found on the companion website.

Pontic Design

Classically, there are four options to consider in evaluating pontic design: hygienic, ridge lap, modified ridge lap, and ovate designs (Fig. 52.7). Regardless of design, the pontic should provide an

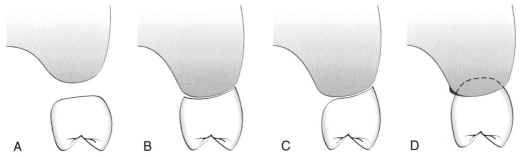

Fig. 52.7 Four Options to Designing the Shape of a Pontic. (A) Hygienic pontic. Tissue surface of the pontic is 3 mm from the underlying ridge. (B) Ridge-lap pontic. Tissue surface of the pontic straddles the ridge in saddle-like fashion. The entire tissue surface of the ridge-lap pontic is convex and very difficult to clean. (C) Modified ridge-lap pontic. Tissue surface on the facial is concave, following the ridge. However, the lingual saddle has been removed to allow access for oral hygiene. (D) Ovate pontic. The pontic form fits into a receptor site within the ridge. This allows the tissue surface of the pontic to be convex and also optimizes aesthetics.

occlusal surface that stabilizes the opposing teeth, allows for normal mastication, and does not overload the abutment teeth. The area of the pontic interfacing with the gingiva can be porcelain, metal, zirconia, lithium disilicate, or some other material with no variation in the biologic response of the tissue provided it has a smooth surface finish.[16,36,45]

The key differences between the four pontic designs relate to the aesthetics and access for hygiene procedures. The primary method for cleaning the undersurface of pontics is to draw dental floss mesiodistally along the undersurface. The shape of this undersurface determines the ease with which plaque and food debris can be removed in the process. The hygienic and ovate pontics have convex undersurfaces, which makes them easiest to clean. The ridge lap and modified ridge-lap designs have concave surfaces, which are more difficult to access with the dental floss. Although the hygienic pontic design provides the easiest access for hygiene procedures, it is much less aesthetic and objectionable by some patients.

The reader is referred to the online material for a brief discussion on ridge modification procedures for ideal pontic contours. Online materials for this chapter are found on the companion website.

OCCLUSAL CONSIDERATIONS IN RESTORATIVE THERAPY

KEY FACT

A mutually protective occlusion is created when all the teeth touch at the same time in a normal closing arc, but when the mandible moves, all contacts are on the anterior teeth.

Chapter 48 presents details on the biology of occlusion and related clinical evaluation procedures. The importance of occlusal trauma as a factor in periodontal disease and its role in orofacial pain have been deemphasized in numerous papers.[a] However, the role that occlusion plays in restorative dentistry has been reemphasized. The increased use of dental implants and nonmetallic restorations has resulted in increased concern over force management. Some of these materials are more sensitive to occlusal trauma, and resulting fracture, than are metal restorations. Consequently, for the clinician who wants a high degree of predictability, understanding occlusion is critical. The reader is referred to Chapter 48 for a more comprehensive overview of occlusal evaluation and therapy.

The reader is referred to the online material for a detailed discussion on special restorative considerations. Online materials for this chapter are found on the companion website.

Case Scenarios are found on the companion website.

REFERENCES

 References for this chapter are found on the companion website www.expertconsult.com.

[a]References 7, 10, 22, 23, 27, 28, 37, 47, 52

53

Supportive Periodontal Treatment[a]

CHAPTER OUTLINE

Preservation of the periodontal health of the treated patient requires a supportive program that is just as important as the therapy used to treat the periodontal disease. After phase I therapy has been completed, patients are placed on a schedule of periodic recall visits for maintenance care to prevent the recurrence of the disease (Figs. 53.1 and 53.2).

> **KEY FACT**
>
> The long-term preservation of the dentition is closely associated with the frequency and quality of recall maintenance.

Transfer of the patient from active treatment status to a maintenance program is a definitive step in total patient care that requires time and effort on the part of the dental team. Patients must understand the purpose of the maintenance program, and the dental hygienist must emphasize that preservation of the teeth depends on maintenance therapy.[5] Patients who are not maintained in a supervised recall program subsequent to active treatment show obvious signs of recurrent periodontitis (e.g., increased pocket depth, bone loss, or tooth loss).[b] The more often patients present for recommended supportive periodontal treatment (SPT), the less likely they are to lose teeth.[c] One study indicated that treated patients who do not return for regular recall have a 5.6 times greater risk for tooth loss than compliant patients.[12] Another study showed that patients with inadequate SPT after successful regenerative therapy have a 50-fold increase

in risk of probing attachment loss compared with those who have regular recall visits.[15]

> **KEY FACT**
>
> Patients who do not return for SPT lose five to six times more teeth than compliant patients.

Motivational techniques and reinforcement of the importance of the maintenance phase of treatment should be considered before performing definitive periodontal surgery.[7] Studies show that few patients display complete compliance with recommended maintenance schedules[d] (Fig. 53.3). *It is meaningless simply to inform patients that they are to return for periodic recall visits without clearly explaining the significance of these visits and describing what is expected of patients between visits.*

The maintenance phase of periodontal treatment starts immediately after the completion of phase I therapy (see Figs. 53.1 and 53.2). While the patient is in the maintenance phase, the necessary surgical and restorative procedures are performed. This ensures that all areas of the mouth retain the degree of health attained after phase I therapy.

RATIONALE FOR SUPPORTIVE PERIODONTAL TREATMENT

Studies indicate that even with appropriate periodontal therapy, some progression of disease is possible.[e] One likely explanation for the recurrence of periodontal disease is incomplete subgingival

---

[a]Adapted from the following chapter of Newman and Carranza's Clinical Periodontology, 13th edition: Chapter 72: Supportive Periodontal Treatment, by Robert L. Merin.

[b]References: 6, 7, 11, 12, 16, 17, 37.

[c]References: 17, 28, 34, 37, 40, 54, 61.

[d]References: 1, 33, 34, 38, 39, 59, 61.

[e]References: 23, 25, 41, 44, 46, 53, 62.

Phase I

↓

Reevaluation

↓

Phase II (periodontal surgery)

↓

Phase III (restorative)

↓

Phase IV (maintenance)

Fig. 53.1 Incorrect Sequence of Periodontal Treatment Phases. Maintenance phase should be started immediately after the reevaluation of phase I therapy.

Phase I

↓

Reevaluation

↓

Phase IV (maintenance)

Phase II   →   Phase III
(periodontal surgery)   (restorative)

Fig. 53.2 Correct Sequence of Periodontal Treatment Phases.

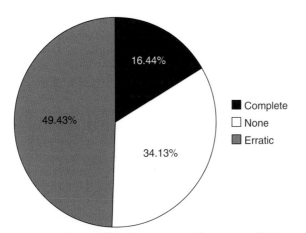

■ Complete
□ None
■ Erratic

16.44%

34.13%

49.43%

Fig. 53.3 Compliance With Maintenance Therapy in 961 Patients Studied for 1 to 8 Years. (Modified from Wilson TG Jr, Glover ME, Schoen J, et al: Compliance with maintenance therapy in a private periodontal practice, *J Periodontol* 55:468, 1984.)

plaque/biofilm and calculus removal.[56,62] If subgingival biofilm is left behind during scaling, it regrows within the pocket. The regrowth of subgingival biofilm is a slow process compared with that of supragingival biofilm. During this period (perhaps months), the subgingival biofilm may not induce inflammatory reactions that can be discerned at the gingival margin. The clinical diagnosis may be further confused by the introduction of adequate supragingival biofilm control because the inflammatory reactions caused by the biofilm in the soft-tissue wall of the pocket are not likely to manifest clinically as gingival erythema and edema.[18] Thus inadequate subgingival biofilm control can lead to continued loss of attachment, even without the presence of clinical gingival inflammation. Scaling and root planing are not always effective at sites with probing depths of 6 mm or greater.[5]

Bacteria are present in the gingival tissues in chronic and aggressive periodontitis cases.[9,14,19,43] Eradication of intragingival microorganisms may be necessary for a stable periodontal result.[19] Scaling, root planing, and even flap surgery may not eliminate intragingival bacteria in some areas.[9] These bacteria may recolonize the pocket and cause recurrent disease.

Bacteria associated with periodontitis can be transmitted between spouses and other family members.[2,55] Patients who appear to be successfully treated can become infected or reinfected with potential pathogens. This is especially likely in patients with remaining pockets.

Another possible explanation for the recurrence of periodontal disease is the microscopic nature of the dentogingival unit healing after periodontal treatment. Histologic studies have indicated that after periodontal procedures, tissues usually heal by the formation a long junctional epithelium instead of new connective tissue attachment to root surfaces.[10,49,50] It has been speculated that this type of dentogingival unit may be weaker and that inflammation may rapidly separate the long junctional epithelium from the tooth. Thus treated periodontal patients may be predisposed to recurrent pocket formation if maintenance care is not optimal.

Subgingival scaling alters the microflora of periodontal pockets.[35,42,47] In one study, a single session of scaling and root planing in patients with chronic periodontitis resulted in significant changes in subgingival microflora.[35] Reported alterations included a decrease in the proportion of motile rods for 1 week, a marked elevation in the proportion of coccoid cells for 21 days, and a marked reduction in the proportion of spirochetes for 7 weeks.

Although pocket debridement suppresses components of the subgingival microflora associated with periodontitis, periodontal pathogens may return to baseline levels within days or months.[3,46] The return of pathogens to pretreatment levels generally occurs in approximately 9 to 11 weeks but can vary dramatically among patients.[3]

KEY FACT

Scaling and root planing are not always effective at sites with probing depths of 6 mm or greater.

Both the mechanical debridement performed by the therapist and the motivational environment provided by the appointment seem to be necessary for good maintenance results. Patients tend to reduce their oral hygiene efforts between appointments.[4,61] Knowing that their hygiene will be evaluated motivates them to perform better oral hygiene in anticipation of the appointment.

In one study, the proportion of spirochetes obtained in baseline samples of subgingival flora was highly correlated with clinical periodontal deterioration over 1 year.[31] However, subsequent reports in the same longitudinal study concluded that the arbitrary assignment of treated periodontitis patients to 3-month maintenance intervals appears to be as effective in preventing recurrences of periodontitis as assignment of recall intervals based on microscopic monitoring of the subgingival flora.[30,31] Microscopic monitoring was found not to be a reliable predictor of future periodontal destruction in patients on 3-month recall programs, presumably because of the alteration of subgingival flora produced by subgingival instrumentation.

In conclusion, there is a sound scientific basis for recall maintenance because subgingival scaling alters the pocket microflora for variable but relatively long periods.

MAINTENANCE PROGRAM

Periodic recall visits form the foundation of a meaningful long-term prevention program. The interval between visits is initially set at 3 months but may vary according to the patient's needs.[5,20,26,27]

Periodontal care at each recall visit comprises three parts (Box 53.1). The first part involves examination and evaluation of the patient's current oral health. The second part includes the necessary maintenance treatment and oral hygiene reinforcement. The third part involves scheduling the patient for the next recall appointment, additional periodontal treatment, or restorative dental procedures. The time required for a recall visit for patients with multiple teeth in both arches is approximately 1 hour.[45]

> ### KEY FACT
> There are three parts to an SPT appointment: (1) examination; (2) treatment; and (3) report and scheduling.

Examination and Evaluation

The recall examination is similar to the initial evaluation of the patient (see Chapter 30). However, because the patient is not new to the office, the dentist or hygienist primarily looks for changes that have occurred since the last evaluation. Analysis of the current oral hygiene status of the patient is essential. Updating of changes in the medical history and evaluation of restorations, caries, prostheses, occlusion, tooth mobility, gingival status, and periodontal and periimplant probing depths are important parts of the recall appointment. The oral mucosa should be carefully inspected for pathologic conditions (Figs. 53.4–53.9).

Radiographic examination must be individualized,[22] depending on the initial severity of the case and the findings during the recall visit (Table 53.1). These are compared with findings on previous radiographs to check the bone height and look for

---

BOX 53.1   Maintenance Recall Procedures

Part I: Examination
(Approximate time: 14 min)
Patient greeting
Medical history changes
Oral pathologic examination
Oral hygiene status
Gingival changes
Pocket depth changes
Mobility changes
Occlusal changes
Dental caries
Restorative, prosthetic, and implant status

Part II: Treatment
(Approximate time: 36 min)
Oral hygiene reinforcement
Scaling
Polishing
Chemical irrigation or site-specific antimicrobial placement

Part III: Report and Scheduling
(Approximate time: 10 min)
Write report in chart.
Discuss report with patient.
Schedule next recall visit.
Schedule further periodontal treatment.
Schedule or refer for restorative or prosthetic treatment.

Fig. 53.4 (A) Hyperplastic gingivitis related to crown margins and plaque accumulation in a 27-year-old woman. (B) Four months after treatment, there is significant improvement. However, some inflammation around crown margins still exists, which cannot be resolved without replacing the crowns.

Fig. 53.5 (A) Patient was 38 years old when these original radiographs were taken and was treated with a combination of surgical and nonsurgical therapy. This individual is a classic class C maintenance patient. (B) Pretreatment photograph. Note the inflammation and heavy calculus deposits. (C) Photograph taken 10 years after treatment. (D) Radiographs taken 5 years after treatment. (E) Radiographs taken 10 years after treatment. The radiographic appearance is as good as can be expected in such a severe case. Teeth #15 and #17 were extracted 8 years after treatment.

Fig. 53.6 This Series of Radiographs Clearly Shows the Importance of Maintenance Therapy. (A) Original radiograph of a 58-year-old male. Note the deep distal bone loss on tooth #18 and the moderate distal lesion of tooth #19. Surgical treatment included osseous grafting. (B) Radiograph 14 months after surgical therapy. The patient had recall maintenance performed every 3 to 4 months. (C) Appearance 3 years after surgery, with regular recalls every 3 to 4 months. (D) Appearance after 2 years without recalls (7 years after surgery). Note the progression of the disease on the distal surfaces of teeth #18 and #19.

Fig. 53.7 Advanced Cases Sometimes Do Better Than Expected When the Patient Complies With Maintenance Therapy. (A) Initial radiographs showing an advanced case. The maxillary arch had extractions and nonsurgical treatment. A plastic partial denture was placed and was expected to grow into a full denture within a few years. The mandibular arch was treated with periodontal surgery, and a permanent, metal and plastic, removable partial denture was placed. (B) Radiographs taken 8 years later. The patient performed good oral hygiene and had 3-month recalls. Teeth #12 and #15 required extraction.

Fig. 53.8 (A) Initial radiographs. The patient was advised to have localized areas of periodontal surgery and periodontal recall every 3 months. However, the patient did not comply and only had dental cleanings once or twice yearly. (B) Radiographs 4 years later. Note the loss of teeth #5 and #15 and the increased bone loss of several premolars and molars.

TABLE 53.1	Radiographic Examination of Recall Patients for Supportive Periodontal Treatment
Patient Condition/Situation	**Type of Examination**
Clinical caries or high-risk factors for caries	Posterior bitewing examination at 6–18-month intervals
No clinical caries and no high-risk factors for caries	Posterior bitewing examination at 24–36-month intervals
Periodontal disease not under good control	Periapical or vertical bitewing radiographs of problem areas every 12–24 months
History of periodontal treatment with disease under good control	Bitewing examination every 24–36 months
Root form dental implants	Periapical or vertical bitewing radiographs after prosthetic placement and at 12 and 24 months, then every 24–36 months unless clinical problems arise
Transfer of periodontal or implant maintenance patients	Full-mouth series if a current set not available; if full-mouth series has been taken within 24 months, radiographs of implants and periodontal problem areas should be taken

Radiographs should be taken when they are likely to affect diagnosis and patient treatment. The recommendations in this table are subject to clinical judgment and may not apply to every patient.
Adapted from *Guide to Patient Selection and Limiting Radiation Exposure.* American Dental Association website, http://ada.org/2760/aspx, 2013.

repair of osseous defects, signs of trauma from occlusion, periapical pathologic changes, and caries.

Checking of Plaque/Biofilm Control

To assess the effectiveness of their plaque control, patients should perform their hygiene regimen immediately before or at the recall appointment. Plaque/biofilm control must be reviewed and corrected until the patient demonstrates the necessary proficiency, even if additional instruction sessions are required. A motivational interviewing technique of teaching may help to produce positive results.[57] Patients instructed in plaque/biofilm control have less biofilm and gingivitis than uninstructed patients,[6,51,52] and because

Fig. 53.9 (A) Initial radiographs. The patient was advised to have localized areas of periodontal surgery and periodontal recall every 3 months. However, the patient did not comply and had no treatment other than emergency care and occasional dental cleanings. (B) Radiographs 7 years later. Note the advanced bone loss and caries on many teeth.

the amount of supragingival plaque/biofilm is less, there is a decrease in the number of subgingival anaerobic organisms.[10,48]

Treatment

Following consultation, examination, consultation, and oral hygiene instruction, the required scaling and root planing are performed (see Chapter 45). Care must be taken not to instrument healthy sites with shallow sulci (1 to 3 mm deep) and an absence of gingival inflammation, because studies have indicated that repeated subgingival scaling and root planing of sites not periodontally involved result in significant loss of attachment and gingival recession, which will affect aesthetics.[29] Irrigation with antimicrobial agents or placement of site-specific antimicrobial devices may be performed in maintenance patients with remaining pockets.[3,24,32]

Recurrence of Periodontal Disease

Occasionally, lesions may recur, which is often due to inadequate plaque/biofilm control on the part of the patient or failure to comply with recommended SPT schedules. It should be understood, however, that it is the responsibility of the dental hygienist to educate and motivate patients to improve their oral hygiene

techniques. Surgery should not be undertaken unless the patient participates in disease prevention and demonstrates proficiency in plaque/biofilm control.[7,53,60]

Other causes for recurrence include the following:

1. Inadequate or insufficient treatment that has failed to remove all of the potential factors favoring biofilm accumulation (see Fig. 53.4). Incomplete calculus removal in areas of difficult access is a common source of problems.
2. Inadequate restorations placed after the periodontal treatment was completed.
3. Failure of the patient to return for periodic maintenance care (see Fig. 53.6). This may be a result of the patient's conscious or unconscious decision not to continue treatment or the failure of the dental hygienist to emphasize the need for periodic supportive therapy.
4. Presence of some systemic diseases that may affect host resistance to previously acceptable levels of biofilm.

A failing case can be recognized by the following:

1. Recurring inflammation revealed by gingival changes and bleeding of the sulcus on probing.
2. Increasing depth of sulci, leading to the recurrence of pocket formation.

TABLE 53.2 Symptoms and Causes of Recurrence of Disease

Symptom	Possible Causes
Increased mobility	Increased inflammation Poor oral hygiene Subgingival calculus Inadequate restorations Deteriorating or poorly designed prostheses Systemic disease-modifying host response to plaque
Recession	Toothbrush abrasion Inadequate keratinized gingiva Frenum pull Orthodontic therapy
Increased mobility with no change in pocket depth and no radiographic change	Occlusal trauma caused by lateral occlusal interference, bruxism, high restoration Poorly designed or worn-out prosthesis Poor crown-to-root ratio
Increased pocket depth with no radiographic change	Poor oral hygiene Infrequent recall visits Subgingival calculus Poorly fitting partial denture Mesial inclination into edentulous space Failure of new attachment surgery Cracked teeth Grooves in teeth New periodontal disease Gingival overgrowth caused by medication
Increased pocket depth with increased radiographic bone loss	Poor oral hygiene Subgingival calculus Infrequent recall visits Inadequate or deteriorating restorations Poorly designed prostheses Inadequate surgery Systemic disease modifying host response to plaque Cracked teeth Grooves in teeth New periodontal disease

3. Gradual increases in bone loss, as determined by radiographs.
4. Gradual increases in tooth mobility, as ascertained by clinical examination.

The decision to retreat a periodontal patient should not be made at the preventive maintenance appointment but should be postponed for 1 to 2 weeks.[11] Often, the mouth appears improved at that time because of the resolution of edema and the resulting improved tone of the gingiva. Table 53.2 summarizes the symptoms of the recurrence of periodontal disease and their probable causes.

CLASSIFICATION OF POSTTREATMENT PATIENTS AND RISK ASSESSMENT

The first year after periodontal therapy is important in terms of indoctrinating the patient in a recall pattern and reinforcing oral hygiene techniques. In addition, it may take several months to evaluate accurately the results of some periodontal surgical procedures. Consequently, some areas may have to be retreated because the results may not be optimal. Furthermore, the first-year patient often has etiologic factors that may have been overlooked and may be amenable to treatment at this early stage. For these reasons, the recall interval for first-year patients should not be longer than 3 months.

Patients who are on a periodontal recall schedule are a varied group. Table 53.3 lists several categories of maintenance patients and a suggested recall interval for each group. Patients can improve or may relapse to a different classification, with a reduction in or exacerbation of periodontal disease. When one dental arch is more involved than the other, the patient's periodontal disease is classified by the arch with the worse condition.

Table 53.3 is a traditional method of assigning the risk of a recurrence of periodontal destruction. A practitioner uses the listed risk factors and his or her own diagnostic and prognostic gestalt to assign a risk category and maintenance schedule. New risk factor assessment tools for the prevention of periodontal destruction have been developed.[21,26,27,36] The Periodontal Risk Assessment (PRA) (Fig. 53.10) and the Periodontal Risk Calculator (PRC) have the most studies documenting their ability to predict the progression of periodontitis and tooth loss.[26] The PRC is marketed by the PreViser Corporation and offers a web-based system for periodontal risk analysis and prognosis.[21] The PRA is offered free of charge by the Clinical Research Foundation and the University of Bern at http://www.perio-tools.com/PRA/en/index.asp. Patient data are entered into the online form, and the program automatically calculates whether the patient is at low risk, moderate risk, or high risk; an appropriate recall interval is then suggested. Fig. 53.9A is a sample assessment from the PRA website. Because the different assessment tools use different risk factors and algorithms, they will not be in complete agreement. In one study, 57 patients were assessed with the PRC and PRA.[36] The PRC classified 14 as low risk, 17 as medium risk, and 26 as high risk, whereas the PRA classified 8 as low risk, 28 as medium risk, and 21 as high risk.[36]

Currently, there is no universally accepted objective method of predicting periodontitis progression, and there has been little research to determine if the risk calculators are more accurate than good clinical judgment.[21] In summary, maintenance care is a critical phase of therapy. The long-term preservation of the dentition is closely associated with the frequency and quality of recall maintenance.

KEY FACT

The dental hygienist should use risk assessment to determine SPT frequency.

REFERRAL OF PATIENTS TO THE PERIODONTIST

General dentist-dental hygienist team can properly manage many periodontal patients, as a greater number of people retain their teeth throughout their lifetime. Another important fact to consider is that as the proportion of older people in the population increases, more teeth will be at risk for periodontal disease.

TABLE 53.3   Recall Intervals for Various Classes of Recall Patients

Merin Classification	Characteristics	Recall Interval
First year	First-year patient: routine therapy and uneventful healing. First-year patient: difficult case with complicated prosthesis, furcation involvement, poor crown-to-root ratios, or questionable patient cooperation	3 months 1–2 months
Class A	Excellent results well maintained for 1 year or longer Patient displays good oral hygiene, minimal calculus, no occlusal problems, no complicated prostheses, no remaining pockets, and no teeth with less than 50% of alveolar bone remaining	6 months to 1 year
Class B	Generally good results maintained reasonably well for 1 year or more, but patient displays some of the following factors: 1. Inconsistent or poor oral hygiene 2. Heavy calculus formation 3. Systemic disease that predisposes to periodontal breakdown 4. Some remaining pockets 5. Occlusal problems 6. Complicated prostheses 7. Ongoing orthodontic therapy 8. Recurrent dental caries 9. Some teeth with less than 50% of alveolar bone support 10. Smoking 11. Positive family history or genetic test 12. More than 20% of pockets bleed on probing	3–4 months (decide on a recall interval based on the number and severity of negative factors)
Class C	Generally poor results after periodontal therapy or several negative factors from the following list: 1. Inconsistent or poor oral hygiene 2. Heavy calculus formation 3. Systemic disease that predisposes to periodontal breakdown 4. Many remaining pockets 5. Occlusal problems 6. Complicated prostheses 7. Recurrent dental caries 8. Periodontal surgery indicated but not performed for medical, psychological, or financial reasons 9. Many teeth with less than 50% of alveolar bone support 10. Condition too far advanced to be improved by periodontal surgery 11. Smoking 12. Positive family history or genetic test 13. More than 20% of pockets bleed on probing	1–3 months (decide on a recall interval based on the number and severity of negative factors; consider retreating some areas or extracting severely involved teeth)

Numerous studies indicate possible links between periodontal disease and systemic diseases, such as heart disease, stroke, diabetes, and adverse pregnancy outcomes. Therefore, the prevalence of patients requiring SPT is likely to increase in the future.

This expected increase in the number of periodontal patients will necessitate a greater understanding of periodontal problems and an increased level of expertise for the solution of such problems on the part of the general practitioner. The general dentist–dental hygienist team must know when co-management with a periodontist is indicated. Specialists are needed to treat difficult periodontal cases, patients with systemic health problems, dental implant patients, and those with a complex prosthetic construction that requires predictable results.

The criteria for cases to be treated in the general dental office and cases to be referred to a specialist vary for different practitioners and patients. The American Academy of Periodontology has issued guidelines to help the general practitioner decide when co-management with a periodontist is indicated.[4] The diagnosis will indicate the type of periodontal treatment required. If periodontal destruction necessitates surgery on the distal surfaces of second molars, extensive osseous surgery, or complex regenerative procedures, the patient is usually best treated by a specialist. Patients who require localized nonsurgical therapy or minor flap surgery can usually be managed by the general practitioner. Dental professionals have a primary responsibility to do what is best in the interest of the patient. According to Christensen, quality dentistry for a complex case requires a team effort partnering with a periodontal specialist to provide optimal care for the patient.[13]

The decision to have the general dentist–dental hygienist team treat a patient's periodontal disease should be guided by consideration of the risk that the patient will lose a tooth or teeth due to periodontal involvement or the periodontal disease negatively affecting the patient's systemic health.

The most important factors in the decision to refer a patient to a periodontist are the severity and location of the periodontal disease. Teeth with pockets of 5 mm or more, as measured from the cementoenamel junction, may have a questionable prognosis, as do teeth with furcation invasions even when more than 50% of bone support remains. Therefore, patients with strategically

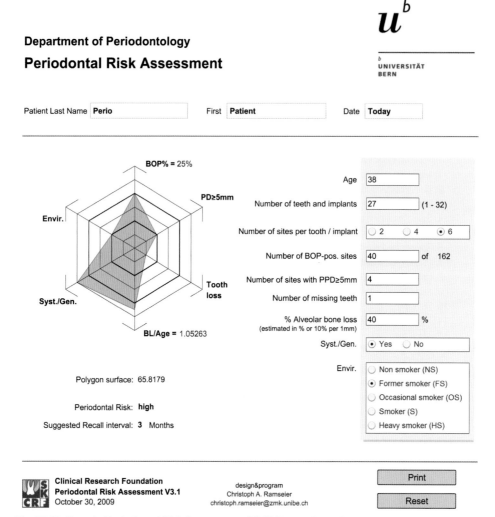

Department of Periodontology

Periodontal Risk Assessment

u^b

b UNIVERSITÄT
BERN

Patient Last Name **Perio**   First **Patient**   Date **Today**

BOP% = 25%

PD≥5mm

Envir.

Tooth loss

Syst./Gen.

BL/Age = 1.05263

Polygon surface: 65.8179

Periodontal Risk: **high**

Suggested Recall interval: **3** Months

Age   38

Number of teeth and implants   27   (1 - 32)

Number of sites per tooth / implant   ○ 2   ○ 4   ⊙ 6

Number of BOP-pos. sites   40   of   162

Number of sites with PPD≥5mm   4

Number of missing teeth   1

% Alveolar bone loss   40   %
(estimated in % or 10% per 1mm)

Syst./Gen.   ⊙ Yes   ○ No

Envir.   ○ Non smoker (NS)
⊙ Former smoker (FS)
○ Occasional smoker (OS)
○ Smoker (S)
○ Heavy smoker (HS)

Print

Reset

Clinical Research Foundation
Periodontal Risk Assessment V3.1
October 30, 2009

design&program
Christoph A. Ramseier
christoph.ramseier@zmk.unibe.ch

Fig. 53.10 Sample Periodontal Risk Assessment (PRA) Report Completed and Downloaded From http://www.perio-tools.com/PRA/en/index.asp.

important teeth that have moderate to severe attachment loss or furcation invasions are usually best treated by specialists.

An important question remains: Should the maintenance phase of therapy be performed by the general practitioner–dental hygienist team or the specialist? This should be determined by the extent and severity of periodontal disease present. Class A recall patients should be maintained by the general dentist–dental hygienist team, whereas class C patients should be maintained by the specialist (see Table 53.3). Class B patients can alternate recall visits between the general practitioner and the specialist (Fig. 53.11). The suggested rule to decide who should maintain the recall therapy is determined by the initial category of the patient's disease and the result of the therapy. Patients with moderate to severe initial bone loss, advanced grades 2 or 3 furcation invasions, or pockets that could not be completely eradicated are those who should be seen by the periodontist. The specialist and the general dentist-dental hygienist team must work together, respect the other's knowledge and skills, and decide on a maintenance schedule that is in the best interest of the patient.

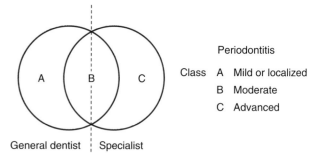

Periodontitis

Class   A   Mild or localized
B   Moderate
C   Advanced

General dentist   Specialist

Fig. 53.11 Scheme for Determining Which Practitioner Should Perform Periodontal Maintenance in Patients With Different Degrees of Periodontitis.

KEY FACT

Quality dentistry for a complex case requires a team effort partnering with a periodontal specialist to provide optimal care for the patient.[13]

TESTS FOR DISEASE ACTIVITY

Periodontal patients, even though they have received effective periodontal therapy, are at risk of disease recurrence for the remainder of their lives.[23,24] In addition, pockets in and around the furcation areas are difficult to eliminate even with surgical therapy. These areas with pockets may continue to lose attachment.[3] Comparison of sequential probing measurements, which may be facilitated by a dental practice management software, gives the most accurate indication of the rate of loss of attachment. A number of other clinical and laboratory variables have been correlated with disease activity.

No accurate method exists to predict disease activity, and clinicians rely on the information obtained from evaluating multiple risk factors.[21,25,30,58] Patients whose disease is clearly refractory are candidates for bacterial culturing and antibiotic therapy in conjunction with additional mechanical therapy.

New methods will undoubtedly be developed in the future to help predict disease activity.[3] The clinician must be able to interpret whether a test may be useful in determining disease activity and future loss of attachment.[8] Tests should be adopted only when they are based on research that includes a critical analysis of the sensitivity, specificity, disease incidence, and predictive value of the proposed test.[21]

CONCLUSION

The long-term preservation of the dentition is closely associated with the frequency and quality of recall maintenance. The therapist should use risk assessment and educate the patient on the need for periodontal maintenance. Supportive periodontal therapy is a lifetime effort to prevent the disease from recurring. Patients who do not return for supportive periodontal therapy lose more teeth than compliant patients.

A Case Scenario is found on the companion website.

REFERENCES

 References for this chapter are found on the companion website.

Results of Periodontal Treatment[a]

Note: In the 2018 Classification of Periodontal and Peri-Implant Diseases and Conditions, "chronic periodontitis" and "aggressive periodontitis" disease categories are grouped under a single category called "periodontitis," and are further characterized based on a multidimensional staging and grading system. In this chapter, the term "aggressive periodontitis" is still used because the related studies were conducted before the 2018 classification. Readers are referred to Chapter 6 for the detailed discussion on periodontal disease classification.

The prevalence of periodontal disease, the resulting high rate of tooth mortality, and the potential for multiple systemic health complications aggravated by chronic periodontitis raise an important question: Is periodontal treatment effective in preventing and controlling the chronic infection and progressive destruction of periodontal disease? Current concepts of evaluating health care require a scientific basis for treatment, referred to as *evidence-based therapy*. Evidence is now overwhelming that periodontal therapy is effective in preventing periodontal disease, slowing the destruction of the periodontium, and reducing tooth loss.

PREVENTION AND TREATMENT OF GINGIVITIS

> **KEY FACT**
>
> Gingivitis is reversible.

For many years, the belief that good oral hygiene is necessary for the successful prevention and treatment of gingivitis has been widespread among periodontists. In addition, worldwide epidemiologic studies have confirmed a close relationship between the incidence of gingivitis and lack of oral hygiene.[8,9]

Löe and coworkers[20,38] provided conclusive evidence on the association between oral hygiene and gingivitis. After 9 to 21

days without performing oral hygiene measures, healthy dental students with previously excellent oral hygiene and healthy gingiva developed heavy accumulations of biofilm and generalized mild gingivitis. When oral hygiene techniques were reinstituted, the biofilm in most areas disappeared in 1 or 2 days, and gingival inflammation in these areas disappeared approximately 1 week after the biofilm was removed. Thus, gingivitis is reversible and can be resolved by daily, effective biofilm removal.

A number of long-term studies have shown that gingival health can be maintained by a combination of effective oral hygiene maintenance and scaling procedures.[b] A 3-year study was conducted on 1248 General Telephone workers in California to determine whether progression of gingival inflammation is reduced in an oral environment in which high levels of hygiene are maintained.[36,37] Experimental and control groups were computer matched based on periodontal and oral hygiene status, past caries experience, age, and gender. During the study period, several procedures were instituted to ensure that the oral hygiene status of the experimental group was maintained at a high level. Subjects were given a series of frequent oral prophylaxis treatments combined with oral hygiene instruction. Subjects in the control group received no attention from the study team except for annual examinations. They were advised to continue their usual daily practices and accustomed visits for professional care. After 3 years, the increase in biofilm and debris in the control group was four times as great as that in the experimental group. Similarly, gingivitis scores were much higher in control subjects than in the matching experimental group. Therefore, chronic marginal gingivitis can be controlled with good oral hygiene and dental prophylaxis.

> **KEY FACT**
>
> A number of long-term studies have shown that gingival health can be maintained by a combination of effective oral hygiene maintenance and scaling procedures.[a]

---

[a]Adapted from the following chapter of Newman and Carranza's Clinical Periodontology, 13th edition: Chapter 73: Results of Periodontal Treatment, by Robert L. Merin.

[a]References 1, 2, 11, 13–15, 22, 24, 36, 37.

[b]References 1, 2, 11, 13–15, 22, 24, 36, 37.

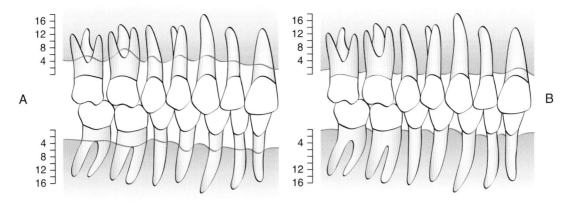

Fig. 54.1 (A) Mean periodontal support of teeth of Sri Lankan tea laborers at approximately 40 years of age. (B) Mean periodontal support of teeth of Norwegian academicians at approximately 40 years of age. (From Löe H, Anerud A, Boysen H, et al: The natural history of periodontal disease in man: the rate of periodontal destruction before 40 years of age. *J Periodontol* 49:607–620, 1978.)

PREVENTION AND TREATMENT OF LOSS OF ATTACHMENT

Although periodontal therapy has been utilized for more than 100 years, it is only since the mid-1970s that a number of studies have been conducted to determine the effect of treatment on reducing the progressive loss of periodontal support for the natural dentition.

Prevention of Loss of Attachment

Löe and coworkers[19,20] conducted a longitudinal investigation to study the natural development and progression of periodontal disease. The first study group, established in Oslo, Norway, in 1969, consisted of 565 healthy male non-dental students and academicians between 17 and 40 years of age. Oslo was selected mainly because this city had an ongoing preschool, school, and post-school dental program offering systematic preventive, restorative, endodontic, orthodontic, and surgical therapy on an annual recall basis for all children and adolescents, complete with a documented attendance record, for the previous 40 years. Members of the study population had experienced maximum exposure to conventional dental care throughout their lives. A second study group, established in Sri Lanka in 1970, consisted of 480 male tea laborers between 15 and 40 years of age. They were healthy and in excellent physical condition by local standards, and their nutritional condition was clinically fair. The workers had never been exposed to any programs relative to the prevention or treatment of dental diseases. Oral care was unknown, and dental caries was virtually nonexistent.

The results of this study are interesting. As the members of the Norwegian group approached 40 years of age, the mean individual loss of attachment was slightly above 1.5 mm and the mean annual rate of attachment loss was 0.08 mm for interproximal surfaces and 0.1 mm for buccal surfaces. As the Sri Lankans approached 40 years of age, the mean individual loss of attachment was 4.5 mm, and the mean annual rate of progression of the lesion was 0.3 mm for interproximal surfaces and 0.2 mm for buccal surfaces. Fig. 54.1 shows a graphic

Classification of 480 Sri Lankan Laborers According to Progression of Periodontal Disease

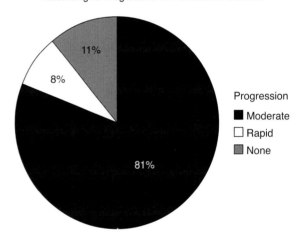

Fig. 54.2 Progression of Periodontal Disease in an Untreated Population. (Data from Löe H, Anerud A, Boysen H, et al: Natural history of periodontal disease in man: rapid, moderate and no loss of attachment in Sri Lankan laborers 14 to 46 years of age. *J Clin Periodontol* 13:431–445, 1986.)

interpretation of the difference between the two groups. This study suggests that without oral care, periodontal lesions progress continually and at a relatively even pace.

Further analysis of the Sri Lankan laborers showed not all were losing attachment at the same rate (Figs. 54.2 and 54.3).[20] Virtually all gingival areas showed inflammation, but attachment loss varied tremendously. Based on interproximal loss of attachment and tooth mortality, three subpopulations were identified as individuals with "rapid progression" (RP) of periodontal disease (8%), individuals with "moderate progression" (MP) (81%), and individuals who exhibited "no progression" (NP) of periodontal disease beyond gingivitis (11%). At age 35, the mean loss of attachment in the RP group was 9 mm; in the MP group, 4 mm; and in the NP group, less than 1 mm. At the age of 45, the mean loss of attachment in the RP group was 13 mm and in the MP group it was 7 mm. Therefore, under natural conditions and in

Mean Loss of Attachment at Various Ages (mm)

Age	Progression Group	
	Rapid	Moderate
35	9	4
45	13	7

Fig. 54.3 Loss of Attachment in Untreated Sri Lankan Laborers. (Data from Löe H, Anerud A, Boysen H, et al: Natural history of periodontal disease in man: rapid, moderate and no loss of attachment in Sri Lankan laborers 14–46 years of age. *J Clin Periodontol* 13:431–445, 1986.)

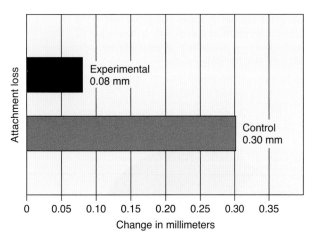

Fig. 54.4 Change in Mean Attachment Level From Baseline to Third-Year Examination for Experimental and Control Groups. (From Suomi JD, Greene JC, Vermillion JR, et al: The effect of controlled oral hygiene procedures on the progression of periodontal disease in adults: results after third and final year. *J Periodontol* 42:152–160, 1971.)

the absence of therapy, 89% of the Sri Lankan laborers had severe periodontitis that progressed at a much greater rate than that observed in the Norwegian group.

In the previously discussed study of General Telephone workers in California, loss of attachment was measured clinically and alveolar bone loss was measured radiographically.[36,37] After 3 years, the control group showed loss of attachment at a rate more than three times that of the matching experimental group during the same period (Fig. 54.4). In addition, subjects who received frequent oral prophylaxis and were instructed in good oral hygiene practices showed less bone loss radiographically after 3 years than did control subjects. It is clear that loss of attachment can be reduced by good oral hygiene and frequent dental prophylaxis.

Treatment of Loss of Attachment

A longitudinal study of patients with moderate-to-advanced periodontal disease conducted at the University of Michigan indicated that the progression of periodontal disease can be terminated for 3 years postoperatively regardless of the modality of treatment.[29–32] With long-term observations, the average loss of attachment was only 0.3 mm over 7 years.[30] These results indicated a more favorable prognosis for treatment of advanced periodontal lesions than previously assumed.

KEY FACT

Patient ability for regular, thorough biofilm removal with periodic maintenance therapy can predictably stop ongoing attachment loss.

Another study was conducted in 75 patients with advanced periodontal disease to determine the effect of biofilm control and surgical pocket elimination on the establishment and maintenance of periodontal health.[16] This study indicated that no further alveolar bone loss occurred during the 5-year observation period. The meticulous biofilm control practiced by the patients in this study was considered a major factor in the excellent results produced. After 14 years, results for 61 of the initial 75 individuals were reported.[14] Repeated examinations demonstrated that treatment of advanced forms of periodontal disease resulted in clinically healthy periodontal conditions and that this state of health was maintained in most patients and sites during the 14-year period. A more detailed analysis of the data, however, revealed that a small number of sites in a few patients lost a substantial amount of attachment. Approximately 43 surfaces in 15 different patients were exposed to recurrent periodontal disease of significant magnitude. The frequency of sites that lost more than 2 mm of attachment during the 14 years of maintenance was 0.8% to 0.1% per year.

Neither of these studies used a control group because failing to treat advanced periodontal patients cannot be justified for ethical reasons. However, in a study in a private practice, an effort was made to find and evaluate patients with diagnosed moderate-to-advanced periodontitis who had not followed through with recommended periodontal therapy.[3] Thirty patients ranging in age from 25 to 71 years were evaluated after periods ranging from 18 to 115 months. All of these untreated patients had progressive increases in pocket depth and radiographic evidence of progressive bone resorption.

In a study of the progression of periodontal disease in the absence of therapy, two different populations were monitored.[18] One group of 64 Swedish adults with mild-to-moderate periodontal disease and one group of 36 American adults with advanced destructive disease were monitored but not treated for 6 years and 1 year, respectively. During the course of 6 years, 11.6% of all sites in the Swedish population (1.9% per year) showed attachment loss of greater than 2 mm, and the corresponding figure for the American population was 3.2% per year. Thus the frequency of sites with disease progression was 20 to 30 times higher in untreated groups of patients than in the treated and well-maintained groups described in the preceding discussion.[18] Thus treatment is effective in reducing loss of attachment.

TOOTH MORTALITY

The ultimate test for the effectiveness of periodontal treatment is whether tooth loss can be prevented. Sufficient studies from both private practice and research institutions are now available to document that therapy reduces or prevents loss of teeth.

The combined effect of subgingival scaling every 3 to 6 months and controlled oral hygiene was evaluated over a 5-year period in 1428 factory workers in Oslo.[22] Tooth loss was significantly reduced in all patients. This study showed that frequent subgingival scaling reduces tooth loss even when oral hygiene is "not good" (Table 54.1).

The previously mentioned longitudinal study conducted at the University of Michigan included 104 patients with a total of 2604 teeth.[29–32] After 1 to 7 years of treatment, 53 teeth were lost for various reasons (Table 54.2). Approximately 32 teeth were lost during the first and second years after the initiation of treatment. The remaining 21 teeth were lost in a random pattern over the next 6 years. Therefore, the loss of teeth caused by advanced periodontal disease after treatment was minimal (1.15%).

Another study was undertaken to test the effect of periodontal therapy in cases of advanced disease.[16–17] The subjects were 75 patients who had lost 50% or more of their periodontal support (Fig. 54.5). Treatment consisted of oral hygiene measures, scaling procedures, extraction of untreatable teeth, periodontal surgery, and prosthetic therapy if indicated. After completion of periodontal treatment, none of the patients showed further loss of periodontal support for the next 5 years. None of the teeth were extracted in the 5-year posttreatment period. Patients in this study were selected because of their capacity to meet the high requirements of biofilm control after repeated instruction in oral hygiene techniques. This fact does not detract from the validity of the study but tends to indicate the etiologic importance of bacterial biofilm. The results indicate that periodontal surgery coupled with a detailed biofilm control program not only temporarily cures the disease but also reduces further progression of periodontal breakdown, even in patients with severely reduced periodontal support.

After 14 years, 61 of the original patients were still in the study.[17] Recurrence of destructive periodontal disease in isolated sites of the dentition resulted in loss of a certain number of teeth during the observation period (Fig. 54.6). In the 6 to 10 years after active therapy, one tooth in each of three different patients was lost, and during the final observation period (11 to 14 years), three teeth in one patient, two teeth in each of three patients, and one tooth in each of four patients had to be extracted because of recurrent periodontal disease. In addition, three teeth

TABLE 54.1 Average Loss of Teeth During a 5-Year Period Compared With Normal Loss of Teeth in 1428 Men and Women Ages 20 Through 59

	GRADE OF ORAL HYGIENE		
	Good	Fairly Good	Not Good
"Normal" loss of teeth[a]	1.1	1.4	1.8
Actual loss of teeth during 5-year period	0.4	0.6	0.9

[a]Estimate based on data recorded at initiation of study period.
From Lovdal A, Arno A, Schei O, et al: Combined effect of subgingival scaling and controlled oral hygiene on the incidence of gingivitis. *Acta Odontol Scand* 19:537–555, 1961.

TABLE 54.2 Tooth Mortality After Treatment of Advanced Periodontitis in 104 Patients With 2604 Teeth Treated Over a 10-Year Period

Teeth Lost[a]	Reason
2	Pulpal disease
3	Accidents
4	Prosthetic considerations
14	Various reasons; for example, one patient wanted a maxillary denture for cosmetic reasons
30	Periodontal
53	All reasons

[a]Two percent of the teeth were lost during the study period. Note that US health surveys conducted in the 1960s indicated that an average of 4.3 teeth were lost after age 35 in the general population.[9]
Data from Ramfjord SP, Knowles JW, Nissle RR, et al: Longitudinal study of periodontal therapy. *J Periodontol* 44:66–77, 1973.

Fig. 54.5 Radiographs Taken 5 Years After Typical Periodontal Treatment. Note the advanced bone loss, despite the teeth retained in a healthy condition for the duration of the study. (From Lindhe J, Nyman S: The effect of plaque control and surgical pocket elimination on the establishment and maintenance of periodontal health: a longitudinal study of periodontal therapy in cases of advanced disease. *J Clin Periodontol* 2:67–79, 1975.)

Cumulative Tooth Loss After 10–14 Years of Therapy in 61 Patients

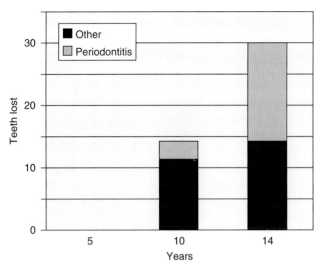

Fig. 54.6 Tooth Loss in Treated Patients With Very Advanced Periodontal Disease. (Data from Lindhe J, Nyman S: Long-term maintenance of patients treated for advanced periodontal disease. *J Clin Periodontol* 11:504–514, 1984.)

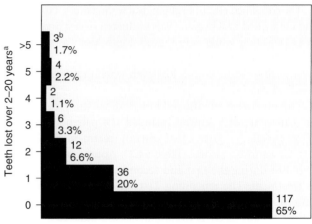

Number of patients (*n* = 180) with percentage of total

[a]Average of 8.6 years.
[b]3 patients lost 35 teeth.

The average tooth loss per patient was 0.9 per 10 years.

Fig. 54.7 Tooth Mortality. Average tooth loss per patient was 0.9 per 10 years. (Modified from Ross IF, Thompson RH, Galdi M: The results of treatment: a long term study of one hundred and eighty patients. *Parodontologie* 25:125–134, 1971.)

in each of three different patients and one tooth in each of five patients were extracted because of the development of extensive caries, periapical lesions, or other endodontic complications. Throughout the course of the study, the total loss was 30 teeth (for all reasons) from the total of 1330 teeth. Therefore, the tooth mortality rate was 2.3%.

University-based studies on the treatment of moderate to severe periodontitis continue to show minimal tooth loss in patients who are able to comply with periodontal maintenance therapy.[5,26]

Several studies in private practice have attempted to measure the frequency of tooth loss after periodontal therapy. In one study, 180 patients who had been treated for chronic destructive periodontal disease were evaluated.[33] The average age of the patients before treatment was 43.7 years. A total of 141 teeth were lost. From the beginning of treatment to the time of the survey, the majority of patients did not lose any teeth (Fig. 54.7). Three of 180 patients (1.7%) lost 35 teeth; approximately 25% of the teeth were lost. Twelve additional patients lost 46 teeth, or 32.6% of the teeth were lost. Many patients in the study had advanced alveolar bone loss, including extensive furcation involvements. However, only a relatively small number (141) of the teeth were lost in the study group of 180 patients between the beginning of periodontal treatment and the time of the study.

The teeth were lost for several reasons, including periodontal disease, caries, and other non-periodontal causes. The length of time after treatment varied from 2 to 20 years, with an average of 8.6 years. Of considerable significance is the large number of teeth (81 teeth, or 57.5%) lost by a few patients (15 patients, or 8.4%). Even when this group is considered with the remaining 165 patients, the periodontal care helped to retain most teeth because the average loss was slightly less than one tooth (0.9) over the 10 years after treatment.

Percentage of Patients (*n* = 211) With Teeth Lost Over 15–34 Years

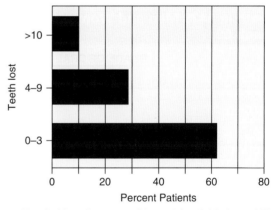

Fig. 54.8 Tooth Mortality 15–34 Years After Initiation of Therapy (Average of 22.2 Years). Average tooth loss per patient was 1.6 teeth per 10 years. Compare with the same study population in Fig. 73.7. As the treated population ages, the rate of bone loss appears to increase. (Modified from Goldman MJ, Ross IF, Goteiner D: Effect of periodontal therapy on patients maintained for 15 years or longer: a retrospective study. *J Periodontol* 57:347–353, 1986.)

In a follow-up study, the long-term results of periodontal therapy were evaluated after 15 to 34 years (average of 22.2 years).[7] The average tooth loss at this time was 1.6 teeth per 10 years. Patients were classified into three groups according to tooth loss. Approximately 62% had an average tooth loss of 0.45 per 10 years and were considered "well maintained"; 28% lost an average of 2.6 teeth per 10 years and were considered "downhill"; and 10% lost an average of 6.4 teeth per 10 years and were considered "extreme downhill" (Fig. 54.8).

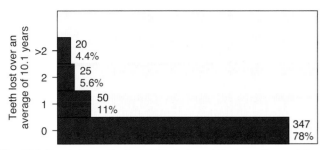

Fig. 54.9 Tooth Mortality in 442 Periodontal Patients Treated Over 10 Years. (Courtesy Dr. R.C. Oliver, Rio Verde, AZ.)

Fig. 54.10 Loss of Teeth With Advanced Periodontal Disease Over 10 Years. (Courtesy Dr. R.C. Oliver, Rio Verde, AZ.)

Another study included all patients in a practice who had been treated 5 or more years previously and had received regular preventive periodontal care since that time.[28] The 442 patients had an average of 10.1 years since treatment. Two-thirds of the patients were older than 40 years of age at the time of treatment. These patients had been seen every 4.6 months, on average, for their preventive periodontal care, which consisted of oral hygiene instruction and prophylaxis (Figs. 54.9 and 54.10).

The total tooth loss resulting from periodontal disease was 178 of more than 11,000 teeth available for treatment. More important, 78% of the patients did not lose a single tooth after periodontal therapy, and 11% lost only one tooth. Considering that more than 600 teeth had furcation involvements at the time of the original treatment and that far more than 1000 teeth had less than half the alveolar bone support remaining, there was minimal tooth loss. During the same average 10-year period after periodontal therapy, only 45 teeth were lost through caries or pulpal involvement. Even more surprising are the statistics over an average 10-year period for teeth with a poor prognosis. Only 85 (14%) of a total of 601 teeth with furcation involvement were lost, and 117 (11%) of 1039 teeth with half or less of the bone remaining were lost. Of the 1043 teeth listed as having a "guarded prognosis" by the clinician performing the initial examination, only 126 (12%) were lost over this 10-year period. The average tooth mortality rate was 0.72 tooth lost per patient per 10 years.

In a third study in a private practice, 600 patients were followed for 15 to 53 years after periodontal therapy (Figs. 54.11 and 54.12).[10] The majority (76.5%) had advanced periodontal disease at the start of treatment. There were 15,666 teeth present, for an average of 26 teeth per patient. During the follow-up period (an average of 22 years), a total of 1312 teeth were lost from all causes. Of this number, 1110 were lost for periodontal reasons. The average tooth mortality rate per patient was 2.2 teeth, and when this is converted to a 10-year rate, an average of one tooth was lost per 10 years in each patient. During this period of observation, 666 teeth with a questionable prognosis were lost out of a total of 2141. This means that 31% of the teeth with a questionable prognosis were lost over 22 years of treatment. A total of 1464 teeth with furcation involvement were treated, and 31.6% were lost during the period of study. Approximately 83% of the patients lost fewer than three teeth over the 22-year average treatment period and were classified as "well maintained." The remaining 17% of the patients were divided

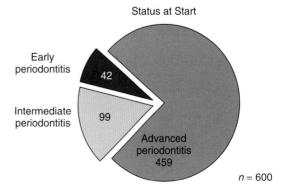

Fig. 54.11 Status at the Start of a Study of 600 Patients. (Data from Hirschfeld L, Wasserman B: A long-term survey of tooth loss in 600 treated periodontal patients. *J Periodontol* 49:225–237, 1978.)

into two groups: "downhill" (4 to 9 teeth lost) or "extreme downhill" (10 to 23 teeth lost). Thus 17% of the patients studied accounted for 69% of the teeth lost from periodontal causes. This study also indicated that relatively few teeth are lost after periodontal therapy. In addition, few teeth with a guarded prognosis, including those with furcation involvement, are lost, and a small percentage of patients lose most of the teeth.

Clinical studies have also indicated a relatively low rate of tooth loss in patients who are involved in a supportive periodontal maintenance program. One study showed that 0.9% of teeth

were lost over 7.8 years, whereas another showed 1.5% were lost over a 9.8-year period after the initiation of active periodontal treatment.[4,6] Another study showed that questionable teeth in patients with aggressive periodontitis can be maintained for longer than 15 years if the patient is compliant.[41]

A study at the University of Bern looked at the outcome of multirooted teeth treated for longer than 11.5 years.[42] The study found that grade 1 furcation status was not a risk factor for tooth loss compared with no furcation bone loss in patients treated for periodontal disease. Risk factors for the loss of multirooted teeth included furcation involvements grades 2 and 3, smoking, and lack of compliance with regular maintenance therapy (Fig. 54.13).

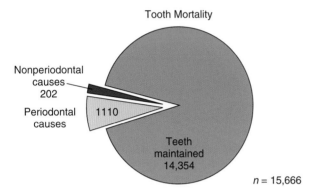

Tooth Mortality

Nonperiodontal causes 202

Periodontal causes 1110

Teeth maintained 14,354

$n = 15,666$

Fig. 54.12 Loss of Teeth in 600 Patients Over 15 to 53 Years From Nonperiodontal and Periodontal Causes. (Data from Hirschfeld L, Wasserman B: A long-term survey of tooth loss in 600 treated periodontal patients. *J Periodontol* 49:225–237, 1978.)

> ### KEY FACT
> Numerous studies indicate the possibility of maintaining teeth in patients with aggressive periodontitis if the patient can perform excellent biofilm removal along with regular supportive periodontal care.

Three studies give insight into tooth mortality in untreated patients. The studies of Löe and coworkers[20,21] in Sri Lankan laborers showed that after age 35, an average of 5 and 16 teeth were lost per 10 years in the "moderate progression" and "rapid progression" groups, respectively (Fig. 54.14). In a previously discussed study in private practice,[3] an effort was made to find

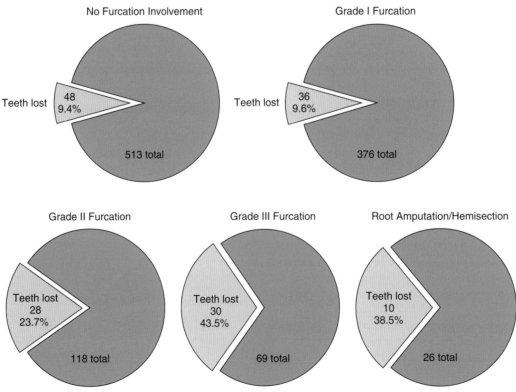

No Furcation Involvement

Teeth lost 48 9.4%

513 total

Grade I Furcation

Teeth lost 36 9.6%

376 total

Grade II Furcation

Teeth lost 28 23.7%

118 total

Grade III Furcation

Teeth lost 30 43.5%

69 total

Root Amputation/Hemisection

Teeth lost 10 38.5%

26 total

Fig. 54.13 Loss of Multirooted Teeth During 11.5 Years of Supportive Periodontal Therapy. (Data from Salvi GE, Mischler DC, Schmidlin K, et al: Risk factors associated with longevity of multi-rooted teeth: long-term outcomes after active supportive periodontal therapy. *J Clin Periodontol* 41:701–707, 2014.)

Tooth Loss in Sri Lankan Laborers

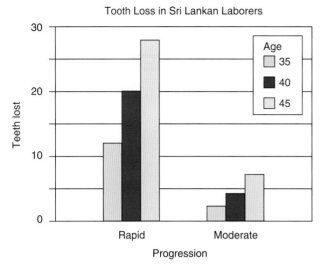

Fig. 54.14 Tooth Loss in a Population With Untreated Periodontal Disease. (Data from Löe H, Anerud A, Boysen H, et al: Natural history of periodontal disease in man: rapid, moderate and no loss of attachment in Sri Lankan laborers 14 to 46 years of age. *J Clin Periodontol* 13:431–445, 1986.)

TABLE 54.3 Tooth Mortality in Treated Periodontitis Patients

Study	Average Number of Teeth Lost Per 10 Years With Periodontal Treatment[a]
Hirschfeld and Wasserman[10]	1.0
Kocher et al.[12]	1.6
McFall[23]	1.4
Oliver[28]	0.7
Ross et al.[33]	0.9
Goldman et al.[7]	1.6
McLeod et al.[24]	1.5
Tsami et al.[39] (nonsmokers)	1.7
Tsami et al.[39] (smokers)	3.7
Ng et al.[26] (compliant with maintenance)	0.8
Ng et al.[26] (noncompliant with maintenance)	2.8
Costa et al.[40] (compliant with maintenance)	1.2
Costa et al.[40] (noncompliant with maintenance)	3.6
Graetz et al.[41] (aggressive periodontitis)	1.4
Graetz et al.[41] (chronic periodontitis)	1.6

[a]Tooth mortality adjusted to 10 years by chapter author.

TABLE 54.4 Tooth Mortality in Untreated Periodontitis Patients

Study	Average Number of Teeth Lost Per 10 Years Without Periodontal Treatment[a]
Becker et al.[3]	6
Kocher et al.[12]	5
Löe et al.[20] (moderate progression)	5
Löe et al.[20] (rapid progression)	16

[a]Tooth mortality adjusted to 10 years by chapter author.

and evaluate patients with diagnosed moderate-to-advanced periodontitis who did not follow through with recommended periodontal therapy. Patients with untreated periodontal disease were losing teeth at a rate greater than 0.61 per year (6.1 teeth per 10 years). A total of 83 teeth were lost in 30 patients, but the investigators excluded 1 patient who had lost 25 teeth. Including this patient would have increased the tooth loss in untreated patients to an even higher rate. In another study, reporting on patients with moderate-to-advanced periodontitis examined at the Department of Periodontology at the University of Kiel in Germany, Kocher and associates[12] found a marked increase in tooth loss in the untreated patients compared with the treated patients when they were examined after 7 years.

When Tables 54.3 and 54.4 are compared, it is obvious that tooth mortality is much greater in untreated groups.

CONCLUSION

The prevalence of periodontal disease and the resulting high rate of tooth mortality have increased the need for effective treatment. Strong evidence now indicates that periodontal disease can contribute to numerous health problems, including pregnancy complications, heart disease, stroke, and diabetes.[25,27,34,35] For patients with periodontitis, treatment effectively prevents periodontal disease and stops the progression of the disease. In addition, overwhelming evidence suggests that periodontal therapy greatly reduces tooth mortality. Every dental practitioner should

be familiar with the philosophy, recognition, and techniques for periodontal therapy. Failure to diagnose and treat periodontal disease or not make periodontal treatment available to patients causes unnecessary dental problems and tooth loss and places the patient at risk for other systemic health problems.

A Case Scenario is found on the companion website.

REFERENCES

 References for this chapter are found on the companion website.

PART 4

Oral Implantology

Peri-Implant Anatomy, Biology, and Function[a]

 For online-only content on endosseous implants, root form (cylindric) implants, transmandibular implants, subperiosteal implants, and implant surface characteristics (microdesign), go to the companion website.

CHAPTER OUTLINE

The history of modern implant dentistry began with the introduction of titanium implants.[41] In the 1950s, Per-Ingvar Brånemark, a Swedish professor of anatomy, had a serendipitous finding while studying blood circulation in bone that became a historical breakthrough in medicine. He discovered an intimate bone-to-implant apposition with titanium that offered sufficient strength to cope with load transfer. He called the phenomenon *osseointegration* and developed an implant system with a specific protocol to predictably achieve it. The implants were used to anchor prosthetic replacement teeth in the edentulous jaw,[27] and the first patient was successfully treated in 1965.[30,71] Subsequent clinical studies proved that commercially pure (CP) titanium implants, placed with a strict protocol, including an unloaded healing period, could predictably achieve osseointegration and retain a full-arch prosthesis in function with long-term success (15 years).[8]

Currently, implant designs, surgical placement techniques, healing times, and restorative protocols continue to evolve with the goal of improving outcomes. It is important for clinicians to know peri-implant anatomy, to understand the biology, and to appreciate the functional capacity of osseointegrated implants. This chapter reviews implant geometry and surface characteristics, as well as the anatomic and biologic relationships of peri-implant tissues.

IMPLANT GEOMETRY (MACRODESIGN)

Numerous implant systems with various geometric (macrodesign) designs have been developed and used before the current implant systems currently in use. Previous implant designs included blade vents (narrow, flat shape; tapped into bony trough prepared with rotary burs),[69] press-fit cylindric (bullet shape; pressed or tapped into prepared hole),[99] subperiosteal (custom-made framework; adapted to the surface of jawbone),[37] and transmandibular (long rods or posts; placed through the anterior mandible).[103] Some of these implant systems were initially stable and appeared to be successful over short-term periods (e.g., 5 years) but failed to remain stable, became symptomatic or loose, and failed over longer periods.[97,120] Lacking predictability, these implant systems are no longer used.

Since the time of the Brånemark studies, millions of patients have been treated worldwide using variations of these techniques with implants of different geometries and surface characteristics. Similar research including that of André Schroeder in Switzerland in the mid-1970s contributed to the success of endosseous dental implants. The serendipitous finding of Brånemark was that when a hole is prepared into bone without overheating or otherwise traumatizing the tissues, an inserted biocompatible implantable device would predictably achieve an intimate bone apposition, as long as micromovements at the interface were prevented during the early healing period. The history of the research endeavors in Sweden provides a better understanding of the relevant biologic parameters involved.[71]

The macroscopic configuration of implants has varied widely; the most common types are listed in Box 55.1. Currently, most endosseous implants have a cylindric or tapered, screw-shaped/

[a]Adapted from the following chapter of Newman and Carranza's Clinical Periodontology, 13th edition: Chapter 74: Peri-implant Anatomy, Biology, and Function, by Joseph Fiorellini, Keisuke Wada, Hector Leonardo Sarmiento, and Perry R. Klokkevold.

threaded design. The disastrous results with other implant configurations were largely responsible for the evolution toward the current popular designs.[13] Detailed description of the various implant designs including blades, pins, discs, root form, transmandibular, and subperiosteal implants is found on the companion Expert Consult website.

HARD-TISSUE INTERFACE

The primary goal of implant installation is to achieve and maintain a stable bone-to-implant connection (i.e., osseointegration).[29,30] Histologically, osseointegration is defined as the direct structural and functional connection between ordered, living bone and the surface of a load-bearing implant without intervening soft tissues (Fig. 55.1).[27,28] Clinically, osseointegration is the asymptomatic rigid fixation of an alloplastic material (implant) in bone with the ability to withstand occlusal forces.[12,122] The hard-tissue interface is a fundamental requirement for and an essential component of implant success.

Initial Bone Healing

The osseointegration process observed after implant insertion can be compared with bone fracture healing. Implant site osteotomy preparation (bone wounding) initiates a sequence of events, including an inflammatory reaction, bone resorption, release of growth factors, and attraction by chemotaxis of osteoprogenitor cells to the site. Differentiation of osteoprogenitor cells into osteoblasts leads to bone formation at the implant surface. Extracellular matrix proteins, such as osteocalcin, modulate apatite crystal growth.[119] Specific conditions, optimal for bone formation, must be maintained at the healing site to achieve osseointegration.

Immobility of the implant relative to the bone must be maintained for bone formation at the surface. A mild inflammatory response enhances the bone healing, but moderate inflammation or movement greater than a certain threshold is detrimental.[6] When micromovements at the interface exceed 150 μm, the movement will impair differentiation of osteoblasts and fibrous

---

> **BOX 55.1**   **Implant Geometry (Macrodesign)**
>
> 1. Endosseous implants
>   - Bladelike
>   - Pins
>   - Root form, cylindric (hollow and full)
>   - Disclike
>   - Screw shaped
>   - Tapered and screw shaped
> 2. Subperiosteal (custom frame) implants
> 3. Transmandibular implants

Fig. 55.1 (A) Three-dimensional diagram of the tissue and titanium interrelationship showing an overall view of the intact interfacial zone around the osseointegrated implant. (B) Physiologic evolution of the biology of the interface over time.

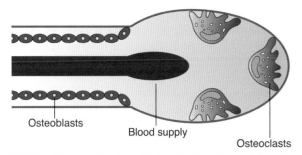

Fig. 55.2 The Basic Multicellular Unit Is the Basic Remodeling Process for Bone Renewal. Osteoclasts are imported by the vascular supply, and the resorption lacunae are soon filled by the lining osteoblasts.

Fig. 55.3 (A) After initial healing, woven bone, as characterized by its irregular pattern, is laid down. (B) After weeks or months, progressively a lamellar bone is laid down, with regular concentric lamellae. *B,* Bone; *I,* implant. (Courtesy Professor T. Albrektsson, Gothenburg, Sweden.)

Fig. 55.4 Once a Steady State Has Been Achieved at the Bone-To-Implant Interface, an Intimate Contact Can Be Observed, With Some Marrow Spaces Seen in Between at the Light Microscopic Level.

scar tissue will form between the bone and implant surface.[89] Therefore it is important to avoid excessive forces, such as occlusal loading, during the early healing period.

Bone tissue damage and debris created by the osteotomy site preparation must be cleared up by osteoclasts for normal bone healing. These multinuclear cells, originating from the blood, can resorb bone at a pace of 50 to 100 μm/day. There is a coupling between bone apposition and bone resorption (Fig. 55.2). Preosteoblasts, derived from primary mesenchymal cells, depend on a favorable oxidation-reduction (redox) potential of the environment. Thus a proper vascular supply and oxygen tension are needed. If oxygen tension is poor, the primary stem cells may differentiate into fibroblasts, form scar tissue, and lead to implant failure (nonintegration).

If bone is overheated or crushed during preparation, it will become necrotic and may lead to nonmineralized (soft tissue) scar formation or be sequestered. The critical temperature for bone cells that should not be exceeded is 47°C (116.6°F) at an exposure time of 1 minute.[6] Thus preparation of implant osteotomy sites requires profuse irrigation (cooling) along with gentle, intermittent, moderate-speed drilling using sharp drills. Another complicating factor, well recognized from open wound fractures, is that microbial contamination jeopardizes the normal bone healing. Accordingly, strict aseptic techniques should be maintained.

> ### KEY FACT
> If micromovements exceed 150 μm, the movement will impair the differentiation of osteoblasts, and fibrous scar tissue will form between the bone and implant surface.

New bone formation follows a specific sequence of events. Woven bone is quickly formed in the gap between the implant and the bone; it grows fast, up to 100 μm/day, and in all directions. Characterized by a random orientation of its collagen fibrils, high cellularity, and limited degree of mineralization, the biomechanical capacity of woven bone is poor (Fig. 55.3A). Thus any occlusal load should be well controlled or avoided in the early phase of healing. After several months, woven bone is progressively replaced by lamellar bone with organized, parallel layers of collagen fibrils and dense mineralization. Contrary to the

fast-growing woven bone, lamellar bone formation occurs at a slow pace (only a few microns per day). Ultimately, after 18 months of healing, a steady state is reached where lamellar bone is continuously resorbed and replaced (see Fig. 55.3B).[27] At the light microscopic level, an intimate bone-to-implant contact has been extensively reported (Fig. 55.4).[95] Once the bone-to-implant interface has reached a steady state, it can maintain itself over decades, as ascertained by human histology from implants retrieved because of hardware fractures.[10]

> ### FLASH BACK
> The biomechanical capacity of woven bone is poor. New bone formation adjacent to an implant follows a specific sequence of events with woven bone forming quickly in the gap; it grows fast (100 μm/day) and in all directions. It is characterized by a random orientation of its collagen fibrils, high cellularity, and a limited degree of mineralization.

Bone Remodeling and Function

Clinically, both primary stability and secondary stability of an implant are critical to success. Primary stability, achieved at the time of surgical placement, depends on the implant geometry (macrodesign), as well as the quality and quantity of bone available for implant anchorage at a specific site. Studies using resonance frequency analysis (RFA) have reported decreased implant stability in the early weeks of postinsertion healing.[18,44,56,90] Secondary stability, achieved over time with healing, depends on the implant surface (microdesign), as well as the quality and quantity of adjacent bone, which will determine the percentage of contacts between the implant and bone.[18,48,93,109] For example, areas such as the anterior mandible have dense cortical bone and provide rigid primary stabilization and good support throughout the healing process. Conversely, areas such as the posterior maxilla have thin cortical bone, and large marrow spaces provide less primary stability. For this reason, the posterior maxilla has been associated with lower success rates compared with other sites with greater bone density and support.[17,60] Interestingly, a new implant with unique knife-edge-wide threads (macrodesign) has been shown, in completely healed sites, to maintain stability without the typical drop in the implant stability quotient (ISQ) through the early bone remodeling phase.[72]

Once osseointegration is achieved, implants can resist and function under the forces of occlusion for many years. Longitudinal biomechanical assessments seem to indicate that during the first weeks after placement of one-stage implants, decreased rigidity is observed.[46] This may be indicative of bone resorption during the initial phase of healing. Subsequently, rigidity increases and continues to increase for years.[108] Thus when a prosthesis is installed immediately (in 1 day) or early (in 1 to 2 weeks), care must be taken to control against overload. It is important to recognize that sites with limited primary stability or less bone-to-implant contact (e.g., posterior maxilla) will likely go through a period of even less bone support in the early stages of bone healing due to the initial phase of bone resorption.

SOFT-TISSUE INTERFACE

Not surprisingly, for two decades, research and clinical interest focused on the bone-to-implant interface of osseointegrated implants, and the overlying soft tissues were largely ignored. Except for a few descriptive sentences, the classic handbook by Brånemark and colleagues[27] presented no data or information about the soft-tissue interface. This may be due in part to the fact that most patients were fully edentulous and the Brånemark system implants had turned (machined) surfaces, which are less likely to be associated with soft-tissue inflammatory problems.[5] Currently, there is greater interest in and appreciation for peri-implant soft tissues and the soft tissue–to-implant interface as a function of aesthetics and maintenance of a seal or barrier against microbial invasion.

Peri-implant soft tissues are similar in appearance and structure to periodontal soft tissues (see Chapter 4).[5] Clearly, both implants and teeth emerge through the soft tissues on the alveolar ridge. The soft tissues consist of connective tissue covered by epithelium. There is a gingival/mucosal sulcus, a long junctional epithelial attachment, and a zone of connective tissue above the supporting bone (Fig. 55.5). Despite the apparent similarities in soft tissues around teeth and implants, the presence of a periodontal ligament around teeth and not around implants is an important, distinct difference. Natural teeth have a periodontal ligament with connective tissue fibers inserting into the cementum and suspending them in the alveolar bone, whereas osseointegrated implants do not. There are no inserting collagen fibers anywhere along the interface of osseointegrated implants. Bone is in direct contact with the implant surface without intervening soft tissues.

> ### FLASH BACK
>
> Sharpey fibers are bundles of collagenous fibers in the periodontal ligament that pass into the outer circumferential lamellae of alveolar bone and the cementum of teeth.

Clinically, the thickness of the peri-implant soft tissues varies from 2 mm to several millimeters (Fig. 55.6). An animal study determined the total height of the peri-implant "biologic width" to be approximately 3 to 4 mm, where approximately 2 mm is the epithelial attachment and approximately 1 to 2 mm is the supracrestal connective tissue zone.[19] Consistent with this finding, a human histologic study determined the height of the peri-implant "biologic width," consisting of an epithelial attachment and supracrestal connective tissue, to be approximately 4 to 4.5 mm (Fig. 55.7).[47]

Epithelium

As in the natural dentition, the oral epithelium around implants is continuous with a sulcular epithelium that lines the inner surface of the gingival sulcus; the apical part of the gingival sulcus is lined with long junctional epithelium.[70] Ultrastructural examination of the long junctional epithelial attachment adjacent to dental implants has demonstrated that epithelial cells attach with a basal lamina and hemidesmosomes (Fig. 55.8).[2,4,49,62,111] Histologic studies indicate that these epithelial structures and the surrounding lamina propria cannot be distinguished from those structures around teeth.[33] In health, the dimension of the sulcular epithelium is approximately 0.5 mm,[92] and the dimension of the epithelial attachment is approximately 2 mm,[19] which is higher than that of the periodontal epithelial attachment.

The apical edge of the epithelial attachment is approximately 1.5 to 2 mm above the bone margin.[87] In healthy peri-implant tissues, progressive epithelial downgrowth does not occur, indicating that factors other than inserted collagen fiber bundles (i.e., Sharpey fibers in natural dentition) prevent it.

Connective Tissue

Peri-implant connective tissue morphology closely resembles that of the natural dentition except that it lacks a periodontal ligament, cementum, and inserting fibers (Fig. 55.9). No significant differences were found at the biochemical level between the peri-implant and the periodontal soft tissues,[34] whereas the dimension of the peri-implant connective tissue is 1 to 2 mm,

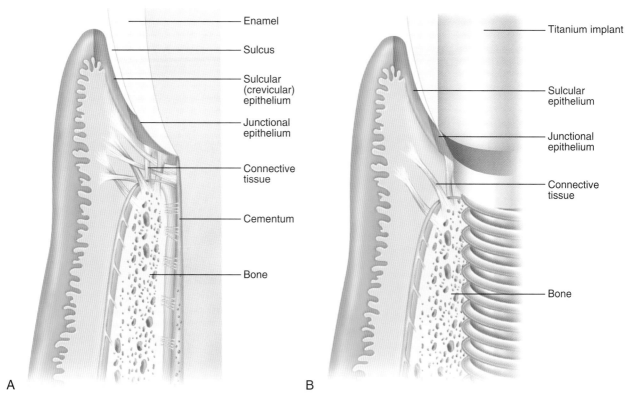

Fig. 55.5 Schematic Illustration of Hard and Soft Tissue Around a Tooth and an Implant. (A) Hard- and soft-tissue anatomy around a natural tooth demonstrates bone support with a periodontal ligament, a connective tissue zone above the crest of bone with connective tissue fibers (Sharpey) inserting into dentin, a long junctional epithelial attachment, a gingival sulcus lined with sulcular epithelium, and oral gingival epithelium (outer surface of gingiva). (B) Hard- and soft-tissue anatomy around an implant demonstrates some similarities and some distinct differences. There is supporting bone in direct approximation to the implant surface without any intervening soft tissues (i.e., no periodontal ligament). A connective tissue zone is present above the level of bone with fibers running parallel to the implant surface and no inserting fibers. There is a long junctional epithelial attachment, a gingival/mucosal sulcus lined with sulcular epithelium, and oral gingival/mucosal epithelium (outer surface of soft tissue). (From Rose LF, Mealey BL: *Periodontics: medicine, surgery, and implants,* St. Louis, 2004, Mosby.)

Fig. 55.6 Clinical Appearance of Normal, Healthy Peri-Implant Tissue With Implant Restoration Removed. Soft-tissue thickness varies from site to site, depending on quantity and quality of tissue, as well as the anatomy of the surrounding area (e.g., adjacent to natural teeth with healthy periodontal attachment versus adjacent to a space). Note that the intrasulcular tissue appears more erythematous as the result of the thin, nonkeratinized layer of epithelium overlying the connective tissue.

which is higher than that of the average periodontal connective tissue.[19,87]

The zone of supracrestal connective tissue has an important function in the maintenance of a stable soft tissue–implant interface and as a seal or barrier to the "outside" oral environment. The orientation of connective tissue fibers adjacent to an implant differs from that of periodontal connective tissue fibers. In the absence of cementum and inserting connective tissue fibers (i.e., as in a natural tooth), most peri-implant connective tissue fibers run in a direction more or less parallel to the implant surface. Even when the fiber bundles are oriented perpendicularly, which occurs more often in the gingiva than in the mucosa surrounding implants, the bundles are never embedded in the implant surface.

FLASH BACK

In the absence of cementum and inserting connective tissue fibers (i.e., as in a natural tooth), most peri-implant connective tissue fibers run in a direction more or less parallel to the implant surface.

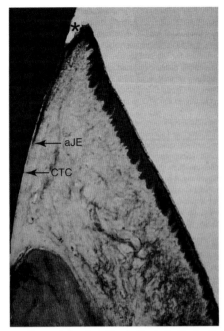

Fig. 55.7 Buccolingual Section (Basic Fuchsin Stain; Original Magnification, ×12.5; One-Part Sandblasted and Acid-Etched (SLA) Implant, 3 Months Unloaded) Showing the Gingiva and the Most Coronal Part of Alveolar Bone. Rete peg formation is only apparent in the area of the keratinized oral gingival epithelium. The oral sulcular epithelium exhibits no keratinization. In the area of the most coronal point of the junctional epithelium, the soft tissues are slightly torn away (artifact) because of nondecalcified histologic processing. The most apical point of the junctional epithelium is indicated (aJE). No rete peg formation is evident adjacent to the basal cell layer of the junctional epithelium, all showing healthy and physiologic soft-tissue structures. In addition, the area of connective tissue contact (CTC) adjacent to the machined titanium surface is marked. A slight round cell infiltrate in the connective tissue indicates a mild inflammation. Note bone remodeling/new bone formation in the crestal bone region indicated by saturated, dark red stained areas*, Sulcus.

Fig. 55.8 (A) Overview of ground section showing peri-implant tissues covered with keratinizing oral epithelium (OE). Junctional epithelium (JE) is interposed between connective tissue and alveolar bone crest (BC). Apical end of junctional epithelium (arrow). Toluidine blue stain. (Bar = 200 μm.) (B) Transmission electron microscopic view of sulcular epithelium showing tightly sealed intercellular spaces by numerous spot desmosomes (arrows), contributing to low permeability of this portion of peri-implant mucosa. Bar = 3 μm.[14]

Fig. 55.9 (A) Scanning electron microscope image of the junctional epithelium. Note the neutrophils located between the cells (red arrows). Bar = 40 μm. (B) Higher magnification of Fig. 55.8 with polarized light showing the apical extent (red arrow) of the junctional epithelium (JE). Note the dense collagen fibers running apicocoronal (i.e., parallel to the implant surface).

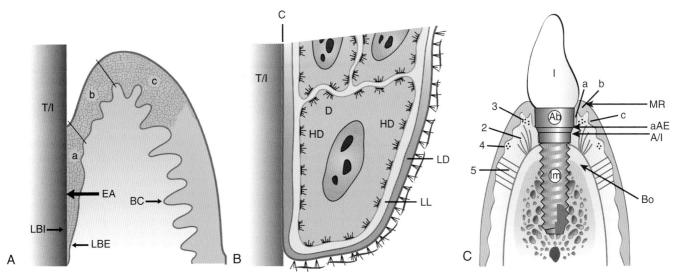

Fig. 55.10 (A) Histologic scheme of epithelial attachment *(EA)* (identical for tooth and implant). *BC,* Basal complex; *LBE,* lamina basalis externa (only location where cell divisions occur); *LBI,* lamina basalis interna; *T/I,* Titanium implant; *a,* long junctional epithelial attachment zone; *b,* sulcular epithelial zone; *c,* oral epithelial zone. (B) At the electron microscopic level, basal complex at the epithelial attachment (three most apical cells) and connection with stroma. *C,* Cuticle; *D,* desmosome; *HD,* hemidesmosomes; *LD,* lamina densa; *LL,* lamina lucida. (C) Implant, abutment *(Ab),* and crown within alveolar bone and soft tissues. *Bo,* Marginal bone level; *Im,* endosseous part of implant; *MR,* margin of gingiva/alveolar mucosa; *1,* implant crown; *2,* vertical alveolar-gingival connective tissue fibers; *3,* circular gingival connective tissue fibers; *4,* circular gingival connective tissue fibers; *5,* periosteal-gingival connective tissue fibers; *a,* junctional epithelium; *b,* sulcular epithelium; *c,* oral epithelium; *A/I,* abutment/implant junction; *aAE,* apical (point) of attached epithelium.

The fiber bundles can also have a cufflike circular orientation.[20,90] The role of these fibers remains unknown, but it appears that their presence helps to create a soft-tissue "seal" around the implant. The adaptation of the connective tissue to an implant surface may also be affected by the mobility of the soft tissue around the implant. The connective tissue in direct contact with the implant surface is characterized by an absence of blood vessels and an abundance of fibroblasts interposed between collagen fibers.[68] Several animal and human studies have shown that the alignments of connective fibers were circular and horizontal around the implants (Fig. 55.10).[b]

More recent studies have shown histologic evidence of connective tissue attachment perpendicular to the microgrooved implant surface on both animal and human studies.[77-79] These laser-microtextured grooves (Fig. 55.11) have been shown to be able to stop the epithelial downgrowth and establish connective tissue insertion right at the most coronal part of the laser microgrooved area. (Fig. 55.12). A prospective controlled clinical study showed that laser-grooved surface resulted in shallower probing depth and less peri-implant crestal bone loss than that seen around implants with machined collars.[25,84]

This connective tissue interface has been examined by probing attachment level measurements in patients. Probing attachment levels were consistently found coronal to the alveolar crest in patients with peri-implant tissue health, indicating the presence

Fig. 55.11 (A) Laser-microtextured surface. (B) Machined collar, original magnification, ×500. (Botos S, Yousef H, Zweig B, et al: The effects of laser microtexturing of the dental implant collar on crestal bone levels and peri-implant health. *Int J Oral Maxillofac Implants* 26:492–498, 2011. With the permission of Dr. Spyros Botos.)

of a zone of direct connective tissue contact to the implant surface. This means that the probing depth measurement performed with a periodontal probe may be approximately 1.5 mm higher above the bone level in healthy tissues. At inflamed sites, the probe may penetrate to the bone, with the probing depth measurement reflecting the total soft-tissue thickness above bone. In cases with inflammatory peri-implant tissue disease, increasing probing depth and reduced attachment levels have been reported.[3,40,85,113]

Keratinized Tissue

Questions emerged decades ago, as it did for the natural dentition, about the need for keratinized tissue to surround implants. Prospective and cross-sectional studies, evaluating screw-shaped implants with a machined surface, suggest that the presence or absence of keratinized gingiva is not a prerequisite for long-term stability.[98] However, it has been suggested that implants surrounded by mucosa only (i.e., nonkeratinized) are more susceptible to peri-implant problems. An animal study observed that ligature-induced peri-implantitis occurs more frequently when alveolar mucosa surrounds the implant as compared with when keratinized mucosa surrounds the implant.[112]

Keratinized mucosa tends to be more firmly anchored by collagen fibers to the underlying periosteum than nonkeratinized mucosa, which has more elastic fibers and tends to be movable relative to the underlying bone. In clinical studies evaluating

intraoral implants, with or without peri-implant keratinized mucosa, no clinically significant difference in implant success was reported.[66,117] However, when there is a lack of keratinized tissue, patients tend to complain about pain and discomfort while performing oral hygiene procedures or other functions in the area. The symptoms are alleviated by increasing the amount of keratinized (firmly bound) tissue around the implant(s) via soft-tissue grafting.[9,66,117] Finally, although it may not be comparable with intraoral implants, mobility of soft tissues surrounding extraoral implants is associated with a higher incidence of implant failure.[9]

Vascular Supply and Inflammation

The vascular supply of the peri-implant gingival or alveolar mucosa may be limited, as compared with periodontal gingiva, due to the lack of a periodontal ligament (Fig. 55.13).[21] This is especially true in the tissue immediately adjacent to the implant surface. However, capillary loops in the connective tissue under the junctional and sulcular epithelium around implants appear to be anatomically similar to those found in the normal periodontium (Fig. 55.14).[110]

Emerging knowledge indicates that the peri-implant gingival or alveolar mucosa has the same morphology as the corresponding tissues around teeth. These soft tissues also react the same way to plaque accumulation. Studies investigating the histology

Fig. 55.12 Laser-Ablated Surface: Epithelial Downgrowth Was Stopped Right at the Coronal-Most Microgrooved Area *(arrow).* Apical to the junctional epithelium, healthy connective tissue fibers attached perpendicularly to the laser-ablated channels. (Courtesy Dr. Myron Nevins.)

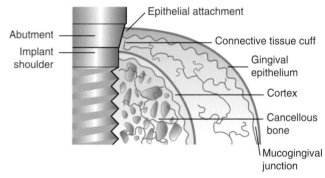

Fig. 55.13 Schematic Illustration of the Blood Supply in the Connective Tissue Cuff Surrounding the Implant/Abutment, Which Is Scarcer Than in the Gingival Complex Around Teeth Because None Originates From a Periodontal Ligament.

Fig. 55.14 (A) Microvascular topography surrounding a tooth. (B) Microvascular topography surrounding an implant. Bar = 5 μm.[101] (Courtesy Drs. N. Selliseth and K. Selvig, Bergen, Norway.)

Fig. 55.15 (A) Histologic slide from healthy gingiva surrounding a well-functioning implant in a human patient. No morphologic characteristics differentiate tissue around implant from that around teeth. (B) When gingivitis occurs, a profuse migration of inflammatory cells through the pocket epithelium can be observed. (Courtesy Professor Mariano Sanz, Madrid, Spain.)

(light microscopic and ultrastructural) of healthy and inflamed tissues surrounding implants in humans have indicated that the inflammatory response to plaque is similar to that observed in periodontal tissues.[92] Polymorphonuclear cells and mononuclear cells transmigrate normally through the peri-implant sulcular epithelium (Fig. 55.15).[92]

CLINICAL COMPARISON OF TEETH AND IMPLANTS

Although the soft tissue–to-implant (abutment) interface offers striking similarities with tissue surrounding the natural dentition, some differences should be considered. At the bone level, the lack of a periodontal ligament is the most striking difference. The following discussion elaborates on the clinical perspectives of these similarities and differences.

At the bone level, the absence of the periodontal ligament surrounding an implant has important clinical consequences. This means that no resilient connection exists between implants and supporting bone. Implants cannot intrude or migrate to compensate for the presence of a premature occlusal contact (as teeth can). Implants and the rigidly attached implant restorations do not move. Thus any occlusal disharmony will have repercussions at either the restoration-to-implant connection, the bone-to-implant interface, or both.

Proprioception in the natural dentition comes from the periodontal ligament. The absence of a periodontal ligament around implants reduces tactile sensitivity[58] and reflex function.[23] This can become even more challenging when osseointegrated, implant-supported, fixed prostheses are present in both jaws.

The lack of a periodontal ligament and the inability of implants to move contraindicates their use in growing individuals. Natural teeth continue to erupt and migrate during growth, whereas implants do not. Implants placed in individuals prior to the completion of growth can lead to occlusal disharmonies with implants.[82] Likewise, it may be problematic to place one or more implants in a location adjacent to teeth that are very mobile from the loss of periodontal support because, as the teeth move in response to or away from the occlusal forces, the implant(s) will bear the entire load.

Overload, because of improper superstructure design, parafunctional habits, or excessive occlusal load, may cause microstrains and microfractures in the bone, which will lead to bone loss and a fibrous inflammatory tissue at the implant interface.[110]

CONCLUSION

A thorough understanding of bone biology is essential for clinicians to fully appreciate the phenomenon and limitations of osseointegration. Many factors can interfere with the predictable establishment and maintenance of a long-term rigid connection between the implant surface and the surrounding bone that is able to sustain occlusal loads. The bone-to-implant interface and its rigidity are a predominant biomechanical aspect of coping with the time and intensity of loading. The quality of the soft tissue-to-implant interface also plays an important role in the long-term maintenance of stable marginal bone levels around implants. Clinicians must familiarize themselves with the underlying molecular and cellular events to evaluate the future evolution of implant design and implant protocols, including surgical placement, restoration, and maintenance.

A Case Scenario is found on the companion website www.expertconsult.com.

REFERENCES

References for this chapter are found on the companion website *www.expertconsult.com.*

56

Clinical Evaluation and Imaging of the Implant Patient[a]

Over the past several decades, following the landmark research and development of osseointegrated dental implants by Bråne-mark and colleagues,[17–19] treatment options and treatment planning in dentistry have evolved tremendously. Initially, prosthetic reconstructions with osseointegrated implants were limited to use in the edentulous patient, with many reports documenting excellent long-term success.[1,2,29]

Shortly thereafter, the original implant treatment protocols were adapted for use in partially edentulous patients. There were some transitional challenges associated with the early use of dental implants being adapted to the partially edentulous patient, but ultimately successes were achieved for this population as well. Modifications in implant design, procedural techniques, and treatment planning greatly improved implant therapy for the partially edentulous patient. Currently, the long-term success of dental implants used to replace single and multiple missing teeth in the partially edentulous patient is very good.[33,47,49,60,67] The implementation of bone augmentation procedures further increased the option for patients with inadequate bone volume to be successfully restored with implant-retained prostheses.[31,38,71] Virtually any patient with an edentulous space could be a candidate for endosseous implants, and studies suggest that success rates of 90% to 95% can be expected in healthy patients with good bone and normal healing capacity.[28]

The ultimate goal of dental implant therapy is to satisfy the patient's desire to replace one or more missing teeth in an aesthetic, secure, functional, and long-lasting manner. To achieve this goal, clinicians must accurately diagnose the dentoalveolar condition, as well as the overall mental and physical well-being of the patient. It is necessary to determine whether implant therapy is possible, practical, and, perhaps most important, whether it is indicated for the particular patient who is seeking implants. Local evaluation of potential jaw sites for implant placement (e.g., measuring available alveolar bone height, width, and spatial relationship) and prosthetic restorability are essential considerations in determining whether an implant(s) is possible. However, making as assessment of the patient and determining whether that patient is a good candidate for implants is an equally important part of the evaluation process. The patient evaluation includes identifying factors that might increase the risk of failure or the possibility of complications, as well as determining whether the patient's expectations are reasonable.

This chapter presents an overview of the clinical aspects of dental implant therapy, including an assessment of possible risk factors and contraindications. It also provides guidelines for the pretreatment evaluation of potential implant patients and the posttreatment evaluation of patients with implants.

CASE TYPES AND INDICATIONS

Edentulous Patients

The patients who seem to benefit most from dental implants are those with fully edentulous arches. These patients can be effectively restored, both aesthetically and functionally, with an implant-assisted removable prosthesis, an implant-supported removable prosthesis, or an implant-supported fixed prosthesis.

The original design for the edentulous arch was a fixed-bone–anchored bridge that used five to six implants in the anterior area of the mandible or the maxilla to support a fixed, hybrid prosthesis. The design is a denture-like complete arch of teeth attached to a substructure (metal framework), which in turn is attached to the implants with cylindrical titanium abutments (Fig. 56.1). The prosthesis is fabricated without flange extensions and does not rely on any soft-tissue support. It is entirely implant supported. Usually, the prosthesis includes bilateral

[a]Adapted from the following chapters of Newman and Carranza's Clinical Periodontology, 13th edition: Chapter 75: Clinical Evaluation of the Implant Patient, by Perry R. Klokkevold and David L. Cochran, and Chapter 76: Diagnostic Imaging for the Implant Patient, by Sotirios Tetradis, Sanjay M. Mallya, and Perry R. Klokkevold.

Fig. 56.1 Clinical Photograph of Patient With a Complete Maxillary Denture Opposing a Full-Arch Implant-Supported Fixed Prosthesis in the Mandibular Arch.

Fig. 56.2 (A) Clinical photograph of acrylic provisional fixed full-arch prosthesis in the maxilla. (B) Clinical photograph of the final ceramometal restoration, anterior view. (C) Occlusal view of final restoration on master cast. (Courtesy Dr. Russell Nishimura, Westlake Village, CA.)

distal cantilevers, which extend to replace posterior teeth (back to premolars or first molars).

Another implant-supported design used to restore an edentulous arch is the ceramic-metal fixed bridge (Fig. 56.2). Some patients prefer this design because the ceramic restoration emerges directly from the gingival tissues in a manner that makes its appearance similar to that of natural teeth.

One limitation of both hybrid and ceramometal implant-supported fixed prostheses is that they provide very little lip support and thus may not be indicated for patients who have lost significant alveolar dimension. This is often more problematic for maxillary reconstructions because lip support is more critical in the upper arch. Furthermore, for some patients, the lack of a complete seal (i.e., spaces under the framework) allows air to escape during speech, thus creating phonetic problems.

Depending on the volume of existing bone, the jaw relationship, the amount of lip support, and phonetics, some patients may not be able to be rehabilitated with an implant-supported fixed prosthesis. For these patients, a removable, complete-denture type of prosthesis is a better choice because it provides a flange extension that can be adjusted and contoured to support the lip, and there are no spaces for unwanted air escape during speech. This type of prosthesis can be retained and stabilized by two or more implants placed in the anterior region of the maxilla or mandible. Methods used to secure the denture to the implants vary from separate attachments on each individual implant to clips or other attachments that connect to a bar, which splints the implants together (Fig. 56.3). It is also possible to design a removable prosthesis to intimately and securely attach to a precision-fit substructure (e.g., milled bar), making it an implant-supported removable prosthesis.

Although the stability of the implant-retained overdenture does not compare with the rigidly attached, implant-supported fixed prosthesis, the increased retention and stability over conventional complete dentures is an important advantage for denture wearers.[77] Additionally, implant-assisted and implant-supported

prostheses are thought to lessen the amount of alveolar bone loss associated with long-term use of removable prostheses that bear directly on the alveolar ridges.

Partially Edentulous Patients
Multiple Teeth

Partially edentulous patients with multiple missing teeth represent another viable treatment population for osseointegrated implants, but the remaining natural dentition (occlusal schemes, periodontal health status, spatial relationships, and aesthetics) introduces additional challenges for successful rehabilitation.[48] The juxtaposition of implants with natural teeth in the partially edentulous patient presents the clinician with challenges not encountered with implants in the edentulous patient. As a result of distinct differences in the biology and function of implants compared with natural teeth, clinicians must educate themselves and use a prescribed approach to the evaluation and treatment planning

Fig. 56.3 (A) Maxillary overdenture bar attached to four implants with anterior clips and posterior extracoronal resilient attachments (ERAs). (B) Clinical view of maxillary overdenture bar. (C) Palateless maxillary complete overdenture. (D) Tissue surface of the same maxillary implant-assisted overdenture showing clips and ERAs. (Courtesy Dr. John Beumer, Maxillofacial Prosthodontics, University of California, Los Angeles, CA.)

of implants for partially edentulous patients. In general, endosseous dental implants can support a free-standing fixed partial denture. Adjacent natural teeth are not necessary for support, but their close proximity requires special attention and planning.[12] The major advantage of an implant-supported restoration in the partially edentulous patient is that it replaces missing teeth without invasion or alteration of adjacent teeth. Preparation of natural teeth becomes unnecessary, and larger edentulous spans can be restored with implant-supported fixed bridges.[61] Moreover, patients who previously did not have a fixed option, such as those with Kennedy class I and II partially edentulous situations, can be restored with an implant-supported fixed restoration (Fig. 56.4).

Early attempts to use endosseous implants to replace missing teeth in the partially edentulous patient were a challenge partly because the implants and armamentarium were designed for the edentulous patient and did not have much flexibility for adaptation and use in the partially edentulous patient. Today, clinicians have many choices in terms of implant length, diameter, and abutment connection to choose for the optimal replacement of any missing tooth, large or small (Fig. 56.5).

The primary challenge with partially edentulous cases is an underestimation of the importance of treatment planning for implant-retained restorations with an adequate number of implants to withstand occlusal loads. For example, one problem that required correction was the misconception that two implants could be used to support a long-span, multiunit

fixed bridge in the posterior area. Multiunit fixed restorations in the posterior jaw are more likely to experience complications or failures (mechanical or biologic) when they are inadequately supported in terms of the number of implants, quality of bone, or strength of the implant material. Better treatment planning with the use of an adequate number and size of implants, particularly in areas of poor-quality bone, has solved many of these problems.

> **FLASH BACK**
>
> The Kennedy Classification refers to a system developed by Dr. Edward Kennedy for the classification of an edentulous jaw and partial dentures. It is based on the distribution of edentulous spaces. Kennedy class I is a bilateral free-end posterior edentulous area. Kennedy class II is a unilateral free-end posterior edentulous area. Kennedy class III is a single bounded edentulous area that does not cross the midline (unilateral). Kennedy class IV is a single anterior bounded edentulous area that crosses the midline (bilateral).

Single Tooth

Patients with a missing single tooth (anterior or posterior) represent another type of patient who benefits greatly from the success and predictability of endosseous dental implants (Video 56.1). Replacement of a single missing tooth with an implant-supported crown is a much more conservative approach than preparing two adjacent teeth for the fabrication of a

Fig. 56.4 (A) Clinical view of a partially edentulous posterior mandible (Kennedy class II distal extension). (B) Occlusal view of the same patient as in part A restored with an implant-supported fixed restoration replacing teeth #18 and #19. Note that the dimensions of the crowns are smaller than typical mandibular molars (i.e., closer to bicuspid size). (C) Buccal view of the same restorations.

Fig. 56.5 Diagram Representing the Use of Wide-, Narrow-, and Standard-Diameter Implants for Molars, Mandibular Incisors, and Other Teeth (Different-Sized Implants Superimposed Over Various Teeth). (A) Maxillary teeth. (B) Mandibular teeth.

tooth-supported fixed partial denture. It is no longer necessary to "cut" healthy or minimally restored adjacent teeth to replace a missing tooth with a nonremovable prosthetic replacement (Fig. 56.6). Reported success rates for single-tooth implants are excellent.[27]

Replacement of an individual missing posterior tooth with an implant-supported restoration has been successful as well. The greatest challenges to overcome with the single-tooth implant restorations were screw loosening and implant or component fracture. Because of the increased potential to generate forces in the posterior area, the implants, components, and screws often failed. Both of these problems have been addressed with the use of wider-diameter implants and internal fixation of components (Fig. 56.7). Wide-diameter implants often have a wider platform (restorative interface) that resists tipping forces and thus reduces screw loosening. The wide-diameter implant also provides greater strength and resistance to fracture as a result of increased wall

thickness (i.e., the thickness of the implant between the inner screw thread and the outer screw thread). Implants with an internal connection are inherently more resistant to screw loosening and thus have an added advantage for single-tooth applications.

Aesthetic Considerations

Anterior single-tooth implants present some of the same challenges as the single posterior tooth supported by an implant, but they also are an aesthetic concern for patients. Some cases are more aesthetically challenging than others because of the nature of each individual's smile and display of teeth. The prominence and occlusal relationship of existing teeth, the thickness and health of periodontal tissues, and the patient's own psychological perception of aesthetics all play a role in the aesthetic challenge of the case. Cases with good bone volume, bone height, and tissue thickness can be predictable in terms of achieving satisfactory aesthetic results (see Fig. 56.6). However, achieving aesthetic results for patients with less-than-ideal tissue qualities poses difficult challenges for the restorative and surgical team.[13] Replacing a single tooth with an implant-supported crown in a patient with a high smile line, compromised or thin periodontium, inadequate hard or soft tissues, and high expectations is probably one of the most difficult challenges in implant dentistry and should not be attempted by novice clinicians.

PRETREATMENT EVALUATION

A comprehensive evaluation is indicated for any patient who is being considered for dental implant therapy. The evaluation should assess all aspects of the patient's current health status, including a review the patient's past medical history, medications, and medical treatments. Patients should be questioned about parafunctional habits, such as clenching or grinding teeth, as well as any substance use or abuse, including tobacco, alcohol, and drugs. The assessment should also include an evaluation of the patient's motivations, level of understanding, compliance, and overall behavior. For most patients, this involves simply observing their demeanor and listening to their comments for an impression of their overall sensibility and coherence with other patient norms.

An intraoral and radiographic examination must be done to determine whether it is possible to place implant(s) in the desired location(s). Properly mounted diagnostic study models and intraoral clinical photographs are useful parts of the clinical examination and treatment-planning process to aid in the assessment of spatial and occlusal relationships. Once the data collection is completed, the clinician will be able to determine whether implant therapy is possible, practical, and indicated for the patient.

Conducting an organized, systematic history and examination is essential to obtaining an accurate diagnosis and creating a treatment plan that is appropriate for the patient. Each treatment plan should be comprehensive and provide several treatment options for the patient, including periodontal and restorative therapies. Then, in consultation, the clinician can agree on the final treatment plan with the patient. Information gathered throughout the process will help the clinician's decision making and determination of whether a patient is a good candidate for dental implants. A thoughtful and well-executed evaluation can

Fig. 56.6 Single-Tooth Replacement. (A) Implant in place. (B) Metalloceramic crown.

Fig. 56.7 (A) Occlusal view of healing abutment, which is attached to a wide-diameter implant used to replace a single missing molar. (B) Radiograph of the same patient depicted in part A, showing the wide-diameter implant supporting the final restoration (molar replaced with a single-tooth implant-supported crown).

also reveal deficiencies and indicate what additional surgical procedures may be necessary to accomplish the desired goals of therapy (e.g., localized ridge augmentation, sinus bone augmentation). Each part of the pretreatment evaluation is briefly discussed here.

KEY FACT

Every treatment plan should be comprehensive. It should provide multiple treatment options, including periodontal and restorative therapies. Then, once presented with correct information, the patient can ask questions and make an informed decision about the final treatment plan. Information gathered throughout the process will help the clinician's decision making and determination of whether a patient is a good candidate for dental implants.

Chief Complaint

What is the problem or concern in the patient's own words? What is the patient's goal of treatment? How realistic are the patient's expectations? The patient's chief concern, desires for treatment, and vision of the successful outcome must be taken into consideration. The patient will measure implant success according to his or her personal criteria. The overall comfort and function of the implant restoration are often the most important factors, but satisfaction with the appearance of the final restoration will also influence the patient's perception of success. Furthermore, patient satisfaction may be influenced simply by the impact that the treatment has on the patient's perceived quality of life. Patients will evaluate for themselves whether the treatment helped them to eat better, look better, or feel better about themselves.

The clinician could consider an implant and the retained prosthesis a success using standard criteria of symptom-free implant function, implant stability, and lack of peri-implant infection or bone loss. At the same time, however, the patient who does not like the aesthetic result or does not think the condition has improved could consider the treatment a failure. Therefore it is critical to inquire, as specifically as possible, about the patient's expectations before initiating implant therapy and to appreciate the patient's desires and values. With this goal in mind, it is often helpful and advisable to invite patients to bring their spouses or family members to the consultation and treatment-planning visits to add an independent "trusted" observer to the discussion of treatment options. Ultimately, it is the clinician's responsibility to determine if the patient has realistic expectations for the outcome of therapy and to educate the patient about realistic outcomes for each treatment option.

CLINICAL CORRELATION

It is essential to listen to a patient's chief concerns. The patient will ultimately decide whether the implant is successful based on his or her personal criteria. The overall comfort and function of the implant restoration are often the most important factors, but satisfaction with the appearance will also influence the patient's perception of success. Patient satisfaction will be influenced by the impact of treatment on their perceived quality of life. Patients will evaluate for themselves whether the implant treatment helped them to eat better, look better, or feel better.

Medical History

A thorough medical history is required for any patient in need of dental treatment, regardless of whether implants are part of the plan. This history should be documented in writing by the patient's completion of a standard health history form and verbally through an interview with the treating clinician. The patient's health history should be reviewed for any condition that might put the patient at risk for adverse reactions or complications.

Patients must be in reasonably good health to undergo surgical therapy for the placement of dental implants. Any disorder that may impair the normal wound-healing process, especially as it relates to bone metabolism, should be carefully considered as a possible risk factor or contraindication to implant therapy (discussed later).

A thorough physical examination is warranted if any questions arise about the patient's health status.[17] Appropriate laboratory tests (e.g., coagulation tests for a patient receiving anticoagulant therapy) should be requested to evaluate further any conditions that may affect the patient's ability to undergo the planned surgical and restorative procedures safely and effectively. If any questions remain about the patient's health status, a medical clearance for surgery should be obtained from the patient's treating physician.

Dental History

A review of a patient's past dental experiences can be a valuable part of the overall evaluation. Does the patient report a history of recurrent or frequent abscesses, which may indicate a susceptibility to infections or diabetes? Does the patient have many restorations? How compliant has the patient been with previous dental recommendations? What are the patient's current oral hygiene practices?

The individual's previous experiences with surgery and prosthetics should be discussed. If a patient reports numerous problems and difficulties with past dental care, including a history of dissatisfaction with past treatment, the patient may have similar difficulties with implant therapy. It is essential to identify past problems and to elucidate any contributing factors. The clinician must also assess the patient's dental knowledge and understanding of the proposed treatment, as well as the patient's attitude and motivation toward implants.

Intraoral Examination

The oral examination is performed to assess the current health and condition of existing teeth, as well as to evaluate the condition of the oral hard and soft tissues. It is imperative that no pathologic conditions are present in any of the hard or soft tissues in the maxillofacial region. All oral lesions, especially infections, should be diagnosed and appropriately treated before implant therapy. Additional criteria to consider include the patient's habits, level of oral hygiene, overall dental and periodontal health, occlusion, jaw relationship, temporomandibular joint condition, and ability to open wide.

After a thorough intraoral examination, the clinician can evaluate potential implant sites. All sites should be clinically evaluated to measure the available space in the bone for the

BOX 56.1 How Much Space Is Required for Placement of One or More Implants?[a]

Alveolar Bone

Assuming an implant is 4 mm in diameter and 10 mm long, the minimal width of the jawbone needs to be 6–7 mm, and the minimal height should be 10 mm (minimum of 12 mm in the posterior mandible, where an additional margin of safety is required over the mandibular nerve). This dimension is desired to maintain at least 1–1.5 mm of bone around all surfaces of the implant after preparation and placement.

Interdental Space

Edentulous spaces need to be measured to determine whether enough space exists for the placement and restoration with one or more implant crowns. The minimal space requirements for the placement of one, two, or more implants are illustrated diagrammatically in Fig. 75.9. The minimal mesial-distal space for an implant placed between two teeth is 7 mm. The minimal mesial-distal space required for the placement of two standard-diameter implants (4-mm diameter) between teeth is 14 mm. The required minimal dimensions for wide-diameter or narrow-diameter implants will increase or decrease incrementally according to the size of the implant. For example, the minimal space needed for the placement of an implant 6 mm in diameter is 9 mm (7 mm + 2 mm). Whenever the available space between teeth is greater than 7 mm and less than 14 mm, only one implant, such as placement of a wide-diameter implant, should be considered. Two narrow-diameter implants could be positioned in a space that is 12 mm. However, the smaller implant may be more vulnerable to implant fracture.

Interocclusal Space

The restoration consists of the abutment, the abutment screw, and the crown (it may also include a screw to secure the crown to the abutment if it is not cemented). This restorative "stack" is the total of all the components used to attach the crown to the implant. The dimensions of the restorative stack vary slightly depending on the type of abutment and the implant-restorative interface (i.e., internal or external connection). The minimum amount of interocclusal space required for the restorative "stack" on an external hex-type implant is 7 mm.

[a]All of the minimal space requirements discussed here are generic averages. The actual space limitations for any particular implant system must be determined according to the manufacturer's specifications.

Fig. 56.8 (A) Clinical photograph of maxillary premolar space with apparently adequate space between the remaining teeth for an implant-supported crown. (B) Radiograph clearly shows a lack of space between the roots of the adjacent teeth as a result of convergence into the space (same patient as in part A).

for standard-, wide-, and narrow-diameter implants placed between natural teeth, and the minimal interocclusal space needed to restore implants.

Hard-Tissue Evaluation

The amount of available bone is the next criterion to evaluate. Wide variations in jaw anatomy are encountered, and it is therefore important to analyze the anatomy of the dentoalveolar region of interest both clinically and radiographically.

A visual examination can immediately identify deficient areas (Fig. 56.10), whereas other areas that appear to have good ridge width will require further evaluation (Fig. 56.11). Clinical examination of the jawbone consists of palpation to feel for anatomic defects and variations in the jaw anatomy, such as concavities and undercuts. If desired, it is possible with local anesthesia to probe through the soft tissue (intraoral bone mapping) to assess the thickness of the soft tissues and measure the bone dimensions at the proposed surgical site.

The spatial relationship of the bone must be evaluated in a three-dimensional view because the implant must be placed in the appropriate position relative to the prosthesis. It is possible that an adequate dimension of bone is available in the anticipated implant site (see Box 56.1), but that the bone and thus the implant placement might be located too lingual or too buccal for the desired prosthetic tooth replacement.[34] Bone augmentation procedures may be necessary to facilitate the placement of an implant in an acceptable prosthetic position despite the availability of an adequate quantity of bone (i.e., the bone is in the wrong location).

Radiographic Examination

Radiographic assessment of the quantity, quality, and location of available alveolar bone in potential implant sites ultimately determines whether a patient is a candidate for implants and if

placement of implants and in the dental space for prosthetic tooth replacement (Box 56.1). The mesial-distal and buccal-lingual dimensions of edentulous spaces can be approximated with a periodontal probe or other measuring instrument. The orientation or tilt of adjacent teeth and their roots should be noted as well. There may be enough space in the coronal area for the restoration but not enough space in the apical region for the implant if roots are directed into the area of interest (Fig. 56.8). Conversely, there may be adequate space between roots, but the coronal aspects of the teeth may be too close for emergence and restoration of the implant. If either of these conditions is discovered, orthodontic tooth movement may be indicated. Ultimately, edentulous areas need to be precisely measured using diagnostic study models and imaging techniques to determine whether space is available and whether adequate bone volume exists to replace missing teeth with implants and implant restorations. Fig. 56.9 diagrams the minimal space requirements

The minimum mesial-distal space (*d*) required for a:
A. Narrow diameter implant (e.g., 3.25 mm) is 6 mm.
B. Standard diameter implant (e.g., 4.1 mm) is 7 mm.
C. Wide diameter implant (e.g., 5.0 mm) is 8 mm.
D. Wide diameter implant (e.g., 6.0 mm) is 9 mm.

The minimum mesial-distal space (*d*) required for two standard diameter implants is 14 mm wide.

Fig. 56.9 (A) Minimum amount of mesial-distal space *(d)* required for placement of single-tooth implant between natural teeth: *A,* 6 mm for narrow-diameter implant (3.25 mm); *B,* 7 mm for standard-diameter implant (4.1 mm); *C* and *D,* 8 mm and 9 mm, respectively, for wide-diameter implants (5 mm and 6 mm). (B) Minimum amount of mesial-distal space *(d)* required for placement of two standard-diameter implants (4.1 mm) between natural teeth is 14 mm. This allows approximately 2 mm between teeth/implants and between implant/implant. Minimum amount of space required between implant/restoration interface and opposing occlusal surfaces for restoration of an implant. This dimension will vary depending on implant design and manufacturer component dimensions. The minimal dimension of 7 mm is based on an externally hexed implant and UCLA abutment.

a particular implant site needs bone augmentation. Appropriate radiographic procedures, including periapical radiographs, panoramic projections, and cross-sectional imaging, can help identify vital structures such as the floor of the nasal cavity, maxillary sinus, mandibular canal, and mental foramen. In addition to the absolute dimensional measurement of the alveolar bone, it is important to determine whether the volume of bone radiographically (as well as clinically) is located in a position to allow for the proper position of the implant to facilitate restoration of the tooth/teeth in proper aesthetic and functional relationship with the adjacent and opposing dentition. The best way to evaluate the relationship of available bone to the dentition is to image the patient with a diagnostically accurate guide using radiopaque markers that are positioned at the proposed prosthetic locations, ideally with appropriate restorative contours (Fig. 56.12).

KEY FACT

Implant planning should be "prosthetically driven." This can be achieved with a diagnostic wax-up of the proposed prosthesis and radiographic imaging with radiopaque markers, ideally tooth-shaped, that show the desired tooth position(s) relative to the available bone.

Fig. 56.10 Clinical photographs of edentulous areas with obvious deficient areas of alveolar dimension noted on visual examination: (A) anterior maxilla, (B) posterior maxilla, (C) anterior mandible, and (D) posterior mandible. These clinical images all represent buccal-lingual deficiencies in the alveolar dimensions.

Fig. 56.11 Clinical photographs of edentulous areas with apparent good alveolar dimension noted on visual examination: (A) anterior maxilla, (B) posterior maxilla, (C) anterior mandible, and (D) posterior mandible. It is likely that these sites have adequate bone volume for implant placement. However, it is also possible to find alveolar deficiencies despite the appearance of wide ridges.

Fig. 56.12 Cone-beam computed tomography images for the evaluation of the edentulous space at the area of missing tooth #4 (A) and missing tooth #30 (B) using a limited field-of-view scan (3D Accuitomo, J. Morita Corporation, Suita City, Osaka, Japan, distributed by J. Morita USA, Inc., Irvine, CA). Sagittal and cross-sectional slices are shown. Although the anatomic area imaged is limited, the resolutions of the images are high. (A) Implant site #4 (maxillary right second premolar) in anterior–posterior (A1) and buccolingual (A2) cross-sectional views. (B) Implant site #30 (mandibular right first molar) in anterior–posterior (B1) and buccolingual (B2) cross-sectional views.

Soft-Tissue Evaluation

Evaluation of the quality, quantity, and location of soft tissue present in the anticipated implant site helps to anticipate the type of tissue that will surround the implant(s) after treatment is completed (keratinized vs. nonkeratinized mucosa). For some cases, clinical evaluation may reveal a need for soft-tissue augmentation (Box 56.2). Areas with minimal or no keratinized mucosa may be augmented with gingival or connective tissue grafts. Other soft-tissue concerns, such as frenum attachments that pull on the gingival margin, should be thoroughly evaluated as well.

RISK FACTORS AND CONTRAINDICATIONS

Clearly, there are numerous indications for the use of endosseous dental implants to replace missing teeth. Most patients who are missing one or more teeth can benefit from the application of an implant-retained prosthesis provided they meet the requirements for surgical and prosthetic rehabilitation. Edentulous patients who are unable to function with complete dentures and who have adequate bone for the placement of dental implants

BOX 56.2   How Much Keratinized Tissue Is Required for the Health and Maintenance of Implants?

Debate continues about whether it is necessary to have a zone of keratinized tissue surrounding implants. Despite strong opinions and beliefs about the need for keratinized mucosa around implants versus this mucosa being unnecessary, neither argument has been proved.

Some studies have concluded that, in the presence of good oral hygiene, a lack of keratinized tissue does not impair the health or function of implants.[72] Others strongly believe that keratinized mucosa has better functional and aesthetic results for implant restorations. Keratinized mucosa is typically thicker and denser than alveolar mucosa (nonkeratinized). It forms a strong seal around the implant with a cuff of circular (parallel) fibers around the implant, abutment, or restoration that is resistant to retracting with mastication forces and oral hygiene procedures. Implants with coated surfaces (i.e., hydroxyapatite or titanium plasma spray coating) demonstrate greater peri-implant bone loss and failures in the absence of keratinized mucosa.[15,43]

can be especially good dental implant candidates. More and more partially edentulous patients are also being treated with dental implant restorations. Many patients, whether they are missing one, several, or all of their teeth, can be predictably restored with implant-retained prostheses.

In this era of high implant success and predictability and thus possible complacency, it is imperative for clinicians to recognize risk factors and contraindications to implant therapy so that problems can be minimized and patients can be accurately informed about risks. As such, the clinician must be knowledgeable in this area and inform patients about risk factors and contraindications before initiating treatment. Contraindications for the use of dental implants, although relatively few and often not well defined, do exist. Some conditions are probably best described as "risk factors" rather than "contraindications" to treatment because implants can be successful in almost all patients; implants may be less *predictable* in some situations, and this distinction should be recognized. Ultimately, it is the clinician's responsibility with the patient to make decisions as to when implant therapy is not indicated.

Table 56.1 lists some conditions and factors that are thought to increase the risk for implant failure or otherwise deem the patient a poor candidate for implant therapy. Some of these conditions are briefly discussed here.

The reader is referred to the online material for more information on the topic of medical and systemic health-related issues considered prior to implant placement. Online materials for this chapter are found on the companion website.

POSTTREATMENT EVALUATION

Periodic posttreatment examination of implants, the retained prosthesis, and the condition of the surrounding peri-implant tissue are important components of successful treatment. Aberrations and complications can often be treated if discovered early, but many problems will go unnoticed by the patient. Thus, periodic examination is essential to discovering problems early and to intervening and preventing problems from getting worse.

TABLE 56.1 Risk Factors and Contraindications for Implant Therapy

	Risk Factor	Contraindication
Medical and Systemic Health–Related Issues		
Diabetes (poorly controlled)	??—Possibly	Relative
Bone metabolic disease (e.g., osteoporosis)	??—Probably	Relative
Radiation therapy (head and neck)	Yes	Relative/absolute
Bisphosphonate therapy (intravenous)	??—Probably	Relative/absolute
Bisphosphonate therapy (oral)	??—Possibly	Relative
Immunosuppressive medication	??—Probably	Relative
Immunocompromising disease (e.g., HIV, AIDS)	??—Possibly	Relative
Psychological and Mental Conditions		
Psychiatric syndromes (e.g., schizophrenia, paranoia)	No	Absolute
Mental instability (e.g., neurotic, hysteric)	No	Absolute
Mentally impaired; uncooperative	No	Absolute
Irrational fears; phobias	No	Absolute
Unrealistic expectations	No	Absolute
Habits and Behavioral Considerations		
Smoking; tobacco use	Yes	Relative
Parafunctional habits	Yes	Relative
Substance abuse (e.g., alcohol, drugs)	??—Possibly	Absolute
Intraoral Examination Findings		
Atrophic maxilla	Yes	Relative
Current infection (e.g., endodontic)	Yes	Relative
Periodontal disease	??—Possibly	Relative

??, Unknown; *AIDS,* acquired immunodeficiency syndrome; *HIV,* human immunodeficiency virus.

Several parameters are available to evaluate the condition of the prosthesis, the stability of the implants, and the health of surrounding peri-implant tissues after implant integration and prosthetic restoration. Intraoral radiographs should be taken at the time of placement (baseline), at the time of abutment connection (to confirm seating and serve as another baseline), at the time of final restoration delivery (loading), and subsequently to monitor marginal or peri-implant bone changes. Periapical radiographs have excellent resolution and provide adequate details for evaluating bone support around implants if taken at a perpendicular direction.

The long-term success of dental implants is dependent on the health and stability of supporting peri-implant tissues. Good oral hygiene and regular professional care are essential to maintaining peri-implant health, and the importance of good oral hygiene should be stressed as early as possible. Patients should

be taught to maintain good oral hygiene. Their performance should be monitored and reinforced at each visit.

See Chapter 59 for a detailed description of important clinical and radiographic monitoring methods as well as oral hygiene and implant maintenance protocols.

DIAGNOSTIC IMAGING FOR THE IMPLANT PATIENT

Several radiographic imaging options are available for the diagnosis and treatment planning of patients receiving dental implants.[13,69,70] Options range from standard projections routinely available in the dental office to more complex radiographic techniques typically available only in radiology centers. Standard projections include intraoral (periapical, occlusal) and extraoral (panoramic, lateral cephalometric) radiographs. More complex imaging techniques include cone-beam computed tomography (CBCT) and multislice computed tomography (MSCT). The CBCT and MSCT image data files can be reformatted and viewed on a personal computer using simulation software, making the diagnosis and treatment-planning process interactive and visually more meaningful. Often, combinations of various modalities are used because no single modality can provide all information pertinent to the radiographic evaluation of the implant patient. Familiarity with the benefits and limitations of various techniques and awareness of the specific clinical questions that need to be answered should guide the decision-making process and selection of radiographic examinations for individual patients.

Multiple factors influence the selection of radiographic technique(s) for a particular case, including cost, availability, radiation exposure, and case type. The decision is a balance between these factors and the desire to minimize risk of complications to the patient. Accurately identifying vital anatomic structures and being able to perform implant placement surgery without injury to these structures are critical to treatment success. Diagnostic imaging must always be interpreted in conjunction with a good clinical examination.

This chapter discusses common imaging techniques used for evaluation of the implant patient. Indications for each technique are outlined, along with the advantages and limitations of each technique.

KEY FACT

Accurate identification of vital anatomic structures is critical to treatment success when performing dental implant surgery. Diagnostic imaging must always be interpreted along with a clinical examination.

STANDARD PROJECTIONS

Standard diagnostic imaging modalities include periapical, panoramic, lateral cephalometric, and occlusal radiographs. Table 56.2 summarizes the advantages and disadvantages of each modality.

Periapical Radiographs

Periapical radiographs are often the first imaging modality used to evaluate the implant patient.[73,74] These radiographs provide

TABLE 56.2   Advantages and Disadvantages of the Various Radiographic Projections

Modality	Advantages	Disadvantages
Periapical and occlusal radiography	High resolution and detail, easy acquisition, low radiation exposure, relatively inexpensive	Unpredictable magnification, small imaged area, 2D representation of anatomy
Panoramic radiography	Easy to acquire, images the full dentoalveolar ridge, low radiation dose, relatively inexpensive	Unpredictable magnification, unequal magnification in vertical and horizontal dimensions, 2D representation of anatomy, not detailed
Lateral cephalometric radiography	Easy to acquire, predictable magnification, low radiation dose, relatively inexpensive	Limited use in area of midline, 2D representation of anatomy
Multislice computed tomography	3D representation, no magnification, sufficient detail, digital format, images whole arch	Requires special equipment, expensive, higher radiation dose
Cone-beam computed tomography	3D representation, no magnification, sufficient detail, digital format, images whole arch, low radiation dose	Requires special equipment, relatively expensive

2D, Two-dimensional; *3D*, three-dimensional.

TABLE 56.3   Radiation Dose (Effective Dose in µSv) Received From Common Projections During Evaluation of the Implant Patient Data

Modality	Effective Dose (µSv)
Full-mouth x-ray (FMX) series	177
Panoramic	20
Limited field-of-view CBCT	47
Medium field-of-view CBCT	98
Large field-of-view CBCT	117
MSCT, Maxillofacial	913

CBCT, Cone-beam computed tomography; *MSCT,* multislice computed tomography.
Adapted from Mallya SM: Principles of cone beam computed tomography. In Fayad M, Johnson BR, editors: *3D imaging in endodontics: a new era in diagnosis and treatment.* Median effective doses for standard exposure protocols were derived from collation of data from several reports in the literature.

Fig. 56.13 The Periapical Radiograph Offers a High-Resolution, Detailed Image of the Edentulous Area. Healing of the extraction socket with dense bone (socket sclerosis) can be seen *(small white arrows).* Some anatomic structures, such as the maxillary sinus *(large white arrow)* and the zygomatic process of the maxilla *(black arrow),* can also be visualized.

an overall assessment of the quantity and quality of the edentulous alveolar ridge and the adjacent teeth. They are easy to obtain in the dental office, are relatively inexpensive, and deliver low radiation dose to the patient (Table 56.3).[52] Dentists are familiar with the depicted anatomy and possible pathology. Because these direct-exposure projections do not use intensifying screens, intraoral radiographs offer the highest detail and spatial resolution of all radiographic modalities (Fig. 56.13). Thus, intraoral radiographs are the projection of choice when subtle, localized pathology, such as a retained root tip, needs to be detected and evaluated.

The most significant disadvantage of periapical radiographs is their susceptibility to unpredictable magnification of anatomic structures, which does not allow reliable measurements.[65] Foreshortening or elongation can be minimized by the use of paralleling technique. However, distortion is particularly accentuated in edentulous areas, where missing teeth and resorption of the alveolus necessitate receptor placement at significant angulation in relation to the long axis of the teeth and alveolar bone. Additionally, periapical radiographs are two-dimensional representations

of three-dimensional objects and do not provide any information of the buccal-lingual dimension of the alveolar ridge. Structures that are distinctly separated in the buccal-lingual dimension appear to be overlapping. Also, the periapical image is limited by the size of film or sensor being used. Often, it is not possible to image the entire height of the remaining alveolar ridge, and when extensive mesial-distal areas need to be evaluated, multiple periapical radiographs are required.

Periapical radiographs are useful screening images that offer a detailed view of a small area of the alveolar arch. Limitations that must be considered include the possibility of distortion and the two-dimensional representation of anatomic structures.

Panoramic Radiographs

Panoramic radiographs are often used in the evaluation of the implant patient because they offer several advantages over other modalities.[68] Panoramic radiographs deliver low radiation doses (see Table 56.3) to provide a broad picture of both arches and

Fig. 56.14 Panoramic Radiograph. Both jaws are visualized on the same image. An overall assessment of superoinferior and mesial–distal dimensions of the alveolar ridge can be formulated. Tooth and root positions relative to planned implant sites can be evaluated. Important anatomic structures, such as the maxillary sinus and mandibular canal, can be identified.

thus allow assessment of longer edentulous spans, angulation of existing teeth and occlusal plane, and important anatomy in implant treatment planning such as the maxillary sinus, nasal cavity, mental foramen, and mandibular canal (Fig. 56.14). Panoramic units are widely available and easy to operate, and dentists are familiar with the anatomy and pathology depicted by the images. Similar to intraoral projections, panoramic images are two-dimensional and thus do not offer diagnostic information for the buccal–lingual width of the alveolar arch.

Panoramic images appear intuitively familiar. However, they combine characteristic physical and radiographic principles that make them distinct from other intraoral and extraoral radiographs. Although outside the scope of this chapter, familiarity with the principles underlying panoramic radiography is central for understanding, and thus compensating for, the limitations and constraints of the images. The reader is referred to other textbooks for detailed discussion of this topic.[46,54] Briefly, the existence of ghost shadows, unpredictable horizontal and vertical magnification, distortion of structures outside the focal trough, projection geometry generated by the negative vertical angulation of the x-ray beam, and the propensity to patient-positioning errors do not allow consistently detailed and accurate measurements to be generated. As a result, panoramic radiographs do not provide the highly detailed images that are generated by intraoral radiographs.

Measurement distortion is more prevalent and varies across the radiographic image. On average, panoramic radiographs are 25% magnifications of actual size. Implant manufacturers often provide transparency sheets with implant size outlines of 25% magnification. However, it is important to appreciate that the 25% magnification is an estimate. The actual magnification may range from 10% to 30% in different areas within the same image and depends greatly on patient positioning during panoramic radiography. For this reason, precise measurements on panoramic projections are not possible. Nonetheless, panoramic radiographs offer an overall view of the maxilla and mandible that can be used to estimate bone measurements and evaluate the approximate relationships between teeth and other anatomic structures. More precise diagnostic imaging should be used to measure the

proximity of critical anatomic structures, such as the maxillary sinus or the mandibular canal, to proposed implant positions.

Panoramic projections provide useful information for the initial assessment of the implant patient. However, because of magnification and distortion errors, panoramic radiographs should not be used for detailed measurements of proposed implant sites.

CROSS-SECTIONAL IMAGING

Cross-sectional diagnostic imaging modalities include MSCT and CBCT. Conventional tomography also provides cross-sectional images with predictable magnification and has been used in the assessment of the implant patient. However, with the introduction and expansion of CBCT imaging, conventional tomography is becoming obsolete and is not described in this chapter.

The reader is referred to the online material for more information on the topic of CBCT and software-guided implant placement. Online materials for this chapter are found on the companion website.

KEY FACT

CBCT offers significant advantages for the evaluation of implant patients. The field of view (FOV) is an important feature that describes the extent of the imaged volume from large FOV (>15 cm) to medium FOV (8 to 15 cm) and limited FOV (<8 cm). Limited FOV units image a small area, delivering less radiation and producing a higher-resolution image.

PATIENT EVALUATION

Evaluation of the implant patient should be disciplined and objective. Specific questions that can affect implant placement and outcome should be considered and examined carefully and explicitly. The advantages and disadvantages of various radiographic projections should be considered and radiographic modalities chosen based on necessary information for the particular patient. The objectives for any radiographic evaluation, regardless of imaging technique used, should include an evaluation to (1) exclude pathology, (2) identify anatomic structures, and (3) measure the quantity, quality, and location of available bone.

CLINICAL CORRELATION

All diagnostic images, regardless of technique, should be evaluated to identify or exclude pathology and to identify normal anatomic structures.

Exclude Pathology

Healthy bone is a prerequisite for successful osseointegration and long-term implant success. The first step in the radiographic evaluation of the implant site is to establish the health of the alveolar bone and other tissues imaged within a particular projection. Local and systemic diseases that affect bone homeostasis

Fig. 56.15 Cone-Beam Computed Tomography Examination of the Posterior Left Maxilla. Top row (A) shows reconstructed "panoramic" and coronal sections of the alveolar ridge. Note the thickened mucoperiosteal lining of the floor of the left maxillary sinus *(white arrow)*. The patient has chronic maxillary sinusitis. Bottom row (B) shows conventional panoramic, reconstructed "panoramic," coronal, and axial sections of the alveolar ridge at the area of the missing first maxillary molar. A large radiolucent lesion at the edentulous alveolar ridge elevates the floor of the maxillary sinus and occupies most of the sinus. Biopsy revealed a keratocystic odontogenic tumor that was an incidental finding in this asymptomatic patient.

can preclude, modify, or alter the placement of implants. Retained root fragments, residual periodontal disease, cysts, and tumors should be identified and resolved before implant placement. Systemic diseases, such as osteoporosis and hyperparathyroidism, alter bone metabolism and might affect implant osseointegration. Areas of poor bone quality should be identified and, if indicated, adjustments to the treatment plan incorporated. Maxillary sinusitis, polyps, or other sinus pathology should be diagnosed and treated when implants are considered in the posterior maxilla, especially if sinus bone augmentation procedures are planned (Fig. 56.15).

Identify Anatomic Structures

Several important anatomic structures are found close to desired areas of implant placement in the maxilla and mandible (Box 56.3). Familiarity with the radiographic appearance of these structures is important during treatment planning and implant placement. Their exact localization is central to prevent unwanted complications and unnecessary morbidity. Important anatomic structures in the maxilla include the floor and anterior wall of the maxillary sinus, incisive foramen, floor and lateral wall of the nasal cavity, and canine fossa. Important anatomic structures in the mandible that should be recognized include the mandibular canal, anterior loop of the mandibular canal, mental foramen, anterior extension of the canal, and submandibular fossa. The existence of anatomic variants, such as incomplete healing of an extraction site, sinus loculation, division of mandibular canal (Fig. 56.16), or absence of a well-defined corticated canal, should also be recognized.

BOX 56.3 **Anatomic Structures Pertinent to Treatment Planning of the Implant Patient**

Maxilla
Maxillary sinus (floor and anterior wall)
Nasal cavity (floor and lateral wall)
Incisive foramen
Canine fossa
Canalis sinuosus

Mandible
Mandibular canal
Anterior loop of the mandibular canal
Anterior extension of the mandibular canal
Mental foramen
Submandibular fossa
Retromolar canal
Lingual inclination of the alveolar ridge

CLINICAL CORRELATION

Several important anatomic structures need to be identified in the jaws prior to implant placement. Violation of structures such as nerves may cause serious complications. Familiarity with the radiographic appearance of vital structures is important, and the existence of anatomic variants should also be recognized.

Assess Bone Quantity, Quality, and Volume

The primary goal of diagnostic imaging for potential implant patients is to evaluate the available bone volume for implant placement in desired anatomic locations. The clinician should

Fig. 56.16 Cone-Beam Computed Tomography Examination of the Area of Missing Tooth #19 Before Implant Placement. (A) Panoramic view of the area of interest depicts an accessory mandibular canal. (B) Same panoramic view with the accessory mandibular canal colored blue and the main canal colored red. (C) Cross-sectional views through the area of missing tooth #19. (D) Same cross-sectional images depicting the blue and red markings. Note that the position of the markings coincides with the position of the accessory and main mandibular canals (compare parts C and D).

estimate and verify exact adequate height, width, and density to the recipient bone while avoiding damage to critical anatomic structures. Failure to accurately assess the location of important anatomic structures can lead to unnecessary complications. For example, inadvertent penetration and damage to the inferior alveolar nerve can result in serious immediate-term (profuse bleeding), short-term, and long-term (nerve paresthesia/anesthesia) complications. The height and width of the alveolar bone should be accurately detailed. Depending on the technique, diagnostic imaging can estimate or measure the coronal–apical height, the buccal–lingual width, and the mesial–distal spacing available for implants that will be placed in proximity to teeth or relative to other planned implants.

This task can be simple in cases with good bone quality and sufficient bone volume in the desired implant location(s). However, in cases with moderate to severe bone resorption, alveolar defects, or recent extraction sites, obtaining a clear and accurate diagnostic image can be more challenging. The diagnostic imaging may reveal inadequate bone volume for the proposed implant(s) and indicate a need for bone augmentation or, depending on the severity of the deficiency, preclude the patient from the possibility of implant therapy (Fig. 56.17). When ridge augmentation is deemed necessary, radiographic evaluation prior to and after surgery informs treatment planning and ensures grafting integrity and quality (Fig. 56.18).

In addition to the amount, the quality of the available bone should also be evaluated. A uniform, continuous cortical outline and a lacy, well-defined trabecular core reflect the normal bone homeostasis necessary for appropriate bone response around the implant. Thin or discontinuous cortex, sparse trabeculation,

Fig. 56.17 Radiographic Evaluation of a Patient With Congenitally Missing Maxillary Lateral Incisors Before Implant Placement. (A) Panoramic radiograph reveals sufficient height and mesial-lateral width of the alveolar ridge. (B) Cross-sectional conventional tomography of the edentulous areas reveals a narrow (<4 mm) buccal-lingual width of the alveolar ridge that needs to be addressed by modifications in the treatment planning, such as bone augmentation.

Fig. 56.18 Radiographic Evaluation of a Patient With Missing Left Maxillary Second Premolar and First Molar. Initial cone-beam computed tomography (CBCT) reveals an atrophic alveolar ridge (A) with inadequate height for implant placement (B). Also note the thickened mucoperiosteum at the floor of the maxillary sinus. CBCT after sinus grafting for ridge augmentation shows the uniformly opaque grafting area blending with alveolar trabeculation and a smooth sinus floor elevation (C), which provides adequate dimensions for implant placement (D).

large marrow spaces, and altered trabecular architecture should be noted because they might predict poor implant stabilization and less desirable response of the bone. Poor bone quality may necessitate modifications of the treatment planning, such as waiting longer for healing (osseointegration) to maximize bone-to-implant contact before loading.

Evaluate Relation of Alveolar Ridge With Existing Teeth and Desired Implant Position

Accurate placement (spatial position and angulation relative to adjacent teeth and occlusal plane) will greatly affect the restorative success and long-term prognosis of the implant. A significant variable during the preimplant evaluation is the relation of the desired implant position relative to the existing teeth, alveolar crest, and occlusal plane. Angled or custom abutments can accommodate slight variations in implant position and implant inclination. However, more significant deviations should be avoided.

Prolonged tooth loss is usually associated with atrophy of the alveolar ridge and, in the case of the maxilla, with pneumatization of the sinus floor toward the alveolar crest. Traumatic extractions can compromise the buccal or lingual cortex and alter the shape and buccolingual ridge dimension. Anatomic variants, such as lingual inclination of the alveolus or narrow ridges, should be considered during treatment planning of the implant patient (Fig. 56.19).

An important part of diagnostic imaging must include an evaluation of the available bone relative to the "prosthetically driven" implant position. This aspect of the patient evaluation is best accomplished with diagnostic models, wax-up of planned tooth replacement, and radiographic markers in the desired tooth positions during imaging. Steel balls, brass tubes,

Fig. 56.19 Radiographic Evaluation of a Patient With an Edentulous Posterior Left Mandible Before Implant Placement. Panoramic (A) and periapical (B) radiographs demonstrate sufficient height of the alveolar ridge with little or no resorption. Cone-beam computed tomography sections (C and D) reveal significant lingual inclination of the alveolar ridge with lingual concavity that is not depicted on conventional radiographs.

Fig. 56.20 (A) Panoramic view of partially edentulous maxilla with tooth-shaped markers in areas of missing teeth (potential implant sites). (B) Cross-sectional views from a cone-beam computed tomography examination before implant placement in the right maxilla. Appropriately sized and shaped tooth markers placed in the prosthetically desired locations of the planned restorations for the missing teeth help evaluate the existing alveolar ridge relative to the prospective tooth positions and contours.

and gutta-percha have all been used to establish the proposed tooth positions relative to the existing alveolar bone. The use of these nonanatomic markers is helpful for evaluating bone height and width in specific anatomic locations. However, they do not accurately represent the tooth contours and do not allow the clinician to estimate variations in implant position and angulation relative to the position and emergence of the planned tooth replacement. Therefore it is more desirable and beneficial to use radiopaque tooth-shaped markers so that the existing alveolar bone can be evaluated relative to the entire tooth position/contours (Fig. 56.20). This is particularly important for anterior, aesthetic implant cases. Patients should always be imaged with radiographic guides (markers).

> **KEY FACT**
>
> An important part of diagnostic imaging must include an evaluation of the available bone relative to the "prosthetically driven" implant position. It is most beneficial to assess the prosthetic position in scans using radiopaque tooth-shaped markers so the proper contours of the proposed restoration can be appreciated.

CLINICAL SELECTION OF DIAGNOSTIC IMAGING

Radiography is an important diagnostic tool for the evaluation of the implant patient. However, radiographic imaging alone is insufficient. It is important to correlate diagnostic information with a good clinical examination. Conversely, a clinical examination is insufficient to provide the information needed to plan implant treatment for a patient without some radiographic imaging.

Clinical Examination

Before taking any radiographs, a complete clinical examination of the implant patient is required. This should include the etiology and duration of tooth loss, any history of traumatic extraction, and a review of records and radiographs, if available. A clinical assessment of the edentulous area, covering mucosa, adjacent and opposing teeth, and occlusal plane, should be performed. Temporomandibular function, mandibular maximal opening, and protrusive and lateral movements should be evaluated.

Screening Radiographs

At this point, an overall assessment of the health of the jaws should be performed. The American Academy of Oral and Maxillofacial Radiology recommends panoramic radiography as the initial evaluation of the dental implant patient, supplemented with periapical radiographs as needed.[69] Periapical radiographs provide a high-resolution image of the alveolus and the surrounding structures, including adjacent teeth. For extended edentulous areas, panoramic, lateral cephalometric, and occlusal radiographs can be used to estimate bone height and width. Any pathology of the bone at the prospective implant site, as well as of the surrounding structures, should be identified and treated as indicated.

KEY FACT

The American Academy of Oral and Maxillofacial Radiology recommends panoramic radiography as the initial evaluation of the dental implant patient, supplemented with periapical radiographs as needed. The organization also recommends that radiographic examination of any potential implant site should include cross-sectional imaging orthogonal to the site of interest.

Fabrication of Radiographic and Surgical Guides

Once the health of the soft and hard tissues is established, casts should be taken and a detailed analysis performed. The clinician should decide on the number of implants and their desired location. Next, a radiographic guide should be fabricated, usually with clear acrylic. The position of the desired implants is indicated by the use of radiopaque objects such as metallic balls, cylinders, or rods; gutta-percha; or composite resin. If CT imaging might be performed, the use of metallic markers should be avoided. The design of such a guide greatly enhances the diagnostic information provided by the radiographs because it correlates the radiographic anatomy with the exact position of the proposed implant location.

Cross-Sectional Imaging

The American Academy of Oral and Maxillofacial Radiology recommends that radiographic examination of any potential implant site should include cross-sectional imaging orthogonal to the site of interest.[69] The potential morbidity of a compromised anatomic structure and the poor performance and potential failure of a misplaced implant, combined with the wide availability of tomographic facilities, favor the use of cross-sectional imaging in most cases of implant treatment planning. It is crucial that the cross sections are perpendicular to the curvature of the mandible and parallel to the planned implant. Improper patient positioning can lead to an overestimation of the height and width of the available bone. If the surgeon believes that sections were performed at the wrong angulation, new images should be requested. This might necessitate reexposure of the patient.

Intraoperative and Postoperative Radiographic Assessment

Various radiographic modalities can provide valuable information during implant placement. Because of the ease of acquisition and high resolution, periapical radiographs are most commonly used. Intraoperative radiographs can be taken during surgery to evaluate proximity to important anatomic structures. Sequential periapical radiographs guide the clinician to visualize changes in direction and depth of the drilling procedure and parallelism to adjacent teeth and other implants (Fig. 56.21). Digital radiographs are particularly advantageous during an intraoperative assessment of implant placement; images appear on the screen almost instantaneously and can be manipulated to extract the most pertinent diagnostic information (see Chapter 31).

Implant osseointegration, and the level of peri-implant alveolar bone are major determinants of implant prognosis. Panoramic

Fig. 56.21 Intraoperative Periapical Radiographs Are Valuable in Assessing the Proximity of Adjacent Teeth. (A) The 2-mm guide pin is used to determine the direction of the osteotomy site and its proximity to the adjacent root. (B) After angle correction, the osteotomy sites are completed to length with the final drill. Here the 3-mm guide pins confirm the correct angulation and spacing of the final osteotomy site preparation before implant placement.

Fig. 56.22 Radiographic Follow-Up After Implant Placement in Three Different Patients. (A) Periapical radiograph of three implants in the posterior right mandible. "Normal" bone remodeling around the anterior two implants and slight horizontal bone loss/remodeling around the molar/posterior implant is present. (B) Periapical radiograph of two implants in the left posterior mandible. Severe bone loss (50% of implant length) is seen around the anterior implant, whereas mild bone loss/bone remodeling is observed around the posterior implant. A moderate buccal cantilever in the restoration likely contributed to an adverse occlusal load and the resultant bone loss observed in this case. (C) Panoramic radiograph of maxillary and mandibular implants in an edentulous patient prior to implant loading. The mandibular implants do not show signs of bone loss and appear to be osseointegrated. All maxillary implants show signs of moderate-to-severe peri-implant bone loss, and the success of osseointegration is questionable.

and periapical radiographs offer a fast, easy, and low-radiation depiction of the implant and surrounding tissues and aid in the assessment of implant success. To obtain an accurate assessment of peri-implant bone height, the x-ray beam should be directed perpendicular to the implant. In the case of threaded implants, the implant threads should be distinguishable and not overlapping (Fig. 56.22A).

A 1.2-mm marginal bone loss during the first year after implant placement and 0.1 mm per year afterward are expected; however, further bone loss is considered abnormal.[13] Pathologic bone loss could be localized along the full extent of the implant (peri-implant bone loss) or around the crestal part of the implant ("saucerization"), and it could reflect poor osseointegration, peri-implantitis, or unfavorable stress distribution (see Fig. 56.22B and C).

In select cases, when poor implant placement (Fig. 56.23) or compromise of vital anatomic structures (Fig. 56.24) is suspected, advanced imaging (CBCT, CT, or conventional tomography) provides a three-dimensional evaluation of the oral structures in relation to the implants. This information can be very important for proper assessment and treatment planning. The treating

dentist should recognize relevant signs and symptoms and order appropriate imaging as soon after implant placement as possible. Implant removal, if necessary, would be less complicated before advanced osseointegration.

CONCLUSION

Today, clinicians are able to predictably replace missing teeth with endosseous dental implants. Whether missing a single tooth, several teeth, or all teeth, many patients can be candidates for dental implant therapy. It is important for clinicians to recognize factors that influence implant success. In addition to the quantity, quality, and location of available bone, the patient's health, risk factors, and contraindications must be assessed. Patients should be informed about risk factors and provided with treatment options both with and without dental implants. Periodic evaluation, good oral hygiene, and regular maintenance are important aspects of care for the long-term success and the prevention of complications with dental implants.

Many radiographic projections are available for the evaluation of implant placement, each with advantages and disadvantages.

Fig. 56.23 Radiographic Follow-Up After Implant Placement. (A) Panoramic radiograph suggests mild-to-moderate bone loss around the neck of all implants. This is especially true for the implants in the left maxilla. These implants appear to be angled, and the distal implant is positioned more apical. The overdenture bar is not completely seated on the left implants. Note that superimposed overlapping anatomic structures in this panoramic radiograph impair the ability to clearly visualize and assess bone loss around implants. (B) Cross-sectional (B1) and sagittal cone-beam computed tomography (B2) images of the anterior implant in the left maxilla. Poor implant placement beyond the buccal cortex of the alveolar ridge (cross section) and peri-implant bone loss (sagittal) are revealed.

Fig. 56.24 Cone-Beam Computed Tomography Sagittal and Cross-Sectional Images Clearly Demonstrate Penetration of the Implant Into the Mandibular Canal.

The clinician must follow sequential steps in patient evaluation, and radiography is an essential diagnostic tool for implant design and successful treatment of the implant patient. Selection of appropriate radiographic modalities will provide the maximum diagnostic information, help avoid unwanted complications, and maximize treatment outcomes while delivering an "as low as reasonably achievable" radiation dose to the patient.[57]

Case Scenarios are found on the companion website.

REFERENCES

 References for this chapter are found on the companion website www.expertconsult.com.

57

Basic Implant Surgical Procedures[a]

The surgical procedures for the placement of nearly all endosseous dental implants currently used are based on the original work of Professor Per-Ingvar Brånemark and colleagues in Sweden in the 1960s and 1970s.[4,5] Their landmark research evaluated the biologic, physiologic, and mechanical aspects of the titanium screw-shaped implant, subsequently known commercially as the Nobelpharma "Brånemark" implant system and currently manufactured by Nobel Biocare. The original Brånemark implant was a parallel-walled, cylindrically shaped, threaded implant with an external hex connection and a machined surface. Since their introduction, many designs of root form implants have been developed, modified, and studied. The same fundamental principles of atraumatic, precise implant site preparation apply to all implant systems. Briefly, this includes a gentle surgical technique and progressive, incremental preparation of the bone for a precise fit of the implant at the time of placement.

This chapter outlines the basic surgical procedures for the placement of endosseous dental implants using either one-stage or two-stage protocols. The principles described here are intentionally generic and meant to serve as guidelines that are applicable to most common implant systems (Video 57.1). Each implant system is designed with specific armamentarium and recommendations for use (e.g., drilling speeds), and it is advisable to follow the detailed protocols provided by the manufacturer. For the presentation of a dental implant case, see Video 57.2.

[a]Adapted from the following chapter of Newman and Carranza's Clinical Periodontology, 13th edition: Chapter 78: Basic Implant Surgical Procedures, by Perry R. Klokkevold.Editors' note: An animation (slide show) has been added by the editors as a supplement to the chapter. It was produced by My Dental Hub as a patient education tool and covers the basic elements in a conceptual manner. It is not intended to be a procedural guide for dental professionals.

GENERAL PRINCIPLES OF IMPLANT SURGERY

Patient Preparation

Most implant surgical procedures can be done in the office using local anesthesia. Conscious sedation (oral or intravenous) may be indicated for some patients. The risks and benefits of implant surgery specific to the patient's situation and needs should be thoroughly explained prior to surgery. A written, informed consent should be obtained for the procedure.

Implant Site Preparation

Some basic principles must be followed to achieve osseointegration with a high degree of predictability (Box 57.1).[3,4,7] The surgical site should be kept aseptic, and the patient should be appropriately prepared and draped for an intraoral surgical procedure. Prerinsing with chlorhexidine gluconate for 1 to 2 minutes immediately before the procedure will aid in reducing the bacterial load present around the surgical site. Every effort should be made to maintain a sterile surgical field and to avoid contamination of the implant surface. Implant sites should be prepared using gentle, atraumatic surgical techniques with an effort to avoid overheating the bone.

Successful osseointegration occurs predictably for submerged[4] and nonsubmerged[11] dental implants when proven clinical guidelines are followed. Well-controlled studies of patients with good plaque control and appropriate occlusal forces have demonstrated that root form, endosseous dental implants show little change in bone height around the implant over years of function.[1] After initial bone remodeling in the first year (1 to 1.5 mm of resorption described as "normal remodeling around an externally hexed implant"),[1] the bone level around healthy functioning implants remains stable for many years afterward. The average annual crestal bone loss after the first year in function is expected to be 0.1 mm or less. Hence, implants offer a predictable solution for tooth replacement.

BOX 57.1 Basic Principles of Implant Therapy to Achieve Osseointegration

1. Implants must be sterile and made of a biocompatible material (e.g., titanium).
2. Implant site should be prepared under sterile conditions.
3. Implant site should be prepared with an atraumatic surgical technique that avoids overheating of the bone during preparation of the recipient site.
4. Implants should be placed with good initial stability.
5. Implants should be allowed to heal without loading or micromovement (i.e., undisturbed healing period to allow for osseointegration) for 2–4 or 4–6 months, depending on the bone density, bone maturation, and implant stability.

Fig. 57.1 One-Stage Implant Versus Two-Stage Implant Surgeries. (A) One-stage surgery with the implant designed so that the coronal portion of the implant extends through the gingiva. (B) One-stage surgery with implant designed to be used for two-stage surgery. A healing abutment is connected to the implant during the first-stage surgery. (C) In the two-stage surgery, the top of the implant is completely submerged under gingiva.

Regardless of the surgical approach, the implant must be placed in healthy bone with good primary stability to achieve osseointegration, and an atraumatic technique must be followed to avoid damage to bone. Drilling of the bone without adequate cooling generates excessive heat, which injures bone and increases the risk of failure.[12] The anatomic features of bone quality (dense compact versus loose trabecular) at the recipient site influences the interface between bone and implant.[9] Compact bone offers a much greater surface area for bone-to-implant contact than cancellous bone. Areas of the jaw exhibiting thin layers of cortical bone and large cancellous spaces, such as the posterior maxilla, have lower success rates than areas of dense bone.[9] The best results are achieved when the bone-to-implant contact is intimate at the time of implant placement.

One-Stage Versus Two-Stage Implant Placement Surgery

Currently, most threaded endosseous implants can be placed using either a one-stage (nonsubmerged) or a two-stage (submerged) protocol. In the one-stage approach, the implant or the abutment emerges through the mucoperiosteum/gingival tissue at the time of implant placement, whereas in the two-stage approach, the top of the implant and cover screw are completely covered with the flap closure (Fig. 57.1). Implants are allowed to heal, without loading or micromovement, for a period of

time to allow for osseointegration. In two-stage implant surgery, the implant must be surgically exposed following a healing period. Some implants, referred to as "tissue level," are specifically designed with the coronal portion of the implant positioned above the crest of bone and extending through the gingival tissues at the time of placement in a one-stage protocol (see Fig. 57.1A). Other implant systems, referred to as "bone level," are designed to be placed at the level of bone and require a healing abutment to be attached to the implant at the time of placement to be used in a one-stage approach (see Fig. 57.1B).[8]

A one-stage surgical approach simplifies the procedure because a second-stage exposure surgery is not necessary. The two-stage, submerged approach is advantageous for situations that require simultaneous bone augmentation procedures at the time of implant placement because membranes can be submerged, which will minimize postoperative exposure. Mucogingival tissues can be augmented if desired at the second-stage surgery in a two-stage protocol or as part of the one-stage protocol. Fundamental differences in flap management for these two surgical techniques are described separately.

TWO-STAGE "SUBMERGED" IMPLANT PLACEMENT

In the two-stage implant surgical approach, the first-stage or implant placement surgery ends by suturing the soft tissues together over the implant cover screw so that it remains submerged and isolated from the oral cavity. In areas with dense cortical bone and good initial implant support, the implants are left to heal undisturbed for a period of 2 to 4 months, whereas in areas of loose trabecular bone, grafted sites, and sites with lesser implant stability, implants may be allowed to heal for periods of 4 to 6 months or more. Longer healing periods are indicated for implants in sites with less bone support. During healing, osteoblasts migrate to the surface and form bone adjacent to the implant (osseointegration).[6] Shorter healing periods are indicated for implants placed in good-quality (dense) bone and for implants with an altered surface microtopography (e.g., acid etched, blasted, or etched and blasted). Readers are referred to online material and other resources for more information about implant surface microtopography.

In the second-stage (exposure) surgery, the implant is uncovered and a healing abutment is connected to allow emergence of the abutment through the soft tissues. Once healed, the restorative dentist then proceeds with the prosthodontic aspects of the implant therapy (impressions and fabrication of prosthesis).

The following paragraphs describe the steps for osteotomy preparation and the first-stage implant placement surgery of the two-stage protocol. Figs. 57.2 and 57.3 illustrate the procedures via diagrams, and Fig. 57.4 depicts the procedures with clinical photographs.

Flap Design, Incisions, and Elevation

Flap management for implant surgery varies slightly, depending on the location and objective of the planned surgery. There are different incision/flap designs, but the most common is the crestal flap design. The incision is made along the crest of

Fig. 57.2 Tissue Management for a Two-Stage Implant Placement. (A) Crestal incision is made along the crest of the ridge, bisecting the existing zone of keratinized mucosa. (B) Full-thickness flap is raised buccally and lingually to the level of the mucogingival junction. A narrow, sharp ridge can be surgically reduced/contoured to provide a reasonably flat bed for the implant. (C) Implant is placed in the prepared osteotomy site. (D) Tissue approximation achieves primary flap closure without tension.

the ridge, bisecting the existing zone of keratinized mucosa (see Figs. 57.2A and 57.4B).

A remote incision with a layered suturing technique may be used to minimize the incidence of bone graft exposure when extensive bone augmentation is planned. The crestal incision, however, is preferred in most cases, because closure is easier to manage and typically results in less bleeding, less edema, and faster healing.[10] A full-thickness flap is raised (buccal and lingual) up to or slightly beyond the level of the mucogingival junction, exposing the alveolar ridge of the implant surgical sites (see Figs. 57.2B and 57.4C).

Implant Site Preparation

Once the flaps are reflected and the bone is prepared (i.e., all granulation tissue removed and knife-edge ridges flattened), the implant osteotomy site can be prepared. A series of drills are used to prepare the osteotomy site precisely and incrementally for an implant (Fig. 57.5). A surgical guide or stent is inserted, checked for proper positioning, and used throughout the procedure to direct the proper implant placement (see Fig. 57.4E).

Round Bur

A small round bur (or spiral drill) is used to make the initial penetration into bone for the implant site. The surgical guide

is removed, and the initial marks are checked for their appropriate buccal-lingual and mesial-distal location, as well as the positions relative to each other and adjacent teeth. Slight modifications may be necessary to adjust spatial relationships and to avoid minor ridge defects. Any changes should be compared with the prosthetically driven surgical guide positions. Each marked site is then prepared to a depth of 1 to 2 mm with a round drill, breaking through the cortical bone and creating a starting point for the 2-mm twist drill (see Fig. 57.3A).

The 2-mm Twist Drill

A small twist drill, usually 2 mm in diameter and marked to indicate various lengths (i.e., corresponding to the implant sizes), is used next to establish the depth and align the long axis of the implant recipient site (see Fig. 57.3B). This drill may be externally or internally irrigated. In either case, the twist drill is used at a speed of approximately 800 to 1500 rpm, with copious irrigation to prevent overheating of the bone. Additionally, drills should be intermittently and repeatedly "pumped" or pulled out of the osteotomy site while drilling to expose them to the water coolant and to facilitate clearing bone debris from the cutting surfaces. In other words, clinicians should pump the drill (up and down) intermittently and avoid using a constant "push" of the drill in the apical direction only.

When multiple implants are being placed next to one another, a guide pin should be placed in the prepared sites to check alignment, parallelism, and proper prosthetic spacing throughout the preparation process (see Fig. 57.3C). The relationship to neighboring vital structures (e.g., nerve and tooth roots) can be determined by taking a periapical radiograph with a guide pin or radiographic marker in the osteotomy site (see Chapter 56). Implants should be positioned with approximately 3 mm between one another to ensure sufficient space for interimplant bone and soft-tissue health and to facilitate oral hygiene procedures. Therefore the initial marks should be separated by at least 7 mm (center to center) for 4 mm standard-diameter implants. Incrementally more space is needed for wide-diameter implants (see Chapter 56).

The 2-mm twist drill is used to establish the final depth of the osteotomy site corresponding to the length of each planned implant. The clinician should also evaluate the bone quality (density) with this drill while preparing the osteotomy to assess the need for modifying subsequent drills used (eBox 57.1). If the vertical height of the bone was reduced during the initial ridge preparation, this must be taken into account when preparing the site for a predetermined implant length. For example, if it appears that the implant will be too close to a vital structure, such as the inferior alveolar nerve canal, the depth of the implant osteotomy site and length of the implant may need to be reduced.

The next step is to use a series of drills to incrementally increase the width of the osteotomy site to accommodate the planned implant diameter. The styles, shapes, and final diameter of the drills will differ slightly among different implant systems, but their general purpose is to prepare a recipient site with a precise diameter (and depth) for the selected implant without unduly traumatizing the surrounding bone. It is important to use copious irrigation and a "pumping" action for all drilling.

Fig. 57.3 Implant Site Preparation (Osteotomy) for a 4-mm Diameter, 10-mm Length Screw-Type, Threaded (External Hex) Implant in a Subcrestal Position. (A) Initial marking or preparation of the implant site with a round bur. (B) Use of a 2-mm twist drill to establish depth and align the implant. (C) Guide pin is placed in the osteotomy site to confirm position and angulation. (D) Pilot drill is used to increase the diameter of the coronal aspect of the osteotomy site. (E) Final drill used is the 3-mm twist drill to finish preparation of the osteotomy site. (F) Countersink drill is used to widen the entrance of the recipient site and allow for the subcrestal placement of the implant collar and cover screw. Note: An optional tap (not shown) can be used following this step to create screw threads in areas of dense bone. (G) Implant is inserted into the prepared osteotomy site with a handpiece or handheld driver. Note: In systems that use an implant mount, it is removed prior to placement of the cover screw. (H) The cover screw is placed and soft tissues are closed and sutured.

KEY FACT

A series of drills will be used (speeds determined by manufacturer) sequentially to prepare osteotomy sites. It is essential to prepare sites with copious irrigation to prevent overheating of the bone. Additionally, drills should be intermittently and repeatedly "pumped" or pulled out of the osteotomy site while drilling to expose them to the water coolant and to facilitate clearing bone debris from the cutting surfaces.

Fig. 57.4 Clinical View of Stage-One Implant Placement Surgery. (A) Partial edentulous ridge; presurgical and prosthodontic treatment has been completed. (B) Mesial sulcular and distal vertical incisions are connected by a crestal incision. Notice that bands of gingival collars remain adjacent to the distal molar tooth. (C) Minimal flap reflection is used to expose the alveolar bone. Sometimes a ridge modification is necessary to provide a flap recipient bed. (D) Buccal flap is partially dissected at the apical portion to provide a flap extension. This is a critical step to ensure a tension-free closure of the flap after implant placement. (E) It is important to use the surgical stent to determine the mesial-distal and buccal-lingual dimensions and proper angulation of the implant placement. (F) Frequent use of the guide pins ensures parallelism of the implant placement. (G) After placement of two Nobelpharma implants, the cover screws are placed. The cover screws should be flush with the rest of the ridge to minimize the chance of exposure. This is especially important if the patient will wear a partial denture during the healing phase. (H) Suturing completed. Both regular interrupted and inverted mattress sutures are used intermittently to ensure tension-free, tight closure of the flaps.

Fig. 57.5 Sequence of Drills Used for Standard-Diameter (4-mm) Implant Site Osteotomy Preparation: Round, 2-mm Twist, Pilot, 3-mm Twist, and Countersink. Bone tap (not shown here) is an optional drill that is sometimes used in dense bone before implant placement.

Pilot Drill

Following the 2-mm twist drill, a pilot drill with a noncutting 2-mm–diameter "guide" at the apical end and a cutting 3-mm–diameter (wider) midsection is used to enlarge the osteotomy site at the coronal end, thus facilitating the insertion of the subsequent drill in the sequence (see Fig. 57.3D).

The 3-mm Twist Drill

The final drill in the osteotomy site preparation for a standard-diameter (4 mm) implant is the 3-mm twist drill. It is the last drill used to widen the site along the entire depth of the osteotomy from the previous diameter (2 mm) to final diameter (3 mm). This final drill in the sequence finishes preparing the osteotomy site and consequently is the step that dictates whether the implant will be stable or not (see Fig. 57.3E). It is critically important that the final diameter drilling be accomplished with a steady hand, without wobbling or changing direction so that the site is not overprepared. Finally, depending on bone density, the diameter of this final drill may be slightly increased or decreased to enhance implant support (see eBox 57.1).

The reader is referred to the online material for information on optional countersinking and bone tapping procedures, prior to implant placement. Online materials for this chapter are found on the companion website.

Implant Placement

Implants are inserted with a handpiece rotating at slow speeds (e.g., 25 rpm) or by hand with a wrench. Insertion of the implant must follow the same path or line as the osteotomy site. When multiple implants are being placed, it is helpful to use guide pins in the other sites to have a visual guide for the path of insertion.

Flap Closure and Suturing

Once the implants are inserted and the cover screws secured (see Fig. 57.4G), the surgical sites should be thoroughly irrigated with sterile saline to remove debris and clean the wound. Proper closure of the flap over the implant is essential. One of the most important aspects of flap management is achieving good approximation and primary closure of the tissues in a tension-free manner (see Fig. 57.3H). This is achieved by incising the periosteum (innermost layer of full-thickness flap), which is nonelastic. Once the periosteum is released, the flap becomes very elastic and is able to be stretched over the implant without tension. One suturing technique that consistently provides the desired result is a combination of alternating horizontal mattress and interrupted sutures (see Fig. 57.4H).

The clinician should choose an appropriate suture for the given patient and procedure. For patient management, it is sometimes simpler to use a resorbable suture that does not require removal during the postoperative visit (e.g., 4-0 chromic gut suture). However, when moderate-to-severe postoperative swelling is anticipated, a nonresorbable suture is recommended to maintain a longer closure period (e.g., 4-0 monofilament suture). These sutures require removal at a postoperative visit.

Postoperative Care

Simple implant surgery in a healthy patient usually does not require antibiotic therapy. However, antibiotics (e.g., amoxicillin, 500 mg three times a day [tid]) can be prescribed if the surgery is extensive or if the patient is medically compromised. Postoperative swelling is likely after flap surgery. This is particularly true when the periosteum has been incised (released). As a preventive measure, patients should apply cold packs over the first 24 to 48 hours. Chlorhexidine gluconate oral rinses can be prescribed to facilitate plaque control, especially in the days after surgery when oral hygiene is typically poorer. Adequate pain medication should be prescribed (e.g., ibuprofen, 600 to 800 mg tid).

Patients should be instructed to maintain a relatively soft diet after surgery. Then, as healing progresses, they can gradually return to a normal diet. Patients should also refrain from tobacco and alcohol use after surgery. Provisional restorations, whether fixed or removable, should be checked and adjusted to minimize trauma to the surgical area.

The reader is referred to the online material for information on second-stage implant exposure surgery. Online materials for this chapter are found on the companion website.

ONE-STAGE "NONSUBMERGED" IMPLANT PLACEMENT

In the one-stage implant surgical approach, a second implant exposure surgery is not needed because the implant is exposed (per gingival) from the time of implant placement (Fig. 57.6). In the standard (classic) implant protocol, the implants are left unloaded and undisturbed for a period similar to that for implants placed in the two-stage approach (i.e., in areas with dense cortical bone and good initial implant support, the implants are left to heal undisturbed for a period of 2 to 4 months, whereas in areas of loose trabecular bone, grafted sites, or minimal implant support, they may be allowed to heal for periods of 4 to 6 months or more).

Fig. 57.6 Tissue Management for a One-Stage Implant Placement. (A) Crestal incision made along the crest of the ridge, bisecting the existing zone of keratinized mucosa. (B) Full-thickness flap is raised buccally and lingually to the level of the mucogingival junction. A narrow, sharp ridge can be surgically reduced or contoured to provide a reasonably flat bed for the implant. (C) Implant is placed in the prepared osteotomy site. (D) Tissues are adapted around the neck of the implant to achieve flap closure with the implant protruding through the soft tissues.

In the one-stage surgical approach, the implant or the healing abutment protrudes approximately 2 to 3 mm from the bone crest, and the flaps are adapted around the implant/abutment. As with the second-stage surgical procedures described, the soft tissues may be thinned, repositioned, or augmented at the implant placement surgery to increase the zone of keratinized tissue surrounding the implant.

Flap Design, Incisions, and Elevation

The flap design for the one-stage surgical approach is always a crestal incision bisecting the existing keratinized tissue (see Fig. 57.6). Vertical incisions may be needed at one or both ends to facilitate access to the bone or osteotomy site. Tissues can be thinned in posterior areas if desired but are generally not thinned in anterior aesthetic areas. Full-thickness flaps are elevated facially and lingually.

Implant Site Preparation

Implant site preparation for the one-stage approach is identical in principle to the two-stage implant surgical approach. The primary difference is that the coronal aspect of the implant or the healing abutment (two-stage implant) is placed approximately 2 to 3 mm above the bone crest and the soft tissues are approximated around the implant/implant abutment.

Flap Closure and Suturing

The keratinized edges of the flap are sutured with single interrupted sutures around the implant. Depending on the clinician's preference, the wound may be sutured with resorbable or nonresorbable sutures. When keratinized tissue is abundant, scalloping around the implant provides better flap adaptation.

Postoperative Care

The postoperative care for the one-stage surgical approach is similar to that for the two-stage surgical approach except that the cover screw or healing abutment is exposed to the oral cavity. Patients are advised to avoid chewing in the area of the implant. Prosthetic appliances should not be used if direct chewing forces can be transmitted to the implant, particularly in the early healing period (first 4 to 8 weeks). When removable prosthetic appliances are used, they should be adequately relieved and a soft-tissue liner should be applied.

CONCLUSION

It is essential to understand the basic guidelines to predictably achieve osseointegration. Fundamental protocols must be followed for implant placement (stage one) and implant exposure surgery (stage two). These fundamentals apply to all implant systems.

A Case Scenario is found on the companion website www.expertconsult.com.

REFERENCES

 References for this chapter are found on the companion website www.expertconsult.com.

58

Implant-Related Complications and Failures[a]

Content on complications related to augmentation procedures and to placement and loading protocols can be accessed on the companion website.

The successful use of osseointegrated dental implants has dramatically changed dentistry and significantly improved dentists' ability to provide tooth replacement options for patients.[3,92] Despite implants' long-term predictability and success, implant-related complications and failures happen in some cases.[4,24] Complications can be surgical, biologic, mechanical, or aesthetic. Some complications are relatively minor and easy to manage, whereas others are more significant and challenging to resolve. The most serious complications can result in failure of prostheses, loss of implants, and severe loss of supporting bone.

Surgical complications are those problems or adverse outcomes that result from surgery, including procedures used for implant site development, implant placement, implant exposure, and tissue augmentation. Implant complications commonly arise from placement of an implant in a nonideal position. Malpositioned implants, which normally result from poor preoperative treatment planning or errors in surgical technique, can lead to an array of implant problems ranging in severity from minor to major. Surgical complications include compromised aesthetic and prosthetic results, soft-tissue and bone dehiscences, impingement on and damage to anatomic structures, and implant failure. Unfortunately, the problems that arise from implant malposition are often not recognized until after osseointegration, when the prosthesis is being fabricated.

Biologic complications involve the hard and soft tissues that support the implant. Peri-implant tissue changes can be limited to inflammation of surrounding soft tissues or be more significant, such as progressive loss of supporting bone. The ultimate biologic complication is implant loss or failure, which can produce soft- and hard-tissue defects. Loss of implants can be caused by failure to achieve osseointegration in the early stages before restoration or by loss of osseointegration as a result of destruction of supporting bone after the restoration is installed and functioning.

Prosthetic or *mechanical complications* and failures typically occur in the form of material failure, such as abutment and prosthetic screw loosening or fractures. The prosthesis can be rescued from many mechanical problems if they are minor and recognized early. However, some complications, such as implant fractures, are devastating and not salvageable.

Aesthetic complications arise when the patient's expectations are not met. Satisfaction with the aesthetic outcome of the implant prosthesis varies from patient to patient. The risk of aesthetic complications is increased among patients with high aesthetic expectations and suboptimal patient-related factors, such as a high smile line, thin gingival tissues, or inadequate bone quantity and quality.

This chapter reviews common implant-related complications. A summary of the literature offers some insight into the prevalence of implant-related complications. Implant failure and surgical complications related to site development and variations in implant placement protocols are discussed.

DEFINITIONS OF IMPLANT SURVIVAL AND SUCCESS

The criteria used to define and report implant success or failure can vary substantially among publications. Selection of success criteria can be based on the author's preference, study population, or some other study objective. Because the level of success reported in an article is based on the criteria used to define success, recognizing the tremendous variation in the way investigators measure and interpret success is crucial. Sometimes, outcomes are measured by the presence or absence of implants

---

[a]Adapted from the following chapter of Newman and Carranza's Clinical Periodontology, 13th edition: Chapter 85: Implant-Related Complications and Failures, by Stuart J. Froum, Perry R. Klokkevold, Sang Choon Cho, and Scott H. Froum.

at the time of the last examination, which is a measure only of implant survival and should not be confused with implant success. In contrast to this simplified reporting, some investigators use detailed criteria to measure implant success and failure, with variations of successful outcomes separated and defined by additional criteria.

Implant survival is defined as an implant that remains in place at the time of evaluation, regardless of any untoward signs, symptoms, or history of problems. There is a difference between implants that are functioning under an implant-retained restoration and those that are not connected to a restoration and not providing support or function. These implants are sometimes referred to as *sleepers*, and they should not be considered successful merely because they remain osseointegrated. Sleeper implants instead should be included in the discussion as surviving but counted as *failures* because they did not fulfill the originally intended treatment objective.

Implant success is defined by the presence of the implant and the criteria evaluating its condition and function at the time of examination. Various criteria for implant success and failure have been published, but not all investigators agree with or use them. In the classic definition, Albrektsson and colleagues[6] defined success as an implant with no pain, no mobility, no radiolucent peri-implant areas, and no more than 0.2 mm of bone loss annually after the first year of loading. Roos-Jansaker and associates[125] added to this by defining a successful implant as one that loses no more than 1 mm of bone during the first year of function.

Sometimes, the criteria are used as proposed, but in other cases, they are used by investigators with modifications and additional criteria. This makes it difficult to compare studies and draw conclusions about any aspect of implant success or failure based on one or a few studies.

Strictly defined, implant success is any implant-retained restoration in which (1) the original treatment plan is performed as intended without complications, (2) all implants that were placed remain stable and functioning without problems, (3) the peri-implant hard and soft tissues are healthy, and (4) the patient and treating clinicians are pleased with the results. When these strict criteria are used, the rate of implant success (i.e., absence of complications) is only approximately 61% after 5 years for implant-supported fixed partial dentures (FPDs) and 50% after 10 years for combined tooth-implant FPDs.[90]

An additional criterion of implant success that is not typically reported but should be considered is the aesthetic success or patient satisfaction with the outcome.

> ## KEY FACT
>
> *Implant survival* indicates that the implant has become osseointegrated but does not consider associated problems. An implant that is not restored can be included in survival percentages while failing to fulfill its intended purpose. *Implant success* is defined by criteria evaluating the condition and function of the implant. Because different criteria have been used to define implant success, it is difficult to make comparisons between studies and often impossible to make conclusions about implant success or failure based on only one or a few studies.

TYPES AND PREVALENCE OF IMPLANT COMPLICATIONS

The prevalence of implant-related complications has been reported in several reviews. However, a systematic review of the incidence of complications in studies of at least 5 years revealed that biologic complications were considered in only 40% to 60% and technical complications in only 60% to 80% of the studies. The review found that the incidence of technical complications related to implant components and suprastructures was higher for overdentures than for fixed restorations.[21]

In a systematic review of reports on the survival and complication rates of implant-supported FPDs, Lang and associates[90] found that the most common technical complication was fracture of veneers (13.2% after 5 years), followed by loss of the screw access hole restoration (8.2% after 5 years), abutment or occlusal screw loosening (5.8% after 5 years), and abutment or occlusal screw fracture (1.5% after 5 years and 2.5% after 10 years). Implant fracture is also a significant yet uncommon complication. Goodacre and colleagues[63] reported a 1.5% incidence in their literature review. The incidence of implant fracture was higher in FPDs supported by only two implants. Consistent with this finding, Rangert and coworkers[120] reported that most implant fractures occurred in single- and double-implant–supported restorations. They also found that most of these fractures were in posterior partially edentulous segments, in which the generated occlusal forces can be greater than in anterior segments (Fig. 58.1).

A critical review of the literature by Esposito and associates[54] included 73 publications reporting early and late failures of Brånemark implants; biologically related implant failures were relatively low at 7.7%. Treatments involved all anatomic areas and all types of prosthetic design. The study authors concluded that the predictability of implant treatment was especially good for partially edentulous patients compared with totally edentulous patients; failures in the latter population were twice as high as those in the other group. The incidence of implant failure was three times higher for the edentulous maxilla than for the edentulous mandible, whereas failure rates for the partially edentulous maxilla were similar to those for the partially edentulous mandible.

Risk factors such as smoking, diabetes, and periodontal disease can contribute to implant failure and complications. Several studies with numerous implants and years of follow-up have concluded that smoking is a definite risk factor for implant survival.[12,43,44,48,108] A systematic review of the effect of risk factors on implant outcomes concluded that smoking had an adverse effect on implant survival and success; the effects were more pronounced in areas of loose trabecular bone (i.e., posterior maxilla).[85] The review suggested that type 2 diabetes could have an adverse effect on implant survival rates but did not have enough studies to permit a definitive conclusion.[85] The same review concluded that although patients with a history of treated periodontitis did not show a decrease in implant survival, they did experience more biologic implant complications and lower success rates, especially with longer-term follow-up.[85]

Fig. 58.1 (A) Radiograph of a three-unit, posterior, fixed partial denture supported by two standard-diameter, screw-shaped threaded implants. Notice the long crown height, relatively short implant length, and bone loss around the posterior implant. (B) Photograph of the ultimate implant-supported restoration failure. The anterior implant fractured between the second and third threads, which resulted in loss of the restoration.

TYPES OF DENTAL IMPLANTS

Analysis of the data on the prevalence of implant complications (i.e., failure, fracture, and peri-implantitis) in published systematic reviews should consider the fact that many of these studies reported on implants with earlier designs (i.e., machined surfaces and external connections). Most current implant systems feature surfaces with an altered microtopography (i.e., rough), and many have internal connections. The prevalence and type of complications associated with the newer implant designs may be different.

Many modifications have been developed to try to improve the long-term success rates of implants. More than 1300 types of dental implants are available with different materials, shapes, sizes, lengths, and surface characteristics or coatings. Although it has been suggested that machined surfaces are more resistant to plaque accumulation and peri-implantitis, there is limited evidence to show that implants with relatively smooth surfaces (i.e., machined) are less prone to bone loss from chronic infection than implants with rough surfaces. To date, there is no evidence showing that any particular type of dental implant has superior long-term success.[50]

Different implant designs and surfaces must be studied in prospective human trials over long periods. Until those data

become available, clinicians should be aware that historical data reporting success rates for earlier implant designs may not reflect the outcomes for current implants. Moreover, new implant surfaces and designs are commonly introduced with limited or no data available on potential complications.[a]

SURGICAL COMPLICATIONS

As with any surgical procedure, implant surgery has risks. Proper precautions must be taken to prevent injuries, including (1) a thorough review of the patient's medical history, (2) a comprehensive clinical and radiographic examination, (3) establishment of a comprehensive interdisciplinary treatment plan, and (4) good surgical techniques.

Surgical complications include perilous bleeding, damage to adjacent structures such as teeth, injury to nerves, and iatrogenic jaw fracture. Postoperative complications include bleeding, hematoma, and infection. They may be minor, transient, and easily managed or more serious and require postoperative treatment.

More information on hemorrhage and hematoma can be found in the expert consult version of the book. Online materials for this chapter are found on the companion website.

CLINICAL CORRELATION

Although the incidence of a life-threatening hemorrhage from implant surgery is extremely low, it is a serious problem that can occur. Implant surgical procedures in the anterior mandible have been associated with potentially fatal complications. Massive internal bleeding in the floor of the mouth from inadvertent injury to lingual arteries can cause an expanding hematoma that displaces the tongue and soft tissues, obstructing the upper airway. Emergency treatment includes airway management and surgical intervention to isolate and stop the bleeding. Clinicians must be aware of this risk and be prepared to act quickly.

Neurosensory Disturbances

One of the more problematic surgical complications is an injury to nerves. Neurosensory alterations caused by damage to a nerve can be temporary or permanent. Neuropathy can be caused by a drilling injury (i.e., cut, tear, or puncture of the nerve) or by implant compression or damage to the nerve (Fig. 58.2). In either case, the injury causes neuroma formation, and two patterns of clinical neuropathy may follow. *Hypoesthesia* is a neuropathy defined by impaired sensory function that is sometimes associated with phantom pain. *Hyperesthesia* is a neuropathy defined by pain with minimal or no sensory impairment.[65] Some neuropathies resolve, whereas others persist. The type of neuropathy does not indicate the potential for recovery.

Implant Malposition

Many of the complications that arise during implant surgery can be attributed to the dental implant being placed in an

---

[a]References 7, 9, 34, 45, 114, 115, 141, 144, 157.

Fig. 58.2 (A) Cross-sectional computed tomography (CT) image shows the implant impinging on the inferior alveolar nerve canal. (B) Panoramic CT scan shows the implant in the lower left first molar area impinging on the inferior alveolar nerve canal. The nerve is marked by tracing with software.

Fig. 58.3 Radiograph of Two Mandibular Anterior Implants Placed Too Close Together (i.e., no proximal space), Resulting in Implants That Are Impossible to Restore.

undesired or unintended position. Malpositioning of dental implants is usually the result of poor treatment planning before surgery, lack of surgical skill, or poor communication between the implant surgeon and the restorative dentist. Optimal implant aesthetics and the avoidance of positional complications can be achieved by placing the implant in a prosthetically driven manner.[99,113] The implant should be placed with reference to the three dimensions dictated by the position of the final restoration and not by the availability of bone.

The implant should be placed at a distance of 1.5 to 2 mm from an adjacent natural tooth and 2 to 3 mm from an adjacent implant to maintain an adequate biologic dimension.[67] Similar to natural teeth, violation of biologic width around an implant can lead to bone loss.[71] Implants that are placed too close to each other (Fig. 58.3) or to natural teeth can be difficult to restore. Impression copings and impression-taking techniques must be modified. Improperly spaced implants invariably lead to chronic inflammation and peri-implantitis.[49,147] Conversely, an implant placed at an excessive distance from an adjacent tooth or implant may require prosthetic compensation in the form of mesial or distal cantilevers, which can predispose the implant to biologic (i.e., bone loss) and mechanical (i.e., screw loosening,[64] screw fracture,[145] and implant fracture[120]) complications and difficulties with hygiene.[147]

Ideally, an implant should be placed buccolingually so there is at least 2 mm of bone circumferentially around it.[140] Implant exposure through the lingual or buccal cortex can predispose an individual to abscess and suppuration.[32] Implants that are placed too palatally or lingually require prosthetic compensation in the form of a buccal ridge lap, which may be difficult for the patient to clean and can lead to tissue inflammation.[20]

To obtain ideal aesthetics, avoid potential aesthetic complications, and correct bodily placement of the dental implant, it must be correctly angulated on insertion. In most anterior cases, it is desirable to have the long axis of the implant directed so it is emerging toward the cingulum. In the posterior region, the implant axis should be directed toward the central fossa or the stamp cusp of the opposing tooth. Implants that are placed with mild to moderate misangulations can often be corrected prosthetically with implant abutments. Minor misangulations (i.e., 15 to 20 degrees) can be corrected with prefabricated or customized angled abutments; moderate misangulations (i.e., 20 to 35 degrees) can usually be managed with customized UCLA-type abutments; and extreme errors in implant angulations (>35 degrees) may make an implant unrestorable and require it to be left submerged (i.e., a sleeper) or be removed (Fig. 58.4).

The ultimate complication of malpositioning is implant or instrument invasion into vital structures. The most common violation of neighboring anatomy is placement of the dental implant into the adjacent tooth root. Surgical procedures used to prepare osteotomy sites and place implants adjacent to teeth can injure them by directly cutting into the tooth structure or by damaging nearby supporting tissues and nerves. Instrumentation (e.g., drills) directed at or near the adjacent tooth can injure the periodontal ligament, tooth structure, and nerve of the tooth. Depending on the extent of the injury, the tooth can require endodontic therapy or extraction.

Fig. 58.4 Clinical Photograph of a Maxillary Anterior Implant (i.e., left central incisor) Placed With an Extreme Facial Angulation, Resulting in an Implant That Emerges Through the Gingiva at a Level That Is More Apical Than the Adjacent Natural Tooth Gingival Margins. (A) Surgical exposure of the malpositioned implant. (B) Surgically removed implant. (C) Alveolar defect resulting from surgical removal of the malpositioned implant.

KEY FACT

Malpositioned implants can be avoided by proper planning, good communication, and meticulous surgical skills. Radiographs taken periodically during implant surgery with guide pins in the osteotomy site can greatly reduce damage to adjacent teeth. Radiographic analysis before implant surgery should include detection of curved, convergent, or dilacerated root structures of adjacent teeth that can limit implant placement.

BIOLOGIC COMPLICATIONS

Biologic complications involve pathology of the surrounding peri-implant hard and soft tissues. Frequently, soft-tissue problems are an inflammatory response to bacterial accumulation around implants. Bacteria can accumulate at the junction of an ill-fitting implant–abutment or abutment–crown connection. Some of the highly textured, macroscopically rough implant surfaces (e.g., titanium plasma–sprayed [TPS] or hydroxyapatite [HA] coating) may also perpetuate the accumulation of bacteria on the implant surface.

Inflammation and Proliferation

Because inflammation of the peri-implant soft tissues is similar to the inflammatory response in gingival and other periodontal tissues, the clinical appearance also is similar. Inflamed

Fig. 58.5 Inflammatory Proliferation Caused by a Loose-Fitting Connection Between the Abutment and the Implant. (Courtesy Dr. John Beumer, UCLA Maxillofacial Prosthetics, Los Angeles, CA.)

peri-implant tissues demonstrate the same erythema, edema, and swelling around teeth. Occasionally, the reaction of peri-implant soft tissues to bacterial accumulation is profound and unusual, with dramatic inflammatory proliferation (Fig. 58.5). This type of lesion is somewhat characteristic around implants and indicates a loose-fitting implant-to-abutment connection or trapped excess cement that remains buried within the soft-tissue space (i.e., pocket).

Fig. 58.6 (A) Clinical photograph of an abscess caused by excess cement trapped within the soft tissues. (B) Radiograph of an implant with a cemented crown (same patient as in A). Notice the subgingival depth of the crown-abutment (cement line) junction, which is below the level of the adjacent interproximal bone and therefore impossible to adequately access with an explorer to remove the excess cement. (Courtesy Dr. John Beumer, UCLA Maxillofacial Prosthetics, Los Angeles, CA.)

Fig. 58.7 Fistula Caused by a Loose Implant-Abutment Connection (i.e., maxillary left lateral incisor).

The precipitating local factor ultimately becomes infected with bacterial pathogens, leading to mucosal hypertrophy or proliferation and possible abscess formation (Fig. 58.6). Correction of the precipitating factors (e.g., loose connection, excess cement) can effectively resolve the lesion. Another type of lesion resulting from a loose abutment connection is a fistula (Fig. 58.7), and correcting the etiologic factor can quickly resolve it.

Dehiscence and Recession

Dehiscence or recession of the peri-implant soft tissues occurs when support for the tissues is lacking or has been lost. Recession is a common finding after implant restoration and should be anticipated, especially when soft tissues are thin and not well supported (Fig. 58.8). Improper implant positioning also

predisposes peri-implant tissues to recession. Placement or angulation of the implant too far buccally causes the buccal plate to resorb, resulting in greater recession.[139]

However, peri-implant soft tissues depend entirely on the surrounding bone for support. Soft-tissue thickness accounts for some soft-tissue height, but there are no supracrestal inserting connective tissue fibers to aid the soft-tissue support around an implant. The soft-tissue height around implants is typically limited to approximately 3 or 4 mm, and bone loss around implants often leads to recession.

FLASH BACK

The peri-implant soft-tissue seal is weaker than the periodontal soft-tissue seal. The soft-tissue seal around implants depends on tissue thickness and a long junctional epithelial attachment with hemidesmosomes. It is inferior to the periodontal attachment around natural teeth because it lacks the inserting connective tissue fibers (i.e., Sharpey fibers) of the periodontium. Periodontal papillae and gingival margins are also supported at a higher supracrestal level compared with peri-implant soft tissues. Periodontal soft tissues are supported by circumferential and transseptal connective tissue fibers that insert into the cementum at a level that is more coronal than the supporting bone.

Peri-Implantitis and Bone Loss

Peri-implantitis is an inflammatory process that affects the tissues around an osseointegrated implant and results in the loss of supporting bone.[104] The reported prevalence of peri-implantitis varies from less than 7% to 37% of implants.[84] The variation can be attributed to differences in studied populations, length of follow-up time, implant variables, and the criteria used to

Fig. 58.8 (A) Clinical photograph of a single-tooth implant crown (maxillary right central) with moderate recession that occurred 1 year after the final restoration. In this case, recession most likely occurred because the labial bone around this wide-diameter implant was very thin or nonexistent. (B) Radiograph of a wide-diameter (6-mm) implant supporting a maxillary central incisor crown (same patient as in A).

Fig. 58.9 Moderately Advanced Bone Loss Around an Implant With the Typical Circumferential Trough Type of Bony Defect. (From Garg AK: *Implant dentistry: a practical approach*, ed 2, Mosby, St. Louis, 2010.)

Fig. 58.10 Severe Horizontal and Vertical Bone Loss Around Several Mandibular Implants.

define peri-implantitis.[87,126] Two systematic reviews concluded that peri-implantitis affected 10% of implants and 20% of patients during the 5 to 10 years after placement.[10,106]

Clinicians should monitor the surrounding tissues for signs of peri-implant disease by observing changes in probing depth and radiographic evidence of bone destruction, suppuration, calculus buildup, swelling, color changes, and bleeding.[105,110] Peri-implantitis can be perpetuated by bacterial infection that has contaminated a rough (e.g., TPS- or HA-coated) implant surface and by excessive biomechanical forces.[154,155] The classic trough-type defect is typically associated with peri-implantitis (Fig. 58.9). In cases with severely reduced bone support

extending into the apical half of the implant (Fig. 58.10) or in cases demonstrating mobility, implant removal should be considered.[6,109]

The number and distribution of implants and the occlusal relationships influence the biomechanical forces applied to implants.[119,122] A review by Lindhe and Meyle from the Consensus Report of the Sixth European Workshop on Periodontology concluded that risk indicators for peri-implantitis included (1) poor oral hygiene, (2) a history of periodontitis, (3) diabetes, (4) cigarette smoking, (5) alcohol consumption, and (6) implant surface.[94] Risk factors 1 to 4 have been recognized and reported in the literature.[85] The report suggests that although data for

Fig. 58.11 (A) Radiograph of an early failed implant caused by lack of osseointegration. In addition to the crestal bone loss, notice the radiolucency along the sides of the implant. (B) Photograph of the failed (nonintegrated) implant (shown in A) that was easily removed along with surrounding connective tissue.

Fig. 58.12 A Four-Unit Fixed Partial Denture in the Posterior Maxilla Was Supported by Only Two Implants. (A) Clinical photograph of implant abutments in the posterior maxilla. (B) Radiograph taken 30 months after restoration. Notice the bone loss around the distal implant. (C) Failed distal implant attached to a failed prosthesis. The biologic failure of one (posterior) implant resulted in a long-span cantilever extension from the other (anterior) implant that ultimately led to its mechanical failure (i.e., abutment screw fracture). (Courtesy Dr. John Beumer, UCLA Maxillofacial Prosthetics, Los Angeles, CA.)

risk factors 5 and 6 are limited, they appear to be relevant to peri-implantitis.[94] One study found little evidence to support smoking as a risk factor for peri-implantitis.[135] Another proposed risk factor involves individual genetic polymorphisms.[28,89] More research is needed to study the relation of this risk factor to the development of peri-implantitis.

Risk factors, including excess and retained cement, have been implicated in peri-implantitis. One article said that excess dental cement was associated with signs of peri-implant disease in 81% of cases evaluated using a dental endoscope.[153] The radiopacity of some commonly used cements affects their detectability.[149] This emphasizes the importance of proper cementation, use of screw-retained rather than cemented restorations when possible, and careful clinical examination after final crown cementation on implants.

Implant Loss or Failure

Implant loss or failure is considered relative to the time of placement or restoration. Early implant failures occur before implant restoration. Late implant failures occur after the implant has been restored. When an implant fails before restoration, it probably did not achieve osseointegration, or the integration was weak or jeopardized by infection, movement, or impaired wound healing (Fig. 58.11). Late implant failures occur after prosthesis installation for a variety of reasons, including infection and implant overload (Fig. 58.12). In a review of the literature to evaluate biologic causes for implant failure, Esposito and colleagues[53] found that infections, impaired healing, and overload were the most important contributing factors. Two systematic reviews of the literature concluded that a single dose of

preoperative antibiotic therapy could decrease the failure rate of dental implants.[51,136]

A review of the reasons for failure of oral implants concluded that several situations increased the failure rate: a low insertion torque on immediately placed or early loaded implants, inexperienced surgeons, implants inserted in the maxilla and posterior regions of the jaws, implants placed in heavy smokers, implant insertion in poor-quality (i.e., type III and IV) bone, lack of initial stability, and prosthetic rehabilitation with implant-supported overdentures.[33]

The risk of implant failure varies among patients, but patterns of loss tend to cluster. A second attempt at dental implant placement should be approached cautiously if placing the implant in the same site as the one that previously failed. It is often challenging to achieve adequate diameter, length, and stability of replacement implants due to the residual defect created by removal of the failed implant. In 2007, Grossmann and Levin reported an overall survival rate of 71% for dental implants that were placed in sites of previously failed single implants. In that study, all of the original implants failed during the early healing phase (mean of 2.3 to 3.2 months after placement).[66] In a 2008 study, Machtei and colleagues[96] reported an overall survival rate of 83.5% for the second attempt at dental implants. They concluded that replacing failed implants resulted in a lower survival rate compared with that for implants placed in pristine sites. This could not be associated with conventional implant- or patient-related factors. They suggested that a site-specific negative effect might be associated with this phenomenon.[96]

In 2011, Machtei and coworkers reported a lower survival rate (60%) for third reimplanted sites.[95] This outcome represents a further diminished prognosis compared with implants in original sites or after a second attempt.[36] Replacement of a failed implant poses a challenge in achieving osseointegration in a healed bone site and can reduce the implant survival rate.[95]

More information on complications related to surgical procedures can be found in the expert consult version of the book. Online materials for this chapter are found on the companion website.

Another method of sinus elevation and bone augmentation involves the use of osteotomes. This technique is indicated when there is enough native bone to stabilize the implant and a minimal need for sinus floor elevation. Bone is added through the crestal osteotomy by means of osteotomes and a mallet, the floor of the sinus is fractured, and the schneiderian membrane is lifted by the bone graft. This method is thought to be a relatively less invasive technique of great utility in certain patients. However, it has been associated with the complication of benign paroxysmal positional vertigo (BPPV),[116] which is a consequence of working the implant bed with osteotomes. During the osteotomy preparation and sinus floor elevation using the osteotome technique, the trauma induced by percussion with the surgical hammer, along with hyperextension of the neck during the operation, can displace otoliths in the inner ear and induce BPPV. It has been reported that 1.25% of the patients treated suffered vertigo when trying to sit up immediately after surgery and were diagnosed with BPPV. Because implant treatment is increasingly being carried out on older patients and because of the widespread use of bone expansion technique with osteotomes, the incidence of BPPV can be expected to increase.[117] In suspected cases of BPPV, the patient should be informed about the condition and then referred to an otoneurologic specialist to determine which semicircular canal is affected and to carry out the appropriate otolithic reinstatement maneuver.

PROSTHETIC OR MECHANICAL COMPLICATIONS

Prosthetic or mechanical complications occur when the strength of materials is no longer able to resist the forces that are being applied. As materials fatigue, they begin to stretch and bend. Ultimately, depending on the applied forces, they will fracture. Material failures lead to prosthetic complications such as loose, broken, and failed restorations.

Screw Loosening and Fracture

Screw loosening has occurred frequently in screw-retained FPDs. Screw-retained single crowns attached to externally hexed implants (i.e., those with narrow- or standard-diameter restorative interface connection surfaces) are particularly prone to this type of mechanical complication. Screw loosening has been reported for 6% to 49% of cases at the first annual checkup.[75,107] Screw loosening was a more prevalent problem with earlier designs. For example, abutment screws were previously made with titanium, which did not offer the clamping forces of current materials. Newer abutment designs and improved abutment screws enable an increased clamping force to be achieved without excessive torque, which has helped to reduce the rate of screw loosening.

Abutment or prosthesis screw loosening is often corrected by retightening the screws, but if screws continue to be stretched over time, they become fatigued and eventually fracture. This problem is evident in the patient with a loose single crown. In the patient with a prosthesis retained by multiple implants, the ability to detect a loose screw is greatly diminished, and the problem may go unnoticed until additional screws stretch, fatigue, and fracture. In either case, the biomechanical support (and resistance) for the restoration must be evaluated and, if possible, changed to prevent recurrence of the problem.

Implant Fracture

The ultimate mechanical failure is implant fracture because it results in loss of the implant and possibly of the prosthesis (Fig. 58.13). Removal of a fractured implant creates a large osseous defect. Factors such as fatigue of implant materials (Fig. 58.14) and weakness in prosthetic design or dimension are the usual causes of implant fractures.[4,15] Balshi[15] listed three categories of causes that may explain implant fractures: (1) design and material, (2) nonpassive fit of the prosthetic framework, and (3) physiologic or biomechanical overload. Patients with bruxism seem to be at higher risk for these events and therefore need to be screened, informed, and treated accordingly.[14,15] These patients should be fitted with occlusal guards in conjunction with placement of the final prostheses.

Fracture of Restorative Materials

Fracture or failure of materials used for implant-retained restorations can be a significant problem. This is particularly true for veneers (i.e., acrylic, composite, or ceramic) that are attached to superstructures (Fig. 58.15).

Fig. 58.13 (A) Radiograph of a fractured standard-diameter implant used to support a molar-sized single crown in the posterior mandible. (B) Crown and coronal portion of the implant (same as shown in A) that fractured between the third and fourth threads.

Fig. 58.14 The Implant Fractured at the Internal Connection Collar. Fracture was caused by rotational forces applied to the implant at the time of placement into dense bone and was likely the result of combined material weakness and density of the prepared site.

Fig. 58.15 Fractured Porcelain From Incisal Edges of an Implant-Supported Fixed Partial Denture.

AESTHETIC AND PHONETIC COMPLICATIONS

Aesthetic Complications

The challenge of modern implant dentistry is achieving an aesthetic and functional implant restoration. Harmonious tooth shape and size and ideal soft-tissue contours are key factors for successful aesthetic outcomes.[86]

Aesthetic complications arise when patient expectations are not met. Patients' degree of satisfaction with the aesthetic outcome of implant prostheses varies. The risk of aesthetic complications is increased for patients with high aesthetic expectations and suboptimal patient-related factors such as a high smile line, thin periodontal soft tissues, or inadequate bone quantity and quality. In addition to the appearance of the final restoration, factors such as a patient's perception and desires determine the acceptance of the results. Aesthetic complications can result from poor implant position, deficiencies in the existing anatomy of edentulous sites that were reconstructed with implants, and prosthetic-related factors such as color mismatch.[13]

Important prerequisites for achieving optimal gingival tissue contour are sufficient peri-implant bone to support the soft tissues and a sufficient zone of keratinized tissue. Soft- and hard-tissue defects can be treated by a variety of augmentation procedures.

Implant placement in the aesthetic zone requires precise three-dimensional tissue reconstruction and ideal implant placement.[67,128] This reconstructive procedure enables the restorative dentist to develop a natural emergence profile of the implant crown. If the amount of available bone does not allow for ideal implant placement and the implant is positioned too far apically or buccally or in the proximal space, an unaesthetic emergence profile can result (Fig. 58.16).

If crown contours and dimensions are not ideal or gingival harmony around the implant restoration is unaesthetic, the patient may consider the implants or restorations to be failures because the outcome does not represent a natural appearance (Fig. 58.17).

> **KEY FACT**
>
> Aesthetic complications arise when a patient's expectations are not met. Satisfaction with the aesthetic outcome varies tremendously among patients, and the increased risk of aesthetic complications correlates with high aesthetic expectations and less than optimal patient-related factors, such as a high smile line, thin periodontal soft tissues, or inadequate bone quantity and quality. Risk factors should be carefully evaluated and discussed with the patient before initiating therapy, and the ability to meet the patient's expectations should be carefully considered.

Fig. 58.16 Poor Implant Position Makes It Impossible to Correct the Problem With an Aesthetic, Natural-Appearing Restoration. (A) Anterior view with the removable partial dentures inserted. (B) Anterior view without the removable partial dentures. Notice the high level of implant cover screw/head exposure (maxillary right lateral incisor) that is significantly apical to the level of the adjacent natural tooth (cuspid) gingival margin. (C) Occlusal view of the same patient. Notice the labial projection of the same implant (maxillary right lateral incisor) and the palatal position of the implant in the premolar area. Any attempt to restore the anterior implants would not be aesthetically acceptable.

Phonetic Problems

Implant prostheses that are fabricated with unusual palatal contours (i.e., restricted or narrow palatal space) or that have spaces under and around the superstructure can create phonetic problems for the patient. This is particularly problematic when full-arch, implant-supported, fixed restorations are fabricated for

Fig. 58.17 High Gingival Margin on Single-Tooth Implant Crown in the Maxillary Lateral Incisor Position, Showing the Discrepancy Between Gingival Margin Levels of the Implant and the Adjacent Natural Teeth.

patients who have a severely atrophied maxilla. Horizontal bone loss in the premaxilla often causes palatal positioning of the dental implants, resulting in the prosthesis covering the incisive papilla region. Because some sounds are formed when the tip of the tongue lightly touches the palate at the incisive papilla region, covering this area can interfere with proper enunciation. Titanium-framed full restorations allow a thinner bulk of material in this region and can minimize phonetic complications.

These complications are exacerbated when using an immediate fixed provisional restoration. Phonetic problems can be common in full-denture cases. However, with dentures, the clinician can figure out many of the speech issues in wax before the final restoration, making it easier to focus on the specific problem area. Ideal tooth setup and multiple adjustments are needed to minimize phonetic problems. These patients are probably best served with an implant-assisted maxillary overdenture because the design facilitates replacement of missing alveolar structure and avoids creating spaces that allow air to escape during speech.

CONCLUSIONS

Although implants offer a highly predictable treatment option for the replacement of single and multiple missing teeth, surgical, biologic, mechanical, prosthetic, and aesthetic complications can occur. Careful diagnosis and treatment planning with the use of diagnostic imaging, surgical guides, meticulous techniques, and adherence to proven principles can prevent many of the problems discussed in this chapter.

A thorough understanding of anatomy, biology, and wound healing can reduce the incidence of complications. There is no substitute for good training, knowledge, and clinical experience. The dentist who places or restores implants must be well prepared to diagnose, prevent, and manage complications.

A Case Scenario is found on the companion website.

REFERENCES

 References for this chapter are found on the companion website.

Supportive Implant Treatment[a]

Dental implant therapy does not end with the final prosthetic restoration of the implant. Predictability and long-term success of a dental implant and its restoration require sound treatment planning, precise surgical and restorative execution, and impeccable long-term maintenance, which depend on patient compliance with home care and professional supportive implant treatment.

Peri-implant maintenance begins as the implant becomes exposed to the oral cavity and continues at regular intervals during the life of the implant. The recall interval is determined by the patient's oral hygiene and susceptibility to biofilm-induced inflammatory diseases. For the first year after treatment, recall maintenance visits should be scheduled at 3-month intervals and then adjusted to suit the patient's needs. Patients who have good oral hygiene, minimal deposits, and disease resistance require infrequent professional hygiene maintenance, whereas those who have poor oral hygiene, heavy deposits, and disease susceptibility require more frequent follow-up care.

RATIONALE FOR SUPPORTIVE IMPLANT TREATMENT

Although dental implants are not vulnerable to dental caries, they are susceptible to mechanical complications and peri-implant, biofilm-induced inflammatory tissue changes. A 10-year retrospective study[46] of 397 fixed-implant reconstructions in 300 patients observed a mechanical complication rate of 24.7%. The most frequent complication was ceramic chipping (20.31%), followed by occlusal screw loosening (2.57%) and loss of retention (2.06%). Although relatively infrequent, occlusal screw loosening can result in a subgingival gap at the implant–abutment junction that retains plaque and stimulates an inflammatory reaction in soft and hard tissues.

Biologically, biofilm accumulation due to inadequate or no access for oral hygiene can result in peri-implant mucositis and peri-implantitis. Peri-implant mucositis is characterized by inflammation confined to the soft tissue and is reported to affect up to 80% of patients with dental implants.[23] Peri-implantitis is characterized by peri-implant inflammation with progressive crestal bone loss beyond the initial remodeling. The prevalence of peri-implantitis among patients is 11.2% to 53%.[25,35,36-38] Poor oral hygiene, residual cement, current or history of periodontitis, cigarette smoking, and diabetes mellitus are important risk factors for peri-implant diseases.[1,9]

The relationship between peri-implant mucositis and peri-implantitis is similar to that between gingivitis and periodontitis. Although peri-implant mucositis does not necessarily progress to peri-implantitis, it is likely the precursor to peri-implantitis.[1] The inflammatory response in peri-implant disease appears to be similar to that in periodontal disease.[39] However, the severity and rate of disease progression appear to be more pronounced around implants. This may be caused by the absence of a self-limiting process, which is observed in periodontitis, around implants that separates the inflammatory cell infiltrate from the bone.[6] Experimental models demonstrated that peri-implant mucositis was reversible at the biomarker level (i.e., matrix metalloproteinase 8 [MMP-8] and interleukin-1β [IL-1β]).[39]

A review of the literature[34] reported that peri-implant mucositis could be effectively treated with nonsurgical mechanical therapies, but these modalities tended to be ineffective against peri-implantitis. Results of surgical treatment for peri-implantitis are not predictable. Prevention, early detection, and early treatment of peri-implant diseases are therefore crucial. Periodic and well-regimented supportive implant treatment is essential to the long-term success of dental implant therapy.

---

[a]Adapted from the following chapter of Newman and Carranza's Clinical Periodontology, 13th edition: Chapter 86: Supportive Implant Treatment, by Jonathan H. Do and Perry R. Klokkevold.

KEY FACT

Implants are susceptible to mechanical complications and biofilm-induced inflammatory diseases, such as peri-implant mucositis and peri-implantitis.

CLINICAL CORRELATION

Implant examination includes evaluation of biofilm control, visual and tactile assessment of peri-implant tissue for inflammatory changes and changes in probing depths, and radiographic examination of the mesial and distal bone level.

EXAMINATION OF IMPLANTS

The supportive implant treatment appointment should include: an inquiry about new concerns, problems, or pain; review of changes in the patient's medical and oral status; evaluation and reinforcement of oral hygiene; examination and evaluation of soft and hard tissue health; evaluation of implants and the associated implant restorations' stability and integrity; and professional supportive treatment. Assessment should determine the appropriate recall interval and plan for the next visit.

Examination begins with visual inspection for biofilm and calculus accumulation; signs of inflammation and swelling; peri-implant soft tissue quality, color, consistency, and contour; and aberrations in the implant prosthesis. Peri-implant soft tissue can be digitally palpated to detect edema, tenderness, exudation, or suppuration. Peri-implant probing can be done to assess the condition and level of soft and hard tissues surrounding implants. When indicated, radiographic images can be obtained to help verify the level of the peri-implant crestal bone. Determination of implant stability or mobility and percussion testing can help verify implant osseointegration (Fig. 59.1).

Peri-Implant Probing

Probing of implants can be done with light force (i.e., 0.25 N) using a traditional steel probe without adverse effects to the peri-implant mucosa.[15] Implant probing should be recorded at the time of final restoration as the baseline measurement and done at least annually thereafter.[23]

Dental hygienists should use caution when evaluating peri-implant probing because these measures cannot be interpreted the same as probing depths around teeth. Although periodontal probing around natural teeth is useful for assessing the health of periodontal tissues, the sulcus or pocket depth, and the level of attachment, probing around implants may not provide comparable results.[7] Due to distinct differences in the tissues that surround and support teeth compared with those that surround and support implants, the probe inserts and penetrates differently. Around teeth, the periodontal probe is resisted by the health of the periodontal tissues and importantly by the insertion of supracrestal connective tissue fibers into the cementum of the root surface. These fibers, which are unique to teeth, are the primary source of resistance to the probe.[3] There is no equivalent

Fig. 59.1 Peri-Implantitis. (A and B) Minimal biofilm accumulation is seen. The peri-implant mucosa exhibits minimal erythema and edema. Notice the buccal placement of the implant in B. (C) Manipulation of tissue indicates a lack of buccal keratinized attached gingiva and exudation from the peri-implant sulcus *(arrow)*. (D) The periapical radiograph shows peri-implant bone loss to the apex of the implant.

fiber attachment around implants. Connective tissue fibers around implants usually run parallel to the implant or restorative surface and do not have perpendicular or inserting fibers (see Chapter 55). The primary source of resistance to the probe depends on the conditions around the implant.[12,22] At noninflamed sites, the most coronal aspect of connective tissue adhesion to the implant resists the probe. At inflamed sites, the probe tip consistently penetrates farther into the connective tissue until less inflamed connective tissue is encountered, which is often close to or at the level of bone.

The value of peri-implant probing is different from periodontal probing and offers comparatively limited information. Probing around implants can measure the level of the mucosal margin relative to a fixed position on the implant or restoration and can also measure the depth of tissue around the implant. The peri-implant probing depth is often a measure of the thickness of the surrounding connective tissues and correlates most consistently with the level of surrounding bone. However, peri-implant probing is affected by several conditions, including the size of the probe, the force and direction of insertion, the health and resistance of peri-implant tissues, the level of bone support, and the features of the implant, abutment, and prosthesis design (Fig. 59.2).

A comparison[43] of probing pocket depth of implants with peri-implantitis before and after the removal of the prosthetic restorations reported similar probing depths in only 37% of sites. In 39% of sites, the difference was ±1 mm; in 15% of sites, it was ±2 mm; and in 9% of sites, it was ±3 mm. Probing measurements can be an accurate measure of soft tissue thickness around an implant (i.e., peri-implant soft tissue above the bone level), but in many cases or sites, the inability to properly angle and direct the probe along the implant can lead to inaccurate assessment of soft tissue thickness. In these situations, the clinician must appreciate the limitations and know that other clinical parameters and radiographs are required to help evaluate the peri-implant's condition.

Probing around implants is likely to vary more than around teeth. Studies have shown that a change in probing force around implants results in more dramatic changes than a similar change in probing force around teeth.[27] The probing depth around implants presumed to be healthy (and without bleeding) has

been documented as about 3 mm around all surfaces.[2,8] The absence of bleeding on probing around teeth has been established as an indicator of health and a predictor of periodontal stability.[19] Studies comparing bleeding on probing around teeth and implants in the same patient have reported that bleeding around implants occurs more frequently.

Bleeding on probing at implant sites can indicate inflammation in the peri-implant mucosa. However, the ability to use bleeding on probing as an indicator for assessing diseased or healthy sites around implants has not been established. Due to the potential for false-positive bleeding (i.e., provoked bleeding) with probing, the use of marginal bleeding, which is a more sensitive indicator of inflammation and is less likely to elicit false-positive bleeding, has been proposed to assess peri-implant inflammation.[48] Marginal bleeding can be evaluated by running a probe circumferentially along the coronal portion in the implant sulcus. Overall, the value of peri-implant probing is in monitoring changes in the probing pocket depth over time rather than the initial value because some implants are placed apically for aesthetics.[1]

CLINICAL CORRELATION

Probing of implants can be accomplished with a traditional steel probe. It is valuable for detecting tactilely inflammatory changes in the tissue, such as loss of tissue to resistance to probe penetration, sponginess of peri-implant mucosa, and bleeding on probing, and for monitoring changes in probing depth over time.

Microbial Testing

Studies in animals and humans have demonstrated the development of peri-implant mucosal inflammation in response to the accumulation of bacterial plaque.[5,31,39,49] Microbiologic studies suggest that greater probing depths (i.e., pockets) around implants harbor higher levels of pathogenic microorganisms.[28,33,41] Studies have also documented similarities in the microbial composition of plaque in healthy periodontal sites compared with healthy peri-implant sites.[29] Evidence indicates that the microbiota of diseased periodontal pockets harbor the same pathogenic microorganisms as those observed in inflamed peri-implant sites (i.e., peri-implantitis).[29,41] However, there is no evidence to prove that periodontal pathogens cause peri-implant disease, and the pathogenesis of inflammatory disease around implants has not been defined.[10]

One report[1] accepted the idea that peri-implant disease, like periodontal disease, occurs primarily as a result of an overwhelming bacterial insult and subsequent host response. Human biopsies indicate that peri-implantitis and periodontitis exhibit similar histologic features, including an inflammatory cell infiltrate in the connective tissue dominated by B lymphocytes and plasma cells and by up-regulation of inflammatory biomarkers. No evidence indicates that laboratory tests for the identification of suspected periodontal pathogens are of use in the evaluation of implants.[14] The usefulness of microbial testing may be limited to the evaluation of peri-implant sites that are showing signs of infection and bone loss, allowing the dentist to prescribe appropriate antibiotics.

Fig. 59.2 Buccal Probing of the Implant Is Impeded by the Implant Restoration.

Stability Measures

The assessment of implant stability or mobility is an important measure for determining whether osseointegration is being maintained. Important as it is, however, this measure has extremely low sensitivity but high specificity. An implant can exhibit significant bone loss and remain stable; the stability measure in this case has a low sensitivity for the detection of bone loss. Conversely, if implant mobility is detected, it is likely that the implant is not surrounded by bone; mobility is highly specific for the detection of implant failure or lack of osseointegration. Mobility demands differentiation of loss of implant osseointegration from a loose implant restoration.

There is great interest in evaluating the stability of bone-to-implant contact in a noninvasive manner. Two noninvasive techniques for evaluating implant stability are impact resistance (e.g., Periotest) and resonance frequency analysis (RFA). Originally designed to evaluate tooth mobility quantitatively, the Periotest (Gulden, Bensheim, Germany) is a noninvasive electronic device that provides an objective measurement of the reaction of the periodontium to a defined impact load applied to the tooth crown. The Periotest value depends to some extent on tooth mobility but mainly on the dampening characteristics of the periodontium. Despite dependence on the periodontium, the Periotest has been used to evaluate implant stability. However, unlike teeth, the movement of implants and surrounding bone is minuscule, and Periotest values therefore fall within a much smaller range compared with those for teeth. Detection of horizontal mobility may be a significant advantage of the Periotest because it is much more sensitive to horizontal movement than similar detection by other means, such as manual assessment.[14]

Another noninvasive method used to measure the stability of implants is RFA,[26] which uses a transducer that is attached to the implant or abutment. A steady-state signal is applied to the implant through the transducer, and the response is measured. The RFA value is a function of the stiffness of the implant in the surrounding tissues. The stiffness is influenced by the implant, the interface between the implant and the bone and soft tissues, and the surrounding bone itself. The height of the implant or abutment above the bone influences the RFA value. Unlike the Periotest, the RFA does not depend on movement in only one direction. The absolute RFA values vary from one implant design to another and from one site to another, but there is high consistency for any one implant or location.

The value of RFA is most appreciated with repeated measures of the same implant over time because it is very sensitive to changes in the bone–implant interface. Small changes in tissue support can be detected using this method. An increase in RFA value indicates increased implant stability, whereas a decrease indicates loss of stability. However, this is a relative measure, and it has not been determined whether RFA is capable of detecting impending failure before the implant fails.

Much interest and research have focused on the use of noninvasive methods to evaluate implant stability. Mobility remains the cardinal sign of implant failure, and detecting mobility is therefore an important parameter.

Implant Percussion

Tapping an implant's healing abutment or restoration with an instrument produces a sound that can help determine its osseointegration. A solid resonating sound and the absence of pain usually indicate osseointegration. A dull sound can indicate that the implant is fibrous encapsulated; radiographic and other clinical findings are needed for diagnosis.

Radiographic Examination

Perpendicular intraoral periapical radiographs should be taken at implant placement, at abutment connection, and at final restoration for baseline documentation of bone levels, and annually[11] thereafter to monitor marginal or peri-implant bone changes. In the setting of peri-implant inflammation, a periapical radiograph is indicated for peri-implant bone evaluation and disease diagnosis. Periapical radiographs have excellent resolution and, when taken perpendicular to an implant, can provide valuable details of the implant-abutment junction, mesial and distal crestal bone level relative to the implant platform, and bone-to-implant interface along the length of the implant (Fig. 59.3). Periapical radiographs are difficult to standardize, and great variation is inherent in the acquisition process, but they are relatively simple, inexpensive, and readily available in the dental office. It is diagnostically important to obtain images that clearly show implant threads (i.e., not blurred by nonperpendicular angulation) and the restorative implant–abutment connection.

The objective of the radiographic examination is to measure the height of bone adjacent to the implant, evaluate the quality of bone along the length of the implant, and detect peri-implant radiolucencies. Although the predictive value of assessing implant stability with radiographs is low, films do offer a reasonable method to measure changes in bone levels.[44] The predictive value of detecting implant failure or loss of stability is good when radiolucent lesions are discovered with periapical radiographs. Identification of unstable implants is reliable when radiographs are obtained as part of an annual examination and when examining patients on a routine long-term basis.[18]

The radiographic examination remains one of the primary tools for detection of failed or failing implants in routine clinical evaluations, although it is not as accurate as mobility tests. In one study designed to evaluate the accuracy and precision of radiographic diagnosis of mobility, the probability of predicting implant mobility in a population with a low prevalence of implant failures was low.[44] Other studies, however, have demonstrated a much higher predictive value for radiographic diagnosis of implant mobility.[17,18] Investigators concluded that the most important factors for making an accurate radiographic diagnosis are the quality of the radiograph and the experience of the clinician.[18,44]

FLASH BACK

Intraoral periapical radiographs of implants must be taken with the x-ray beam perpendicular to the implant fixture to enable clear visualization of implant threads and the mesial and distal crestal bone levels.

Fig. 59.3 (A) A periapical radiograph captures the whole implant. (B) A second perpendicular periapical radiograph is necessary to assess the crestal bone level. Platform switching is seen at the implant–abutment junction.

ASSESSMENT OF PERI-IMPLANT HEALTH

Evaluation of Biofilm Control

Impeccable biofilm control is crucial to peri-implant tissue health. Poor biofilm control is associated with peri-implant disease (odds ratio = 14.3).[23] It is advantageous to evaluate biofilm control before tissue manipulation. The amount and location of biofilm and calculus accumulation should be assessed visually. Poor control is typically associated with biofilm and calculus retention and with erythematous and edematous gingival tissue. When biofilm control is inadequate, the patient should be asked to demonstrate his or her oral hygiene routine in front of a mirror so that the dental hygienist can evaluate the patient's technique. If the patient fails to remove biofilm in any areas, the patient's attention should be directed to the location of the biofilm. An instrument can be used to remove the biofilm, with the patient paying attention so that he or she can see its color and consistency. At this time, oral hygiene instruction should be demonstrated and reinforced.

Evaluation of Peri-Implant Health and Disease

Peri-implant mucosal health is characterized by pink, firm, and well-adapted gingival tissue. Peri-implant disease is associated with clinical erythema, edema, and loss of tissue tightness around the implant. Peri-implant mucosa can be nonkeratinized and unattached (see Fig. 59.1C) or keratinized and attached (Fig. 59.4C). In the setting of keratinized, attached mucosa, a gingival seal or gingival cuff is established around the implant.[4] The gingival cuff can protect the underlying bone and reduce subgingival plaque formation. Due to the mobile nature of oral mucosa, the protective function of nonkeratinized, unattached peri-implant mucosa may not be as effective. However, the presence of keratinized, attached gingiva, which can facilitate oral hygiene, is not a requisite for peri-implant health if biofilm is well controlled.[42,47] Nonetheless, sites deficient in keratinized, attached tissue typically exhibit vertical or horizontal ridge deficiencies, shallow vestibular depths, and long or bulky restorations. All of these factors can impede oral hygiene access and contribute to biofilm accumulation and peri-implant inflammation.

KEY FACT

Peri-implant health is characterized by pink, firm, and well-adapted peri-implant mucosa. Peri-implant disease is associated with erythema, edema, and loss of tissue tightness around the implant.

In cases of inflammation, the peri-implant tissue must be palpated for tenderness and suppuration, the implant must be probed, and periapical radiographs must be obtained and compared with baseline images to determine peri-implant bone loss. Suppuration often indicates peri-implantitis.[23] Radiographic crestal bone loss beyond the implant baseline level at the time of final prosthesis delivery in conjunction with bleeding on probing is characteristic of peri-implantitis.[20] Due to potential measurement errors, a threshold of detectable bone loss of 1.0 to 1.5 mm is recommended for the diagnosis of peri-implantitis.[40] In the absence of a baseline radiograph, a vertical distance of 2 mm from the expected marginal bone level after the initial crestal bone remodeling is recommended as the threshold for diagnosing peri-implantitis.[40]

The amount of initial marginal bone remodeling depends on the design of the implant–abutment junction. Platform-switched implants (Fig. 59.5C; see also Fig. 59.3), in which the abutment is internally offset relative to the implant fixture at the implant–abutment junction, may exhibit less crestal bone remodeling than non–platform-switched implants (see Fig. 59.4), in which the abutment is flush or even with the implant fixture at the implant–abutment junction.

Evaluation of Implant Osseointegration

Implant osseointegration must be determined before fabrication and delivery of the final implant prosthesis. Implant osseointegration can be definitively determined only histologically, which requires the implant and the surrounding bone to be removed. A combination of radiographic and clinical parameters are used to assess implant osseointegration or to rule out lack of osseointegration. They include absence of peri-implant

Fig. 59.4 (A) Subcrestal placement of an implant with adequate buccal and lingual bone thickness. (B) Periapical radiograph at the time of implant placement. (C) Implant at the 5-month osseointegration check exhibits adequate peri-implant keratinized attached tissue. (D) It also shows crestal bone remodeling to the first thread. *(Arrows)* indicate the mesial crestal bone level.

inflammation and pain in response to palpation and percussion, a solid resonating sound in reaction to percussion, complete radiographic bone-to-implant contact along the implant surface (i.e., absence of radiolucencies along the bone–implant interface), and implant stability.

Evaluation of Implant Restorations

Implant superstructures, frameworks, and restorations should be fabricated to accommodate and facilitate oral hygiene (e.g., embrasure spaces made to allow passage of a proxy brush) (see Fig. 59.4). Occlusal schemes of implant restorations should provide adequate posterior support, maximize axial loading, and minimize incline contacts, nonaxial loading, and interferences in excursive movements.

During delivery, radiographs perpendicular to the implant should be obtained for baseline documentation and to verify complete seating of the restorations. After delivery, cement-retained implant restorations should be thoroughly evaluated for residual excess cement, which must be removed. During follow-up visits, implant restorations should be carefully examined for heavy contacts, fractures, loose screws, and in removable

prostheses, worn-out retentive components (i.e., Hader clips and locator attachment inserts). Occlusion should be adjusted accordingly to prevent implant overload and fractures of implant parts. Loose abutment and set screws must be evaluated, possibly replaced, and properly torqued down. Worn-out retentive components must be replaced periodically to ensure proper retention, stability, and function of the removable prosthesis. Occlusal wear of teeth and fit of tissue-borne surfaces of an implant prosthesis should be assessed and corrected as indicated. In patients with oral parafunctions and heavy occlusal forces, occlusal guards are recommended to protect implants and restorations.

IMPLANT MAINTENANCE

Methods for Patient Oral Hygiene

The importance of good oral hygiene should be stressed even before implants are placed, and peri-implant oral hygiene for biofilm control should begin as early as possible after the implant is exposed to the oral cavity. A cotton tip, cotton gauze, or soft toothbrush can be used to gently remove biofilm from healing abutments or provisional restorations during the early

Fig. 59.5 Restoration Is Designed With Adequate Hygiene Access. (A) Lingual view. (B) Mesial view of the buccal contour. (C) The periapical radiograph shows a gradual transition from the implant fixture to the restoration. Platform switching is seen at the implant–abutment junction.

postoperative phase of healing. Before implant osseointegration, the use of powered toothbrushes should be avoided.

After implant osseointegration has been achieved and verified, brushing with dentifrice can help remove deposits and increase smoothness of exposed implant and restoration surfaces.[30] Other dental hygiene aids, such as dental floss, rubber tips, and interdental brushes, can be employed (Fig. 59.6). Oral hygiene should emphasize removal of biofilm and deposits along the gingival margin. Evidence for the use of a powered oral irrigator around implants is limited. One study reported that subgingival irrigation of 0.06% chlorhexidine gluconate with a Waterpik device (Water Pik, Inc., Fort Collins, CO) was more effective at reducing biofilm and gingival inflammation and produced fewer stains than rinsing with 0.12% chlorhexidine gluconate once daily.[16]

Methods for Professional Recall Maintenance

Professional maintenance consists of the removal of dental biofilm and calculus from implant components exposed to the oral environment.[24] Like root surfaces, the transmucosal surfaces of implants should be smooth to minimize plaque accumulation and to facilitate oral hygiene practices.[21] At sites with excellent biofilm control and peri-implant health, the need for professional instrumentation is minimal, and instrumentation should be limited to prevent iatrogenic damage to implant components that can contribute to plaque and calculus accumulation. In the

setting of biofilm, calculus, and tenacious deposits, care should be taken to minimize damage to transmucosal implant surfaces. However, priority should be placed on the complete removal of implant surface deposits.

All metal instruments, including metal curettes and scalers, and ultrasonic scalers increase the surface roughness of polished titanium.[24] The use of carbon and gold-coated curettes and nonmetal ultrasonic tips have been advocated to protect the titanium implant surface and the titanium abutment from contamination by other metals and to reduce the likelihood of scratching the surface. Unfortunately, the large size and flexibility of nonmetal curettes may not allow effective biofilm and calculus removal,[32] and Teflon- and gold-coated curettes cannot be sharpened.

Most implant prostheses are made with gold alloys or ceramic materials, which are usually identical to the materials used in restorations for the natural dentition. The location of the connection between the restorative material and the implant is typically below the mucosa and often near the crest of bone; most calculus removal is done above this level. The fear of contaminating the titanium implant is therefore unwarranted. Gold alloy or ceramic surfaces can be debrided with most scalers and curettes (e.g., plastic, gold-coated, stainless steel) without damaging the surface. Rubber cups and polishing paste can be used to remove biofilm and to enhance the smoothness of machined and polished surfaces. Magnetostrictive and piezoelectric ultrasonic instruments

Fig. 59.6 Methods for Patient Oral Hygiene Are Shown. (A) Flossing. (B) Bass method of brushing with an extra-soft toothbrush. (C) Interproximal brushing. (D) Removal of biofilm with a rubber tip. Hygiene methods remove biofilm along the gingival margin.

with metal tips (e.g., Cavitron) should be used with caution because of irregularities that can easily be created in the surface.

TREATMENT OF PERI-IMPLANT DISEASES

The goals of treatment are elimination of all peri-implant infectious and inflammatory processes, prevention of disease progression, and preservation and restoration of function and aesthetics. Treatment begins with patient education about the causes, pathogenesis, and prevention of peri-implant diseases, along with oral hygiene instruction. Although bacteria are the main etiologic factor, systemic (e.g., smoking, poorly controlled diabetes) and local (e.g., residual excess cement, poorly designed restorations that inhibit hygiene access) factors should be identified and modified.

Peri-Implant Mucositis

Peri-implant mucositis can be effectively treated with nonsurgical mechanical therapy.[34] Treatment requires complete removal of supramucosal and submucosal biofilm, calculus, and deposits using curettes, ultrasonic scalers, and polishing cups with prophy paste. Antimicrobials (e.g., chlorhexidine irrigation, mouth rinse) can be used with mechanical debridement to enhance treatment outcome.[34]

Peri-Implantitis

The treatment of peri-implantitis includes nonsurgical and surgical interventions, which can be combined with the adjunctive use of antimicrobials. Nonsurgical interventions consist of antimicrobial rinse and irrigation, local antibiotics, ultrasonic debridement, mechanical debridement with air-abrasive devices, and laser therapy. Surgical treatment includes full-thickness flap elevation for access, followed by degranulation, surface debridement by laser or mechanical instruments, surface decontamination with laser or antimicrobials, and bone augmentation. The data from two systematic reviews[13,45] are insufficient to suggest which intervention for peri-implantitis is most effective or to allow specific recommendations for the use of locally or systematically administered antibiotics.

Implant surface decontamination or disinfection remains challenging, especially for implants with roughened surfaces. For some treatment modalities, recurrence of peri-implantitis appears to be high (up to 100%) after one or more years of treatment, and retreatment may be necessary. Surgical access appears to be necessary to arrest peri-implant bone loss. Surgical treatment can result in gingival recession and compromised aesthetics. At sites with high aesthetic demands, definitive treatment of peri-implantitis can include the removal of the implant, grafting of the site, and placement of another implant.

KEY FACT

Treatment of peri-implant mucositis is effective, whereas treatment of peri-implantitis is unpredictable. Prevention, early detection, and treatment of peri-implant inflammatory diseases are essential for successful outcomes.

REFERRAL OF PATIENTS TO THE PERIODONTIST

The previously described guidelines allow many implants to be maintained quite well by primary dental care providers (i.e., general dentists and dental hygienists). Referral to a periodontist should be considered if peri-implantitis or peri-implant mucositis is diagnosed and cannot be resolved with improved oral hygiene and professional maintenance care. Early referral is advantageous to stop progression and limit the extent of bone loss.

A Case Scenario is found on the companion website.

REFERENCES

 References for this chapter are found on the companion website.

Results of Implant Treatment[a]

CHAPTER OUTLINE

The landmark Göteborg study and the replica study at the University of Toronto supported expectations for the success and predictability of root-form dental implants. The study, conducted over a 15-year period at the University of Göteborg, Sweden, by P.I. Bränemark and coworkers, began in 1965 and concluded in 1980. The results, which were reported in several articles, defined the concept of osseointegration, described protocols for success, and shared clinical experiences.

The most significant article from the study, published in 1981, was on osseointegrated implants in the treatment of the edentulous jaw.[2] The Göteborg study included 2768 root-form implants placed into 410 edentulous jaws in 371 consecutive patients. The data were most often reported in subsets according to the three study phases (i.e., initial, developmental, and routine). Cases treated in the routine period with standardized procedures and an observation time of 5 to 9 years were thought to reflect the potential of the method and were the basis of data reported in that historic publication. The subset consisted of 895 implants placed in 130 jaws. The implant survival rate was 81% in the maxilla and 91% in mandible. The prosthesis survival (i.e., continuous stability) rate was 89% in the maxilla and 100% in the mandible.

The replica study, which was conducted at the University of Toronto, demonstrated that comparable results could be predictably achieved using the same implant design and treatment protocols.[5,78–80] Together, these studies demonstrated that implant survival of 81% or more and prosthesis survival of 89% or more could be expected in the edentulous patient.

In the decades since the landmark discovery of osseointegration and the documentation of its clinical effectiveness, clinicians have had tremendous success in replacing missing teeth with endosseous root-form dental implants in both partially edentulous and edentulous patients.[1,48] Despite the high level of success and long-term predictability, a 100% success rate cannot be achieved. Complications and implant failures do occur.[2,12] Some implants fail to achieve osseointegration; some achieve osseointegration but lose bone progressively over time, leading to failure; and other implants rapidly lose bone and fail in a short time. Some implants achieve and maintain osseointegration but fail because they do not meet the aesthetic expectations of the patient or clinician.

The reporting of implant success varies widely in the literature, which makes defining an absolute implant success rate impractical. This chapter considers implant treatment results in light of the factors that influence implant survival and success. The intent is to outline important aspects that need to be considered in evaluating implant outcomes and offer guidelines for understanding published results.

DEFINING IMPLANT OUTCOMES

Implant outcomes are reported in a variety of ways in the literature. Various levels of implant success and failure are described in case reports, case series, retrospective studies, controlled studies, and prospective studies. The type of study and method of reporting are decided by the authors and often influenced by the data collected and the study objectives. Each type of study or report has recognized limitations, but because of tremendous variation that exists in the ways individual investigators measure, interpret, and report implant outcomes, differences in the results from one study to another may not be obvious.

Some implant outcomes are reported as the presence or absence of the implant at the time of the last examination, regardless of whether the implant was functional, suffered from bone loss, or had other problems. This type of assessment is a measure of implant *survival* and should not be confused with implant *success*. In contrast to such an overly simplified assessment, some investigators report implant outcomes using specific criteria to determine implant success.

Implant success is defined by specific criteria used to evaluate the condition and function of the implant. Criteria for implant success have been proposed in the literature but have not been used consistently. The problem is that a universally accepted definition of implant success has not been established. In the classic definition, Albrektsson and colleagues[3] defined success as

---

[a]Adapted from the following chapter of *Newman and Carranza's Clinical Periodontology*, 13th edition: Chapter 87: Results of Implant Treatment, by Perry R. Klokkevold.

an implant with no pain, no mobility, no radiolucent peri-implant areas, and less than 0.2 mm of bone loss annually after the first year of loading.[3] Bone loss in the first year was recognized, but it was not defined or quantified as part of the success criteria until later in a separate definition by Roos and associates.[61]

The challenge in comparing reported data between studies is that investigators use different criteria for success in their work. As a result, it is difficult or impossible to make comparisons between studies, and drawing conclusions about implant success or failure from data reported in different studies is tenuous.

Success rates are dramatically affected by variations in the criteria used to define them. In strict terms, if implant success is considered to be an outcome without adverse effects or problems, the treatment would be performed as planned, implants would remain stable and functioning without problems, peri-implant tissues would be stable and healthy, and the patient and treating clinician would be pleased with the outcome (Fig. 60.1).

Use of strict criteria would produce implant success rates lower than those determined using less stringent criteria.

Table 60.1 illustrates the powerful effect that small changes in success criteria have on reported success rates. The data demonstrate that changing the criteria of success to include a probing pocket depth (PPD) of 5 mm or less to 6 mm or less changed the implant success rates from 52.4% to 62% and from 79.1% to 81.3% for patients with and without a history of periodontitis, respectively.[42] This also shows that implant survival is quite different from implant success.

> ## KEY FACT
>
> Implant success is defined by specific criteria used to evaluate the condition and function of the implant. Criteria for implant success have been proposed in the literature but not used consistently. Depending on the criteria used, the rates of implant success reported in studies can vary substantially.

Fig. 60.1 Clinical Implant Success Was Demonstrated When a Single Implant Was Placed in the Mandible to Replace the Lower Second Premolar (as Planned). The implant osseointegrated, and function was successfully restored. The patient and clinicians were pleased with the outcome. (A) Photograph of the dentition in occlusion (from the left side). (B) Close-up photograph of the dentition in occlusion. The mandibular second premolar is an implant-supported crown. (C) Occlusal view of an implant-supported crown in the second premolar position. Replacement of the mandibular second premolar with an implant is a conservative treatment, obviating the need to prepare adjacent teeth. (D) Periapical radiograph of the posterior mandibular teeth and implant in the second premolar position. Bone support is good, and bone loss is minimal and consistent with expectations for this implant design.

TABLE 60.1 **Effect of Slight Modifications of Implant Success Criteria on Successful Outcomes**[a]

Group	PPD ≤5 mm, No BOP, BL <0.2 mm/year (%)	PPD ≤6 mm, No BOP, BL <0.2 mm/year (%)	PPD ≤5 mm, No BOP (%)	PPD ≤6 mm, No BOP (%)	Implant Survival (%)
Group A	52.4	62	71.4	81	90.5
Group B	79.1	81.3	94.5	96.7	96.5

[a]The initial success criteria at 10 years were set as a PPD ≤5 mm, no BOP, and BL <0.2 mm annually. The implant success rates for group A (i.e., patients with a history of periodontitis) and group B (i.e., patients with periodontal health) using these initial criteria are listed in the first column. Notice how dramatically the success rates change when the criteria used to define success are modified to include PPD ≤6 mm (i.e., second column). The next two columns show the success rates for each group using PPD ≤5 mm and ≤6 mm when the criteria are modified to omit bone loss as a determinant. The last column shows the implant survival rate for each group, which demonstrates that the survival rate is different than the success rate.

BL, Bone loss; *BOP,* bleeding on probing; *PPD,* probing pocket depth.

Data from Karoussis IK, Salvi GE, Heitz-Mayfield LJ, et al: Long-term implant prognosis in patients with and without a history of chronic periodontitis: a 10-year prospective cohort study of the ITI Dental Implant System, *Clin Oral Implant Res* 14:329–339, 2003.

Fig. 60.2 Panoramic Radiograph Shows an Implant Placed in the Position of a Missing Maxillary Right Central Incisor. The implant appears to be placed in a nonrestorable position. It is osseointegrated and could technically be counted as a surviving implant, but it must be considered a failure because it does not meet the intended goal and function has not been restored.

Implant survival is defined as an implant that remains in place at the time of evaluation, regardless of untoward signs and symptoms or a history of problems. Extant implants that are healthy and functioning under an implant-retained restoration are different from those that are suffering from peri-implant bone loss or those that are not connected to a restoration and not functioning (Fig. 60.2), but these operational differences do not affect calculations of implant survival. Implants that are osseointegrated but not functional are referred to as *sleepers* and should not be considered successful merely because they are present and osseointegrated.

Implant survival and implant success are different outcome measures. Consider the dramatic difference between survival and success rates for implants reported in a systematic review (21 studies included) of implants supporting fixed partial dentures.[59] The 5-year implant survival rate was 95.4%, whereas the

overall 5-year success rate (individual implant success rates were not calculated), defined as free of complications, was only 61.3%.[59]

In a 10-year retrospective study of 397 fixed implant reconstructions in 300 patients, the observed mechanical complication rate was 24.7%.[77] The most frequent complication was ceramic chipping (20.31%), followed by occlusal screw loosening (2.57%) and loss of retention (2.06%).[77] Although relatively uncommon, occlusal screw loosening can result in a subgingival gap at the implant–abutment junction that retains plaque and stimulates an inflammatory reaction in the soft and hard tissues, leading to bone loss around the implant. Although surviving, these implants would fail to meet optimal success criteria.

Defining implant results in absolute terms is difficult and confusing. Implant survival, which typically is reported in studies, can overestimate good implant outcomes. Implant success, which is less often reported, could offer a better measure if specific success criteria were universally defined, accepted, and used. Implant success is difficult or impossible to compare across studies because of differences in evaluation criteria used by investigators. Implant success in a single study or series of studies using the same success criteria is meaningful only in the context of that study or series.

Currently, the usefulness of implant success rates from different studies is limited. Implant survival is important but is only an indicator of surviving implants and does not reveal whether they are functioning or had problems associated with them over time. The incidence of peri-implant problems is more significant than once thought. A systematic review of the literature evaluating the prevalence of peri-implant disease reported that peri-implant mucositis and peri-implantitis occurred in 19% to 65% and 1% to 47% of cases, respectively.[22]

FACTORS THAT INFLUENCE IMPLANT OUTCOMES

Many issues influence implant outcomes, including available bone, implant design, placement and loading protocols, and host-related factors.

Anatomic Location

Osseointegration depends on the availability of an adequate quantity and quality of bone at the implant site. Areas with abundant bone volume in the desired location are better than those with deficient bone volume. Areas with good bone density provide more predictable outcomes than those with poor bone density.

The bone classification system described by Lekholm and Zarb[49] defines bone with different levels of support for implants and the likely impact on survival and success. The quality of bone support is greatly influenced by the anatomic location, and implant outcomes are sometimes categorized according to location. Extreme examples are the anterior mandible and the posterior maxilla. The anterior mandible typically consists of dense cortical bone, which offers great support and high bone-to-implant contact, whereas the posterior maxilla is often limited in volume because of alveolar resorption and sinus pneumatization and typically consists of a loose, trabecular structure and a thin cortical bone shell.

Implants placed in the posterior maxilla are less well supported compared with implants placed in the anterior mandible. Jaffin and Berman[36] demonstrated the significance of bone quality on implant survival in a report of 1054 Bränemark implants. Ninety percent of the implants were placed in type I, II, or III bone, with a failure rate of only 3%. Of the 10% that were placed in type IV bone, 35% failed.[36] Excluding those placed in the mandible, 23 (44%) of 52 implants placed in type IV bone in the maxilla failed, for a dismal survival rate of 56%. The study authors concluded that bone quality was the single greatest determinant of implant loss.

Anatomic location has a significant effect on implant outcome, particularly for the posterior maxilla. The implants used in the study by Jaffin and Berman[36] had machined surfaces, and current implants with altered microtopography are thought to perform better in the posterior maxilla owing to increased bone-to-implant contact. When all 1054 implants (placed in all types of bone) are considered together, the combined implant survival rate (93.9%) in the study is within or slightly higher than the reported range in the Göteborg study (done with similar implants).

Implant Design

Implant design influences outcome. Hundreds of companies manufacture and market dental implants worldwide, and the number continues to grow. Implant dimensions, geometries, and surface characteristics vary tremendously and continue to evolve as innovation and research findings pave the way for changes that are thought to improve outcomes. Very few implant designs have been studied. They instead rely on being clinically similar to researched and approved designs without additional studies or documentation to support their effectiveness. In most cases, it is impossible to appreciate the effect of a particular implant design features on outcomes. Nonetheless, novel implant designs are being used, and outcomes are being reported in studies that evaluate other aspects of treatment that are not specific to the design, which makes comparisons and assessments more confusing and unreliable.

The studies that have documented the success of dental implants on the basis of design characteristics have shaped current standards for selection and use. For example, many clinicians adhere to the premise that longer implants, threaded implants, and rough-surfaced implants are better than shorter, unthreaded, and smooth designs. As changes in design and use have evolved over time, some beliefs have been disproved, and continued advances and research will undoubtedly refute other firmly held beliefs.

Clinicians would like to know whether one implant design performs better than the rest, but it is almost impossible to determine which design characteristics are important, because there are many variables to consider, and implants are successful most of the time. Given the generally high rate of success, it appears that subtle differences in implant design are probably not significant for most patients and situations.[24,28] However, in patients with inadequate sites or challenging circumstances, certain implant designs may perform better than others. An example is the effect of implant surface characteristics. Implants with altered surface microtopography (i.e., acid-etched or blasted) enhance the bone-to-implant interface[44,45] and can improve outcomes, especially in compromised sites.[71,72] Lower success rates have been associated with smooth-surface (i.e., machined) implants.[37,60,64]

Implant length is another consideration. Many studies have supported the dogma that longer is better for implant success,[65,66] but later studies have challenged it.[31] Another important feature is the macro-thread design of implants. Clinical research[52] evaluating the stability (assessed by resonance frequency analysis) of a novel implant designed with a wide thread depth and increased pitch found that it did not cause the typical decrease in stability in the early postoperative healing period. This finding may have an impact on early and immediate loading protocols.

> **KEY FACT**
>
> Many features influence outcomes, including available bone, implant design, placement and loading protocols, and host-related factors. Defining implant results in absolute terms can be difficult and confusing.

Placement and Loading Protocols

The traditional placement protocol required a healed edentulous ridge into which implants were placed and allowed to osseointegrate for a period without occlusal loading (see Chapter 57). The nonloading period after implant placement was empirically determined to be 3 to 4 months in the mandible and 6 months in the maxilla.[10] A strongly held belief was that early loading would lead to higher failure rates.[11]

In contrast to the early standards, some current protocols advocate dramatically different approaches, including implant placement immediately after tooth extraction and implant occlusal loading immediately or shortly after placement. Each of these approaches has distinct advantages, but they are accompanied by challenges that have the potential to adversely affect outcomes.

Immediate Implant Placement

The immediate implant placement protocol describes the procedure in which an implant is placed in an extraction socket after tooth removal and socket debridement. This procedure, described by Schulte and colleagues[68] in 1978 and by Lazzara in 1989,[47] has been reported with survival rates equivalent to those of implants placed into healed ridges.[14,51] The advantages of immediate placement include decreased surgery, cost, and healing time.[69] Immediate implant placement introduces an additional risk of complications, including poor implant position, compromised aesthetic outcome, and implant failure (see Chapter 58). Despite the increased risk, a high long-term (1- to 16-year) survival rate of 96% has been reported for implants immediately placed into extraction sockets.[74]

Immediate Occlusal Loading

Bränemark established the concept of the osseointegrated dental implant as a predictable treatment modality for the edentulous patient on the empirically based requirement that the implant remain submerged and unloaded for a healing period of 3 to 6 months.[10] This original protocol, requiring the implant to remain stress free, was based on the concern that premature loading would cause micromotion of the dental implant, leading to fibrous encapsulation and implant failure. However, studies have shown this assumption to be incorrect, demonstrating that immediately loaded implants can achieve success rates (>90%) similar to those for conventionally loaded dental implants.[15,19,29,33,40] The long-term predictability of immediately loaded implants requires strict surgical and prosthodontic protocols.[7]

Bone Augmentation

A common problem encountered in implant dentistry is insufficient bone quantity to allow implant placement. Deficiencies in alveolar bone result from developmental defects, periodontal disease, tooth loss, or trauma.[6,13,67] For most cases with alveolar ridge resorption, bone regenerative procedures are required to correct the defects before or simultaneously with implant placement. The question is whether implants placed in sites that are reconstructed with bone augmentation procedures can achieve the same survival and success rates as implants placed in native bone sites.

The results of implants and bone augmentation procedures reported in the literature have been assessed by expert clinicians in several workshops.[16,30,34,35] One systematic review of the literature (2003 Workshop on Contemporary Science in Clinical Periodontics), including 13 studies (i.e., guided bone regeneration) with 1741 patients and 5 studies (i.e., distraction osteogenesis) with 92 patients, found that survival rates of dental implants in augmented bone achieved a high level of predictability that was similar to that for implants placed in natural (nongrafted) bone.[30]

Another systematic review of the literature (2008 Consensus Report of the Sixth European Workshop on Periodontology[73]) pointed out that bone augmentation procedures can fail and that implants placed in these areas do not enjoy the high long-term survival rates of dental implants placed in pristine sites.[73] The 2003 systematic review did not include an assessment of whether bone augmentation procedures failed; it intentionally focused on implants placed in sites that were successfully treated with bone augmentation. More research is needed to determine the long-term performance of dental implants placed in augmented bone and the clinical benefits of bone augmentation with respect to alternative treatments (e.g., use of short implants).

Risk Factors

Most patients enjoy similar rates of survival and success with dental implants. Only a few patients experience implant failure.

In addition to the factors previously discussed, host-related factors can adversely affect healing, osseointegration, and maintenance of dental implants. Smoking, diabetes, and periodontitis have been identified as risk factors that can adversely affect implant outcomes. In a systematic review of the literature, Klokkevold and Han[43] evaluated the influence of smoking, diabetes, and periodontal disease on outcomes and found that smoking has an adverse effect on implant survival and success, with the effects being more pronounced in areas of loose trabecular bone (e.g., posterior maxilla).

The review also suggested that type 2 diabetes had an adverse effect on implant survival rates, but the limited number of included studies did not permit a definitive conclusion.[43] The review did conclude that although patients with a history of treated periodontitis did not show a decrease in implant survival, they did experience more complications and lower success rates, especially when the implants were followed over longer periods (10+ years).[43]

Smoking

Above all other risk factors, smoking has a significant negative impact on implant survival and success. In a study of 2194 implants, Bain and Moy reported a significantly greater rate of failure among smokers (11.28%) than nonsmokers (4.76%).[8] De Bruyn and Colleart reported an early failure rate of 9% among smokers compared with 1% among nonsmokers.[18] Two other studies, 1 of 10 years[25] and the other with follow-up assessment of 6 months to 21 years,[56] concluded that smoking was a definite risk factor for implant survival.[20,21]

Diabetes

The role of diabetes mellitus as a risk factor for implant outcomes is less clear. Although a metabolic disease such as diabetes was expected to have an adverse effect on bone healing[75] and tissue support for implants, the research has not definitively determined that diabetes has a negative impact on implant survival or success.[4]

Moy and coworkers[56] reported a significantly lower success rate (68.7%) for patients with diabetes compared with the success rate (85.1%) for the entire study population (1140 patients with 4680 implants); individual implant survival and success rates were not reported. However, the low success rate (i.e., high failure rate) may be an overestimate of the actual implant failure rate for patients with diabetes because it counts the number of patients with failures regardless of how many implants they had (i.e., implants successfully inserted and maintained in these patients are not counted). There were 48 patients with diabetes in the study, 4.2% of the 1140 total. Of these, 15 patients experienced implant failures.

Conversely, in a systematic review of the literature (33 studies), Javed and Romanos found that patients with good metabolic control (i.e., glycated hemoglobin [HbA1c] levels in the normal range) achieve success rates with osseointegrated implants that are similar to those for patients without diabetes.[38] Dowell and coworkers[23] also found similar success for implants placed in patients with controlled diabetes.

Periodontitis

A limited number of studies have assessed the prognosis of implant treatment in patients with a history of periodontitis.[41] Most of these studies suggest that implants are equally successful in patients with a history of chronic periodontitis. Short-term studies demonstrate 90% to 100% implant survival in patients with a history of chronic periodontitis.[53,55] Long-term studies report 90% to 97% implant survival rates for patients with a history of chronic periodontitis.[42,50,62,76] Short-term implant survival rates for patients treated for aggressive periodontitis are 95% to 100%.[53,54] One long-term study reported an 88.8% implant survival rate over 5 years for patients treated for aggressive periodontitis.[55]

Implant survival in patients with a history of periodontitis appears to be highly predictable. However, the lack of long-term studies to support implant survival in patients treated for aggressive periodontitis leaves the prognosis for these patients open to question.[41]

Long-term studies evaluating implant treatment in periodontally compromised patients suggest that they may experience more peri-implant problems.[42] When these patients are followed for extended periods, there appear to be more complications (i.e., peri-implantitis) associated with implants than in periodontally healthy patients. In a 10-year prospective study of patients with and without a history of chronic periodontitis, the rate of biologic complications (i.e., peri-implantitis) was higher for those with a history of chronic periodontitis (28.6%) than those with periodontal health (5.8%).[42] This controlled study by Karoussis and coworkers[42] found a statistically significant difference in mean peri-implant bone loss between patients with a history of chronic periodontitis and patients who were periodontally healthy.

Peri-implant problems may be attributed to a continuous increase in the percentage of implants exhibiting PPDs of 4 mm or deeper over time.[26] A systematic review of implant outcomes in patients treated for periodontitis concluded that these individuals had a greater incidence of biologic complications and lower success and survival rates compared with periodontally healthy subjects.[70]

> ### KEY FACT
> Smoking, diabetes, and periodontitis are risk factors that can adversely affect implant outcomes.

AESTHETIC RESULTS AND PATIENT SATISFACTION

The ultimate goal of treatment is to achieve natural-appearing, optimally functioning, implant-supported tooth replacements.

Fig. 60.3 Clinical Photograph Shows a Maxillary Anterior Fixed Restoration Supported by Two Malpositioned Implants in the Central Incisor Positions. The patient was dissatisfied with the aesthetic outcome. The left implant was positioned between the central and lateral incisor and angled toward the facial surface at a level above the gingival margin. A tooth-colored material was used to mask the exposed framework in the gingival area.

Proper tooth dimensions and contours and ideal soft tissue support are key factors for successful aesthetic outcomes.[46] If crown form, dimension, and shape and gingival harmony around the implants are not ideal, the patient may consider the implant restoration unacceptable, because the result does not represent a natural dental profile (Fig. 60.3). For some patients, such as those with severe alveolar deficiency, an ideal aesthetic outcome may be impossible because reconstructive surgical procedures are complex, require extensive time, and remain unpredictable. For others, a less-than-ideal aesthetic outcome may be acceptable.

Aesthetic problems and patient dissatisfaction happen when results are inferior to what was expected. Satisfaction with the aesthetic outcome of the implant prosthesis varies from patient to patient, depending on a number of factors. The risk for aesthetic failure is increased for patients with high aesthetic expectations. The risk is also higher when patients present with patient-related risk factors such as a high smile line, thin periodontal soft tissues, and compromised bone support. Two recent systematic reviews reported that the patient's perceptions and desires greatly influence and determine how well he or she accepts the implant outcome.[17,57]

Although infrequently reported, aesthetic success and patient satisfaction need to be included when considering the results of implant therapy. Despite several proposed methods for evaluating aesthetic results, reports of aesthetic parameters in the scientific literature are scarce.[9] A restorative index appraises the white aesthetics of the final restoration,[39] a soft tissue or pink aesthetic score considers soft tissue parameters,[32] and an aesthetic index uses a combination of pink and white aesthetic scores, focusing on the visible part of the implant restoration.[8] These indices quantify the aesthetic result, providing an objective method of judging aesthetic success.

In a survey of patient satisfaction, more than 90% of patients were completely satisfied in terms of function and aesthetics.[58]

TABLE 60.2 **Patient Satisfaction With Implant Treatment**

Implant Experience	Highly Satisfied or Satisfied (%)[a]
Function or chewing	97
Phonetics	96
Aesthetics	97
Oral hygiene ease	93
Complete fulfillment	92
Would do treatment again	94
Would recommend to friend or relative	89
Reasonable or justified cost	87

[a]Percentage of patients subjectively responding with *highly satisfied* or *satisfied* to survey questions about their implant experience. More than 90% responded favorably and thought implant treatment was a positive experience.

Data from Pjetursson BE, Karoussis I, Burgin W, et al: Patients' satisfaction following implant therapy. A 10-year prospective cohort study, *Clin Oral Implants Res* 16:185–193, 2005.

A questionnaire was given to 104 patients 5 to 15 years (mean, 10.2 years) after implant placement to assess subjective perceptions of treatment. Of these patients, 48% were treated with single implant crowns and 52% were treated with fixed partial dentures. The survival rate for all implants was 93%. Most patients had favorable responses to the questions regarding function, aesthetics, hygiene, and cost. Table 60.2 lists the percentage of patients responding as highly satisfied or satisfied for each category. Comparing chewing comfort for teeth or implants, 72.1% perceived no difference, 17.3% felt more secure chewing on teeth, and 7.7% felt more secure chewing on implants.

In another survey, patient satisfaction with implant-supported prostheses in totally edentulous jaws was evaluated.[63] Experience with an implant-supported prosthesis was assessed over a period of 10 years, and 97% of the 135 patients reported overall satisfaction with treatment. Chewing satisfaction was reported as good or very good by all but one patient (99.3% positive response rate). Improved lifestyle and greater self-confidence in public were reported by 75% and 82% of patients, respectively.

A systematic review of the literature, which included all randomized controlled trials published in English or French up to April 2007 comparing conventional mandibular dentures and implant overdentures in adult edentulous patients, identified eight publications for meta-analysis.[27] The study reported that patients were more satisfied with implant overdentures than with conventional mandibular dentures. However, there was a lack of evidence to show a patient's perception of the impact of mandibular implant overdentures on general health.

CLINICAL CORRELATION

Aesthetic problems and dissatisfaction happen when results do not match a patient's expectations. Satisfaction with the aesthetic outcome of an implant prosthesis varies among patients. The risk of failure is greater among those with high aesthetic demands and risk factors such as a high smile line, thin periodontal soft tissues, or compromised bone support.

CONCLUSIONS

The use of dental implants to replace missing teeth is highly predictable, advantageous, and beneficial for patients. Because of variations in implant designs, study protocols, and populations studied, results are difficult to compare, and an absolute definition of implant success remains elusive. The results of implant treatment are reported using a wide range of criteria from being present (i.e., survival) to being functional without complications (i.e., success).

It is challenging to compare the results of studies because the number of variables continues to change. Clinical research suggests that certain risk factors can decrease success rates for some patients. Understanding what is being reported in the literature helps patients and clinicians appreciate implant treatment results.

A Case Scenario is found on the companion website.

REFERENCES

 References for this chapter are found on the companion website.

Atlas of Periodontal Diseases[a]

This chapter provides several additional illustrations for Chapter 25, and some from Chapters 4 to 39. The presentation of cases follows the classification of periodontal diseases and conditions developed by the 1999 International Workshop for the Classification of Periodontal Diseases, which was organized by the American Academy of Periodontology (see Chapter 6). All illustrations are from the Archives of the Department of Periodontology, School of Dentistry, Cukurova University, Adana, Turkey (Box A.1).

[a]Adapted from the following chapter of *Newman and Carranza's Clinical Periodontology*, 13th edition: Chapter 88: Atlas of Periodontal Diseases, by M. Cenk Haytac and Onur Ucak Turer.

BOX A.1   Gingival Diseases

Plaque-Induced Gingival Diseases

I. Gingivitis associated with dental plaque only
 A. Without local contributing factors
 B. With local contributing factors (see Figs. A.1–A.32)
II. Gingival diseases modified by systemic factors
 A. Associated with endocrine system
  1. Puberty-associated gingivitis (see Fig. A.33)
  2. Menstrual cycle–associated gingivitis (see Fig. A.34)
  3. Pregnancy-associated gingivitis (see Figs. A.35–A.37)
   a. Gingivitis
   b. Pyogenic granuloma
  4. Diabetes mellitus–associated gingivitis
 B. Associated with blood dyscrasias
  1. Leukemia-associated gingivitis (see Figs. A.38–A.40)
  2. Other (see Figs. A.41–A.46)
III. Gingival diseases modified by medications
 A. Drug-induced gingival diseases
  1. Drug-influenced gingival enlargement (see Figs. A.47–A.51)
  2. Drug-influenced gingivitis
   a. Oral contraceptive–associated gingivitis
   b. Other
IV. Gingival diseases modified by malnutrition
 A. Ascorbic acid–deficiency gingivitis
 B. Other

Non–Plaque-Induced Gingival Lesions

I. Gingival diseases of specific bacterial origin
 A. Neisseria gonorrhoeae
 B. Treponema pallidum
 C. Streptococcus species (see Fig. A.52)
 D. Other
II. Gingival diseases of viral origin
 A. Herpesvirus infection (see Fig. A.53)
  1. Primary herpetic gingivostomatitis
  2. Recurrent oral herpesvirus infection
  3. Varicella zoster
 B. Other (see Fig. A.54)
III. Gingival diseases of fungal origin
 A. *Candida* species infections: generalized gingival candidiasis (see Figs. A.55 and A.56)
 B. Linear gingival erythema
 C. Histoplasmosis
 D. Other (see Figs. A.57 and A.58)
IV. Gingival lesions of genetic origin
 A. Hereditary gingival fibromatosis (see Figs. A.59–A.61)
 B. Other
V. Gingival manifestations of systemic conditions
 A. Mucocutaneous lesions
  1. Lichen planus (see Figs. A.62–A.65)
  2. Pemphigoid
  3. Pemphigus vulgaris (see Fig. A.66)
  4. Erythema multiforme
  5. Lupus erythematosus
  6. Drug induced
  7. Other (see Figs. A.67–A.73)
 B. Allergic reactions
  1. Dental restorative materials
   a. Mercury
   b. Nickel
   c. Acrylic
   d. Other
  2. Reactions attributable to the following
   a. Toothpastes or dentifrices
   b. Mouthrinses or mouthwashes
   c. Chewing gum additives
   d. Foods and additives (see Fig. A.74)
  3. Other
VI. Traumatic lesions: factitious, iatrogenic, or accidental (see Figs. A.75–A.92)
 A. Chemical injury
 B. Physical injury
 C. Thermal injury
VII. Foreign body reactions
VIII. Not otherwise specified
 A. Cysts and tumors (see Figs. A.93–A.102)

Chronic Periodontitis (See Figs. A.103–A.108)

I. Localized
II. Generalized
III. Chronic periodontitis modified by systemic disorders
 A. Diabetes mellitus (see Figs. A.109–A.113)

Aggressive Periodontitis (See Figs. A.114–A.119)

I. Localized
II. Generalized

Periodontitis as a Manifestation of Systemic Diseases

I. Hematologic disorders
 A. Acquired neutropenia
 B. Leukemias (see Figs. A.120–A.122)
 C. Other
II. Genetic disorders
 A. Familial and cyclic neutropenia (see Fig. A.123)
 B. Down syndrome
 C. Leukocyte adhesion deficiency syndromes (see Figs. A.124 and A.125)
 D. Papillon-Lefèvre syndrome (see Figs. A.126 and A.127)
 E. Chediak-Higashi syndrome
 F. Histiocytosis syndromes
 G. Glycogen storage disease
 H. Infantile genetic agranulocytosis
 I. Cohen syndrome
 J. Ehlers-Danlos syndrome (types 4 and 8)
 K. Hypophosphatasia (see Fig. A.128)
 L. Other
III. Not otherwise specified

Necrotizing Periodontal Diseases

I. Necrotizing ulcerative gingivitis (NUG) (see Figs. A.129–A.131)
II. Necrotizing ulcerative periodontitis (NUP) (see Fig. A.132)
III. Bisphosphonate-related osteonecrosis (see Figs. A.133 and A.134)

Abscesses of the Periodontium

I. Gingival abscess
II. Periodontal abscess (see Figs. A.135–A.137)
III. Pericoronal abscess (see Fig. A.138)

Periodontitis Associated With Endodontic Lesions

I. Endodontic-periodontal lesions (see Figs. A.139 and A.140)
II. Periodontal-endodontic lesions
III. Combined lesions

Developmental or Acquired Deformities and Conditions

I. Localized tooth-related factors
II. Mucogingival deformities around teeth
III. Mucogingival deformities on edentulous ridges
IV. Occlusal trauma

Fig. A.1 In the Healthy Gingiva of a 17-Year-Old Girl, Notice the Demarcation (Mucogingival Line) *(Arrows)* Between the Attached Gingiva and the Darker Alveolar Mucosa.

Fig. A.2 Two Views Show Prominent Stippling of the Healthy Gingiva in a 21-Year-Old Man.

Fig. A.3 Bright-Red Color and Loss of Stippling of the Gingiva Are Seen in a 21-Year-Old Woman With Gingivitis.

Fig. A.4 Two Views Show Bleeding on Probing in a 24-Year-Old Man With Gingivitis and Inflammatory Enlargement.

Fig. A.5 Plaque Accumulation and Red Color of the Gingiva Are Seen in a 17-Year-Old Girl With Gingivitis.

Fig. A.6 Bluish Red Color of the Gingiva Is Seen in a 46-Year-Old Man With Advanced Chronic Periodontitis.

Fig. A.7 Two Views Show Melanin Pigmentation That Caused Aesthetic Problems in a 21-Year-Old Woman and the Gums 6 Months After Treatment With a Carbon Dioxide Laser.

Fig. A.8 Two Views Show Diffuse Melanin Pigmentation That Caused Aesthetic Problems for a 34-Year-Old Woman and the Gums 2 Months After Treatment With Conventional Gingivectomy.

Fig. A.9 Two Views Show Localized Melanin Pigmentation in a 26-Year-Old Woman and the Result 1 Month After Treatment With a Carbon Dioxide Laser.

Fig. A.10 Two Views Show Diffuse Localized Melanin Pigmentation in a 33-Year-Old Woman and the Result 1 Month After Carbon Dioxide Laser Treatment.

Fig. A.11 Severe Plaque Accumulation and Gingivitis Occurred in a 13-Year-Old Boy With Neglected Hygiene.

Fig. A.12 Extensive Plaque Formed in a 46-Year-Old Man With Chronic Periodontitis. Darker shades of gingiva are seen in areas with subgingival calculus.

Fig. A.13 Three Views Show Extreme Plaque Formation and Periodontitis in a 52-Year-Old Woman With Prolonged Neglect of Oral Hygiene Procedures.

Fig. A.16 Advanced Plaque and Calculus Formed Around Implants in a 72-Year-Old Woman.

Fig. A.14 Plaque Formation Was Caused by Habitual One-Sided Chewing in a 9-Year-Old Boy. The patient had avoided chewing on the right side because of the mobility of deciduous teeth.

Fig. A.17 Plaque and Calculus Formed Around Implants in a 55-Year-Old Man.

Fig. A.15 There Is Extensive Plaque Accumulation and Severe Inflammation in a 35-Year-Old Male Smoker.

Fig. A.18 Three Views Show Calculus Formation on Teeth #26 and #27 Where the Parotid Gland Duct (i.e., Stensen Duct) Opens in a 47-Year-Old Man. These teeth had lost their functional antagonists. Calculus also covered the occlusal surfaces.

Fig. A.20 Anterior Open-Bite Malocclusion and the Loss of Functional Antagonist Teeth Caused Extensive Calculus Formation on the Left Maxillary Teeth in This 35-Year-Old Woman.

Fig. A.19 Calculus Formed on Upper Molars Adjacent to the Parotid Duct in a 44-Year-Old Man. Notice the divergence of the roots of the first molar.

Fig. A.21 Bridgelike Formations of Calculus Resulted From Malocclusion, Loss of an Antagonist Tooth, Tilting of the Remaining Teeth, and Avoidance of Chewing on the Affected Site in a 49-Year-Old Woman.

Fig. A.22 Two Views Show Extensive Calculus That Formed Adjacent to the Parotid Duct in a 53-Year-Old Man.

Fig. A.23 Extensive Bridgelike Calculus Formed on the Lingual Surfaces of the Lower Anterior Teeth Where the Sublingual and Bartholin Ducts Empty in a 36-Year-Old Man.

Fig. A.24 (A) Extensive bridgelike calculus formed on the lingual surfaces of the lower anterior teeth where the sublingual and Bartholin ducts empty in a 42-year-old woman. (B) In the same patient seen in A after extraction of the left central incisor, calculus has covered almost all surfaces of the tooth.

Fig. A.25 A Radiograph Shows the Radiopaque Projection of Extensive Calculus, Which Is Compared With Its Appearance After Extraction in a 62-Year-Old Man.

Fig. A.27 Extensive Plaque and Calculus Formation Was Associated With Crowding of the Teeth in a 21-Year-Old Woman.

Fig. A.28 Periodontal Destruction Was Associated With Class III Malocclusion in a 35-Year-Old Man.

Fig. A.26 Three Views Show the Extreme Plaque and Calculus Formation That Was Caused by Habitual One-Sided Chewing in a 35-Year-Old Woman. The patient had avoided chewing on the left side for 10 years.

Fig. A.29 Four Views Show Extensive Calculus Formation in a 9-Year-Old Child With an Open Bite and Lack of Hygiene.

Fig. A.30 Two Views Show Plaque Formation and Gingival Inflammation With Crowding and Supernumerary Teeth in a 14-Year-Old Boy.

Fig. A.32 Two Views Show Extensive Plaque and Calculus Formation in a 27-Year-Old Woman and the Same Patient After 2 Months of Receiving Initial Debridement and Oral Hygiene Instruction. Although the patient still has hygiene problems, the inflammation, redness, and contour of the gingiva are greatly reduced.

Fig. A.31 Gingival Inflammation and Enlargement Was Associated With Chronic Habitual Mouth Breathing in a 16-Year-Old Boy. There is clear demarcation of the affected gingiva.

Fig. A.33 Puberty Gingivitis in a 14-Year-Old Girl Was Associated With Poor Hygiene, Crowding of Teeth, and Mouth Breathing. Gingival hyperplasia was confined to the anterior regions.

Fig. A.34 Periodic Localized Color Changes of the Gingiva Around Maxillary Anterior Teeth Were Associated With Menstruation in a 29-Year-Old Woman.

Fig. A.35 Localized Gingival Enlargement Occurred in a 24-Year-Old Woman Who Was in the Seventh Month of Pregnancy. The lesion was first noticed in the fourth month by the patient.

Fig. A.36 Severe Gingival Enlargement Occurred in a 29-Year-Old Woman Who Was 8 Months Pregnant.

Fig. A.37 Gingival Enlargement in a 32-Year-Old Woman in the (A) Seventh, (B) Eighth, and (C) Ninth Months of Pregnancy, and (D) at 1 Month After Delivery. Notice the progression of the dimensions and the increase of the vascularization of the lesion. (E) The extraoral view shows the lesion interfering with occlusion and aesthetics.

Fig. A.38 Two Views Show Gingival Hyperplasia and Spontaneous Bleeding *(Left)* in a 6-Year-Old Boy With Newly Diagnosed Acute Myelogenous Leukemia and After One Course of Chemotherapy and Periodontal Treatment *(Right)*.

Fig. A.39 Enlargement of the Gingiva and Floor of the Mouth Occurred in an 8-Year-Old Boy With Acute Myelogenous Leukemia.

Fig. A.41 Pale Gingiva and Apparent Vascular Structures Are Seen in a 22-Year-Old Woman With Iron Deficiency Anemia.

Fig. A.40 Severe Gingival Inflammation, Hyperplasia, and the Results of Poor Hygiene Are Seen in a 46-Year-Old Man With Chronic Myelogenous Leukemia.

Fig. A.42 Severe Malocclusion and Gingival Recession Occurred in an 18-Year-Old Boy With Thalassemia.

Fig. A.43 Skeletal Disturbance of the Thumb *(Left)* and Severe Gingival Inflammation With Spontaneous Bleeding *(Right)* Occurred in a 12-Year-Old Boy With Fanconi Anemia.

Fig. A.44 Localized Bleeding *(Black Arrows)* Occurred in the Tissue in a 24-Year-Old Woman With Glanzmann Thrombasthenia.

Fig. A.46 Spontaneous Bleeding and Clot Formation Occurred in a 22-Year-Old Man With von Willebrand Disease.

Fig. A.45 Plaque Accumulation and Spontaneous Bleeding Occurred in a 28-Year-Old Patient With Hemophilia A Who Neglected Oral Hygiene Procedures Due to Severe Bleeding.

Fig. A.47 Gingival Enlargement Was Associated With Phenytoin Use in a 20-Year-Old Patient With Epilepsy.

Fig. A.48 Amlodipine-Associated Gingival Enlargement Was Seen in a 47-Year-Old Man With Hypertension.

Fig. A.49 Gingival Enlargement Occurred in a 44-Year-Old Man Receiving Cyclosporine After Kidney Transplantation.

Fig. A.50 (A) In a case of cyclosporine-associated gingival enlargement, the clinical crowns are covered and enlargement reaches up to the occlusal plane. (B) Intraoperative view of the enlargement. Views of the patient after (C) 6 and (D) 12 months. (From Haytac CM, Ustun Y, Essen E, et al: Combined treatment approach of gingivectomy and CO_2 laser for cyclosporine-induced gingival overgrowth, *Quintessence Int* 38(1):e54–e59, 2007.)

Fig. A.51 Gingival Thickening and Hyperplasia Occurred in a 25-Year-Old Male Bodybuilder Who Had Been Using Steroid Injections for 3 Years.

Fig. A.52 Lesions on the Lip and Gingiva Are Seen in a 7-Year-Old Child With Acute Streptococcal Gingivostomatitis.

Fig. A.53 Ruptured and Unruptured Herpetic Vesicles *(Arrows)* Are Seen in a 19-Year-Old Male With Herpetic Gingivostomatitis.

Fig. A.54 Two Views Show Recurrent Aphthous Ulcers in a 27-Year-Old Woman.

Fig. A.55 Four Views Show Severe Mucositis on the Gingiva, Cheek, Palatal Mucosa, and Tongue of a 7-Year-Old Boy With Acute Myelogenous Leukemia After Remission Induction Chemotherapy. These lesions are very prone to candidal infections.

Fig. A.56 Candidal Infection of the Oral Cavity Occurred After Chemotherapy in a 3-Year-Old Boy With Acute Myelogenous Leukemia.

Fig. A.57 Mucormycosis Caused Soft and Hard Tissue Destruction in a 9-Year-Old Patient With Acute Myelogenous Leukemia.

Fig. A.58 (A) Two views show rapid gingival and alveolar bone destruction caused by mucormycosis infection in a 14-year-old boy with acute myelogenous leukemia. The lesions started on the third day of chemotherapy, and breakdown occurred within 1 week. (B) Histologic analysis used Gomori methenamine silver staining, which showed fungal hyphae. (Courtesy Dr. M. Cem Dogan and Dr. M. Cenk Haytac.)

Fig. A.59 Hereditary Gingival Fibromatosis Occurred in a Family. Intraoral views of the father were obtained in (A) 2000, (B) 2003, and (C) 2005.

Fig. A.60 Hereditary Gingival Fibromatosis Occurred in a Family. In four views of the father in 2000, notice the severe enlargement of the tuberosities contacting the mandibular ridges and the root fragments in the overgrown tissue.

Fig. A.61 Hereditary Gingival Fibromatosis Occurred in a Family. Intraoral views of the younger son show his condition when he was (A) 10 days and (B) 2 years old. (From Haytac MC, Ozcelik O: The phenotypic overlap of syndromes associated with hereditary gingival fibromatosis: follow-up of a family for five years, *Oral Surg Oral Med Oral Pathol Oral Radiol Endodontol* 103:521–527, 2007.)

Fig. A.63 Two Views Show Reticular Lichen Planus in a 63-Year-Old Woman Who Was Referred Because of a Complaint of a Burning Sensation in Her Mouth.

Fig. A.62 Severe Desquamation and Positive Nikolsky Sign Were Seen in a 56-Year-Old Woman With Lichen Planus. Desquamation leaves the connective tissue exposed and painful in response to stimulant agents.

Fig. A.64 Two Views Show Desquamation and Spontaneous Bleeding in a 62-Year-Old Woman With Erosive Lichen Planus. The patient was extremely sensitive to temperature changes and foods.

Fig. A.65 Two Views Show Atrophic Lichen Planus That Exposed Connective Tissue in a 62-Year-Old Man.

Fig. A.66 Three Views Show Pemphigus Vulgaris Characterized by Desquamation, Pain, and Bleeding in a 56-Year-Old Woman. The suprabasal and subepithelial separation of cells can be detected in the histologic analysis.

Fig. A.67 Four Views Show Developmental Deformities of the Fingers and Limited Mouth Opening in an 18-Year-Old Boy With Scleroderma. Insufficient attached gingival width complicates oral hygiene procedures, and advanced gingival recession is seen on the lower central incisor.

Fig. A.68 Gingival Enlargement Occurred in a 9-Year-Old Boy With Juvenile Hyaline Fibromatosis.

Fig. A.69 Four Views Show Atopic Dermatitis Characterized by Pruritic Lesions on the Extremities and Lips of a 22-Year-Old Woman. Notice the inadequate vestibular depth and gingival recession.

Fig. A.70 Five Views Show Fibrous Dysplasia Characterized by Unilateral Fibroosseous Expansion of the Bones in a 17-Year-Old Girl. Notice the facial asymmetry, advanced malocclusion, migration of teeth starting from the midline, and gingival enlargement in accordance with expansion of the underlying bones. The radiograph shows unilateral increases of the dimensions of mandible and maxilla.

Fig. A.71 Three Views Show Sturge-Weber Syndrome Characterized by Unilateral Cavernous Hemangiomas on the Face and Neck of a 35-Year-Old Man. Notice the unilateral soft tissue and easily bleeding gingival enlargement with high vascularization on the affected site.

Fig. A.72 Three Views Show Rothmund-Thomson Syndrome Characterized by Photosensitivity and Hypopigmentation and Hyperpigmentation on the Skin of a 16-Year-Old Girl. Notice the decreased keratinization and spontaneous bleeding of the gingiva. Histologic analysis showed discontinuity of the basement membrane. (From Haytac MC, Oztunç H, Mete UO, et al: Rothmund-Thomson syndrome: a case report, *Oral Surg Oral Med Oral Pathol Oral Radiol Endodontol* 94:479–484, 2002.)

Fig. A.73 Four Views Show Recurrent Major Aphthous Lesions on the Cheek and Lip Mucosa, Tongue, and Alveolar Mucosa in a 42-Year-Old Man With Behçet Disease.

Fig. A.74 Four Views Show Results of the Oral Challenge Test for the Diagnosis of an Allergic Reaction of the Gingiva to Apples in a 48-Year-Old Woman. Notice the formation of blisters, desquamation, and subepithelial bleeding. (From Haytac MC, Ozcelik O: Oral challenge test for the diagnosis of gingival hypersensitivity to apple: a case report, *Oral Surg Oral Med Oral Pathol Oral Radiol Endodontol* 101:317–321, 2006.)

Fig. A.75 Inadequate Margins, Design, and Shape of the Restoration Violating the Biologic Width Caused Severe Gingival Inflammation in a 32-Year-Old Woman.

Fig. A.76 Overhanging Margins and Injury Were Caused by the Self-Curing Acrylic Used for Restoration in a 49-Year-Old Woman.

Fig. A.77 Three Views Show Extensive Calculus Formation and an Ill-Fitting Restoration on the Lower Anterior Teeth of a 51-Year-Old Man. Notice the trauma caused by the deposits on the sublingual soft tissue seen after the restoration was removed.

Fig. A.79 Subgingival Margin Locations and Lack of Interproximal Embrasures of the Crowns Caused Gingival Inflammation in a 29-Year-Old Man.

Fig. A.78 Two Views Show Extensive Calculus Formation Under the Restoration on the Lower Anterior Teeth of a 44-Year-Old Man. Notice the trauma caused by calculus on the sublingual soft tissue seen after removal.

Fig. A.80 Two Views Show the Results of Misuse of Ferric Sulfate During Gingival Retraction, Which Caused Burns and Desquamation in a 30-Year-Old Man.

Fig. A.81 Two Views Show Iatrogenic Use of a Bonding Agent for the Treatment of Dentinal Hypersensitivity, Causing Gingival Recession in a 32-Year-Old Woman.

Fig. A.84 Gingival Recession Was Associated With Vigorous Tooth-brushing in a 48-Year-Old Man.

Fig. A.82 Trauma and Inflammation of the Soft Tissues Was Caused by the Brackets in a 14-Year-Old Orthodontic Patient.

Fig. A.85 Gingival Desquamation After a 21-Year-Old Woman Rinsed With Cologne.

Fig. A.83 Gingival Trauma Was Caused by the Ligature Wire in a 12-Year-Old Girl.

Fig. A.86 Hyperkeratosis Was Associated With Smokeless Tobacco Use in a 42-Year-Old Man.

Fig. A.87 Desquamation Was Associated With Toothbrushing With Soap in a 55-Year-Old Man.

Fig. A.90 Gingival Recession Was Associated With Habitual Cleansing With Tissue in a 42-Year-Old Woman.

Fig. A.88 Trauma and Desquamation Occurred After Placing Plant Seeds on the Gingiva for a Toothache in a 41-Year-Old Man.

Fig. A.91 Desquamation and Burn Occurred After a 50-Year-Old Man Rinsed With Raki, a Turkish Drink With 40% to 50% Alcohol Content.

Fig. A.89 Gingival Recession Was Associated With Habitual Scratching of the Gingiva With a Nail in a 26-Year-Old Woman.

Fig. A.92 A Traumatic Lesion Resulted From Placing Fresh Garlic Onto the Aching Third Molar in a 26-Year-Old Man.

Fig. A.93 A Fibroma in a 45-Year-Old Man Had a Firm and Nodular Character.

Fig. A.95 A Papilloma Occurred in a 27-Year-Old Woman.

Fig. A.94 Two Views Show a Fibroma in a 56-Year-Old Man. (Courtesy Dr. Burcu Cam and Dr. Onur Ozcelik.)

Fig. A.96 A Papilloma Developed on the Palatal Tissue in a 42-Year-Old Woman.

Fig. A.98 A Peripheral Giant-Cell Granuloma Was Seen in a 31-Year-Old Woman.

Fig. A.97 Two Views Show Severe, Generalized Human Papillomavirus–Associated Warts in a 7-Year-Old Child.

Fig. A.99 An Ameloblastoma Occurred in a 54-Year-Old Woman.

Fig. A.101 Squamous Cell Carcinoma Was Detected in a 62-Year-Old Patient.

Fig. A.100 An Ameloblastoma Was Seen in a 49-Year-Old Patient.

Fig. A.102 Malignant Melanoma Was Seen in a 52-Year-Old Woman.

Fig. A.103 Two Views Show Plaque and Calculus That Caused Chronic Periodontitis in a 42-Year-Old Man Without Any Systemic Diseases. Notice the generalized radiographic bone loss.

Fig. A.104 Two Views Show Gingival Recession, Mobility, Migration, and Extrusion of Teeth Due to Alveolar Bone Loss in a 48-Year-Old Man With Chronic Periodontitis.

Fig. A.105 Advanced Chronic Periodontitis Was Seen in a 54-Year-Old Man Who Had Hygiene Neglect and Smoking as Contributing Factors.

Fig. A.107 Two Views Show Generalized Bone Loss That Occurred in a 45-Year-Old Male Smoker With Advanced Chronic Periodontitis.

Fig. A.106 Generalized Bone Loss Occurred in a 38-Year-Old Woman With Moderate Chronic Periodontitis.

Fig. A.108 (A) Cone-beam computed tomography shows generalized bone loss in a 39-year-old man with advanced chronic periodontitis. (B) Two views show the patient before and 4 months after initial periodontal therapy and extraction of mandibular incisors (*bottom*). There is closure of the diastema between the maxillary central incisors after therapy.

Fig. A.109 Severe Gingival Inflammation and Periodontal Abscess Occurred in a 26-Year-Old Woman With Type 1 Diabetes Mellitus. Notice the extrusion of the maxillary left central incisor caused by alveolar bone loss.

Fig. A.110 Severe Inflammation, Pus Formation, and Periodontal Breakdown Occurred in a 34-Year-Old Man With Uncontrolled Type 1 Diabetes Mellitus.

Fig. A.111 Two Views Show the Dentition of a 14-Year-Old Girl Who Was Referred With a Complaint of Tooth Mobility. She had spontaneous loss of teeth #11, #31, #41, and #46 in the past 2 years. The patient had advanced bone loss despite a minimal amount of bacterial plaque and degree 3 mobility of many teeth. She was diagnosed with type 1 diabetes mellitus on consultation.

Fig. A.112 Three Views Show Alveolar Bone Loss and Severe Inflammation With Spontaneous Bleeding, Pus Formation, and Abscess in a 56-Year-Old Man With Type 2 Diabetes Mellitus Who Used External Insulin for 12 Years.

Fig. A.113 A 28-Year-Old Woman With Uncontrolled Type 1 Diabetes Mellitus Was Referred With Complaints of Rapid Mobility of Teeth, Severe Pain, Spontaneous Pus, and Several Abscesses. Her fasting glucose level was 486 mg/dL on the day of referral. (A) Although the lesions resembled abscesses of periodontal origin, the pocket depths and attachment levels were within normal levels. (B) The computed tomography findings and consultation with the infection department confirmed the diagnosis of osteomyelitis. (C) View of the patient after 1 week of blood glucose control in the intensive care unit and hyperbaric oxygen therapy. (D) Although the lesions healed uneventfully, severe malocclusion was evident at the 1-year follow-up examination.

Fig. A.114 Three Views Show Aggressive Periodontitis in a 3-Year-Old Boy Without Systemic Diseases. There is severe alveolar bone destruction of deciduous molar teeth.

Fig. A.115 Two Views Show Extrusion of the Left Central Incisor in a 21-Year-Old Man With Localized Aggressive Periodontitis. There is severe breakdown of alveolar bone of the incisor and mandibular first molar.

Fig. A.116 Three Views Show Advanced Bone Loss in an 18-Year-Old Boy With Aggressive Periodontitis.

Fig. A.117 Two Views Show Intrabony Defects in a 24-Year-Old Woman With Aggressive Periodontitis.

Fig. A.118 Five Clinical and Cone-Beam Computed Tomography Views Show Advanced Alveolar Bone Resorption Around the Incisors and First Molar in a 24-Year-Old Man With Aggressive Periodontitis.

Fig. A.119 Clinical and radiographic views of a 27-year-old man show generalized aggressive periodontitis at (A) the initial visit and (B) the 5-year follow-up examination after therapy. Cone-beam computed tomography views show (C, D, and F) advanced alveolar bone resorption around incisors, (E) premolars, and (G) first molar.

Fig. A.120 A 12-year-old girl was referred with complaints of rapid swelling on (A) the face and (B) the gingiva, and (C) spontaneous bleeding. The patient also had persistent fever and general malaise for 2 weeks. (D) Radiographic analysis revealed alveolar bone loss and separation of the roots of the maxillary right lateral and canine. Consultation with the hematology department and histologic analysis of the lesion confirmed the diagnosis of granulocytic sarcoma, which can precede acute myelogenous leukemia. (E) Histologically, infiltration of atypical myeloid cells into the gingival tissues was evident (hematoxylin and eosin; original magnification ×100). (F) The lesion regressed significantly after two courses of chemotherapy. (From Antmen B, Haytac MC, Sasmaz I, et al: Granulocytic sarcoma of gingiva: an unusual case with aleukemic presentation, *J Periodontol* 74:1514–1519, 2003.)

Fig. A.121 A 14-Year-Old Boy Was Referred With Complaints of Rapid Mobility of Teeth, Gingival Swelling, Persistent Fever, and Joint Pain. (A) Clinical examination revealed gingival hyperplasia in accordance with the expansion of jawbones and third-degree mobility in many teeth despite minimal bacterial plaque. (B) Bone marrow aspiration biopsy revealed cytoplasmic vacuolization of lymphoblasts specific for acute lymphoblastic leukemia type L3 (May-Grünwald Giemsa stain; original magnification ×100). (C) Radiographically, there was severe bone loss, abnormal trabeculation, and radiolucent areas around roots, which were more prominent on the molar teeth. (From Haytac MC, Antmen B, Dogan MC, et al: Severe alveolar bone loss and gingival hyperplasia as initial manifestation of Burkitt cell type acute lymphoblastic leukemia, *J Periodontol* 74:547–551, 2003.)

Fig. A.122 Two Views Show Alveolar Bone Destruction and Gingival Enlargement Around Teeth #41, #42, and #43 in a 15-Year-Old Boy With Acute Lymphocytic Leukemia.

Fig. A.123 A 16-Year-Old Girl Who Had Been Receiving Treatment for Neutropenia for 8 Years Was Referred for Gingival Inflammation. Two views show severe malocclusion and gingival inflammation, spontaneous bleeding, deep periodontal pockets up to 15 mm, and advanced radiographic alveolar bone loss.

Fig. A.124 An 11-Year-Old Girl With Leukocyte Adhesion Deficiency (LAD) Was Referred to the Periodontology Department. She had recurrent skin, ear, upper respiratory tract, and lung infections since early childhood and was diagnosed with LAD 4 years earlier. She had one kidney surgically removed due to infection. Two views show severe periodontal breakdown with spontaneous loss of many teeth and advanced bone loss, deep pockets up to 15 mm, and mobility for the remaining teeth. The patient's elder sister, who was 14 years old, also had LAD and was diagnosed during the same period. The elder sister's periodontal status is shown in Fig. A.125.

Fig. A.125 Two Views Show Leukocyte Adhesion Deficiency in a 14-Year-Old Girl.

Fig. A.126 Three Views Show Hyperkeratosis of the Palms, Loss of Anterior Teeth, Gingival Recession, and Extensive Radiographic Alveolar Bone Loss of Deciduous Teeth in a 3-Year-Old Boy With Papillon-Lefèvre Syndrome.

Fig. A.127 Three Views Show Effects of Papillon-Lefèvre Syndrome in a 12-Year-Old Girl, Including Hyperkeratosis of the Palms and Soles. The patient had spontaneous loss of many teeth and deep pockets ranging from 4 to 12 mm on the remaining teeth. Severe alveolar bone destruction is seen in the panoramic radiograph.

Fig. A.128 Three Views Show Skeletal Deformities and Gingival Inflammation in a 14-Year-Old Girl With Hypophosphatasia.

Fig. A.129 Typical Punched-Out Appearance of the Gingiva *(Arrow)* in Necrotizing Ulcerative Gingivitis Is Seen in a 25-Year-Old Man.

Fig. A.130 Two Views Show a Necrotizing Ulcerative Gingivitis Lesion Before and After Removal of Pseudomembrane in a 27-Year-Old Woman.

Fig. A.131 Two Views Show a Crater-Like Lesion and Pseudomembrane Formation on the Palatal Gingiva in a 31-Year-Old Man With Necrotizing Ulcerative Gingivitis.

Fig. A.132 Three Views Show Severe Necrotizing Ulcerative Gingivitis and a Necrotizing Ulcerative Periodontitis Infection That Caused Extreme Pain in a 22-Year-Old Woman on the First, Third, and Seventh Day of Referral. Rapid soft tissue destruction exposed the alveolar bone.

Fig. A.133 Zoledronic Acid–Related Osteonecrosis Occurred in a 54-Year-Old Woman Who Had Been Using the Drug Intravenously for Breast Cancer. The lesion occurred 1 month after extraction of tooth #36.

Fig. A.134 Three Views Show Rapid Gingival and Bone Necrosis 1 Month *(Top Left)*, 2 Months *(Top Right)*, and 7 Months *(Bottom)* After Scaling and Root Planing in a 52-Year-Old Woman Receiving Intravenous Zoledronic Acid After Breast Cancer Treatment.

Fig. A.135 Two Views Show a Periodontal Abscess of the Left Central Incisor in a 21-Year-Old Woman With Aggressive Periodontitis.

Fig. A.136 Periodontal Abscess of the Maxillary First Molar Occurred in a 35-Year-Old Man With Chronic Periodontitis.

Fig. A.137 Two Views Show a Periodontal Abscess in a 39-Year-Old Woman Before and After Treatment.

Fig. A.138 Pericoronitis Is Seen Around a Partially Erupted Mandibular Third Molar in a 19-Year-Old Girl.

Fig. A.139 Two Views Show an Endodontic-Periodontal Lesion in a 36-Year-Old Man.

Fig. A.140 Two Views Show an Endodontic-Periodontal Lesion in an 18-Year-Old Girl.

INDEX

A

ABCA1, 122.e2t–122.e150t
ABCA4, 122.e2t–122.e150t
ABCB11, 122.e2t–122.e150t
ABCC6, 122.e2t–122.e150t
ABCC8, 122.e2t–122.e150t
Abfraction, 371, 371f
ABP1, 122.e2t–122.e150t
Abrasion, 371, 371f
Abscesses
   acute *versus* chronic abscess, 466, 467f, 467b
   classification of, 465–466
   gingival, 465, 467f
   pericoronal, 466
   periodontal. *see* Periodontal abscess
Absorbable hemostatic agents, 558t
ACACB, 122.e2t–122.e150t
ACADL, 122.e2t–122.e150t
ACAN, 122.e2t–122.e150t
AcceleDent, 548.e9
Accessory pathogens, 149
ACE, 122.e2t–122.e150t
ACE2, 122.e2t–122.e150t
Acellular cementum, 49–50, 50f
ACE.LTA, 122.e2t–122.e150t
Acoustic streaming, 516
Acoustic turbulence, 516
Acquired immunodeficiency syndrome (AIDS).
   see HIV/AIDS
ACSM3, 122.e2t–122.e150t
Actinomyces spp., 127f–128f
Active eruption, 43
Activity, periodontal infection and, 221
Acute gingival disease, treatment of, 459–464
   case scenario, 464.e1, 464.e1f
   necrotizing ulcerative gingivitis as, 459–462
   pericoronitis as, 463–464
   primary herpetic gingivostomatitis as, 462–463,
      463f, 463b
Acute inflammation, 163–165, 163f
   lipoxins, 164–165
   resolvins, 165, 165b
   specialized pro-resolving mediators, 164, 164f
Acute necrotizing gingivitis, 279
Acute periodontal abscess, 370.e3
   chronic abscess *versus*, 466, 467f, 467b
   treatment of, 466–469, 468f, 468b
Acute respiratory distress, 430.e2
Acute respiratory infections, periodontal disease
   and, 226.e4–226.e5
Acute-phase proteins, 223
ADA, 122.e2t–122.e150t
ADAMTS8, 122.e2t–122.e150t
Adaptation, periodontal instruments and, 515.e6,
   515.e6f, 515.e6b
Adaptive immunity, 113t, 115–118
   antibodies, 118–119
   antigen-presenting cells, 116
   T cells, 116–118, 116b, 117f
ADCY3, 122.e2t–122.e150t
ADCY6, 122.e2t–122.e150t

ADCY9, 122.e2t–122.e150t
ADD1, 122.e2t–122.e150t
ADD2, 122.e2t–122.e150t
Addison disease, 245
Additive processes, 604.e3–604.e4, 604.e4f–604.e5f
Adhesion, initial, 138.e1
Adhesive surface proteins, 160
Adjusted association, 24.e1
ADO22, 122.e2t–122.e150t
Adolescents, gingivitis in, 274
ADORA2A, 122.e2t–122.e150t
Adrenal crisis, 428.e1, 428.e1b
Adrenal insufficiency, 428.e1–428.e2, 428.e1b
β-Adrenergic receptor antagonists, hypertension
   and, 420–421, 421t
Adrenocorticotropic hormone (ACTH)
   stimulation test, 428.e1
Advanced glycation end products (AGEs), 326
Aerosol, production of, power-driven instruments
   and, 519, 519b
Aesthetic surgery techniques, for periodontal
   disease, 551
Age
   chronic adult periodontitis and, 533
   periodontal disease and, 395
   in prognosis determination, 397
   supragingival dental plaque formation and,
      143, 144b
AGER, 122.e2t–122.e150t
Aggregatibacter actinomycetemcomitans, 106, 110,
   114, 118, 127f–128f, 394, 523
Aggressive periodontitis, 83, 83b, 85f–86f, 159.e1,
   329–337, 451–457, 452b, 452.e1f, 452.e2b,
   453f–454f
   case scenario on, 337.e1f, 337.e1b–337.e3b,
      337.e3f, 457.e1f, 457.e1b
   characteristics of, 329–330
   in children, 277–278, 278f
   classification of, 329–330
   diagnostic criteria for, 330t
   epidemiology of, 330–333
      case definition in, 331–332, 331f
      current understanding of, 333
   generalized, 330, 330t, 331f–332f, 451
   host response to, 335
   localized, 159.e1, 159.e1f, 330, 330t, 333f–334f,
      451, 453.e1f–453.e2f
   microbiology of, 335
   pathobiology and risk factors for, 333–336
   periodontal maintenance in, 455–456
   prognosis for, 405
   therapeutic considerations for, 336–337, 336b
   therapeutic modalities of, 451–455
      antimicrobial therapy as, 452–455,
         453f–454f
      conventional periodontal therapy as, 452,
         452b
      full-mouth disinfection as, 455
      regenerative therapy as, 452.e1–452.e2,
         452.e1f
      surgical resective therapy as, 452

Aggressive periodontitis (Continued)
   treatment planning and restorative
      considerations for, 455, 455b
Aging, 62–66, 62b. *see also* Older adults
   effects on periodontium, 62–65
      alveolar bone, 64–65
      bacterial plaque, 65
      case scenario on, 66.e1f, 66.e1b
      cementum, 64
      gingival connective tissue, 63
      gingival epithelium, 62–63, 63f–64f, 63b
      immune response, 65
      inflammatory responses, 65
      periodontal ligament, 63–64
      response to treatment, 66, 66b
   effects on progression of periodontal diseases,
      65–66
Agranulocytosis, 203, 204f, 265, 430.e1
AGT, 122.e2t–122.e150t
AGTR1, 122.e2t–122.e150t
AIRE, 122.e2t–122.e150t
Air-powder polishing, 514, 514f–515f, 514b–515b
Albright syndrome, 245
Albucasis, 2, 2f
ALCAM, 122.e2t–122.e150t
Alcohol consumption, in older adults,
   449.e4–449.e5
ALDH2, 122.e2t–122.e150t
ALDH3A1, 122.e2t–122.e150t
ALDH3A2, 122.e2t–122.e150t
Allogenic succession, 150
ALOX15, 122.e2t–122.e150t
Al-Tasrif, 1
Alternative pathway, 161.e6–161.e7, 161.e8f
Alveolar bone
   aging and, 64–65
   area between base of pocket and, 299
   development of attachment apparatus and, 59
   height, orthodontic therapy and, 189
   loss of, in periodontal charting, 370.e1–370.e3,
      370.e3f
   normal variation in, 308, 308f
   relationship of pocket to, 299, 299b, 300f–301f
   resorption, 112
Alveolar bone proper, 53
Alveolar crest fibers, 45, 45f
Alveolar process, 53–58, 53f–55f
   bone marrow, 56
   cells and intercellular matrix, 55
   endosteum, 56
   fenestration and dehiscence in, 57–58
   interdental septum, 56, 57f
   osseous topography, 56–57, 57f–58f
   periosteum, 56
   remodeling of, 58
   socket wall, 55–56, 55f–56f
Alveolar ridge
   implant position and, 627–628, 627f–628f, 628b
   reconstruction of, 575.e4, 575.e5f–575.e6f
AMACR, 122.e2t–122.e150t
Amine fluoride, for oral malodor, 499

Note: Page numbers followed by "*f*" refer to illustrations; page numbers followed by "*t*" refer to tables; page numbers followed by "*b*" refer to boxes.